NUTRITIONAL ANTHROPOLOGY

Nutritional Anthropology

Biocultural Perspectives on Food and Nutrition

Second Edition

EDITED BY

DARNA L. DUFOUR
University of Colorado

ALAN H. GOODMAN
Hampshire College

GRETEL H. PELTO
Cornell University

New York   Oxford
OXFORD UNIVERSITY PRESS

Oxford University Press, Inc., publishes works that further Oxford University's
objective of excellence in research, scholarship, and education.

Oxford New York
Auckland Cape Town Dar es Salaam Hong Kong Karachi
Kuala Lumpur Madrid Melbourne Mexico City Nairobi
New Delhi Shanghai Taipei Toronto

With offices in
Argentina Austria Brazil Chile Czech Republic France Greece
Guatemala Hungary Italy Japan Poland Portugal Singapore
South Korea Switzerland Thailand Turkey Ukraine Vietnam

For titles covered by Section 112 of the US Higher Education
Opportunity Act, please visit www.oup.com/us/he for the latest
information about pricing and alternate formats.

Published by Oxford University Press, Inc.
198 Madison Avenue, New York, New York 10016
http://www.oup.com

Oxford is a registered trademark of Oxford University Press

Library of Congress Cataloging-in-Publication Data
Nutritional anthropology : biocultural perspectives on food and nutrition / edited by Darna L. Dufour,
Alan H. Goodman, Gretel H. Pelto. —
2nd ed.
  p. cm.
ISBN 978-0-19-973814-4
1. Nutritional anthropology.   I. Dufour, Darna L.   II. Goodman, Alan H.   III. Pelto, Gretel H.
GN407.N878 2012
306.4–dc23   2012017135

Printing number: 9 8 7 6 5 4 3 2

Printed in the United States of America
on acid-free paper

CONTENTS

v

PREFACE

In the dozen years since the first edition of this book appeared, interest in food and nutrition has grown worldwide and especially in North America. Food now occupies—we think correctly—a more central place in our thinking, not as background but more in the foreground. As we begin to consider more deeply the importance of food in a variety of ways, including how it is produced, where it comes from, and how it impacts our bodies, brains, and environments, we see that producing, distributing, and consuming food are arguably the most fundamental roles of a society. The growth in thinking about food has deepened the need for a second edition of *Nutritional Anthropology: Biocultural Perspectives on Food and Nutrition*.

Whether you are a professor, student, expert, or novice, we hope that this book will contribute to your enthusiasm for good food and your appreciation for anthropological approaches to food and nutrition. The anthropological study of food and nutrition is both rewarding and important for understanding ourselves and others. Such studies bridge diverse parts of the human experience—past and present, theoretical and applied, biological and cultural, the personal and the political. Anthropological studies are extremely holistic, drawing on subdisciplines of anthropology from studies of language, the past, and legal systems and between anthropology and other disciplines concerned with nutrition, such as nutritional science, nursing, and public health. An anthropological perspective on nutrition offers great potential for understanding the multifaceted nature of human relationships to food. Food is "good to think" and "good to eat." Food is richly symbolic; nutrition is essential. We hope this book helps the reader to better understand the intertwined symbolic and material webs and systems of food.

Food and nutrition studies have changed dramatically since the first edition was published in 2000. This edition reflects many of those changes. There have been important new developments in the study of nearly every aspect of food and nutrition including, for example, our understanding of early hominid diets, the nutritional ecology of hunter-gatherers, the globalization of food, food and political power, technologies for food production, local responses to food quality, and an ever-growing pandemic of diet-related chronic disease and obesity. While various forms of undernutrition remain prevalent, our collective concerns are increasingly focused on the problem of consuming too much food.

Nutritional anthropology came into being as a distinct area of inquiry in the 1970s. Before that time, anthropologists, including such notables as Margaret Mead and Audrey Richards, had studied food and nutrition, particularly from a food systems perspective, with a main focus on ethnographic field work in small-scale societies. In the 1970s, interests in the evolution of diets and contemporary nutrition problems coalesced. Since that time, the field of nutritional anthropology has continually expanded. Courses in nutritional anthropology are now regularly taught on many college campuses, under various names, including "Nutritional Anthropology," "The Anthropology of Food and Nutrition," "Food and Culture," and so on.

We sense that the students who take these courses come from diverse backgrounds and have diverse aspirations. Where once nutritional anthropology seemed to be an anthropological child, it is now frequently a means to introduce nutritionists to culture and anthropological perspectives, and it is even making inroads into public health, nursing, and medical school curricula. Indeed, a variety of colleges and universities have begun to offer certificate programs and minors in food studies.

As the field has grown, the foremost challenge we faced in designing the new edition stemmed from the great variability of topics and approaches found across the spectrum of nutritional anthropology courses. Our goal is to bring together a core set of readings that would provide a foundation for the field and, at the same time, be appropriate for students of different backgrounds and for instructors with various needs and foci. Here is how we went about doing it.

Theoretical Perspective

The dominant perspective of the book is a biocultural one. As anthropologists, we are predominantly interested in how biology and culture intersect. As foods are consumed and processed in the gastrointestinal system, the meal is transformed to nutrients. On a more theoretical level, we can say that culture blends into biology. How food tastes is a matter of both culture and biology. What is culturally defined as food and what is eaten may have reverberations in domains as diverse as ethnic identity, growth, and health. Nutritional anthropology from the start has been an arena in which ecology, biology, and culture come together.

Our chief aim is to ensure that *Nutritional Anthropology: Biocultural Perspectives on Food and Nutrition* was not only concerned with contemporary foodways, but also included chapters on how foodways have come together, mixed, and evolved. It is about the state of nutrition today, and also about what our ancestors ate, what problems they encountered, and what their nutrition might mean for us.

Finally, learning comes from reading and from doing. Thus, our goal was to integrate theory and learning with doing and implementing. Many of the chapters have been selected because they show "nutritional anthropology in action," and this perspective is further supplemented by our "suggestions for thinking and doing nutritional anthropology." This focus on linking theory to action reflects the emerging situation in which an anthropological perspective is an increasingly valued component of public health and international nutrition programs. From these readings and the optional activities, students may gain a better sense of how nutritional anthropologists work, and hence a deeper appreciation of issues in this evolving field of inquiry.

Topical Coverage and Organization

After a brief introductory section that provides a "taste of nutritional anthropology," this book is divided into 12 sections of three to six readings each. In a semester-long course, the topic of each section may be used as a weekly focus. The section introductions are intended to provide a sense of the area of inquiry, how questions have evolved, and some of the current key areas of concern. In the introductions we briefly note the purpose and salient points of each chapter and explain some of the more difficult parts. Sometimes we raise questions that may also provide the basis for class discussions. We end each introduction with suggestions for further reading and for "thinking and doing nutritional anthropology."

The chapters in the book are grouped into four main parts:

- Part I provides an introduction and a taste of the topics to follow.
- Part II focuses on key aspects of the evolution of human food procurement and an overview of contemporary human food systems. The chapters in this part focus on the role of food in human evolution and the importance of the development of agriculture and provide examples of food systems in contemporary populations.
- Part III covers diverse theoretical perspectives that are used to analyze food systems. Included are sections on materialist perspectives, symbolism and the power of symbols, food as medicine, adapting to foods, and cultural modifications of food.
- Part IV takes on the issues of under- and over-nutrition in the contemporary world. The specific areas addressed include the consequences of undernutrition, the significance of globalization and ongoing dietary transitions, infant feeding as a critical nexus, nutritional issues in developed nations, and the search for solutions to global nutritional problems.

The Selection of Chapters

The process of selecting chapters to include in *Nutritional Anthropology: Biocultural Perspectives on Food and Nutrition* was our most difficult and most rewarding task. We relied on the wisdom of many colleagues, as well as our own experiences. Selecting chapters involved a great deal of give and take because tastes in reading, like tastes in food, are individualistic. One of the rewards of the selection process was discovering little-known "gems." Our selections were guided by the following criteria.

- Clarity and readability. Even if the material is detailed or technically difficult, it must be clearly presented.
- Current issues. A few of the chapters were originally published in the 1960s, 1970s, and 1980s. We include these as historical pieces because of the issues they addressed and because of the fact that their means of addressing them are still timely. The majority of the chapters are more recent.
- Representation of diverse perspectives. Although the dominant perspective is biocultural, we wish to show that there is much variety in how one might approach various nutrition and food issues.
- Ethnographic and geographic spread. We have selected chapters to maximize geographic diversity and, at the same time, have endeavored to provide a focus on the nutritional anthropology of the United States.
- A spectrum of types of chapters. We have intentionally selected chapters that were written for different audiences and with different purposes. Some of the chapters are written for general audiences, others are reviews for specialists, and others are primary research chapters written for professional anthropologists, nutritionists, medical doctors, or epidemiologists. The variety provides a sense of the goals and purposes of different types of writings, as well as the complexity of the issues addressed. As Susan Blum said in her preface to *Making Sense of Language* (Oxford University Press, 2009), it is a bit like getting your vitamin C from a juicy orange rather a tablet.
- This revision also gave us the opportunity to include seven essays specifically commissioned

for this volume. These essays were written to summarize the authors' current work and/or interests in ways that are more appropriate for the audience than some of their other published work. They provide the most current and up-to-date analysis of rapidly changing areas of inquiry.

Using This Reader

Our aim is for this book to be flexibly included in a variety of courses on food and nutrition. For example, in an anthropology course we expect that it could be supplemented with a monograph that provides more ethnographic detail. Conversely, in a more nutritionally oriented course it may be supplemented with a nutrition text.

Many of the chapters we selected were included to provoke discussion. Was cooking the key to the evolution of our genus, *Homo*? Is the international response to famine misguided? Does it really matter how much meat people in wealthier countries eat or how many miles an apple has traveled from harvest to consumption? We hope that these controversial areas will provide students with a sense of the currency of important debates.

The section introductions and appendices in this second edition contain links to reference materials that we have found useful. For example, the Centers for Disease Control (CDC) website provides a body mass index (BMI) calculator for adults that allows students to estimate their own and their classmates' BMI, one of the central methodologies of nutritional anthropology. The CDC website also provides a summary of key issues in nutrition for those who have not taken a course in nutrition and in classes that are not supplemented with a nutrition text.

Finally, we apologize if we have left out any of your favorite topics or chapters. We have not, for example, focused on eating disorders, because this topic is well covered in other edited books and monographs. We have not included fictional writing that focuses on food, although there are many excellent examples. These may be assigned alongside the reader.

We hope this volume will mark a new stage in the continued development of nutritional anthropology. We also hope readers will provide feedback on chapters that did not meet their expectations and offer suggestions of new ones to consider. Good reading!

Acknowledgments

As foods systems are often wide and intricate, a similarly wide network of colleagues provided support and advice.

In addition to all the contributors, we would particularly like to thank George Armelagos, Richard Bender, Susan Blum, Barry Bogin, Miriam Chaiken, Debra Crooks, Elliot Fratkin, Jean-Pierre Habicht, Chaia Heller, David Himmelgreen, Sol Katz, Thomas Leatherman, Leslie Sue Lieberman, Lynn Morgan, Suzanne Nelson, Barbara Piperata, R. Brooke Thomas, Andrea Wiley, and Heather Williams. Students, particularly those at the University of Colorado, University of Massachusetts, Amherst, and Hampshire College, "pretested" many of the chapters, and we thank them for their good advice. Thanks to Richard Bender and Keegan Patmore for handling requests for permissions, Heather Williams for updating the glossary, and Paul Patmore, Valerie McBride, and Karen Lund for help with manuscript preparation. Thank you also to those whose comments contributed to the revision process for the second edition:

- Ryan Thomas Adams, Indiana University–Purdue University Indianapolis
- James R. Bindon, University of Alabama
- Elaine Gerber, Montclair State University
- Tom Leatherman, University of Massachusetts, Amherst
- Lois Stanford, New Mexico State University
- Susan deFrance, University of Florida

We owe a great debt of gratitude to individuals associated with Oxford University Press who helped bring this second edition to reality. We are especially grateful to Sherith Pankratz, Theresa Stockton, and Cari Heicklen. Finally, we want to thank Jan Beatty, who has been an unwavering source of great advice and encouragement from the beginning of the first edition to the present.

New for the Second Edition

- Expanded coverage: 55 chapters covering a wide range of topics
- Two-thirds (67%) of the chapters are new to this edition
- Inclusion of 7 original essays
- Major new section entitled "Looking for Solutions" was added to make students aware of current approaches to solving food and nutrition problems
- Appendices provide links to important websites

Darna L Dufour
Alan H. Goodman
Gretel Pelto

CONTRIBUTORS OF ORIGINAL CHAPTERS

Richard L. Bender, *Department of Anthropology, University of Colorado at Boulder, Boulder, Colorado.*

Barry Bogin, *Centre for Global Health & Human Development, School of Sport, Exercise & Health Sciences, Loughborough University, United Kingdom.*

Alexandra A. Brewis, *School of Human Evolution and Social Change, Arizona State University, Tempe, Arizona.*

Rachel Casiday, *Department of Voluntary Sector Studies, University of Wales, Lampeter, United Kingdom.*

Katherine Hampshire, *Department of Anthropology, Durham University, United Kingdom.*

David A. Himmelgreen, *Department of Anthropology, University of South Florida, Tampa, Florida.*

Kate Kilpatrick, *Development Consultant, Bonn, Germany.*

Charlotte A. Noble, *Department of Anthropology, University of South Florida, Tampa, Florida.*

Catherine Panter-Brick, *Jackson Institute and Department of Anthropology, Yale University, New Haven, Connecticut.*

Nancy Romero-Daza, *Department of Anthropology, University of South Florida, Tampa, Florida.*

CHAPTER 1

The Biocultural Perspective in Nutritional Anthropology

Gretel H. Pelto, Darna L. Dufour, and Alan H. Goodman
(2012)

Scenario 1. Jane and Frank are discussing the house renovations their neighbors, Jeff and Carol, are doing. Jane reports to Frank the sum of money that is being spent on the kitchen, an amount that vastly exceeds the amount that they themselves would be willing to spend. Frank reacts, "That's nuts—just for the kitchen? Think what else they could do with that money; they could even put in a tennis court." Jane replies, "Well, dear, you have to remember that Jeff lives to eat."

Scenario 2. Bill and Joe have finished lunch and are lingering over coffee and a fruit tart before they return to their offices to continue work. Peter, another colleague, walks into the café and orders a "sandwich to go." While it is being prepared, he comes over to the table to greet Bill and Joe, and they chat amiably for a few minutes. "Number 10, peanut butter and jelly," the clerk announces. "That's me," says Peter, who proceeds to pay for the sandwich and then turns to wave as he leaves. "Does that guy ever sit down to lunch?" Bill asks. "Not likely," Joe replies. "Peter eats to live, you know."

"He lives to eat."

"He eats to live."

These two variations of an aphorism that describes the relationship between some individuals and their food have become commonplace in popular American discourse. The first is often intended as a thinly veiled accusation of gluttony. It good-naturedly caricatures an individual whose interest in food exceeds a level that is "seemly" (that is, culturally appropriate). Food is slow in preparation and maximally social. The second is also often used with a mildly pejorative intent. It carries the implication that the individual being described is insufficiently interested in the "finer" (that is, culturally valued) aspects of food. It conjures up an image of someone who "wolfs down" food and is oblivious to the sensory and social pleasures of eating. Food is fast; in and out as quickly as possible. Together, these two variations of the aphorism capture the extremes of an implicit cultural dimension about how people should relate to food, and in so doing they reveal the varied significance of food in American culture.

As is true of many aphorisms, the characterization in the "eat-to-live" and "live-to-eat" observations derive their punch

from the fact that they rest on an underlying truism. In this case, the truism is that humans, like all living organisms, must eat food to obtain the nutrients that are essential to life, and, at the same time, we humans invest food with a host of symbolic and social qualities that enhance its meaning beyond that of sustaining physical functioning. A tacit recognition of the interplay of these two elements is invoked in the popular aphorism.

This interplay between food as a biological necessity and the social and cultural factors that condition its availability and consumption is the focus of a number of fields of research. Nutrition and/or food are the subjects of study in many disciplines, from biochemistry and molecular biology to philosophy, folklore, and history. Contemporary scholarship on food and nutrition covers the full range from questions that are exclusively biological to ones that are exclusively about social issues. Some disciplines, including nutritional epidemiology, public health nutrition, community nutrition, and nutritional anthropology, focus on the middle ground in the spectrum from biological to social aspects of food and nutrition. Each of these "middle-of-the-spectrum" disciplines has its own identity and orientation, which are determined to a large extent by the types of questions with which it is concerned.

As a field of study, *nutritional anthropology is fundamentally concerned with understanding the interrelationships*

Adapted from GH Pelto, AH Goodman, DL Dufour, "The Biocultural Perspective in Nutritional Anthropology." *Nutritional Anthropology*. Goodman AH, Dufour DL, and Pelto GH, eds. Mountain View, CA: Mayfield Publishing Company, pp. 1–9, 2000.

of biological and social forces in shaping human food use and the nutritional status of individuals and populations. Food, or what is bioculturally defined as edible, contains nutrients and other substances. Once food is consumed, the human digestive tract begins to convert food to its chemical constituents. One result of variation in the amount and quality of foods consumed is variation in nutritional status, or the state of balance resulting from the supply and expenditure of nutrients. Nutritional status is important because it is linked to a host of health and functional consequences. A simplified flow of the process linking food to function is presented below.

Culture/Environment→Food→Nutrients→
Nutritional Status→Functional Outcomes

In pursuing knowledge of this important process, nutritional anthropologists use theory from both biological and social sciences and employ research methods from biological sciences, from cultural anthropology, and from other social sciences. In addition, they also draw on humanistic scholarship as a source of insights into the cultural and historical aspects of food. In this essay, we outline key elements of the concepts and approaches that characterize the field of nutritional anthropology.

AN ECOLOGICAL MODEL OF FOOD AND NUTRITION

The ecological model of food and nutrition, published a number of years ago by Jerome, Kandel, and Pelto (1980), is a conceptual model that has been invaluable in helping us think about the myriad of factors and forces that shape human food use and nutritional status. This model

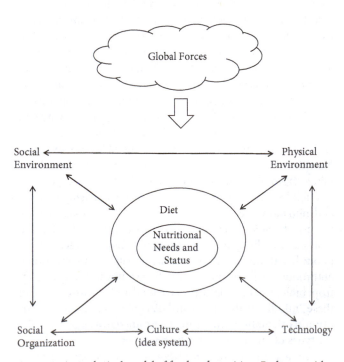

Figure 1 *An ecological model of food and nutrition. Redrawn with modifications from Jerome, Kandel, and Pelto (1980).*

(Figure 1) identifies the main social and environmental sectors in a truly holistic analysis of the factors that affect the nutrition of a population. In any particular study, investigators may focus their attention primarily on one of these sectors, but *the hallmark of a biocultural approach is the examination of interactions* among them. Augmented with a chronological perspective and attention to interactions of genetics, disease, and the biological characteristics of foods, the ecological model provides a framework for a biocultural approach to understanding food systems and nutrition.

The sectors in the model are defined as follows. The *physical environment* includes climate, water resources, soil characteristics, naturally occurring flora and fauna, and other features that establish the conditions for food procurement and production. The *social environment* refers to the larger, external environment (other societies, regions, and communities) whose food production and distribution behavior can have profound effects on the society or social group in question. *Social organization* encompasses a large set of social institutions and arrangements, from the structure and organization of the household to the political and economic structures that relate to the production, distribution, and consumption of food. *Technology* includes the entire range of tools and techniques that are used for production, distribution, acquisition, storage, and preparation of food. *Culture* (systems of thought and ideology) refers to ideas and concepts related to food, such as food preferences and restrictions, the use of food in social interactions, religious beliefs involving food, and ideas about food and health. In our own society the knowledge that we refer to under the rubric of "nutritional science" would be part of the *cultural systems* component of the ecological model.

In the center of the model is *diet,* which includes everything that is consumed. Nested within *diet* are *nutritional needs* and *nutritional status.* The latter refers to the biological status, or health of the population, as determined by dietary intake.

To the original model we have added a "cloud" to represent the global forces that impinge on local populations to a much greater extent today than they did when the model was first published. These forces include things like food commodity prices, multinational trade agreements, and the marketing behavior of multinational food processing companies.

The bidirectional arrows in the diagram are intended to indicate the dynamic, interactive nature of the model. Only some of the interrelationships are shown because the diagram would be difficult to decipher if all the sectors were connected to each other with two-way arrows. In theory, however, there are multiple ways in which these sectors are linked, and changes and developments in each affect all of the others. To illustrate, consider the effects of global warming—an aspect of the physical environment. This phenomenon can be examined in terms of not only its immediate effects on the food supply in specific locations but also changes in idea systems (culture) as new language, new concepts, and even new fears enter the vocabulary of daily life. The effects of global warming are identifiable in the invention of new technologies and in alterations in economic exchanges and in the policies and organizational structures that facilitate these exchanges. No sector in the ecological model is unaffected by a change in the physical environment, and each of these changes influences dietary intakes to some degree. The same principle of "interconnectedness" holds for changes that begin in other sectors of the model. In other words, the ecological model on which research in nutritional anthropology is based is fundamentally a *systems model*.

FOOD SYSTEMS IN NUTRITIONAL ANTHROPOLOGY

The concept of food as a dynamic system is one of the most central concepts in nutritional anthropology. Anthropologists use food systems in at least two different ways. The phrase "food system" can be used to refer to the totality of activities, social institutions, material inputs and outputs, and cultural beliefs *within* a social group that are involved in the production, distribution, and consumption of food. This holistic definition is clearly related to the ecological model described previously. The different components of physical and social actions that are concerned with food are seen as constituting an interactive and interdependent system. An important trend in human history is toward increasing "delocalization" of food systems, by which food production and consumption are geographically separated. And, of course, the local foods movement has developed as an effort to reverse this trend. Many of the chapters in this book examine the internal workings of specific food systems (for examples, see sections on "Explaining Food Ways" and "Dietary Transitions and Globalization").

A second, less common definition of "food systems" is based on the means of food acquisition and in this usage is synonymous with subsistence system. The food quest is so central to the functioning of societies that anthropologists have made extensive studies of subsistence systems. The differences in the ways that human groups obtain and use food resources have powerful effects on social organization, kinship structure, religious practices, child rearing practices, and many other aspects of life. In the most simplified form, the categorization distinguishes among (1) hunting-gathering subsistence systems; (2) pastoralist systems; (3) agricultural systems, which are subdivided into horticultural (or gardening) systems and more intensive (or plow) agricultural systems; and (4) industrialized agricultural systems. Before we turn to an overview of these different types of food systems, we should review the fundamental similarities that have characterized human food use throughout our evolution as a species, regardless of the type of systems we create.

Universals in Human Food Use

The wide variation that one finds in contemporary and historical food systems is a function of interactions among ecological/cultural determinants in relation to the plasticity and flexibility of the human biological template. Compared with those of other animals, human food systems are distinctive in a number of ways, and despite their great diversity, it is possible to identify core characteristics of basic human biocultural food patterns:

- *Homo sapiens* are omnivores. Unlike many species that are adapted to specific foods, humans can derive all of their nutrients from an extremely wide spectrum of sources.
- Moreover, humans cook. All human groups prepare at least some of their food by cooking, which includes boiling, roasting, frying, and steaming, usually with the addition of various flavoring elements, including salt, sweeteners, or other substances that modify the taste of the prepared foods.
- Humans use fire. The use of fire and other food preparation techniques means that humans spend more time in the preparation and alteration of foods than do other animals.
- Foods are meaningful. Humans everywhere have elaborate systems of food distribution, sharing, and exchange. These systems of food sharing have resulted in complex ideologies of meaning.
- Humans select their foods. From the process of selecting goods to eat from the larger pool of potentially edible plants and animals, all human groups have created food prohibitions as well as food preferences. Together with the symbolic structures that have developed through the regulation of social exchanges around food, these ideological elements of preference and prohibition have powerful influences on dietary intakes.

Variations in the Food Quest

Hunting-Gathering Subsistence Systems. For most of our history, humans lived as hunter-gatherers, collecting food from land and water, but not cultivating plant foods or raising animals. In most environments, the distribution of food resources was such that human groups were small, seminomadic bands, utilizing fairly large land areas. Population density was low, and population growth was slow. Only in unusually rich environments, especially riverine and coastal areas, were food resources sufficiently concentrated to allow for permanent settlement and the development of more complex social organizations.

A review of hunting-gathering, or foraging subsistence systems, reveals a wide range in the types of food consumed and in the ratio of animal to vegetable foods. Several chapters in this book examine the evidence concerning diet and nutritional status in hunting-gathering adaptations to food acquisition (see chapters 6, 12, and 28). Data from archaeological research, as well as studies of foraging peoples who maintained this form of subsistence into the twentieth century, suggest that in general nutritional status was good. Seasonal food shortage was a problem in many environments, but chronic malnutrition and deficiency diseases were rare.

Pastoral Subsistence Systems. These are subsistence systems based on herd animals like cattle, goats, camels, and reindeer. Most pastoralists are nomadic and move with their herds from one area of pasture to another within a defined territory. Others live in settlements and cultivate some crops. The diets of pastoralists are highly dependent on the animals they herd, with milk products playing a central role. However, all pastoralist diets contain foods from local agricultural systems, especially grains. The chapter in this book by McCabe and colleagues (chapter 14) examines characteristics of "the pastoralist strategy." Today, fewer and fewer peoples are able to pursue this subsistence strategy as economic and political forces push them into permanent villages and other forms of obtaining food. However, for more than 3000 years, pastoralists inhabited areas from the Atlantic shore of the Sahara to the steppes of Mongolia, as well as parts of South America.

Agricultural Food Systems. Beginning approximately 12,000 to 15,000 years ago in several different parts of the world, human groups developed ways of cultivating and, hence, domesticating a variety of plants. All over the world the transition from hunting and gathering to cultivation and animal keeping appears to have developed through a process of interactions between increased population pressures and technological-environmental factors. The "idea" of plant and animal domestication spread widely, and by 2000 years ago a very large proportion of the world's peoples were dependent on agricultural production to supply most of their food. The transitions from hunting and gathering came about rather gradually, over many centuries, but their impact on human lifeways was profound. The effects of the "agricultural revolution" not only radically altered diet, nutrition, and health but also brought about social and technological changes that altered the nature of human societies in very fundamental ways (see chapters 10 and 12).

The earliest forms of agricultural food systems, which have continued to the present day, are referred to as "horticultural" or "gardening" systems (for an example see chapter 13) These systems, which rely on relatively simple technology and human labor and rain for irrigation, produce foods for household consumption rather than for commercial sale. Typically, the production unit is a household, which functions as a self-provisioning entity (Wolf, 1966). There is relatively little interdependence with external groups, and expanded market networks are generally not present. Instead, the social relations around food are played out through ceremonial and ritual interactions.

More intensive forms of agriculture that involved only some members of a society in food production (albeit a substantial proportion) arose with the development of the plow, irrigation, and the emergence of a class of producers commonly referred to as peasants. Wolf (1966) described *peasants* as rural cultivators who raise crops and livestock in the countryside for household consumption, while the surplus production of their more efficient methods is transferred to a dominant group in the city who use it to underwrite other activities, including a higher standard of living for themselves. Because peasants often lack control over their agricultural production, they often are not able to keep adequate amounts to meet their own nutritional needs. The malnutrition that plagues rural food producers in many developing countries today is not new but came about with the development of state societies that were built on intensive agriculture. In Mesoamerica, for example, there is substantial evidence from archaeological data to suggest that the average stature of Mayan males decreased from the Early Classic Period (A.D. 250–550) to the Late Classic Period, as intensive cultivation proceeded and rural producers experienced increasing nutritional stress. The decrease in dietary adequacy was due to a number of factors, including increasing environmental degradation under the pressure of overproduction. The reasons for overproduction are also complex, but there is little doubt that the demand of the ruling class for food to support their own nonfood production activities played a significant role. Thus, the class differences in diet that are found in Mexico and Guatemala today represent the continuation of long-standing patterns of dietary inequality.

Industrialized Agriculture and Cash Crops. In modern times in developing countries, the production of nonfood crops (such as tobacco and sisal) and nonnutritive foods (such as coffee and tea) has come to play an increasingly important role as household food production has shifted away from subsistence food needs to the production of crops for sale in the market place. For example, in the Kolli Hills of India farmers have shifted from the cultivation of millet, the traditional basis of the diet, to the cultivation of cassava, which can be sold for cash (see chapter 15). Changes in household production patterns are just one aspect of the vast social, cultural, and environmental changes that are associated with the "delocalization" of food production and the globalization of economies. In nutritional anthropology, the dietary and nutritional consequences of cash cropping at the community, household, and individual level have been a particular focus of research.

During the second half of the twentieth century in many areas of developed countries, the industrialization of food production has transformed farming from a lifestyle for family groups embedded in local communities to factory-like enterprises focused on crops with high profit margins and "durable" enough to be transported long distances. This transformation has gone hand in hand with the industrialization of food processing and the proliferation of the processed and "ready-to-eat" foods found on supermarket shelves. Understanding the short-term and long-term consequences of this new stage in the evolution of human food systems claims the attention of anthropologists as well as researchers across a range of social science disciplines and the humanities.

Chapters 15–17, 23, and 40–42 provide some examples of anthropologically informed work on these contemporary processes.

RESEARCH APPROACHES IN NUTRITIONAL ANTHROPOLOGY

We suggested previously that one of the features that distinguish disciplines concerned with food and nutrition research is the type of questions that the members of each discipline address in their work. Together with the theoretical approaches that they draw on in forming their hypotheses about "how the world works," and the methods they use to investigate these hypotheses, the types of questions that investigators ask tend to have a different cast, depending on their disciplinary orientation. Thus, sociologists, psychologists, anthropologists, political scientists, economists, epidemiologists, humanists, and individuals whose basic training is in the biological or medical sciences frame their questions in different ways. Here we focus on some of the main research orientations of work in nutritional anthropology (see Pelto, 1966).

The evolution of human lifeways in terms of both long- and short-term "sociocultural processes" has always been of interest. In nutritional anthropology, the most significant long-term evolutionary change was the transition from hunting-gathering subsistence to settled, agriculturally based societies. The large-scale sociocultural processes that are currently ongoing, which are also the subject of study by nutritional anthropologists, are often subsumed under the labels of globalization, modernization (including the growth of cities and the importance of mass media), delocalization of energy resources, and industrialization.

The basic structure of the questions that nutritional anthropologists ask about the relationship of sociocultural processes to nutrition is: "What is the impact of X on nutrition?" The X in this question is a particular sociocultural process or set of events, such as the transformation of a subsistence system from one form to another, the introduction of a new technology, or migration from rural to urban areas. For example, anthropologists have studied the impact of the shift from hunting-gathering to agriculture for human nutrition and health (see chapter 12), as well as the effects of recent social processes, such as tourism, on nutrition (see chapter 41).

Another common mode of research in nutritional anthropology is to focus on a specific factor or set of factors in a particular place to understand how they relate to food intake and nutrition. In this case the basic structure of the question is: "How is factor(s) X related to diet and nutrition?" For example, the well-known studies of the !Kung San (represented in this book by Lee's chapters 2 and 7) describe the linkages between the social organization of the group, the environment, and dietary intake in hunting-gathering food systems. Studies of dietary changes associated with cross-national migration caused by warfare and political upheaval are another example of this mode of question.

A slightly different approach is to put the initial focus on a nutritional condition and seek to identify the role of social factors in the etiology of that condition. The general structure of the research question is: "What are the determinants of (or the factors associated with) outcome Y?" The Y in this question is a nutritional condition, such as iron deficiency anemia, short stature in children, marasmus (a protein-energy deficiency disease), or obesity (see chapters 33–37 and 48–50).

The study of cultural systems of belief as they relate to nutritional outcomes is another focus of research for nutritional anthropology. The structure of questions takes the form: "What is the relationship of X [beliefs] to Y [nutritional outcome]?" In this statement, the word "beliefs" is used broadly to cover the range from specific elements of knowledge, such as the concept of "vitamins" or "iron-rich foods," to more general cultural constructs. An example of the latter is the humoral medical system of "hot/cold" beliefs, which imputes qualities of "hot" or "cold" to individual food items as well as to illnesses. In this book, Dubisch (chapter 32) applies this perspective to the health foods movement.

Finally, a larger question concerns the analysis of the factors that lead to a particular food ideology. What is, for example, the context and conditions under which the hot/cold belief system originated? Why do some individuals in a society value local foods and other value fast foods? The answers to these questions come slowly through systemic analyses of the flows of knowledge and relations of power. Soft drinks are offered to guests of Yucatecan Mayans because they are high status, but why are they high status? Could it be because they are associated with the West or that they are widely advertised on billboards throughout the Yucatan?

Nutritional anthropologists also pursue studies in which they apply principles of human adaptation to guide the development of hypotheses about how the nutritional history of a population has shaped or influenced its physiological or genetic characteristics. Adaptation refers to the beneficial responses or adjustments that organisms, humans included, make to environmental conditions including nutritional conditions. The general form of the research question is: "What is the role of X [biochemical feature of a food or a pattern of food availability and/or use] in explaining the distribution of Y [physiological or genetic trait or condition] in this *population*?" A classic example of this type of research interest is the study of lactose tolerance in adults, a genetic trait found in populations with a long history of animal husbandry (see chapter 26). Another example would be the nutritional status of !Kung hunter-gatherers living under conditions of food scarcity (see chapter 28).

The concept of adaptation has also been used to frame questions about the beneficial aspects of behavioral and technological innovations rather than biological adjustments. The development of maize-processing techniques that prevent pellagra (see chapter 25) and manioc-processing techniques that make it possible to use bitter manioc (see chapter 24) are examples of cultural adaptations that improve people's ability to successfully exploit food resources.

Commonalities in Method and Theory

A notable characteristic of nutritional anthropology is its eclecticism. The ecological model leads investigators to draw from methods and theories in nutritional biochemistry, physiology, genetics, and epidemiology, as well as the social and policy sciences. At the same time, there are several commonalities in the research approach of nutritional anthropologists. These not only cut across the specific questions that are the topics of study, but also reflect an anthropological approach to these questions. These commonalities include the following:

- Studies generally focus on a *population* rather than studying individual subjects without consideration of the population of which they are a part. Often the population is defined in terms of a specific *community,* although larger, geographically delimited units may also be used.
- Many studies select the *household* as the primary unit of analysis, which permits the investigation of nutrition and food use within the context of household organization.
- Most studies examine multiple aspects of family characteristics (for example, economic status, demographic and social characteristics), even when the focus is on a particular factor—that is, the approach tends to be "holistic."
- Most studies include both qualitative, descriptive data and quantitative data, which are obtained by using several different data collection methods. These range from informal and open-ended interviews and observations to highly structured formats for interviews and physical measurements, which yield data that are amenable to statistical analysis.

NUTRITIONAL ANTHROPOLOGY IN ACTION

Another aspect of nutritional anthropology is the work carried out by anthropologists who are working in applied settings and conducting studies that are intended to assist programs to function more effectively. Because this kind of work is designed to serve the immediate needs of an organization, agency, or other clients, it is usually more difficult to access through academically oriented publishing sources. Some of it appears in newsletters, project reports, and other similar media. The fact that some of this work is never presented in printed form and that much of it is in widely scattered sources makes it more difficult to characterize. However, the following three categories appear to be the main areas in which applied nutritional anthropologists are currently working:

- Formative research to obtain a better definition of a general nutritional problem that will be the focus of programs or other actions to improve that problem. For example, anthropologists have conducted community studies of infant and young child feeding to provide programs with information to better define the specific problems that families face in a community or region where a new program will be started. A related goal is to identify common problematic behaviors that are negatively affecting child health and growth.
- Research to improve communication strategies and the content of nutrition and health education. Applied nutritional anthropologists work with programs and community members to identify local concepts and beliefs and determine what methods are most appropriate for providing people with the information they need in a manner that will enable them to accept and use it. In the best situations, the anthropologist also provides information and advice from the community back to programs so that the agencies can learn and profit from community knowledge.
- Qualitative ethnographic evaluation of nutrition and health interventions. Some public health agencies and NGOs (nongovernmental organizations) have become interested in obtaining qualitative evaluations that provide insights into how communities are responding to their programs, including what community members perceive to be the goals, purposes, strengths, and weaknesses of the activities and services that have been introduced (see chapter 37).

In recent years, the number of anthropologists working in applied settings has greatly increased. Among this growing body of applied scientists are individuals who specialize in nutrition. Some of them have advanced training in the biological aspects of nutrition, while others come into food and nutrition programs with training in public health, in policy and program evaluation, or in cultural anthropology. As the opportunities for comparative analysis of their studies and experiences increase, applied nutritional anthropology will be in a strong position to make significant contributions to our understanding of human behavior related to food and nutrition. This, in turn, will help to create new knowledge for action to address the pressing problems that currently threaten the health and well-being of people all over the globe.

References

Jerome NW, Kandel RF, Pelto GH. 1980. An ecological approach to nutritional anthropology. In NW Jerome, RF Kandel, GH Pelto, eds. *Nutritional Anthropology: Contemporary Approaches to Diet and Culture.* Pleasantville, NY: Redgrave Publishing, pp. 13–45.

Pelto GH. 1966. Nutritional anthropology. In D Levinson, M Ember, eds. *Encyclopedia of Cultural Anthropology.* Vol. 3. New York: Henry Holt and Co, pp. 881–884.

Wolf ER. 1966. *Peasants.* Englewood Cliffs, NJ: Prentice Hall.

PART I

A Taste of Nutritional Anthropology

Nutritional anthropology encompasses many types of studies and food is fundamental to most of them. Foods fulfill nutritional functions in that they nourish the body, but anthropologists often start with the assumption that humans make choices about what to eat, and these choices are not necessarily governed by the physiological need for nourishment. Rather, humans make choices governed by the social, cultural, aesthetic, and even moral meaning of food, coupled with the realities of availability and cost. The clearest examples are the extremes. North Americans do not classify dogs, pigeons, or grasshoppers as "food" even though they have nutritional value and are consumed by other groups. They do not consider the small intestine of sheep as food either, but willingly consume it disguised as the natural casing of hotdogs, and they willingly consume hotdogs at picnics but not at formal dinner parties. In contrast, native peoples in the Amazon consider leaf cutter ants a delicacy and find cow's milk quite repulsive. Because of the social dimensions that underlie food consumption, limiting the study of nutrition to aspects of nourishment determined by physiological needs is, well, limiting.

The four chapters in this section illustrate the meanings of foods in different times and places (Figure 1). In his classic article, "Eating Christmas in the Kalahari," Richard Lee relates a lesson learned about humility in providing a gift of food. In "No Heads, No Feet, No Monkeys, No Dogs," Miriam Chaiken provides a personal story of encounters with foods of different kinds and because of their differences finds them difficult to eat. In "From Hunger Foods to Heritage Foods," Penny Van Esterik emphasizes the fact that the meaning of a food is context specific and can be very different at local and global levels. In "Rough Food," a brief introduction to a book of the same name, John Omohundro provides a glimpse of the traditional winter diet in the northernmost reaches of Newfoundland. All four chapters were written by cultural anthropologists. Together they provide a sense of some of the issues to be addressed in greater depth in the section introductions and chapters to follow.

Richard Lee, the author of "Eating Christmas in the Kalahari," undertook a long-term study of the economy of the !Kung San in the Kalahari Desert of southern Africa in the 1960s and 1970s (see chapter 7, "What Hunters Do for

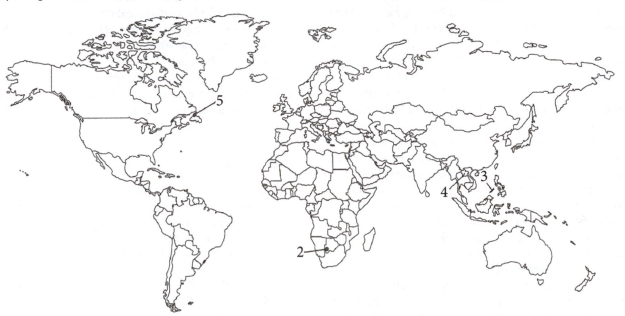

Figure 1 *Map shows the location of the groups referred to in the chapters in this section by chapter number: 2 = !Kung Bushmen of the Dobe area of Botswana; 3 = village, Palawan Island in the Philippines; 4 = Lao People's Democratic Republic; 5 = northern Newfoundland.*

7

a Living, or, How to Make Out on Scarce Resources"). Lee relates a story of his own foibles in deciding to purchase an ox as a gift for his community of informants. Lee imparts a lesson about the power of food, the symbolism that is embedded in important "gifts," and other forms of exchange.

In the second paper, "No Heads, No Feet, No Monkeys, No Dogs," cultural anthropologist Miriam Chaiken shares some of the food-related challenges she faced in doing field research on the pacific island of Palawan in the early 1980s. She and her husband lived in a small, isolated village where there were no food stores and people ate largely what they were able to grow in their garden or catch in the sea. Hence, a fundamental challenge was simply securing food for herself and her husband in an environment where the nearest food market was two and a half to seven hours away depending on the number of "jeepney" breakdowns and flat tires. There was also the challenge of graciously declining local foods that she was uncomfortable eating, including the dog she had thought of as a pet. Miriam Chaiken's story is an example of the challenge that anthropologists often face in accommodating to local food habits.

The third paper, "From Hunger Foods to Heritage Foods: Challenges to Food Localization in Lao PDR" by Penny Van Esterik, is a longer and more complex paper, but a highly provocative one. Van Esterik highlights the contrasts in the meaning of a food that grows wild in a local place, northern Laos, with the meaning of that same food in the global market place. The food, *khai*, is a variety of green algae collected from rivers in northern Laos and eaten in water-based soups in times of food scarcity, when the availability of rice, the basis of the diet, is inadequate. It is what is known as a "hunger food," a food eaten to satisfy the gnawing stomach discomfort that is physical hunger. The same green algae, *khai*, is also collected and sold in the global market to be processed into delicacies for elite diners in North America to satisfy the "hunger" for the exotic.

Van Esterik sets the story of *khai* within the larger nutritional context of Laos, a developing country with alarmingly high rates of adult and child undernutrition. According to a recent report from the World Food Programme (WFP 2011) only 16% of children under 5 years of age have diets that are adequate in terms of quantity and diversity. In poorer households rice is the basis of the diet; meat and oils may only be eaten once or twice a month and vegetables are only available seasonally. As a result of their generally poor diet, over 40% of children suffer from iron deficiency anemia as well as vitamin A deficiency. Deficiencies of other micronutrients (vitamins and minerals) are also likely. As some of the other papers in this volume note, these kinds of deficiencies can lead to physical and cognitive impairments.

The paper raises many questions. Why do farmers run short of rice? Who are these farmers? What could be done to help them be more self-sufficient? Why don't people include iron and vitamin A-rich foods in their diets, or the diets of their children? Is it poverty and/or beliefs about what constitutes a "good" diet? These are the kinds of questions nutritional anthropologists, working in a variety of different societies, attempt to answer.

The fourth paper, "Rough Food," is from the first pages of an ethnography by John Omohundro, in which he describes subsistence practices and diet in northern Newfoundland at the very northern edge of where agriculture is possible in North America. This was a place where people lived far from food markets until the 1970s, but did not find the remoteness of the setting a problem because they could grow, hunt, and fish much of what they needed. Theirs was a diet attuned to the rhythm of the seasons and the resources of the local environment. As romantic as that might seem, it was also a simpler diet than most readers of this book can probably imagine. In the winter it was "rough food," a diet based on the staple foods that had been harvested in the fall and preserved: potatoes, carrots, cabbage and salt beef, supplemented with moose, caribou, rabbit or fish, and some store-bought staples like flour and butter. It is a diet from a time not too long ago, before the word "locavore" (one who eats from the local area) was invented, but a time during which being a locavore was the norm, not the exception. It was the only option.

So what can we learn from the four papers in this section? One thing is that there are, and have been, very different food systems in different places. In some we can clearly see how local subsistence practices connect to diet. Another is that a food can have a different meaning in the local food system, to the anthropologist, and in the global market place. A final example is açai, a palm fruit that grows wild in the eastern Amazon. In rural areas, açai is an ordinary part of the diet and consumed as a thick oil-rich drink alongside *farinha* (a toasted meal made from manioc roots) and grilled fish (Piperata et al., 2011). Exported to North America it becomes an exotic food, a "berry" with properties that verge on the magical. Its advertised role in promoting weight loss comes as a great surprise to rural Amazonians who say that the season of açai is the season when everyone gets fat! Interesting. How can people attribute such different attributes to the same food?

References

Piperata BA, Ivanova SA, Da-Gloria P, Veiga G, Polsky A, Spence JE, Murrieta RSS. 2011. Nutrition transition: Dietary patterns of rural Amazonian women during a period of economic change. American Journal of Human Biology 23:458–469.

World Food Programme. WPF Lao PDR Country Strategy. Accessed on May 5, 2011 at http://www.wfp.org/sites/default/files/WFP%20Lao%20PDR%20Country%20Strategy_ENG.pdf

CHAPTER 2

Eating Christmas in the Kalahari

Richard Borshay Lee

(1969)

The !Kung Bushmen's knowledge of Christmas is third-hand. The London Missionary Society brought the holiday to the southern Tswana tribes in the early nineteenth century. Later, native catechists spread the idea far and wide among the Bantu-speaking pastoralists, even in the remotest corners of the Kalahari Desert. The Bushmen's idea of the Christmas story, stripped to its essentials, is "praise the birth of white man's god-chief"; what keeps their interest in the holiday high is the Tswana-Herero custom of slaughtering an ox for his Bushmen neighbors as an annual good-will gesture. Since the 1930's, part of the Bushmen's annual round of activities has included a December congregation at the cattle posts for trading, marriage brokering, and several days of trance-dance feasting at which the local Tswana headman is host.

As a social anthropologist working with !Kung Bushmen, I found that the Christmas ox custom suited my purposes. I had come to the Kalahari to study the hunting and gathering subsistence economy of the !Kung, and to accomplish this it was essential not to provide them with food, share my own food, or interfere in any way with their food-gathering activities. While liberal handouts of tobacco and medical supplies were appreciated, they were scarcely adequate to erase the glaring disparity in wealth between the anthropologist, who maintained a two-month inventory of canned goods, and the Bushmen, who rarely had a day's supply of food on hand. My approach, while paying off in terms of data, left me open to frequent accusations of stinginess and hard-heartedness. By their lights, I was a miser.

The Christmas ox was to be my way of saying thank you for the cooperation of the past year; and since it was to be our last Christmas in the field, I determined to slaughter the largest, meatiest ox that money could buy, insuring that the feast and trance-dance would be a success.

Through December I kept my eyes open at the wells as the cattle were brought down for watering. Several animals were offered, but none had quite the grossness that I had in mind. Then, ten days before the holiday, a Herero friend led an ox of astonishing size and mass up to our camp. It was

solid black, stood five feet high at the shoulder, had a five-foot span of horns, and must have weighed 1,200 pounds on the hoof. Food consumption calculations are my specialty, and I quickly figured that bones and viscera aside, there was enough meat—at least four pounds—for every man, woman, and child of the 150 Bushmen in the vicinity of /ai/ai who were expected at the feast.

Having found the right animal at last, I paid the Herero £20 ($56) and asked him to keep the beast with his herd until Christmas day. The next morning word spread among the people that the big solid black one was the ox chosen by /ontah (my Bushman name; it means, roughly, "whitey") for the Christmas feast. That afternoon I received the first delegation. Ben!a, an outspoken sixty-year-old mother of five, came to the point slowly.

"Where were you planning to eat Christmas?"

"Right here at /ai/ai," I replied.

"Alone or with others?"

"I expect to invite all the people to eat Christmas with me."

"Eat what?"

"I have purchased Yehave's black ox, and I am going to slaughter and cook it."

"That's what we were told at the well but refused to believe it until we heard it from yourself."

"Well, it's the black one," I replied expansively, although wondering what she was driving at.

"Oh, no!" Ben!a groaned, turning to her group. "They were right." Turning back to me she asked, "Do you expect us to eat that bag of bones?"

"Bag of bones! It's the biggest ox at /ai/ai."

"Big, yes, but old. And thin. Everybody knows there's no meat on that old ox. What did you expect us to eat off it, the horns?"

Everybody chuckled at Ben!a's one-liner as they walked away, but all I could manage was a weak grin.

That evening it was the turn of the young men. They came to sit at our evening fire. /gaugo, about my age, spoke to me man-to-man.

"/ontah, you have always been square with us," he lied. "What has happened to change your heart? That sack of guts and bones of Yehave's will hardly feed one camp, let alone all the Bushmen around ai/ai." And he proceeded to enumerate the seven camps in the /ai/ai vicinity, family by

Richard Borshay Lee, "Eating Christmas in the Kalahari." *Natural History,* December 1969:14–22. Copyright 1969 by the American Museum of Natural History. Reprinted with permission.

9

family. "Perhaps you have forgotten that we are not few, but many. Or are you too blind to tell the difference between a proper cow and an old wreck? That ox is thin to the point of death."

"Look, you guys," I retorted, "that is a beautiful animal, and I'm sure you will eat it with pleasure at Christmas."

"Of course we will eat it; it's food. But it won't fill us up to the point where we will have enough strength to dance. We will eat and go home to bed with stomachs rumbling."

That night as we turned in, I asked my wife, Nancy: "What did you think of the black ox?"

"It looked enormous to me. Why?"

"Well, about eight different people have told me I got gypped; that the ox is nothing but bones."

"What's the angle?" Nancy asked. "Did they have a better one to sell?"

"No, they just said that it was going to be a grim Christmas because there won't be enough meat to go around. Maybe I'll get an independent judge to look at the beast in the morning."

Bright and early, Halingisi, a Tswana cattle owner, appeared at our camp. But before I could ask him to give me his opinion on Yehave's black ox, he gave me the eye signal that indicated a confidential chat. We left the camp and sat down.

"/ontah, I'm surprised at you: you've lived here for three years and still haven't learned anything about cattle."

"But what else can a person do but choose the biggest, strongest animal one can find?" I retorted.

"Look, just because an animal is big doesn't mean that it has plenty of meat on it. The black one was a beauty when it was younger, but now it is thin to the point of death."

"Well I've already bought it. What can I do at this stage?"

"Bought it already? I thought you were just considering it. Well, you'll have to kill it and serve it, I suppose. But don't expect much of a dance to follow."

My spirits dropped rapidly. I could believe that Ben!a and /gaugo just might be putting me on about the black ox, but Halingisi seemed to be an impartial critic. I went around that day feeling as though I had bought a lemon of a used car.

In the afternoon it was Tomazo's turn. Tomazo is a fine hunter, a top trance performer…and one of my most reliable informants. He approached the subject of the Christmas cow as part of my continuing Bushman education.

"My friend, the way it is with us Bushmen," he began, "is that we love meat. And even more than that, we love fat. When we hunt we always search for the fat ones, the ones dripping with layers of white fat: fat that turns into a clear, thick oil in the cooking pot, fat that slides down your gullet, fills your stomach and gives you a roaring diarrhea," he rhapsodized.

"So, feeling as we do," he continued, "it gives us pain to be served such a scrawny thing as Yehave's black ox. It is big, yes, and no doubt its giant bones are good for soup, but fat is what we really crave and so we will eat Christmas this year with a heavy heart."

The prospect of a gloomy Christmas now had me worried, so I asked Tomazo what I could do about it.

"Look for a fat one, a young one…smaller, but fat. Fat enough to make us //gom ('evacuate the bowels'), then we will be happy."

My suspicions were aroused when Tomazo said that he happened to know of a young, fat, barren cow that the owner was willing to part with. Was Tomazo working on commission, I wondered? But I dispelled this unworthy thought when we approached the Herero owner of the cow in question and found that he had decided not to sell.

The scrawny wreck of a Christmas ox now became the talk of the /ai/ai water hole and was the first news told to the outlying groups as they began to come in from the bush for the feast. What finally convinced me that real trouble might be brewing was the visit from u!au, an old conservative with a reputation for fierceness. His nickname meant spear and referred to an incident thirty years ago in which he had speared a man to death. He had an intense manner; fixing me with his eyes, he said in clipped tones:

"I have only just heard about the black ox today, or else I would have come here earlier. /ontah, do you honestly think you can serve meat like that to people and avoid a fight?" He paused, letting the implications sink in. "I don't mean fight you, /ontah; you are a white man. I mean a fight between Bushmen. There are many fierce ones here, and with such a small quantity of meat to distribute, how can you give everybody a fair share? Someone is sure to accuse another of taking too much or hogging all the choice pieces. Then you will see what happens when some go hungry while others eat."

The possibility of at least a serious argument struck me as all too real. I had witnessed the tension that surrounds the distribution of meat from a kudu or gemsbok kill, and had documented many arguments that sprang up from a real or imagined slight in meat distribution. The owners of a kill may spend up to two hours arranging and rearranging the piles of meat under the gaze of a circle of recipients before handing them out. And I also knew that the Christmas feast at /ai/ai would be bringing together groups that had feuded in the past.

Convinced now of the gravity of the situation, I went in earnest to search for a second cow; but all my inquiries failed to turn one up.

The Christmas feast was evidently going to be a disaster, and the incessant complaints about the meagerness of the ox had already taken the fun out of it for me. Moreover, I was getting bored with the wisecracks, and after losing my temper a few times, I resolved to serve the beast anyway. If the meat fell short, the hell with it. In the Bushmen idiom, I announced to all who would listen:

"I am a poor man and blind. If I have chosen one that is too old and too thin, we will eat it anyway and see if there is enough meat there to quiet the rumbling of our stomachs."

On hearing this speech, Ben!a offered me a rare word of comfort. "It's thin," she said philosophically, "but the bones will make a good soup."

At dawn Christmas morning, instinct told me to turn over the butchering and cooking to a friend and take off with Nancy to spend Christmas alone in the bush. But curiosity kept me from retreating. I wanted to see what such a scrawny ox looked like on butchering and if there *was* going to be a fight, I wanted to catch every word of it. Anthropologists are incurable that way.

The great beast was driven up to our dancing ground, and a shot in the forehead dropped it in its tracks. Then, freshly cut branches were heaped around the fallen carcass to receive the meat. Ten men volunteered to help with the cutting. I asked /gaugo to make the breast bone cut. This cut, which begins the butchering process for most large game, offers easy access for removal of the viscera. But it also allows the hunter to spot-check the amount of fat on the animal. A fat game animal carries a white layer up to an inch thick on the chest, while in a thin one, the knife will quickly cut to bone. All eyes fixed on his hand as /gaugo, dwarfed by the great carcass, knelt to the breast. The first cut opened a pool of solid white in the black skin. The second and third cut widened and deepened the creamy white. Still no bone. It was pure fat; it must have been two inches thick.

"Hey /gau," I burst out, "that ox is loaded with fat. What's this about the ox being too thin to bother eating? Are you out of your mind?"

"Fat?" /gau shot back, "You call that fat? This wreck is thin, sick, dead!" And he broke out laughing. So did everyone else. They rolled on the ground, paralyzed with laughter. Everybody laughed except me; I was thinking.

I ran back to the tent and burst in just as Nancy was getting up. "Hey, the black ox. It's fat as hell! They were kidding about it being too thin to eat. It was a joke or something. A put-on. Everyone is really delighted with it!"

"Some joke," my wife replied. "It was so funny that you were ready to pack up and leave /ai/ai."

If it had indeed been a joke, it had been an extraordinarily convincing one, and tinged, I thought, with more than a touch of malice as many jokes are. Nevertheless, that it was a joke lifted my spirits considerably, and I returned to the butchering site where the shape of the ox was rapidly disappearing under the axes and knives of the butchers. The atmosphere had become festive. Grinning broadly, their arms covered with blood well past the elbow, men packed chunks of meat into the big cast-iron cooking pots, fifty pounds to the load, and muttered and chuckled all the while about the thinness and worthlessness of the animal and /ontah's poor judgment.

We danced and ate that ox two days and two nights; we cooked and distributed fourteen potfuls of meat and no one went home hungry and no fights broke out.

But the "joke" stayed in my mind. I had a growing feeling that something important had happened in my relationship with the Bushmen and that the clue lay in the meaning of the joke. Several days later, when most of the people had dispersed back to the bush camps, I raised the question with Hakekgose, a Tswana man who had grown up among the

!Kung, married a !Kung girl, and who probably knew their culture better than any other non-Bushman.

"With us whites," I began, "Christmas is supposed to be the day of friendship and brotherly love. What I can't figure out is why the Bushmen went to such lengths to criticize and belittle the ox I had bought for the feast. The animal was perfectly good and their jokes and wisecracks practically ruined the holiday for me."

"So it really did bother you," said Hakekgose. "Well, that's the way they always talk. When I take my rifle and go hunting with them, if I miss, they laugh at me for the rest of the day. But even if I hit and bring one down, it's no better. To them, the kill is always too small or too old or too thin; and as we sit down on the kill site to cook and eat the liver, they keep grumbling, even with their mouths full of meat. They say things like, 'Oh this is awful! What a worthless animal! Whatever made me think that this Tswana rascal could hunt!'"

"Is this the way outsiders are treated?" I asked.

"No, it is their custom; they talk that way to each other too. Go and ask them."

/gaugo had been one of the most enthusiastic in making me feel bad about the merit of the Christmas ox. I sought him out first.

"Why did you tell me the black ox was worthless, when you could see that it was loaded with fat and meat?"

"It is our way," he said smiling. "We always like to fool people about that. Say there is a Bushman who has been hunting. He must not come home and announce like a braggard, 'I have killed a big one in the bush!' He must first sit down in silence until I or someone else comes up to his fire and asks, 'What did you see today?' He replies quietly, 'Ah, I'm no good for hunting. I saw nothing at all [pause] just a little tiny one.' Then I smile to myself," /gaugo continued, "because I know he has killed something big."

"In the morning we make up a party of four or five people to cut up and carry the meat back to the camp. When we arrive at the kill we examine it and cry out, 'You mean to say you have dragged us all the way out here in order to make us cart home your pile of bones? Oh, if I had known it was this thin I wouldn't have come.' Another one pipes up, 'People, to think I gave up a nice day in the shade for this. At home we may be hungry but at least we have nice cool water to drink.' If the horns are big, someone says, 'Did you think that somehow you were going to boil down the horns for soup?'

"To all this you must respond in kind. 'I agree,' you say, 'this one is not worth the effort; let's just cook the liver for strength and leave the rest for the hyenas. It is not too late to hunt today and even a duiker or a steenbok would be better than this mess.'

"Then you set to work nevertheless; butcher the animal, carry the meat back to the camp and everyone eats," /gaugo concluded.

Things were beginning to make sense. Next, I went to Tomazo. He corroborated /gaugo's story of the obligatory insults over a kill and added a few details of his own.

"But," I asked, "why insult a man after he has gone to all that trouble to track and kill an animal and when he is going to share the meat with you so that your children will have something to eat?"

"Arrogance," was his cryptic answer.

"Arrogance?"

"Yes, when a young man kills much meat he comes to think of himself as a chief or a big man, and he thinks of the rest of us as his servants or inferiors. We can't accept this. We refuse one who boasts, for someday his pride will make him kill somebody. So we always speak of his meat as worthless. This way we cool his heart and make him gentle."

"But why didn't you tell me this before?" I asked Tomazo with some heat.

"Because you never asked me," said Tomazo, echoing the refrain that has come to haunt every field ethnographer.

The pieces now fell into place. I had known for a long time that in situations of social conflict with Bushmen I held all the cards. I was the only source of tobacco in a thousand square miles, and I was not incapable of cutting an individual off for non-cooperation. Though my boycott never lasted longer than a few days, it was an indication of my strength. People resented my presence at the water hole, yet simultaneously dreaded my leaving. In short I was a perfect target for the charge of arrogance and for the Bushmen tactic of enforcing humility.

I had been taught an object lesson by the Bushmen; it had come from an unexpected corner and had hurt me in a vulnerable area. For the big black ox was to be the one totally generous, unstinting act of my year at /ai/ai, and I was quite unprepared for the reaction I received.

As I read it, their message was this: There are no totally generous acts. All "acts" have an element of calculation. One black ox slaughtered at Christmas does not wipe out a year of careful manipulation of gifts given to serve your own ends. After all, to kill an animal and share the meat with people is really no more than Bushmen do for each other every day and with far less fanfare.

In the end, I had to admire how the Bushmen had played out the farce—collectively straight-faced to the end. Curiously, the episode reminded me of the *Good Soldier Schweik* and his marvelous encounters with authority. Like Schweik, the Bushmen had retained a thorough-going skepticism of good intentions. Was it this independence of spirit, I wondered, that had kept them culturally viable in the face of generations of contact with more powerful societies, both black and white? The thought that the Bushmen were alive and well in the Kalahari was strangely comforting. Perhaps, armed with that independence and with their superb knowledge of their environment, they might yet survive the future.

CHAPTER 3

No Heads, No Feet, No Monkeys, No Dogs: The Evolution of Personal Food Taboos

Miriam S. Chaiken

(2010)

Every fledgling anthropologist who is preparing to conduct first fieldwork is formally trained in research methods, and informally prepared by the anecdotes shared by friends and mentors who have already successfully navigated the rite of passage that "fieldwork" represents for anthropologists. My training was no different than this scenario: while a graduate student at University of California-Santa Barbara I took research methods from the esteemed Paul Bohannan (then President of the American Anthropological Association), classes on theory from other faculty, and delved into southeast Asian cultures with Donald Brown (and previously as an undergraduate with James Eder at Arizona State). All of these professors set the bar high for us, challenging us to do excellent qualitative and quantitative field work and to continue this important tradition of anthropologists. The informal transmission of knowledge needed during this apprenticeship was shared by the senior grad students, who had returned from "the field" full of wisdom and amusing tales of what not to do in conducting fieldwork, stories that remain vivid in my memory now decades later. Nowhere in all of this excellent preparation did anyone warn me about chicken head soup. But I get ahead of myself.

In the early 1980s I began to prepare for dissertation field research in Southeast Asia, and ultimately Palawan Island in the Philippines was the destination for my work. Palawan was an ideal choice because many of my interests could be pursued in this one locale. I had become interested in the process of spontaneous relocations of populations, which were happening all over Asia, paralleling a process of government managed relocation schemes that were also moving people from areas of population density to frontier regions. I had originally envisioned exploring this issue in Indonesia, where the government-planned "transmigrations" were well established and well documented, but political difficulties in that nation at the time made this a problematic location.

While there was a smaller scale process underway in the Philippines, and Palawan Island was the site of a notoriously badly managed relocation project near the town of Narra (both of which factored into my choice of Palawan for research), the real reasons for the selection of this site boiled down to personal choices. My friend and undergraduate mentor, Jim Eder, had been working in Palawan for many years and generously provided contacts and networks to help establish plans for working there as well. Secondly, my then boyfriend and now husband, Tom, went to Palawan in 1979 to scout for possible locations for both of our dissertation research projects. While my intent is not to expose my romances indiscreetly, my encounter with chicken head soup was directly a result of my attachment to Tom.

During the summer that Tom was in Palawan, he received a great deal of support from a family I'll call Flores, who had been great friends of Jim, and this couple generously gave Tom advice and a place to stay while he scouted locations for our field work. They knew that Tom was unmarried at the time, and although he referred to me and indicated I would be joining him when it came time for our full stint of fieldwork, Mrs. Flores apparently thought she had a better plan for his future. She had an unmarried friend from a prominent local family who she thought would make an ideal wife for Tom, and the chance to live in the United States was a welcome prospect for this woman. In spite of her valiant efforts, Mrs. Flores' matchmaking efforts were not successful. When Tom returned to begin fieldwork in 1980 with a wife (me), she was obviously disappointed that her friend was not destined to be betrothed to the handsome American anthropologist.

All of this is a roundabout introduction to the chicken head soup encounter. When we arrived in the Philippines, after months of preparation, we spent the first few days living in luxury with good friends Bob and Gina Cowell, who were working at the International Rice Research Institute (IRRI) on the Philippines main island of Luzon. This was a way to make an easy transition to the heat and humidity and to begin our tentative efforts to speak the national language, Tagalog. While our visit to IRRI was wonderful in many ways, we also experienced our first episode of food

Miriam Chaiken, "No Heads, No Feet, No Monkeys, No Dogs: The Evolution of Personal Food Taboos." *Adventures in eating*. Hanes HR and Sammells CA, eds. Boulder, CO: University of Colorado Press, pp. 181–190, 2010. Reprinted with permission.

poisoning, ironically, from a lavish country-club like party at IRRI. We left Luzon and arrived in Palawan still wobbly from that illness.

The morning we arrived in Palawan we traveled to the Flores' home where Mrs. Flores had prepared lunch for us, which she called chicken noodle soup. Although my constitution had not yet adjusted to the high heat and humidity, and I was still reeling from the IRRI illness, the thought of the Philippine version of my grandmother's "Jewish penicillin" sounded like just the right meal. As we sat down to eat our chicken soup, I noticed something peeking at me from my bowl, partially obscured by a fat noodle. Upon brief exploration it became apparent that Tom's bowl contained noodles, chicken pieces, and broth, and mine contained a chicken head (or more precisely rooster as the cockscomb clearly indicated) and two chicken feet, as well as my share of noodles. Hmmm, what to do? To this day I do not know whether my bowl contained those body bits just by chance, or whether Mrs. Flores thought these were special and intended to share them with me...or whether this was her expression of displeasure of my role in botching her matchmaking plans. Even after 2 years of fieldwork in Palawan I'm not sure how to interpret the body bits in my bowl. While most families include heads and feet in the cooking pot, it is odd that I would receive them all in a random portioning of soup. Heads and feet aren't special delicacies that I was singled out to receive, so what was the symbolism of my soup?

As I was new to the practice of ethnographic fieldwork, I was concerned about not offending my host, but I was also pretty sure I could not bring myself to chew on a chicken head, and so I sipped broth and a few noodles, but kept some in the bowl to hide the remnants of the soup I had not been able to bring myself to eat. In that first meal in Palawan, I had discovered the first two of the food taboos that I would later codify for myself: no heads, no feet.

Within a few days after our arrival we had located a house in the village of Napsaan, on the remote and isolated west coast of Palawan, where we settled in for our fieldwork. Palawan has long been considered the Philippines' frontier, as it is remote, sparsely settled, and the destination for prospectors and pioneers seeking to claim lands and a new life. The west coast of Palawan where we lived is the most inaccessible area of the island, where most travel is still done on foot or by boat along the coast of the South China Sea. The coastline is dotted with small villages of subsistence farmers who cultivate upland rice in slash and burn fields. The mountainous terrain and relatively easy access to land have permitted this very traditional system of cultivation to flourish, and very little area has been developed into the irrigated rice padi that is found most commonly elsewhere in Asia.

The village where we lived was only about 35 miles as the crow flies from the capital city of Puerto Princesa, but it was worlds away in a practical sense. Access was difficult at all times and impossible during the worst of the rainy season—getting to Napsaan required driving through several big rivers, the largest in the middle of the island in the Iwahig penal colony. If weather permitted, once or twice a day a jeepney, converted weapons carriers that were remnants of World War II, made the bumpy journey to Napsaan, bringing people and cargo in each direction. One's journey was equally likely to be shared with live pigs and chickens as with fellow passengers, and we soon learned the maxim that there is no such thing as a full jeepney; there is always room for another person or two. On a good day the journey from Napsaan to Puerto took about two and a half hours; on a bad one the journey could take as long as seven hours, depending on the number of break downs and flat tires. Given the difficulty and relative expense of travel for our meager research budget, trips to Puerto were fairly rare, but welcome respites from life in our village.

Our house was a typical rural Philippine house on stilts, bamboo slats woven into panels for the wall, and widely spaced slats for the floor. Complete with thatch roof, living in this house was like living in a giant basket, and the loosely woven walls and slats in the floors allowed the air to circulate and the whole building to breathe. We soon adjusted to life in our village: we made friends with our neighbors; we learned to sleep soundly with a mosquito net that also prevented bats, mice, and lizards from sharing our bed; and we learned how to manage a house lacking both electricity and running water.

Over the next 2 years in the field, we also encountered many wonderful foods, I learned to use many exotic ingredients that I had never encountered growing up in suburban Phoenix, but we also had a few challenges in the food department. We quickly, and fortunately, learned that local people were very familiar with the concept of allergies, and when food that was offered was too far out of our comfort level, a claim of being allergic to said food gave us a gracious way to refuse. Tom's polite fiction of being "allergic" to shellfish, which he really dislikes, was usually greeted with other people recounting the food allergies that they or a family member experienced. We invoked the allergy excuse quite rarely, as most of the foods we encountered proved to be tasty and enjoyable treats. Although I had never cleaned and prepared a whole fish prior to my life in Palawan, I eventually learned how to grill over an open fire the incredibly fresh fish we could sometimes buy from neighbors, who had been fishing in the sea. This produced some delicious meals of grouper and red snapper, though the first effort at cooking fish was disastrous and resulted in tossing it out in the woods for cats to scrap over in the night. In general, our consumption of protein largely rested on neighbors' success at fishing.

Most of the fieldwork we have conducted over the years were in communities like Napsaan where obtaining fresh food was a big challenge, and in our isolated village on Palawan that was because of the absence of a market. The few local *sari-sari* stores, windows in the wall of someone's home where we could purchase items, stocked only very basic durable and dry goods such as matches and kerosene, sugar and instant coffee. Every household grew their own vegetables, most of the men went fishing occasionally, and people gathered shellfish during low tides. Surplus foods, such as extra fish that were caught, were processed at home for storage and consumption at a later date, usually by packing them in salt and air drying. We compensated for difficult access to food by buying rice in bulk, which was our staple three times per day, as was the local custom. We would purchase dried, salted fish or fresh fish from neighbors when they had some to spare, and we occasionally splurged and bought a chicken for the pot. When we visited the capital city we would purchase a few canned goods to provide occasional relief from the monotony of our rice-based diet.

A few months into our stay we began to grow a vegetable garden, but our inexperience resulted in poor yields of everything except zucchini and yellow squash, so this was only marginally successful in bringing home dinner. During one three week period during the rainy season, the seas were too rough for local men to venture out fishing, and our diet during that time consisted *only* of rice and yellow squash (*kalabasa*) for three meals a day. Once back in the United States, it was many years before I could face yellow squash with any enthusiasm. We also tried raising our own chickens and found our skills with animal husbandry were as pathetic as our farming. One hen was enticed away into the forest by the wild roosters that inhabited the hinterland, another was killed in the night by a snake and her chicks scattered and were lost. Clearly we were not cut out to be subsistence farmers like our neighbors. During our 2 years in Napsaan, it was frequently difficult to count on access to foods to provide the *ulam*, or savory side dish to accompany rice.

As part of my research involved collecting data on household food consumption and child nutrition, I was well aware that most local people's diet was far better than what we were consuming. Despite this awareness, we had neither the time nor the skill to become full time subsistence cultivators as were our neighbors, and so we had to make do with the limited food resources at our disposal. There were a few important interludes that gave us a respite from our dietary monotony, the most common of which was when someone had reason to throw a party. In rural Palawan instead of the person who has a birthday to celebrate being treated by their friends and family, the person who had the birthday celebrated by throwing a party, preparing lots of food, and inviting everyone around to help them mark the occasion. Poor families had very modest celebrations that may involve only their closest family members and consist of noodles cooked with vegetables (*pancit*) or tinned mackerel in sauce, but wealthier households would mark the occasion by slaughtering a pig as the centerpiece of the feast. Both the best and worst dishes we encountered were served at these feasts.

Slaughter of a pig for cooking at a party necessitated cooperation by people from neighboring households, as the butchering process was complicated, and no part of the pig was allowed to go to waste. The butchering was usually performed by the men, who would collect the blood and offal and turn it over to the women for preparation; then they would build a spit and start a fire to slowly roast the whole pig over a low fire to prepare the famous dish *lechon*.

In this preparation the meat remains very succulent as it is naturally basted by the rendering fat of the pig as it cooked, and the outer skin became a crispy counterpoint to the meat. Preparing *lechon* was expensive and time consuming, as the properly prepared pig required hours of slow roasting and rotation to be ideal. It represented the finest in Philippine cooking, and was a dish highly anticipated by all guests at a party.

The second most popular dish that was usually served at parties was made from the innards of the pig that the women cleaned and prepared. This dish, known as *dinuguan*, came from the root word, *dugo* or blood. In a nutshell, *dinuguan* was pigs' intestines cooked in pig blood with vinegar to prevent the blood from coagulating. While this is a local favorite, and a dish that I ate on many occasions, I never grew to share my neighbors' love of this concoction. I may have been channeling my Jewish grandmother when I faced this dish with revulsion, as I imagined my kosher-keeping grandmother rolling over in her grave at the thought of eating something so *treyf* (unclean).

In addition to birthday parties or celebration of saint's days, smaller gatherings of men were occasionally held, during which they would typically drink and play cards. Women were not normally included in these parties, but if they happened to be close at hand, they would be invited to share in whatever food the men had prepared. There was a special classification for food served at these events, termed *pulutan*, which are finger foods to be eaten while drinking. Instead of the store-bought chips or pretzels that might be the fare for such occasions in the United States, *pulutan* was generally a strongly seasoned meat or seafood dish that counterbalanced the flavor of the beer or *ginebra San Miguel*, a Philippine gin. I have had *pulutan* that consisted of squid cooked in soy sauce and vinegar (*adobo*-style), or strongly seasoned fried chicken that were delicious treats, but on one memorable occasion I was offered *pulutan* that led to my third food taboo.

In some parts of the Philippines, notably in the north of Luzon Island, far from Palawan, eating dogs is considered a delicacy. In Palawan dogs were not common fare, nor were dogs coddled house pets. Most dogs were fairly mangy beasts that largely fended for themselves, but were kept by households with the expectation that they provided protection. For this reason, dogs were given names that made them sound ferocious, such as *matapang* (brave, fierce) and, notably, Hitler. The risk of rabies in dogs was also well known, and this too led to people's ambivalent attitudes towards keeping dogs in the home.

There were a very few households that seemed to treat their dogs more like the family pet that I had grown up with, where the dogs lived in the house and were shown affection by their owners. One such exception was the household of Jose and Linda Alvarez, a couple who ran a small *sari-sari* store and several small businesses. Jose and Linda became our good friends and their store window was in the central part of the village, so it was a frequent gathering place for people as they walked through the area. I recall many happy conversations on the benches outside the window of their store and many language lessons as local people coached me to become proficient in the national language, Tagalog. Another reason I liked to visit Jose and Linda was because their friendly black dog, Perla, would greet all comers with a wagging tail and plea to be petted—this was a couple I could relate to.

One day, well into my second year in Palawan, I walked by the Alvarez's store and saw Linda sitting outside, obviously in a foul mood. Jose and his companions were close by, sitting on the verandah of their house, obviously very inebriated and in high spirits as a rousing card game was underway. I was invited to come to join them, and as I greeted them they offered to share their *pulutan*, which was on a platter in the middle of the table. Linda then piped up, with alarm, that I should not eat this *pulutan* because Jose had killed and cooked Perla and was serving her to the guests. She was clearly very angry with Jose, and was upset about what he had done to Perla, a dog who was her faithful companion at home while she tended the store. Linda was not about to share in partaking of this *pulutan*. Obviously I was not alone in my shock at the prospect of eating the family pet! In fact, on earlier occasions, I had heard my neighbors refer to northerners disparagingly as dog-eating people, so I came to learn that my taboo against eating dog (especially Perla) was considered acceptable by many people. In Palawan eating dog is a guilty pleasure that usually only men engage in, and eating dog as *pulutan* has macho qualities. My polite refusal to share the dog meat was generally ignored, and I joined Linda outside to sit in silence, reflecting on the fate of the friendly black dog.

The fact that Jose and his *barkada*, or pals, could blithely eat Perla may not be attributable to insensitivity, so much as scarcity of meat and animal protein. Fish was consumed when available, and on special occasions families would cook a chicken, but meat was rarely consumed because it was rarely available. There was no equivalent of a butcher or meat market, so everyone felt pangs of "meat hunger" as Richard Lee so poignantly discusses among the San people (Lee 1993).

Many families raised pigs, but these were intended as investments to be sold for profit when they reached maturity. These pigs were shipped to Puerto Princesa to be sold at market for a better price than they could ever fetch in the village. Other livestock were intended as working animals—there were a few oxen and water buffalos that were used to pull plows in cultivating irrigated rice fields or to pull a sledge or a cart. Unless an animal died of natural causes, such valuable animals would never be considered fair game for the cooking pot, so meat consumption was a rare and special treat.

In some ways it is ironic that meat was so seldom available, as Philippine cooking is replete with recipes that effectively preserve and season meat in the absence of refrigeration. Efficiently using up a pig butchered and sold locally would not have been a problem. Perhaps the most famous national dish, *adobo*, differs from Spanish and Latino versions of the same name. It is a blend of soy sauce, rice wine vinegar, and lots of garlic and black pepper that is used as a marinade and preservative for raw meat. Even very tough cuts of ancient animals become tender and delicious prepared in this way. Other preservations involve slicing meat into thin strips and smoking it over a fire, resulting in a bacon-like flavor, or salting and drying it in the air, similar to the preparation of hams and cured meat found in so many cultures.

The only occasions when meat might be available to purchase were when someone had luck with hunting, either with conventional weapons or with a "pig bomb." Our time in Palawan coincided with President Ferdinand Marcos' imposition of martial law, and guns and bullets were illegal. While a few households might have owned a hunting gun, these were kept under wraps and never used (to my knowledge). Hunting was a macho affair; groups of men would track and kill a formidable wild pig in the forest using a traditional spear as a weapon. Hunting was only successfully carried out by a few men, all of whom were members of the ethnic minority Tagbanua people, who had a stronger hunting and gathering tradition than the majority population of lowland Filipino farmers. When these Tagbanua men returned to the village carrying the carcass of a wild pig, everyone, including the local anthropologists, would line up to try to buy some of the precious meat to satisfy their "meat hunger."

The other strategy to obtain wild pig involved an ingenious explosive device called a "pig bomb," borrowing the English words to name this device. These were perhaps the original improvised explosive device (IED), not intended for targeting enemy humvees, but rather for marauding wild pigs. For farmers who planted upland rice close to the forest margins, protecting the crop from the threat of wild pigs was a constant challenge. Pigs would root around these fields just as the rice was ripening, and one pig's raid in the middle of the night could do tremendous damage to a farmer's annual harvest. To combat these porcine threats many farmers rigged pig bombs, which were made of a mixture of extremely ripe mashed bananas and shards of broken glass wrapped in banana leaves. The smell of ripe bananas would attract the pigs to these baited bombs and as they bit into them it set off a detonation. The home-made detonators were made from phosphorous scraped from match heads as the incendiary material, as gun powder was illegal under martial law. The shards of glass would be propelled through the pig's face and head, killing the animal.

Most pig bombs detonated just before dawn. We recall waking up with the sound of the explosion during the pre-harvest season and happily anticipating the first light, so we could go inquire whose pig bomb had been successful, and whether there was any fresh meat to purchase. While pig bombs were very ingenious, these were generally only used during the few weeks before and during the rice harvest, as these were the only times the wild pigs were lured out of the remote forests by the promise of cultivated foods to ravage.

The other wild animals that threatened to wreak havoc on farmers' fields were the monkeys and birds that also lived in the forests. Birds were only active during daylight hours, so for the few weeks of the harvest season many families would build a lean-to in their fields and camp there for the duration of the season. Children were out of school during this harvest holiday and would be put to work in the fields, scaring birds by waving their arms, and using slingshots to pelt birds with pebbles.

Monkeys, like pigs, were active during the night hours and presented a more serious threat to the harvest. We found monkeys to be very ingenious when it came to experimenting with human food; they routinely raided the farm fields to feast on ripening rice. Once while we were hiking on another island, a curious monkey found Tom's backpack sitting on the ground, unzipped it, and helped himself to a peanut butter sandwich that was wrapped in plastic. Local farmers had equally ingenious ways to combat these monkeys, as they devised snares that were baited with the ripening rice. The bait was placed on top of a long pole cut from a variety of thorny tree, which the sensible monkeys would not climb because they would be impaled. The snare was placed on an adjacent pole that the monkey could climb and, as he reached out to grab the rice, it tripped a counterweight and noose, and snapped the poor monkeys' necks.

Some local people, as with the eating of dogs, found these snared monkeys acceptable game for the cooking pot. Others, however, commented that they too closely resembled humans and had qualms about eating them—so I was safe in my fourth food taboo as they understood some peoples' reticence to partake of monkey meat.

Other wild animals did not rate dietary deference as far as I was concerned. On one sojourn we traveled on foot a long day's walk away to the more remote village of Bubusawen, also on the west coast of Palawan. Bubusawen was one of the coastal villages settled by lowland, Christian farmers who were homesteading land not occupied by one of the indigenous ethnic minorities of Palawan. We were accompanying our friend who was the parish priest, and he had planned to visit Bubusawen to say Mass in this remote community that had no formal church, in celebration of a saint's day. We were joined on our adventure by a number of young people who volunteered for the local church, and by our landlord and father-figure, our neighbor Mang Luis, who was a Tagbanua, a member of a tribal minority group indigenous to Palawan. We camped on the floor of local porches for the few days that we were in Bubusawen, and were well cared for by the local villagers, who were pleased to have visitors, as this was a rare experience. As we shared the festivities and honors intended for our friend Father Erning, we sat down to a dinner of rice and a flavorful stew. As we chatted over dinner my husband thanked our hosts and commented that the chicken was delicious, to which I replied, "I've cut up a lot of chickens, these are not chicken bones." As the conversation continued we were informed that we were eating a stew of monitor lizard, a huge lizard common in the area that often exceeded 4 feet in length. Mang Luis dropped his plate and looked appalled! He said that for the Tagbanua people, monitor lizard was strictly taboo, and that he could not continue eating this food that clearly now repelled him. This was a little lesson to us—*to each her own food taboos.* While sympathizing with Mang Luis' reaction, we did not share his dislike of eating lizards, and to the delight of our hosts, we happily cleaned our plates.

ACKNOWLEDGMENTS

I am grateful to our editors for helpful suggestions in revising this paper, and to many students over the years who have been regaled with our tales of adventures in eating. I received very helpful feedback and comments on this paper from James and Pia Eder, Gina Cowell, Billy Garrett, David Brokensha, and my aunt and prolific author Miriam Chaikin.

Reference

Lee RB. 1993. The Dobe Ju/'hoansi. Fort Worth, TX: Harcourt Brace College Publishers.

CHAPTER 4

From Hunger Foods to Heritage Foods: Challenges to Food Localization in Lao PDR

Penny Van Esterik

(2006)

"A commodity chain is a series of interlinked exchanges through which a commodity and its constituents pass from extraction or harvesting through production to end use" (Ribot 1998:307). The end of the commodity chain for a small basket of crisps made of Lao river algae purchased for 40,000 kip (around $4.00 U.S.) at a local market in Vientiane, Lao People's Democratic Republic (Lao PDR), is my kitchen. But before I simply consume the algae chips, and their sweet counterparts, cassava chips, I want to place them in a broader interpretive framework than commodity chains and use them to interrogate the ethics of exotic foods. I do this first by placing these two food items in the context of Lao national food security, and then in the context of Southeast Asian culinary traditions. But the story of these chips is neither linear nor unambiguous. Nor are these food products centrally important to anyone's diet. They are marginal in the Lao diet where the chain begins and in the North American diet where it ends—marginal in multiple ways and in multiple contexts. It is their marginality I want to reflect upon in this chapter.

Under conditions of food insecurity and seasonal scarcity, Lao cooks—usually women—rely heavily on collecting wild foods from the forest. They make ingenious use of wild foods considered exotic by outsiders, such as crickets, green tree ant eggs, river algae, wild cassava, and wild yams. These regionally specific seasonal foods are not always part of the regular diet of the lowland Lao; we might refer to them as *hunger foods*—foods that act as insurance against hunger in times of seasonal or catastrophic food shortages.

This chapter argues that the rarer and harder these foods are for the Lao to obtain, the more valued they have become to North American and European chefs. How have seasonal hunger foods become heritage foods in the gourmet boutiques of Europe and North America? In the quest for new ingredients and new tastes for chefs and consumers, some importers have discovered elements of the Lao cuisine that can be sold as specialties in niche markets. These include products that are produced in the northern region of Luang Prabang, Lao PDR, like *khai pen* (river algae sheets), and products created out of cassava such as *khao kiep* (cassava crisps). These items have been redesigned to meet Western tastes. In California, where food boutiques and food banks stand side by side, these two Lao food items have begun to appear in specialty food shops and online shopping services, provisioners of yuppie chow.

BEING FOOD INSECURE

Lao People's Democratic Republic (Lao PDR), a landlocked country in Southeast Asia, is classified as a low-income, food deficit country. After decades of war, including fighting for independence from French colonial control and surviving the bombing inflicted by the American secret war in Laos, the country remains food insecure.

With a per capita income of around $400, Lao PDR is one of the poorest and least developed countries in Asia. This poverty is reflected in the nutritional status of its population. Forty percent of children under five are underweight, 41 percent stunted, and 15 percent wasted (Health Status of the People in Lao PDR, 2001). The prevalence of wasting among children increased to 15 percent in 2000, and the presence of chronic energy deficiency among adults was "alarmingly high (19 percent), even higher than reported during a previous survey in 1995 (14 percent)" (FAO country profile). According to the Food and Agriculture Organization (FAO) country profile on Lao PDR, "the daily dietary energy supply per capita increased from 2030 kcal in 1968 to 2400 kcal in 1995." Almost 30 percent of the population is below the minimal level of dietary energy consumption. Household food insecurity is defined by the government as the inability to provide 2,100 calories per person per day. To reduce the number of poverty households, the government reduced the minimal dietary energy requirements to 1,983 calories per day (Millennium Development Goals 2004:6). Clearly there is a poor fit between the measurement of calories nationally and the hunger and malnutrition experienced by individuals in households.

Penny Van Esterik, "From Hunger Foods to Heritage Foods: Challenges to Food Localization in Lao PDR." In *Fast Food/Slow Food: The Cultural Economy of the Global Food System*, R. Wilk, ed. Lanham, MD: Altamira, pp. 83–96, 2006. Reprinted with permission.

Local and national food shortages are not relieved by trade in food items. Food imports and exports are minimal, government controlled, and directed toward urban markets. Lao PDR is a closed, protected trading system—but one where informal and nonformal trade with China, Vietnam, and Thailand thrives. Stocks of stored rice are available neither nationally nor locally, as most households do not produce enough rice to meet their needs and have to purchase it. About half the provinces regularly fail to reach rice self-sufficiency because of drought, flooding, or underproduction related to irrigation problems. Since rice provides over 80 percent of total calorie intake (UNDP 2003), many households are food insecure and have to stretch rice with other foods. In Lao PDR, as in Vietnam, gruels made from broken rice grains, rice flour, and tubers such as cassava or yam "saved a lot of people from famine" (Nguyen 2001:94). In short, for some households in some communities in some seasons, food itself is a scarce commodity.

In response, the Lao government has developed policies to improve the nutritional status of Lao families by enhancing Lao food self-sufficiency and encouraging the production and export of cash crops. Lao government planning gives highest priority to reducing poverty especially in rural areas, by improving the food security and nutrition situation through diversification of the Lao diet. Integration into global markets is part of this plan: "The Lao government believes in the globalization process since it considers that it will create a propitious environment for achieving the over-arching goal of alleviating poverty and creating a more prosperous and peaceful society" (Lao PDR 2000:29).

But has Lao PDR always been food insecure? Recently (2001) the Asian Development Bank concluded that poverty in Lao PDR is "new poverty," produced by the process of development. The policy imperative driving market integration has made things worse for most Lao, and better for a few. Efforts to increase market integration are increasing this policy-induced new poverty, so that the more remote communities are actually more food secure than communities close to roads (EU 1997:20). Yet, government policies operate on the assumption that remoteness and lack of market integration is a cause of poverty. This chapter provides one example of what happens when the market comes to remote locations where food insecurity is common. Market integration makes possible the movement of some food products out of the Lao food system and into the North American, and the constant devaluation of the Lao currency (kip) makes some food products more valuable outside the country than inside.

CULINARY COMPLEXES OF SOUTHEAST ASIA

That poverty and food shortages may be recent experiences for the Lao explains why the country retains its self-identity around concepts of hospitality and food sharing. A Lao proverb states: "You can live in a narrow space, but it's hard to live with a narrow heart" (Rakow 1992:54); failure

to share food is evidence of a narrow heart. Southeast Asian cuisines, including the Lao, are born of festive meals, communally prepared and eaten (Ho 1995:8).

Food as a focus of interest in Southeast Asia has been a matter of praxis not analysis, unless by analysis we consider the endless evaluations of food, flavors, and eating experiences that dominate discussions in rural and urban communities. Food matters to people at many levels, but it has rarely figured analytically in the work of anthropologists of Southeast Asia. However, the area is favored by food writers such as Alford and Duguid, whose award-winning books on Asian foods (*Hot Sour Salty Sweet: A Culinary Journey through Southeast Asia*, 2002; *Seductions of Rice*, 1998) easily delineate the boundaries and characteristics of Southeast Asia as a culinary area.

In addition to cookbook authors, linguists have also provided clues that suggest food is something worth talking and thinking about throughout Southeast Asia. Different Southeast Asian language families make similar distinctions between cooked and uncooked rice and contain multiple verbs for drying and cutting (Matisoff 1992), hinting about the existence of a regional culinary complex. Culinary terms are critical to aligning otherwise distinct cultures, even before globalization made *pad Thai* (Thai fried noodles) a household word (cf. Van Esterik 1992).

For economic anthropologists, using food systems as a means of defining ethnic and agricultural boundaries within a Southeast Asian culture area suggests an outmoded theoretical concern with classification, diffusion, and typologies. But without a perspective on the structure of typical meals, we are more likely to consider food items such as river weed and wild cassava in isolation, rather than as parts of historically produced complexes. O'Connor's (1995) model of agricultural change in Southeast Asia calls for a regional anthropology that situates agro-cultural complexes within regional history. In our admiration for fieldwork-driven empiricism, he argues, we have avoided regional comparisons, lest we be accused of returning to a theoretically antiquated culture area concept, unsuitable for addressing questions of globalization and transnational migration. Although only the broadest outlines of the regional food system are provided here, Lao food systems emerged out of past systems and bear some relation to comparable systems elsewhere in the region.

Southeast Asian culinary complexes include: rice as the central source of calories and a dominant cultural symbol of feminine nurture, fermented fish products, soups, local fresh vegetables and herbs, spicy dipping sauces to add zest to bland rice, and meat or fish in variable amounts. Most meal formats feature rice in a common bowl with side dishes presented simultaneously. Throughout Southeast Asia, and particularly in Lao PDR, we taste the rural roots of the cuisine.

LAO FOOD SYSTEM

The Lao government recognizes sixty-five distinct ethnic groups, although it stresses "unity in diversity" among all ethnic groups. The food system discussed here is characteristic of lowland Lao *Lum* groups, the dominant majority making up 68 percent of the population. Lao PDR is a country of subsistence rice farmers, with some minority groups growing maize and cassava in addition to rice. As elsewhere in the world, rice as the key staple is valued far beyond its nutritional value (Bray 1986; Ohnuki-Tierney 1993; Goody 1982; Hanks 1972). The key marker of the collective identity of lowland Lao is the use of glutinous or sticky rice. Only more recent arrivals to the country such as the Yao and Hmong prefer nonglutinous rice (Schiller et al. 1998:228). Recent rice surveys have found over 3,200 varieties in the country, 85 percent of them glutinous (Rao et al. 2001). Most glutinous rice is consumed less than fifty kilometers from its place of production (Nguyen 2001:112). And no rice tastes better than the rice grown at home. While Lao and Vietnamese who use glutinous rice as their daily staple celebrate the taste of their local rice varieties, a European visitor in 1877 did not like the "stickiness" of glutinous rice, referring to it as that "ghastly rice of Laotians" (Nguyen 2001:64).

Glutinous rice is by far the preferred rice for the lowland Lao. It is an understatement to say that the Lao appreciate the qualities of glutinous rice; like the Vietnamese, they deeply believe that glutinous rice is more nutritious and more aromatic than any other kind of rice. In Vietnam, contests were held to perfect glutinous rice steaming skills for young girls and men (Nguyen 2001:57). Lao are very conscious of the aromatic and cooking qualities of glutinous rice, as well as its keeping quality (Schiller et al. 1998:234). This is equally true of families with adequate rice and families who must buy rice because their own fields have not produced enough, or because they have no access to rice fields.

Accompanying most rice meals is a sauce or paste made from fermented local fish or shellfish. The fish are salted, dried, pounded, and packed with toasted rice and rice husk in jars for a month or more. Fish sauce (*nam pa*) is a crucial ingredient in many dishes. In its thicker form (*padek*), it is served as a dish with rice. The strong-smelling product is not appealing to many westerners who have little tolerance for fermented, fishy foods, but overseas Lao speak longingly of the taste of local versions recalled nostalgically from their homeland.

Fresh greens and herbs are available from household gardens and local markets. Recent development projects on home gardens have dramatically increased the amount of fresh vegetables available to households. In pilot projects, families participating in these projects consumed three times more vegetables than they sold. However, households need land, labor, and seeds to benefit from these initiatives. Vegetables are served in soups; stir fried with onion, garlic, meat, or fish; or served raw with fermented fish products or dipping sauces (*jeaw*).

There is a clear continuity between medicinal and culinary use of herbs and other forest products. Ginger, coriander root, and aromatic woods play important roles in both medicinal and culinary systems. Elders, both male and

female, generally know where to locate these products if they still live in the same localities where they were taught to locate and process these items when they were young. However, relocated individuals and households may not know where to obtain wild foods, particularly medicinal herbs, and may not know how to process them to remove toxins. Correct processing and prescribing requires specialized knowledge. For example, wild cassava needs to be carefully processed to remove toxins; elders report that young people may have no idea how to find or process wild cassava, although they recall eating it mixed with rice when rice supplies were low. In other parts of the world knowledge of how to process toxic tubers has already been lost, resulting in deaths from cyanide poisoning (Cardoso et al. 2005).

In Lao PDR, as elsewhere in Southeast Asia, dipping sauces add zest to bland rice, stimulating appetites, and tempting intemperate eaters to consume more calories from starchy staples. With the early adoption of chili peppers, originally from America, Lao developed local sauces (*jeaw*) made from ingredients such as peppers, garlic, lime, sugar, fish sauce, onions, and coriander—each combination unique to a region, community, or household. Some dry *jeaw* consist primarily of salt and chili peppers and are not given to children.

Meat and fish are valued parts of Lao diets. Variable amounts of fish or meats are mixed with herbs and spices in stews and soups; large amounts of meat or fish are grilled mainly for communal festive meals. Meat or fish may also be used in soups served in communal or individual dishes. Soups are particularly valued as they allow cooks to stretch ingredients, make use of bones, and generally expand the meal to serve more people.

Squirrels, snakes, frogs, crickets, and insects also supply protein, along with freshwater fish, although there is clear preference for chicken, pork, duck, or beef, should cash be available to purchase meat. Domestic animals in Lao communities do not fare well without regular vaccinations, although development projects attempt to increase domestic livestock and poultry. Most projects fail unless external aid projects are able to provide extension support.

Fermented rice liquor (*laolao*) plays a key role in all celebrations, as consumption of alcohol creates links between the living and the dead, humans and spirits, and guests and hosts. Among minority groups living north of Luang Prabang, rice alcohol is kept in heirloom jars (Nguyen 2001:73), and in the past was a necessary ingredient for oath taking and other rituals. Producing *laolao* used to be a household enterprise in the past, but more recently, liquor is purchased from local enterprises where glutinous rice is grown specifically for this purpose. Steamed sticky rice is fermented with balls of yeast for about a week, when it is distilled and consumed (Schiller et al. 2001:236).

FOOD IN MOTION

Describing the structure of the Lao food system as I have done above overstresses the continuity of traditional food items and meal formats. But the structure of systems of food production and consumption in Lao PDR may provide valuable opportunities for examining diversity and continuities, including historical transformations brought about through processes of colonization, development, and globalization.

Colonialism affected the Lao food system in many ways: French bread, pâté, and salads clearly came from the French colonial experience. Many urban and overseas Lao substitute baguettes for glutinous rice for breakfast. What is known as Luang Prabang salad exemplifies the fusion of French salad traditions and the Lao practice of providing plates of raw or steamed vegetables and herbs to go with dipping sauces. Foo (2002:18, 88) describes Lao long lunches as a colonial remnant, and notes that the popularity of French baguettes endured longer than the bricks of colonial buildings. However, apart from freshly baked baguettes, the French had less impact on the Lao food system than on the Vietnamese (cf. Norindr 1996).

Other changes can be linked to development processes within Lao PDR. Because of government policies to reduce slash-and-burn upland agriculture and to increase production of cash crops, Lao farmers with access to irrigated fields have been encouraged to produce nonglutinous rice for sale. The few new varieties of glutinous and nonglutinous rice grown in irrigated fields in the central region of Lao PDR since 1993 require fertilizers, mechanical threshers, and hand tractors in order to make a profit (Schiller et al. 1998:226). The small amount of glutinous rice exported for use by overseas Lao comes from northeastern Thailand, and overseas Lao find Thai rice less flavorful than the rice they remember from home villages.

While Lao make distinctions between people who eat glutinous rice and those who eat nonglutinous rice, in fact, the distinction is somewhat arbitrary and is breaking down rapidly. Ordinary or nonglutinous rice can become glutinous, and glutinous rice can become ordinary rice, as the glutinous character of the rice endosperm is reversible (Nguyen 2001:26). Lao have selected for glutinous characteristics that increase with domestication (Nguyen 2001:20). Just as the product itself can change over time, so too is the way rice is served. Several Hmong and lowland Lao households I visited in 2005 had both glutinous and nonglutinous rice in their kitchens, and rural restaurants served both kinds of rice in the same meal. Glutinous rice can no longer be considered unambiguously as the primary marker of Lao ethnic identity.

Conversion of forests to agricultural land and the expansion of commercial logging have reduced forests in many parts of Lao PDR. Villagers complain that it is now more difficult to collect wild greens from these shrinking forest reserves. In addition, the valuable nontimber forest products (NTFP) that have provided both emergency food for poor households and income for many more households can now be sold more conveniently by locals or, more often, by middlemen who are able to access NTFP and new markets more directly, thanks to new roads.

Wild Meat and Fish

Forest animals are harder to find now than in the past. To obtain meat, Lao villagers now need to go deeper into the forest and become even more skilled hunters. Where a dozen years ago, villagers in Champassak province in southern Laos reported an abundance of animals and fish close to their villages, now many species have disappeared; a two-day trek might yield nothing and an hour fishing might yield half a kilogram of fish (UNDP 2003:82).

Villagers speak with nostalgia of the days when the giant Mekong catfish (*Pangasianodon gigas*), now close to extinction, could still be caught (Heldke 2003:74; Davidson 1975; Levy 1986). Like river algae, the rarity of the giant catfish makes it doubly appealing to Western food adventurers. After eating Lao catfish soup, food writer Levy comments: "Certainly, a local fisherman did catch one of the huge creatures some time that week. It's a horrible thought, but it could have been the last one. And, readers, we ate it" (1986:190).

There is a well-developed trade in endangered species across the borders to Thailand and Vietnam. Eating exotic animals, including eating uncustomary parts of customary animals, and eating animals rarely consumed in North America such as bears, dogs, and cats, as well as wild animals that are dangerous to catch or process, is thrilling for a food adventurer (Heldke 2003:71).

The wild animals are not always eaten but rather may be traded for the body parts with medicinal value (horn, antler, teeth, bone, gallbladder, shell, blood, excrement, urine [Baird 1995]) as part of systems of contagious magic. Lao healers report that an animal part used for medicine can "last a lifetime" (Baird 1995:22), and some claim that the overharvesting of endangered species is driven by the demand for these products in Vietnam, China, and Thailand.

Exports for Gourmets

Globalization has brought in new stakeholders who are looking at Lao food resources from very different perspectives. In spite of national food insecurity—or perhaps because of it—Lao PDR has become a site for agricultural, pharmaceutical, and gastronomic bioprospecting. Agribusinesses want to patent the incredibly diverse rice varieties found in different regions of Lao PDR. "The development of 'boutique rices' that combine the glutinous endosperm and aromatic character of many traditional Lao rices is regarded as having the greatest potential for the export market," concludes a report from the Lao-IRRI project and the National Agricultural Research Institute (Schiller et al. 2001:240). Pharmaceutical companies want access to the herbs and other plant resources (most are wild NTFP), along with the specialized knowledge of traditional healers, in order to discover, develop, and patent new drugs to combat malaria, cancer, and HIV/AIDS. Lao communities have used these products for centuries as medicinal cures and ingested them in soups and tonic drinks in the absence of adequate primary health care.

These products are now being exported to make medicinal tonics in China, Vietnam, and Thailand, endangering the herbal resources available for future generations of Lao.

Khai Pen and *Khao Kiep*

Culinary bioprospecting in Lao PDR has attracted new entrepreneurs—both Lao and non-Lao—who want rare ingredients and new tastes for chefs and Western consumers. This brings me back to the seasonal hunger foods mentioned at the beginning of the chapter. Few Westerners have the opportunity to visit exotic Luang Prabang, the former royal capital. But they can consume rare foods that come from there—foods like *khai pen* (river algae sheets) and *khao kiep* (cassava crisps) that have been romanticized by association with the former royal palace. The recipe book of the former royal chef includes a dish made from river algae mixed with ground pork (Sing 1981:235).

A few well-traveled individuals discovered these foods and publicized their features, while others developed the products, arranged their export, and introduced them into new markets. The sale of these rare, exotic food items is neither a large nor a particularly profitable business, but it requires a great deal of culinary capital on the part of the distributors and their customers.

Khai pen is made from a river weed (*khai*), as it is known in the north of the country, a variety of green algae (*chlorophyceae*) collected from the fast-flowing rivers of northern Laos and Thailand. It is harvested in winter, from November to January; the algae identified as *thao* was also collected from stagnant water in the rainy season (Sing 1981:25). Although it was used in royal households, it was more common in poor households: "Households that routinely suffer from food insecurity in the form of insufficient rice often depend on wild aquatic resources to compensate for this deficiency" (Meusch et al. 2003:22). River algae was consumed two to four times a week by more than half the households surveyed in a study of the value of aquatic resources in southern Attapeu province (Meusch et al. 2003:31). It was probably consumed in simple water-based soups rather than used to make *khai pen*.

Families, including children, collect the bright green algae that looks like fine seaweed from rocks on the sides of rivers. To make *khai pen*, the algae is spread in the sun to dry and processed by pressing dried tomatoes, garlic, chilies, sesame seeds, and salt into the dried sheets. The sheets are held together with tamarind paste. They can be cut into strips and used as flavoring in vegetable dishes or fried rice (Alford and Duguid 2000:165) or grilled and served as a snack with drinks. In Lao PDR, it is primarily served to men in town bars. According to *New York Times* food writer Florence Fabricant, *khai pen* has a "pleasantly earthy, slightly spinach-like flavor that is both nutty and peppery" (Fabricant 2002:D3).

Once the algae is removed from the subsistence system, commodified, and reintroduced into Lao markets as *khai pen*, it is expensive to purchase; it costs approximately one dollar for four large sheets in the markets of Luang Prabang and $7.49 (reduced from $9.99) for four very small sheets from a California-based, online food boutique.

One Lao couple in Vientiane has been producing Lao algae chips for three years; they estimate they have sold between three and five hundred kilos in that period. They developed and marketed the product because they are interested in preserving traditional Lao recipes. The algae is collected by networks of women who gather it by hand, helped by their children, from fast-flowing rivers around Vang Vieng and Luang Prabang. They could also collect river algae from the southern provinces, and thus expand their market without endangering the river environment. Locals, they say, are not yet aware of the possibility of collecting and selling the algae.

In order to control the quality, insure the cleanliness of the product, regulate its taste, and insure proper preservation, they process the product themselves in their house in Vientiane. They have increased its shelf life up to six months by drying it in special ovens to remove the moisture and destroy the germs. The algae chips are distributed through a few outlets in the capital frequented by foreigners, where four small sheets are sold in a Lao basket for forty thousand kip (with five thousand kip profit for the company). It is also sold at the airport, where Japanese visitors and visiting Lao expatriates buy it in great quantities—forty to fifty boxes at a time—often for gifts. They complain that few local shops are interested in their products because of the demand for imported food.

In some parts of Southeast Asia, cassava is collected wild as an emergency food; in other areas, it is planted in upland fields as a dry season crop; in Thailand, it is grown for animal fodder. But wherever root crops are grown in Southeast Asia, they are freely given up for the more prestigious rice: "Rice advances across Southeast Asia as if it were addictive" (O'Connor 1995:986). But root crops are never entirely abandoned. In the forests of Lao PDR, wild yams, cassava, and taro are collected by women who know where to find them and how to process them to remove poisons, if necessary, by soaking, cooking, and drying the roots. Once harvested, cassava tubers are very perishable and hard to store. Cassava tubers have a high carbohydrate content and are a good source of potassium, iron, magnesium, vitamin C, and other vitamins. Currently, the same entrepreneurs who are marketing *khai pen* are also marketing sweet and savory cassava cakes for sale in California and online. Their household-based production involves forming the flat cakes in a simple wooden press and sun-drying them. Cassava crisps—semi-savory or sweet—are also available from Lotus foods for $7.49 (reduced from $9.99) per package. These products are too expensive for Lao families to purchase in either country.

The products were promoted by a luncheon presentation in New York on May 30, 2002, where well-known chefs from New York and Chicago prepared them in specialties such as "grilled *kaipen* wrapped seabass with somen noodles and cilantro vinaigrette," "*kaipen* with Asian guacamole," "smoked corn and *kaipen* fritters," and "cassava sesame crisp tacos with grilled shrimp, rice noodles, bean sprouts and tangy dipping sauce."

New roads in Lao PDR made it possible for these products to leave the localities where they were produced; the newly integrated market economy made it possible for them to make their way to food boutiques in San Francisco and Toronto.

CONCLUSION

Foods and their meanings are increasingly mobile in a globalized food market. But the same foods have very different meanings in different contexts—river algae in soup as a side dish with sticky rice for a Lao subsistence farmer, or as grilled *kaipen*-wrapped sea bass with noodles and cilantro vinaigrette in an upscale Chicago restaurant; wild cassava to stretch sticky rice in a Lao community, or as the base for cassava sesame crisp baskets with lobster, chorizo, and lobster stock emulsion in that same Chicago restaurant.

Lao farmers use these products as part of their seasonal subsistence strategies and as insurance against crop failure. North American chefs use them to experiment with new taste combinations and perhaps to attract new admirers. Further examination of the commodity chain linking Lao river algae chips and cassava cakes to North American specialty food markets requires close attention to the meaning of *scarce*, *rare*, and *exotic*. The Oxford English Dictionary defines *scarce* as "restricted in quantity, size or amount, accessible in deficient quantity or limited number" (2658); *rare* denotes "seldom appearing, infrequent, uncommon, exceptional, unusual in respect to some good quality, of uncommon excellence" (2417). These foods are scarce to Lao farmers who harvest them, but rare to the North American chefs who cook them. It is their rarity that makes them exotic to the latter group.

Hunger foods and heritage foods represent disconnected discourses. My task here has been to identify these discourses and link them together, acting as the broker of these stories, just as food importers act as business brokers to provide exotic foods to North American consumers. Yet it would be a mistake to overstate the obvious binaries inherent in this story: slow food in Lao PDR becoming fast food snacks in North America; hunger over there, abundance over here; traditional food being given new life in another locale; poverty food necessities used as exotic expensive luxuries; here and there, then and now.

Such binaries force us to make moral judgments about the interconnections between food systems. On the one hand, a few Lao households are making extra income by providing these products to local entrepreneurs. On the other, the export of these products might destroy the scarce resource base both locals and exporters depend on. But the products are of interest in California and Toronto only as long as they remain exotic and rare. These particular items are no longer found in Toronto gourmet shops but must be ordered on the internet. In fact, the long-term demand for river weed and wild cassava would reduce their availability to Lao households as emergency hunger foods.

This chapter also questions the contrast between poverty foods and luxury foods. Lao villagers might well prefer pork loin to boiled pork backs, chicken breast to chicken feet, shrimp to crickets. Chicken feet and crickets are not the poverty foods that become exotic rare treats for foodies, notwithstanding the craze for chocolate-covered insects in the 1960s—foods used by teens to "gross people out." These latter products were food fads of short duration. Similarly, the interest in *khai pen* and *khao kiep* in North America is unlikely to last long.

The slow-fast distinction makes little sense in the Lao case. Lao food is unusually slow in preparation compared to Thai and other Asian cuisines. Rice must be soaked and steamed, fish products fermented, vegetables, fruits, and herbs collected and eaten fresh, or sun dried. But this is not the slow food envisioned by the Italian Slow Food movement.

When hunger foods, whose origins are inextricably linked to a place or tradition, are taken out of such traditions, away from their roots, their *terroir* (flavor unique to a particular region and soil), they no longer function as seasonal insurance and become instead markers of elite consumption in very different food systems. This decoupling of food from people and culture, of production from consumption, raises a question for future research: What are the boundaries between fascination with food—its taste and textures—and food fanaticism, with its prescriptive rules and border patrolling of what is ingested? How do these boundaries shift during globalization and the development of transnational commodity chains when the food deprived and the food obsessed eat the same food? *Bon appetit!*

Note

I would like to thank Richard Wilk for encouraging me to attend my first Society for Economic Anthropology meeting and to transform my poster presentation into a paper. His insights into what I wanted to say through my Lao food poster combined with his critical commentary about how to get there shaped this final chapter. I have benefited from participating in a project on community-based natural resource management at the Department of Forestry, National University of Laos, giving me an opportunity to meet others interested in Lao food. In addition, I recorded details about most meals I consumed in the country, and I thank those who fed me and ate with me for their patience with my questions. In the end, this chapter emerged more from trips to the table and the market than from trips to the library.

References

Alford, J., and N. Duguid. 1998. Seductions of Rice. New York: Artisan.

———. 2000. Hot Sour Salty Sweet: A Culinary Journey through Southeast Asia. Toronto: Random House.

Asian Development Bank (ADB). 2001. Participatory Poverty Assessment: Lao People's Democratic Republic. Manila: ADB.

Baird, Ian. 1995. Lao PDR: An Overview of Traditional Medicines Derived from Wild Animals and Plants. A TRAFFIC Southeast Asia Consultancy Report.

Bray, Francesca. 1986. The Rice Economies: Technology and Development in Asian Societies. Berkeley: University of California Press.

Cardoso, P., E. Mirione, M. Ernesto, F. Massaza, J. Cliff, M. Rezaulttaquei, and J. Bradbury. 2005. Processing of Cassava Roots to Remove Cyanogens. Journal of Food Composition and Analysis 18(5):451–60.

Davidson, Alan. 1975. Fish and Fish Dishes of Laos. Rutland, VT: Charles Tuttle and Co.

EU (European Union). 1997. Micro-projects. Unpublished report, Luang Prabang, Vientiane.

Fabricant, Florence. 2002. In Laos, a Regional Specialty Goes Global. New York Times, May 22:D3.

Food and Agriculture Organization (FAO). 2005. Nutrition Country Profiles: Lao Peple's Democratic Republic. Rome: FAO.

Foo Check Teck. 2002. No Cola, Pepsi Only. Bangkok: White Lotus.

Goody, Jack. 1982. Cooking, Cuisine and Class. New York: Cambridge University Press.

Hall, Michael, E. Sharples, R. Mitchell, B. Cambourne, and N. Macionis, eds. 2003. Food Tourism around the World: Development, Management and Markets. Oxford: Butterworth Heinemann.

Hanks, Lucien. 1972. Rice and Man: Agricultural Ecology in Southeast Asia. Chicago: Aldine Atherton.

Harrison, Julia. 2003. Being a Tourist: Finding Meaning in Pleasure Travel. Vancouver: UBC Press.

Heldke, Lisa. 2003. Exotic Appetites: Ruminations of a Food Adventurer. New York: Routledge.

Ho, Alice Yen. 1995. At the Southeast Asian Table. Kuala Lumpur: Oxford University Press.

Lao PDR. 2000. Fighting Poverty through Human Resource Development, Rural Development and People's Participation. Government report, Vientiane.

Levy, Paul. 1986. Out to Lunch. New York: Harper and Row.

Matisoff, James A. 1992. International Encyclopedia of Linguistics. Oxford: Oxford University Press.

Meusch, E., J. Yhoung-Aree, R. Friend, and S. Funge-Smith. 2003. The Role and Nutritional Value of Aquatic Resources in the Livelihoods of Rural People. Bangkok: FAO.

Millenium Development Goals. 2004. Progress Report. Vientiane, Lao PDR.

Ministry of Health. 2001. Health Status of the People in Lao PDR. Vientiane, Lao PDR.

Nguyen Xuan Hien. 2001. Glutinous-Rice-Eating Tradition in Vietnam and Elsewhere. Bangkok: White Lotus.

Norindr, Panivong. 1996. Phantasmatic Indochina. Durham: Duke University Press.

O'Connor, Richard. 1995. Agricultural Change and Ethnic Succession in Southeast Asian States: A Case for Regional Anthropology. Journal of Asian Studies 54(4): 968–96.

Ohnuki-Tierney, Emiko. 1993. Rice as Self: Japanese Identities through Time. Princeton: Princeton University Press.

Oxford English Dictionary. 1971. Oxford: Oxford University Press.

Rakow, Meg. 1992. Women in Lao Morality Tales. Southeast Asia Paper No. 35, Center for Southeast Asian Studies, Schools of Hawaiian, Asian and Pacific Studies, University of Hawaii at Manoa.

Rao, A., C. Bounphanonsay, J. Schiller, and M. Jackson. 2001. Collection of Rice Germplasm in the Lao PDR between 1995 and 2000. National Rice Research Program (NAFRI), Vientiane, Lao PDR.

Ribot, Jesse. 1998. Theorizing Access: Forest Profits along Senegal's Charcoal Commodity Chain. Development and Change 29:307–341.

Schiller, J., A. Rao, and P. Inthapanya. 1998. Glutinous Rice Varieties of Laos: Their Improvement, Cultivation, Processing and Consumption. In Specialty Rices of the World. R. Duffy, ed. Rome: FAO.

Sing, Phia. 1981. Traditional Recipes of Laos. Devon: Prospect Books.

Trankell, Ing-Britt. 1995. Cooking, Care and Domestication: A Culinary Ethnography of the Tai Yong, Northern Thailand. Uppsala Studies in Cultural Anthropology 21, Uppsala, Sweden.

Trubek, Amy. 2003. Food from Here. Expedition 45(2):22–25.

UNDP (United Nations Development Program). 2003. Human Development Report.

Van Esterik, Penny. 1992. From Marco Polo to McDonalds: Thai Cuisine in Transition. Food and Foodways 5(2):177–93.

CHAPTER 5

Rough Food

John T. Omohundro
(1994)

One afternoon in October 1992 Meg and Peter were serving us tea in their kitchen in Conche, a fishing outport on the Great Northern Peninsula. On the table were home-made bread and squashberry jam, cabbage pickles, some crackers, and molasses for Peter's tea. "Do you like this rough food?" Peter wondered. I asked what that meant. "Rough food is your staples, your winter's diet," Meg said, "the things you got in the fall to see you through 'til spring." Before the road was built into Conche in 1969, Meg and Peter bought nearly all their staples in bulk using the income Peter made selling salt fish and salmon. "When the schooner came in the fall you bought your flour, sugar, and salt in sacks, Barbados molasses in butts, puncheons of butter, big chests of tea, barrels of salt meat [beef] and salt pork," Meg said. These few essentials were supplemented with produce from large gardens, wild fruits, meat and dairy products from sheep, fowl, and cows, and game and fish. Dried, pickled, hung, frozen, bottled or cellared, these victuals fed Peter's family of seven until another schooner could nose through the ice in the harbor in April or May.

"That's all gone now," Peter said. "The pasture fences are down and the young people aren't taking up gardening. Now, even in the winter you can just climb aboard your truck, drive to Roddickton and buy whatever you need. People are getting lazy. If unemployment checks stopped we'd starve." While Peter had a point, home production was not defunct, either. We spent the next hour sipping tea while Meg and Peter explained how they still caught and cooked whelks, rabbits, moose, and sea ducks, and the fine points of curing salt cod and salmon. And when the tea was over, Peter got up to cut firewood and Meg headed over the hills into the marsh to pick "blackberries." Peter's sister next door was doing the same, and in his new house on the high road to Roddickton, where so many groceries were available, Peter's son Barry was also planting a garden and hunting moose and ducks, with every bit as much enthusiasm as his parents. The old times were gone, perhaps, but the new times looked familiar in many ways.

Excerpted from John T. Omohundro, *Rough Food: The seasons of subsistence in northern Newfoundland*. Institute of Social and Economic Research, Memorial University of Newfoundland. Copyright 1994. Reprinted with permission.

PART II

The Quest for Food: Evolutionary and Comparative Perspectives

UNIT I

THE BIOLOGICAL BASELINE

What foods did our ancestors eat? How did they manage to obtain an adequate supply of nutrients? How do we know what they ate and why should we contemporary humans care about the answer to these questions?

Not surprising, most scientists now agree that our ancestors' diets have changed dramatically from the time we were small rodent-like primates in the Eocene, some 50 million years ago. Changes in how we got our food and what we ate changed us. We may have become upright to grab foods with our hands, carry foods, and communicate with others. Later on, the use of fire may have protected us from other predators and helped along the evolution of our big brains. Furthermore, knowing more about ancestral diets and nutrition—the science called paleonutrition—may provide insights into what we might best consume today. Knowing what our recent ancestors ate may provide lessons or even a blueprint for what we ought to eat.

The early primates that we evolved from tended to eat fruits and insects and have stomachs and gastrointestinal tracts that were designed to process these different dietary staples. When the great apes appeared, perhaps 20 million years ago, diets shifted to include foods found on the ground as well as in trees. Although these new foods appear to have been mostly vegetarian and fibrous, dietary generalizations across time and species are bound to be difficult. Variety was, and is, always on the menu.

Our proto-human ancestors separated from the evolutionary line leading to our closest living relatives, gorillas and chimpanzees, about 6 million years ago. From that time and until about 12,000 years ago, all humans obtained food by what we call foraging, a combination of hunting, fishing, gathering, and scavenging (consumption of animals that died from causes unrelated to humans). Thus, for well over 99 percent of our time as an evolutionary lineage, we have subsisted by foraging. Conversely, we adopted agriculture and became food producers in the last blink of an evolutionary eye. Do our gastrointestinal systems and other aspects of our species reflect the history of our dietary adaptations as foragers? How did our ancestors' guts, hands, teeth, brains, and social behaviors evolve over this long history of foraging? What is the biobehavioral legacy of the long history of foraging?

Foods, and the nutrients they contain, were doubtlessly key regulators of the lives of animals now extinct, just as they are for living species. It is likely that pre-agricultural humans focused on foods that were both easily obtained and nutritious, and their biology and behavior evolved over time as they continued to use these foods. For example, the hominid line that includes individuals identified as *Australopithecus robustus* developed huge molar teeth (the relatively flat-surfaced teeth toward the back of the mouth; see chapter 6). The locations of the bony attachments of their chewing muscles are clear signs that the muscles were long and that they were powerful chewers. These anatomical changes suggest an increased reliance on bulky and/or hard-to-chew foods, such as hard nuts and palm fronds. These hominids may have been vegetarians.

By comparison, a contemporaneous group of hominids, identified as *Australopithecus africanus*, appears to have been less specialized in their food quest. It is this group that may have developed tools, perhaps to transport food, to dig for roots, or to kill and consume animals. Understanding what foods were consumed leads to knowledge about behavior as well as biology.

But how can we know the past without written records? In general, there are three sources of data that one can use to make inferences. One is archaeological and paleontological information—that is, information from fossils, human cultural remains such as evidence of fire or tools, and their ecological contexts. These are the most direct sources of information. A second source is the information available from the study of nonhuman primates (and other closely related species), and a third source is information available from the study of the few remaining foragers. We call the second and third sources of information inferential because one must carefully consider the validity of the inference that the information from primates or contemporary foragers is applicable to our ancestors. As chapter 6 by Ungar and Sponheimer warns, inferences from existing primates may or may not be useful because the human diet, and our biological adaptations to it, have changed many times. Contemporary foragers may have the same suite of biobehavior adaptations, but their ecological conditions are very different from Paleolithic foragers.

In different ways, the chapters to follow show how fascinating it is to try to reconstruct prehistoric foodways. The selections also highlight a number of fundamental issues, such as the relative importance of hunting and meat eating versus gathering other food sources, the importance of fire and food preparation, and the nutritional linkages among food sources, food preparation and brain evolution. As a group, these selections illustrate how behavior may be inferred from analogy and from the study of material remains (stones and bones).

In the lead chapter, "The Diet of Early Hominins," biological anthropologists Peter Ungar and Matt Sponheimer highlight results from newly developed methods that are adding complexity and even more variability to our picture of the evolution of human diets. For the longest time, archeologists and human paleontologists attempted to reconstruct what our human ancestors ate from ecological contexts and the few archaeological remains, and from the size and shape of human bones and teeth. For example, large flat teeth and large chewing muscles suggested a coarse diet; this is evident in the remains known as *Australopithecus robustus* (also *Paranthropus*). They also employed ecological reconstruction to provide information of what might have been available to eat, which of course is not necessarily what was actually consumed. Archaeological remains have also provided a number of clues, such as the use of fire and other food preparation techniques, but these clues are clearer only toward the end of the human career.

Ungar and Sponheimer bring together their combined analysis of two newer techniques: dental microwear and stable carbon isotopes. Microwear is the analysis of the pits and scratch marks left on the occlusal (biting) surfaces of teeth. They are studied using an electron microscope and indicate what was consumed close to death, a sort of snapshot of "the last meal" or the last few meals. On the other hand, carbon isotopes (chemically distinctive forms of carbon) provide evidence of the relative importance of different types of food consumed (i.e., tropical grasses versus tree fruits) over a range of time. Isotopes found in the enamel of teeth provide a dietary record during the time of tooth development early in life, whereas isotopes in bones provide a window into diets of the last years of life. Because they are incorporated into tissue, chemicals such as carbon isotopes are a concrete example of the adage that "you are what you eat." Together, these new methods provide direct evidence of what was actually consumed: the meal versus the ecological menu.

Ungar and Sponheimer argue that a review of this direct evidence demonstrates that there is more variation in the diets of early hominins across species and time than we might have previously realized. As is true today, variation is everywhere.

In "Eating Christmas in the Kalahari" (chapter 2), Richard Lee recounts his lessons learned about symbolic meanings associated with food exchange among the Dobe !Kung San of the Kalahari. In "What Hunters Do for a Living, or, How to Make Out on Scarce Resources" (chapter 7), Lee reports on the details of the diets of the Dobe !Kung. The chapter is included here as an excellent and intensely interesting study of the details of the diet of modern hunters and one of great historical significance.

Lee aims to answer the question "How difficult is it for the San to meet their daily food needs?" Lee's work was a pioneering energy input-output analysis. He observed and measured the amount of time expended in subsistence activities and calculated the amounts of energy and protein that were obtained. To the surprise of many, the time that the !Kung San spent foraging for plant foods averaged only a couple of hours a day and energy return was high relative to energy expended. Lee particularly highlights the importance of mongongo nuts as sources of energy and protein. Finally, Lee estimated that vegetable rather than animal products provided the majority of nutrients. Could Lee's results hold true for most or all foragers? His observation that the San "eat as much vegetable food as they need and as much meat as they can" gives us another perspective on "Eating Christmas in the Kalahari."

In "Food for Thought" (chapter 8), science writer Ann Gibbons reports on a set of studies on the importance of fire in human evolution. Our big brains undoubtedly lead us to do many of the things that mark our species. Our infants are born immature because a head could not fit through a mother's birth canal. Therefore, we have particularly long infancies that allow for great socialization and bonding with mothers and groups of individuals. Our large brains have allowed for language, more social discourse, and planning hunts and countless other activities. And, finally, our large brains are energetically costly. How do we afford the high cost?

Tracking the work of Harvard primatologist Richard Wrangham and his colleagues, Wrangham provides a convincing argument that fire and cooking foods may have allowed for an important shift in human evolution. Fire allowed humans to stay on the ground, safe from predators, sleeping in groups, and increased reliance on others and socialization. Cooking foods with fire also allowed for the digestion of more animal protein. Our dietary tracts needed to work less and allowed more energy to go to our brains.

In the last chapter in this section (chapter 9), "Paleolithic Nutrition: A Consideration of Its Nature and Current Implications," S. Boyd Eaton and Melvin Konner outline what Paleolithic humans may have eaten and what their diet may portend for individuals today. This chapter first appeared in the *New England Journal of Medicine*, with the obvious readership of physicians. The authors assess the diets of contemporary foragers such as the !Kung San (chapters 2 and 7) and prehistoric foragers such as those studied by Ungar and Sponheimer (chapter 6), as well as Goodman and Armelagos (chapter 12). They estimate that the diet of Paleolithic humans consisted of about 35% animal product.

How secure is this generalization? Is it likely that meat consumption, for example, was as high as they proposed? How constant was the food supply? Is any generalization possible given the diversity of forager lifestyles and diets?

Lastly, is it any more valid to think we are adapted to a Paleolithic rather than an Eocene primate's insect-rich diet? Might we just as easily point to the healthiness of eating fruits and insects as our primate cousins do?

In summary, this section aims to explore the scientific methods used to infer prehistoric diets, as well as arguments for the role of diet and nutrition in human evolution, and the importance of ancient diets for contemporary humans. Ungar and Sponheimer highlight the findings made possible by newer methods. Gibbon reports on the once controversial role of fire and the evolution of large human brains. Lee's data call into question the importance placed on hunting over gathering, meat over fruits and vegetables, male-centered activities over female-centered activities. Finally, Eaton and Konner bring together multiple sources and speculate on the importance of ancestral diets in preventing modern diseases.

How much of the diet of our ancestors was based on hunting, gathering, or scavenging? How much came from meats, vegetables, and fruits? Do we have the guts, teeth, and brains of an omnivore and the psychology of a carnivore? Although the precise mix remains unknown, what seems certain is that the methods of procurement and the types of foods changed over time and place. Thankfully, we are a flexible species.

SUGGESTIONS FOR THINKING AND DOING NUTRITIONAL ANTHROPOLOGY

1. Compare teeth. Look in a mirror at the chewing surfaces of your teeth. Compare your teeth to those of your cat or dog. Go to a local natural history museum (or any place you might be able to observe the teeth of different animals) and describe the differences. What are the functions of teeth? How are variations in typical diets reflected in variations in size and shape?

2. Write an essay on the importance of meat in human evolution. Were we born to be meat eaters, vegetarians, or omnivores? What data can be brought to this question? A variety of sources may be used, such as evidence from human anatomy and physiology (lengths of intestines) and epidemiological studies of diet and health. In class, compose essays and debate the importance of meat. A useful first source is *Food and Evolution* (Harris and Ross, 1987).

3. Study your own food quest using the techniques of observation that are employed by Lee. Over the course of a week, record the amount of time you spend in your quest for food. How much time do you spend "shopping" and "preparing"

food? Calculate the amount that your food costs. How long did it take you or your parents to earn that money? Did you spend more or less time than the San?

4. The raw foods movement is about not cooking foods. They claim that cooking can rob foods of vital nutrients. Go for a day without cooking or eating processed foods. What did you eat? Any meat or fish?

Suggested Further Reading

Eaton SB, Shostak M, Konner M. 1989. The Paleolithic Prescription. HarperCollins: New York. One of a number of books that recommend eating like our ancestors.

Harris M, Ross E, eds. 1987. Food and Evolution. Philadelphia: Temple University Press. Selections by Katharine Milton and others further explore the significance of the diet of hominids and nonhuman primates.

Hill K, Hurtado AM. 1996. Ache Life History: The Ecology and Demography of a Foraging People. Hawthorne, NY: Aldine de Gruyter. An exceptional comparative analysis of South American foragers based on a long-term study.

Lee R. 1979. The !Kung San: Men, Women, and Work in a Foraging Society. Cambridge: Cambridge University Press. An update and expansion of Lee's seminal work.

Lee R, DeVore I, eds. 1968. Man the Hunter. Chicago: Aldine. A. A classic book, and the source of the article by Richard Lee.

Lee-Thorp JA. 2001. Chemistry and hominid fossils. How to extract information about diet from those ancient teeth and bones. Science in Africa Dec: http://www.science inafrica.co.za/2001/december/hominids.htm. Very accessible source on the use of chemical methods for extracting dietary information from bones and teeth.

Leonard WR, Snodgrass JJ, Robertson ML. 2007. Effects of Brain Evolution on Human Nutrition and Metabolism. Annual Review of Nutrition 27:311–327. Excellent overview on the relationship between brain evolution and nutrition.

Sponheimer M, Ungar P, Reed K, Lee-Thorp J, eds. In press. Early Hominin Paleoecology. Boulder: The University of Colorado Press.

Ungar PS, Teaford MF, eds. 2006. Human Diet: Its Origins and Evolution. London and Westport, CT., Bergen & Garvey. Technically written series of articles on the evolution of human diets.

Ungar PS, ed. 2007. Early Hominin Diets: The Known, the Unknown and the Unknowable. New York, Oxford University Press. An addition technical source on human diets.

CHAPTER 6

The Diets of Early Hominins

Peter S. Ungar and Matt Sponheimer

(2011)

Diet is fundamental to an organism's ecology and, unsurprisingly, changes in diet have been hailed as key milestones in human evolution. Our understanding of the diets of our distant forebears, the early hominins, has been honed over much of the past half century given new methods for dietary inference, the discovery of new fossil species and additional specimens, and improved reconstructions of the environments in which they evolved. In this review we focus on recent contributions from dental microwear and stable isotope analyses, two approaches that have challenged traditional thinking about early hominin dietary ecology over the past few years.

There are four principal groups of interest in early hominin evolution: the Mio-Pliocene probable hominins (*Sahelanthropus, Orrorin, Ardipithecus*), the Plio-Pleistocene "gracile" australopiths (genus *Australopithecus*), the "robust" australopiths (genus *Paranthropus*), and the earliest members of our own genus, *Homo*. The first group dates from about 7 Ma, though the best-known species, *Ar. ramidus*, lived about 4.4 Ma. The earliest recovered *Australopithecus* dates to approximately 4.2 Ma, whereas *Paranthropus* and *Homo* have first known appearances shortly before and after 2.5 Ma respectively, presumably from *Australopithecus* or *Australopithecus*-like ancestors. All of these groups are represented in eastern Africa, the first two are also known from Chad, and the latter three are found in South Africa (1).

WHAT WE THOUGHT ABOUT EARLY HOMININ DIETS

The earliest probable hominins are not all well known, but in some cases their molars are smaller and more thinly enameled than those of later australopiths and more like those of extant chimpanzees (1), suggesting a diet of fleshy fruits and soft, young leaves. According to conventional wisdom, the craniodental morphology of later *Australopithecus* (e.g., thickly enameled, large, flat cheek teeth and heavily-built crania and mandibles compared

with living apes) reflects an adaptive shift from diets dominated by soft, sugary forest fruits to hard, brittle nuts or seeds, or to those with adherent abrasives, such as underground storage organs that were readily available in increasingly open Plio-Pleistocene landscapes (2–3) (Fig. 1). The larger teeth with well-buttressed skulls and massive chewing muscles of *Paranthropus* have led to the notion that "robust" australopiths relied on more hard foods than did *Australopithecus*. The eastern African "hyper-robust" *P. boisei* has been considered the quintessence of this "nut-cracking" morphology (4) (Fig. 1).

The earliest members of our own genus are believed to have had tools to acquire and process a broad range of foods, such as meat and underground storage organs, bespeaking a generalized and versatile diet (5). Morphological evidence suggests that early *Homo* had smaller cheek teeth, thinner dental enamel, and greater occlusal relief than did their *Australopithecus* predecessors or their *Paranthropus* contemporaries (6–8) (Fig. 1). This may indicate changing selective pressures due to extraoral food processing with tools, but also suggests that early *Homo* teeth could more efficiently shear tough foods (such as leaves and meat) than could those of the australopiths. The possession of larger brains in some cases has also been used to argue that *Homo* required high-energy-yielding foods (9–10).

Much research on early hominin diets has focused on archaeological and morphological data, but like all lines of evidence for subsistence of fossil species, they have limitations. Stone tools and butchered bones tell us little about the plant foods that likely dominated early hominin diets. Moreover, the earliest known stone tools and cut-marked bones date to at least 2.6 Ma and possibly earlier (11–12), but still postdate the earliest hominins by millions of years. And though tooth and jaw size, shape, and structure offer important clues to the fracture properties of foods and associated masticatory stresses and strains to which a species is adapted (13–16), they indicate what early hominins were capable of eating and suggest the selective pressures faced by their ancestors rather than what specific individuals ate. For direct evidence of the diets of fossil specimens recovered, we need other sources of information, such as dental microwear and stable light isotope analyses of teeth.

Peter S. Ungar and Matt Sponheimer, "The Diets of Early Hominins." *Science* 334(6053):190–93, 2011. Reprinted with permission.

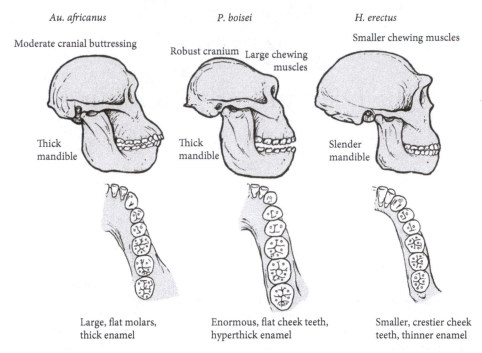

Figure 1 *Skulls and teeth of early hominins. Differences between species and genera have been used to infer differences in their feeding adaptations.*

DENTAL MICROWEAR

Mammals show a strong and consistent association between dental microwear pattern and food fracture properties. Those that crush hard, brittle foods (e.g., nuts, bones) typically have occlusal microwear dominated by pits, whereas those that shear tough items (e.g., leaves, meat) more often show long, parallel striations on their wear surfaces (*17*) (supporting online text). These pits and scratches are traces of actual chewing events; they record activities during a moment in the life of an individual, much like footprints. And like footprints, microwear is fleeting; individual features turnover and are replaced by others as a tooth wears down (*18*). Indeed, microwear textures reflect diet in the days or weeks before death. This "last-supper" phenomenon (*19*) can be an asset, as large samples provide a sense of variation in diet within a species. Taxa with more catholic diets should evince a broader range of microwear textures than those that consume a more limited variety of foods. Several integrated metrics of microwear have proven useful: surface fractal complexity, or change in apparent roughness with scale of observation, is used as a proxy for food hardness; and anisotropy, or directionality of the wear fabric, is used as a proxy for food toughness. High complexity and anisotropy values roughly correspond to surfaces with heavy pitting and highly-aligned scratches respectively.

Dental microwear texture data have not yet been collected for the earliest probable hominins, but results have been published for cheek teeth of 73 specimens of *Australopithecus* (*Au. anamensis, Au. afarensis, Au. africanus*), *Paranthropus* (*P. boisei, P. robustus*), and early *Homo* (*H. habilis*, African *H. erectus, Homo* specimens

from Sterkfontein Member 5 and Swartkrans Member 1) (*20–23*) (Figs. 2, 3). None of the *Australopithecus* specimens have the high complexity values or heavily pitted surfaces of a hard-object feeder as originally expected given their morphology. And the two eastern African species, *Au. anamensis* and *Au. afarensis*, have similar and homogenous microwear complexity (within and between taxa) despite a sample distribution spanning more than 1 million years and 1500 km and habitats ranging from closed woodland to grassland (*24*). The South African *Au. africanus* has higher average complexity, but this is still lower than that expected of a hard-object feeder. *Australopithecus* spp. also have low to moderate anisotropy, with few values extending into the upper ranges of living folivorous primates. This indicates that they did not shear tough leaves as do modern folivores, perhaps because such foods were not an important part of their diet. However, it is also possible that they ground tough foods like a mortar and pestle might mill grist, as their flat teeth might have posed fewer masticatory constraints than those of modern folivores (*22*).

The eastern African "robust" australopith, *P. boisei*, has low microwear texture complexity and low-to-moderate anisotropy values, suggesting a diet dominated by foods with similar fracture properties to those eaten by *Au. anamensis* and *Au. afarensis* (*21–22*). The South African *P. robustus*, on the other hand, has the highest average complexity and lowest anisotropy of any early hominin (*20*). Complexity in South African "robust" australopiths also shows high variance, with a distribution most comparable to hard-object fallback feeders such as grey-cheeked mangabeys (*Lophocebus albigena*) and brown capuchins (*Cebus apella*),

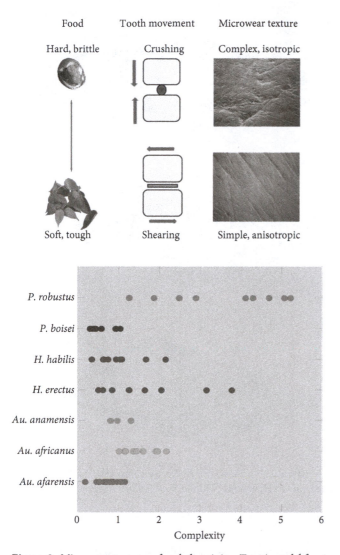

Figure 2 *Microwear textures of early hominins. Top: A model for microwear formation, wherein hard and brittle foods are crushed between opposing teeth, causing pitting with complex, isotropic surface textures; in contrast, soft and tough foods are sheared between opposing teeth that slide past one another, causing parallel scratches and simpler, anisotropic surfaces (see supporting online text). Bottom: microwear texture complexity values for individual fossil hominins by species [data from (20–23)].*

which tend to "fallback" on harder items when softer, more preferred foods are unavailable (20). This could indicate that their anatomy evolved to cope with infrequently eaten but fracture resistant foods (see 15).

Microwear textures of early *Homo* suggest that all species had fairly generalized diets lacking specialization for either extremely hard or tough foods (23). Of note, *H. erectus* has substantially more variation in microwear complexity values than *H. habilis*, or indeed than that of any other hominin examined to date except *P. robustus*. This suggests that *H. erectus* had a comparatively broad-based diet, spanning a range of fracture properties including some hard and perhaps tough foods, which may also produce small pits through adhesive wear (25).

STABLE ISOTOPES

Stable isotope analysis of ancient tissues is based on the principle "you are what you eat" (26). Stable isotopes in foodstuffs become incorporated into the growing teeth and bones of consumers. These tissues then acquire an isotopic composition related to that of the source food that can reveal much about paleodiets (27–29). While dietary studies can be undertaken with bone mineral in some cases, dental enamel is preferred as it is more highly mineralized and thus less susceptible to post-depositional chemical alteration than bone (30); it is also an incremental tissue that may allow investigation of intra-individual diet change through time.

Carbon isotopes are particularly useful for hominin paleodietary studies because they tell us about the relative proportions of plants using the C_3 (trees, bushes, forbs) and C_4 (tropical grasses and some sedges) photosynthetic pathways that were consumed by herbivores, or in the case of faunivores, the proportions of these foods consumed by their prey (27) (Fig. 4). This allows a variety of questions to be addressed. For instance, did the early members of our lineage have diets similar to those of our closest living kin, the chimpanzee (*Pan troglodytes*)? We know that chimpanzees have diets dominated by C_3 tree foods (especially fleshy fruits) whether in their preferred forest habitats or fairly open savannas with abundant grasses (31–32). Carbon isotope ratios ($^{13}C/^{12}C$) have been analyzed for more than 75 hominin specimens from sites in Ethiopia, Kenya, Tanzania, and South Africa, ranging in age from about 4.4 to possibly 0.8 Ma (Fig. 4).

The broad view of these data is that early hominins did not have diets like extant African apes; but this conclusion belies the complexity of the varied results. For instance, the earliest taxon analyzed to date, *Ardipithecus ramidus*, had in aggregate a C_3 diet much like savanna chimpanzees (33). Other taxa, such as *Au. africanus*, *P. robustus*, and early *Homo*, were more middling, as they ate more than 50% C_3 foods but also consumed significant quantities of C_4 foods (32, 34–37) that became increasingly available in the Plio-Pleistocene (38–39). In marked contrast, *P. boisei* had a diet of about 75–80% C_4 plants, unlike any other fossil hominin, but similar to grass-eating warthogs, hippos, and zebras (supporting online text) (36, 40). Carbon isotopic variability between these taxa is also marked, with *Au. africanus* ranging from pure C_3 to nearly pure C_4 diets, while other taxa, such as *P. boisei*, have much reduced ranges.

Thus, carbon isotopes suggest marked dietary diversity within the hominins. This is not surprising given their temporal and ecogeographic ranges and the variation in masticatory morphology they manifest; however, the isotope data also suggest enormous and unanticipated differences between contemporaneous taxa with strong morphological similarities, notably the "robust" australopiths *P. robustus* and *P. boisei*. Despite their attribution to the same genus, there is no overlap in their carbon isotope compositions (40), which is a rarity for congeners among extant mammals.

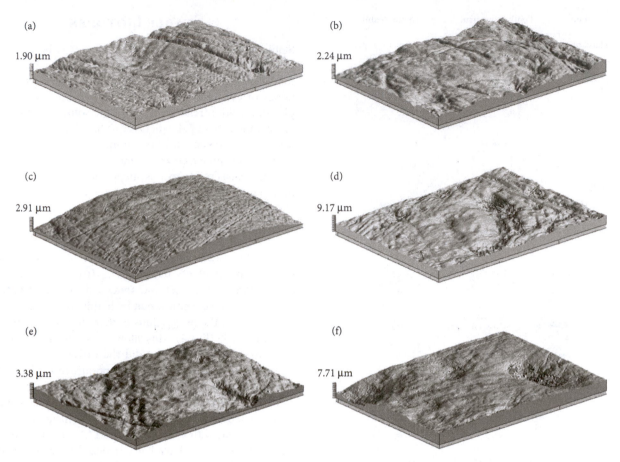

Figure 3 *Photosimulations of microwear surfaces representing A) Au. afarensis (AL 333w-1a), B) Au. africanus (Sts 61), C) P. boisei (KNM-CH1B), D) P. robustus (SK 16), E) H. habilis (OH 16), and F) H. erectus (KNM-ER 807). Each represents an area 102 × 139 μm on facet 9 and vertical scales are as indicated.*

All told, the early hominins analyzed to date fall roughly into three groups: (i) those with carbon isotope compositions indicating strong C_3 diets similar to those of savanna chimpanzees, (ii) those with variably mixed C_3/C_4 diets, and (iii) those with carbon isotope compositions indicating diets of chiefly C_4 vegetation as is typically seen for grass-eating ungulates in tropical climes.

INTEGRATING AND MOVING FORWARD

Microwear and stable carbon isotope studies have challenged long-held assumptions about early hominin diets. The simple, textbook model of hominin craniodental functional morphology evolving for increasing consumption of hard, brittle foods as savannas spread is incorrect, or at least too simplistic. None of the *Australopithecus* or even *Paranthropus* specimens examined from eastern Africa show microwear patterns of a hard-object feeder (supporting online text). And while the *Ardipithecus* carbon isotope composition is consistent with a diet similar to those of savanna chimpanzees as might be expected, that of *P. boisei* indicates that C_4 plant foods such as grasses or sedges provided the vast majority of dietary energy for this taxon. This was almost completely unanticipated [but see (*41*)] and

raises the intriguing possibility that earlier eastern African australopiths may have had a similar penchant for C_4 foods, especially given the similarities of their dental microwear to that of *P. boisei*.

Both the microwear and carbon isotope data offer other surprises. First, there seems to be a geographic influence on australopith diets; microwear texture complexity of eastern African *Australopithecus* and *Paranthropus* are lower than those of their South African congeners. Likewise, *P. boisei* and *P. robustus* have different carbon isotope compositions, with the South African "robust" australopiths consuming a much higher fraction of C_3 foods, like most other early hominins (though not to the extent seen in *Ardipithecus*). This might indicate that a specialized morphological complex can serve more than one function and reflect more than one type of diet; perhaps "robust" morphology functions in high-stress hard-object feeding for *P. robustus*, but in repetitive loading during grinding of tough foods for *P. boisei*.

The apparent continuity of microwear pattern through the putative lineage *Au. anamensis* to *Au. afarensis* to *P. boisei* could even suggest that morphological changes reflect increasing efficiency for grinding large quantities of tough food. Although living primates that eat tough items typically have sharp shearing crests, eastern African australopiths,

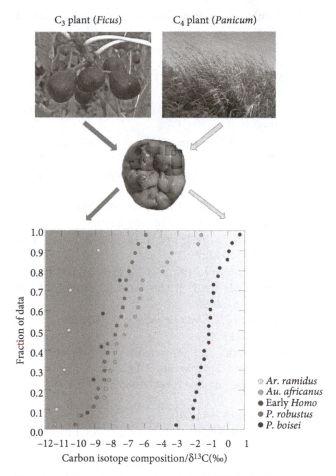

Figure 4 *Carbon isotope compositions ($^{13}C/^{12}C$) of early hominins. Top: carbon flows from C_3 and C_4 plants (dark and light arrows respectively) into the tooth enamel of the consumer (in this case* P. robustus, *SK 1), and its resulting carbon isotope composition reveals the proportions of these plant types consumed. Bottom: quantile plot with carbon isotope ratio data for all early hominins analyzed to date (data from 33–37, 48). Darker shading indicates a greater degree of C_3 plant consumption. Each data point reflects a hominin's diet for a period ranging from months to years depending on the sampling procedure used (rectangles represent hypothetical sampling areas). Carbon isotope ratios ($^{13}C/^{12}C$) are expressed as δ values in parts per thousand (‰) relative to the V-PDB standard.*

and especially *P. boisei*, may have evolved a different solution for processing such foods given the flattened, thickly enameled teeth of their close ancestors (*22*). Natural selection must work with the raw materials available to it. Thus, the present day ecomorphological diversity within the primates may not be sufficient for making some paleoecological inferences, which is not surprising considering that the vast majority of all primates, especially apes, that have ever lived are now extinct.

The microwear and isotope evidence also give insights into food choices and foraging strategies. The *P. robustus* microwear complexity distribution suggests that individuals ate hard objects only on occasion, perhaps in a manner akin to the lowland gorilla's (*Gorilla gorilla*) falling back

on lower quality, tough foods during times when preferred soft, sugar-rich items are unavailable (*42*). Laser ablation analysis, which allows isotopic sampling along the rough growth trajectory of teeth, also reveals significant variation in within-tooth carbon isotope compositions of *P. robustus* at inter- and intra-annual timescales (*43*). In contrast, the teeth of *Au. afarensis* show little variance in microwear texture complexity despite a range of samples across time and space. In this case, a model involving increased foraging ranges for foods with given fracture or nutritional properties, such as observed for some chimpanzees (*44*), might be more appropriate.

The above evidence challenges certain aspects of our understanding of hominin biology, biogeography, and evolution. For instance, if *P. boisei* was a C_4 sedge consumer (*36*), its distribution was likely limited to the periphery of permanent sources of water. Its eventual extinction might then be linked to the difficulty of dispersing away from water sources despite the vaunted energetic efficiency of bipedalism (*45*). On the other hand, if *P. boisei* was a C_4 grass consumer, it might have thrived in the emerging savannas of the Pleistocene, demanding an explanation other than habitat change for its extinction.

Our understanding of the paleoecology of these organisms is in flux, and a great deal of directed, integrative research remains to be done (e.g., *46*). Microwear and stable isotope analyses are needed for all relevant species, and these results must be integrated with data on masticatory biomechanics, plant distributions and nutritional/mechanical properties, and primate ecology/digestive physiology. An important role for microwear and isotope analyses within contemporary paleodietary research is to focus on underlying processes rather than outcomes, and to recognize evolutionary novelties, such as grazing giraffes (*47*) and grass- or sedge-eating apes (*36*). When these behavioral proxies are linked to morphological and paleoenvironmental datasets through time, yoking habitat and dietary change to morphological response, it should greatly augment our understanding of the patterns and processes of hominin evolution.

Notes

Supported by the U.S. National Science Foundation, the Leakey Foundation, and the Wenner-Gren Foundation. We thank C. Campbell, J. Leichliter, O. Paine, Yasmin Rahman, C. Ross, and P. Sandberg for comments; and T. Cerling, D. Codron, D. de Ruiter, F. Grine, J. Lee-Thorp, R. Scott, M. Teaford, and N. van der Merwe for discussions over the years. All raw data referred in this paper are published in references *20–23, 33–37,* and *48*.

References

1. B. Wood, N. Lonergan, *J. Anat.* **212**, 354–376 (2008).
2. M. F. Teaford, P. S. Ungar, *Proc. Nat. Acad. Sci. USA* **97**, 13506 (2000).
3. G. Suwa *et al.*, *Science* **326**, 94 (2009).

4. B. Wood, P. Constantino, *Yrbk. Phys. Anthropol.* **50**, 106 (2007).

5. P. S. Ungar, F. E. Grine, M. F. Teaford, *Ann. Rev. Anthropol.* **35**, 209 (2006).

6. A. D. Beynon, B. A. Wood, *Am. J. Phys. Anthropol.* **70**, 177 (1986).

7. P. S. Ungar, J. Hum. Evol. **46**, 605 (2004).

8. H. M. McHenry, K. Coffing, *Ann. Rev. Anthropol.* **29**, 125 (2000).

9. L. C. Aiello, P. Wheeler, *Curr. Anthropol.* **36**, 199 (1995).

10. K. Milton, *Evol. Anthropol.* **8**, 11 (1999).

11. S. Semaw, *J. Archaeol. Sci.* **27**, 1197 (2000).

12. S. P. McPherron *et al., Nature* **466**, 857 (2010).

13. D. J. Daegling, F. E. Grine, *Am. J. Phys. Anthropol.* **86**, 321 (1991).

14. W. L. Hylander, in F. E. Grine, Ed. (Aldine de Gruyter, New York, 1988), pp. 55–83.

15. D. S. Strait *et al., Proc. Nat. Acad. Sci. USA* **106**, 2124 (2009).

16. P. W. Lucas, (Cambridge University Press, New York, 2004), pp. 1–355.

17. P. S. Ungar, (Johns Hopkins University Press, Baltimore, 2010), pp. 1–304.

18. M. F. Teaford, O. J. Oyen, *Am. J. Phys. Anthropol.* **75**, 279 (1988).

19. F. E. Grine, *J. Hum. Evol.* **15**, 783 (1986).

20. R. S. Scott *et al., Nature* **436**, 693 (2005).

21. P. S. Ungar, F. E. Grine, M. F. Teaford, *PLoS ONE* **3**, e2044:1 (2008).

22. P. S. Ungar, et al., *Phil. Trans. Roy. Soc. Lond. Ser. B* **365**, 3345 (2010).

23. P. S. Ungar, et al., *J. Hum. Evol.* doi:10.1016/j.jhevol. 2011.04.006 (2011).

24. F. E. Grine, P. S. Ungar, M. F. Teaford, *S. Afr. J. Sci.* **102**, 301 (2006).

25. M. F. Teaford, J. A. Runestad, *Am. J. Phys. Anthropol.* **88**, 347 (1992).

26. M. J. Deniro, S. Epstein, *Geochim.Cosmochim. Acta* **42**, 495 (1978).

27. J. A. Lee-Thorp, J. C. Sealy, N. J. van der Merwe, *J. Archaeol. Sci.* **16**, 585 (1989).

28. P. L. Koch, K. A. Hoppe, S. D. Webb, *Chem. Geol.* **152**, 119 (1998).

29. T. E. Cerling, J. M. Harris, M. G. Leakey, *Oecolog.* **120**, 364 (1999).

30. J. A. Lee-Thorp, N. J. van der Merwe, *J. Archaeol. Sci.* **18**, 343 (1991).

31. M. J. Schoeninger, J. Moore, J. M. Sept, *Am. J. Primatol.* **49**, 297 (1999).

32. M. Sponheimer et al., *J. Hum. Evol.* **51**, 128 (2006).

33. T. D. White et al., *Science* **326**, 67 (2009).

34. J. Lee-Thorp, J. F. Thackeray, N. van der Merwe, *J. Hum. Evol.* **39**, 565 (2000).

35. N. J. van der Merwe, et al., *J. Hum. Evol.* **44**, 581 (2003).

36. N. J. van der Merwe, F. T. Masao, M. K. Bamford, *S. Afr. J. Sci.* **104**, 153 (2008).

37. J. A. Lee-Thorp, N. J. van der Merwe, C. K. Brain, *J. Hum. Evol.* **27**, 361 (1994).

38. P. B. DeMenocal, *Earth Planet. Sci. Lett.* **220**, 3 (2004).

39. R. Bobe, *J. Arid. Environ.* **66**, 564 (2006).

40. T. E. Cerling et al., *Proc. Nat. Acad. Sci. USA* **108**, 9337 (2011).

41. C. J. Jolly, *Man* **5**, 5 (1970).

42. P. S. Ungar, in T. Koppe, G. Meyer, K. W. Alt, Eds. (Karger, Basel, 2009), pp. 38–43.

43. M. Sponheimer *et al., Science* **314**, 980 (2006).

44. W. C. McGrew, P. J. Baldwin, C. E. G. Tutin, *J. Hum. Evol.* **10**, 227 (1981).

45. P. S. Rodman, H. M. McHenry, *Am. J. Phys. Anthropol.* **52**, 103 (1980).

46. N. Dominy, et al., *Evol. Biol.* **35**, 159 (2008).

47. N. Solounias, M. Teaford, A. Walker, *Paleobiol.* **14**, 287 (1988).

48. M. Sponheimer *et al., J. Hum. Evol.* **48**, 301 (2005).

CHAPTER 7

What Hunters Do for a Living, or, How to Make Out on Scarce Resources

Richard B. Lee

(1968)

The current anthropological view of hunter-gatherer subsistence rests on two questionable assumptions. First is the notion that these peoples are primarily dependent on the hunting of game animals, and second is the assumption that their way of life is generally a precarious and arduous struggle for existence.

Recent data on living hunter-gatherers (Meggitt, 1964; Service, 1966) show a radically different picture. We have learned that in many societies, plant and marine resources are far more important than are game animals in the diet. More important, it is becoming clear that, with a few conspicuous exceptions, the hunter-gatherer subsistence base is at least routine and reliable and at best surprisingly abundant. Anthropologists have consistently tended to underestimate the viability of even those "marginal isolates" of hunting peoples that have been available to ethnographers.

The purpose of this article is to analyze the food getting activities of one such "marginal" people, the !Kung Bushmen of the Kalahari Desert. Three related questions are posed: How do the Bushmen make a living? How easy or difficult is it for them to do this? What kinds of evidence are necessary to measure and evaluate the precariousness or security of a way of life? And after the relevant data are presented, two further questions are asked: What makes this security of life possible? To what extent are the Bushmen typical of hunter-gatherers in general?

BUSHMAN SUBSISTENCE

The !Kung Bushmen of Botswana are an apt case for analysis.[1] They inhabit the semi-arid northwest region of the Kalahari Desert. With only six to nine inches of rainfall per year, this is, by any account, a marginal environment for human habitation. In fact, it is precisely the unattractiveness of their homeland that has kept the !Kung isolated from extensive contact with their agricultural and pastoral neighbors.

Field work was carried out in the Dobe area, a line of eight permanent waterholes near the South-West Africa border and 125 miles south of the Okavango River. The population of the Dobe area consists of 466 Bushmen, including 379 permanent residents living in independent camps or associated with Bantu cattle posts, as well as 87 seasonal visitors. The Bushmen share the area with some 340 Bantu pastoralists largely of the Herero and Tswana tribes. The ethnographic present refers to the period of field work: October, 1963–January, 1965.

The Bushmen living in independent camps lack firearms, livestock, and agriculture. Apart from occasional visits to the Herero for milk, these !Kung are entirely dependent upon hunting and gathering for their subsistence. Politically they are under the nominal authority of the Tswana headman, although they pay no taxes and receive very few government services. European presence amounts to one overnight government patrol every six to eight weeks. Although Dobe-area !Kung have had some contact with outsiders since the 1880's, the majority of them continue to hunt and gather because there is no viable alternative locally available to them.[2]

Each of the fourteen independent camps is associated with one of the permanent waterholes. During the dry season (May–October) the entire population is clustered around these wells. Table 1 shows the numbers at each well at the end of the 1964 dry season. Two wells had no camp resident and one large well supported five camps. The number of camps at each well and the size of each camp changed frequently during the course of the year. The "camp" is an open aggregate of cooperating persons which changes in size and composition from day to day. Therefore, I have avoided the term "band" in describing the !Kung Bushman living groups.[3]

Each waterhole has a hinterland lying within a six-mile radius which is regularly exploited for vegetable and animal foods. These areas are not territories in the zoological sense, since they are not defended against outsiders. Rather they constitute the resources that lie within a convenient walking distance of a waterhole. The camp is a self-sufficient subsistence unit. The members move out each day to hunt and gather, and return in the evening to pool the collected foods

Richard B. Lee, "What Hunters Do for a Living, or, How to Make Out on Scarce Resources." In *Man the Hunter*, R. Lee and I. Devore, eds. Aldine, pp. 30–48, 1968. Reprinted with permission.

Table 1 Numbers and Distribution of Resident Bushmen and Bantu by Waterhole[*]

Name of Waterhole	No. of Camps	Population of Camps	Other Bushmen	Total Bushmen	Bantu
Dobe	2	37	—	37	—
!angwa	1	16	23	39	84
Bate	2	30	12	42	21
!ubi	1	19	—	19	65
!gose	3	52	9	61	18
/ai/ai	5	94	13	107	67
!xabe	—	—	8	8	12
Mahopa	—	—	23	23	73
Total	14	248	88	336	340

[*]Figures do not include 130 Bushmen outside area on the date of census.

Table 2 The Bushman Annual Round

	Jan.	Feb.	Mar.	April	May	June	July	Aug.	Sept.	Oct.	Nov.	Dec.
Season	Summer Rains			Autumn Dry			Winter Dry			Spring Dry	First Rains	
Availability of Water	Temporary summer pools everywhere			Large summer pools			Permanent waterholes only				Summer pools developing	
Group Moves	Widely dispersed at summer pools			At large summer pools			All population restricted to permanent waterholes				Moving out to summer pools	
Men's Subsistence Activities	1. Hunting with bow, arrows, and dogs (Year-round) 2. Running down immatures 3. Some gathering (Year-round)					Trapping small game in snares					Running down newborn animals	
Women's Subsistence Activities	1. Gathering of mongongo nuts (Year-round) 2. Fruits, berries,					Roots, bulbs, melons					Roots, leafy resins greens	
Ritual Activities	Dancing, trance performances, and ritual curing (Year-round) Boys' initiation[*]											†
Relative Subsistence Hardship	Water-food distance minimal					Increasing distance from water to food					Water-food distance minimal	

[*]Held once every five years; none in 1963–64.
†New Year's: Bushmen join the celebrations of their missionized Bantu neighbors.

in such a way that every person present receives an equitable share. Trade in foodstuffs between camps is minimal; personnel do move freely from camp to camp, however. The net effect is of a population constantly in motion. On the average, an individual spends a third of his time living only with close relatives, a third visiting other camps, and a third entertaining visitors from other camps.

Because of the strong emphasis on sharing, and the frequency of movement, surplus accumulation of storable plant foods and dried meat is kept to a minimum. There is rarely more than two or three days' supply of food on hand in a camp at any time. The result of this lack of surplus is that a constant subsistence effort must be maintained throughout the year. Unlike agriculturalists who work hard during the planting and harvesting seasons and undergo "seasonal unemployment" for several months, the Bushmen hunter-gatherers collect food every third or fourth day throughout the year.

Vegetable foods comprise from 60–80 per cent of the total diet by weight, and collecting involves two or three days of work per woman per week. The men also collect plants and small animals but their major contribution to the diet is the hunting of medium and large game. The men are conscientious but not particularly successful hunters; although men's and women's work input is roughly equivalent in terms of man-day of effort, the women provide two to three times as much food by weight as the men.

Table 2 summarizes the seasonal activity cycle observed among the Dobe-area !Kung in 1964. For the greater part of the year, food is locally abundant and easily collected. It is only during the end of the dry season in September and October, when desirable foods have been eaten out in the immediate vicinity of the waterholes that the people have to plan longer hikes of 10–15 miles and carry their own water to those areas where the mongongo nut is still available. The important point is that food is a constant, but distance required to reach food is a variable; it is short in the summer, fall, and early winter, and reaches its maximum in the spring.

This analysis attempts to provide quantitative measures of subsistence status including data on the following topics: abundance and variety of resources, diet selectivity, range size and population density, the composition of the work force, the ratio of work to leisure time, and the caloric and protein levels in the diet. The value of quantitative data is that they can be used comparatively and also may be useful in archeological reconstruction. In addition, one can avoid the pitfalls of subjective and qualitative impressions; for example, statements about food "anxiety" have proven to be difficult to generalize across cultures (see Holmberg, 1950; and Needham's critique, 1954).

Abundance and Variety of Resources

It is impossible to define "abundance" of resources absolutely. However, one index of *relative* abundance is whether or not a population exhausts all the food available from a given area. By this criterion, the habitat of the Dobe-area Bushmen is abundant in naturally occurring foods. By far the most important food is the mongongo (mangetti) nut (*Ricinodendron rautanenii* Schinz). Although tens of thousands of pounds of these nuts are harvested and eaten each year, thousands more rot on the ground each year for want of picking.

The mongongo nut, because of its abundance and reliability, alone accounts for 50 per cent of the vegetable diet by weight. In this respect it resembles a cultivated staple crop such as maize or rice. Nutritionally it is even more remarkable, for it contains five times the calories and ten times the proteins per cooked unit of the cereal crops. The average daily per-capita consumption of 300 nuts yields about 1,260 calories and 56 grams of protein. This modest portion, weighing only about 7.5 ounces, contains the caloric equivalent of 2.5 pounds of cooked rice and the protein equivalent of 14 ounces of lean beef (Watt and Merrill, 1963).

Furthermore the mongongo nut is drought resistant and it will still be abundant in the dry years when cultivated crops may fail. The extremely hard outer shell protects the inner kernel from rot and allows the nuts to be harvested for up to twelve months after they have fallen to the ground. A diet based on mongongo nuts is in fact more reliable than one based on cultivated foods, and it is not surprising, therefore, that when a Bushman was asked why he hadn't taken to agriculture he replied: "Why should we plant, when there are so many mongongo nuts in the world?"

Apart from the mongongo, the Bushmen have available 84 other species of edible food plants, including 29 species of fruits, berries, and melons and 30 species of roots and bulbs. The existence of this variety allows for a wide range of alternatives in subsistence strategy. During the summer months the Bushmen have no problem other than to choose among the tastiest and most easily collected foods. Many species, which are quite edible but less attractive, are bypassed, so that gathering never exhausts *all* the available plant foods of an area. During the dry season the diet becomes much more eclectic and the many species of roots, bulbs, and edible resins make an important contribution. It is this broad base that provides an essential margin of safety during the end of the dry season when the mongongo nut forests are difficult to reach. In addition, it is likely that these rarely utilized species provide important nutritional and mineral trace elements that may be lacking in the more popular foods.

Diet Selectivity

If the Bushmen were living close to the "starvation" level, then one would expect them to exploit every available source of nutrition. That their life is well above this level is indicated by the data in Table 3. Here all the edible plant species are arranged in classes according to the frequency with which they were observed to be eaten. It should be noted, that although there are some 85 species available, about 90 per cent of the vegetable diet by weight is drawn from only 23 species. In other words, 75 per cent of the listed species provide only 10 per cent of the food value.

In their meat-eating habits, the Bushmen show a similar selectivity. Of the 223 local species of animals known and named by the Bushmen, 54 species are classified as edible, and of these only 17 species were hunted on a regular basis.[4] Only a handful of the dozens of edible species of small mammals, birds, reptiles, and insects that occur locally are regarded as food. Such animals as rodents, snakes, lizards, termites, and grasshoppers, which in the literature are included in the Bushman dietary (Schapera, 1930), are despised by the Bushmen of the Dobe area.

Range Size and Population Density

The necessity to travel long distances, the high frequency of moves, and the maintenance of populations at low densities are also features commonly associated with the hunting and gathering way of life. Density estimates for hunters in

Table 3 !Kung Bushman Plant Foods

Food Class	Part Eaten								Totals (Percentages)		
	Fruit and Nut	Bean and Root	Fruit and Stalk	Root, Bulb	Fruit, Berry, Melon	Resin	Leaves	Seed, Bean	Total Number of Species in Class	Estimated Contribution by Weight to Vegetable Diet	Estimated Contribution of Each Species
I. *Primary*											
Eaten daily throughout year (mongongo nut)	1	—	—	—	—	—	—	—	1	c. 50	c. 50*
II. *Major*											
Eaten daily in season	1	1	1	1	4	—	—	—	8	c. 25	c. 3
III. *Minor*											
Eaten several times per week in season	—	—	—	7	3	2	2	—	14	c. 15	c. 1
IV. *Supplementary*											
Eaten when classes I–III locally unavailable	—	—	—	9	12	10	1	—	32	c. 7	c. 0.2
V. *Rare*											
Eaten several times per year	—	—	—	9	4	—	—	—	13	c. 3	c. 0.1
VI. *Problematic*											
Edible but not observed to be eaten	—	—	—	4	6	4	1	2	17	nil	nil
Total species	2	1	1	30	29	16	4	2	85	100	—

*1 species constitutes 50 per cent of the vegetable diet by weight.
†23 species constitute 90 per cent of the vegetable diet by weight.
‡62 species constitute the remaining 10 per cent of the diet.

western North America and Australia have ranged from 3 persons/square mile to as low as 1 person/100 square miles (Kroeber, 1939; Radcliffe-Brown, 1930). In 1963–65, the resident and visiting Bushmen were observed to utilize an area of about 1,000 square miles during the course of the annual round for an effective population density of 41 persons/100 square miles. Within this area, however, the amount of ground covered by members of an individual camp was surprisingly small. A day's round-trip of twelve miles serves to define a "core" area six miles in radius surrounding each water point. By fanning out in all directions from their well, the members of a camp can gain access to the food resources of well over 100 square miles of territory within a two-hour hike. Except for a few weeks each year, areas lying beyond this six-mile radius are rarely utilized, even though they are no less rich in plants and game than are the core areas.

Although the Bushmen move their camps frequently (five or six times a year) they do not move them very far. A rainy season camp in the nut forests is rarely more than ten or twelve miles from the home waterhole, and often new campsites are occupied only a few hundred yards away from the previous one. By these criteria, the Bushmen do not lead a free-ranging nomadic way of life. For example, they do not undertake long marches of 30 to 100 miles to get food, since this task can be readily fulfilled within a day's walk of home base. When such long marches do occur they are invariably for visiting, trading, and marriage arrangements, and should not be confused with the normal routine of subsistence.

Demographic Factors

Another indicator of the harshness of a way of life is the age at which people die. Ever since Hobbes characterized life in the state of nature as "nasty, brutish and short," the assumption has been that hunting and gathering is so rigorous that members of such societies are rapidly worn out and meet an early death. Silberbauer, for example, says of the Gwi Bushmen of the central Kalahari that "life expectancy…is difficult to calculate, but I do not believe that many live beyond 45" (1965, p. 17). And Coon has said of the hunters in general:

> The practice of abandoning the hopelessly ill and aged has been observed in many parts of the world. It is always done by people living in poor environments where it is necessary to move about frequently to obtain food, where food is scarce, and transportation difficult.…Among peoples who are forced to live in this way the oldest generation, the generation of individuals who have passed their physical peak is reduced in numbers and influence. There is no body of elders to hand on tradition and control the affairs of younger men and women, and no formal system of age grading (1948, p. 55).

The !Kung Bushmen of the Dobe area flatly contradict this view. In a total population of 466, no fewer than 46 individuals (17 men and 29 women) were determined to be over 60 years of age, a proportion that compares favorably to the percentage of elderly in industrialized populations.

The aged hold a respected position in Bushman society and are the effective leaders of the camps. Senilicide is extremely rare. Long after their productive years have passed, the old people are fed and cared for by their children and grandchildren. The blind, the senile, and the crippled are respected for the special ritual and technical skills they possess. For instance, the four elders at !gose waterhole were totally or partially blind, but this handicap did not prevent their active participation in decision-making and ritual curing.

Another significant feature of the composition of the work force is the late assumption of adult responsibility by the adolescents. Young people are not expected to provide food regularly until they are married. Girls typically marry between the ages of 15 and 20, and boys about five years later, so that it is not unusual to find healthy, active teenagers visiting from camp to camp while their older relatives provide food for them.

As a result, the people in the age group 20–60 support a surprisingly large percentage of non-productive young and old people. About 40 per cent of the population in camps contribute little to the food supplies. This allocation of work to young and middle-aged adults allows for a relatively carefree childhood and adolescence and a relatively unstrenuous old age.

Leisure and Work

Another important index of ease or difficulty of subsistence is the amount of time devoted to the food quest.[5] Hunting has usually been regarded by social scientists as a way of life in which merely keeping alive is so formidable a task that members of such societies lack the leisure time necessary to "build culture."[6] The !Kung Bushmen would appear to conform to the rule, for as Lorna Marshall says:

> It is vividly apparent that among the !Kung Bushmen, ethos, or "the spirit which actuates manners and customs," is survival. Their time and energies are almost wholly given to this task, for life in their environment requires that they spend their days mainly in procuring food (1965, p. 247).

It is certainly true that getting food is the most important single activity in Bushman life. However this statement would apply equally well to small-scale agricultural and pastoral societies too. How much time is *actually* devoted to the food quest is fortunately an empirical question. And an analysis of the work effort of the Dobe Bushmen shows some unexpected results. From July 6 to August 2, 1964, I recorded all the daily activities of the Bushmen living at the Dobe waterhole. Because of the coming and going of visitors, the camp population fluctuated in size day by day, from a low of 23 to a high of 40, with a mean of 31.8 persons. Each day some of the adult members of the camp went out to hunt and/or gather while others stayed home or went visiting. The daily recording of all personnel on hand made it possible to calculate the number of man-days of work as a percentage of total number of man-days of consumption.

Although the Bushmen do not organize their activities on the basis of a seven-day week, I have divided the data this way to make them more intelligible. The work-week was calculated to show how many days out of seven each adult spent in subsistence activities (Table 4, Column 7). Week II has been eliminated from the totals since the investigator contributed food. In week I, the people spent an average of 2.3 days in subsistence activities, in week III, 1.9 days, and in week IV, 3.2 days. In all, the adults of the Dobe camp worked about two and a half days a week. Since the average working day was about six hours long, the fact emerges that !Kung Bushmen of Dobe, despite their harsh environment, devote from twelve to nineteen hours a week to getting food. Even the hardest working individual in the camp, a man named ≠oma who went out hunting on sixteen of the 28 days, spent a maximum of 32 hours a week in the food quest.

Because the Bushmen do not amass a surplus of foods, there are no seasons of exceptionally intensive activities such as planting and harvesting, and no seasons of unemployment. The level of work observed is an accurate reflection of the effort required to meet the immediate caloric needs of the group. This work diary covers the mid-winter dry season, a period when food is neither at its most plentiful nor at its scarcest levels, and the diary documents the transition from better to worse conditions (see Table 2). During the fourth week the gatherers were making overnight trips to camps in the mongongo nut forests seven to ten miles distant from the waterhole. These longer trips account for the rise in the level of work, from twelve or thirteen to nineteen hours per week.

If food getting occupies such a small proportion of a Bushman's waking hours, then how *do* people allocate their time? A woman gathers on one day enough food to feed her family for three days, and spends the rest of her time resting in camp, doing embroidery, visiting other camps,

Table 4 Summary of Dobe Work Diary

Week	(1) Mean Group Size	(2) Adult-Days	(3) Child-Days	(4) Total Man-Days of Consumption	(5) Man-Days of Work	(6) Meat (lbs.)	(7) Average Work Week/Adult	(8) Index of Subsistence Effort
I (July 6–12)	25.6 (23–29)	114	65	179	37	104	2.3	.21
II (July 13–19)	28.3 (23–27)	125	73	198	22	80	1.2	.11
III (July 20–26)	34.3 (29–40)	156	84	240	42	177	1.9	.18
IV (July 27–Aug. 2)	35.6 (32–40)	167	82	249	77	129	3.2	.31
4-wk. total	30.9	562	304	866	178	490	2.2	.21
Adjusted total*	31.8	437	231	668	156	410	2.5	.23

* See text.
KEY: Column 1: Mean group size = total man-days of consumption/7.
Column 7: Work week = the number of work days per adult per week.
Column 8: Index of Subsistence Effort = man-days of work/man-days of consumption (e.g., in Week I, the value of "S" = .21, i.e., 21 days of work/100 days of consumption or 1 work day produces food for 5 consumption days).

or entertaining visitors from other camps. For each day at home, kitchen routines, such as cooking, nut cracking, collecting firewood, and fetching water, occupy one to three hours of her time. This rhythm of steady work and steady leisure is maintained throughout the year.

The hunters tend to work more frequently than the women, but their schedule is uneven. It is not unusual for a man to hunt avidly for a week and then do no hunting at all for two or three weeks. Since hunting is an unpredictable business and subject to magical control, hunters sometimes experience a run of bad luck and stop hunting for a month or longer. During these periods, visiting, entertaining, and especially dancing are the primary activities of men. (Unlike the Hadza, gambling is only a minor leisure activity.)

The trance-dance is the focus of Bushman ritual life; over 50 per cent of the men have trained as trance-performers and regularly enter trance during the course of the all-night dances. At some camps, trance-dances occur as frequently as two or three times a week and those who have entered trances the night before rarely go out hunting the following day. Accounts of Bushman trance performances have been published in Lorna Marshall (1962) and Lee (1968). In a camp with five or more hunters, there are usually two or three who are actively hunting and several others who are inactive. The net effect is to phase the hunting and non-hunting so that a fairly steady supply of meat is brought into a camp.

Caloric Returns

Is the modest work effort of the Bushmen sufficient to provide the calories necessary to maintain the health of the population? Or have the !Kung, in common with some agricultural peoples (see Richards, 1939), adjusted to a permanently substandard nutritional level?

During my field work I did not encounter any cases of kwashiorkor, the most common nutritional disease in the children of African agricultural societies. However, without medical examinations, it is impossible to exclude the possibility that subclinical signs of malnutrition existed.[7]

Another measure of nutritional adequacy is the average consumption of calories and proteins per person per day. The estimate for the Bushmen is based on observations of the weights of foods of known composition that were brought into Dobe camp on each day of the study period. The per-capita figure is obtained by dividing the total weight of foodstuffs by the total number of persons in the camp. These results are set out in detail elsewhere (Lee, in press) and can only be summarized here. During the study period 410 pounds of meat were brought in by the hunters of the Dobe camp, for a daily share of nine ounces of meat per person. About 700 pounds of vegetable foods were gathered and consumed during the same period. Table 5 sets out the calories and proteins available per capita in the !Kung Bushman dietary from meat, mongongo nuts, and other vegetable sources.

This output of 2,140 calories and 93.1 grams of protein per person per day may be compared with the Recommended Daily Allowances (RDA) for persons of the small size and stature but vigorous activity regime of the !Kung Bushmen. The RDA for Bushmen can be estimated at 1,975 calories and 60 grams of protein per person per day (Taylor and Pye, 1966, pp. 45–48, 463). Thus it is apparent that food output exceeds energy requirements by 165 calories and 33 grams of protein. One can tentatively conclude that even a modest subsistence effort of two or three days' work per week is enough to provide an adequate diet for the !Kung Bushmen.

Table 5 Caloric and Protein Levels in the !Kung Bushman dietary, July–August, 1964

Class of Food	Percentage Contribution to Diet by Weight	Per-Capita Consumption			Percentage Caloric Contribution of Meat and Vegetables
		Weight in Grams	Protein in Grams	Calories per Person per Day	
Meat	37	230	34.5	690	33
Mongongo nuts	33	210	56.7	1,260 ⎫	
Other vegetable foods	30	190	1.9	190 ⎭	67
Total all sources	100	630	93.1	2,140	100

THE SECURITY OF BUSHMAN LIFE

I have attempted to evaluate the subsistence base of one contemporary hunter-gatherer society living in a marginal environment. The !Kung Bushmen have available to them some relatively abundant high-quality foods, and they do not have to walk very far or work very hard to get them. Furthermore this modest work effort provides sufficient calories to support not only the active adults, but also a large number of middle-aged and elderly people. The Bushmen do not have to press their youngsters into the service of the food quest, nor do they have to dispose of the oldsters after they have ceased to be productive.

The evidence presented assumes an added significance because this security of life was observed during the third year of one of the most severe droughts in South Africa's history. Most of the 576,000 people of Botswana are pastoralists and agriculturalists. After the crops had failed three years in succession and over 100,000 head of cattle had died on the range for lack of water, the World Food Program of the United Nations instituted a famine relief program which has grown to include 180,000 people, over 30 per cent of the population (Government of Botswana, 1966). This program did not touch the Dobe area in the isolated northwest corner of the country and the Herero and Tswana women there were able to feed their families only by joining the Bushman women to forage for wild foods. Thus the natural plant resources of the Dobe area were carrying a higher proportion of population than would be the case in years when the Bantu harvested crops. Yet this added pressure on the land did not seem to adversely affect the Bushmen.

In one sense it was unfortunate that the period of my field work happened to coincide with the drought, since I was unable to witness a "typical" annual subsistence cycle. However, in another sense, the coincidence was a lucky one, for the drought put the Bushmen and their subsistence system to the acid test and, in terms of adaptation to scarce resources, they passed with flying colors. One can postulate that their subsistence base would be even more substantial during years of higher rainfall.

What are the crucial factors that make this way of life possible? I suggest that the primary factor is the Bushmen's strong emphasis on vegetable food sources. Although hunting involves a great deal of effort and prestige, plant foods provide from 60–80 per cent of the annual diet by weight. Meat has come to be regarded as a special treat; when available, it is welcomed as a break from the routine of vegetable foods, but it is never depended upon as a staple. No one ever goes hungry when hunting fails.

The reason for this emphasis is not hard to find. Vegetable foods are abundant, sedentary, and predictable. They grow in the same place year after year, and the gatherer is guaranteed a day's return of food for a day's expenditure of energy. Game animals, by contrast, are scarce, mobile, unpredictable, and difficult to catch. A hunter has no guarantee of success and may in fact go for days or weeks without killing a large mammal. During the study period, there were eleven men in the Dobe camp, of whom four did no hunting at all. The seven active men spent a total of 78 man-days hunting, and this work input yielded eighteen animals killed, or one kill for every four man-days of hunting. The probability of any one hunter making a kill on a given day was 0.23. By contrast, the probability of a woman finding plant food on a given day was 1.00. In other words, hunting and gathering are not equally felicitous subsistence alternatives.

Consider the productivity per man-hour of the two kinds of subsistence activities. One man-hour of hunting produces about 100 edible calories, and of gathering, 240 calories. Gathering is thus seen to be 2.4 times more productive than hunting. In short, hunting is a *high-risk, low-return* subsistence activity, while gathering is a *low-risk, high-return* subsistence activity.

It is not at all contradictory that the hunting complex holds a central place in the Bushman ethos and that meat is valued more highly than vegetable foods (Marshall, 1960). Analogously, steak is valued more highly than potatoes in the food preferences of our own society. In both situations the meat is more "costly" than the vegetable food. In the Bushman case, the cost of food can be measured in terms of time and energy expended. By this standard, 1,000 calories of meat "costs" ten man-hours, while the "cost" of 1,000 calories of vegetable foods is only four man-hours. Further, it is to be expected that the less predictable, more expensive food source would have a greater accretion of myth and ritual built up around it than would the routine staples of life, which rarely if ever fail.

Eskimo-Bushman Comparisons

Were the Bushmen to be deprived of their vegetable food sources, their life would become much more arduous and precarious. This lack of plant foods, in fact, is precisely the situation among the Netsilik Eskimo, reported by Balikci (Chapter 8, R. Lee and I. DeVore, 1968, *Man the Hunter*). The Netsilik and other Central Arctic peoples are perhaps unique in the almost total absence of vegetable foods in their diet. This factor, in combination with the great cyclical variation in the numbers and distribution of Arctic fauna, makes Eskimo life the most precarious human adaptation on earth. In effect, *the kinds of animals that are "luxury goods" to many hunters and gatherers, are to the Eskimos, the absolute necessities of life.* However, even this view should not be exaggerated, since most of the Eskimos in historic times have lived south of the Arctic Circle (Laughlin, Chapter 25a, R. Lee and I. DeVore, 1968, *Man the Hunter*) and many of the Eskimos at all latitudes have depended primarily on fishing, which is a much more reliable source of food than is the hunting of land and sea mammals.

What Hunters Do for a Living: a Comparative Study

I have discussed how the !Kung Bushmen are able to manage on the scarce resources of their inhospitable environment. The essence of their successful strategy seems to be that while they depend primarily on the more stable and abundant food sources (vegetables in their case), they are nevertheless willing to devote considerable energy to the less reliable and more highly valued food sources such as medium and large mammals. The steady but modest input of work by the women provides the former, and the more intensive labors of the men provide the latter. It would be theoretically possible for the Bushmen to survive entirely on vegetable foods, but life would be boring indeed without the excitement of meat feasts. The totality of their subsistence activities thus represents an outcome of two individual goals; the first is the desire to live well with adequate leisure time, and the second is the desire to enjoy the rewards, both social and nutritional, afforded by the killing of game. In short, *the Bushmen of the Dobe area eat as much vegetable food as they need, and as much meat as they can.*

It seems reasonable that a similar kind of subsistence strategy would be characteristic of hunters and gatherers in general. Wherever two or more kinds of natural foods are available, one would predict that the population exploiting them would emphasize the more reliable source. We would also expect, however, that the people would not neglect the alternative means of subsistence. The general view offered here is that gathering activities, for plants and shellfish, should be the most productive of food for hunting and gathering man, followed by fishing, where this source is available. The hunting of mammals is the least reliable source of food and should be generally less important than either gathering or fishing.

In order to test this hypothesis, a sample of 58 societies was drawn from the *Ethnographic Atlas* (Murdock, 1967). The basis for inclusion in the sample was a 100 per cent dependence on hunting, gathering and fishing for subsistence as rated in Column 7–11 of the Atlas (Murdock, 1967, pp. 154–55).[8,9]

The *Ethnographic Atlas* coding discusses "Subsistence Economy" as follows:

> A set of five digits indicates the estimated relative dependence of the society on each of the five major types of subsistence activity. The first digit refers to the gathering of wild plants and small land fauna; the second, to hunting, including trapping and fowling; the third, to fishing, including shell fishing and the pursuit of large aquatic animals; the fourth, to animal husbandry; the fifth, to agriculture (Murdock, 1967, pp. 154–55).

Two changes have been made in the definitions of subsistence. First, the participants at the symposium on Man the Hunter agreed that the "pursuit of large aquatic animals" is more properly classified under hunting than under fishing. Similarly, it was recommended that shellfishing should be classified under gathering, not fishing. These suggestions have been followed and the definitions now read: *Gathering*—collecting of wild plant, small land fauna and shellfish; *Hunting*—pursuit of land and sea mammals; *Fishing*—obtaining of fish by any technique. In 25 cases, the subsistence scores have been changed in light of these definitions and after consulting ethnographic sources.[10]

The percentage dependence on gathering, hunting, and fishing, and the most important single source of food for each society…can be at best only rough approximations; however, the results are so striking that the use of these scores seems justified. In the Old World and South American sample of 24 societies, sixteen depend on gathering, five on fishing, while only three depend primarily on mammal hunting: the Yukaghir of northeast Asia, and the Ona and Shiriana of South America. In the North American sample, thirteen societies have primary dependence on gathering, thirteen on fishing, and eight on hunting. Thus for the world as a whole, half of the societies (29 cases) emphasize gathering, one-third (18 cases) fishing, and the remaining one-sixth (11 cases) hunting.

On this evidence, the "hunting" way of life appears to be in the minority. The result serves to underline the point made earlier that mammal hunting is the least reliable of the subsistence sources, and one would expect few societies to place primary dependence on it. As will be shown, most of the societies that rely primarily on mammals do so because their particular habitats offer no viable alternative subsistence strategy.

The Relation of Latitude to Subsistence

The peoples we have classified as "hunters" apparently depend for most of their subsistence on sources *other* than meat, namely, wild plants, shellfish and fish. In fact the present sample over-emphasizes the incidence of hunting and fishing since some three-fifths of the cases (34/58) are drawn from North America (north of the Rio Grande), a region which lies entirely within the temperate and arctic zones. Since the abundance and species variety of edible plants decreases as one moves out of the tropical and temperate zones, and approaches zero in the arctic, it is essential that the incidence of hunting, gathering, and fishing be related to latitude.

Table 6 shows the relative importance of gathering, hunting, and fishing within each of seven latitude divisions. Hunting appears as the dominant mode of subsistence *only* in the highest latitudes (60 or more degrees from the equator). In the arctic, hunting is primary in six of the eight societies. In the cool to cold temperate latitudes, 40 to 59 degrees from the equator, fishing is the dominant mode, appearing as primary in 14 out of 22 cases. In the warm-temperate, subtropical, and tropical latitudes, zero to 39 degrees from the equator, gathering is by far the dominant mode of subsistence, appearing as primary in 25 of the 28 cases.

For modern hunters, at any rate, it seems legitimate to predict a hunting emphasis only in the arctic, a fishing emphasis in the mid-high latitudes, and a gathering emphasis in the rest of the world.[11]

The Importance of Hunting

Although hunting is rarely the primary source of food, it does make a remarkably stable contribution to the diet. Fishing appears to be dispensable in the tropics, and a number of northern peoples manage to do without gathered foods, but, with a single exception, *all* societies at all latitudes derive at least 20 per cent of their diet from the hunting of mammals. Latitude appears to make little difference in the amount of hunting that people do. Except for the highest latitudes, where hunting contributes over half of the diet in many cases, hunted foods almost everywhere else constitute 20 to 45 per cent of the diet. In fact, the mean, the median, and the mode for hunting all converge on a figure of 35 per cent for hunter-gatherers at all latitudes. This percentage of meat corresponds closely to the 37 per cent noted in the diet of the !Kung Bushmen of the Dobe area. It is evident that the !Kung, far from being an aberrant case, are entirely typical of the hunters in general in the amount of meat they consume.

CONCLUSIONS

Three points ought to be stressed. First, life in the state of nature is not necessarily nasty, brutish, and short. The Dobe-area Bushmen live well today on wild plants and meat, in spite of the fact that they are confined to the least productive portion of the range in which Bushman peoples were formerly found. It is likely that an even more substantial subsistence base would have been characteristic of these hunters and gatherers in the past, when they had the pick of African habitats to choose from.

Second, the basis of Bushman diet is derived from sources other than meat. This emphasis makes good ecological sense to the !Kung Bushmen and appears to be a common feature among hunters and gatherers in general. Since a 30 to 40 per cent input of meat is such a consistent target for modern hunters in a variety of habitats, is it not reasonable to postulate a similar percentage for prehistoric hunters? Certainly the absence of plant remains on archeological sites is by itself not sufficient evidence for the absence of gathering. Recently abandoned Bushman campsites show a similar absence of vegetable remains, although this article has clearly shown that plant foods comprise over 60 per cent of the actual diet.

Finally, one gets the impression that hunting societies have been chosen by ethnologists to illustrate a dominant theme, such as the extreme importance of environment in the molding of certain cultures. Such a theme can be best exemplified by cases in which the technology is simple and/or the environment is harsh. This emphasis on the dramatic may have been pedagogically useful, but unfortunately it has led to the assumption that a precarious hunting subsistence base was characteristic of all cultures in the Pleistocene. This view of both modern and ancient hunters ought to be reconsidered. Specifically I am suggesting a shift in focus away from the dramatic and unusual cases, and toward a consideration of hunting and gathering as a persistent and well-adapted way of life.

Notes

1. These data are based on fifteen months of field research from October, 1963, to January, 1965. I would like to thank the National Science Foundation (U.S.) for its generous financial support. This article has been substantially revised since being presented at the symposium on Man the Hunter.

2. The Nyae Nyae !Kung Bushmen studied by Lorna Marshall (1957, 1960, 1965) have been involved in a settlement scheme instituted by the South African government. Although closely related to the Nyae Nyae !Kung, the Dobe !Kung across the border in Botswana have not participated in the scheme.

3. Bushman group structure is discussed in more detail in Lee (1965, pp. 38–53; and Chapter 17c, R. Lee & I. DeVore (eds.) (1968). *Man the Hunter*: Chicago: Aldine).

4. Listed in order of their importance, the principal species in the diet are: wart hog, kudu, duiker, steenbok, gemsbok, wildebeeste, springhare, porcupine, ant bear, hare, guinea fowl, francolin (two species), korhaan, tortoise, and python.

5. This and the following topic are discussed in greater detail in Lee, "!Kung Bushman Subsistence: An Input-Output Analysis" (in press).

Table 6 Primary Subsistence Source by Latitude

| Degrees from the Equator | Primary Subsistence Source | | | |
	Gathering	Hunting	Fishing	Total
More than 60°	—	6	2	8
50°–59°	—	1	9	10
40°–49°	4	3	5	12
30°–39°	9	—	—	9
20°–29°	7	—	1	8
10°–19°	5	—	1	6
0°–9°	4	1	—	5
World	29	11	18	58

6. Lenski, for example, in a recent review of the subject, states: "Unlike the members of hunting and gathering societies [the horticulturalists] are not compelled to spend most of their working hours in the search for food and other necessities of life, but are able to use more of their time in other ways" (1966, p. 121). Sahlins (Chap. 9b, R. Lee and I. DeVore, 1968, *Man the Hunter*) offers a counter-argument to this view.

7. During future field work with the !Kung Bushmen, a professional pediatrician and nutritionist are planning to examine children and adults as part of a general study of hunter-gatherer health and nutrition sponsored by the U.S. National Institutes of Health and the Wenner-Gren Foundation for Anthropological Research.

8. Two societies, the Gwi Bushmen and the Walbiri of Australia, were not coded by the *Ethnographic Atlas*. Their subsistence base was scored after consulting the original ethnographies (for the Gwi, Silberbauer, 1965; for the Walbiri, Meggitt, 1962, 1964).

9. In order to make more valid comparisons, I have excluded from the sample mounted hunters with guns such as the Plains Indians, and casual agriculturalists such as the Gê and Siriono. Twenty-four societies are drawn from Africa, Asia, Australia and South America. This number includes practically all of the cases that fit the definition. North America alone, with 137 hunting societies, contains over 80 per cent of the 165 hunting societies listed in the *Ethnographic Atlas*. The sampling procedure used here was to choose randomly one case from each of the 34 "clusters" of North American hunter-gatherers.

10. For their useful suggestions, my thanks go to Donald Lathrap, Robin Ridington, George Silberbauer, Hitoshi Watanabe, and James Woodburn. Special thanks are due to Wayne Suttles for his advice on Pacific coast subsistence.

11. When severity of winter is plotted against subsistence choices, a similar picture emerges. Hunting is primary in three of the five societies in very cold climates (annual temperature less than 32° F.); fishing is primary in 10 of the 17 societies in cold climates (32°–45° F.); and gathering is primary in 27 of the 36 societies in mild to hot climates (over 50° F.).

References

Anderson JN, Balikci A, Helm J, Laughlin WS, Lee RB, Marshall MD, Slobodin R, Woodburn SL. 1968. Analysis of group composition. IN: RB Lee and I DeVore, editors. Man the Hunter. Chicago: Aldine. pp. 150–155.

Coon, Carleton S. 1948. *Reader in general anthropology*. New York: Henry Holt.

Holmberg, Allan R. 1950. *Nomads of the long bow: the Siriono of eastern Bolivia*. Smithsonian Institution, Publications of the Institute of Social Anthropology, no. 10.

Kroeber, AL. 1939. *Cultural and natural areas of native North America*. University of California Publications in American Archaeology and Ethnology (Berkeley), 38.

Laughlin WS. 1968. The demography of hunters: an Eskimo example. IN: RB Lee and I DeVore, editors. Man the Hunter. Chicago: Aldine. pp. 241–243.

Lee, Richard B. 1965. *Subsistence ecology of !Kung Bushmen*. Unpublished doctoral dissertation, University of California, Berkeley.

———1968. The sociology of Bushman trance performances. In Raymond Prince (Ed.), *Trance and possession states*. Montreal, pp. 35–54.

Lenski, Gerhard. 1966. *Power and privilege: a theory of social stratification*. New York: McGraw-Hill.

Marshall, Lorna. 1957. The kin terminology system of the !Kung Bushmen. *Africa*, 27: 1–25.

———1960. !Kung Bushman bands. *Africa*, 30: 325–55.

———1962. !Kung Bushman religious beliefs. *Africa*, 32: 221–52.

———1965. The !Kung Bushmen of the Kalahari Desert. In James Gibbs (Ed.), *Peoples of Africa*. New York: Holt, Rinehart, and Winston.

Meggitt MJ. 1962. *Desert people: a study of the Walbiri aborigines of central Australia*. Sydney: Angus and Robertson.

———1964. Pre-industrial man in the tropical environment: aboriginal food-gatherers of tropical Australia. *Proceedings and Papers of the Ninth Technical Meeting I.U.C.N., Nairobi, Kenya, 1963*. Morges (Vaud), Switzerland: International Union for the Conservation of Nature and Natural Resources.

Murdock, George Peter. 1967. The ethnographic atlas: a summary. *Ethnology*, 6(2).

Needham, Rodney. 1954. Siriono and Penan: a test of some hypotheses. *Southwestern Journal of Anthropology*, 10(3): 228–32.

———1961. An analytical note on the structure of Siriono society. *Southwestern Journal of Anthropology*, 17(3): 239–55.

Radcliffe-Brown AR. 1930. Former numbers and distribution of the Australian aborigines. *Official Yearbook of the Commonwealth of Australia*, 23: 671–96.

Richards, Audrey I. 1939. *Land, labour and diet in Northern Rhodesia*. London: Oxford University Press.

Sahlins MD. 1968. Notes on the original affluent society. IN: RB Lee and I DeVore, editors. Man the Hunter. Chicago: Aldine. pp. 85–89.

Schapera, Isaac. 1930. *The Khoisan peoples of South Africa: Bushmen and Hottentots*. London: Routledge and Kegan Paul.

Service, Elman R. 1966. *The hunters*. Englewood Cliffs, N. J.: Prentice-Hall.

Silberbauer GB. 1965. *Report to the Government of Bechuanaland on the Bushman survey*. Gaberones, Bechuanaland: Government of Bechuanaland.

Taylor, Clara M, and Orrea F Pye. 1966. *Foundations of nutrition*. (6th ed.) New York: Macmillan.

Watt, Bernice K, and Annabel L Merrill. 1963. *Composition of foods: raw, processed, prepared*. Agricultural Handbook no. 8. U.S. Department of Agriculture, Agricultural Research Service.

CHAPTER 8

Food for Thought

Did the first cooked meals help fuel the dramatic evolutionary expansion of the human brain?

Ann Gibbons

(2007)

Richard Wrangham was lying beside a fire at home on a cold winter night in Boston 10 years ago when his mind wandered to the first hominids to cook food. He imagined a small group of *Homo erectus* huddled around a campfire in Africa, roasting a leg of wildebeest and sharing a morsel of singed potato or manioc.

As a Harvard University primatologist who studies wild chimpanzees in Africa, Wrangham knew that cooking is one of the relatively few uniquely human abilities. He also knew that our habit of predigesting our food by heating it allows us to spend less energy on digestion. And he suddenly realized that cooking is not merely the basis of culinary culture. It would have given our ancestors a big evolutionary advantage. "With cooking, we should see major adaptive changes," says Wrangham. He argues that cooking paved the way for the dramatic expansion of the human brain and eventually fueled cerebral accomplishments such as cave painting, writing symphonies, and inventing the Internet. In fact, Wrangham presents cooking as one of the answers to a long-standing riddle in human evolution: Where did humans get the extra energy to support their large brains?

Expanding the brain demands a new supply of energy, because human brains are voracious. The brain consumes 60% of the energy expended by a resting newborn baby. And a resting adult's brain uses 25% of its energy, as opposed to 8% used on average by ape brains. But humans consume about the same amount of calories as smaller-brained mammals of similar body size—for example, small women have the same basal metabolic rate as large chimpanzees.

One classic explanation for this phenomenon is that humans saved energy by shrinking their gastrointestinal organs, effectively trading brains for guts as they shifted to a higher quality diet of more meat. That theory is now gathering additional support (Box 1).

Wrangham thinks that in addition, our ancestors got cooking, giving them the same number of calories for less effort. He floated his hypothesis back in the late 1990s (Pennisi E 1999), but now he's championing it with a slew of new data, some of which he presented at a recent symposium.[1] "Even small differences in diet can have big effects on survival and reproductive success," he says.

Other researchers are enthusiastic about the new results. They show "the fundamental importance of energy budgets in human evolution," says paleoanthropologist Robert Foley of Cambridge University in the U.K. But many aren't convinced by Wrangham's arguments that the first cooked meal was prepared 1.9 million to 1.6 million years ago, when the brain began to expand dramatically in *H. erectus*. They think that although saving energy by shrinking the gut may have been important at this time, the culinary explosion came later, perhaps during the evolution of our own species less than half a million years ago. "What all these adaptations are about is increasing the bang for the buck nutritionally," says William R. Leonard, a biological anthropologist at Northwestern University in Evanston, Illinois. "The challenge ultimately is to work out the exact timing of what led to what."

BOOSTING BRAINPOWER

Even those unsure about the role of cooking in human evolution agree that something crucial must have happened to our ancestors' energy budget. Line up the skulls of early hominids and you'll see why: From 1.9 million to 200,000 years ago, our ancestors tripled their brain size.

The earliest members of the human family, including the australopithecines that lived from 4 million to 1.2 million years ago (Fig. 1), had brains about the size of chimpanzees. The brain didn't expand dramatically until just after *H. erectus* appeared in Africa about 1.9 million years ago (where it is also known as *H. ergaster*), with a brain that eventually averaged 1000 cubic centimeters (cc), or about twice the size of a chimpanzee's. The next leap in brain capacity came 500,000 to 200,000 years ago with the evolution of our own species, whose brains average 1300 cc, and of Neandertals (1500 cc).

Ann Gibbons, "Food for thought: did the first cooked meals help fuel the dramatic evolutionary expansion of the human brain?" *Science* 316(2007):1558–1560. Reprinted with permission.

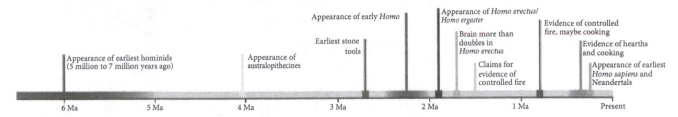

Figure 1 *Human events.*

What spurred this dramatic growth in the *H. erectus* skull? Meat, according to a longstanding body of evidence. The first stone tools appear at Gona in Ethiopia about 2.7 million years ago, along with evidence that hominids were using them to butcher scavenged carcasses and extract marrow from bones. But big changes don't appear in human anatomy until more than 1 million years later, when a 1.6-million-year-old skull of *H. erectus* shows it was twice the size of an australopithecine's skull, says paleoanthropologist Alan Walker of Pennsylvania State University in State College. At about that time, archaeological sites show that *H. erectus* was moving carcasses to campsites for further butchering and sharing; its teeth, jaws, and guts all got smaller. The traditional explanation is that *H. erectus* was a better hunter and scavenger and ate more raw meat than its small-brained ancestors.

But a diet of wildebeest tartare and antelope sashimi alone isn't enough to account for these dramatic changes, says Wrangham. He notes that *H. erectus* had small teeth—smaller than those of its ancestors—unlike other carnivores that adapted to eating raw meat by increasing tooth size. He argues that whereas earlier ancestors ate raw meat, *H. erectus* must have been roasting it, with root vegetables on the side or as a fallback when hunters didn't bring home the bacon. "Cooking produces soft, energy-rich foods," he says.

To find support for his ideas, Wrangham went to the lab to quantify the nutritional impact of cooking. He found almost nothing in food science literature and began to collaborate with physiologist Stephen Secor of the University of Alabama, Tuscaloosa, who studies digestive physiology and metabolism in amphibians and reptiles. Secor's team fed 24 Burmese pythons one of four diets consisting of the same number of calories of beef: cooked ground beef, cooked intact beef, raw ground beef, or raw intact beef. Then they estimated the energy the snakes consumed before, during, and after they digested the meat, by measuring the declining oxygen content in their metabolic chambers. Pythons fed cooked beef spent 12.7% less energy digesting it and 23.4% less energy if the meat was both cooked and ground. "By eating cooked meat, less energy is expended on digestion; therefore, more energy can be used for other activities and growth," says Secor.

Secor also helped Wrangham and graduate student Rachel Carmody design a pilot study in which they found that mice raised on cooked meat gained 29% more weight than mice fed raw meat over 5 weeks. The mice eating cooked food were also 4% longer on average, according to preliminary results. Mice that ate raw chow weighed less even though they consumed more calories than those fed cooked food. "The energetic consequences of eating cooked meat are very high," says Wrangham.

The heat from cooking gelatinizes the matrix of collagen in animal flesh and opens up tightly woven carbohydrate molecules in plants to make them easier to absorb. This translates into less time spent chewing: Chimpanzees spend 5 hours on average chewing their food whereas hunter-gatherers who cook spend 1 hour chewing per day. In fact, Western food is now so highly processed and easy to digest that Wrangham thinks food labels may underestimate net calorie counts and may be another cause of obesity.

The immediate changes in body sizes in the mice also suggest that our ancestors would have been able to get rapid benefits out of cooking, says Wrangham. That's why he thinks there would be little lag time between learning to cook and seeing anatomical changes in humans—and why he thinks early *H. erectus* must have been cooking. Less chewing and gnawing would lead to smaller jaws and teeth, as well as to a reduction in gut and rib cage size—all changes seen in *H. erectus*. Those changes would be favored by selection: Dominant chimpanzees that nab the biggest fruit in a tree, for example, have more offspring, says Wrangham. "It seems to me that groups that cook would have much higher reproductive fitness," he says.

UNDER FIRE

Wrangham's synthesis of nutritional, archaeological, and primatological data adds up to a provocative hypothesis that hot cuisine fueled the brain. "It's such a nice explanation," says paleoanthropologist Leslie Aiello, president of the Wenner-Gren Foundation in New York City. She says the smaller teeth in *H. erectus* indicate to her that it wasn't chewing much tough raw food: "Something must be going on. If only there were evidence for fire."

And that's the stumbling block to Wrangham's theories: Cooking requires fire. Irrefutable evidence of habitual cooking requires stone hearths or even clay cooking vessels. Solid evidence for hearths, with stones or bones encircling patches of dark ground or ash, has been found no earlier than 250,000 years ago in several sites in southern Europe.

Charred bones, stones, ash, and charcoal 300,000 to 500,000 years ago at sites in Hungary, Germany, and France have also been assigned to hearths. And burned flints, seeds, and wood found in a hearthlike pattern have been cited as signs of controlled fire 790,000 years ago in Israel (Goren-Inbar N et al. 2004).

But even the earliest of those dates are long after the dramatic anatomical changes seen in *H. erectus*, says Wrangham. He notes that evidence for fire is often ambiguous and argues that humans were roasting meat and tubers around the campfire as early as 1.9 million years ago.

Indeed, there are a dozen claims for campfires almost that ancient. At the same meeting, paleoanthropologist Jack Harris of Rutgers University in New Brunswick, New Jersey, presented evidence of burned stone tools 1.5 million years ago at Olduvai Gorge in Tanzania and at Koobi Fora in Kenya, along with burned clay. *H. erectus* has been found at both sites. Claims by other researchers include animal bones burned at high temperatures 1.5 million years ago at Swartkrans, South Africa, and clay burnt at high temperatures 1.4 million years ago in the Baringo basin of Kenya.

But where there is smoke there isn't necessarily cooking fire: None of these teams can rule out beyond a doubt that the charring comes from natural fires, although Harris argues that cooking fires burn hot at 600° to 800°C and leave a trail different from that of bush fires, which often burn as low as 100°C.

All the same, those most familiar with *H. erectus* aren't convinced they were chefs. Walker says that if the species was cooking with fire, he and others should have found a trail of campfires associated with its bones and stone tools. Others agree: "I think Wrangham's timing is wrong; cooking is associated with the rapid expansion of the brain in Neandertals and modern humans in the past half-million years," says neurobiologist John Allman of the California Institute of Technology in Pasadena. Paleoanthropologist

---

BOX 1 SWAPPING GUTS FOR BRAINS

Cooking is the latest theory to explain how humans can feed their voracious brains enough calories to survive (see main text), but there's another, classic explanation: As our ancestors began to eat more meat, they took in enough calories at each meal to permit their guts to shrink, saving energy from digestion that in turn helped fuel the brain. Called the expensive tissue hypothesis, this theory was proposed back in 1995 when paleoanthropologist Leslie Aiello, then of University College, London, and physiologist Peter Wheeler of Liverpool John Moores University discovered the tradeoff in guts and brains in 18 species of primates. They found that our gastrointestinal tract is only 60% of the size expected for a primate of similar size (Gibbons 1998).

Now, after a decade of stasis, the idea is getting new support from studies of birds, fish, and primates. Researchers are also expanding the theory by showing that these energetic tradeoffs only happen in animals that grow up slowly, suggesting that a slowdown in juvenile development set the stage for a large brain. "I'm extremely happy that people are taking this up," says Aiello. "Now we're going to get somewhere with it."

Aiello's hypothesis languished in the late 1990s, after researchers sought an energetic tradeoff in other animals—and didn't find it. Small-brained birds such as chickens don't have big guts, for example. And pigs have small brains and small guts.

But more nuanced animal studies are now shoring up the theory. Last year, Carel van Schaik and Karin Isler of the University of Zurich clarified the situation in birds. Most birds, streamlined for long flights, already possess relatively small guts, they explained in the *Journal of Human Evolution*. So the energetic tradeoff happens instead between brains and pectoral or breast muscles: Bigger birds such as turkeys need bigger pectoral muscles to get airborne, and they have smaller brains—these are "the dumb ones we like to eat," says van Schaik. Those with bigger brains have smaller pecs.

The hypothesis also "holds up very well" in six other species of primates, based on preliminary data on wild monkeys and apes, says van Schaik. Brainy capuchin monkeys, for example, eat a high-quality diet of insects and bird eggs and have tiny guts. Howler monkeys have tiny brains and big guts to digest bulky leaves and fruit. "The new data beautifully show the tradeoff, gram for gram, between the brain and gut," says neurobiologist John Allman of the California Institute of Technology in Pasadena.

In another paper in press in the *Journal of Human Evolution*, van Schaik and Duke University graduate student Nancy Barrickman confirm earlier reports that primates can grow a big brain only if they adopt a particular life history strategy. Van Schaik's team shows that 28 species of primates, from tiny mouse lemurs to great apes, have slowed their metabolic rates, thus prolonging their juvenile years, postponing the age at which their first offspring are born, and living longer. This kind of life history is thought to be an adaptation for decreasing infant mortality and boosting maternal health in animals in which the adults have good chances for survival, says paleoanthropologist Jay Kelley of the University of Illinois, Chicago. It also allows primate brains time to grow larger and more complex before adulthood. "Once they slowed down life history, the big brain was inevitable," says Kelley.

Preliminary evidence from the eruption of molars in three *Homo erectus* juveniles, including the Nariokotome skeleton from Kenya, fits with this idea: The teeth suggest that this species had just begun a particularly dramatic developmental slowdown during childhood, a slowdown that reached an extreme in modern humans, says Christopher Dean of University College London.

In this scenario, our ancestors slowed down their development even more as their brains got larger, which required additional energy from a smaller gut and better diet. Thus, the expensive-tissue hypothesis works in primates and other mammals whose young grow up slowly, but not in animals that grow up fast and die young, such as pigs. The energetic tradeoff with the brain can only happen if brains have enough time during development to grow big. "It turns out Leslie [Aiello] was exactly right—with a footnote," says van Schaik.

C. Loring Brace of the University of Michigan, Ann Arbor, agrees. He notes that less than 200,000 years ago, the lower faces of Neandertals and modern humans became smaller, and this is about the same time evidence appears for earth-oven cookery: "While fire has been under control back near 800,000 years, its use in the systematic preparation of food has only been over the last 100,000-plus years."

Others, such as Carel van Schaik of the University of Zurich, think that cooking may have played an important role early on, along with other adaptations to expand human brainpower. As Aiello observes, the big brain was apparently the lucky accident of several converging factors that accentuate each other in a feedback loop. Critical sources of energy to fuel the brain came from several sources—more meat, reduced guts, cooking, and perhaps more efficient upright walking and running. The order in which our ancestors adopted these energy-saving adaptations is under hot debate, with the timing for cooking hardest to test. Regardless, "it's all beginning to come together," says Aiello.

Note

1. "Primatology Meets Paleoanthropology Conference," 17–19 April 2007, University of Cambridge, United Kingdom.

References

Gibbons A. 1998. Solving the brain's energy crisis. Science 280(5368):1345–1347.

Goren-Inbar N, Alperson N, Kislev ME, Simchoni O, Melamed Y, Ben-Nun A, Werker E. 2004. Evidence of hominin control of fire at Gesher Benot Ya'aqov, Israel. Science 304(5671):725–727

Pennisi E. 1999. Did cooked tubers spur the evolution of big brains? Science 283(5410):2004–2005. DOI: 10.1126/science.283.5410.2004.

CHAPTER 9

Paleolithic Nutrition: A Consideration of Its Nature and Current Implications

S. Boyd Eaton and Melvin Konner

(1985)

Humanity has existed as a genus for about 2 million years, and our prehuman hominid ancestors, the australopithecines, appeared at least 4 million years ago (Table 1). This phase of evolutionary history made definitive contributions to our current genetic composition, partly in response to dietary influences at that time. The foods available to evolving hominids varied widely according to the paleontological period, geographical location, and seasonal conditions, so that our ancestral line maintained the versatility of the omnivore that typifies most primates. Natural selection has provided us with nutritional adaptability; however, human beings today are confronted with diet-related health problems that were previously of minor importance and for which prior genetic adaptation has poorly prepared us. Chronic illnesses affecting older, postreproductive persons could have had little selective influence during evolution, yet such conditions are now the paramount cause of morbidity and mortality in Western nations.

The human genetic constitution has changed relatively little since the appearance of truly modern human beings, *Homo sapiens sapiens*, about 40,000 years ago.[2,3] Even the development of agriculture 10,000 years ago has apparently had a minimal influence on our genes. Certain hemoglobinopathies and retention of intestinal lactase into adulthood are "recent" genetic evolutionary trends, but very few other examples are known. Such developments as the Industrial Revolution, agribusiness, and modern food-processing techniques have occurred too recently to have had any evolutionary effect at all. Accordingly, the range of diets available to preagricultural human beings determines the range that still exists for men and women living in the 20th century—the nutrition for which human beings are in essence genetically programmed.[4]

Differences between the dietary patterns of our remote ancestors and the patterns now prevalent in industrialized countries appear to have important implications for health,

and the specific pattern of nutritional disease is a function of the stage of civilization.[5] Physicians and nutritionists are increasingly convinced that the dietary habits adopted by Western society over the past 100 years make an important etiologic contribution to coronary heart disease, hypertension, diabetes, and some types of cancer. These conditions have emerged as dominant health problems only in the past century and are virtually unknown among the few surviving hunter-gatherer populations whose way of life and eating habits most closely resemble those of preagricultural human beings.[6] The longer life expectancy of people in industrialized countries is not the only reason that chronic illnesses have assumed new importance. Young people in the Western world commonly have developing asymptomatic forms of these conditions, but hunter-gatherer youths do not.[7–10] Furthermore, the members of technologically primitive cultures who survive to the age of 60 years or more remain relatively free from these disorders, unlike their "civilized" counterparts.[9,11,12]

NUTRITIONAL EVOLUTION

The ancestral mammals were insectivores, and invertebrate predation was thus the basis from which primate feeding behavior evolved.[13] However, as the primate order expanded and body size increased, vegetable foods became increasingly important for most species. During the Miocene era (from about 24 to about 5 million years ago) fruits appear to have been the main dietary constituent for hominids,[14] but their fossilized dental remains seem suitable for mastication of both animal and vegetable material.[15] After the divergence of the human and ape lines (now thought to have occurred between 7.5 and 4.5 million years ago)[1] our ancestral feeding pattern included increasing amounts of meat, although it is uncertain whether this change reflects hunting, scavenging, or both.[16,17] It is now thought that *Homo habilis* began to manufacture stone tools about 2 million years ago and that the succeeding species, *Homo erectus*, began to consume a much larger amount of meat between 1.8 and 1.6 million years ago.[18–20] It is clear that thereafter early human beings consumed a considerable

S. Boyd Eaton and Melvin Konner, "Paleolithic Nutrition: A Consideration of Its Nature and Current Implications." *The New England Journal of Medicine* 312(1985):283–289. Reprinted with permission.

Table 1 The Main Events of Human Evolution[*]

Millions of Years Ago	Epoch	Development	
0.0002		Industrial revolution	
	Holocene		
0.01		Agricultural revolution	
	Latest Pleistocene		
0.045		*Homo sapiens sapiens* (anatomically modern) appears	
	Late Pleistocene		Paleolithic period (from first manufacture of stone tools to shortly before the development of agriculture)
0.080		*H. sapiens neanderthalensis* appears	
	Middle Pleistocene		
0.400		Archaic *H. sapiens* appears	
1.6	Early Pleistocene	*H. erectus* present	
2.0		*H. habilis* present	
	Pliocene	Australopithecine divergence	
4.5		Bipedal *Australopithecus afarensis* present	
	Late Miocene		
7.5		Hominid–pongid divergence (inferred from molecular data)	
11			
	Middle Miocene	African and Asian hominoids diverge	
17			
	Early Miocene	Hominoid radiation begins	
24			

[*]Modified slightly from the "1984 consensus" of paleontologists, as presented by Pilbeam.[1]

amount of meat: large accumulations of animal remains are found where they lived, the tools they used were mainly geared toward processing game, and their living sites were selectively located in areas where there was a relatively substantial biomass of large grazing animals. The importance of vegetable foods is harder to assess, since plant remains are poorly preserved. Fossilized fruit pits and nuts are commonly found, but tools for processing plant foods are conspicuously absent in comparison with their widespread proliferation in later prehistory.[21] Shells and fish bones are unknown in archaeological material dating from before 130,000 years ago[22] and are found infrequently in material dating from before 20,000 years ago, so that, in paleontological terms, widespread use of aquatic foods is a recent phenomenon.[23]

Several authorities have estimated that *Homo erectus* and early *Homo sapiens* obtained over 50 per cent of their diet from plant sources.[24,25] However, when the Cro-Magnons and other truly modern human beings appeared, concentration on big-game hunting increased; techniques and equipment were fully developed while the human population was still small in relation to the biomass of

available fauna.[26] In some areas during this time meat probably provided over 50 per cent of the diet.[27] But because of overhunting, climate changes, and population growth, the period shortly before the inception of agriculture and animal husbandry was marked by a shift away from big-game hunting and toward a broader spectrum of subsistence activities. Remains of fish, shellfish, and small game are all more common at sites dating from this period, as well as tools that are useful for processing plant foods, such as grindstones, mortars, and pestles.[23] In at least two Middle Eastern sites, trace-element analysis for strontium levels in bone reveals a definite increase in the amount of vegetable material in the diet together with decreased meat consumption at this time.[28] Modern hunter-gatherers most closely resemble the human beings of this relatively recent period.

Agriculture markedly altered human nutritional patterns: over the course of a few millennia the proportion of meat declined drastically while vegetable foods came to make up as much as 90 per cent of the diet.[27] This shift had prominent morphologic consequences: early European *Homo sapiens sapiens*, who enjoyed an abundance of animal protein 30,000 years ago, were an average of six inches taller than their descendants who lived after the development of farming.[29] The same pattern was repeated later in the New World: the Paleoindians were big-game hunters 10,000 years ago, but their descendants in the period just before European contact practiced intensive food production, ate little meat, were considerably shorter,[30] and had skeletal manifestations of suboptimal nutrition,[31-34] which apparently reflect both the direct effects of protein–calorie deficiency and the synergistic interaction between malnutrition and infection.[35] Since the Industrial Revolution, the animal-protein content of Western diets has become more nearly adequate, as indicated by increased average height: we are now nearly as tall as were the first biologically modern human beings. However, our diets still differ markedly from theirs, and these differences lie at the heart of what has been termed "affluent malnutrition."[6]

RECENT HUNTER-GATHERER NUTRITION

Over 50 hunter-gatherer societies have been studied extensively enough to justify some nutritional generalizations about them,[36-38] but only a handful have survived into the second half of the 20th century and have had their diets thoroughly analyzed. In general, groups of hunter-gatherers who, like the earliest human beings, live in an inland, semitropical habitat derive between 50 and 80 per cent of their food (by weight) from plants, with animal sources providing between 20 and 50 per cent.[38] These generalizations hold true for the Hadza of Tanzania[39] (who obtain 20 per cent of their diet from animals), the !Kung[37] (37 per cent) and ≠Kade[40] (20 per cent) San (Bushmen) of the Kalahari, and the Philippine Tasaday[41] (42 per cent), though before contact with Western civilization, the Tasaday were probably less successful hunters. The recently investigated Aché of Paraguay[42] (80 per cent) represent a possible exception, but their setting is so unusual and so affected by contact with more modern economies that they are very unlikely to be representative. Coastal and riverine peoples derive from 10 to 50 per cent of their food from fishing; for example, the Australian Aborigines of Arnhem Land get about 40 per cent of their total intake from fish and shellfish, whereas only a quarter comes from plants.[43,44] Because of their harsh environment, Arctic hunters, such as the aboriginal Eskimos, obtain less than 10 per cent of their food from vegetation.[45] In comparison with the majority of paleolithic human beings, existing hunter-gatherers occupy marginal habitats,[26] and their lives differ in many ways from those of people living before the advent of agriculture. Nevertheless, the range and content of foods they consume are similar (in the sense that they represent wild game and uncultivated vegetable foods) to those that our ancestors ate for up to 4 million years. Thus, an analysis of the nutritional content of these foods can provide a rational basis for estimating what human beings are genetically "programmed" to eat, digest, and metabolize.

MEAT

Paleolithic populations obtained their animal protein from wild game, especially gregarious ungulate herbivores, such as deer, bison, horses, and mammoths. The nutritional quality of such meat differs considerably from that of meat available in the modern American supermarket; the latter has much more fat—in subcutaneous tissue, in fascial planes, and as marbling within the muscle itself.[46] Domesticated animals have always been fatter than their wild ancestors because of their steady food supply and reduced physical activity, but recent breeding and feeding practices have further increased the proportion of fat to satisfy our desire for tender meat.[47-49] These efforts have succeeded: modern high-fat carcasses are 25 to 30 per cent fat or even more.[47] In contrast, a survey of 15 different species of free-living African herbivores revealed a mean carcass fat content of only 3.9 per cent.[50] Not only is there more fat in domesticated animals, its composition is different; wild game contains over five times more polyunsaturated fat per gram than is found in domestic livestock.[51,52] Furthermore, the fat of wild animals contains an appreciable amount (approximately 4 per cent) of eicosapentaenoic acid (C20:5), a long-chain, polyunsaturated, ω3 fatty acid currently under investigation because of its apparent antiatherosclerotic properties.[53,54] Domestic beef contains almost undetectable amounts of this nutrient.[53]

Meat from free-living animals has fewer calories and more protein per unit of weight than meat from domesticated animals,[40,51,55,56] but the amino acid composition of muscle tissue from each source is similar.[51] Since the cholesterol content of fat is roughly equivalent to that of lean tissue,[57] the cholesterol content of game would not be expected to differ substantially from that of commercially available meat. A detailed list of selected nutritional characteristics of 25 wild animal species is available from us.

VEGETABLE FOODS

Except for Eskimos and other high-latitude peoples, hunter-gatherers typically use many species of wild plants for food.[36,39,40] Roots, beans, nuts, tubers, and fruits are the most common major dietary constituents, but others, ranging from flowers to edible gums, are occasionally consumed. Small cereal grains, which have been staples for "civilized" peoples since the Agricultural Revolution, make a surprisingly minor contribution overall; however, the wide range of vegetable foods eaten by foragers contrasts with the relatively narrow variety of crops produced by horticulturists and traditional agriculturists. Furthermore, many domesticated food plants have higher ratios of starch to protein than do their wild forms.[58] The nutrient composition of the wild vegetable foods most commonly consumed by the !Kung,[59] and ≠Kade[40] San, Hadza,[60] Australian Aborigines,[61-63] and Tasaday[41] has been determined. A detailed list of the individual nutritional contents of all 44 items is available from us; average values of selected nutrients are shown in Table 2.

Table 2 Nutritional Values (mean ± S.E.) of 44 Wild Vegetable Foods[*] Consumed by the !Kung[59] and ≠Kade[40] San, Hadza,[60] Tasaday,[41] and Australian Aborigines[61–63]

Content	Nutritional Value
Protein (g/100 g)	4.13 ± 1.04
Fat (g/100 g)	2.84 ± 1.54
Carbohydrate (g/100 g)	22.79 ± 3.15
Fiber (g/100 g)	3.12 ± 0.62
Energy (kcal)	128.76 ± 21.17

[*]The foods include 2 beans, 2 nuts, 11 roots, 1 rhizome, 2 leaf buds, 1 stalk, 2 melons, 1 seed pod, 2 berries, 1 truffle, 7 tubers, 11 fruits, and 1 corm.

Probable Daily Nutrition for Paleolithic Human Beings

Representative nutrient values for wild game and vegetable foods consumed by recent hunter-gatherers can be derived from the literature.[40,41,50,51,55,56,59–71] In turn, these figures can be used to estimate the daily nutrient intake for paleolithic human beings. Estimates of energy intake and various animal:vegetable ratios in subsistence patterns can be generated. Although the specific dietary constituents used by any particular group of preagricultural human beings must have varied with ambient conditions, average nutrient values should reflect central tendencies transcending these effects.

Energy Sources

Game and wild plants yield an average of 1.41 and 1.29 kcal per gram, respectively.[40,41,50,51,55,56,59–71] We can estimate the weight of animal and plant food consumed by assuming a daily energy intake of, say, 3000 kcal,[72] and a subsistence pattern of 35 per cent meat[36,73] and calculating as follows. The daily weight of animal food, in grams, multiplied by 1.41 kcal per gram plus the daily weight of plant food multiplied by 1.29 kcal per gram must equal 3000 kcal. In this model, animal food is 35 per cent and plant food is 65 per cent of the total weight of food eaten. If x is the total weight of food, then:

$$1.41\,(0.35x) + 1.29\,(0.65x) = 3000$$
$$x = 2252\text{ g}$$

(These figures suggest a degree of precision that is of course unwarranted. They are presented simply as the results generated by this particular model.) Under these idealized and probably intermittent isocaloric conditions, the total daily food intake of 2252 g would have been provided by 788.2 g of game and 1463.8 g of vegetable food. On the basis of these calculations and mean nutrient values, the average daily nutrient intake for paleolithic human beings can be reconstructed as shown in Table 3.

Table 3 Proposed Average Daily Macronutrient Intake for Late Paleolithic Human Beings Consuming a 3000-kcal Diet Containing 35 per cent Meat and 65 per cent Vegetable Foods

	Intake (g)
Protein	251.1
Animal	190.7
Vegetable	60.4
Fat	71.3
Animal	29.7
Vegetable	41.6
Carbohydrate	333.4
Fiber	45.7

Fat and Fatty Acids

The fat from Cape buffalo is 30 per cent polyunsaturated, 32 per cent monounsaturated, and 38 per cent saturated.[51] Assuming a similar ratio for wild game in general, the animal fat in a reconstructed paleolithic diet would provide 8.91 g of polyunsaturated fatty acids and 11.29 g of saturated fatty acids. The fat in 36 wild vegetable foods used by the Hadza,[60] San (Bushmen),[74] and other African tribal groups[75] is 38.7 per cent polyunsaturated, on average. If a similar figure can be assumed for wild vegetable fat generally, then the plant foods in this paleolithic dietary example would yield 16.1 g of polyunsaturated fatty acids. In 24 American vegetable foods saturated fatty acids constitute 15.6 per cent of total fat.[56] If the proportion in wild plants is similar, then a paleolithic diet containing 35 per cent meat and 65 per cent vegetables would contribute 6.49 g of saturated vegetable fat, and the overall ratio of polyunsaturated to saturated fats for a day's total (animal and vegetable) fat intake would be 1.41.

Cholesterol

Meat from modern domesticated animals has an average of 75 mg of cholesterol in each 100-g portion.[56] The cholesterol content of meat from wild game should be similar, since the proportion of cholesterol in meat is surprisingly unaffected by the fat content.[57] Thus, paleolithic human beings consuming 788.2 g of meat in a day would have ingested 591.2 mg of cholesterol.

Sodium and Potassium

The sodium and potassium content for 14 vegetable foods used by recent hunter-gatherers is known.[40,41,59] These foods have an average of 10.1 mg of sodium and 550 mg of potassium, respectively, for each 100-g portion. If these values are representative, the daily average of 1463.8 mg of paleolithic vegetable food would have yielded 147.8 mg of sodium. Data on the sodium and potassium content of wild game are unavailable, but if the average values for beef, lamb, pork, and veal (68.75 mg of sodium and 387.5 mg of potassium per 100 g)[56] are assumed to be comparable to those for meat from wild animals, then the 788.2 g of meat in a 35:65 (meat:vegetable) paleolithic diet would have provided 541.9 mg of sodium, for a daily total of 689.7 mg. The overall ratio of dietary potassium to sodium would have been 16.1 to 1.0.

Calcium

The calcium content of 37 plant foods consumed by recent foragers averages 102.5 mg for each 100 g,[40,59,61,62] so the daily provision of calcium from vegetable sources would have been 1500.4 mg in the paleolithic diet. Venison and the meat of most domesticated animals contain about 10 mg of calcium per 100 g of tissue,[56] so meat in a 35:65 paleolithic diet would have yielded an additional 78.8 mg, for a daily grand total of 1579.2 mg of calcium.

Ascorbic Acid

The mean ascorbic acid content of 27 vegetables eaten[40,59-62] by recent hunter-gatherers is 26.8 mg per 100 g, so that the average vitamin C intake would have been 392.3 mg each day in paleolithic diets conforming to this pattern. (This calculation excludes the Australian green plum,[62] which has the highest known vitamin C content [3150 mg per 100 g] and would tend to inflate the estimate.)

Other Nutrients

Even at the lowest estimate of the ratio of meat to plant food (20:80), by modern standards, the estimated paleolithic diet would have been adequate in animal protein, iron, vitamin B_{12}, and folate, whereas agricultural populations of the underdeveloped world in the 20th century have widespread deficiencies in these nutrients.

Because of seasonal and local variation, among other factors, populations that subsist by collecting food invariably have a greater variety of plant foods than is typical for agricultural populations.[13] This variety would have ensured a gradual accumulation of most of the necessary trace elements found in plant foods, despite differing concentrations in different sources. However, the possibility of geographically limited deficiencies in certain nutrients (e.g., iodine) cannot be ruled out.

Fiber

Because of the relatively high proportion of vegetable foods and the primitive character of food processing, paleolithic diets must have included substantially more nondigestible fiber than do typical Western diets. The average fiber content of 37 wild plant foods for which information on fiber content is available is 3.12±0.62 g per 100 g (mean ±S.E.). For a paleolithic diet containing 65 per cent vegetable foods, the estimated fiber content would have been 45.7 g.

Shortages

The majority of preindustrial societies, including those based on hunting and gathering, experience seasonal nutritional stress and occasional (less frequent than annual) severe shortages. Although the paleolithic period was almost certainly characterized by conditions of greater abundance, both in game and plant foods, than those experienced by recent hunter-gatherers,[26] it is nevertheless likely that paleolithic populations experienced infrequent shortages sufficient to produce weight loss and to threaten survival in persons with inadequate adipose reserves. It would have been adaptive to consume more calories than the minimal daily requirement and to store fat during periods of relative abundance. This pattern is in fact observed among recent hunter-gatherers,[76,77] although its magnitude is not known.[37]

Subsistence data from 58 technologically primitive societies reveal that the mean, median, and mode for recent foragers converge on a dietary ratio of 35 per cent meat and 65 per cent vegetable foods.[36,73] Of course, the paleolithic diet was not fixed; it varied in its individual components, as well as in its relative proportions of animal and vegetable foodstuffs. For these reasons, the use of average nutrient values derived from items used by different groups of contemporary hunter-gatherers is more helpful than an analysis of any one group's diet. The mean values can be used to estimate nutritional characteristics for widely varying subsistence patterns (Table 4).

Table 4 Estimated Nutritional Characteristics for Various Animal:Vegetable Subsistence Patterns

	Animal:Vegetable Ratio			
	20:80	40:60	60:40	80:20*
Total dietary energy (%)				
Protein	24.5	37	49	61
Carbohydrate	55	41	28	14
Fat	20.5	22	23	25
P:S ratio†	1.72	1.33	1.08	0.91
Cholesterol (mg)	343	673	991	1299

*For a 3000-kcal diet, an 80:20 subsistence pattern would require an intake of 437 g of protein per day. Urea synthesis and its accompanying obligate water loss place an approximate upper limit of about 400 g of protein per day for a steady diet. This suggests that with animal:vegetable subsistence patterns of this magnitude, the animals eaten were probably fatter (e.g., for hibernation or cold insulation) than those described in the text. This inference, in turn, is consistent with high proportions of meat consumed only by hunter-gatherers in the higher latitudes.
†P:S denotes polyunsaturated:saturated fats.

THE PALEOLITHIC DIET IN MODERN PERSPECTIVE

Whether based on as much as 80 per cent or as little as 20 per cent meat, the paleolithic diet differed substantially from the typical diet in the United States today, and it also differed, although much less so, from that currently advocated by nutritionists and by the U.S. government[78] (Table 5). The foods we eat are usually divided into four basic groups: meat and fish, vegetables and fruit, milk and milk products, and breads and cereals. Two or more daily servings from each are now considered necessary for a balanced diet, but adults living before the development of agriculture and animal husbandry derived all their nutrients from the first two food groups; they apparently consumed cereal grains rarely, if at all, and they had no dairy foods whatsoever. Nevertheless, with a diet containing 35 per cent meat, their calcium intake would have far exceeded the highest estimate of the minimal daily requirement. Neanderthals and Cro-Magnons who inhabited subarctic Eurasia and whose diet is considered to have been most like that of the Eskimos, among recent populations, had massive bones, indicating that they obtained sufficient calcium. The probable paleolithic intake of dietary fiber was much higher than ours and approached that common in rural Africa, where disease conditions linked with deficient dietary fiber rarely occur,[79] although paleolithic human beings obtained their fiber predominantly from fruits and vegetables rather than grain. A paleolithic diet consisting of 35 per cent meat would have contained only a sixth of the sodium in the typical American diet—a third of the level most recently recommended.[80] Even in a diet with 80 per cent meat, the sodium intake would have just reached the lowest recommended level and would have been markedly below the lowest estimate of current intake. Given the typically wide variety of collected plant foods and assuming ascorbic acid to be representative, the vitamin intake of paleolithic human beings would have substantially exceeded ours, irrespective of the proportion of meat in the diet.

In the hunting society of our ancestors meat provided a large fraction of each day's food, ensuring high iron and folate levels. Protein contributed twice to nearly five times the proportion of total calories that it does for Americans. Their high-meat diet contained a high level of cholesterol—similar to or even higher than the level in our diet; most paleolithic human beings must have greatly exceeded the U.S. Senate Select Committee's recommended cholesterol level.[78] Conversely, they ate much less fat than we do, and the fat they ate was substantially different from ours. Whether subsistence was based predominantly on meat or on vegetable foods, the paleolithic diet had less total fat, more essential fatty acids, and a much higher ratio of polyunsaturated to saturated fats than ours does. In comparison with us, our paleolithic ancestors consumed more structural and less depot fat.

The extent to which some of the major chronic diseases of industrialized society are related to the typical Western diet is controversial, but evidence for an important linkage is steadily accumulating. Medical researchers in diverse fields are beginning to define a generally preventive diet—one of benefit against conditions ranging from atherosclerosis to cancer. Such investigations are converging in several ways with the studies of paleontologists and anthropologists. Ultimately, of course, only experimental and clinical studies can confirm hypotheses about the medical consequences of dietary choices. Nevertheless, it

Table 5 Comparison of the Late Paleolithic Diet,[*] the Current American Diet, and U.S. Dietary Recommendations

	Late Paleolithic Diet	Current American Diet[78]	U.S. Senate Select Committee Recommendations[78]
Total dietary energy (%)			
Protein	34	12	12
Carbohydrate	45	46	58
Fat	21	42	30
P:S ratio[†]	1.41	0.44	1.00
Cholesterol (mg)	591	600	300
Fiber (g)	45.7	19.7[‡]	30–60[79]
Sodium (mg)	690	2300–6900[80]	1100–3300[80]
Calcium (mg)	1580	740$	800–1200¶
Ascorbic acid (mg)	392.3	87.7$	45¶

[*]Assuming the diet contained 35 per cent meat and 65 per cent vegetables.
[†]P:S denotes polyunsaturated:saturated fats.
[‡]British National Food Survey, 1976.
$U.S. Department of Agriculture Food Consumption Survey, 1977–1978.
¶Recommended Daily Dietary Allowance, Food and Nutrition Board, National Academy of Sciences–National Research Council.

is both intellectually satisfying and heuristically valuable to estimate the typical diet that human beings were adapted to consume during the long course of our evolution. Points of convergence between this estimate and modern recommendations are encouraging, and points of divergence suggest new lines of research. The diet of our remote ancestors may be a reference standard for modern human nutrition and a model for defense against certain "diseases of civilization."

Note

We are indebted to Denis Burkitt, George Cahill, Irven DeVore, Richard Lee, John R. K. Robson, Margaret J. Schoeninger, Pat Shipman, Marjorie Shostak, and Alan Walker for helpful comments, and to Debra Fey for assistance in preparing it.

References

1. Pilbeam D. The descent of hominoids and hominids. Sci Am 1984; 250:84–96.
2. Rendel JM. The time scale of genetic change. In: Boyden SV, ed. The impact of civilization on the biology of man. Canberra, Australia: Australian National University Press, 1970:27–47.
3. Cavalli-Sforza, LL. Human evolution and nutrition. In: Walcher DN, Kretchmer N, eds. Food, nutrition and evolution: food as an environmental factor in the genesis of human variability. New York: Masson, 1981:1–7.
4. Yudkin J. Archaeology and the nutritionist. In: Ucko PJ, Dimbley GW, eds. The domestication and exploitation of plants and animals. Chicago: Aldine, 1969:547–52.
5. Mayer J. Nutrition and civilization. Trans NY Acad Sci 1967; 29:1014–32.
6. Trowell H. Hypertension, obesity, diabetes mellitus and coronary heart disease. In: Trowell HC, Burkitt DP, eds. Western diseases: their emergence and prevention. Cambridge, Mass.: Harvard University Press, 1981:3–32.
7. Enos WF, Holmes RH, Beyer J. Coronary disease among United States soldiers killed in action in Korea. JAMA 1953; 152:1090–3.
8. Schaefer O. Medical observations and problems in the Canadian arctic. Can Med Assoc J 1959; 81:386–93.
9. Moodie PM. Aboriginal health. Canberra, Australia: Australian National University Press, 1973:92.
10. Velican D, Velican C. Atherosclerotic involvement of the coronary arteries of adolescents and young adults. Atherosclerosis 1980; 36:449–60.
11. Truswell AS, Hansen JDL. Medical research among the !Kung. In: Lee RB, DeVore I, eds. Kalahari hunter-gatherers. Cambridge, Mass.: Harvard University Press, 1976:166–94.
12. Arthaud JB. Cause of death in 339 Alaskan natives as determined by autopsy. Arch Pathol 1970; 90:433–8.
13. Hladik CM. Diet and the evolution of feeding strategies among forest primates. In: Harding RSO, Teleki G. Omnivorous primates: gathering and hunting in human evolution. New York: Columbia University Press, 1981: 215–54.
14. Kay R. Diets of early Miocene African hominoids. Nature 1977; 268:628–30.
15. Stini WA. Body composition and nutrient reserves in evolutionary perspective. In: Walcher DN, Kretchmer N, eds. Food, nutrition, and evolution: food as an environmental factor in the genesis of human variability. New York: Masson, 1981:107–20.
16. Hill K. Hunting and human evolution. J Hum Evolut 1982; 11:521–44.
17. Shipman P. Early hominid lifestyle: hunting and gathering or foraging and scavenging? In: Clutton-Brock J, Grigson C, eds. Animals and archaeology: hunters and their prey. Oxford: BAR, 1983:31–49.
18. Bunn HT. Archaeological evidence for meat-eating by Plio-Pleistocene hominids from Koobi Fora and Olduvai Gorge. Nature 1981; 291:574–7.
19. Potts R, Shipman P. Cutmarks made by stone tools on bones from Olduvai Gorge, Tanzania. Nature 1981; 291: 577–80.
20. Walker A, Zimmerman MR, Leakey REF. A possible case of hypervitaminosis A in Homo erectus. Nature 1982; 296:248–50.
21. Kraybill N. Preagricultural tools for the preparation of foods in the old world. In: Reed CA, ed. Origins of agriculture. The Hague: Mouton, 1977:485–521.
22. Klein RG. Stone age exploitation of animals in Southern Africa. Am Sci 1979; 67:151–60.
23. Cohen MN. The food crisis in prehistory: over population and origins of agriculture. New Haven, Conn.: Yale University Press, 1977.
24. Howell FC, Clark JD. Acheulian hunter-gatherers of sub-Saharan Africa. In: Howell FC, Bourliere F, eds. African ecology and human evolution. Chicago: Aldine, 1963: 458–533.
25. Isaac GLI, Crader DC. To what extent were early hominids carnivorous?: an archaeological perspective. In: Harding RSO, Teleki G, eds. Omnivorous primates: gathering and hunting in human evolution. New York: Columbia University Press, 1981:37–103.
26. Foley R. A reconsideration of the role of predation on large mammals in tropical hunter-gatherer adaptation. Man 1982; 17:393–402.
27. MacNeish RS. A summary of the subsistence. In: Byers DS, ed. The prehistory of the Tehuacan Valley. Vol. 1. Austin. Tex.: University of Texas Press, 1967:290–309.
28. Schoeninger MJ. Diet and the evolution of modern human form in the Middle East. Am J Phys Anthropol 1982; 58:37–52.
29. Angel JL. Paleoecology, paleodemography and health. In: Polgar S, ed. Population, ecology and social evolution. The Hague: Mouton, 1975:167–90.
30. Nickens PR. Stature reduction as an adaptive response to food production in Mesoamerica. J Archaeol Sci 1976; 3:31–41.
31. Buikstra JE. Biocultural dimensions of archaeological study: a regional perspective. In: Blakely RL, ed.

Biocultural adaptations in prehistoric America. Athens, Ga.: University of Georgia Press, 1977:67–84.

32. Larsen CS. Skeletal and dental adaptations to the shift to agriculture on the Georgia coast. Curr Anthropol 1981; 22:422–3.

33. Cassidy CM. Nutrition and health in agriculturalists and hunter-gatherers: a case study of two prehistoric populations. In: Jerome RF, Pelto GH, eds. Nutritional anthropology: contemporary approaches to diet and culture. Pleasantville, N.Y.: Redgrave, 1980:117–45.

34. Cook DC. Subsistence base and health in prehistoric Illinois Valley: evidence from the human skeleton. Med Anthropol 1979; 3:109–24.

35. Scrimshaw NS, Taylor CE, Gordon JE. Interactions of nutrition and infection. Am J Med Sci 1959; 237:367–403.

36. Lee RB. What hunters do for a living, or, how to make out on scarce resources. In: Lee RB, DeVore I, eds. Man the hunter. Chicago: Aldine, 1968:30–48.

37. *Idem.* The !Kung San: men, women, and work in a foraging society. New York: Cambridge University Press, 1979.

38. Gaulin SJC, Konner M. On the natural diet of primates, including humans. In: Wurtman RJ, Wurtman JJ, eds. Nutrition and the brain. Vol. 1. New York: Raven Press. 1977:1–86.

39. Woodburn J. An introduction to Hadza ecology. In: Lee RB, DeVore I, eds. Man the hunter. Chicago: Aldine, 1968:49–55.

40. Tanaka J. The San, hunter-gatherers of the Kalahari: a study in ecological anthropology. New York: Columbia University Press, 1980.

41. Robson JRK, Yen DE. Some nutritional aspects of Philippine Tasaday diet. In: Robson JRK, ed. Food, ecology and culture. New York: Gordon Breech, 1980:1–7.

42. Hawkes K, Hill K, O'Connell JF. Why hunters gather: optimal foraging and the Aché of eastern Paraguay. Am Ethnol 1982; 9:379–98.

43. McArthur M. Food consumption and dietary levels of groups of Aborigines living on naturally occurring foods. In: Mountford CP, ed. Records of the American-Australian scientific expedition to Arnhem Land. Vol. 2. Melbourne: Melbourne University Press, 1960:90–135.

44. Meehan B. Hunters by the seashore. J Hum Evolut 1977; 6:363–70.

45. Draper HH. The aboriginal Eskimo diet in modern perspective. Am Anthropol 1977; 79:309–316.

46. Wittwer SH. Altering fat content of animal products through genetics, nutrition, and management. In: National Research Council. Fat content and composition of animal products. Washington, D.C.: National Academy of Sciences, 1976:80–4.

47. Byerly TC. Effects of agricultural practices on foods of animal origin. In: Harris RS, Karmas E, eds. Nutritional evaluation of food processing. 2nd ed. Westport, Conn.: Avi, 1975:58–97.

48. Smith GC, Carpenter ZL. Eating quality of meat animal products and their fat content. In: National Research Council. Fat content and composition of animal products. Washington, D.C.: National Academy of Sciences, 1976:147–82.

49. Allen CE, Mackey MA. Compositional characteristics and the potential for change in foods of animal origin. In: Beitz DC, Hansen RG, eds. Animal products in human nutrition. New York: Academic Press, 1982:199–224.

50. Ledger HP. Body composition as a basis for a comparative study of some East African mammals. Symp Zool Soc Lond 1968; 21:289–310.

51. Crawford MA. Fatty-acid ratios in free-living and domestic animals. Lancet 1968; 1:1329–33.

52. Wo CKW, Draper HH. Vitamin E status of Alaskan Eskimos. Am J Clin Nutr 1975; 28:808–13.

53. Crawford MA, Gale MM, Woodford MH. Linoleic acid and linolenic acid elongation products in muscle tissue of *Syncerus caffer* and other ruminant species. Biochem J 1969; 115:25–7.

54. Dyerberg J, Bank HO, Stoffersen E, Moncada ES, Vane JR. Eicosapentaenoic acid and prevention of thrombosis and atherosclerosis? Lancet 1978; 2:117–9.

55. Deethardt D. The best of bison. Brookings, S.D.: South Dakota State University Press, 1973.

56. Watt BK, Merrill AL. Composition of foods. (Agriculture handbook no. 8). Washington, D.C.: United States Department of Agriculture, 1975.

57. Feeley RM, Criner PE, Watt BK. Cholesterol content of foods. J Am Diet Assoc 1972; 61:134–49.

58. Harris RS. Effects of agricultural practices on foods of plant origin. In: Harris RS, Karmas, E., eds. Nutritional evaluation of food processing. 2nd ed. Westport, Conn.: Avi, 1975:33–57.

59. Wehmeyer AS, Lee RB, Whiting M. The nutrient composition and dietary importance of some vegetable foods eaten by the !Kung Bushmen. S Afr Med J 1969; 43:1529–30.

60. Wehmeyer AS. The nutrient composition of some edible wild fruits found in the Transvaal. S Afr Med J 1966; 40:1102–4.

61. Fysch CF, Hodges KJ, Siggins LY. Analysis of naturally occurring foodstuffs of Arnhem Land. In: Mountford CP, ed. Records of the American-Australian scientific expedition to Arnhem Land. Vol. 2. Melbourne: Melbourne University Press, 1960:136–9.

62. Brand JC, Cherikoff V, Lee A, McDonnel J. Nutrients in important bush foods. Proc Nutr Soc Austr 1982; 7:50–4.

63. Harris DR. Subsistence strategies across Torres Strait. In: Allen J, Jones R, eds. Sunda and Sahul: prehistoric studies in Southeast Asia, Melanesia and Australia. London: Academic Press, 1977:421–63.

64. Crawford MA, Gale MM, Woodford MH. Muscle and adipose tissue lipids of the warthog, *Phacochoerus aethiopicus*. Int J Biochem 1970; 1:654–8.

65. Ashbrook FG. Butchering, processing, and preservation of meat. New York: Van Nostrand Reinhold, 1955:37.

66. Cook BB, Witham LE, Olmstead M, Morgan AF. The influence of seasonal and other factors on the acceptability

and food value of meat of two subspecies of California deer and of antelope. Hilgardia 1949; 19:265–84.

67. Berkes F, Farkas CS. Eastern James Bay Cree Indians: changing patterns of wild food use and nutrition. Ecol Food Nutr 1978; 7:155–72.

68. Wilber CG, Gorski TW. The lipids in *Bison bison*. J Mammol 1955; 36:305–8.

69. Morris EA, Witkind WM, Dix RL, Jacobson J. Nutritional contents of selected aboriginal foods in northeastern Colorado: buffalo (*Bison bison*) and wild onions (*Allium spp.*) J Ethnobiol 1981; 1:213–20.

70. Smith NS. Appraisal of condition estimation methods for East African ungulates. East Afr Wildlife J 1970; 8:123–9.

71. McCulloch JSG, Talbot LM. Comparison of weight estimation methods for wild animals and domestic livestock. J Appl Ecol 1965; 2:59–69.

72. Montgomery E. Towards representative energy data: the Machiguenga Study. Fed Proc 1978; 37:61–4.

73. Hayden B. Subsistence and ecological adaptations of modern hunter-gatherers. In: Harding RDS, Teleki G, eds. Omnivorous primates: gathering and hunting in human evolution. New York: Columbia University Press, 1981:344–421.

74. Engelter C, Wehmeyer AS. Fatty acid composition of oils of some edible seeds of wild plants. J Agric Food Chem 1970; 18:25–6.

75. Busson F. Plantes alimentaires de l'Ouest Africain. Marseilles: Lecont, 1965.

76. Wilmsen EN. Seasonal effects of dietary intake on Kalahari San. Fed Proc 1978; 37:65–72.

77. Speth JD, Spielmann KA, Energy source, protein metabolism, and hunter-gatherer subsistence strategies. J Anthropol Archaeol 1983; 2:1–31.

78. Select Committee on Nutrition and Human Needs, United States Senate. Dietary goals for the United States. Washington, D.C.: Government Printing Office, 1977.

79. Mendeloff AI. Dietary fiber and human health. N Engl J Med 1977; 297:811–4.

80. Marsh AC, Klippstein RN, Kaplan SD. The sodium content of your food. Washington, D.C.: United States Department of Agriculture, 1980.

UNIT II

AGRICULTURE: THE GREAT REVOLUTION

By evolutionary standards, the adoption of agriculture happened quickly. The available archaeological evidence points to the first domesticated crops and animals appearing around 12,000 years ago. The Middle East was the first home to domesticated animals—dogs, sheep, goats, and cattle—and crops such as barley, wheat, peas, and lentils (Figure 1). Following soon after, and probably as independent inventions, other domesticates appeared in other areas: rice, millet, and pigs in China; peppers, squash, beans, and corn in Mesoamerica; potatoes in the Andes; sugarcane in the Pacific Islands. Wherever these crops thrived, agriculture and agricultural peoples increased in numbers and spread themselves and their lifestyle across the continents. Agriculture may now seem to be humdrum and mundane,

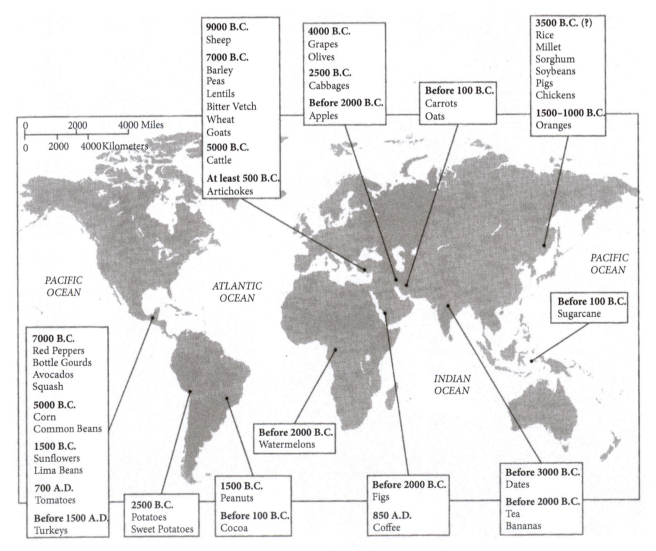

Figure 1 *Origin of main domesticates.*

yet after agriculture human life would never be the same. We domesticated crops and our crops domesticated us.

The archaeologist V. Gordon Childe wrote in the 1930s that agriculture was the most important of human revolutions. First, it is implicit that agriculture changed what individuals do: Instead of looking for food, farmers and herders tend to their crops and animals. As obvious as this might seem, the consequences for biology and culture are dramatic. Changes in activity patterns led to new diseases, new selective pressures, the reorganization of societies, and ideas about the relationship between us and our environments. Second and equally implicit, what individuals eat changed. Wild fruits, nuts, leaves, and wild animals were replaced with cultivated grains and plants and meats and the products of domesticated animals. Do agricultural foods provide more or less energy, protein, and micronutrients? What is the consequence of the aforementioned changes in activity patterns?

Agriculture has a number of obvious advantages over foraging. First, crops may be eaten or destroyed by a variety of means, but they are to be found invariably where they were planted. Agriculture brings a sense, if not necessarily a reality, of stability, regularity, predictability, and control. Second, the amount of time and energy put into growing food is generally less than that spent foraging for food. Therefore, in addition to providing for a family, a successful farmer can produce a surplus that can be traded for other goods. The result is that time is freed up for others to pursue secondary tasks: make works of beauty, build monuments, fight battles, pay tributes.

The second revolution of agriculture involves dramatic changes in demography, ecology, and culture. Because agriculture is based on maintaining fixed fields, mobility is decreased. Groups develop greater attachment and sense of "ownership" of lands, and the way people think about the land changes. Also, agriculture, by providing a greater density of food per unit area, permitted more people to live in a given area. In fact, population increase and agricultural intensification almost always occur simultaneously. As Cohen argues, population increase may have forced humans to adopt agriculture, and agriculture, by providing more food, may have allowed populations to increase. Agriculture was more a necessity than an invention.

With agriculture, the first cities developed. With agriculture came food surpluses. Roles were invented to harness agricultural surpluses, and social classes developed in relationship to production. Agriculture, then, appears to have been a mixed blessing. It allowed for a quickened pace of technological, social, and ideological development, but at what cost? On one side are progressivists such as Hobbes. Agriculture made all things possible from the Parthenon and the B-minor Mass to the computer with which we write and the cup of coffee by its side, no less the coffeemaker and the electricity to run it. It is hard to imagine a foraging society that would have invented any of these things! On the other hand, the central compromise of agriculture, greater food quantity, may have come with costs. Because agriculture changed ecology, culture, and ideology, it is the root cause of a great deal of social ills, such as warfare and inequality between the sexes and classes.

The first of the chapters in this section, Origins of Agriculture, was written by archaeologist Mark Cohen, an expert on this topic. As noted above, Cohen makes the point that agriculture likely had multiple origins. Furthermore, it should be thought of less as an "invention" or bright idea than an option that was always available. It was adopted when it needed to be, or so it seems. Interestingly, once human groups went down the road to agriculture, it was hard to turn back.

Cohen outlines in detail some of the consequences of the turn from foraging to farming. Although these do differ depending on the location, the other variables that changed, and the actual cultivated crops, Cohen argues for an increased caloric efficiency (more calories per work effort) with a decreased spectrum of crops. Cohen also makes the point that population growth took off with agriculture. He provocatively concludes that since health and nutrition seem to have declined with agriculture, the main advantages might have been political and controlling resources.

Biological anthropologists Alan Goodman and George Armelagos are experts in paleopathology, reading signs of undernutrition and poor health from the bones and teeth of past groups. They wondered what the health and nutritional consequences would be of the shift to an agricultural economy, and it is this question that they explore in "Disease and Death at Dr. Dickson's Mounds." To answer the question, they studied the bones and teeth of more than 500 individuals who were buried at Dickson Mounds near Lewiston, Illinois. They were able to identify individuals who grew up before and after people began practicing agriculture (an analysis of the location and manner of burial made this possible). By comparing the rates of disease and malnutrition in the pre- and postagricultural groups, they were able to conduct a naturalistic study of the consequences of agriculture.

Goodman and Armelagos discovered that those who lived before the transition to agriculture exhibited fewer signs of disease and poor nutrition and that they lived longer. What is their evidence? Why would agriculture lead to a decline in health and nutrition? Is it simply that agriculture does not provide a healthy diet? Can one separate the effect of population increase from the effects of agriculture? Finally, is the decline in health related to socioeconomic changes (such as increasing classlike differentiation) that tend to follow agricultural intensification?

The other chapter in this section, "Bread and Beer," was written by the biological anthropologist/archaeologist team of Solomon Katz and Mary Voigt. They ask the biocultural question of why make bread or beer, two products of agricultural grains? They note that as the number of plant varieties decreased, the width of cuisine increased. Furthermore, fermented products are not exclusive to agricultural societies. However, their production certainly increased. Most of the alcoholic products we consume today are, indeed, grain based.

While most attention has been placed on the production of grains to make gruels and breads and other forms of starchy carbohydrates, Katz and Voigt mount a case for the widespread importance of beer. Fermented grains are richer in nutrition than non-fermented grains; thus, one advantage of beer over bread. Another obvious advantage is that beer tastes good and provides alcohol, something we humans enjoy. Finally, after this chapter was written a group of anthropologists lead by George Armelagos (Emory University) discovered that the antibiotic tetracycline is found in Egyptian grains and beers, leading to yet another possible advantage of beer—its antibiotic properties. Their closing question is a simple test. If you are given the choice of gruel, bread, or brew, which would you choose?

Today, in this postagricultural/postindustrial world of mass transportation and "McDonald's-ization" of the far corners of the world, fewer families grow the foods they consume. The closest most of us will come to foraging occurs when we exercise our power to choose among the 100-plus varieties of breakfast cereals in the safe and well-lighted confines of the local supermarket. But what we eat is still based on agriculture. What did agriculture bring us? Knowing how our ancestors managed to get their daily supplies of vegetables, fruits, and meats and the social and biological consequences of this "struggle for food" can provide a window into their lives. Perhaps, too, it can tell us much about ourselves.

SUGGESTIONS FOR THINKING AND DOING NUTRITIONAL ANTHROPOLOGY

1. Cohen and Armelagos (1984) include nearly twenty case studies of the health and nutritional consequences of the change from foraging to farming. Using this book or other sources, what generalizations about the consequences of agriculture can be supported? Under what conditions does agriculture appear to do the greatest harm to human health?

2. A cartoon shows a group of hunters roasting their recent kill. One hunter asks, "Why is our life expectancy so short if our diet is so healthy?" Can you answer this apparent paradox?

3. Eat a Paleolithic diet for a day. How was it different from your usual diet? Was it difficult to find suitable food?

Suggested Further Reading

Cohen M, Armelagos G, eds. 1984. Paleopathology at the Origins of Agriculture. New York: Academic Press. This edited volume includes a large number of examples of the skeletal evidence for change in health and nutrition with agriculture.

Eaton B, Shostak M, Konner M. 1988. The Paleolithic Prescription. New York: Harper & Row. A recommended follow-up to the article by Eaton and Konner. This book helped to launch the field of Darwinian medicine.

Heiser C. 1990. Seed to Civilization. Cambridge: Harvard University Press. Easy-to- read overview of agricultural developments in different parts of the world.

Larsen CS. 1997. Bioarchaeology: Interpreting Behavior from the Human Skeleton. New York: Cambridge University Press. Excellent summary of methods of reconstructing behavior, diet, nutrition, and health from bones and teeth.

McGovern PE. 2009. Uncorking the Past: The Quest for Wine, Beer and Other Alcoholic Beverages. Berkeley: University of California Press.

McNally J. 2010. Ancient Nubians Made Antibiotic Beer. Wired Science. http://www.wired.com/wiredscience/2010/09/antibiotic-beer/

Nesse R, Williams G. 1994. Why We Get Sick: The New Science of Darwinian Medicine. New York: Times Books. An easy-to-read summary of Darwinian medicine from two of its founding fathers.

Sobolik K, ed. 1994. Paleonutrition: The Diet and Health of Prehistoric Americans. Carbondale: Southern Illinois University Press. An excellent compilation of articles on the variety of methods and sources of information used to infer past diets.

CHAPTER 10

Origins of Agriculture

Mark N. Cohen

(2003)

The last thirty years have seen a revolution in our understanding of the origins of agriculture. What was once seen as a pattern of unilateral human exploitation of domesticated crops and animals has now been described as a pattern of coevolution and mutual domestication between human beings and their various domesticates. What was once seen as a technological breakthrough, a new concept, or "invention" (the so-called Neolithic revolution) is now commonly viewed as the adoption of techniques and ultimately an economy long known to foragers in which "invention" played little or no role. Since many domesticates are plants that in the wild naturally accumulate around human habitation and garbage, and thrive in disturbed habitats, it seems very likely that the awareness of their growth patterns and the concepts of planting and tending would have been clear to any observant forager; thus, the techniques were not "new." They simply waited use, not discovery. In fact, the concept of domestication may have been practiced first on nonfood crops such as the bottle gourd or other crops chosen for their utility long before the domestication of food plants and the ultimate adoption of food economies based on domesticates (farming).

The question then becomes not how domestication was "invented" but why it was adopted. What was once assumed to depend on cultural diffusion of ideas and/or crops is now seen by most scholars as processes of independent local adoption of various crops.

PATTERNS OF DOMESTICATION

The domestication of the various crops was geographically a very widespread series of parallel events. Some scholars now recognize from seven to twelve independent or "pristine" centers in which agriculture was undertaken prior to the diffusion of other crops or crop complexes (although many of these are disputed) scattered throughout Southwest, South, Southeast, and East Asia; North Africa and New Guinea; North, Central, and South America; and possibly North America. As the earliest dates for the first appearance of cultigens are pushed back; as individual "centers" of domestication are found to contain more than one "hearth" where cultivation of different crops first occurred; as different strains of a crop, for example, maize or rice, are found to have been domesticated independently in two or more regions; as an increasing range of crops are studied; and, as little-known local domestic crops are identified in various regions in periods before major crops were disseminated, the number of possible independent or "pristine" centers of domestication is increasing, and the increase seems likely to continue.

EARLY DOMESTICATION OF CROPS

Combining patterns provided by various scholars suggest that major domesticates appear in Southwest Asia or in the Near East (wheat barley, lentils) by 9,000–12,000 B.P. or even earlier; in Thailand (rice) between 12,000 and 8,000 B.P.); in China (millet, soybeans, rice) ca. 9,500 B.P.; in Mesoamerica (squash, beans, and maize) between 10,000 B.P. and 5,500 B.P.; in South America (lima beans and peppers) by ca. 8,000–10,000 B.P. and, with less certainty, potatoes and manioc by 6,000 B.P.; and in North America north of Mexico (sunflowers, may grass, chenopods, sump weed, and marsh elder) by 4000–5000 B.P.; in North Africa (pearl millet, sorghum) by 5500–6800 B.P.; in Southeast Asia (taro) by 8000 B.P. and possibly much earlier. (Root crops are presumed to have had even longer histories of domestication in the moist tropics but they are poorly preserved and difficult to document archaeologically.)

As an example of the regional complexity of incipient domestication, there may have been three centers of domestication at three altitudes in South America: a lowland complex involving manioc and sweet potato; a mid-elevation complex involving amaranth, peanut, jicama, and coca; and a high-elevation group including potato and other lesser tubers such as *ullucu*.

The agriculture of particular preferred crops also spread widely by diffusion or population movement in some areas in the prehistoric period. In perhaps the best known patterns of diffusion of agricultural economies (or displacement of indigenous hunter-gatherer populations), Middle Eastern farming economies had spread to Bulgaria by 7500 B.P.; to Italy by 7000 B.P.; and to Britain by 6000–5000 B.P. Maize

Mark N. Cohen, "Origins of Agriculture." In *Encyclopedia of food and culture*, Vol. 1, ed. by S. E. Katz. Thomson Gale, 2003, pp. 49–54. Reprinted with permission.

diffused very widely in North and South America from Mesoamerica (apparently without the significant spread of people); and rice cultivation diffused throughout South, East, and Southeast Asia.

Despite its geographical dispersal, the adoption of the various domestic crop economies occurred within a narrow time span, between about 10,000 and 3,000 B.P. The human population entered a relationship with many different plants at about the same time, implying that human activities were the prime motivator of major economic change and entry into mutual domestication in each instance.

Domestication (genetic manipulation of plants) and the adoption of agricultural economies (primary dependence on domestics as food), once seen as an "event," are now viewed as distinct from one another, each a long process in its own right. There is often a substantial time lag between incipient domestication of a crop and actual dependence on it. That is, the adoption of farming was a gradual quantitative process more than a revolutionary rapid adoption—a pattern of gradually increasing interaction, and degrees of domestication and economic interdependence.

Moreover, the adoption of agriculture was, by all accounts, the coalescence of a long, gradual series of distinctive and often independent behaviors. Techniques used by hunter-gatherers to increase food supplies, long before farming, included the use of fire to stimulate new growth; the protection of favorite plants; sowing seeds or parts of tubers without domestication; preparing soils; eliminating competitors; fertilizing; irrigating; concentration of plants; controlling of growth cycles; expansion of ranges; and ultimately domestication. By this definition, domestication means altering plants genetically to live in proximity to human settlements, enlarging desired parts, breeding out toxins, unpleasant tastes, and physical barriers to exploitation—in short, getting plants to respond to human rather than natural selection.

DEPENDENCE ON CROPS

Almost all authorities describe a gradual increase in the quantitative dependence on domesticated crops. Most also see a quantitative shift from high-quality to low-quality resources (a reduction in the variety and density of essential nutrients, calories, protein, vitamins, minerals, and fatty acids per unit of bulk, desirability of foods, and ease of exploitation). Most also describe a movement downward in the trophic levels of foods exploitated A common theme in almost all discussions of the origins of agriculture is the idea of increasingly "intensive" exploitation of foods (the use of increased labor to exploit smaller and smaller areas of land).

This sequence of events commonly first involved a focus on an increasing range (a "broad spectrum") of low-priority wild resources, increasing the efficiency in which space was utilized—a shift from economies focused on comparatively scarce but otherwise valuable large animals and high-quality vegetable resources to one in which new resources

or different emphases included smaller game, greater reliance on fish and shellfish, and a focus on low-quality starchy seeds. There is a clear and widespread appearance of and increase in apparatus (grindstones for processing small seeds, fishing equipment, small projectile points) in most parts of the world before the adoption of agriculture, which cannot be a function of differential preservation.

Ultimately the spectrum of exploitation seems to have narrowed again as populations shifted toward more complete modification of landscapes to permit increased dependence on particular low-priority but calorically productive starches that could be obtained in large quantities per unit of space and then stored. Such modification of the land to focus on the quantity of calories per unit of space by promoting staple crops would then eliminate some calorically marginal foods, resulting in a loss of dietary variety and of some nutrients. (The major staples—rice, maize, wheat, barley, potatoes, sweet potatoes, manioc, and taro—all cause dietary deficiencies when relied on too heavily as the sole basis of a diet. The deficiencies are likely to be exacerbated by dry storage, which destroys C and B-complex vitamins.)

INTENSIFICATION OF RESOURCE USE

The intensification can probably be seen best through the eyes of optimal foraging theory, much of which has focused on caloric returns for each unit of labor provided by various foods, and has argued that human groups will go first for high-ranking resources (those that yield high returns for a unit of work including preparation). Repeated studies of comparative efficiency of food-gathering techniques in various parts of the world have routinely reported that human populations should prefer resources such as large game, which, when available, can be exploited with great efficiency. Populations turn to increasing reliance on lower-ranking, that is, less efficiently exploited, resources (small game, shellfish, most nuts, individually caught fish, and small seeds) only as those of higher rank disappear or become so scarce that the time involved in finding them becomes prohibitively high (for example, as large game becomes scarce). Such calculations by scientists do not predict the behavior of individual populations perfectly (presumably because other factors such as local food preferences or inertia come into play). But they do dramatically conform to the broad trends in prehistory relating to a Paleolithic-Mesolithic-Neolithic sequence or its equivalents in the New World. And they suggest that this sequence of economic changes is one of declining efficiency in resource exploitation.

Resources used increasingly in the intensification of individual units of land—the so-called broad-spectrum revolution—typically provided fewer calories per unit of labor than the comparative emphasis on large animal exploitation that preceded them. Small seeds such as wheat, barley rice, and maize typically are among the least productive resources (and among the lowest priority as well in taste and quality) and would presumably have come into use only as preferred resources disappeared or became prohibitively scarce. Seasonal seeds, although potentially harvested quickly and in large quantity, typically involved intensive processing and the labor of storage as well as significant storage losses. A significant point is that the adoption of low-ranking resources depended not on their availability but on the declining availability of higher resources. Cereals were adopted not because they were or had become available but because preferred resources such as large game were becoming less available.

The major cereals are relatively inefficient to exploit and process, as demonstrated by Kenneth Russell with specific reference to the Middle Eastern cradle of wheat and barley cultivation. Agriculture, therefore, may not have been "invented" so much as adopted and dropped repeatedly as a consequence of the availability or scarcity of higher-ranked resources. This pattern may in fact be visible among Natufian, or Mesolithic, populations in the Middle East whose patterns of exploitation sometimes appear to defy any attempt to recognize, naively, a simple sequence of the type described above.

Technological changes were motivated by necessity or by demand, not by independent invention or technological advance. In a trend toward declining efficiency, one does not adopt new technologies simply because they are available. Such innovations may well be held in reserve until changing conditions render them the best remaining alternatives. Demand-side economics seems to have powered most of economic history; Malthusian or supply-side economics, with supply independent from demand, became the predominant pattern only when the rise of social classes prevented the needs of the poor from generating any economic "demand"—which implies not only need but entitlement (the ability to command resources).

Various sources point out, however, that such "intensification" occurred in parallel among incipient farmers and populations such as those of the West Coast of the United States, which developed an intense focus on storing starchy staples (such as acorns) but never domesticated them. The two activities may be distinguished, and centers of origin of domestication may be defined, less by human knowledge or intent as by the flexibility or recalcitrance of the intensively harvested plants toward incipient domestication. Some resources such as wheat respond readily to human manipulation; others such as acorns/oak trees defy it.

Increased demand results from population growth, climate change, and socially induced demand. Mark Cohen argues that population growth and increasing population density—or a combination of population growth and declining availability of preferred foods, which result in "population pressure" or an imbalance between population, resources, and prevalent food choices and extractive strategies—may be the main trigger of relevant economic changes. Such increasing density is ultimately traceable to the Pleistocene with the gradual density-dependent closing of cultural systems as increased density permitted groups to switch from exogamy to endogamy. According to this model, the widespread parallelism of different regions is based on the power of population flux (movement between groups) to equalize population pressure from region to region. The model has been criticized for, among other reasons, relying too much on flux as an explanatory necessity, for having the wrong time scale, and for underplaying the role of climate change.

A second category emphasizes the role of post-Pleistocene climate change in both facilitating and demanding exploitation of plants amenable to domestication. It has been argued, in fact, that farming would have been essentially impossible during the Pleistocene, but almost mandatory, at least in a competitive sense, in the Holocene. This model may provide a more powerful explanation of the regional parallelism of intensification in time than a purely population growth/flux model. The climate-based model has been criticized, however, as ignoring the fact that climate and environmental changes are zonal and therefore could not, of themselves, produce parallel economic changes in different environments undergoing different kinds of change.

A third major category that explains increased demand suggests that it resulted from enhanced social and political demand preceding and accompanying intensification. The problem is that such explanations, unless combined with data on population growth or climate change, fail to explain the parallel emergence of complex social forms.

AGRICULTURE AND THE DECLINE IN HEALTH, NUTRITION, AND FOOD SECURITY

Agriculture commonly has been associated with a number of social features: reduced territories, more marked social boundaries, further closing of mating systems; greater territoriality and formal definitions of property; complex social and political organization; more defined concepts of property; food storage; and sedentism. Moreover, agriculture has until recently been considered the cause or enabler of these altered social institutions. These features are only loosely bound, may be separated by long spans of time, and may occur in any of various sequences. For example, sedentism in many regions occurs long before domestication (as in parts of the Middle East), but in the New World the reverse often occurs—domesticates appearing long before settled reliance on those domesticates. Social complexity may commonly follow the origins of agriculture but precedes it in many parts of the world and, as mentioned above, occurs without domestication in some parts of the world.

CHANGES IN HEALTH

What was once interpreted by researchers as a transition toward improving human health, nutrition, reliability of the food supply, greater ease of food procurement, and greater longevity is now viewed as the start of declining health, nutrition, and efficiency of labor, probably declining longevity, and perhaps even declining security of food supplies.

It is now commonly accepted that the adoption of farming economies and sedentism resulted in declining health and nutrition. The conclusion is based on triangulation from three sources: contemporary observation of hunting and gathering versus farming societies; theoretical patterns of nutrients and parasites in nature; and paleopathology, the analysis of health and nutrition in prehistoric skeletons representing different periods of prehistory. Many sources have found parallel trends toward declining health in prehistoric populations but challenges to quantitative methods, interpretations of some evidence, and some specific conclusions in paleopathology have been offered. Observed paleopathological trends commonly accord with expectations from other lines of evidence.

It seems probable from epidemiological considerations—and it is clear from paleopathology—for example, that farming, large concentrations of population and sedentism, the accumulation of human feces, and the attraction of stored foods to potentially disease-bearing animals markedly increased parasite loads on human populations. The increase in the prevalence of visible periostitis, osteomyelitis, treponemal infection, and tuberculosis in skeletal populations conforms both to ethnographic observations and models of probable disease history. The reduction of wild animal meat in the diet with the increasing focus on vegetable foods may initially have reduced the likelihood of food-borne diseases (of which animals are the major source). But the domestication of animals, their crowding, and their continuing proximity to human populations are likely to have raised meat-borne infections to new highs and seems responsible for epidemic diseases in human populations, many of which began as zoonotic (animal-borne) disease shared by people and domestic animals.

CONSEQUENCES OF AGRICULTURE

Sedentism and farming resulted in declining quality of nutrition (or at least in the decline in the quality of nutrients available to the human populations). Indeed, some researchers have extolled the virtue of hunter-gatherer diets. Agriculture is likely to have resulted in a marked downturn in food diversity and food quality, and ultimately to a decline in nutrition. An increase in cumulative neurotoxins may have occurred as farming was adopted, the latter despite the fact that domestication itself may have bred toxic substances out of foods.

Agriculture also seems to have resulted in a change in the texture of foods toward softer foods, resulting in a decline in tooth wear but an increase in dental caries and a reduction in jaws and jaw strength. A significant advantage of soft foods based on boiling in ceramic pots, a practice largely restricted to sedentary populations, may have been the increasing potential for early weaning of children and improved food for toothless elders. But early weaning to cereals as opposed to a diet of mother's milk is well known to have serious negative effects on childhood nutrition, infection, and survival.

A dramatic increase in iron deficiency anemia (porotic hyperostosis and cribra orbitalia) is associated everywhere in the archaeological record with both sedentism, infection, and new crops. The trend is also predictable in nature, and may be observed in contemporary populations. The increased anemia probably resulted primarily from a large increase in iron-robbing hookworm associated with sedentism and with the sequestering by the body of its own iron as protection against bacterial disease.

The declining health that came with the advent of farming is also reflected in (but not universally) childhood declines in stature, osteoporosis in children, decreases in tooth size (as a result of declining maternal nutrition), and tooth defects.

Whether the adoption of broad-spectrum foraging, agriculture, storage, and sedentism increased or decreased the reliability of food supplies (and whether sedentism is itself a consequence of choice permitted by new resources or necessitated by them) is a matter of some debate. For example, it is not clear whether broad-spectrum foraging increased reliability by expanding the resource base, or decreased reliability by focusing exploitation on what had once been emergency resources.

Domestication, sedentism, and storage appear to have evened out potential seasonal shortages in resources, but they may also have reduced the reliability of the food supply by decreasing the variety of foods consumed; by preventing groups from moving in response to shortages; by creating new vulnerability of plants selected for human rather than natural needs; by moving resources beyond their natural habitats to which they are adapted for survival; and by the increase in post-harvest food loss through storage—not only because stored resources are vulnerable to rot, or theft by animals, but stores are subject to expropriation by human enemies. One possible biological clue to the resolution of this problem is that signs of episodic stress (enamel hypoplasia and microdefects in teeth in skeletal populations) generally become more common after agriculture was adopted.

Sedentary agriculture seems likely to have increased human fertility through a variety of mechanisms, including the shifting work loads for women; calorically richer diets; sedentism; and the increased marginal utility of children or the increased availability of weaning foods. Some researchers estimate that during the Mesolithic-Neolithic transition in the Iberian Peninsula fertility may have increased as much as from four to six live births per mother, which would imply very rapid acceleration of population growth. If, in fact, fertility on average increased (possibly significantly) but population growth on average accelerated only by the trivial amount calculated below, then life expectancy must on average have declined (since growth rates are a balance of both fertility and mortality). (There is little evidence from paleopathology that the adoption of sedentary farming increased on average human life expectancy and little reason to expect that it did.)

For whatever reasons, essentially all estimates of average post-domestication population growth suggest an increase in rates of population growth (calculated as compound interest rates). But on average, the increase can have been no more than from about .003 percent per year for pre-Neolithic hunter-gatherers to about 0.1 percent for Neolithic and post-Neolithic farmers. (In both cases the averages are simple mathematical calculations of what is possible based on all reasonable estimates of world population at the period of adoption of agricultural (about 5–25 million) to estimated population in 1500 C.E. (about five hundred million). Average population growth even after the onset of agriculture would therefore have been trivial to the point where it would have been almost imperceptible to the populations involved. It would have taken such populations about one thousand years to double in size. Growth and dispersal of agricultural populations and/or diffusion of domestic crops were hardly likely to have been exuberant in most locations for that reason, particularly if arguments about declining health and very low average growth rates are considered. Owing to their low rank as resources, crops would presumably have diffused only to populations facing similar levels of demand or pressure but lacking good local domesticates of their own.

On the other hand, population growth might have been comparatively quite rapid in some areas because of increased fertility and improved life expectancy. Exuberant growth in some areas, such as Europe, must have been balanced by the decline of other populations, including those of other farmers. Exuberant growth, or diffusion, perhaps based on the relative quality of some cereals such as wheat and barley among otherwise low-ranking, intensively exploited resources, is observable in areas (such as the expansion of the Middle Eastern farming complex and probable expansion of agriculture populations into Europe). But even there, in contrast to old models assuming population expansion of hunter-gatherer "bands" into areas of very low population density, expansion would, based on observed intensity of exploitation, have been expanding into areas occupied by hunter-gatherers, who would by this time have had population densities and social complexity almost equal to their own. The preexisting size and structure of groups of hunter-gatherers in areas of agricultural spread suggests that diffusion may have played a bigger role in the process than was once assumed.

Since health and nutrition seem to have declined, the primary advantage to farmers seems to have been both political and military because of the ability to concentrate population and raise larger armies. This would have conferred a considerable advantage in power at a time when few if any weapons were available that were capable of offsetting numerical superiority.

CHAPTER 11

Disease and Death at Dr. Dickson's Mounds

Alan H. Goodman and George J. Armelagos

(1985)

Clustered in west-central Illinois, atop a bluff near the confluence of the Illinois and Spoon rivers, are twelve to thirteen poorly defined earthen mounds. The mounds, which overlap each other to some extent, cover a crescent-shaped area of about an acre. Since at least the middle of the nineteenth century, local residents have known that prehistoric Native Americans built these mounds to bury their dead. But it was not until the late 1920s that Don Dickson, a chiropractor, undertook the first systematic excavation of the mounds, located on farmland owned by his father. Barely into his thirties at the time, Dickson became so involved in the venture that he never returned to his chiropractic practice. Apparently, he was intrigued by the novel undertaking of unearthing skeletons and trying to diagnose the maladies of long-dead individuals. Later on, he became more concerned with the patterns of disease and death in this extinct group in order to understand how these people lived and why they often died at an early age.

The "Dickson Mounds" (the site also includes two early, unmounded burial grounds) quickly attracted the attention of professional anthropologists. In the early 1930s, a team of University of Chicago archeologists exposed about 200 of the estimated 3,000 burials and identified a number of settlement sites in a 100-square-mile area. A second phase of excavation at Dickson began in the 1960s under the direction of Alan Harn, an archeologist working for the state of Illinois, whose crew excavated many of the local living sites and more than 800 additional burials. The archeological research revealed that these prehistoric people had taken part in an important transition, from hunting and gathering to an agricultural way of life.

About A.D. 950, hunter-gatherers lived along the Illinois River valley area near Dickson, subsisting on a wide range of local plants and animals, including grasses and seeds, fruits and berries, roots and tubers, vines, herbs, large and small mammals, migratory waterfowl and riverine birds, and fish. The moderate climate, copious water supply, and rich soil made this a bountiful and attractive area for hunter-gatherers. Groups occupied campsites that consisted of a few

small structures, and the debris scattered around these sites suggests seasonal use. The population density was low, perhaps on the order of two to three persons per square mile. Then, about 1050, broken hoes and other agricultural tools, as well as maize, began to form part of village refuse, evidence of the introduction of maize agriculture. At the same time, the population grew. By 1200 the population density may have increased by a factor of ten, to about twenty-five persons per square mile. Living sites became larger and more permanent. The largest settlement in the area, Larson, was a residential and ceremonial center where some 1,000 inhabitants lived, many behind a palisaded wall.

Trade also flourished. Dickson became part of what archeologists call the Mississippian tradition, a network of maize-growing, mound-building societies that spread throughout most of the eastern United States. More and more, items used at the village sites or deposited as grave offerings were not of local origin. Some, such as marine shell necklaces, came from as far away as the Gulf of Mexico and Florida, one thousand miles to the south. Everyday objects such as spoons and jars were received from peoples of the eastern plains and the western prairies, while luxury items of ceremonial or decorative value arrived in trade from the south, probably coming upriver to Dickson through Cahokia, a Mississippian center some 110 miles away. Cahokia is a massive site that includes some 120 mounds within a six-square-mile area. As many as 30,000 persons lived at Cahokia and in the surrounding villages.

What we know about Dickson might have ended at this point, but continues because the skeletal remains that Harn excavated have been used to evaluate how the health of these prehistoric people fared following the adoption of agriculture and other changes in their life style. Interest in this issue stems from the writings of the eminent British archeologist V. Gordon Childe (1892–1957), who believed that the development of agriculture prompted the first great revolution in human technology, ushering in fundamental changes in economy, social organization, and ideology. Archeologists continue to debate the causes of agricultural revolutions. For example, some believe that in various regions of the world, increased population pressure, leading to food shortages and declining health, spurred the switch to agricultural food production. Others believe population increase was one of the consequences of agricultural revolutions. More

Alan H. Goodman and George J. Armelagos, "Disease and death at Dr. Dickson's Mounds." *Natural History*, September 1985: 12–18. Reprinted with permission.

important to us are the effects of an agricultural revolution on the health of people who lived at the time of such change.

Three circumstances have made it possible to test the effects agriculture had upon health at Dickson. First, Harn and those working with him valued the potential information to be gained from skeletons and therefore paid close attention to their excavation. Ultimately, the skeletal remains were sent to the University of Massachusetts at Amherst for analysis by George Armelagos and many of his graduate students (this is how we became involved). Second, the recovered remains include both individuals who lived before the development of maize agriculture (Late Woodland, or pre-Mississippian) and after (Mississippian). The two groups of individuals could be distinguished according to the mounds they were buried in, their placement within each mound, and their burial position (in earlier burials the bodies tend to be in a flexed or semi-flexed position; in later burials they tend to be extended). The third enabling condition was provided by Janice Cohen, one of Armelagos's graduate students. Her analysis of highly heritable dental traits showed that although Dickson was in contact with persons from outside the central Illinois River valley area during the period of rapid cultural change, outside groups did not replace or significantly merge with the local groups. It is therefore possible to follow the health over time of a single population that, for all intents and purposes, was genetically stable.

As a doctoral student working under Armelagos in the early 1970s, John Lallo, now at Cleveland State University, set out to test whether health at Dickson improved, got worse, or remained the same with the advent of agriculture and its accompanying changes. Lallo argued that intensification of maize agriculture most likely resulted in a poorer diet. Although a common assumption is that the adoption of agriculture should have provided a prehistoric people with a better diet, there are good reasons to predict just the opposite. Heavy reliance on a single crop may lead to nutritional problems. Maize, for example, is deficient in lysine, an essential amino acid. Furthermore, agricultural societies that subsist on a few foodstuffs are more vulnerable to famines brought about by drought and other disasters. Finally, increased population density, a more sedentary life style, and greater trade, all of which are associated with agriculture, provide conditions for the spread and maintenance of infectious diseases.

The skeletons of individuals who lived before and after the introduction of maize agriculture were examined for a number of different health indicators, in order to provide a balanced picture of the pattern of stress, disease, and death that affected the Dickson population. The indicators that proved most sensitive to health differences were: bone lesions (scars) due to infection, nutritional deficiencies, trauma, and degenerative conditions; long bone growth; dental developmental defects; and age at death. To avoid unconscious bias, we and the other researchers involved measured these seven traits without knowing in advance which skeletons came from each of the two cultural periods.

Persistent bacterial infection leaves its mark on the outer, or periosteal, layer of bone. Tibias (shinbones) are the most frequently affected bones because they have relatively poor circulation and therefore tend to accumulate bacteria. Toxins produced by bacteria kill some of the bone cells; as new bone is produced, the periosteal bone becomes roughened and layered. Lallo and his co-workers found that following the introduction of agriculture there was a threefold increase in the percentage of individuals with such lesions. Eighty-four percent of the Mississippian tibias had these "periosteal reactions," as compared with only 26 percent of pre-Mississippian tibias. The lesions also tended to be more severe and to show up in younger individuals in the Mississippian population.

A second type of lesion, more easily seen in the thinner bones of the body (such as those of the skull), is a sign of anemia. In response to anemia, the body steps up its production of red blood cells, which are formed in the bone marrow. To accomplish this the marrow must expand at the expense of the outer layer of bone. In severe cases, this expansion may cause the outer layer of bone to disappear, exposing the porous, sievelike inner bone. This lesion, called porotic hyperostosis, can occur with any kind of anemia. In the Dickson Mounds populations, the lesions are not severe, are restricted to the eye sockets and crania, and occur mainly in children and young adult females. This pattern suggests anemia resulting from a nutritional deficiency, specifically an iron deficiency. (A hereditary anemia, such as sickle-cell anemia, would have been more severe in its manifestation and would have affected all ages and both sexes in the population.)

There is a significant increase in the frequency of porotic hyperostosis during the Mississippian period. Half the Mississippian infants and children had porotic hyperostosis, twice the rate found for pre-Mississippian infants and children. Individuals with both periosteal reactions and porotic hyperostosis tend to have suffered more severely from each condition. This may be evidence of a deadly synergism of malnutrition and infection, like that often reported among contemporary populations.

Traumatic lesions were measured by diagnosis of healed fractures of the long bones of the legs and arms. Adult males had the highest frequency of such fractures. Approximately one out of three Mississippian males had at least one fracture, twice the frequency of their predecessors. These fractures often occurred at the midshaft of the ulna and radius, the bones of the lower arm. Fractures at this location are called parry fractures because they are typically the result of efforts to ward off a blow.

The frequency of degenerative pathologies, including arthritic conditions found on joints and the contacting surfaces of the vertebral column, also increased through time. One or more degenerative conditions were diagnosed in 40 percent of pre-Mississippian adults but in more than 70 percent of Mississippian adults.

In addition to the studies of the changing pattern of disease and trauma, we, along with Lallo and Jerome Rose, now at the University of Arkansas, assessed differences in skeletal growth and developmental timing. Skeletal growth and development are susceptible to a wide variety of stressful conditions and therefore reflect overall health. We found that in comparison to pre-Mississippians of the same age, Mississippian children between the ages of five and ten had significantly shorter and narrower tibias and femurs (the major long bones of the legs). This difference may be explained by a decreased rate of growth before the age of five. The Mississippians apparently were able to catch up in growth after age ten, however, since adult Mississippians are only slightly smaller than pre-Mississippians.

A more detailed exploration of developmental changes came from studying defects in enamel, the hard white coating of the crowns of teeth. Ameloblasts, the enamel-forming cells, secrete enamel matrix in ringlike fashion, starting at the biting surface and ending at the bottom of the crown. A deficiency in enamel thickness, called a hypoplasia, may result if the individual suffers a systemic physiological stress during enamel formation. Since the timing of enamel secretion is well known and relatively stable, the position of such a lesion on a tooth corresponds to an individual's age at the time of stress.

We examined the permanent teeth—teeth that form between birth and age seven. For skeletons with nearly complete sets of permanent teeth, 55 percent of pre-Mississippians had hypoplasias, while among Mississippians the figure rose to 80 percent. In both groups, hypoplasias were most frequently laid down between the ages of one and one-half and four. However, the hypoplasias in the Mississippian group peak at age two and one-half, approximately one-half year earlier than the pre-Mississippian peak. The peak is also more pronounced. This pattern of defects may indicate both an earlier age at weaning and the use of cereal products as weaning foods.

The repeated occurrence of hypoplasias within individuals revealed an annual cycle of stress. Most likely there was a seasonal food shortage. This seems to have worsened in the period just before the population becomes completely "Mississippianized," suggesting that it provided a rationale for intensifying agriculture.

All the above six indicators point toward a decrease in health associated with cultural change at Dickson. However, they are not meaningful apart from an analysis of the pattern of death in these populations. Healthy-looking skeletons, for example, may be the remains of young individuals who died outright because their bodies were too weak to cope in the face of disease, injury, and other forms of stress. Conversely, skeletons that show wear and tear may be those of individuals who survived during stressful times and lived to a ripe old age.

At Dickson, however, the trend is unambiguous. Individuals whose skeletons showed more signs of stress and disease (for example, enamel hypoplasias) also lived shorter lives, on average, than individuals with fewer such

indications. For the population as a whole, life expectancy at birth decreased from twenty-six years in the pre-Mississippian to nineteen years in the Mississippian. The contrast in mortality is especially pronounced during the infant and childhood years. For example, 22 percent of Mississippians died during their first year as compared to 13 percent of the pre-Mississippians. Even for those who passed through the dangerous early years of childhood, there is a differential life expectancy. At fifteen years of age, pre-Mississippians could expect to live for an average of twenty-three more years, while Mississippians could expect to live for only eighteen more years.

What caused this decline in health? A number of possibilities have been proposed. Lallo and others have emphasized the effect of agriculture on diet. Most of the health trends may be explained by a decline in diet quality. These include the trends in growth, development, mortality, and nutritional disease, all four of which have obvious links to nutrition. The same explanation may be offered for the increase in infectious diseases, since increased susceptibility may be due to poor nutrition. Furthermore, a population subject to considerable infectious disease would be likely to suffer from other conditions, including increased rates of anemia and mortality and decreased growth rates.

The link between diet and infectious disease is bolstered by an analysis of trace elements from tibial bone cores. Robert Gilbert found that the Mississippian bones contain less zinc, an element that is limited in maize. Building on this research, Wadia Bahou, now a physician in Ann Arbor, Michigan, showed that the skeletons with the lowest levels of zinc had the highest frequency of infectious lesions. This is strong evidence that a diet of maize was relied on to a point where health was affected.

The population increase associated with the changeover to agriculture probably also contributed to the decline in health. We do not believe that the population ever threatened to exceed the carrying capacity of the bountiful Dickson area (and there are no signs of the environmental degradation one would expect to find if resources were overexploited). However, increased population density and sedentariness, coupled with intensification of contact with outsiders, create opportunities for the spread of infectious disease. George Milner of the University of Kentucky, while still a graduate student at Northwestern University, argued this point in comparing Dickson with the Kane Mounds populations. Kane is located near Cahokia, the major center south of Dickson. Despite Kane's proximity to this large center, its population density was much lower than at Larson, the major agricultural village of the Dickson population. Of the two, Kane had the lower rate of infectious diseases.

While the "agricultural hypothesis," including the effects of population pressure, offers an explanation for much of the health data, it doesn't automatically account for the two remaining measures: degenerative and traumatic pathologies. Poor nutrition and infectious disease may make people more susceptible to degenerative disease. However, the arthritic conditions found in the Dickson skeletons, involving movable joints, were probably caused by strenuous physical activity. The link, then, is not with the consumption of an agricultural diet but, if anything, with the physically taxing work of agricultural production. An explanation for the increase in traumatic injuries is harder to imagine. Possibly, the increased population density caused social tension and strife to arise within communities, but why should this have happened?

A curious fact makes us think that explanations based only on agricultural intensification and population increase are missing an important contributing factor. Recent archeological research at Dickson suggests that hunting and gathering remained productive enterprises and were never completely abandoned. Many of the local Mississippian sites have a great concentration of animal bones and projectile points used for hunting. A balanced diet apparently was available. The health and trace element data, however, suggest that the Mississippian diet was deficient. There is a disparity between what was available and what was eaten.

At present our search for an explanation for this paradox centers on the relationship between Dickson and the Cahokia population. The builders of the Dickson Mounds received many items of symbolic worth from the Cahokia region, such as copper-covered ear spools and marine shell necklaces. Much of the health data would be explained if Dickson had been trading perishable foodstuffs for these luxury items. In particular, the diversion of meat or fish to Cahokia would explain the apparent discrepancy between diet and resources.

To have a food surplus to trade, individuals from the Dickson area may have intensified their agricultural production while continuing to hunt and gather. The increase in degenerative conditions could have resulted from such a heavy workload. The system may also have put social strain on the community, leading to internal strife. And the accumulation of wealth in terms of ceremonial or other luxury items may have necessitated protection from outside groups. This would explain why the Larson site was palisaded. Both internal and external strain may have led to the increase in traumatic pathologies.

To test the validity of this scenario, we are hoping to gather additional evidence, concentrating on an analysis of trade. The flow of perishable goods such as meat is hard to trace, but we can study the sets of animal bones found at Cahokia and at Dickson village and butchering sites. The distribution of animal bones at the archeological sites can then be compared with examples of bone distributions in areas where trading has been ethnographically recorded. Further evidence is provided by data such as Milner's, which showed that health at Kane—a community that shared in Cahokia's power—was better than at Dickson.

The trading of needed food for items of symbolic value, to the point where health is threatened, may not seem to make sense from an objective, outsider's perspective. But it is a situation that has been observed in historic and modern times. An indigenous group learns that it can trade something it has access to (sugar cane, alpacas, turtles) for something it greatly admires but can only obtain from outside groups (metal products, radios, alcohol). The group's members do not perceive that the long-term health and economic results of such trade are usually unfavorable. Nor are all such arrangements a result of voluntary agreement. The pattern of health observed at Dickson is seen in most situations where there is a decline in access to, and control over, resources. For example, lower classes in stratified societies live shorter lives and suffer more from nearly all major diseases.

Agriculture is not invariably associated with declining health. A recent volume edited by Mark N. Cohen and George J. Armelagos, *Paleopathology and the Origins of Agriculture*, analyzed health changes in twenty-three regions of the world where agriculture developed. In many of these regions there was a clear, concurrent decline in health, while in others there was little or no change or slight improvements in health. Perhaps a decline is more likely to occur when agriculture is intensified in the hinterland of a political system. Groups living far away from the centers of trade and power are apt to be at a disadvantage. They may send the best fruits of their labors to market and receive little in return. And during times of economic hardship or political turmoil, they may be the ones to suffer the most, as resources are concentrated on maintaining the central parts of the system.

Suggested Further Reading

Paleopathology and the Origins of Agriculture, edited by Mark N. Cohen and George J. Armelagos (New York: Academic Press, 1984), compares the health of prehistoric farmers with their hunter-gatherer forebears. A chapter by Alan H. Goodman et al., "Health Changes at Dickson Mounds, Illinois (A.D. 950–1300)," chronicles the effects of economic and cultural change on the health of pre-historic populations in this area. Robert Gilbert, Jr., and James Mielke edited *Analysis of Prehistoric Diets* (New York: Academic Press, 1985), a report on the methods used to interpret prehistoric nutritional stress. For a review of humankind's first three million years, see Robert J. Wenke's *Patterns in Prehistory* (New York: Oxford University Press, 1980).

CHAPTER 12

Bread and Beer: The Early Use of Cereals in the Human Diet

Solomon H. Katz and Mary M. Voigt

(1986)

This article has an intellectual history that begins with a fascinating exchange in the early 1950s. Robert Braidwood's field work at Jarmo led the botanist Jonathan D. Sauer to suggest that the earliest use of wheat and barley may not have been as flour for bread, but for beer. Braidwood posed Sauer's question to his colleagues as follows:

"Could the discovery that a mash of fermented grain yielded a palatable and nutritious beverage have acted as a greater stimulant toward the experimental selection and breeding of the cereals than the discovery of flour and bread making? One would assume that the utilisation of *wild* cereals (along with edible fruits and berries) as a source of collected food would have been in existence for millennia before their domestication...took place. Was the subsequent impetus to this domestication bread or beer?" (1953:515).

The respondents to this question read like a Who's Who of anthropology and archaeology at that time. These scholars looked at the topic from almost every angle, and tentatively concluded that people never lived by beer alone, but must have lived first by gruel, then by bread, and finally by bread and beer. In the past thirty-five years, much new evidence has come not only from archaeology, but also from the field of human nutrition, and especially from the study of what Katz has called the "biocultural evolution of cuisine." This information provides new insights into the relationship between people and food in prehistory, as well as a somewhat different answer to Braidwood's question.

A NEW PARADIGM: THE BIOCULTURAL EVOLUTION OF CUISINE

There are thousands of plants that humans could consume. Yet the number for which there is actual evidence of consumption, either now or in the past, is only in the hundreds, and approximately thirty plants provide over 95 percent of the vegetable calories consumed by the world's human population today. These staple crops include grasses such as wheat, rice, corn, millet, and sorghum, and root crops such as yams, manioc, taro, potato, and sweet potato. A third group of cultivated plants, the legumes or pulses (lentils, many varieties of peas and beans), are eaten in smaller quantities than the staples, but play an important role because of the high quality of their protein nutrients and the variety that they provide.

The plants we now eat connect us in some remarkable ways with our past. Most of the plants we prepare as foods today are domesticated varieties of the wild plants that our ancestors consumed thousands of years ago. Over the last twenty years Katz has worked on a number of problems that integrate the past and present by examining how traditional peoples select diets and prepare foods that satisfy their nutritional needs. By studying the ways in which natural nutritional limitations present in some modern food plants are overcome by their consumers, and by combining this knowledge with what we know of the history and archaeology of the edible plants, we can obtain new insights into a wide range of problems. For example, we can begin to piece together plausible explanations of how domestication might have occurred, to develop new understandings about the evolutionary basis of styles of cooking or "cuisine," and, more broadly, to develop new models of the processes of human biological and cultural evolution.

Let us start on the most general level, that of the relationship between biological and cultural evolution. Plants, like all other biological organisms, have various kinds of naturally evolved defenses against predation. Most plants are protected by chemical substances ("secondary compounds"), located in the seeds and to a lesser extent in the leaves. These compounds discourage predators by producing a toxic response in any organism that ingests them. Before the plants can become useful food, some process must be evolved to neutralize the toxins. One process is biological change: certain organisms have genetically evolved so that they are exquisitely adapted to specific plant defenses, and as a result can subsist on these plants without harm from the toxins.

Humans have been subject to this biological process. This can be demonstrated by a study of the distribution of

Solomon H. Katz and Mary M. Voigt, "Bread and beer: the early use of cereals in the human diet." *Expedition* 28 (1986): 23–34. Some figures have been omitted. Reprinted with permission.

certain genetic traits throughout the world. Depending on the importance of a specific food within the diet, different human populations vary in their ability to consume it without harm. For example, one well-known adaptation that is at least partially genetically controlled involves the ability of adults to digest fresh milk. Nearly all newborn mammals have an enzyme (lactase) in their small intestine that breaks down and permits the absorption of the sugar in milk (lactose). In most mammals this enzyme is reduced with age. For example, in many human individuals the amount of lactase present has decreased greatly by the age of four, so that drinking any quantity of fresh milk will result in cramps and diarrhea. Within populations that practice dairying, however, a high proportion of the adults continue to produce lactase and thus can utilize the energy present in milk sugars. Thus the ability to secrete lactase beyond childhood is apparently the result of a mutation that became "established" because it gave an advantage to those that carried it, allowing them to convert a readily available but potentially harmful substance into a nutritionally beneficial one.

Another biological adaptation can be inferred from the effect of wheat on human groups that have only recently begun to use this crop as food. Such groups have higher frequencies of a genetic trait that is associated with an inability to digest gluten, a substance that occurs in high concentrations in most modern varieties of wheat. Within groups that have relied on wheat as a staple for a long period of time, individuals with such genetic traits would have been at a nutritional disadvantage, and their descendants presumably declined in number until the gene became rare or totally eliminated from the population.

Such examples of human biological adaptation appear to be rare. The majority of cases where natural plant defense mechanisms have been overcome by humans involve cultural adaptations rather than biological ones. Any change in behavior that can be transmitted by learning can be more rapidly established than a change that is genetically based. Katz has suggested that the learned behavior that is most effective in rendering plants nontoxic takes the form of food processing, or practices of cuisine. There are, of course, other ways of culturally overcoming plant defenses. For example, suppose that experiments in cultivation and propagation of a particular plant led to the discovery of a variant that lacked the toxic effects that protected the wild form. While new nontoxic varieties might seem desirable at first glance, the investment of time and labor in such crops would have been self-defeating: the plant's defenses would have been lowered not only to humans but also to *all of the other organisms that competed with humans* for this food source. These competitors, including insects, birds and other mammals, would have outnumbered and out-eaten humans.

So the evolution of cuisine made certain plants accessible to humans, but *only* to humans. No other organism could acquire the complex behavior necessary to transform marginally nutritious and outright toxic substances into high-quality nutritious foods; instead they required

elaborate genetically based digestive and metabolic adaptations. Hence Katz has proposed that our ancestors, like us, overcame plant defenses in the proverbial "cooking pot" (Fig. 3). This process will probably continue into the future. With modern scientific understanding of this largely empirical process, it is possible that plants not yet edible will be consumed in the future, once we learn their chemical "secrets."

The study of processes of adaptation such as those described above has led to a basic change in the way that many anthropologists view the process of human evolution. A new "paradigm" or conceptual approach has developed that does not treat biological and cultural evolution as isolated phenomena, but instead examines the relationship between the biologically evolved capacities of the human species and the culturally evolved factors that complement and supplement these biological adaptations.

One way to consider the process of biocultural evolution is in terms of the transfer of information. The heritable macromolecule DNA provides for the transfer of biological information from one generation to the next; cultural information is transmitted by language and precepts. Both bodies or "pools" of information become part of the process by which humans have adapted to their particular environment. The bridge between the biological and cultural information pools exists in the human central nervous system. Biologically, the central nervous system has highly specialized capacities; these capacities permit the transfer of cultural information that in turn helps to "program" the central nervous system. Thus the specific form that human behavior takes is the result of both biological and socio-cultural factors. Both systems of information evolve and are critical for the survival of a particular human population in the environment that it exploits.

Given this feedback process, one important aspect of the biobehavioral evolutionary process is the unusually long time that humans take to reach full maturity. It is widely accepted that this extended period of growth and development (a strictly biological characteristic) is necessary to provide enough time for the transfer of the cultural information needed for survival by the new generation. This information transfer requires stability. In all probability, myths, stories, and legends, some of which were woven into ritual practices, all play a critical role in the process of stabilizing the content of traditions that are passed from one generation to the next, as well as the social context through which they flow. Once stability has been achieved, the trial and error process that must originally lead to the evolution of specific traditions is no longer necessary.

Among the most crucial traditions are those related to subsistence: the acquisition, processing, and consumption of food. One general pattern in the evolution of subsistence traditions can be observed worldwide. The domestication of plants marks a turning point in the relationship between foods and food-processing techniques. Plants that came under cultural control tended to become more and more important in the diet. At the same time, the allocation of time to agricultural tasks (seeding, weeding, harvesting) led to the neglect of a wide range of seasonal wild foods that were once collected. The net result is summarized in Figure 1: as the number of plant species consumed has decreased over the past millennia, the number of recipes to prepare plants has increased. This has led to the formation of elaborate food traditions and rituals that have been passed down as cultural adaptations from one generation to the next, just as genetic adaptations to wheat and dairy products were biologically transmitted between generations (Figs. 2–3). So variety was maintained and the nutrients necessary for healthy human survival were stabilized.

THE ORIGINS OF FOOD PRODUCTION

The model of biocultural evolution provides us with insights that are useful in attempting to answer a question that still confronts archaeologists: How did the "Neolithic

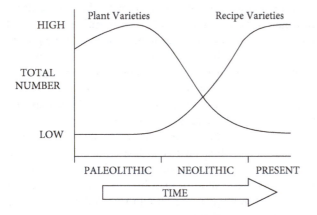

Figure 1 *During the Paleolithic period, hunters and gatherers utilized a wide variety of plant species. With the beginning of food production in the Neolithic, certain plants began to increase in importance, gradually becoming dominant. But while the number of plant species consumed declined, variety was maintained within the diet through an increase in the numbers of recipes used to prepare plant foods.*

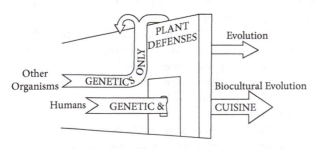

Figure 2 *Plant defenses present an enormous wall that blocks potential predators. Over time, some organisms are able to scale this wall through long-term genetic changes, evolving specializations to overcome the plant defenses. The key to human evolution is the presence of both cultural and biological adaptations, carefully balanced to unlock plant defenses. The result is a biocultural phenomenon, a set of traditions concerning food preparation that we call "cuisine."*

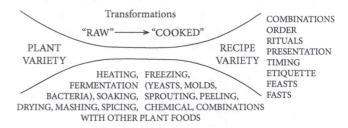

Figure 3 *Food preparation processes transform "raw" or unmodified plant products into "cooked" or culturally modified foods. Variety exists not only in the techniques used to transform foods, but also in the ways in which they are eaten.*

Revolution" ever get started in the first place? The complex processes by which people domesticated plants and animals occurred independently in several regions of the world. In this article we will consider only the Near East, and specifically the factors that led to the domestication of cereals.

At present, the earliest known domesticated plants in this region have been found at sites in the Levant, the area that is now Syria, Jordan, and Israel. Rare seeds of wheat, barley, and lentils that differ in shape from their wild ancestors appear at settlements such as Tell Aswad, Jericho, and Nahal Oren by ca. 8000 B.C. (Fig. 4). At earlier sites occupied by hunters and gatherers (known collectively as the Natufian "culture" or tradition), the presence of sickle blades, grinding tools, storage pits, and seeds indicates that wild cereals were harvested at many locations.

Over the last two decades, many archaeologists have favored environmental factors as causal elements leading to experimentation with the cultivation of wild cereals. Briefly, they theorized that as climatic conditions changed at the end of the last glaciation or Pleistocene period, groups in the Near East, and especially in the Levant, gradually became more dependent on one wild resource—the easily collected and stored wild cereals. (The extent to which cereals were present within this region during the Pleistocene is not certain; evidence from pollen cores as well as from archaeological sites does indicate that wheat and barley were more widespread and abundant during the warmer, wetter Holocene [beginning ca. 9000 B.C. in the Levant].) In some very favorable locations, wild foods were so readily available that groups such as the Natufians were able to remain year round in the same location, either in caves or in large open sites, e.g., villages such as Ain Mallaha (Eynan) in Israel and Mureybit in Syria. With sedentary life came a growth in population that eventually put pressure on the supply of major food sources, including the wild cereals. This pressure resulted in the migration of part of the population into less favorable areas, without good stands of wild wheat and barley. In order to obtain a sufficiently large quantity of these staple foods, the migrants began to experiment with the propagation of these species. Need eventually led to the practice of keeping seeds and planting them.

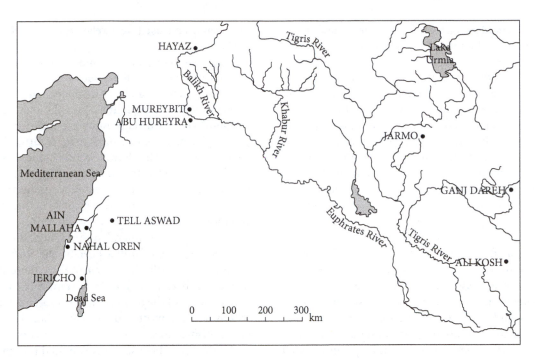

Figure 4 *Map of the Near East showing archaeological sites mentioned in the text.*

Current archaeological evidence does not support this hypothesis. Not only was there an apparent *decrease* in the consumption of wild cereals during the period when the initial experiments with their cultivation and propagation must have taken place, but domestication apparently took place within areas with an abundance of wild resources. Moreover, even after cereals and pulses were fully domesticated, they formed only a very minor part of the diet. A heavy dependence on crops such as wheat, barley, lentils, and vetch is not evident archaeologically until hundreds of years after their initial appearance. For example, at the site of Ali Kosh in southwestern Iran, a large and well-preserved sample of carbonized plant remains was recovered from settlements occupied from ca. 7000 to ca. 6000 B.C. Domesticated cereals (barley and emmer wheat) made up only 3.4 percent of the plant fragments during the initial phase of settlement and were still rare a thousand years later (Helbaek 1969:Table 3).

Scholars have therefore swung away from deterministic models that emphasize environmental factors and strictly biological needs, and turned instead to the investigation of cultural factors. In a recent publication dedicated to Robert Braidwood, many of the contributors suggested that social conditions and motives may have been critical in the shift from hunting and gathering to food production. This point of view was summarized by Robert McC. Adams:

"[I find] it hard to escape the impression that throughout the entire Near Eastern prehistoric sequence, there was a lot of room to rattle around in. Where, and how densely, people settled, then, is more likely to reflect a culturally constrained choice among subsistence or other locational preferences than a decision imposed by an uncontrollable decline in the net balance of resources over needs" (Young et al. 1983:371).

Our own explanation for the beginnings of cereal cultivation is consistent with the biocultural model for the evolution of cuisine. The key element in this explanation, the event that "primed the pump" and led people to choose to invest energy in the collection and propagation of wild wheat and barley, was the discovery of new food processing techniques—the sprouting and fermentation of these grains.

FERMENTATION: THE KEY TO ALCOHOL AND NUTRITION

Suppose that the consumption of a food produced an altered state of awareness or consciousness that was noticeable, but that did not have serious toxic side effects such as motor impairment. Now suppose that this food also had a second, imperceptible effect, a substantial improvement in nutritional value over the unprocessed cereal grains. This is exactly what happens when barley and wheat are fermented into beer.

We suggest that among the factors that led to the domestication of wild cereals were the following. First, the motivation for a change in behavior (an allocation of time and labor to the collection and eventually to the propagation of cereals) was provided by a noticeable phenomenon—the "high" that people obtained from beer. Second, individuals and groups who consumed beer were better nourished than those who consumed wheat and barley as gruel or who ignored these wild resources. Beer would have had sustaining powers well beyond any other food in their diet except animal proteins. In biological terms, beer drinkers would have had a "selective advantage" in the form of improved health for themselves and ultimately for their offspring. Third, cereals were a desirable resource because of the ease with which they could be harvested, transported, and stored from year to year. In the following section we will examine the first two factors.

If we start with the assumption that people consciously modify their behavior and make choices as individuals and as groups concerning the kinds of activities they pursue, then the question of motivation for the shift in food-getting behavior that is involved in the process of domestication is critical. It is important to note that many of the traditions surrounding successful food strategies become highly ritualized. One consistent pattern is the inordinate amount of ritual practice and attention given to foods which have a mind-altering or psychopharmacological effect. Almost invariably, individuals and societies appear to invest enormous amounts of effort and even risk to pursue the continued consumption of a food with a mind-altering property. Because the behavior associated with the search for such foods is so intense, however, it can lead to social disorder. Thus, religious and social traditions have developed that serve to control these foods by prescribing and proscribing them as a part of ritual practices and specified social occasions. Given the importance of mind-altering foods during historic times, it seems highly likely that they were

discovered and used at a relatively early point in human evolution.

The most consistently sought-after beverage with psychopharmacological effects seems to be alcohol. The combination of its initial elevating effects on the emotions, its perception-altering qualities, and the fact that it is easily metabolized and usually nontoxic make alcohol an ideal psychopharmacological substance, or drug. In traditional societies, beer with a low alcoholic content is characteristically associated with a number of secular and nonsecular occasions. These include the formation of groups for labor (harvesting, large-scale construction tasks); ritual ceremonies, including those marking rites of passage such as a marriage or a funeral; and social gatherings (see, for example, the use of millet beer by the Kofyar in Nigeria; Netting 1964). Within the Near East, there is ample evidence that beer played an important role in the economy and ideology of the Sumerians, the most ancient people for whom we have written documents (Box 1). If the discovery of fermentation was made by collectors of wild cereals, and if the use of beer was incorporated into the social and/ or religious system of these people, then any disruption in the supply of these wild foods would have posed a serious

---

BOX 1 BEER IN MESOPOTAMIA

The most ancient documentary evidence for beer production comes from Mesopotamia, written in the Sumerian language on tablets that date to the 3rd millennium B.C. The world's oldest recipe is for beer! A highly detailed description of the brewing process is related as part of a myth that tells how Enki, the third-ranked god in the Sumerian pantheon, prepared a banquet for his father, Enlil, the second-ranked god. A second recipe is found in a hymn to the beer goddess Ninkasi, whose name is translated as "the lady who fills the mouth." Lexical texts contain long lists of very specific terms related to brewing techniques. Rations of beer (as well as barley) were issued to those attached to the estates of Sumerian temples and palaces, ordinary laborers receiving about one liter per day. In general, we can say that beer was an important food that was integrated into the mythology, religion, and economy of the Sumerians.

The purely personal pleasure that these people took in beer drinking is summed up in the following song, written to celebrate the building of a tavern. The toast in the second verse quoted here is addressed to the tavern keeper, who is apparently a woman:

"Let the heart of the gakkul [fermenting] *vat be our heart!*
What makes your heart feel wonderful,
Makes also our heart feel wonderful.
Our liver is happy, our heart is joyful.
You poured a libation over the brick of destiny,
You placed the foundations in peace and prosperity,
May Ninkasi live together with you!
Let her pour for you beer and wine,
Let the pouring of the sweet liquor resound pleasantly for you!
In the...reed buckets there is sweet beer,
I will make cupbearers, boys, and brewers stand by,

While I turn around the abundance of beer,
While I feel wonderful, I feel wonderful,
Drinking beer, in a blissful mood,
Drinking liquor, feeling exhilarated,
With joy in the heart and a happy liver—
While my heart full of joy,
And my happy liver I covered with a garment fit for a queen!

(Civil 1964)

Pictorial representations show the vessels used to brew and store Sumerian beer. All have a similar shape, with long narrow necks and a pointed base. This form also appears on the most ancient (pictographic) tablets, and is translated as "clay container" by Margaret Green of The University Museum's Babylonian Section. A clay container sign with dashes inside refers to beer. The beer was consumed from goblets, or from jars through long straws. The earliest example of this kind of scene, on a stamp seal, is from Tepe Gawra, and extends the period for which we have direct evidence of beer drinking to ca. 4000 B.C.

The use of straws has sometimes puzzled modern authors. One expert on the history of technology interprets them as evidence that the beer was of "doubtful quality" (Hodges 1970:115). Leaving aside the question of what constitutes a good-tasting beer, a study of traditional methods of brewing in Africa provides a very practical explanation of the straws. The Sumerian texts describe both filtered and unfiltered beers. In drinking unfiltered beer, a straw would have been necessary to penetrate below a layer of hulls and yeast floating on the surface. Most straws were probably made from reeds, but the wealthy used pure gold straws such as the one found in the tomb of the lady Pu-abi at Ur. Pu-abi's straw was lying next to a silver vessel that presumably contained her daily ration of beer.

problem, and the transition from Epipaleolithic food collectors to Neolithic cultivators would thus be accounted for.

The enormous nutritional potential provided by cereal proteins and vitamins made the cultivation of these crops biologically as well as economically profitable. Both wheat and barley are largely composed of complex carbohydrates, with approximately 13–20 percent protein and a small amount of fat. As a source of food they are limited in several ways. First, both of these cereals have low levels of the essential amino acid lysine; without lysine, most of the remaining amino acids in wheat and barley cannot be synthesized into usable protein by the human body. Second, barley (but not wheat) has low levels of the essential sulfur-containing amino acids (see below). Third, B vitamins (riboflavin, niacin, and thiamine) are present in both wheat and barley, but not in sufficiently high levels to meet basic nutritional needs. Fourth, these grains, in particular wheat, are high in the concentration of substances called phytates that bind essential minerals like calcium and prevent their absorption in the digestive tract.

It is yeast that converts the cereal grains from a nutritionally limited source of proteins and vitamins into an outstanding source of human nutrition. Both brewing and the making of many types of bread involve the growth of yeast cells. Yeast produces a rich source of lysine, significantly improves the B-vitamin content of the mixture, and decreases the concentration of phytates, thereby permitting the absorption of more essential minerals such as calcium. Some of the vitamins that are enhanced are not available from other plant sources. The major disadvantage of yeast is that the adult human can consume only about 20–25 grams of yeast nucleic acid per day. Beyond that level, a build-up of serum uric acid occurs that may cause high blood pressure, gout, and kidney abnormalities.

Wild yeast is present in the air. The simple exposure of a mixture of cereals and water, whether in the form of a thin gruel or a thicker dough, will result in the implantation and growth of yeast cells. For example, the sourdough used by pioneers in the American West and Alaska was made by combining flour with milk or water and keeping it in a warm place until it began to bubble from the activity of the airborne yeast. Once established, a yeast strain can be saved and used as a starter to ensure the quality of the next batch of bread or to speed up the fermentation process in beer.

The critical step that differentiates bread from beer is the addition of diastase enzymes that convert the cereal starches into sugar, which is used by the yeast to be eventually turned into alcohol. Traditional brewing techniques increase diastase levels through the addition of malt, or sprouted grain (Box 2). The first step of the malting process is to soak the cereals in water. A substantial amount of diastase enzymes form in the root tips. Wheat is not as efficient as barley in this respect, but barley produces enough diastase to break down the starch of an almost equal quantity of wheat. The value of a mixture of wheat and barley is that wheat adds the sulfur-containing essential amino acids that barley is low in. If the process of growth is allowed to continue, the amount of diastase present begins to decline. The sprouted cereal is therefore left to parch in the sun or is artificially heated until lightly toasted; as a result the rootlet dies, but the diastase enzyme levels remain high.

Once the cereal has dried out, the softened hull is easily ground. When the ground malt is added to a mixture of cereal and water, the conversion from starch to sugar begins; this process is known as "mashing." Hydrolized starches, obtained from heating water and raw cereal grains into a porridge, are most susceptible to the effects of the diastases, so that the barley diastases are often mixed into a cooked porridge of water and cereal grains.

During fermentation, the maltose feeds the yeast so that it grows. This process will produce alcohol (rather than some other metabolic product) if two other conditions are met: the fermentation medium must be both acidic and anaerobic (without oxygen). Acid conditions can be maintained by allowing the porridge to sour overnight through the introduction of lactic-acid-producing bacteria found in the air. Once such bacteria are found, they can be kept alive as a starter along with the yeast, and transferred from an old brew to a new one. Anaerobic conditions are also relatively easy to obtain. When the yeast begins to grow, carbon dioxide forms and bubbles up to the surface. If the beer is in a container shielded from the air, the carbon dioxide will itself shut off enough oxygen to ensure alcohol production.

It should be noted that beer and bread are not nutritionally equivalent. The optimum growth of yeast requires the full transformation of sugar into carbon dioxide and water. If alcohol is produced, yeast growth declines; there is, therefore, an inverse relationship between the amount of sugar converted to alcohol and the nutritional value of the resulting cereal product. Under optimal conditions for brewing, the oxygen supply is carefully regulated and the resulting beer will contain about 15 to 18 percent alcohol. Traditional brewing methods, however, are less controlled, allowing air to reach the mixture. As a result, the alcohol concentration is only 5 percent or less, leaving plenty of sugar to be converted into protein. For example, Sotho sorghum beer (Box 2) contains about 3.5 percent alcohol. On the other hand, bread production requires heat, which kills the yeast and stops the enhancement of the protein content.

Within the context of the argument presented here, the fact that bread may represent a *more* efficient way to enhance the nutritional value of cereals, and eventually became the primary way of preparing and consuming wheat, is not strictly relevant. Relative quantities of vitamins and proteins are not immediately perceptible to consumers, and could not serve as a factor in conscious decision-making in 10,000 B.C. Traditional unfiltered beer with a low alcohol content *is* a nutritionally valuable food; but more importantly, the presence of alcohol significantly enhanced a second aspect of its consumption, its cultural value.

A HYPOTHETICAL RECONSTRUCTION

Although few seeds have been recovered from Natufian sites in the southern Levant, the presence of sickle blades, storage pits, and stone pounding and grinding tools from sites dating ca. 10,000 B.C. (the Terminal or Epipaleolithic period) has been interpreted as evidence for the collection of wild cereals by groups of hunters and gatherers. At contemporary and probably related sites in northern Syria, large quantities of wild wheat and barley as well as legumes have been recovered. But how were these wild cereals prepared as food? The first step was probably to pound the seeds in a stone mortar. Both wild wheat and wild barley (as well as early domesticated varieties) are husked: the seeds are encased in glumes and are not freed by threshing. Epipaleolithic groups could have broken up the husks by placing the grain in mortars and pounding them with pestles—tools that are usually very common at these sites. Alternatively the cereal could have been "parched" or roasted on an open hearth. (At this time, neither pottery vessels nor ovens with closed firing chambers were in use.)

It is generally agreed that the simplest method of cooking cereals is to prepare a gruel, a mixture of the broken-up cereal particles (probably including the husks) and water. The container used by the Natufians would have been of an organic material, a skin bag or perhaps a basket or wooden vessel. A second method of preparation might involve sprouting the cereal by soaking it in water. The process of soaking has been widely used to make toxic plants palatable (for example, acorns in the Near East), and it seems highly likely that it was in common use during Paleolithic times. If cereals were steeped, the germination process would have broken the seed coat, made it easier to grind up the cereal for gruel, and enhanced the taste as well.

The key step in making beer would have been the addition of sprouted and ground cereals to water. If this special gruel was heated and then allowed to stand overnight or longer, wild yeasts would have started the process of fermentation. In the Middle East, where daily summer temperatures can reach 120° F or more, there would have been little need to heat the brew. Even in winter, putting the mixture in a sunny spot would provide adequate heat for the yeast to work during the day, and at night it might have been placed near a fire.

Given the steps involved in preparation, the making of gruel must have preceded the invention of bread as well as beer. Unleavened breads require only that a thick mixture of pounded cereal and water be heated. Such breads are,

---

BOX 2 TRADITIONAL METHODS OF BREAD AND BEER MAKING

Bread—In the Middle East today, most of the bread eaten by town or city dwellers is made by specialized bakers. Produced in a great variety of forms, these breads are usually relatively thick and resemble European loaf breads in texture and flavor. Traditional flat breads are, however, still made by village housewives for their own families. The following recipe is from Iran, but is typical of breads produced from Turkey to India, usually on a domed metal plate over an open fire. It has been modified for the American kitchen.

Lavash
1 package active dry yeast
2 cups warm water
1½ tsp. salt
3 cups all-purpose white flour
flour for rolling

Dissolve yeast in warm water. Add salt and mix well. Mix in flour and knead using an electric mixer with a dough hook or by hand for 10 minutes. Cover with a damp cloth and let dough rise for 2 hours. Divide the dough into 20 equal size balls. Roll as thin as possible and place on a cookie sheet that has been warmed and sprinkled with flour. Bake for 1 minute in a 500° oven. Serve hot, or cool for a few minutes and store in an airtight container. Can be easily reheated in a toaster. (Traditionally, *lavash* is freshened by sprinkling it with water.) (Ghanoonparvar 1982)

Beer—The production of beers in Africa today has been studied by Rebecca Huss-Ashmore, who has collected detailed recipes for brewing. The processes used in making unfiltered sorghum beers with properties quite similar to beers made of barley are remarkably simple. They do not require elaborate technology, although considerable knowledge is necessary to carry out the process successfully. In the mid-1950s, when traditional beers were still very popular, the average amount consumed by the Sotho people was two liters per person per day.

Joala, Strong Bantu (Sotho) Beer
Use 1–2 parts maize to 1 part sorghum. Place all or part of the sorghum in a pot of water. Leave it until it starts to sprout. Then spread it out to dry in the sun on mats or sacks. It should be in a very thin layer. Turn it frequently to make sure it dries thoroughly and doesn't mold. This is the malt.

Put the rest of the grain in hot water, enough to make a thin gruel. Leave it to set overnight, or until it sours. It may take up to 2 days if the weather is cool. Then boil the sour gruel for approximately 2 hours. At this stage, the mixture is a sour porridge called *setoto*, which can be drunk. To make *joala*, cool the *setoto* and add the malted sorghum (usually ground first on a stone). (To speed up this second fermentation, modern housewives add dried yeast at this point.) Leave for several days in a large pot or bucket. The mixture should become sparkly and noticeably alcoholic. It is usually filtered through a sieve or a woven grass bag before drinking.

however, rather tasteless, and lack the nutritional advantages of leavened bread. Their popularity in the Middle East and India in recent times may be related to the spread of religions that prohibit the consumption of alcohol: the baking of unleavened breads provides a means of preventing *any* fermentation from occurring. In any case, as cereals formed a higher proportion of the diet we can be sure that they were consumed in a variety of forms, since the amount of beer a person can consume is usually limited by social norms, if not by physiology.

Again, the key to a more nutritious as well as a tastier meal lies in exposure of the dough to wild yeasts before heating it. Early leavened breads would have been quite dense, since the earliest varieties of wheat, as well as all varieties of barley, contain little gluten. Gluten is a protein substance that gives dough elasticity so that it produces a light, porous loaf. The earliest high gluten wheat, a complex hybrid appropriately called "breadwheat," appeared in the Near East after 7000 B.C. (Tell Aswad II), and was distributed from Greece to Iran by 5500 B.C.

THE CRITICAL ROLE OF BEERMAKING IN DOMESTICATION

The essential difference between bread and beer as a means of exploiting cereal grains is that brewing yields alcohol. One major advantage of bread (in addition to the fact that it does *not* contain alcohol) is that it can be made faster than beer. It is also more portable, and can be carried on long journeys. Both foods may well have been used by Epipaleolithic hunters and gatherers, but in unknown quantities. Trace element studies of human skeletons from the southern Levant (the area in which domestication first took place, on present evidence) indicate that cereals were only a minor part of the Natufian diet. A low dependence on cereals might also be inferred from the near absence of charred cereal grains at Natufian camps and villages in this region and from sites where domesticated cereals have been found. For example, the "Pre-Pottery Neolithic A settlement" at Jericho (ca. 8000 B.C.) produced only six grains of domesticated barley, two of domesticated wheat, and three pieces of unidentified legume(s). On the other hand, charred seeds are common at Natufian Abu Hureyra and Mureybit in the north. This differentiation suggests either that our picture of Natufian diets is distorted by accidents of preservation, or that the amount of wild cereal consumed varied significantly between regions.

Bearing in mind these uncertainties, we can return to our initial question: Under what conditions would the consumption of a wild plant resource be sufficiently important to lead to a change in behavior (experiments with cultivation) in order to ensure an adequate supply of this resource? If wild cereals were in fact a minor part of the diet, any argument based on caloric need is weakened. It is our contention that the desire for alcohol would constitute a perceived psychological and social need that might easily prompt changes in subsistence behavior. This type of need would be present whether beer was but one of a series of cereal-based foods that made up a significant part of the diet, or was an occasional food in a diet composed primarily of animal and/or other plant foods.

Although we cannot now directly determine whether beer preceded bread in time, there is some archaeological evidence that suggests the relative importance of these substances for Neolithic peoples in the Near East. Barley appears without wheat at one early site with a good sample of seeds. In the Zagros mountains, where Braidwood's Jarmo is located, the earliest evidence for domesticated plants comes from Ganj Dareh, where both wild and domesticated barley (as well as peas, lentils, and other wild seeds) were found in contexts dated to ca. 7000 B.C. The only Neolithic site that has produced wheat but no barley is Hayaz Hüyük in southeastern Turkey. Hayaz is, however, atypical. It seems to represent a specialized camp for flint working, rather than a village where the entire range of domestic activities was carried out.

Direct evidence that beer consumption led to the domestication of barley and wheat is lacking. Such evidence might eventually be found in the form of sprouted cereal grains from an Epipaleolithic or early Neolithic site, but the chances for preservation of cereals in this form are low, given the fragility of seeds with a broken hull. Beer drinking may also prove to be detectable in human skeletons. As noted above, one physiological disadvantage of yeast is that consumption above a certain level causes a build-up of serum uric acid. The inflammation of the joints associated with gout is in fact caused by the deposition of urates (uric acid salts) in and around the joints. *If* the urates leave any kind of permanent mark on the bone itself, it may eventually be possible to identify Neolithic beer drinkers from their skeletal remains, especially in the case of the older members of a population.

The argument for beer making is compatible with one aspect of the archaeological record that has long puzzled scholars: the rarity of carbonized seeds at sites that have abundant chipped and ground stone artifacts associated with cereal cultivation and processing. Beer making does not *necessarily* include any process that exposes cereal grains to fire; it could be an everyday activity and yet produce not a single carbonized seed. In fact, given the present evidence, we would have to argue that the wild and early cultivated cereals were most likely to have been consumed either as uncooked gruel or as beer. The hulls must have been removed by mechanical action before mixing the cereal with water. Parching, a process that is much more likely to produce carbonized cereal grains, was probably a later invention. In fact, it could be argued that the appearance of numerous charred grains after ca. 7000 B.C. is related specifically to the invention of parching.

The historical and ethnographic records provide evidence of the value placed on beer. Within the area where cereal domestication took place, the Near East, the earliest written records as well as representational art testify to its importance. Studies of modern traditional groups in the Old World demonstrate the simplicity of the technology, and the ease by which critical steps might have been discovered. Ethnography also indicates the extent to which alcohol and other drugs were prized and incorporated into the social, economic, and religious systems of most cultures.

A brief hypothetical sequence for the domestication process might include the following steps.

1. The scattered but sometimes abundant wild cereals were gathered by groups living in the natural habitat zone of wheat and barley.

2. After initial use of the cereals in a gruel or porridge, the technology of brewing was developed in a series of steps including: the accidental sprouting and drying of the cereal, which assisted in the removal of the hull or seed coat; discovering the sweet taste of the sprout; the use of sprouted, dried, and ground cereals in a gruel that was left to stand for some period; the observation that the "old" gruel did not spoil, but instead tasted sweet and had distinct effects on the mind and emotions.

3. Alcohol gained importance to the society because of its social uses. Of course, alcohol could have been made from other foods such as honey or fruit. A cereal-based brew, however, would have had two benefits, one readily observable by the members of the community and one hidden: it would have allowed the rare and seasonally restricted sweetening agents to have been used for foods other than alcoholic beverages, and it would have added a new high-value food to the diet.

4. Once alcohol had been incorporated into specific social and/or ritual events, maintaining a supply of the plants necessary for the preparation of this beverage would have some importance. When the supply of wild cereal was inadequate, experimentation with these plants (cultivation, propagation) was begun in order to increase yields. Thus cultural values and traditions would have encouraged behavior that maintained the cereals from generation to generation until they were fully under human control, or "domesticated." Based on present archaeological evidence, this process probably occurred *within* the natural habitat zone, when the supply of wild cereals was disrupted for an unknown reason. Should new excavations securely place the earliest domesticates *outside* the natural habitat zone, such experimentation would have served to ensure a supply of cereals in the immediate vicinity of new settlements.

To summarize, it is possible with a careful assessment of the facts about nutrition to propose behavioral sequences that could parsimoniously explain the facts discovered by archaeologists. Careful analysis of nutritional biochemistry can lead to generalizations about the human diet and its relations to biocultural evolutionary processes. This yields the hypothesis that the early intensification in the use of barley and wheat, leading eventually to their domestication, could have stemmed from the desirability of alcohol-containing beers. Under controlled circumstances, alcohol could provide a cultural and social advantage. Unlike other alcohol-yielding brews that were probably available to people at this time, beer would have also had an enormous biological advantage. It enhanced the original nutritional quality of a readily available plant to a level almost comparable with that of meat. Finally, we leave each reader with one last test of any hypothesis, its plausibility. Given a choice of gruel, bread, or brew, which would you rather have with your next meal?

References

Aucamp, M. C., et al. 1961. "Kaffircorn Malting and Brewing Studies. Part 8—Nutritive Value of Some Kaffircorn Products." *Journal of the Science of Food and Agriculture* 12:449–456.

Braidwood, Robert J., et al. 1953. "Did Man Once Live by Beer Alone?" *American Anthropologist* 55:515–526.

Ghanoonparvar, M.R. 1982. *Persian Cuisine*. Book 1. Lexington, KY: Mazda Publications.

Helbaek, Hans. 1969. "Plant Collecting, Dry-Farming, and Irrigation Agriculture in Prehistoric Deh Luran." In *Prehistory and Human Ecology of the Deh Luran Plain*, ed. Frank Hole, Kent V. Flannery, and James Neely, 383–426. Museum of Anthropology of the University of Michigan, Memoir No. 1. Ann Arbor.

Hesseltine, C. W. 1979. "Some Important Fermented Foods of Mid-Asia, the Middle East, and Africa." *Journal of the American Oil Chemists' Society* 56:367–374.

Katz, Solomon. In press. "Food and Biocultural Evolution: A Model for the Investigation of Modern Nutritional Problems." In *Nutritional Anthropology*, ed. Frank E. Johnston. New York: Alan I. Liss.

Netting, Robert. 1964. "Beer as a Locus of Value among the West African Kofyar." *American Anthropologist* 66:375–384.

Nicholson, B.E., et al. 1969. *The Oxford Book of Food Plants*. Oxford: Oxford University Press.

Renfrew, Jane M. 1973. *Paleoethnobotany: The Prehistoric Food Plants of the Near East and Europe*. New York: Columbia University Press.

Young, T. Cuyler, P.E.L. Smith, and Peder Mortensen, eds. 1983. *The Hilly Flanks and Beyond: Essays on the Prehistory of Southwestern Asia*. Studies in Ancient Oriental Civilization No. 36. Chicago: The Oriental Institute.

Beer in Ancient Times

Civil, Miguel. 1964. "A Hymn to the Beer Goddess and a Drinking Song." In *Studies Presented to A.*

Leo Oppenheim, 67–69. Chicago: The Oriental Institute.

Forbes, R. J. 1955. *Studies in Ancient Technology*, Vol. 3 (sections on Food and Alcoholic Beverages). Leiden: E. J. Brill.

Hodges, Henry. 1970. *Technology in the Ancient World*. New York: Knopf.

Oppenheim, A. Leo, and Louis F. Hartman. 1950. *On Beer and Brewing Techniques in Ancient Mesopotamia*. Journal of the American Oriental Society Supplement 10.

UNIT III

VARIATION IN CONTEMPORARY FOOD SYSTEMS: PLUSES AND MINUSES

Anthropologists are interested in what our ancestors foraged for lunch, as well as how contemporary peoples living in different parts of the world obtain an adequate diet. How do native peoples in small villages deep in the rain forests of the Amazon find enough to eat? There are no markets to buy food. How could it be that small-scale farmers in some developing countries do not get enough to eat? How could that happen when they are the ones growing the crops? What led to the rise in food prices in 2008 that spurred protests in major cities in the Middle East? These kinds of questions are fundamental to our understanding, and precisely the kinds of questions nutritional anthropologists are particularly interested in.

The following chapters provide examples of food acquisition strategies in groups living in different places (Figure 1) and making a living in different ways. The examples we have chosen include subsistence agriculture in the Amazon and pastoralism in East Africa as practiced by people who produce almost all of their own food, and subsistence agriculture in rural India embedded in a market economy in which people produce some portion of their own food. For contrast we include an example of industrialized food production in the United States—few producing for many. The last paper in the section provides an overview of the current food crisis, i.e., the rise in global food prices that has made it difficult for some people to get enough to eat. The chapter by Darna Dufour, "Use of Tropical Rainforests by Native Amazonians," focuses on Tukanoan Indians in the Amazon who produce virtually all of their own food. Their agricultural system is based on swidden or shifting cultivation, an ancient agricultural system and one still prominent in the tropics. They supplement their agricultural production with hunting and fishing and some collecting of wild plants and small animals such as insects. Interestingly, although Tukanoans live in one of the most diverse ecosystems on the planet, their diet is not very diverse. It is based

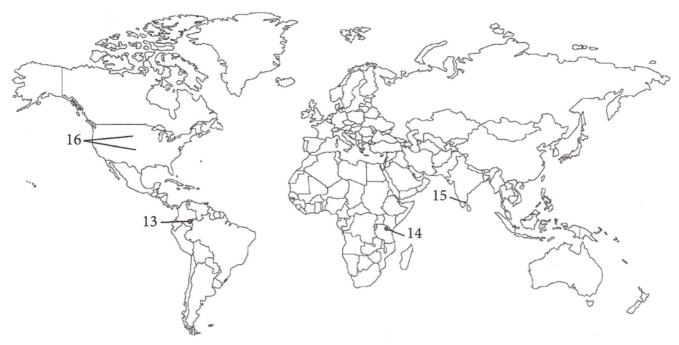

Figure 1 *Map shows the location of the groups referred to in the chapters in this section by chapter number: 13 = Tukanoans, Vaupes region, Colombia; 14 = Maasai pastoralists, Northern Tanzania; 15 = farmers, Kolli Hills region, Tamil Nadu, India; 16 = ranchers and feedlot operators in South Dakota and Kansas, United States.*

on cassava (manioc, a root crop), which is prepared primarily as a bread, and fish. Some 80 percent or more of all the food energy in the diet comes from cassava. For an average adult woman or man living in the United States, that would be equivalent to eating 1.5 to 2 pounds of bread a day.

The chapter by McCabe, Leslie, and DeLuca, "Adopting Cultivation to Remain Pastoralists" is based on their research with the Maasai, one of a number of pastoralist groups living in the dry grassland environments of Africa. The Maasai have traditionally derived much of their sustenance from the milk, blood, and meat of their herd animals and maize, which they obtained by selling animals. The animals they herd are primarily cattle, and the Maasai move frequently within their territory to find adequate pasture and water for their cattle and water for themselves. In essence, pastoralism functions as a system to convert plant foods unsuitable for human consumption (grasses and shrubs) to milk and meat. From the point of view of human nutrition, this is a conversion of low-quality plant food to high-quality animal foods.

The diet of pastoralist groups like the Maasai varies seasonally because their livestock produce more milk in the wet (rainy) season when pasture is abundant. When their diet was studied in the 1980s, the Maasai obtained 74% of their calories from milk in the wet season and only 48% in the dry season (Galvin, 1992). In the dry season when their livestock produced less milk they relied more heavily on meat, blood, and fat (12% of calories in the dry season versus 2% in the wet), and on cereal grains (60% of calories in the dry season versus 24% in the wet). For the average adult female in the United States consuming 2000 kcal per day, a diet similar to the Maasai wet season diet would be roughly equal to 7.5 cups of milk (almost 2 quarts), 1.2 ounces of meat (a very small portion), and 3.4 cups of cooked maize meal (such as grits or polenta). In the dry season it would be roughly equivalent to about 2.8 cups of milk, 7 ounces of meat, and 8.4 cups of cooked maize meal. This is not a very diverse diet!

McCabe and his co-authors discuss changes over time in Maasai subsistence strategies that involve diversification into maize agriculture. As McCabe and colleagues note, the Maasai have long consumed maize, but before the 1970s they purchased it with money from the sale of animals and animal products. In interviews with the Maasai people, the authors found that the diversification of their subsistence strategy to include maize agriculture has been driven by a number of factors including desires to consume more maize, have more food available, and to protect themselves against the need to sell livestock to buy grain and other necessities.

The chapter by Elizabeth Finnis, " 'Now It Is an Easy Life': Women's Accounts of Cassava, Millets, and Labor in South India," also describes a change in subsistence strategies. In this case it is the Malaiyalis, small-scale farmers in rural India who have replaced their traditional staple crop, millet, with rice. Interestingly, people said they preferred millet for its taste and healthful qualities, but changed to rice because it could be processed (hulled and polished) mechanically, whereas millet had to be pounded by hand,

a labor intensive process. This chapter reminds us that subsistence agriculture requires considerable physical work to grow crops as well as to process them for consumption. This paper also makes one wonder if the tradition of consuming millet, and benefiting from its higher micronutrient (vitamins and minerals) content, could be preserved by introducing mechanical milling.

How does the current food production system in the United States compare with the three chapters above? Most striking is the fact that little food seems to make it directly from farmers' fields or herds to the table. How could this be? The reality is that most of the food is produced by relatively few farmers on large mechanized farms and animal facilities. It is then sold directly to food processing facilities, which often take foods apart and remake them in novel ways before inserting them into elaborate packages. The packages are then transported to markets throughout the country, and sometimes the world. Think about a box of breakfast cereal like Kellogg's Corn Pops. It could have been made from maize grown in Nebraska, but "puffed" and sugarcoated in a General Mills factory in Illinois with sugar from sugar beets grown in Colorado and processed in Michigan.

Michael Pollan's chapter, "Power Steer," describes one segment of the industrialized food production system in the United States: beef. The first part of the system, allowing cattle to graze on natural grasslands, has not been industrialized. The industrialized portion begins when the animals are about 7 months old, weaned and moved to feed lots for fattening where they are fed on grain produced in the agricultural segment of the system. From there, at 14 to 16 months of age, they move to meat packing plants and end up in tidy packages on supermarket shelves throughout the country. Contrasts with the Maasai system of animal husbandry are striking.

A plus of the industrialized food production system is that it can produce very large amounts of food. A minus is the energy cost. Because the entire system runs on fossil fuel (farm machinery, fertilizers, pesticides, and processing machines) it is not efficient in terms of energy inputs relative to outputs. For example, in California in the 1980s the ratio of energy inputs to output was about 1 to 2.1 (Pimentel and Pimentel, 2008); that is, for every calorie of energy put into the system, we get 2.1 calories of rice. The Tukanoan, Maasai, and Malaiyalis food production systems, on the other hand, produce much less food but are more efficient in terms of energy use. For example, if the Malaiyalis cultivate rice like farmers in the Philippines or Borneo they may have an input/output ratio of 1 to 3.3 or as high as 1 to 7 (Pimentel and Pimentel, 2008). These traditional farmers can provide diets that are adequate, even though they have little diversity. A real plus of the Tukanoan, Maasai, and Malaiyalis food production systems is that they are probably sustainable over the long term, whereas our industrialized system may not be.

Industrialized food production systems in the United States and other developed countries funnel some of their production into trade networks that carry staple cereal grains, sugar, vegetable oils, and other products to all parts of the globe. Given the access to foods that these trade networks provide, local populations can and sometimes do abandon the production of staple food crops like cereal grains, and instead rely on trade networks. The inherent danger of this arrangement is that rapid increases in the global price of cereal grains can lead to crisis situations in which people cannot afford the cost of grains. On the other hand, local populations that continue to produce their own food are insulated against the shock of food price increases on the global market.

The last paper in the section is really about the trade networks that move foods from one place to another. These trade networks allow us to overcome environmental factors that are limiting in a particular place. For example, it is nearly impossible to grow maize in Scotland because of the limited sunlight, and probably impossible to grow a cool climate crop, like wheat, in the Amazon. Trade networks also allow us to move food to people suffering famine conditions due to natural disasters like drought and human-made disasters like warfare. They are, however, costly in terms of fossil fuel and countries that become dependent on them for their dietary staples are vulnerable to price fluctuations. It is precisely this vulnerability that is the focus of the paper by David Himmelgreen and colleagues, "Anthropological Perspectives on the Global Food Crisis." In it they describe some of the causes and consequences of the dramatic increases in food prices in 2006–2008 that were spawned by the global economic recession. During this period the prices of cereal grains (wheat, maize, rice) increased three to five times, and led to crisis situations in which people in some countries could not afford to feed themselves, and their nutritional situation deteriorated. Himmelgreen and coauthors end their paper with ideas of the ways in which anthropologists can contribute to finding solutions to food crises.

The first four chapters in this section provide brief descriptions of four very different food production systems. What insights do they offer? The Tukanoan and Maasai systems, and likely the Malaiyalis system as well, are powered by human labor and the sun energy necessary for plant growth. They are probably sustainable but offer limited dietary variety. Do we have to choose between sustainability and dietary variety? Could we develop a livestock production system in the United States based on solar energy? Would it produce enough beef to satisfy current demand, or would people need to be willing to eat less beef? Could global food networks be reimagined to optimize for sustainable production systems and at the same time ensure that all people had access to adequate food?

SUGGESTIONS FOR THINKING AND DOING NUTRITIONAL ANTHROPOLOGY

1. Recall the foods you ate yesterday. How many different types of foods did you eat? Did you eat a lot of similar foods, like different types of starches?
2. How many of these foods were grown within 10 or 20 miles of where you live? If you could only eat foods grown with 50 miles of where you live, what would your diet be like?
3. Take a walk around your local supermarket. How many types of foods look like they came directly from a farmer's field or dairy barn? What percentage are they of all foods in the supermarket?
4. Look at the labels on your foods. How many of them contain corn, high fructose corn syrup, or some other type of food? Is your diet truly diverse?
5. Eat a Maasai diet for day. Describe the experience. Could you manage? How did it make you feel?

References

Galvin KA. 1992. Nutritional ecology of pastoralists in dry tropical Africa. American Journal of Human Biology 4:209–221.

Pimentel D, Pimentel MH. 2008. Food Energy and Society. Third edition. Boca Raton: CRC Press.

Suggested Further Reading

Adams C, Murrieta R, Neves W, Harris M. 2006. Amazonian Peasant Societies in a Changing Environment. Springer. A comprehensive collection of papers describing sustainable development, diet and health in the Amazon.

Finnis E. 2007. The Political Ecology of Dietary Transitions: Agricultural Change, Environment, and Economics in the Kolli Hills, India. Agriculture and Human Values 24:343–353. An article that provides a look at the broader context of agricultural changes in the Kolli Hills of India.

Pollan M. 2006. The Omnivore's Dilemma. New York: Penguin Press. An eye-opening account of food production and marketing in the United States.

CHAPTER 13

Use of Tropical Rainforests by Native Amazonians

Darna L. Dufour

(1990)

Indigenous peoples have lived in the rainforests of Amazonia for a long time, probably thousands of years. They were once more numerous and occupied more of Amazonia than they do today. Those groups known ethnographically live in interfluvial regions and share a broadly similar subsistence pattern based on horticulture, hunting, fishing, and collecting. They provide the best example of sustainable use of tropical rainforests under low population densities.

Of the ways in which Amerindians use the rainforest, the best documented are their diverse, multistoried agricultural plots, or swiddens. More recently studied is their management of swidden fallows, in which annual crops are combined with perennial tree crops and the natural process of reforestation. Some groups also modify what appears to be primary forest by planting along trailsides and campsites. The result of their agricultural practices is a mosaic of vegetational patches in different stages of succession and under differing degrees of management. This vegetational mosaic is then used for food, materials, and medicinals, as well as for hunting game animals.

The objectives of this article are briefly to summarize the history of indigenous peoples, describe some of the contributions anthropology and allied disciplines have made to understanding how these peoples use tropical rainforests, and, finally, to compare this knowledge briefly with patterns of use characteristic of other populations. Many examples are drawn from the Tukanoan Indians in the Colombian Vaupes region in Northwest Amazonia, the area with which I am most familiar.

HISTORY OF NATIVE AMAZONIANS

When the Europeans arrived, the indigenous population of Amazonia was much greater than it is today. One estimate is that the Amerindians numbered approximately 6.8 million in an area of almost 10 million km[2] (Denevan 1976)[1]. Population density was highest in the floodplains of the major rivers, or what is referred to as *várzea*, and along the Atlantic coast. Early explorers such as G. Carvajal and F. Orellana reported dense settlements along the banks of the Amazon in the 1540s and a level of social organization

Darna L. Dufour, "Use of tropical rainforests by Native Amazonians." *BioScience* 40 (1990): 652–659. Reprinted with permission.

referred to as a chiefdom (Roosevelt 1989). The remains of large middens (refuse heaps), as well as the extent and depth of *terra preta do indio*[2] (Indian black earth) provide additional evidence that the riparian zones of major rivers were heavily populated (Roosevelt 1989, Smith 1980). The interior forests and savannas, or *terra firme*, appear to have been much more sparsely populated (Denevan 1976).

The indigenous population in the floodplain declined rapidly, and, by only 150 years after Orellana's expedition, the chiefdoms were extinct (Roosevelt 1989). The severe depopulation that followed this contact is assumed to have been the result of a combination of disease, slavery, and warfare. The rate of population decline in the more isolated interior forest areas was probably lower than in the floodplain, because many of these groups had only sporadic contact with outsiders until well into this century (Denevan 1976).

In the early 1970s, the indigenous population of Amazonia was estimated at less than 500,000 (Denevan 1976). In Brazil alone, the population dropped between 1900 and 1957 from approximately 1 million to less than 200,000 (Ribeiro 1967). Amerindians are now confined to interior forests and savannas, and the once densely populated floodplain is home to *caboclos*, the descendants of detribalized Indians and early European immigrants (Moran 1974, Parker et al. 1983). However, even in *terra firme*, it is clear that no present-day indigenous villages are as large as some of the villages were in the past (Nimuendajú 1939, Smith 1980). Understanding of indigenous use of Amazonian ecosystems is limited to *terra firme* forests, and these forests themselves may have been more heavily used in the past.

AMERINDIAN USE OF FORESTS FOR AGRICULTURE

Swidden Plots

The traditional indigenous agricultural system is based on swidden cultivation (also known as slash-and-burn or shifting cultivation). In essence, this system involves felling and burning a patch of forest, cultivating and harvesting crops for a period of several years, and then allowing the forest to regrow for 15 years or more before the site is cleared again (Beckerman 1987). The felling and burning releases

Table 1 Number of Crop Species, Cassava Varieties, and Varieties of Other Crops in Sample Units of Four Tukanoan Swidden Plots in Northwest Amazonia

Swidden	Size (ha)	Sample units	Crop species	Cultivars Cassava	Other
Primary forest*	0.35	20	17	48	25
Primary forest	0.15	10	2	17	1
Rastrojo[†] (60-year)	0.78	29	10	39	11
Rastrojo (25-year)	0.70	25	6	37	5

Unpublished data from 1986. Sampling units were randomly selected circles of 2-meter radius. All plants in each circle were tagged and then identified by the garden owner. Names of cassava cultivars were systematically checked for overlap with each garden owner, but naming of cultivars between swidden plots was not cross-checked.
*Tall forests, not cut in the memory of current inhabitants, is assumed to be primary forest.
†*Rastrojo* is local Spanish for successional forest. Ages are estimated from informants' histories of use.

the nutrients stored in the forest biomass and makes them available to cultivated crops. The long fallow restores soil fertility, protects the physical properties of the soil, allows time for nutrient accumulation in the biomass, and helps control agricultural pest populations.

Amerindian swiddens are typically small, 0.4–0.6-hectare (Beckerman 1987), polycultural plots (i.e., they are planted in more than one crop simultaneously). Multiple varieties of the staple crops are planted in each swidden. Most groups of Amerindians also have monocrop swidden plots devoted to the dietary staple. The predominate staples are cassava (*Manihot esculenta* Crantz), plantains and bananas (*Musa* sp.).

Cassava, or manioc, is a perennial shrub grown for its starchy roots. It is native to the neotropics, and well adapted to the low-fertility, acidic soils common in *terra firme* (Cock 1985). Cassava is cyanogenic, and varieties are recognized as being either bitter or sweet (i.e., containing high or low amounts of cyanide). The bitter-sweet distinction determines culinary use: bitter varieties are elaborately processed to reduce cyanide levels before being consumed, whereas the sweet varieties can simply be peeled and boiled (Dufour 1988).

The agricultural plots of Tukanoan Indians in northwestern Amazonia provide a good example of traditional swidden cultivation. Swidden plots are felled by individual households in well-drained soils in both primary and successional forests. Most households fell swiddens in both types of forest. Bitter cassava, the dietary staple, is densely planted over nearly the entire garden surface. Other crops, such as taro (*Colocasia* spp.), sweet potato (*Ipomoea* sp.), arrowroot (*Maranta ruiziana*), pineapple (*Anana sativa*), chili peppers (*Capsicum annuum*), mafafa (*Xanthosoma mafafa*), lulo (*Solanum* sp.), bananas, and plantains, are interplanted where microenvironmental conditions (such as drainage and ash concentration) are deemed most suitable. They are planted toward the center of the garden where the regrowth of the forest will be most easily delayed by weeding. Coca (*Erythroxylum coca*), which is a shrub, and tree crops such as guama (*Inga* sp.), uvilla (*Pourouma cercropiaefolia*), and peachpalm (*Bactris gasipaes*) are also interplanted with cassava toward the center of the garden.

Tukanoan swidden plots are polycultural. They are polyvarietal as well, but the diversity of cassava varieties is much greater than the diversity of the other crop species. For example, in identifying cultivated plants in subsample units in four Tukanoan swiddens[3] (Table 1), we found that each contained between 2 and 16 different crops, but as many as 17 to 48 different cassava varieties. On average, the four most common cassava varieties in each swidden accounted for only 38% of all cassava plants identified. We also found that, of all the cassava varieties reported, only the one or two sweet varieties in each swidden were planted in a recognizable patch. The remaining varieties were all interplanted. We found 4 to 17 bitter varieties per sampling unit (12.57 m^2), with a mean of 7.8 ± 3.72 (Figure 1).

Tukanoan swiddens are most intensively used and managed from approximately the 12th through the 24th month after burning. During this time, the first cassava crop is being harvested and some areas of the swidden are weeded for replanting. A second, smaller cassava crop is planted in swiddens with good yields as the first is being harvested, so that cassava harvesting continues through approximately the 36th month. Other crops are harvested as they mature and are needed. Tree crops such as uvilla and peachpalm

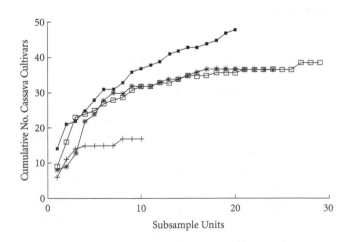

Figure 1 *Cumulative number of cassava varieties in subsample units in four Tukanoan swiddens. Subsample units were randomly placed circles, 2 meters in radius.*

mature in approximately three years and are harvested until forest regrowth dominates the plot.

Households establish one or two new swidden plots each year, and therefore they have access to a number of swiddens in different stages at any time: a newly planted swidden with immature crops, a cassava-producing swidden, and one or more older swidden or fallows with fruit trees, fish poisons, and medicinal plants. Some of the plots are contiguous and form a mosaic of patches of successional vegetation. Others are widely dispersed to take advantage of areas of particularly good agricultural soil and/or serve as bases for hunting and fishing.

Swidden Fallows

The transition between a swidden and a swidden fallow is not sharp, and, certainly from the Amerindian point of view, the plot is not abandoned after the principal crop has been harvested. Denevan and Padoch (1988) examined the swiddens of Bora Indians living in the humid tropical rainforests of Peru at different stages of regrowth from the time of cutting. They found a continuum from a swidden dominated by cultivated grasses, forbs, and shrubs; to an orchard fallow phase, in which there was a combination of fruit trees, smaller cultigens, and natural vegetation; to a forest fallow that still contained economically useful plants, but became progressively more and more like the surrounding forest (Table 2). Some of the useful plants were non-domesticated plants that appeared in the natural reforestation sequence and were protected.

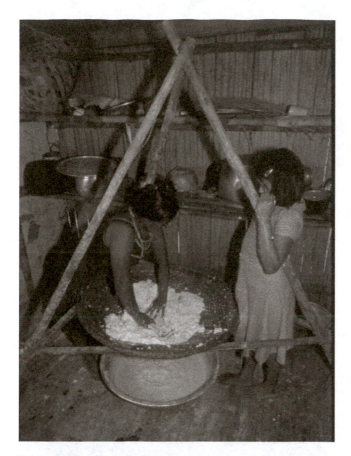

Tukanoan woman sieving grated cassava roots to extract the starch. This extraction is part of the process used to make cassava bread, the dietary staple in Northwest Amazonia. Photograph courtesy of Paul N. Patmore.

Table 2 Harvestable Plants Found in Bora Fields and Fallows at Different Stages of Regrowth after Cutting

Stage	Cultigens	Other useful plants
Newly planted field (0–3 mo)	None	Dry firewood
New field (3–9 mo)	Maize, rice, cowpeas	Various useful early successional species
Mature field (9 mo–2 yr)	Manioc, some tubers,* bananas, cocona, other quick-maturing crops	Some useful vines and herbs in abandoned edge
Transitional field (1–5 yr)	Replanted manioc, peanuts, pineapple, guava, caimito, uvilla, avocado, cashew, coca, barbasco, chili peppers, miscellaneous tubers	Useful medicinals and other plants within field; on edges, seedlings of useful trees appear; saplings of *Cercropia* and *Ochroma lagopus* in abandoned edges
Transitional fruit field (4–6 yr)	Peach palm, bananas, uvilla, caimito, guava, annatto, coca, some tubers, propagules of pineapple, other crops	Many useful soft construction woods and firewoods, palms (including *Astrocaryum*), useful vines, and understory aroids
Orchard fallow (6–12 yr)	Peach palm, some uvilla, macambo, propages	Useful plants as above and self-seeding *Inga*
Forest fallow (12–30 yr)	Macambo, umari, breadfruit, copal	Self-seeding macambo and umari; high forest successional species appearing; some hardwoods becoming harvestable (e.g., *Iriartea* sp.); many large palms (*Astrocarym hunicungo, Euterpe* sp., *Jessenia bataua*)
Old fallow (30+ yr)	Macambo, umari	Numerous construction, medicinal, handicraft, and food plants

Plant identifications are as follows: Annatto (*Bixa orellana*), avocado (*Persea americana*), banana (*Musa* sp.), barbasco (*Lonchocarpus* sp.), breadfruit (*Artocarpus incisa*), caimito (*Pouteria caimito*), cashew (*Anacardium occidentale*), chili pepper (*Capsicum* sp.), coca (*Erythroxylon coca*), cocona (*Solanum* sp.), copal (*Hymenaea courbaril*), cowpeas (*Vigna unguiculata*), guava (*Inga* sp.), macambo (*Theobroma bicolor*), maize (*Zea mays*), manioc (*Manihot esculenta*), peach palm (*Bactris gasipaes*), peanut (*Arachis hypogaea*), pineapple (*Ananas comosus*), rice (*Oryza sativa*), umari (*Poraqueilba sericea*), uvilla (*Pourouma cercropiaefolia*).
*These tubers include cocoyams (*Xanthosoma* sp.), sweet potatos (*Ipomoea batatas*), and yams (*Dioscorea trifida macrocarpa*)
(Adapted from Denevan et al. 1984.).

The Bora, therefore, practice a form of agroforestry in which perennial tree crops are combined with natural forest regrowth (Denevan et al. 1984). Similar practices have been reported for other Amerindians and appear to be widespread (Balée and Gély 1989, Eden and Andrade 1987, Harris 1971, Posey 1984).

Forest-Fields and Trailside Plantings

Posey (1984) has documented among Kayapo Indians in Brazil a much broader system of forest management, which he refers to as *nomadic agriculture*. Traditionally the Kayapo were seminomadic and spent much of the year trekking along an extensive system of trails between the Tocantins and Araguaya rivers and the north-south limits of the Planalto and Amazon rivers.

Anthropologists had assumed that the Kayapo lived by hunting and collecting wild plant foods during these treks. However, Posey (1984) found that the trailsides and campsites were actually planted with "numerous varieties of yams, sweet potatoes, Marantacea, Cissus, Zingiberaceae, Araceae, Cannaceae, and other unidentified, edible, tuberous plants," as well as fruit trees and medicinal plants. This planting was a conscious attempt to replicate naturally occuring concentrations of resources in primary forest. The plants used included both domesticates and semidomesticates (i.e., plants transplanted from primary and successional forest). These semidomesticates were also transplanted to old swiddens and naturally occuring forest gaps.

Ecological Effects of Traditional Agricultural Practices

The ecological effects of traditional Amerindian agricultural practices are still poorly understood. Swidden cultivation, as practiced by Amerindians with short cropping and long fallows, is considered a relatively benign disturbance (Herrera et al. 1981), and it does not seriously impair ecosystem function (Uhl 1987).

At the level of the individual swidden plot, a number of traditional farming practices are considered beneficial. For example, the use of shade trees, mixed cropping of species that differ in phenology, dense spacing of crops, and fallowing all help preserve soil organic matter, which is a critical factor in the maintenance of soil fertility in the deeply weathered and leached soils common in Amazonia (Ewel 1986). The species richness of the plots is assumed to confer pest protection and decrease the risk of complete crop failure (Ewel 1986; c.f. Brown and Ewel 1987). Planting many varieties of a staple crop may fulfill the same functions (Balée and Gély 1989, Beckerman 1983, Boster 1983, Parker et al. 1983).

Forest regeneration during the fallow is considered a key to the sustainability of swidden systems (Ewel 1986). Amerindian management of the successional process, by

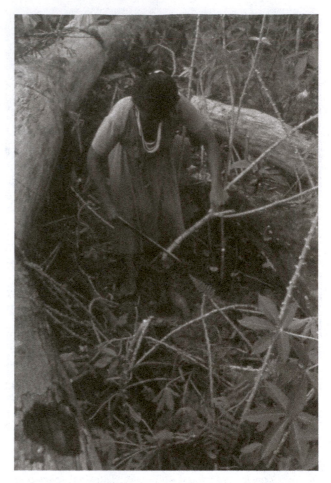

Tukanoan woman harvesting cassava roots in a representative swidden in Northwest Amazonia. The palmate-leafed plant at lower right is cassava. Photograph courtesy of Paul N. Patmore.

the selective weeding out of certain trees and the protecting and planting of others, appears to have a greater impact on species diversity than it does on forest regrowth in stature and biomass (Uhl 1987). Uhl (1983) has suggested that heavily managed successions in areas such as house gardens may grow to forest stature as fast or faster than natural ones (Uhl 1983).

Recovery to primary forest in terms of biomass and species diversity, however, is slow. Current estimates are that in areas like San Carlos de Rio Negro it will take 100 years or more for traditionally farmed sites to return to primary forest, and sites suffering greater disturbance will take even longer (Saldarriaga 1985, Uhl and Murphy 1981).

Given this long period of recovery, and the practice of cutting swidden plots yearly, it is clear that human settlements will be surrounded by a complex mosaic of agricultural and agroforestry plots, as well as forest in various stages of regrowth. In addition, in some areas, the species composition of the forests themselves will be the result of human endeavors to increase the density of useful plants. Such vegetational mosaics may offer advantages in terms of pest protection and be a way of risk spreading (Eden and Andrade 1987, Ewel 1986). For indigenous populations, these landscapes offer clear advantages in hunting and collecting.

AMERINDIAN USE OF FORESTS FOR HUNTING, FISHING, AND COLLECTING

Hunting, fishing, and collecting are integral components of the subsistence pattern of Amerindians that cannot be considered apart from swidden agriculture (Balée and Gély 1989). In nutritional terms, these activities provide the sources of dietary protein, fat, and other nutrients that are critical supplements to the high-carbohydrate staples.

Faunal Resources

Amerindians hunt a wide variety of animals, the numerically most important of which are primates and rodents (Redford and Robinson 1987). One of the explicitly recognized functions of swidden plots is to attract game animals for hunting. The roots, tubers, and low-successional vegetation of swidden are attractive to such game animals as rodents, peccary, and deer.

Crop losses due to predation are routinely compensated for by over-planting (Balée and Gély 1989, Carneiro 1983). Tukanoan women, for example, plant extra sweet-cassava for a small rodent, boo (*Dasyprocta punctada*, which averages approximately 2 kg in weight), and only complain when "he" seems to be eating more than "his" share. This rodent

accounted for more than 20% of all animals killed during three-month-long observation periods in 1977, and women hunting in gardens with dogs were responsible for almost half of all kills (Dufour 1981).

The fruit trees in swidden fallows are attractive to a number of large game animals, especially tapir (*Tapirus terrestris*) and peccary (*Tayassu* spp.; Balée and Gély 1989, Chagnon and Hames 1979, Denevan et al. 1984, Dufour 1981, Posey 1984). The Kayapo purposefully disperse their gardens so as to attract game animals over a large area (Parker et al. 1983, Posey 1982, 1983, 1984). For this reason, Posey (1984) suggests that old swiddens be called "game-farm-orchards."

The effect of indigenous hunting practices on animal biomass and diversity is a complex question. Posey (1982) has argued that certain game species would not occur in forest unmodified by humans, and several of the important mammals such as deer, tapir, and collared peccary may reach higher densities in modified areas. Further, not all animals that frequent the swiddens are taken for food (Ross 1978), and researchers have described a number of ways in which the Amerindians may be regulating their hunting of game animals (Balée 1985, Beckerman 1980, Reichel-Dolmatoff 1976).

The only long-term study of the effects of indigenous hunting is Vickers' (1988) documentation of the hunting returns in a Siona-Secoya village in northeastern Ecuador over a 10-year period. His data suggest that some species were being depleted locally. These included the woolly monkey (*Lagothrix lagotricha*), a large forest understory bird called the curassow (*Mitu salvini*), and a large ground-dwelling bird, the trumpeter (*Psophia crepitans*). Other

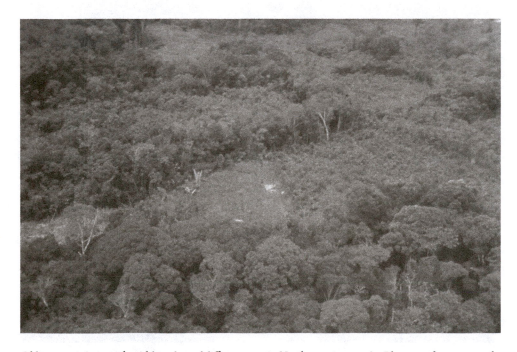

Oblique aerial view of swidden plots of different ages in Northwest Amazonia. Photograph courtesy of Paul N. Patmore.

species, such as peccaries, tapir, deer, other primates, other birds, rodents, and reptiles, did not, however, show evidence of depletion. These data support the suggestion that the patches of successional vegtation created in swidden cultivation may allow some game species to survive near human settlements (Redford and Robinson 1987).

Fishing. The majority of the Amerindians in Amazonia rely on fish, rather than game, as their principal source of animal protein. In blackwater areas where rivers are small, such as northwestern Amazonia, fish can be considered part of the forest ecosystem, because nonpredatory fish feed primarily on forest products (Knöppel 1970). Tukanoan Indians recognize the importance of forests to fish (Chernela 1985, Dufour 1981). The flood forest, or igapo, is an important feeding ground for fish. The Indians have protected it from deforestation (Chernela 1985).

Other Tukanoan practices, such as the use of fish poisons, may negatively affect the local fish populations, but it is not clear to what extent. The fish poisons are the crushed roots, stems, and/or leaves of a variety of wild and cultivated plants. Their use was traditionally controlled by the village shaman (Reichel-Dolmatoff 1976) and typically restricted to small forest streams that could be temporarily dammed. The effects of these poisons appear to be temporary (several hours) and highly localized.

Collecting. Small vertebrates, such as frogs, as well as invertebrates, are important faunal resources that are collected. The use of insects for food is widespread (Dufour 1987, Posey 1978). The more commonly collected and consumed insects appear to be ants (especially *Atta* spp.), termites, and larvae of both Coleoptera (especially Buprestidae, Curculionidae, and Scarabaeidae) and Lepidoptera. Tukanoans harvest ants and termites at low but constant rates. Nests are never destroyed, and some colonies in favorable locations are actively protected. Palm grubs (Curculionidae) are a managed resouce: palms are cut with the expectation that they will be invaded by weevils and the larvae can be harvested at a later date.

Floral resources

Amerindians collect a wide range of plants and plant products as food and for use in housing, tool manufacture, craft production, and medicine. The role of collected plant foods in the diet ranges from trail snacks and emergency foods to important sources of nutrients. Palm fruits and Brazil nuts are well-known examples of wild plant foods. Less well-known are oil seeds such as *Erisma japura* and the legume *Monopteryx angustifolia*, which are seasonally important in the diets of some groups (Dufour and Zarucchi 1979).

Plant foods are collected from the entire range of successional vegetation types, from nondomesticated herbs such as *Phytolacca rivinoides*, which grow in newly burnt swiddens, to the seeds of the rubber trees, *Hevea* sp., which grow in primary forests (Dufour 1981). In collecting plant parts (fruits, nuts, and seeds) from the litter on the forest floor or from living trees, humans are competing with other herbivores, but the impact of their activity on the forest is minimal. When trees are felled to harvest fruit or other parts, the impact is greater. Localized depletion of products such as cedar (*Cedrela odorata*) for canoes and palms for roof thatch has been documented (Vickers 1988).

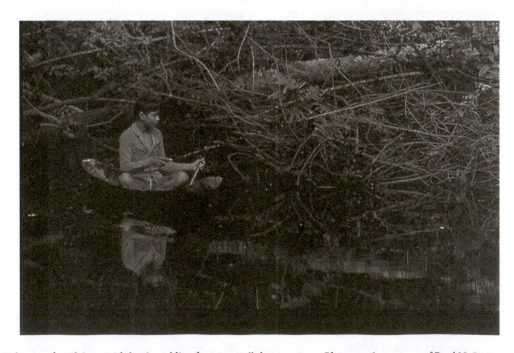

Tukanoan boy fishing with hook and line from a small dugout canoe. Photograph courtesy of Paul N. Patmore.

Some of the more important collected plant foods appear to be from anthropogenic forests, that is, forests that are the result of human disturbance. Balée (1989) has argued that babassu palm (*Orbignya phalerata*) forests and Brazil nut (*Bertholletia excelsa*) forests, among others, should be considered anthropogenic, because the predominance of these trees in the forest is associated with evidence of human settlement. Babassu palms tend to be the dominant, or at least an important species in burned forest clearings because of the manner in which they germinate: the apical meristem grows downward, rather than upward, and remains protected underground for a year or more (Anderson and Anderson 1985, Balée 1989). Brazil nut forests, at least in some areas, appear on or near *terra preta* sites (Balée 1989). Furthermore, Kayapo actually plant Brazil nuts as a source of food for themselves and the game they hunt (Posey 1985). Balée (1989) estimates that at least 11.8% of *terra firme* in the Brazilian Amazon is covered by anthropogenic forests.

CONTRASTS WITH NONINDIGENOUS FARMERS

Indigneous peoples are not the only ones who have a detailed knowledge of the local Amazonian ecosystems in which they live. The long-term residents of Amazonia, the *caboclos* (also *riberenos*, *mestizos*, or *campesinos*), do as well. The *caboclos* are the rural peasantry of Amazonia, and they are now the principal inhabitants of the *várzea*, the narrow but productive floodplain of Amazonian rivers (Parker et al. 1983). Their use of resources resembles that of Amerindians, from whom many are descended, but they are more oriented to market economies and typically quick to respond to market opportunities (Padoch 1988, Parker et al. 1983).

For example, the *caboclos*, studied by Padoch (1988) along the Ucayali River in Peru, recognized a complex set of ecological zones in the riparian environment and used them to advantage. They cash-cropped rice on the seasonally flooded mud flats of the river and cultivated subsistence and market crops on the *restingas* (river levees). On the poorer soils of the higher areas, they had intensively managed for subsistence crops the swidden plots, which gradually turned into orchards and then forest fallows. Some orchards were used for as long as 30 years, and the forest fallows were weeded selectively to maintain a high proportion of useful species.

Like Amerindians, *caboclos* use a wide variety of forest products as food, medicinals, fiber, and building materials. They also collect nontimber forest products such as palm fruits, Brazil nuts, and rubber for commercial sale (Padoch 1988, Parker et al. 1983). At least for Brazil nuts and rubber, their collection practices are productive and environmentally conservative, and they provide examples of the sustainable use of Amazonian forests (Fearnside 1988).

The newest immigrants to Amazonian rainforests are the *colonos*, or colonists. *Colonos* are the subsistence farmers who went and still go to the Amazon as part of resettlement schemes promoted by government agencies (Moran 1988). The majority see the rainforest for the first time when they arrive in the Amazon, and, understandably, they have little knowledge of how to make a living in it.

In his study of Brazil's Transamazon Resettlement Scheme in the 1970s, Moran (1988) found that the *colonos* treated the forest as an enemy rather than a resource. They cleared more land per year, but cultivated less, and they were

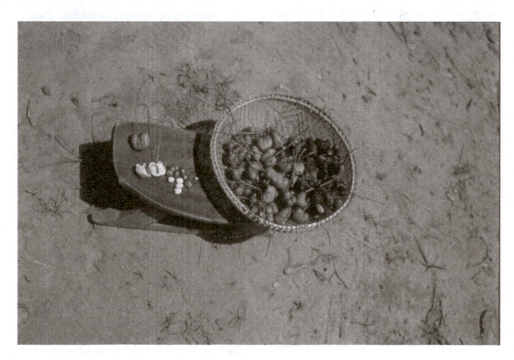

Seeds of Heavea brasiliensis, *a seasonally important wild plant food in Northwest Amazonia. Photograph courtesy of Paul N. Patmore.*

less successful agriculturally than *caboclos* living in the same area. They gradually learned, however, to clear less land, work it more intensively, and use some of the resources of the forest.

CHANGING VIEWS OF NATIVE AMAZONIAN RESOURCE USE

Recent studies have considerably refined understanding of the ways in which Amerindians use the tropical rainforest. Originally anthropologists and ecologists envisioned swiddens, fallows, and forests as more or less separate entities. Now, however, we understand more clearly the process of swiddens becoming forests, the length of time involved, and the degree to which human management is part of the transition.

The distinctions between domesticated and wild plants, or natural and managed forest, are also not as sharp as we thought they were. Much of what has been considered natural forest in Amazonia is probably the result of hundreds of years of human use and management (Posey 1984, Smith 1980). We are not certain how specific human activities may have changed Amazonian ecosystems over the long term, but they were certainly an essential component. Future research will have to take into account the long history of occupation and use of these forests by Amerindians.

The agricultural systems of Amerindians and *caboclos* have proven to be more sophisticated and complex than we imagined. There is a growing recognition that these agricultural systems have a great deal to offer in the design of sustainable agroecosystems (Denevan et al. 1984, Ewel 1986, Hart 1980). Further study of these systems that explicitly recognizes and incorporates the detailed knowledge and long experience of Amerindians and *caboclos* is needed. Such study will require the collaboration of anthropologists and ecologists.

Notes

Funding for research in the Northwest Amazon was provided by the National Science Foundation (BSN-8519490). I am very grateful to R. Wilshusen for his invaluable assistance in mapping and sampling Tukanoan swiddens and his helpful comments on the manuscript. W. Balée kindly provided prepublication copies of two of his papers.

1. The use of Amazonia in this article follows that of Denevan (1976). It refers to greater Amazonia, which includes the tropical lowlands and plateaus east of the Andes and north of the Tropic of Capricorn, except for the Gran Chaco region. It is an area considerably larger than the drainage of the Amazon and its tributaries.

2. *Terra preta do indio* is a soil darkened by the residue of repeated fires. It characterizes ceramics and other remains of human activity (Smith 1980).

3. D. L. Dufour and R. Wilshusen, 1986, unpublished data.

References

Anderson, A., and S. Anderson. 1985. A "tree of life" grows in Brazil. *Nat. Hist.* 94(12): 40–47.

Balée, W. 1985. Ka'apor ritual hunting. *Hum. Ecol.* 13: 485–510.

———. 1989. The culture of Amazon forests. In D. A. Posey and W. Balée, eds. Special issue: *Resource Management in Amazonia: Indigenous and Folk Strategies. Adv. Econ. Bot.* 7: 1–21.

Balée, W., and A. Gély. 1989. Managed forest succession in Amazonia: the Ka'apor case. In D. A. Posey and W. Balée, eds. *Resource Management in Amazonia: Indigenous and Folk Strategies. Adv. Econ. Bot.* 7: 129–158.

Beckerman, S. 1980. Fishing and hunting by the Barí of Colombia. Pages 67–109 in R. B Hames, ed. *Studies in Hunting and Fishing in the Neotropics.* Bennington College, VT.

———. 1983. Barí swidden gardens: crop segregation patterns. *Hum. Ecol.* 11: 85–101.

———. 1987. Swidden in Amazonia and the Amazon rim. Pages 55–94 in B. L. Turner and S. B. Brush, eds. *Comparative Farming Systems.* Guilford Press, New York.

Boster, J. 1983. A comparison of the diversity of Jivaroan gardens with that of the tropical forest. *Hum. Ecol.* 11: 47–68.

Brown, B. J., and J. J. Ewel. 1987. Herbivory in complex and simple tropical successional ecosystems. *Ecology* 68: 108–116.

Carneiro, R. 1983. The cultivation of manioc among the Kuikuru of the upper Xingu. Pages 65–111 in R. B. Hames and W. T. Vickers, eds. *Adaptive Responses of Native Amazonians.* Academic Press, New York.

Chagnon, N., and R. B. Hames. 1979. Protein deficiency and tribal warfare in Amazonia: new data. *Science* 20: 910–913.

Chernela, J. 1985. Indigenous fishing in the neotropics: the Tukanoan Uanano of the blackwater Uaupes River basin in Brazil and Colombia. *Interciencia* 10: 78–86.

Cock, J. H. 1985. *Cassava: New Potential for a Neglected Crop.* Westview Press, Boulder, CO.

Denevan, W. M. 1976. The aboriginal population of Amazonia. Pages 205–234 in W. M. Denevan, ed. *The Native Population of the Americas.* University of Wisconsin Press, Madison.

Denevan, W. M., and C. Padoch. 1988. The Bora agroforestry project. In W. M. Denevan and C. Padoch, eds. Special issue: *Swidden-Fallow Agroforestry in the Peruvian Amazon. Adv. Econ. Bot.* 5: 1–7.

Denevan, W. M., J. M. Treacy, J. B. Alcorn, C. Padoch, J. Denslow, and S. F. Paitan. 1984. Indigenous agroforestry in the Peruvian Amazon: Bora Indian management of swidden fallows. *Interciencia* 9: 346–357.

Dufour, D. L. 1981. Household variation in energy flow in a population of tropical forest horticulturalists. Ph.D dissertation, State University of New York, Binghamton.

———. 1987. Insects as food. *Am. Anthropol.* 89: 383–397.

———. 1988. Cyanide content of Cassava (*Manihot esculenta*, Euphorbiaceae) cultivars used by Tukanoan Indians in Northwest Amazonia. *Econ. Bot.* 42: 255–266.

Dufour, D. L., and J. L. Zarucchi. 1979. Monopteryx Angustifolia and Erisma Japura: their use by indigenous peoples in the northwest Amazon. *Bot. Mus. Leaf. Harv. Univ.* 27: 69–91.

Eden, M. J., and A. Andrade. 1987. Ecological aspects of swidden cultivation among the Andoke and Witoto Indians of the Colombian Amazon. *Hum. Ecol.* 15: 339–359.

Ewel, J. J. 1986. Designing agricultural ecosystems for the humid tropics. *Annu. Rev. Ecol. Syst.* 17: 245–271.

Fearnside, P. M. 1989. Extractive reserves in Brazilian Amazonia. *BioScience* 39: 387–393.

Hames, R. B. 1979. A comparison of the efficiencies of the shotgun and the bow in neotropical forest hunting. *Hum. Ecol.* 7: 219–252.

Harris, D. R. 1971. The ecology of swidden cultivation in the Upper Orinoco rain forest, Venezuela. *Geogr. Rev.* 61: 475–495.

Hart, R. D. 1980. A natural ecosystem analog approach to the design of a successional crop system for tropical forest environments. *Biotropica* 12: 73–83.

Herrera, R., C. F. Jordan, E. Medina, and H. Klinge. 1981. How human activities disturb the nutrient cycles of a tropical rainforest in Amazonia. *Ambio* 10: 109–114.

Knöppel, H. 1970. Food of central Amazonian fishes: contribution to the nutrient ecology of Amazonian rain forest streams. *Kiel Amazoniana* 2: 257–352.

Moran, E. F. 1974. The adaptive system of the Amazonian Caboclo. Pages 136–159 in C. Wagley, ed. *Man in the Amazon*. University of Florida Press, Gainsville.

———. 1988. Following the Amazon highways. Pages 155–162 in J. S. Denslow and C. Padoch, eds. *People of the Tropical Rainforest*. University of California Press, Berkeley.

Nimuendajú, C. 1939. *The Apinaye*. Anthropological series no. 8. Catholic University of America, Washington, DC.

Padoch, C. 1988. People of the floodplain and forest. Pages 127–140 in J. S. Denslow and C. Padoch, eds. *People of the Tropical Rainforest*. University of California Press, Berkeley.

Parker, E., D. A. Posey, J. Frechione, and L. F. Da Silva. 1983. Resource exploitation in Amazonia: ethnoecological examples from four populations. *Ann. Carnegie Mus.* 52: 163–203.

Posey, D. A. 1978. Ethnoentomological survey of Amerind groups in lowland Latin America. *Fla. Entomol.* 61: 225–229.

———. 1982. Keepers of the forest. *Garden* 6: 18–24.

———. 1983. Indigenous ecological knowledge and development of the Amazon. Pages 225–256 in E. Moran, ed. *The Dilemma of Amazonian Development*. Westview Press, Boulder, CO.

———. 1984. A preliminary report on diversified management of tropical forest by the Kayapó Indians of the Brazilian Amazon. In G. T. Prance and J. A. Kallunki, eds. *Ethnobotany in the Neotropics. Adv. Econ. Bot.* 1: 112–126.

———. 1985. Indigenous management of tropical forest ecosystems: the case of the Kayapó Indians of the Brazilian Amazon. *Agroforestry Systems* 3: 139–158.

Posey, D. A., J. Frechione, J. Eddins, L. Francelino da Silva, D. Myers, D. Case, and P. Macbeath. 1984. Ethnoecology as applied anthropology in Amazon development. *Hum. Organ.* 43: 95–107.

Redford, K. H., and J. G. Robinson. 1987. The game of choice: patterns of Indian and colonist hunting in the neotropics. *Am. Amthropol.* 89: 650–667.

Reichel-Dolmatoff, G. 1976. Cosmology as ecological analysis: a view from the forest. *Man* 11: 307–318.

Ribeiro, D. 1967. Indigenous cultures and languages of Brazil. Pages 69–76 in J. H. Hopper, ed. *Indians of Brazil in the Twentieth Century*. Institute for Cross-Cultural Research, Washington, DC.

Roosevelt, A. 1989. Lost civilizations of the lower Amazon. *Nat. Hist.* 98(2): 75–83.

Ross, E. 1978. Food taboos, diet, and hunting strategy: the adaptation to animals in Amazon cultural ecology. *Curr. Anthropol.* 19: 1–19.

Saldarriaga, J. G. 1985. Forest succession in the upper Rió Negro of Colombia and Venezuela. Ph.D. dissertation, University of Tennessee, Knoxville.

Smith, N. J. H. 1980. Anthrosols and human carrying capacity in Amazonia. *Annals of the Association of American Geographers* 70: 553–566.

Uhl, C. 1983. You can keep a good forest down. *Nat. Hist.* 92(4): 71–79.

———. 1987. Factors controlling succession following slash and burn agriculture in Amazonia. *Ecology* 75: 377–407.

Uhl, C., and P. Murphy. 1981. A comparison of productivities and energy values between slash and burn agriculture and secondary succession in the upper Rió Negro region of the Amazon. *Agro-Ecosystems* 7: 63–83.

Vickers, W. T. 1988. Game depletion hypothesis of Amazonian adaptation: data from a native community. *Science* 239: 1521–1522.

CHAPTER 14

Adopting Cultivation to Remain Pastoralists: The Diversification of Maasai Livelihoods in Northern Tanzania

J. Terrence McCabe, Paul W. Leslie, and Laura DeLuca

(2010)

There are two dominant images of East African pastoral peoples. One is an image of young men—warriors—living in a pristine wilderness, moving their beloved livestock from one seasonal pasture to another, coping with the vagaries of nature and the danger of attack from wild animals. The other is of destitute families barely able to survive and most likely walking to, or living in, refugee or famine camps. One or the other of these images is promoted by NGOs, governments or tourist companies appealing to particular constituencies in the attempt to promote a product or encourage a donation. What is not often projected is an image of an African pastoralist swinging a hoe, guarding someone else's house, driving oxen in front of a plow, or, heaven forbid, driving a tractor. But it is a combination of these latter images that more accurately reflects the current reality of modern day pastoralists throughout much of Africa.

Pastoral peoples in Africa, and in fact in many areas around the world, have been rapidly diversifying their economies. Although the public images of pastoral peoples may not have kept up with this transition, those who have been studying pastoral peoples have been writing about the causes and consequences of adopting cultivation (e.g., O'Malley 2000; Brockington 2001; McCabe 2003; Homewood et al. 2005; Fratkin and Roth 2005). Anthropologists and geographers, among others, have also been writing about men, and to some extent women, migrating to find work (Batterbury 2001; May and McCabe 2004; Homewood et al. 2009) and entering the livestock trade or petty business (Little et al. 2001; Little 2003).

We (JTM and PWL) have been working with East African pastoralists for almost thirty years (first with the Turkana of Kenya and later with Maasai in northern Tanzania) and have witnessed many of the changes mentioned above. However

it was during the time that the ban on cultivation was lifted in the Ngorongoro Conservation Area (NCA) in Tanzania that we realized the importance, and potentially overwhelming rapidity, of the transition. Within a two year period following the lifting of the ban in 1992, approximately 90% of the families living in the NCA had adopted cultivation. The adoption of cultivation in the NCA had important implications for the nutrition of children, the break of a downward spiral of impoverishment due to the overselling of livestock to purchase grain, and a long-term perspective of being in control of their livelihoods, as well as for wildlife conservation (McCabe 2003). We were able to document that the human population there has been steadily increasing while the livestock population fluctuated around a long-term mean, and hypothesized that this disarticulation of human population dynamics from that of the livestock population, was the principal factor driving the transition from pure pastoralism to agro-pastoralism (McCabe 2003).

The policy restrictions on cultivation in the NCA so strongly shaped livelihood diversification that the NCA case is of limited utility for understanding the historical roots of diversification among the Maasai elsewhere. In this paper we present the results of a multi-year study of the process of livelihood diversification among the Maasai in the Loliondo area, just north of the NCA. We argue that the process is more complex than has previously been appreciated, including in some of our own publications (McCabe 1997; McCabe 2003). We support the conclusions reached by others that the motivations for adopting cultivation differed among people of different wealth categories, but further argue that those decisions were part of a larger cultural shift and were also influenced by power differentials among Maasai age sets and by government policies.

LIVELIHOOD DIVERSIFICATION

Although people like the Maasai have been primarily understood as practicing "pure pastoralism",[1] the advent of a livelihood strategy based exclusively on livestock is probably a

J. Terrence McCabe, Paul W. Leslie, and Laura DeLuca, "Adopting cultivation to remain pastoralists: the diversification of Maasai livelihoods in northern Tanzania." *Human Ecology* 38 (2010): 321–334. Reprinted with permission.

relatively recent development (Marshall 1990; Spear 1993). Marshall has argued quite convincingly that there was a change in climate approximately 2,000–3,000 years ago that resulted in a bi-modal rainfall pattern. The resulting environmental conditions permitted people in East Africa to depend on the year-round availability of milk for food (Marshall 1990). Prior to this climatic shift, pastoral peoples in East Africa combined livestock keeping with small scale cultivation, hunting and gathering, and fishing. However, even in the recent past, people like the Maasai have been divided into sections that were purely pastoral, such as the Kisongo, and sections that practiced cultivation in addition to livestock keeping, like the Parakuyu and Arusha.

During the last thirty years most of the region's purely pastoral peoples have diversified their economies. Reasons advanced to explain this change in livelihood strategies have included the alienation of rangelands due to the expansion of parks and protected areas (Homewood and Brockington 1999; McCabe 2003; Brockington 2001; Igoe 2003a, b; Goldman 2003), changes in land tenure and the privatization of land held as common property (Galaty 1994; Homewood 2004; Burnsilver 2007; Leserogol 2008), the penetration of the market economy (Ensminger 1992; Little 2003), the loss of livestock due to drought and disease (Western 1997; O'Malley 2000), and the increase in the human population while the livestock population remained steady or declined (McCabe 2003). A common theme in this literature has been that poor people are pushed into alternative livelihood strategies due to poverty, while wealthy pastoralists diversify as a risk avoidance strategy (Homewood *et al.* 2009; Brockington 2001; Little *et al.* 2001). The poor are seen as adopting cultivation, but also migrating for wage labor, selling milk (almost exclusively by women), and engaging in petty trade. The more wealthy people may move into commercial agriculture, livestock trading or even real estate.[2] Homewood and colleagues (2009) have argued that the diversification process affects all segments of pastoral society, while Little *et al.* (2001) have argued that wealthy and poor pastoralists diversify but those in the middle wealth category do not. Little has further argued that the economic diversification is cyclical and reflects the life histories of individuals and the developmental cycle of families, while others (e.g., Homewood *et al.* 2009; McCabe 2003) have argued that the process tends to be linear, permanent, and will eventually define the livelihood strategy of most, if not all East African pastoral peoples.

Another common theme has been that livelihood diversification has been accompanied by reduced mobility and this is associated with increasing impoverishment. However, Fratkin and colleagues present a more complex picture of pastoral sendentarization and the adoption of cultivation among the Rendille and Ariaal pastoralists in northern Kenya (Fratkin and Roth 2005).

This transition to a more diversified pastoral economy has also been observed for other peoples in the African rangelands. For example, Hampshire and Randall (2000) note that Fulbe livelihoods, in the West African Sahel, diversified following the 1973 drought. Individual men began migrating to cities to find seasonal work and families also began to adopt cultivation. They argue that this diversification encourages the persistence of large families as more people are needed to undertake the various necessary economic activities. Thebaud and Batterbury (2001) and LaRovere *et al.* (2005) have also published on the diversification and intensification of livelihood strategies among Sahelian pastoralists. Further, investigation of pastoral livelihood diversification has not been restricted to Africa—see for example the work of Mearns and others for Mongolia (Fernandez-Gimenez 2002; Fratkin and Mearns 2003; Marin 2008).

THE SETTING

The research reported here took place in the Loliondo Division of Ngorongoro District in northern Tanzania (see Fig. 1). The area is bounded to the north by the Kenyan border, to the south by the Ngorongoro Conservation Area, to the west by Serengeti National Park, and to the east by Lake Natron. The major towns in the area are Loliondo (the District headquarters) and Wasso, a short distance to the south. Research was conducted in smaller villages of the Division, including Olorien/Magaiduru, Ololosokwan, Arash, Maloni, and Soitsambu.

The northern part of Loliondo Division forms the southern extremity of the Loita Hills, while to the west the land drops off to the Serengeti plains. In the south the topography includes hills, plains and Arash mountain. Precipitation in the area varies from a high of approximately 1,400 mm/yr in the highest elevations to 500 mm/yr in the very low areas. Rainfall is generally bimodal with a short rainy season during the months of November and December and a longer more intense rainy season in late March, April and May. However, as is typical of arid and semi-arid areas, precipitation is highly variable, both spatially and temporally, and drought is a common feature of the climatic pattern. Wildlife is abundant in the area, especially during the months of January and February when the migrating wildebeest move through the eastern plains on their way to calf in the short grass plains of the Ngorongoro Conservation Area and the Serengeti.

THE PEOPLE

The Maasai occupy approximately 150,000 km^2 spanning northern Tanzania and southern Kenya. The Maasai in Kenya have experienced more development and changes in land tenure than the Maasai of Tanzania. In Kenya, group ranch schemes initially fragmented the common property regimes that were the basis of the traditional system of resource management; and more recently many of the group ranches have undergone subdivision into individually held properties (Galaty 1999; Burnsilver 2007). In Tanzania, common property has remained the core for the management of grazing resources, although many villages

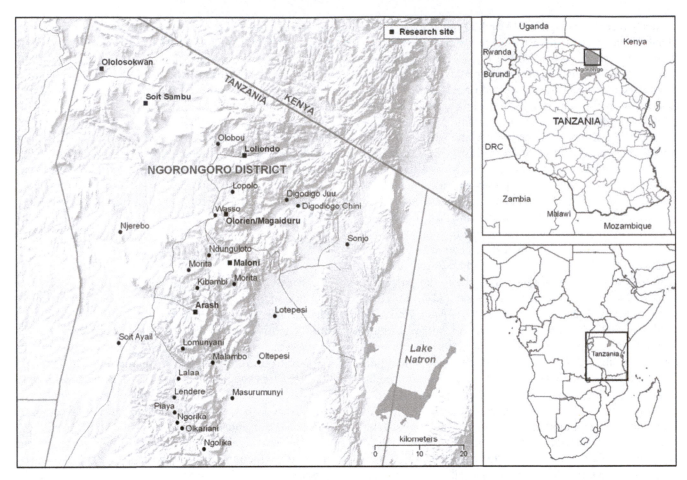

Figure 1 *Map of study area.*

are experiencing significant shifts as individuals are being allocated private[3] holdings and villages are designing land use plans that include areas for cultivation, livestock keeping, and sometimes wildlife conservation.

The people living in the study area are primarily Maasai of the Purko, Loita, and Laitoyoka sections. Town populations are more mixed and another agricultural ethnic group of Bantu origins, the Sonjo or Watemi, live in the hills to the east of the study area. There are also small pockets of other cultivating peoples with whom the Maasai have interacted, in particular the Iraqw (or Mbulu); as well as hunting and gathering peoples generally referred to as Dorobo. The different Maasai sections migrated into the study area sometime during the last 200–250 years and by the late 1800s had evicted the former occupants, the Barabaig (or Datoga, *Il Tatwa* in Maa), from the entire region including the Ngorongoro Conservation Area (O'Malley 2000).

Although there are significant differences among the three sections of the Maasai living in the study area (O'Malley 2000), the important point for the purposes of this paper is that during the first half of the 20th century all three Maasai groups practiced a form of pure pastoralism, based on the raising of cattle, goats, and sheep.

Maasai social organization is based on three interlinking institutions: marriage and family relationships,

territory, and the age set organization. The smallest social unit is the house or *enkaji*, consisting of a wife and her children. A man, his wives and dependents form the next organizational unit, referred to as *enkishomi* (translated as gate) or *olmarei*. This is the basic family unit responsible for the management of livestock. In the past it was typical for a number of *enkishomi* living together in a unit to be referred to as an *enkang*. One rather recent development is that there is a trend for an *enkang* to consist of a single *enkishomi*, but this varies across Maasailand, and appears to be less common in the Loliondo area than in other Maasai areas. All Maasai men are members of a clan (*olgilata*), and this forms the basic unit for mutual aid and redistribution of livestock.

Maasai are organized into territorial sections (*olosho*) in which all members have access to the grazing resources. This is the largest political unit for the Maasai, and in the past, sections have engaged each other in war. The age/grade, age/set system is the other basic unit of Maasai social organization. Together with other members of his cohort or age set, each male member of the society goes through a series of age grades (boy, warrior, junior elder, senior elder, retired elder), each with its own set of norms and responsibilities. During the warrior age grade members acquire a name that identifies them as an age set and remains with them throughout their life. Age sets have leaders (*olenguinani*), and constitute the political basis of the society. As senior elders they may wield significant power and authority over decisions relating to what is right or wrong with respect to the management of natural resources and articulating with outside entities (see results section).

Historically, few events influenced the current Maasai as much as the period known as *Emutai* that occurred in the 1880's and 1890's (Waller 1988). This period was characterized by a series of disasters beginning with an outbreak of contagious bovine pleuropneumonia, followed by an outbreak of rinderpest which was unknown in East Africa prior to that time and which devastated the cattle population. This was followed by an outbreak of small pox among the human population. The last stage of these disasters entailed internecine warfare among many of the Maasai sections, as people attempted to rebuild herds by raiding any group that managed to prevent wholesale losses due to disease. One important impact of these events, for the study presented here, was that many people migrated to live with agricultural peoples who were much less affected by the disease outbreaks. Many men ended up living and marrying within these groups (Kikuyu, WaArusha, WaMeru). Eventually most of these men returned to Maasailand and brought their wives with their agricultural knowledge back with them.

METHODS

The methods used in this research included open ended interviews with household heads, group interviews, and a survey of 93 household heads. The open ended interviews were conducted by the authors and served to provide a qualitative understanding of the process by which households adopted cultivation. Group interviews were conducted in a number of villages where the individual surveys were conducted, with the same goal in mind. We conducted additional group interviews after initial analysis of some of the surveys to clarify some points, especially with respect to the initial phase of cultivation. The household surveys were conducted by the authors, as well as by two research assistants who were hired from the local area. Both had been trained in survey techniques and were also supervised by DeLuca. The individuals interviewed during the survey phase of the research were all household heads and were chosen opportunistically. Although the sampling was not random we tried to ensure that those surveyed included all wealth and age classes. All age sets that had achieved elder status were represented in the sample, but only 5% of the household heads interviewed were in the youngest age set. These men, and the majority of the next youngest age set, were in the warrior age grade at the time that their family adopted agriculture. They were for the most part living in their father's *olmarei*, where they were responsible for much of the day-to-day herd management, but are reporting their understanding of decisions made by their father or other household members.

In addition to the interviews, we were able to draw on the work of Elizabeth O'Malley who had conducted earlier fieldwork on similar issues in the area under the supervision of McCabe (O'Malley 2000).

This analysis depends on the ability of informants to recall past events, situations, and decisions. There are potential difficulties inherent in dependence on retrospective data. We are confident that the data presented in the following sections accurately depict the decision-making process regarding the adoption of cultivation. However, we also recognize the difficulties in trying to reconstruct family histories that may go back a number of decades. Problems might arise from 1) imperfect recall and/or 2) selection bias.

Recall

Our confidence in the accuracy of our informants' memories is grounded in part on the fact that the central topics here entail the composition and dynamics of herds and families. These are two of the most persistently prominent concerns of Maasai life and figure centrally in their discussions and planning. Further, we endeavored to enhance recall accuracy in several ways. In our experience, tying questions and discussion to salient events is an effective means of aiding recall related to life histories (e.g., Leslie and Dyson-Hudson 1999; Bernard 2006). We coupled the questions in our interviews to major events in the Maasai calendar—in particular, the opening and closing of age sets. These events are highly significant to the Maasai and are marked by important, memorable ceremonies and rituals; we believe that most people remember those who were living in their household at those particular times. Thus, with each household head we probed for each person present in the household at the times that these ceremonies were taking place, including their wives and children and others who may have been living in the *olmarei* at the time; we also asked married or widowed women about the number of children present.

The number of livestock reported by each family at these points in time is not likely to be precise, but should be quite sufficiently accurate to serve as an indication of wealth, useful for identifying trends, distributions of wealth, and the general economic context in which families were making livelihood decisions.

Selection Bias

Our analysis is based on the histories of a cross sectional sample of households present in 2001. If these households are not representative of those present at some point in the past, because households with certain characteristics (e.g., wealth) were less likely to persist long enough to be included in the sample, conclusions about that characteristic (or others associated with it) in the past may be distorted. The likelihood and implications of such bias are best addressed in the context of the presentation and discussion of specific results, as we do below. However, it is well to keep in mind that our results reflect the experience of the 93 families in our sample. We believe that they are representative of the Maasai living in the study area at the time of the study; if substantial numbers of families left the pastoral sector and area because of impoverishment or other reasons (and at this time we have no good indication of how common this was), some of our results may not fully represent the situation at earlier times.

RESULTS

One of the first challenges we faced was to identify the time period that each family adopted cultivation. Based on the open ended and group interviews we were able to ascertain that the process usually involved two steps. The first was the planting of a small garden (*bustani* in KiSwahili), and the second was to expand to a farm (*shamba* in KiSwahili). The garden was usually planted by the wife or wives of a household head and the crops included pumpkins (squash), some other vegetables, and small plots of maize and sometimes beans. These were planted adjacent to the *enkang*, and most if not all work was done by women. The farm may or may not have been planted adjacent to the *enkang*, and was usually in excess of an acre in size. The crops planted were predominantly maize, sometimes intercropped with beans. For some families the transition from garden to farm was slow and gradual as the garden expanded. For other families the transition was rapid and may have occurred in a single year.

We determined the time that each family initially adopted cultivation, and their livestock holdings and family (*olmarei*) size at that time. We were able to do this by asking what age set were warriors at this time and how close the time of adoption was to the opening or closing of the age set (opening and closing defines the span of years during which all boys become members of a given age set as they are circumcised). This gave us a good idea about the timing of adoption but the dates are not precise. We thus collapsed them into decades, as represented in Fig. 2. Numbers of cattle, goats and sheep were recalculated as Tropical Livestock Units.[4] We used the same procedure for the time period when the garden became a farm and for the time of the survey, 2001. This gives us data at three points in time for each household—adoption of cultivation (start of garden), expansion to farm, and 2001. Note that the first two of these points are not fixed in time but refer to events in each family's history. With these data we can track economic and demographic change in families over time as well as examine the relationship between wealth and family size and the adoption and expansion of cultivation.

INITIAL ADOPTION OF CULTIVATION

Figure 2 summarizes the timing of the initial planting of gardens.

The data clearly show that the peak of adoption occurred during the 1970s. Approximately 45% of the families interviewed adopted cultivation during this decade, and more

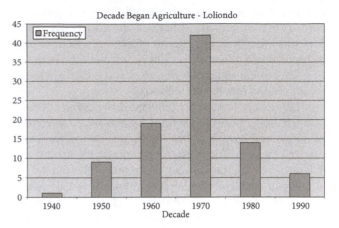

Figure 2 *Number of households starting gardens, by decade.*

than a third of these did so within a two to three year period (1975–1977). No other time period comes close to that for initiation of first planting a garden. By the 1990s, 100% of families were cultivating.

One of the first tasks was to describe the sample population in terms of wealth at each of the three time periods (adoption, expansion, and 2001). In previous publications McCabe (2003) has defined wealth using Potkanski's (1997) classification based on Tropical Livestock Units (TLU) per capita. They are: destitute, below 0.5; very poor, 0.5–1.25; poor, 1.25–2.50; medium, 2.5–5.0; rich, above 5. However because it takes between 4 and 5 TLU per capita to sustain a livelihood as a pastoralist (Fratkin and Roth 1990) the above 5 TLU per capita does not appear rich to us. Therefore we have divided the rich category into moderately wealthy: (5.0–10 TLU per capita); and wealthy (above 10 TLU per capita). There has also been much recent discussion about the proper assets to include in a categorization of wealth among pastoral people (e.g., Homewood 2008). Considering that at the time of adoption of cultivation the families in this study were purely pastoral and had experienced very little migration of young men or others outside the pastoral sector, the definition used here captures the differences in wealth among families and allows us to explore the dynamics of wealth change over time.

We began this research project with the hypothesis that a growing human population and a livestock population that fluctuated around a long-term mean would eventually push people into a diversified economy. The data on household wealth at the time of the adoption of cultivation do not support that hypothesis (see Table 1).

Although the year that families adopted cultivation varied, it is clear that the great majority of people started gardens at a time when they had enough livestock to support their families—given our assumption about how many TLU per capita are needed to support pure pastoralism.

Table 2 summarizes the responses that people gave to an open ended question concerning their decision to begin cultivation. Both "push" factors and "pull" factors are involved in the diversification, and both categories are represented

Table 1 Household Wealth at the Time That Cultivation Was Adopted

Wealth category	Number	Percent
Destitute	2	2.2
Very poor	2	2.2
Poor	6	6.5
Medium	11	11.8
Moderately wealthy	15	16.1
Wealthy	57	61.3
Total	93	

Table 2 Reasons for Adopting Cultivation

Reasons	Number	Percentage[a]
Push factors		
Not enough livestock	27	20%
Not enough milk	15	11%
Sharp decline in livestock—disease	14	10%
Not enough food	9	7%
Need to increase food	8	6%
Sharp decline in livestock—drought	7	5%
Pull factors		
[b]Influence of neighbors	16	12%
Want to diversify	16	12%
[b]Want to eat more maize	13	10%
To avoid selling livestock	9	7%
[b]Dislike blood	7	5%
[b]Influence of government	2	1%

[a]Some people gave more than one reason, so the total is greater than 100%.
[b]Reasons that suggest change in norms.

among the most commonly cited reasons. The push factors (those forcing people to cultivate in order to survive) are: not enough livestock, not enough milk, not enough food, the need to increase food, and sharp declines in livestock due to drought and disease.[5] The pull factors (those that decrease risk or provide other benefits, but are not necessary for survival) are: the wish to diversify and to avoid selling livestock, the influence of neighbors, wanting to taste or eat more maize, the dislike of blood, and the influence of government. The reasons given also indicate some strong shifts in cultural norms. These include the influence of neighbors,

wanting to eat more maize, the dislike of blood, and to some extent the influence of government.

The breakdown of the reasons given for adopting cultivation by wealth category demonstrates the different priorities of poorer and wealthier families. These data are presented in Table 3.

Although the push factors are represented in all wealth categories, the pull factors are seen primarily among the more wealthy households. This is somewhat consistent with what others have reported (Brockington 2001; Little *et al.* 2001). One difference here is that "not enough milk" and "not enough food" are identified as separate reasons from "not enough livestock." This is an indication that there may be enough milking animals but they are not producing as much milk as might have been expected in the past. The explanation for this is twofold. First, there was a very high rate of calf mortality in the area due to tick borne disease, primarily East Coast Fever (Field *et al.* 1997); and second, there was a high disease load carried by cattle, again primarily from tick borne disease. Our interviews suggest that the decades of the 1970s and 1980s saw a significant increase in the amount of tick borne disease, especially East Coast Fever (ECF—*ndigana* in Maa). One potential reason for the rise in the incidence of ECF was that the Tanzanian government ceased providing acaricides. This left cattle with little resistance, and was particularly devastating to calves, with death rates often exceeding 50% (Field *et al.* 1997).

The spread of maize in many parts of East Africa was associated with the attraction of consuming a food eaten by people of higher status—in particular the Indians working on the railroad (hence the KiSwahili word for maize—*mahindi*), but this does not appear to be the case here. Unlike many other "purely pastoral" peoples, the Maasai have traditionally incorporated maize into their diet. Prior to the 1970s maize was bought from shops or by barter with traders in the form of ground maize meal. However, many Maasai said that they had not known what plant the maize that they were eating came from. When they saw people from other ethnic groups cultivating the plants, harvesting the maize, then grinding or pounding it into maize flour, some were interested in cultivating the plants themselves. Some of these "neighbors" included small groups of Mbulu or Iraqw living in the area, people hired as laborers working for the regional government, some Indian shop keepers, and some women from agricultural groups who had married Maasai men. Thus, the attraction of maize was not the wish to emulate others, including high status groups. Rather, Maasai wanted to cultivate maize in order to have access to more food and to reduce the pressure on their livestock. At the same time, they had developed a taste for maize and wanted to have readier access to it.

Despite this history of maize consumption, the Maasai have often been presented as the archetypical pastoralists, scorning cultivation and denigrating those who "scratch the earth". The fact that Maasai household heads emulated neighbors (many of whom were non-Maasai) in cultivating indicates a major change in Maasai thinking about which

Table 3 Reasons for Adopting Cultivation, by Wealth

Reasons	Wealth category at time cultivating was begun					
	Destitute	Very poor	Poor	Medium	Moderately wealthy	Wealthy
Push factors						
Not enough livestock	2 (7%)[a]	2 (7%)	4 (15%)	6 (22%)	4 (15%)	9 (33%)
Not enough milk	–	–	–	3 (20%)	3 (20%)	9 (60%)
Sharp decline in livestock—disease	–	1 (7%)	1 (7%)	1 (7%)	2 (14%)	9 (64%)
Not enough food	–	1 (11%)	1 (11%)	–	–	7 (78%)
Need to increase food	–	–	2 (25%)	–	2 (25%)	4 (50%)
Sharp decline in livestock—drought	–	–	1 (14%)	–	2 (29%)	4 (57%)
Pull factors						
Influence of neighbors	–	1 (6%)	2 (13%)	–	2 (13%)	11 (67%)
Want to diversify	–	–	–	–	2 (22%)	7 (78%)
Want to eat more maize	–	–	–	–	–	13 (100%)
To avoid selling livestock	–	–	–	–	–	9 (100%)
Dislike blood	–	–	–	–	–	7 (100%)
Influence of government	–	–	–	–	1 (50%)	1 (50%)

[a]Percent of those offering a given reason that is in each wealth category.

livelihood practices are acceptable and which are not. The responses "the influence of neighbors" and "wanting to eat more maize" suggest an important shift in cultural norms.

An additional response that frequently came out in the group interviews but that was not expressed in the individual interviews was the notion that people could no longer depend on livestock. This also suggests an important shift in how people view future livelihoods, a dramatic change from the past. We will explore this topic in more detail in a later section.

Our data suggest that the decision to cultivate was generally made by the male household head. 54% of those interviewed said that the male household head made the decision alone. The decision to cultivate was made primarily by the household head's mother in 23% of the cases and by the household head's wife in 6.5% of the cases. Joint decisions were also reported: 14% of household heads said the decision was made in consultation with their father; 14% in consultation with their mother. None were reported to be made in consultation with their wife. The influence of mothers in individual and joint decisions is not surprising; it is often the case that a Maasai man will have his mother living with him after his father has died or has separated from his mother. These figures are based on the interviews with men; women might have a somewhat different view of decision making.

The apparent dominance of the household heads in the decision to adopt cultivation does not mean that these men invested their own labor in cultivation, especially in the case of small gardens, where women do most of the work. In the larger fields, men do often hoe or plow with oxdrawn plows.

REASONS FOR ADOPTING CULTIVATION AT DIFFERENT TIMES

We have discussed how the various push and pull factors related to the adoption of cultivation varied by wealth category. Here we consider how they may vary according to the time at which cultivation was adopted. We have divided the time of adoption into three periods: prior to 1970, during the 1970s, and from the 1980s on (see Table 4).

One issue that immediately becomes apparent in these data is the increased importance of disease-driven declines in livestock during the 1970s. As discussed below (see Tables 6 and 7), our data reveal a distinct trend of declining livestock numbers per person over time among the households included in this study. As the livestock numbers were holding steady or declining many of the study families were growing, and as mentioned in the section on wealth, livestock disease also depressed milk production. As will be discussed further in a later section there was a decrease in nomadic mobility in the 1970s and some herd-owners said that this led to an increase in livestock disease.

The change in cultural norms brought up in the section on the relationship of wealth to the adoption of cultivation

Table 4 Reasons for Adopting Cultivation by Time of Adoption

Reason[a]	Early (*N*=29)[b] (before 1970)	Middle (*N*=42) (1970s)	Late (*N*=20) (1980s and later)
Push factors			
Not enough livestock	7 (24%)	9 (21%)	6 (30%)
Not enough milk	8 (28%)	4 (10%)	3 (15%)
Sharp decline in livestock (disease)	2 (7%)	8 (19%)	3 (15%)
Not enough food	3 (10%)	2 (5%)	1 (5%)
Need to increase food	1 (3%)	7 (17%)	3 (15%)
Sharp decline in livestock (drought)	2 (7%)	3 (7%)	3 (15%)
Pull factors			
Influence of neighbors	4 (14%)	8 (19%)	2 (10%)
Want to diversify	0 –	7 (17%)	4 (20%)
Want to eat more maize	3 (10%)	11 (26%)	0 –
To avoid selling livestock	2 (7%)	3 (7%)	4 (20%)
Dislike blood	0 –	0 –	5 (25%)
Influence of government	0 –	2 (5%)	0 –

[a]Some information concerning the time of adoption is missing or questionable in the data set so the numbers included here may not match those presented in Table 3.
[b]N refers to the number of households in each time period. Percentages in table refer to percent of households offering a given reason. Sum of reasons in any period is greater than N and sum of percentages is greater than 100 because an informant could cite more than one reason.

is clearly seen in these data as well. "Wanting to eat more maize", and "the influence of neighbors" peak during the 1970's, and is rarely mentioned following this period. The "dislike of blood" is only mentioned in the latest period. For the early adopters the lack of livestock and lack of milk are clearly the predominant reasons given for the adoption of cultivation. There is no mention of the desire to diversify the household economy and little mention of wanting to avoid selling livestock. Some of the cultural issues mentioned above are reflected by the early adopters but they become prominent in the middle and late adopters. The changing cultural norms and their importance to this livelihood shift will be discussed further in the concluding sections.

THE EXPANSION OF GARDENS TO FARMS

The distinction between garden (*bustani*) and farm (*shamba*) is not absolute, but farms are considered to be agricultural plots of one acre or larger and gardens are smaller in size. Farms are also devoted primarily to maize, sometimes intercropped with beans, while gardens may have a mixture of maize, beans, pumpkins, and greens. A few individuals experimented with growing sunflowers on farms but this was relatively rare.

For the most part people gradually expanded their gardens each year and after a number of years the garden was large enough to be considered a farm. Our data show that this process took about ten years. While the peak period for adopting cultivation was in the 1970s, the peak period

for expansion began in the 1970s and extended into the 1980s (see Fig. 3). Very few (3%) of the families interviewed expanded cultivation to a farm before the 1970s. The decline in number after the 1980s is a function of the dwindling numbers of families who had not yet adopted agriculture.

Not all families gradually expanded their gardens—some expanded rapidly, in a single season. In our sample, 13 of the 93 households rapidly shifted from a garden to a farm. We will discuss this below.

The most common reasons given for the gradual expansion from gardens to farms, summarized in Table 5, were: (1) that the household head did not want to sell any more livestock in order to purchase food; (2) that the

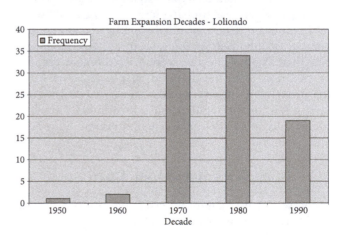

Figure 3 *Number of households expanding garden to farm, by decade.*

Table 5 Reasons Given for the Expansion of Gardens to Farms, by Wealth Category

Reasons	Wealth category						
	Destitute	Very poor	Poor	Medium	Moderately wealthy	Wealthy	Total
Avoid selling livestock	0	0	0	3	8	9	20
Family growth	0	1	2	3	5	6	17
Hunger	2	0	0	1	7	4	14
Higher standard of living	0	0	3	3	0	3	9
Wanted alternative foods	0	0	0	0	4	5	9
Decreased livestock	0	1	2	2	2	0	7
For money to buy livestock	0	0	1	0	1	1	3
Influenced by others	0	0	0	0	1	1	2
Preferred maize	0	0	0	0	0	2	2
To get money for household	1	0	0	0	0	0	1
Give to friend	0	0	1	0	0	0	1
Was raided	1	0	0	0	1	0	2
In case of drought	0	0	0	0	0	1	1
Interested in cultivation	0	0	0	0	1	0	1
Total	4	2	9	12	30	32	89

family was growing in size and needed more food; and (3) they faced decreased food availability, associated with declining livestock numbers and depressed milk production, so more land needed to be cultivated. The reasons given varied by wealth as was the case for initial adoption of cultivation. The poorer households tended to give reasons related to economic necessity while the more wealthy households tended to explain the transition from gardens to farms in terms of not selling livestock, to improving the standard of living, and to diversifying the household economy.

For the 13 families who expanded rapidly from a garden to a farm, a similar picture emerges. Six of the 13 herdowners who expanded rapidly said they did so because of the need for more food. Of these, four were classified as poor and two were of medium wealth. Five of the remaining seven rapid responders were from the moderately or very wealthy categories and the reasons given for the rapid expansion included wanting to increase livestock, the influence of others and just being able to do so.

Wealth Over Time

In this section we examine the economic histories of households over time. In terms of absolute numbers of livestock the households classified as poor, medium and moderately wealthy all showed steady increases over time (see Table

6). The very wealthy steadily lost livestock; the very poor increased livestock from the time of adopting cultivation to expansion but then experienced a decrease. The small numbers in the destitute, very poor and poor categories make the analysis somewhat problematic. Overall, these data do not support a marked or consistent decrease in livestock numbers as time progressed.

This situation is quite different when we divide the number of TLUs by the number of people depending on them. These data are presented in Table 7 and Fig. 4, which reflect the number of livestock in TLUs divided by the number of people depending on them—the size of the *olmarei*. Figure 4 illustrates the changes in overall wealth for the study population at the 3 time periods. Figure 5 shows the changing percentages of households in the different wealth categories at the 3 points in those households' histories.

The data clearly demonstrate a progressive impoverishment of households in terms of TLU per person. The data also show a steady increase in the proportion of households in the destitute, very poor, poor and medium wealth categories at each time period, with a concomitant decline in the percentage in the very wealthy category. Only the households in the moderately wealthy category do not follow this trend; the proportion in this category increased from the adoption of cultivation to the expansion to farms, but then declined by 2001.

As noted in the Methods section, it is possible that some poorer families lost so many livestock that they had

Table 6 Changes in Livestock Holdings Over Time, in TLUs

Wealth category	When adopted cultivation	Time of expansion	2001
Wealthy	13,088	9,586	8,933
Moderately wealthy	730	1,583	1,871
Medium	347	902	1,173
Poor	89	242	680
Very poor	11	49	26
Destitute	0	4	0.3
TOTAL	14,265	12,366	12,683

Table 7 Changes in Wealth Over Time, by Wealth Category Measured in TLU per Capita

Wealth category	When adopted agriculture		When expanded to farm		In 2001	
	Number	Percent	Number	Percent	Number	Percent
Wealthy	57	61.3	35	37.6	25	26.9
Moderately wealthy	15	16.1	30	32.3	24	25.8
Medium	11	11.8	13	14.0	23	24.7
Poor	6	6.5	9	9.7	10	10.8
Very poor	2	2.2	3	3.2	8	8.6
Destitute	2	2.2	3	3.2	3	3.2
Total	93	100[a]	93	100[a]	93	100[a]

[a]Allowing for rounding.

to leave the area altogether, and their histories would not be included in the sample. It is thus worth considering the possibility that selection bias has affected the results of this analysis. If poorer families are more likely to fall out of the system, then the wealth distribution of families in earlier periods, judged by the experience of the present (2001) sample, would be biased toward greater wealth, and estimates of TLU/capita might be biased upward in the earlier periods. However, we argue that the apparent decline in wealth per capita over time is real. Families in the sample declined in wealth; for this result to be a product of selection bias, the unascertained families would had to have increased in wealth, but it is reasonable to assume that the poorest households were unascertained because they became even more impoverished. Therefore, inclusion of "failed" households (families not ascertained in the present sample) would if anything strengthen the conclusion that per capita wealth has declined. The absolute decline in the sample might not accurately reflect the absolute amount of decline that actually occurred in the population as a whole, but the trend detected remains correct. Note that many, perhaps most, of the members of failed households would have been taken in by other families to whom they were related. This may

have contributed to the decline in per capita wealth of those receiving families.

There is little doubt that the overall decline in economic status is strongly influenced by the growth of household sizes over time. The average size of the *olmarei* for the study families at the time that cultivation was adopted was 7.4 individuals; at the time that gardens expanded to farms—10.5; and as of 2001—15.3. It should also be noted that as time progressed and families grew, significant increases in necessary expenses were also accruing. This is reflected in the following statement from one of the household heads during the interviews: "Life is expensive these days. There is a high demand in families for food, money for education, money for medical care—the livestock are not enough to fulfill these life requirements." What these data demonstrate is that the livestock population taken as a whole experienced a modest decrease, while at the same time the households depending on those herds were undergoing significant growth. In addition, the households' need for additional income was growing rapidly in response to the changing cultural, social, and political contexts in which they were living.

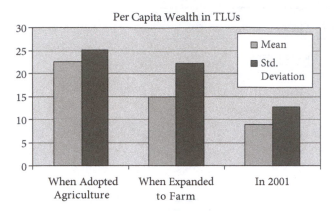

Figure 4 *Changes in per capita wealth for three time periods, in TLUs.*

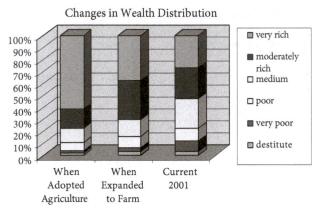

Figure 5 *Changes in percentage of households in each wealth category over time.*

THE LARGER CONTEXT

The Environmental Context

During the interviews people often mentioned drought as playing a role in livestock mortality. Precipitation records show declines in rainfall occurring between 1975 and 1979, 1981 to 1984, and 1994 to 1997. The extent to which these dry periods contributed directly to a decline in livestock numbers is difficult to assess, but it was certainly the perception of many of those interviewed that it did. It was also the case that the incidence of tick-borne disease was increasing from the 1970s. In addition to the decreases in livestock numbers, the increase in livestock disease depressed milk production. The combination of periods of low rainfall, increased livestock mortality, and lower productivity resulted in many people losing confidence in livestock as a sole means of support. This signifies an important shift for the "people of the cattle." The periods of reduced rainfall were not unusual for this region; droughts are a longstanding, recurrent feature of the environment. The larger environmental context consisted of a combination of periods of reduced rainfall, increases in livestock disease, a slowly growing livestock population, and an expanding human population.

The Political Context

The most important political events relevant to this paper were the sweeping changes throughout Tanzania associated with Ujamaa or the Villagization Program, part of Tanzania's social and economic development policy following independence in 1961. This program required the development of village centers based around schools, clinics and shops. Homesteads were moved both voluntarily and forcibly around these centers, and each household was supposed to build permanent structures. Tanzania's single political party (the CCM) became the major decision-maker in terms of land management and the use of natural resources and did not recognize local customs or institutions. In Maasailand this program was called "Operation *Imparnati*" based on the Maasai word for permanent structure, *emparnat* (O'Malley 2000). For the Loliondo area, the influence of the villagization program began to be seen in the mid 1970s and was officially implemented in 1978. People were required to leave rural areas and live in permanent structures in proximity to village centers. They were also encouraged to cultivate.

According to O'Malley the program was both ill suited to the area and short lived. The pastoral people who moved into the villages knew that they would have to move with their livestock as conditions became drier and the government would have to allow for that. In addition, the Kagera War (in which Tanzania invaded Uganda and overthrew Idi Amin) was a major financial drain on the Tanzanian economy and made the monitoring of movement impossible. Within a few months of implementing Operation *Imparnati* most Maasai pastoralists returned to livestock herding. One of the long-term consequences was the exposure to cultivation and this had both direct and indirect influences on the decision to begin cultivation.

The Social and Cultural Context

We have mentioned the changing cultural norms as people became more involved in the modern world. We asked male elders what household heads needed now in order to be successful. Not surprisingly livestock, especially cattle, and the knowledge of livestock management were seen as extremely important. But new needs—for education, land for cultivation, and a way to make money—were also viewed as important.

Other changes that were mentioned by elders were increased sedentarization associated with cultivation and potential strains on social relationships with some people having access to cultivated maize while others did not. One man mentioned adopting cultivation because his children liked the taste of maize and they were stealing it from the fields of a neighbor. In order to reduce the potential for conflict, he began to cultivate himself. Reduced mobility was also mentioned as a possible contributor to increased livestock disease as this increased the exposure of animals to disease vectors, especially ticks. Finally, O'Malley (2000) mentions how plowing techniques changed as those Maasai men in the senior age grades retired. The older Maasai men did not feel that it was appropriate for cattle to be used as beasts of burden, but that this attitude was not shared by those in the younger age grades. She noted a distinct increase in use of animal traction for plowing fields as the senior elders retired.

CONCLUSIONS

In this paper we have examined the process by which Maasai pastoral people in northern Tanzania diversified their economy through the adoption of cultivation. We found that the process generally involved two stages: planting a garden first, and later expanding the garden to a farm. We found that some households adopted cultivation out of necessity, but far more households adopted cultivation by choice. For some of these households cultivation was a means to reduce risk, while for others it was a reflection of changing cultural and social norms. To some extent this supports the findings of Brockington, Homewood and Little, but not completely. We found the process to be more complex and influenced by a variety of factors other than just economic ones. Eventually, Maasai from all wealth categories adopted cultivation, supporting the argument put forward by Homewood and her colleagues.

The changes observed during the period of fieldwork were couched within rapidly changing political and cultural contexts. Policy changes ranging from the implementation of the socialist villagization program in the 1970s to the decision to stop supporting the delivery of acaricides in subsequent decades had direct and indirect effects. The presence of non-Maasai cultivators—Indian shopkeepers, Kikuyu farmers, and Iraqw laborers—also influenced families to adopt cultivation. Changing norms, from diet to the roles that livestock play in the household, were also being contested and debated as families planted for the first time and expanded their gardens to farms. We hope that this paper will contribute to our understanding of livelihood diversification and the responses of pastoral peoples to a rapidly changing world.

Notes

This research was supported by NSF Grants BCS-0351462, BCS-0349825, BCS-0624343, BCS-0624265, and a grant from the John D. and Catherine T. MacArthur Foundation. Reviewers of the manuscript made several useful suggestions and forced us to make aspects of our argument clearer.

1. Pure pastoralism is generally understood as meaning that the human population depends exclusively on livestock as their means of subsistence—this may mean that the people consume only livestock products or that livestock provide the means for acquiring grains and other goods through trade, in addition to providing livestock based foods.
2. Although East African pastoralists have only very recently begun to invest in real estate, this process was reported on as typical for wealthy Middle Eastern pastoral peoples decades ago (Barth 1961).
3. In many villages plots of land are being allocated to individuals, often in 3–10 acre allotments. Although individuals have rights to use these allocations they are legally not allowed to sell them.
4. Tropical Livestock Units were derived by multiplying total cattle numbers by 0.72 and small stock numbers by 0.17. This follows the procedure used by Grandin 1988 and Homewood et al. 2009.
5. The sharp decline in livestock numbers could also be considered a pull factor, especially if herd-owners witnessed sharp declines in others herds but were not personally affected.

References

Barth, F. (1961). Nomads of South Persia: The Basseri Tribe of the Khamseh Confederacy. Little Brown and Company, Boston.

Batterbury, S. (2001). Landscapes of Diversity: A Local Political Ecology of Livelihood Diversification in South-Western Niger. Ecumene 8(4): 437–463.

Bernard, H. R. (2006). Research Methods in Anthropology. Qualitative and Quantitative Approaches, 4th ed. Altamira, New York.

Brockington, D. (2001). Fortress Conservation. The Preservation of the Mkomazi Game Reserve. James Currey, African Issues series.

Burnsilver, S. (2007). Pathways of Continuity and Change: Diversification, Intensification and Mobility in Maasailand Kenya. Ph.D dissertation. Graduate Degree Program in Ecology. Colorado State University.

Ensminger, J. (1992). Making a market: The Institutional Transition of an African Society. Cambridge University Press, Cambridge.

Fernandez-Gimenez, M. (2002). Spatial and Social Boundaries and the Paradox of Pastoral Land Tenure: A Case Study for Postsocialist Mongolia. Human Ecology 30(1): 49–78.

Field, C. R., Moll, G., and ole Sonkoi, C. (1997). Livestock development. In Thompson, S. M. (ed.), Multiple Land Use: The Experience of the Ngorongoro Conservation Area Tanzania. IUCN, Geneva, pp. 181–199.

Fratkin, E., and Mearns, R. (2003). Sustainablity and pastoral livelihoods: Lessons from East African Maasai and Mongolia. Human Organization 62(2): 112–122.

Fratkin, E., and Roth, E. (1990). Drought and Economic Differentiation among Ariaal Pastoralists of Kenya. Human Ecology 18(4):385–402.

Fratkin, E., and Roth, E. (2005). As Pastoralists Settle: Social, Health, and Economic Consequences of the Pastoral Sedentarization in Marsabit District. Kluwer Academic, Kenya.

Galaty, J. (1994) Rangeland Tenure and Pastoralism in Africa. In Fratkin, E., Galvin, K., & Roth, E. A. (eds.), 1994. African Pastoral Systems: an integrated approach. Lynne Rienner, pp 185–204.

Galaty, J. (1999). Grounding Pastoralists: Law, Politics and Dispossession in East Africa. Nomadic Peoples 3(2): 56–73.

Goldman, M. (2003). Partitioned nature, privileged knowledge: community based conservation in Tanzania. Development and Change 34(5): 833–862.

Grandin, B. (1988). Wealth and Pastoral Dairy Production: A Case Study of Maasailand. Human Ecology 16: 1–21.

Hampshire, K., and Randall, S. (2000). Pastoralists, Agropastoralists and Migrants: Interactions Between Fertility and Mobility in Northern Burkina Faso. Population Studies 54: 247–261.

Homewood, K. (2004). Policy, Environment and development in African rangelands. Environmental Science and Policy 7: 125–143.

Homewood, K. (2008). Ecology of African Pastoral Societies. James Currey Ltd., Oxford.

Homewood, K., and Brockington, D. (1999). Biodiversity, Conservation And Development in Mkomazi Game Reserve, Tanzania. Global Ecology and Biogeography 8: 301–313.

Homewood, K. M., Thompson, P. T., Kiruswa, S., and Coast, E. (2005). Community- and State-based Natural Resource Management and Local Livelihoods in Maasailand. Special issue on Community Based Natural Resource Management. Afriche e Orienti 2: 84–101.

Homewood, K., Patti, K., and Pippa, T. (eds.) (2009). Staying Maasai: Livelihoods, Conservation and Development in East African Rangelands. Springer, New York.

Igoe, J. (2003a). Scaling Up Civil Society: Donor Money, NGOs and the Pastoralist Land Rights Movement in Tanzania. Development and Change 34(5): 863–885.

Igoe, J. (2003b). Conservation and Globalization: A Study of National Parks and Indigenous Communities from East Africa to South Dakota. Wadsworth, Belmont.

LaRovere, R., Hieraux, P., Van Keulen, H., Schiere, J. B., and Szonyo, J. A. (2005). Co-evolutionary Scenarios of Intensification and Privatization of Resource use in Rural Communities of South-Western Niger. Agricultural Systems 83(3): 251–276.

Leserogol, C. (2008). Contesting the Commons: Privatizing Pastoral Lands in Kenya. University of Michigan Press, Ann Arbor.

Leslie, P., and Dyson-Hudson, R. (1999). People and herds. In Little, M. A., and Leslie, P. W. (eds.), Turkana Herders of the Dry Savanna. Ecology and Biobehavioral Response of Nomads to an Uncertain Environment. Oxford University Press, Oxford, pp. 233–247.

Little, P. (2003). Somalia: Economy Without a State. Indiana University Press, Bloomington.

Little, P., Smith, K., Cellarius, B., Coppock, D., and Barrett, C. (2001). Avoiding Disaster: Diversification and Risk Management Among East African Herders. Development and Change 32: 410–433.

Marin, A. (2008). Between Cash Cows and Golden Calves: Adaptations of Mongolian Pastoralism in the "Age of the Market". Nomadic Peoples 12(2): 75–101.

Marshall, F. (1990). Origins of Specialized Pastoral Production in East Africa. American Anthropologist 92: 873–894.

McCabe, J. T. (1997). Risk and Uncertainty Among the Maasai of the Ngorongoro Conservation Area in Tanzania: A Case Study in Economic Change. Nomadic Peoples 1(1): 54–65.

McCabe, J. T. (2003). Sustainability and Livelihood Diversification Among the Maasai of Northern Tanzania. Human Organization 62(3): 100–111.

May, A., and McCabe, J. T. (2004). City Work in a Time of AIDS: Maasai Labor Migration in Tanzania. Africa Today 51(2): 3–32.

O'Malley, M. E. (2000). Cattle and Cultivation: Changing Land Use Patterns in Pastoral Maasai Livelihoods, Loliondo Division, Ngorongoro District, Tanzania. Ph.D dissertation, Department of Anthropology, University of Colorado.

Potkanski, T. (1997). Pastoral Economy, Property Rights and Traditional Assistant Mechanisms Among the Ngorongoro and Salei Maasai of Tanzania. London: International Institute for Environment and Development, Pastoral Land Tenure Series Monograph 2.

Spear, T. (1993). Being "Maasai" but not "People of the Cattle." Arusha Agricultural Maasai in the Nineteenth Century. In Spear, T., and Waller, R. (eds.), Being Maasai: Ethnicity and Identity in East Africa. James Currey, London.

Thebaud, B., and Batterbury, S. (2001). Sahel Pastoralists: Opportunism, Struggle, Conflict and Negation. A Case Study from Eastern Niger. Global Environmental Change 11: 69–78.

Waller, R. D. (1988) *Emutai*: Crisis and Response in Maasailand 1883–1902. In Johnson, D., and Anderson, D. (eds.), The Ecology of Survival: Case Studies from Northeast African History. Lester Crook Academic Publishing/Westview Press, pp 73–114.

Western, D. (1997). In the Dust of Kilimanjaro. Island, Washington.

CHAPTER 15

"Now It Is an Easy Life": Women's Accounts of Cassava, Millets, and Labor in South India

Elizabeth Finnis

(2009)

Since the 1960s, coarse grain cultivation in India has been declining, falling from 29.45% of the total cultivated land in the 1960s, to 15.76% by 2000 (MSSRF 2004:29). There are numerous reasons for this decrease, including Green Revolution technology that focused on wheat and rice cultivation, pressures to grow cash crops, and the devaluation of coarse grains on the market. Yet, in the last several years, coarse grains have gained increasing attention as underused crops that have the potential to improve food security and positively affect the income of small farmers (King et al. 2008; Padma 2005; Padulosi et al. 2003). This realization, along with the reality that coarse grains continue to be abandoned in locales across India (Finnis 2007; Mehta 1996; Rao and Hall 2003; Shiva 2004), offers the opportunity to examine the specific ways that contemporary declines in coarse grains are understood at the local level, which in turn provides insights into the possibilities for local-level coarse grain projects. This local-level understanding is particularly important given that the positioning of different actors can affect their attitudes toward coarse grain cultivation. In this brief paper, I examine the decline of millet varieties in the Kolli Hills, Tamil Nadu, through the lens of the experiences and workloads of women. While the decline in coarse grain cultivation may be part of a wider process of ongoing crop commercialization, biodiversity decreases, a loss of culinary practices, and changes to livelihood practices (see Rajamma 1993; Shiva 2004) throughout India, it is necessary to consider how women in specific locales and at specific times view these agricultural and dietary transitions in terms of their impacts on everyday workloads and time demands.

The Kolli Hills, one of a range of hill stations along India's Eastern Ghats, is home to over 37,000 Malaiyali small farmers. Although the Hills are not precisely isolated, limited road networks mean that they can be considered geographically marginal; inhabitants are typically considered economically marginalized due to limited income-earning opportunities. As small-scale farmers, Malaiyalis grow subsistence and cash crops, although crop preferences, and profit and debt cycles, vary among over 240 communities in the Hills. Since 2003, I have worked with community members, and in particular with women, from villages in Thakkali Nadu,[1] one of the more isolated areas of the Kolli Hills. I have examined changes in agricultural and dietary practices along with the economic implications of the shift from subsistence to commercial agriculture. Households in this area typically farm less than five acres of land, generally a mix of some wetlands for rice and some drylands for other crops. Irrigation is minimal to nonexistent, and farmers rely on regular rainfall for dryland crop success.

MOVING AWAY FROM MILLET CULTIVATION

Minor millets, including *samai, thenai, varagu,* and *panivaragu,* have traditionally been central to the diets and livelihoods of Thakkali Nadu villagers, as well as of small farmers across India (Bohle 1992; Rajamma 1993; Shiva 2004). In the Kolli Hills, millets were dietary staples and the ideal pattern was to consume a different variety for each meal of the day. Yet millets have become increasingly scarce throughout the Hills. This decline reflects changes to local livelihood practices that focus on increasing engagements with the market economy, as well as government attempts to improve food security through the introduction of rice cultivation (Bohle 1992; Finnis 2006; Rajasekaran and Warren 1994). Results have been twofold. First, rice now plays a central role in everyday household consumption, having replaced millets as the staple grain. Rice may be purchased from government ration shops, or it might be grown on household wetlands. Most families are able to produce a portion of their annual household rice needs, relying on purchased rice as supplements.

Second, drylands have increasingly been converted to cash crops. Cash crops may include coffee, bananas, citrus fruits, pineapple, and sweet cassava. In Thakkali Nadu, the cash crop of choice is sweet cassava. As I have discussed elsewhere (Finnis 2006), farmers articulate this preference

Elizabeth Finnis, " 'Now it is an easy life': women's accounts of cassava, millets, and labor in South India." *Culture & Agriculture* 31 (2009): 88–94. Reprinted with permission.

in two primary ways. Cassava is constructed as a crop that can be grown during a time of rainfall uncertainty, providing some degree of livelihood security; as farmers put it, cassava allows them to "have a job," even when rainfall patterns are erratic, and even if the crop and harvests are not ideal.[2] Sweet cassava also brings unprecedented income to most households. This has allowed farmers in Thakkali Nadu villages to undertake a number of projects, including improvements to houses and paying for further education for their children. This income has also led increased access to commodity goods, including kitchen items, televisions, bicycles, and the occasional motorcycle. Given perceptions of environmental uncertainty and the reality that the market demand for millets is limited, men and women frequently stated that they were wary of returning to growing traditional grain varieties.

Amidst discussions of environmental changes and economic aspirations, issues of labor loads emerged during interviews, focus groups, and casual conversations with women. While it might be tempting to focus solely on environmental and economic reasons for the agricultural transition in Thakkali Nadu, the changes to labor loads—specifically in terms of labor decreases—provides an important facet to understanding the ways that women experience different crops. In India and other locales, cash crops have been found to have numerous potential negative implications for women. A shift to cash cropping might devalue women's traditional knowledge about once-important tasks such as seed saving, might increase household tensions, or might require that women work harder to make viable livelihoods (Carney 1993; Chancellor 2005; Dey 1981; Dolan 2001; Mehta 1996; Rajamma 1993). Yet cash crops may not have wholly negative effects on women's lives and workloads (Hamilton and Fischer 2005; Lim et al. 2007; Paolisso et al. 2002). In working with women in Thakkali Nadu, it became clear that women are experiencing what they perceive to be positive changes in their everyday workloads, both in the field and in the home. They associate these changes with sweet cassava, both in terms of growing the crop, as well as the relative work associated with the current reliance on rice as the staple food.

CASSAVA VERSUS MILLETS, IN THE FIELD AND IN THE HOME

In terms of the work required in agricultural fields, millet cultivation was described as more arduous, with millets requiring "more care" throughout the growing season. In contrast, cassava was discussed as an "easier" crop, requiring fewer sessions of the laborious weeding that is the responsibility of women.[3] It also means less difficulty finding workers willing to participate in field labor. As sweet cassava has made inroads into Thakkali Nadu, women and men are increasingly uninterested in working with other crops. As one elderly man, who is now heavily dependent on the assistance of others, put it, "For millets we need a lot of people for work, to cut and all. So many we have to call.

[But] because everybody is growing cassava, they will only go for that work. If we grow millets, we won't get enough workers." Beyond this, cassava has another advantage in that it is sent to market in an unprocessed state. Tubers are harvested, cut from the stems, bagged and packed on trucks to be transported to sago-starch factories located in the lowlands surrounding the Hills. Processing takes place at the factories, and farmers need only worry about ensuring that their harvests arrive in good condition.[4]

While women consistently raised the issue of working in the fields, it quickly became clear that work in the home is a far more important concern. Millets, like most grains, require a considerable amount of preparation before consumption. They must be harvested and dried before grains can be removed and hulled. While locally grown rice undergoes the same basic process, a key difference is that rice husks can be removed with the privately owned electric rice mill enterprises located in three Thakkali Nadu villages. These mills are not equipped to handle millets. Furthermore, rice purchased from ration shops and markets comes premilled and does not require precooking preparation beyond the searching out of grit and stray husks.

In the absence of mechanical millet hullers, women must rely on two manual methods for processing before cooking. The first entails pounding the grains, while standing, with a heavy pestle. This is a repetitive action that requires strength and stamina and it results in whole grains ready to be boiled. Millets can also be processed with a large, heavy stone grinder, which is somewhat less difficult than pounding due to the fact that grinding takes place while sitting down. It is nevertheless labor intensive. The end result is flour used to make balls for frying or boiling.

Women of all ages in Thakkali Nadu consistently made reference to the strength and endurance required to process millets. For example, one woman stated that one kilogram of *samai* can take up to half a day of manual processing before it is ready to cook, while King et al. (2008) have found that approximately five kilograms of *thenai* may take an hour or more. Across generations, women were unwilling or unable to undertake the drudgery of manual processing. One 60-year-old grandmother put it this way, "I don't grow millets...if I grow millets, I have to pound it. If we can't pound, what to do?" while a woman in her mid-forties demonstrated her appreciation of the changes in labor patterns that came with the arrival of rice when she said, "Before we were eating only millets. We had to wake up at 4 a.m. to pound them. By 7 a.m. we had to finish the cooking and go to work in the field." She later continued, "Before we used to pound millets, then cook them. It was too hard to make food for a day. Now it is an easy life." A woman in her twenties pointed out that her generation is not necessarily interested in a return to the older ways of work, "Samai, thenai have to be hand beaten before being cooked...in the past, the people did that work. They didn't have any hand pain. Now the younger girls feel hand pain, so we stopped beating it." It should be noted that while there are a variety of mechanical millet hullers available in general, women in Thakkali Nadu do not currently have access to this technology. Private mechanical rice mills may be available in some Thakkali Nadu villages, but these are profit-driven enterprises and there is currently no capital or impetus for the purchasing and running of even a small-scale millet huller.

LESS WORK, MORE FREE TIME

The replacement of millets by cassava in the fields and rice in the cookpot has real implications for women's day-to-day workloads, particularly given that they are responsible for a range of time-consuming household and agriculture tasks. Workdays typically begin between 5 and 6 a.m., and women's responsibilities include childcare, daily house-cleaning and water collection, all cooking related activities, animal care, fuelwood gathering, and laundry. Women weed fields, plant rice and cassava, and play an important, central part of harvesting and packing cassava, as well as harvesting, drying, sorting, and packing locally grown rice. Even if they are not working in their own fields, they are generally exchanging labor or earning money by working in the fields of neighbors, extended family members, and larger landowners.[5] Many research participants also help with the household and cooking needs of their extended families, including their own parents.

Given these numerous responsibilities, it is not surprising that women would appreciate food crops that might reduce their relative workloads, minimize drudgery, and offer the opportunity for some free time. There are a number of ways that women make use of this time, both in terms of public and community participation, and private activities. For example, there is increasing interest in participating in self-help savings and loans groups, and in late 2006, a group in one Thakkali Nadu village came together to begin evening literacy classes. One of the most vibrant uses of free time was the organizing of groups to learn and practice traditional songs and dances, part of a self-help initiative. These are fun, lively and laughter-filled sessions that women value and enjoy. Socializing in other ways, including sitting and talking with friends, is popular and valued. Additionally, cassava income means that many households have access to commodity goods such as televisions. Televisions and related serials, news stories, and cultural programming have become increasingly popular, and those households with a television set are destinations for afternoon breaks or evening get-togethers. As one young woman said, "Planting cassava is less work. Monthly or bimonthly we will work in the field. Other times we are free. So I can watch TV."

COMPLEX THINKING ABOUT MINOR MILLETS

While women might view rice as an appealing food in terms of labor loads, the loss of minor millets crops and dishes has not been wholeheartedly embraced. Many women lament the loss of millets in the diet, even as they speak with relief about labor requirements. Millet varieties are described as tastier than rice. They are discussed as filling and as helping to build strength, in contrast to rice, which was tellingly described by a woman in her late twenties as something that does not keep hunger away for very long.

As I have discussed in detail elsewhere (Finnis 2008), women also increasingly express concerns about the health effects of eating a rice-based diet, particularly when they eat ration rice. As one 23-year-old mother said, "The ration rice is not good for health. It's making health problems. In the past, *samai, thenai* made good health. Because in the past they didn't put [chemical] fertilizers or pesticides. But in the shop and the ration shop, they use pesticides and fertilizers."[6]

These complex attitudes toward millets cannot be ignored in attempts to gain a detailed understanding of the decline of millet cultivation in Thakkali Nadu. Indeed, when presented with scenarios about the reintroduction of millets, women were not necessarily convinced. While some felt they would try the grains again if rainfall returned to expected patterns,[7] others were less willing. When asked if she would switch back to millets if growing and market conditions were right, one young woman thought briefly and answered, "I wouldn't plant them. If *ragi* and [other millets] are planted, it is much work. I am not interested in doing so much work," while a 60-year-old grandmother stated, "It takes a lot of hard work to prepare it for eating. I am not able, and there is no one else to do that. They are not interested."

LESSONS

Although women have commented on the labor intensiveness associated with millets, there are also several important reasons to advocate a return to millet cultivation in Thakkali Nadu and the Kolli Hills. Millet varieties, considered neglected and underused species, have been recognized as having the potential to play an important role in income generation, food security, and improved nutritional status (King et al. 2008; Padulosi et al. 2003). Although millets and milled rice are similar in terms of energy and carbohydrates, in almost all other cases millet varieties exceed rice in other available nutrients, including iron, calcium, and protein. For example, per 100 grams of cooked grain, *thenai* and *pani-varagu* contain almost twice the amount of protein, *ragi* contains over 38 times the amount of calcium, and *samai* contains over nine times the amount of iron than cooked, mill-processed rice (Gopalan et al. 2004), making millets a more nutritionally appealing staple grain. Moreover, the loss of minor millets represents a loss to the pool of Indian agricultural biodiversity; as global food crises escalate, increasing attention to underused and neglected food plant species may play a crucial role in food security (King et al. 2008; Padma 2005; Padulosi et al. 2003). As Shiva (2004) has noted, increased millet cultivation may also have key implications for Indian food sovereignty.

Yet calls for an increase in the cultivation and consumption of coarse grains need to also consider the experiences and preferences of the individuals who are responsible for preparing the grains to eat; this requires working closely with farmers on a very local level in order to grasp differences between and within different locales. While Thakkali Nadu farmers stress economic and environmental reasons for a shift from millet to cassava cultivation, labor loads and time demands have also emerged as central to the ways women think about millets. A reading of dietary and agricultural changes in Thakkali Nadu that focuses on economic and environmental reasons alone might suggest that a widespread reintroduction of millets to the area would primarily be a matter of improved irrigation and better millet marketing opportunities. However, a gendered consideration of household resource use and labor (Quisumbing and McClafferty 2006) allows for a more complex understanding of the question of millets; another dimension of agricultural transitions and crop preferences is revealed when women's agriculture and household labor constraints are considered, particularly because women have been able to rely on local electric rice mills and premilled rice for several years now. Given other work demands, and the time and strength needed to prepare millets, it is not surprising that Thakkali Nadu women would welcome the easy practicalities of rice.

Nevertheless, while millets might be a nonpreference in terms of workloads, women still consider millet varieties the preferred food in terms of flavor, variety, and perceptions of health. The lingering longing for millet varieties strongly suggests that there is a place for millets in Thakkali Nadu in the future. While irrigation and a market for coarse grains might be important in returning millet biodiversity to the Kolli Hills, the workloads millets place on women suggest that even more importantly, it is access to mechanical processing facilities that would play a central role in encouraging small farmer households to consider growing minor millets again particularly for household use. By reducing processing times from hours to minutes, small-scale mechanical hullers, similar to those available for locally grown rice, have the potential to minimize or eliminate millet-processing drudgery, allowing women to take advantage of both their preferences for reduced labor loads and for the taste of millets in their everyday diets.

Notes

This work would not have been possible without the support of the villagers of Thakkali Nadu, Dr. Tina Moffat, Dr. T. Vasantha Kumaran, Sister Francina, Ms. N. Annammadevi, Ms. A. Chitra, Ms. Gracie Sevariammal, and Ms. Vimala Mathew. Research funding gratefully acknowledged from the Social Sciences and Humanities Research Council (Canada), the International Development Research Centre (Canada), the Wenner-Gren Foundation, and the Canadian Anthropology Society.

1. This is a pseudonym.

2. It should be noted that sweet cassava is not without numerous problems. These include the depletion of soil and the subsequent need to clear new land and purchase chemical fertilizers. Crop quality has been declining over the years, and

farmers state that crop diseases are developing. The reliance on one crop means that if harvests are poor, most households have little in the way of security. Moreover, market gluts mean that farmers may not obtain good prices for their harvests.

3. Research elsewhere has suggested that cassava cultivation is not necessarily viewed in similar ways. Avotri and Walters (1999), for example, have found that cassava cultivation is viewed as part of the drudgery of everyday life for women in the Volta region of Ghana.

4. If farmers were required to process the cassava tubers in some way, this would likely radically change how the crop is perceived. As of yet, however, there are neither sago-starch factories in the Hills, nor are there any discussions of processing cassava in Thakkali Nadu.

5. When there is little local work, some men and women may travel to the lowlands to harvest rice or other crops. Others migrate for factory work or construction, coming home during key agricultural seasons.

6. Rajamma (1993) has found similar concerns about eating crops treated with pesticides in other areas of South India where small farmers have shifted from growing subsistence to cash crops.

7. In early 2007, I observed several fields of *ragi* millet being cultivated in one community. This was a stark contrast to earlier fieldwork visits. When asked, I was told that rainfall had seemed promising enough that a few households had decided to try growing a small amount of *ragi* for their own use.

References

Avotri, Joyce Yaa, and Vivienne Walters. 1999. You Just Look at Our Work and See if You Have Any Freedom on Earth: Ghanaian Women's Accounts of their Work and their Health. Social Science and Medicine 48: 1123–1133.

Bohle, Hans G. 1992. Disintegration of Traditional Food Systems as a Challenge to Food Security: A Case Study of Kollimalai Hills in South India. *In* Development and Ecology. Mehdi Raza, ed. Pp. 139–146. Jaipur: Rawat Publications.

Carney, Judith. 1993. Converting the Wetlands, Engendering the Environment: The Intersection of Gender with Agrarian Change in the Gambia. Economic Geography 69(4):329–348.

Chancellor, Felicity. 2005. Enabling Women to Participate in African Smallholder Irrigation Development and Design. *In* Gender, Water and Development. Anne Coles and Tina Wallace, eds. Pp. 155–173. Oxford: Berg Publishers.

Dey, Jennie. 1981. Gambian Women: Unequal Partners in Rice Development Projects? The Journal of Development Studies 17(3):109–122.

Dolan, Catherine S. 2001. The 'Good Wife': Struggles Over Resources in the Kenyan Horticultural Sector. The Journal of Development Studies 37(3):39–73.

Finnis, Elizabeth. 2006. Why Grow Cash Crops? Environmental Uncertainty and Economic Aspiration in the Kolli Hills, South India. American Anthropologist 108(2):363–369.

Finnis, Elizabeth. 2007. The Political Ecology of Dietary Transitions: Agricultural Change, Environment, and Economics in the Kolli Hills, India. Agriculture and Human Values 24: 343–353.

Finnis, Elizabeth. 2008. Economic Wealth, Food Wealth and Millet Consumption: Shifting Notions of Food, Identity and Development in South India. Food, Culture, and Society. 11(4):463–485.

Gopalan, C., B. V. Rama Sastri, and S. C. Balasubramanian. 2004. Nutritive Value of Indian Foods. Hyderabad: National Institute of Nutrition.

Hamilton, Sarah, and Edward F. Fischer. 2005. Maya Farmers and Export Agriculture in Highland Guatemala: Implications for Development and Labor Relations. Latin American Perspectives 32(5):33–58.

King, E. D., Israel Oliver, V. Arivudai Nambi, and Latha Nagarajan. 2008. Integrated Approaches in Small Millets Conservation – A Case from Kolli Hills, India. Presentation at the International Symposium on Underutilized Plant Species for Food, Nutrition, Income and Sustainable Development, Arusha, Tanzania, March 4, 2008.

Lim, Sung Soo, Alex Winter-Nelson, and Mary Arends-Kuenning. 2007. Household Bargaining Power and Agricultural Supply Response: Evidence from Ethiopian Coffee Growers. World Development 35(7):1204–1220.

Mehta, Manjari. 1996. Our Lives are no Different from that of Our Buffaloes: Agricultural Change and Gendered Spaces in a Central Himalayan Valley. In Feminist Political Ecology: Global Issues and Local Experiences. D. Rocheleau, B. Thomas-Slayter, and E. Wangari, eds. pp. 180–208. London: Routledge.

M.S. Swaminathan Research Foundation. 2004. Atlas of the Sustainability of Food Security. Chennai: Nagaraj & Company Private Ltd.

Padma, T. V. 2005. Beating World Hunger: the Return of 'Neglected' Crops. Electronic document, http://www.scidev.net/en/features/beating-world-hunger-the-return-of-neglected-cr.html, accessed July 10, 2008.

Padulosi, S., J. Noun, A. Giuliani, F. Shuman, W. Rojas, and B. Ravi. 2003. Realizing the Benefits in Neglected and Underutilized Plant Species through Technology Transfer and Human Resources Development. UN Conference on Technology Transfer and Capacity Building, Norway 2003. Electronic document, http://www.bioversityinternational.org/Themes/Neglected_and_Underutilized_Species/Publications/index.asp, accessed July 7, 2008.

Paolisso, Michael J., Kelly Hallman, Lawrence Haddad, and Shibesh Regmi. 2002. Does Cash Crop Adoption Detract from Child Care Provision? Evidence from Rural Nepal. Economic Development and Cultural Change 50: 313–337.

Quisumbing, Agnes R., and Bonnie McClafferty. 2006. Using Gender Research in Development: Food Security in Practice. Food Security in Practice Technical Guide Series 2. Washington, DC: International Food Policy Research Institute (IFPRI).

Rajamma, G. 1993. Changing from Subsistence to Cash Cropping. Gender and Development 1(3):19–21.

Rajasekaran, B., and D. M. Warren. 1994. IK for Socioeconomic Development and Biodiversity: The Kolli Hills. Indigenous Knowledge and Development Monitor 2(2). Electronic document, http://www.nuffic.nl/ciran/ikdm/2-2/articles/rajasekaran.html, accessed May 12, 2005.

Rao, P. Parthasarathy, and A. J. Hall. 2003. Importance of Crop Residues in Crop-Livestock Systems in India and Farmers' Perceptions of Fodder Quality in Coarse Cereals. Field Crops Research 84: 189–198.

Shiva, Vandana. 2004. The Future of Food: Countering Globalization and Recolonization of Indian Agriculture. Futures 36: 715–732.

CHAPTER 16

Power Steer

Michael Pollan

(2002)

Garden City, Kan., missed out on the suburban building boom of the postwar years. What it got instead were sprawling subdivisions of cattle. These feedlots—the nation's first—began rising on the high plains of western Kansas in the 50's, and by now developments catering to cows are far more common here than developments catering to people.

You'll be speeding down one of Finney County's ramrod roads when the empty, dun-colored prairie suddenly turns black and geometric, an urban grid of steel-fenced rectangles as far as the eye can see—which in Kansas is really far. I say "suddenly," but in fact a swiftly intensifying odor (an aroma whose Proustian echoes are more bus-station-men's-room than cow-in-the-country) heralds the approach of a feedlot for more than a mile. Then it's upon you: Poky Feeders, population 37,000. Cattle pens stretch to the horizon, each one home to 150 animals standing dully or lying around in a grayish mud that it eventually dawns on you isn't mud at all. The pens line a network of unpaved roads that loop around vast waste lagoons on their way to the feedlot's beating heart: a chugging, silvery feed mill that soars like an industrial cathedral over this teeming metropolis of meat.

I traveled to Poky early in January with the slightly improbable notion of visiting one particular resident: a young black steer that I'd met in the fall on a ranch in Vale, SD. The steer, in fact, belonged to me. I'd purchased him as an 8-month-old calf from the Blair brothers, Ed and Rich, for $598. I was paying Poky Feeders $1.60 a day for his room, board, and meds and hoped to sell him at a profit after he was fattened.

My interest in the steer was not strictly financial, however, or even gustatory, though I plan to retrieve some steaks from the Kansas packing plant where No. 534, as he is known, has an appointment with the stunner in June. No, my primary interest in this animal was educational. I wanted to find out how a modern, industrial steak is produced in America these days, from insemination to slaughter.

Eating meat, something I have always enjoyed doing, has become problematic in recent years. Though beef consumption spiked upward during the flush 90s, the longer-term trend is down, and many people will tell you they no longer eat the stuff. Inevitably they'll bring up mad-cow disease (and the accompanying revelation that industrial agriculture has transformed these ruminants into carnivores—indeed, into cannibals). They might mention their concerns about E. coli contamination or antibiotics in the feed. Then there are the many environmental problems, like groundwater pollution, associated with "Concentrated Animal Feeding Operations." (The word "farm" no longer applies.) And of course there are questions of animal welfare. How are we treating the animals we eat while they're alive, and then how humanely are we "dispatching" them, to borrow an industry euphemism?

Meat-eating has always been a messy business, shadowed by the shame of killing and, since Upton Sinclair's writing of "The Jungle," by questions about what we're really eating when we eat meat. Forgetting, or willed ignorance, is the preferred strategy of many beef eaters, a strategy abetted by the industry. (What grocery-store item is more silent about its origins than a shrink-wrapped steak?) Yet I recently began to feel that ignorance was no longer tenable. If I was going to continue to eat red meat, then I owed it to myself, as well as to the animals, to take more responsibility for the invisible but crucial transaction between ourselves and the animals we eat. I'd try to own it, in other words.

So this is the biography of my cow.

The Blair brothers ranch occupies 11,500 acres of short-grass prairie a few miles outside Sturgis, SD, directly in the shadow of Bear Butte. In November, when I visited, the turf forms a luxuriant pelt of grass oscillating yellow and gold in the constant wind and sprinkled with perambulating black dots: Angus cows and calves grazing.

Ed and Rich Blair run what's called a "cow-calf" operation, the first stage of beef production, and the stage least changed by the modern industrialization of meat. While the pork and chicken industries have consolidated the entire life cycles of those animals under a single roof, beef cattle are still born on thousands of independently owned ranches. Although four giant meatpacking companies (Tyson's subsidiary IBP, Monfort, Excel and National) now slaughter and market more than 80 percent of the beef cattle born in this country, that concentration represents the narrow end of a funnel that starts out as wide as the great plains.

Michael Pollan, "Power Steer." *The New York Times*, 31 March 2002. Reprinted with permission.

The Blairs have been in the cattle business for four generations. Although there are new wrinkles to the process—artificial insemination to improve genetics, for example—producing beef calves goes pretty much as it always has, just faster. Calving season begins in late winter, a succession of subzero nights spent yanking breeched babies out of their bellowing mothers. In April comes the first spring roundup to work the newborn calves (branding, vaccination, castration); then more roundups in early summer to inseminate the cows ($15 mail-order straws of elite bull semen have pretty much put the resident stud out of work); and weaning in the fall. If all goes well, your herd of 850 cattle has increased to 1600 by the end of the year.

My steer spent his first six months in these lush pastures alongside his mother, No. 9,534. His father was a registered Angus named GAR Precision 1,680, a bull distinguished by the size and marbling of his offspring's rib-eye steaks. Born last March 13 in a birthing shed across the road, No. 534 was turned out on pasture with his mother as soon as the 80-pound calf stood up and began nursing. After a few weeks, the calf began supplementing his mother's milk by nibbling on a salad bar of mostly native grasses: western wheatgrass, little bluestem, green needlegrass.

Apart from the trauma of the April day when he was branded and castrated, you could easily imagine No. 534 looking back on those six months grazing at his mother's side as the good old days—if, that is, cows do look back. ("They do not know what is meant by yesterday or today," Friedrich Nietzsche wrote, with a note of envy, of grazing cattle, "fettered to the moment and its pleasure or displeasure, and thus neither melancholy or bored." Nietzsche clearly had never seen a feedlot.) It may be foolish to presume to know what a cow experiences, yet we can say that a cow grazing on grass is at least doing what he has been splendidly molded by evolution to do. Which isn't a bad definition of animal happiness. Eating grass, however, is something that, after October, my steer would never do again.

Although the modern cattle industry all but ignores it, the reciprocal relationship between cows and grass is one of nature's underappreciated wonders. For the grasses, the cow maintains their habitat by preventing trees and shrubs from gaining a foothold; the animal also spreads grass seed, planting it with its hoofs and fertilizing it. In exchange for these services, the grasses offer the ruminants a plentiful, exclusive meal. For cows, sheep, and other grazers have the unique ability to convert grass—which single-stomached creatures like us can't digest—into high-quality protein. They can do this because they possess a rumen, a 45-gallon fermentation tank in which a resident population of bacteria turns grass into metabolically useful organic acids and protein.

This is an excellent system for all concerned: for the grasses, for the animals, and for us. What's more, growing meat on grass can make superb ecological sense: so long as the rancher practices rotational grazing, it is a sustainable, solar-powered system for producing food on land too arid or hilly to grow anything else.

So if this system is so ideal, why is it that my cow hasn't tasted a blade of grass since October? Speed, in a word. Cows raised on grass simply take longer to reach slaughter weight than cows raised on a richer diet, and the modern meat industry has devoted itself to shortening a beef calf's allotted time on earth. "In my grandfather's day, steers were 4 or 5 years old at slaughter," explained Rich Blair, who, at 45, is the younger of the brothers by four years. "In the 50s, when my father was ranching, it was 2 or 3. Now we get there at 14 to 16 months." Fast food indeed. What gets a beef calf from 80 to 1200 pounds in 14 months are enormous quantities of corn, protein supplements—and drugs, including growth hormones. These "efficiencies," all of which come at a price, have transformed raising cattle into a high-volume, low-margin business. Not everybody is convinced that this is progress. "Hell," Ed Blair told me, "my dad made more money on 250 head than we do on 850."

Weaning marks the fateful moment when the natural, evolutionary logic represented by a ruminant grazing on grass bumps up against the industrial logic that, with stunning speed, turns that animal into a box of beef. This industrial logic is rational and even irresistible—after all, it has succeeded in transforming beef from a luxury item into everyday fare for millions of people. And yet the further you follow it, the more likely you are to wonder if that rational logic might not also be completely insane.

In early October, a few weeks before I met him, No. 534 was weaned from his mother. Weaning is perhaps the most traumatic time on a ranch for animals and ranchers alike; cows separated from their calves will mope and bellow for days, and the calves themselves, stressed by the change in circumstance and diet, are prone to get sick.

On many ranches, weaned calves go directly from the pasture to the sale barn, where they're sold at auction, by the pound, to feedlots. The Blairs prefer to own their steers straight through to slaughter and to keep them on the ranch for a couple of months of "backgrounding" before sending them on the 500-mile trip to Poky Feeders. Think of backgrounding as prep school for feedlot life: the animals are confined in a pen, "bunk broken"—taught to eat from a trough—and gradually accustomed to eating a new, unnatural diet of grain. (Grazing cows encounter only tiny amounts of grain, in the form of grass seeds.)

It was in the backgrounding pen that I first met No. 534 on an unseasonably warm afternoon in November. I'd told the Blairs I wanted to follow one of their steers through the life cycle; Ed, 49, suggested I might as well buy a steer, as a way to really understand the daunting economics of modern ranching. Ed and Rich told me what to look for: a broad, straight back, and thick hindquarters. Basically, you want a strong frame on which to hang a lot of meat. I was also looking for a memorable face in this Black Angus sea, one that would stand out in the feedlot crowd. Almost as soon as I started surveying the 90 or so steers in the pen, No. 534 moseyed up to the railing and made eye contact. He had a wide, stout frame and was brockle-faced—he had three distinctive white blazes. If not for those markings, Ed said, No.

534 might have been spared castration and sold as a bull; he was that good-looking. But the white blazes indicate the presence of Hereford blood, rendering him ineligible for life as an Angus stud. Tough break.

Rich said he would calculate the total amount I owed the next time No. 534 got weighed but that the price would be $98 a hundredweight for an animal of this quality. He would then bill me for all expenses (feed, shots, et cetera) and, beginning in January, start passing on the weekly "hotel charges" from Poky Feeders. In June we'd find out from the packing plant how well my investment had panned out: I would receive a payment for No. 534 based on his carcass weight, plus a premium if he earned a USDA grade of choice or prime. "And if you're worried about the cattle market," Rich said jokingly, referring to its post-Sept. 11 slide, "I can sell you an option too." Option insurance has become increasingly popular among cattlemen in the wake of mad-cow and foot-and-mouth disease.

Rich handles the marketing end of the business out of an office in Sturgis, where he also trades commodities. In fact you'd never guess from Rich's unlined, indoorsy face and golfish attire that he was a rancher. Ed, by contrast, spends his days on the ranch and better looks the part, with his well-creased visage, crinkly cowboy eyes and ever-present plug of tobacco. His cap carries the same prairie-flat slogan I'd spotted on the ranch's roadside sign: "Beef: It's What's for Dinner."

My second morning on the ranch, I helped Troy Hadrick, Ed's son-in-law and a ranch hand, feed the steers in the backgrounding pen. A thickly muscled post of a man, Hadrick is 25 and wears a tall black cowboy hat perpetually crowned by a pair of mirrored Oakley sunglasses. He studied animal science at South Dakota State and is up on the latest university thinking on cattle nutrition, reproduction, and medicine. Hadrick seems to relish everything to do with ranching, from calving to wielding the artificial-insemination syringe.

Hadrick and I squeezed into the heated cab of a huge swivel-hipped tractor hooked up to a feed mixer: basically, a dump truck with a giant screw through the middle to blend ingredients. First stop was a hopper filled with Rumensin, a powerful antibiotic that No. 534 will consume with his feed every day for the rest of his life. Calves have no need of regular medication while on grass, but as soon as they're placed in the backgrounding pen, they're apt to get sick. Why? The stress of weaning is a factor, but the main culprit is the feed. The shift to a "hot ration" of grain can so disturb the cow's digestive process—its rumen, in particular—that it can kill the animal if not managed carefully and accompanied by antibiotics.

After we'd scooped the ingredients into the hopper and turned on the mixer, Hadrick deftly sidled the tractor alongside the pen and flipped a switch to release a dusty tan stream of feed in a long, even line. No. 534 was one of the first animals to belly up to the rail for breakfast. He was heftier than his pen mates and, I decided, sparkier too. That morning, Hadrick and I gave each calf six pounds of corn mixed with seven pounds of ground alfalfa hay and a quarter-pound of

Rumensin. Soon after my visit, this ration would be cranked up to 14 pounds of corn and 6 pounds of hay—and added two and a half pounds every day to No. 534.

While I was on the ranch, I didn't talk to No. 534, pet him or otherwise try to form a connection. I also decided not to give him a name, even though my son proposed a pretty good one after seeing a snapshot. ("Night.") My intention, after all, is to send this animal to slaughter and then eat some of him. No. 534 is not a pet, and I certainly don't want to end up with an ox in my backyard because I suddenly got sentimental.

As fall turned into winter, Hadrick sent me regular e-mail messages apprising me of my steer's progress. On Nov. 13 he weighed 650 pounds; by Christmas he was up to 798, making him the seventh-heaviest steer in his pen, an achievement in which I, idiotically, took a measure of pride. Between Nov. 13 and Jan. 4, the day he boarded the truck for Kansas, No. 534 put away 706 pounds of corn and 336 pounds of alfalfa hay, bringing his total living expenses for that period to $61.13. I was into this deal now for $659.

Hadrick's e-mail updates grew chattier as time went on, cracking a window on the rancher's life and outlook. I was especially struck by his relationship to the animals, how it manages to be at once intimate and unsentimental. One day Hadrick is tenderly nursing a newborn at 3 a.m., the next he's "having a big prairie oyster feed" after castrating a pen of bull calves.

Hadrick wrote empathetically about weaning ("It's like packing up and leaving the house when you are 18 and knowing you will never see your parents again") and with restrained indignation about "animal activists and city people" who don't understand the first thing about a rancher's relationship to his cattle. Which, as Hadrick put it, is simply this: "If we don't take care of these animals, they won't take care of us."

"Everyone hears about the bad stuff," Hadrick wrote, "but they don't ever see you give C.P.R. to a newborn calf that was born backward or bringing them into your house and trying to warm them up on your kitchen floor because they were born on a minus-20-degree night. Those are the kinds of things ranchers will do for their livestock. They take precedence over most everything in your life. Sorry for the sermon."

To travel from the ranch to the feedlot, as No. 534 and I both did (in separate vehicles) the first week in January, feels a lot like going from the country to the big city. Indeed, a cattle feedlot is a kind of city, populated by as many as 100,000 animals. It is very much a premodern city, however—crowded, filthy and stinking, with open sewers, unpaved roads, and choking air.

The urbanization of the world's livestock is a fairly recent historical development, so it makes a certain sense that cow towns like Poky Feeders would recall human cities several centuries ago. As in 14th-century London, the metropolitan digestion remains vividly on display: the foodstuffs coming in, the waste streaming out. Similarly, there is the crowding together of recent arrivals from who knows where, combined with a lack of modern sanitation. This combination has always been a recipe for disease; the only reason contemporary animal cities aren't as plague-ridden as their medieval counterparts is a single historical anomaly: the modern antibiotic.

I spent the better part of a day walking around Poky Feeders, trying to understand how its various parts fit together. In any city, it's easy to lose track of nature—of the connections between various species and the land on which everything ultimately depends. The feedlot's ecosystem, I could see, revolves around corn. But its food chain doesn't end there, because the corn itself grows somewhere else, where it is implicated in a whole other set of ecological relationships. Growing the vast quantities of corn used to feed livestock in this country takes vast quantities of chemical fertilizer, which in turn takes vast quantities of oil—1.2 gallons for every bushel. So the modern feedlot is really a city floating on a sea of oil.

I started my tour at the feed mill, the yard's thundering hub, where three meals a day for 37,000 animals are designed and mixed by computer. A million pounds of feed passes through the mill each day. Every hour of every day, a tractor-trailer pulls up to disgorge another 25 tons of corn. Around the other side of the mill, tanker trucks back up to silo-shaped tanks, into which they pump thousands of gallons of liquefied fat and protein supplement. In a shed attached to the mill sit vats of liquid vitamins and synthetic estrogen; next to these are pallets stacked with 50-pound sacks of Rumensin and tylosin, another antibiotic. Along with alfalfa hay and corn silage for roughage, all these ingredients are blended and then piped into the dump trucks that keep Poky's eight and a half miles of trough filled.

The feed mill's great din is made by two giant steel rollers turning against each other 12 hours a day, crushing steamed corn kernels into flakes. This was the only feed ingredient I tasted, and it wasn't half bad; not as crisp as Kellogg's, but with a cornier flavor. I passed, however, on the protein supplement, a sticky brown goop consisting of molasses and urea.

Corn is a mainstay of livestock diets because there is no other feed quite as cheap or plentiful: thanks to federal subsidies and ever-growing surpluses, the price of corn ($2.25 a bushel) is 50 cents less than the cost of growing it. The rise of the modern factory farm is a direct result of these surpluses, which soared in the years following World War II, when petrochemical fertilizers came into widespread use. Ever since, the USDA's policy has been to help farmers dispose of surplus corn by passing as much of it as possible through the digestive tracts of food animals, converting it into protein. Compared with grass or hay, corn is a compact and portable foodstuff, making it possible to feed tens of thousands of animals on small plots of land. Without cheap corn, the modern urbanization of livestock would probably never have occurred.

We have come to think of "cornfed" as some kind of old-fashioned virtue; we shouldn't. Granted, a cornfed cow develops well-marbled flesh, giving it a taste and texture American consumers have learned to like. Yet this meat is demonstrably less healthy to eat, since it contains more saturated fat. A recent study in The European Journal of Clinical Nutrition found that the meat of grass-fed livestock not only had substantially less fat than grain-fed meat but that the type of fats found in grass-fed meat were much healthier. (Grass-fed meat has more omega 3 fatty acids and fewer omega 6, which is believed to promote heart disease; it also contains betacarotine and CLA, another "good" fat.) A growing body of research suggests that many of the health problems associated with eating beef are really problems with cornfed beef. In the same way ruminants have not evolved to eat grain, humans may not be well adapted to eating grain-fed animals. Yet the USDA's grading system continues to reward marbling—that is, intermuscular fat—and thus the feeding of corn to cows.

The economic logic behind corn is unassailable, and on a factory farm, there is no other kind. Calories are calories, and corn is the cheapest, most convenient source of calories. Of course the identical industrial logic—protein is protein—led to the feeding of rendered cow parts back to cows, a practice the FDA banned in 1997 after scientists realized it was spreading mad-cow disease.

Make that mostly banned. The FDA's rules against feeding ruminant protein to ruminants make exceptions for "blood products" (even though they contain protein) and fat. Indeed, my steer has probably dined on beef tallow recycled from the very slaughterhouse he's heading to in June. "Fat is fat," the feedlot manager shrugged when I raised an eyebrow.

FDA rules still permit feedlots to feed nonruminant animal protein to cows. (Feather meal is an accepted cattle feed, as are pig and fish protein and chicken manure.) Some public-health advocates worry that since the bovine meat and bone meal that cows used to eat is now being fed to chickens, pigs and fish, infectious prions could find their way back into cattle when they eat the protein of the animals that have been eating them. To close this biological loophole, the FDA is now considering tightening its feed rules.

Until mad-cow disease, remarkably few people in the cattle business, let alone the general public, comprehended the strange semicircular food chain that industrial agriculture had devised for cattle (and, in turn, for us). When I mentioned to Rich Blair that I'd been surprised to learn that cows were eating cows, he said, "To tell the truth, it was kind of a shock to me too." Yet even today, ranchers don't ask many questions about feedlot menus. Not that the answers are so easy to come by. When I asked Poky's feedlot manager what exactly was in the protein supplement, he couldn't say. "When we buy supplement, the supplier says it's 40 percent protein, but they don't specify beyond that." When I called the supplier, it wouldn't divulge all its "proprietary ingredients" but promised that animal parts weren't among them. Protein is pretty much still protein.

Compared with ground-up cow bones, corn seems positively wholesome. Yet it wreaks considerable havoc on bovine digestion. During my day at Poky, I spent an hour or two driving around the yard with Dr. Mel Metzen, the staff veterinarian. Metzen, a 1997 graduate of Kansas State's vet school, oversees a team of eight cowboys who spend their days riding the yard, spotting sick cows and bringing them in for treatment. A great many of their health problems can be traced to their diet. "They're made to eat forage," Metzen said, "and we're making them eat grain."

Perhaps the most serious thing that can go wrong with a ruminant on corn is feedlot bloat. The rumen is always producing copious amounts of gas, which is normally expelled by belching during rumination. But when the diet contains too much starch and too little roughage, rumination all but stops, and a layer of foamy slime that can trap gas forms in the rumen. The rumen inflates like a balloon, pressing against the animal's lungs. Unless action is promptly taken to relieve the pressure (usually by forcing a hose down the animal's esophagus), the cow suffocates.

A corn diet can also give a cow acidosis. Unlike that in our own highly acidic stomachs, the normal pH of a rumen is neutral. Corn makes it unnaturally acidic, however, causing a kind of bovine heartburn, which in some cases can kill the animal but usually just makes it sick. Acidotic animals go off their feed, pant and salivate excessively, paw at their bellies and eat dirt. The condition can lead to diarrhea, ulcers, bloat, liver disease and a general weakening of the immune system that leaves the animal vulnerable to everything from pneumonia to feedlot polio.

Cows rarely live on feedlot diets for more than six months, which might be about as much as their digestive systems can tolerate. "I don't know how long you could feed this ration before you'd see problems," Metzen said; another vet said that a sustained feedlot diet would eventually "blow out their livers" and kill them. As the acids eat away at the rumen wall, bacteria enter the bloodstream and collect in the liver. More than 13 percent of feedlot cattle are found at slaughter to have abscessed livers.

What keeps a feedlot animal healthy—or healthy enough—are antibiotics. Rumensin inhibits gas production in the rumen, helping to prevent bloat; tylosin reduces the incidence of liver infection. Most of the antibiotics sold in America end up in animal feed—a practice that, it is now generally acknowledged, leads directly to the evolution of new antibiotic-resistant "superbugs." In the debate over the use of antibiotics in agriculture, a distinction is usually made between clinical and nonclinical uses. Public-health advocates don't object to treating sick animals with antibiotics; they just don't want to see the drugs lose their efficacy because factory farms are feeding them to healthy animals to promote growth. But the use of antibiotics in feedlot cattle confounds this distinction. Here the drugs are plainly being used to treat sick animals, yet the animals probably wouldn't be sick if not for what we feed them.

I asked Metzen what would happen if antibiotics were banned from cattle feed. "We just couldn't feed them as hard," he said. "Or we'd have a higher death loss." (Less than 3 percent of cattle die on the feedlot.) The price of beef would rise, he said, since the whole system would have to slow down.

"Hell, if you gave them lots of grass and space," he concluded dryly, "I wouldn't have a job."

Before heading over to Pen 43 for my reunion with No. 534, I stopped by the shed where recent arrivals receive their hormone implants. The calves are funneled into a chute, herded along by a ranch hand wielding an electric prod, then clutched in a restrainer just long enough for another hand to inject a slow-release pellet of Revlar, a synthetic estrogen, in the back of the ear. The Blairs' pen had not yet been implanted, and I was still struggling with the decision of whether to forgo what is virtually a universal practice in the cattle industry in the United States. (It has been banned in the European Union.)

American regulators permit hormone implants on the grounds that no risk to human health has been proved, even though measurable hormone residues do turn up in the meat we eat. These contribute to the buildup of estrogenic compounds in the environment, which some scientists believe may explain falling sperm counts and premature maturation in girls. Recent studies have also found elevated levels of synthetic growth hormones in feedlot wastes; these persistent chemicals eventually wind up in the waterways downstream of feedlots, where scientists have found fish exhibiting abnormal sex characteristics.

The FDA is opening an inquiry into the problem, but for now, implanting hormones in beef cattle is legal and financially irresistible: an implant costs $1.50 and adds between 40 and 50 pounds to the weight of a steer at slaughter, for a return of at least $25. That could easily make the difference between profit and loss on my investment in No. 534. Thinking like a parent, I like the idea of feeding my son hamburgers free of synthetic hormones. But thinking like a cattleman, there was really no decision to make.

I asked Rich Blair what he thought. "I'd love to give up hormones," he said. "If the consumer said, We don't want hormones, we'd stop in a second. The cattle could get along better without them. But the market signal's not there, and as long as my competitor's doing it, I've got to do it, too."

Around lunch time, Metzen and I finally arrived at No. 534's pen. My first impression was that my steer had landed himself a decent piece of real estate. The pen is far enough from the feed mill to be fairly quiet, and it has a water view—of what I initially thought was a reservoir, until I noticed the brown scum. The pen itself is surprisingly spacious, slightly bigger than a basketball court, with a concrete feed bunk out front and a freshwater trough in the back. I climbed over the railing and joined the 90 steers, which, en masse, retreated a few steps, then paused.

I had on the same carrot-colored sweater I'd worn to the ranch in South Dakota, hoping to jog my steer's memory. Way off in the back, I spotted him—those three white blazes. As I gingerly stepped toward him, the quietly shuffling mass of black cowhide between us parted, and there No. 534 and I stood, staring dumbly at each other. Glint of recognition? None whatsoever. I told myself not to take it personally. No. 534 had been bred for his marbling, after all, not his intellect.

I don't know enough about the emotional life of cows to say with any confidence if No. 534 was miserable, bored or melancholy, but I would not say he looked happy. I noticed that his eyes looked a little bloodshot. Some animals are irritated by the fecal dust that floats in the feedlot air; maybe that explained the sullen gaze with which he fixed me. Unhappy or not, though, No. 534 had clearly been eating well. My animal had put on a couple hundred pounds since we'd last met, and he looked it: thicker across the shoulders and round as a barrel through the middle. He carried himself more like a steer now than a calf, even though he was still less than a year old. Metzen complimented me on his size and conformation. "That's a handsome looking beef you've got there." (Aw, shucks.)

Staring at No. 534, I could picture the white lines of the butcher's chart dissecting his black hide: rump roast, flank steak, standing rib, brisket. One way of looking at No. 534—the industrial way—was as an efficient machine for turning feed corn into beef. Every day between now and his slaughter date in June, No. 534 will convert 32 pounds of feed (25 of them corn) into another three and a half pounds of flesh. Poky is indeed a factory, transforming cheap raw materials into a less-cheap finished product, as fast as bovinely possible.

Yet the factory metaphor obscures as much as it reveals about the creature that stood before me. For this steer was not a machine in a factory but an animal in a web of relationships that link him to certain other animals, plants and microbes, as well as to the earth. And one of those other animals is us. The unnaturally rich diet of corn that has compromised No. 534's health is fattening his flesh in a way that in turn may compromise the health of the humans who will eat him. The antibiotics he's consuming with his corn were at that very moment selecting, in his gut and wherever else in the environment they wind up, for bacteria that could someday infect us and resist the drugs we depend on. We inhabit the same microbial ecosystem as the animals we eat, and whatever happens to it also happens to us.

I thought about the deep pile of manure that No. 534 and I were standing in. We don't know much about the hormones in it—where they will end up or what they might do once they get there—but we do know something about the bacteria. One particularly lethal bug most probably resided in the manure beneath my feet. Escherichia coli 0157 is a relatively new strain of a common intestinal bacteria (it was first isolated in the 1980s) that is common in feedlot cattle, more than half of whom carry it in their guts. Ingesting as few as 10 of these microbes can cause a fatal infection.

Most of the microbes that reside in the gut of a cow and find their way into our food get killed off by the acids in our stomachs, since they originally adapted to live in a neutral-pH environment. But the digestive tract of the modern feedlot cow is closer in acidity to our own, and in this new, manmade environment acid-resistant strains of E. coli have developed that can survive our stomach acids—and go on to kill us. By acidifying a cow's gut with corn, we have broken down one of our food chain's barriers to infection. Yet this process can be reversed: James Russell, a USDA microbiologist, has discovered that switching a cow's diet from corn to hay in the final days before slaughter reduces the population of E. coli 0157 in its manure by as much as 70 percent. Such a change, however, is considered wildly impractical by the cattle industry.

So much comes back to corn, this cheap feed that turns out in so many ways to be not cheap at all. While I stood in No. 534's pen, a dump truck pulled up alongside the feed bunk and released a golden stream of feed. The animals stepped up to the bunk for their lunch. The $1.60 a day I'm paying for three giant meals is a bargain only by the narrowest of calculations. It doesn't take into account, for example, the cost to the public health of antibiotic resistance or food poisoning by E. coli or all the environmental costs associated with industrial corn.

For if you follow the corn from this bunk back to the fields where it grows, you will find an 80-million-acre monoculture that consumes more chemical herbicide and fertilizer than any other crop. Keep going and you can trace the nitrogen runoff from that crop all the way down the Mississippi into the Gulf of Mexico, where it has created (if that is the right word) a 12,000-square-mile "dead zone."

But you can go farther still, and follow the fertilizer needed to grow that corn all the way to the oil fields of the Persian Gulf. No. 534 started life as part of a food chain that derived all its energy from the sun; now that corn constitutes such an important link in his food chain, he is the product of an industrial system powered by fossil fuel. (And in turn, defended by the military—another uncounted cost of "cheap" food.) I asked David Pimentel, a Cornell ecologist who specializes in agriculture and energy, if it might be possible to calculate precisely how much oil it will take to grow my steer to slaughter weight. Assuming No. 534 continues to eat 25 pounds of corn a day and reaches a weight of 1,250 pounds, he will have consumed in his lifetime roughly 284 gallons of oil. We have succeeded in industrializing the beef calf, transforming what was once a solar-powered ruminant into the very last thing we need: another fossil-fuel machine.

Sometime in June, No. 534 will be ready for slaughter. Though only 14 months old, my steer will weigh more than 1,200 pounds and will move with the lumbering deliberateness of the obese. One morning, a cattle trailer from the National Beef plant in Liberal, Kan., will pull in to Poky Feeders, drop a ramp and load No. 534 along with 35 of his pen mates.

The 100-mile trip south to Liberal is a straight shot on Route 83, a two-lane highway on which most of the traffic consists of speeding tractor-trailers carrying either cattle or corn. The National Beef plant is a sprawling gray-and-white complex in a neighborhood of trailer homes and tiny houses a notch up from shanty. These are, presumably, the homes of the Mexican and Asian immigrants who make up a large portion of the plant's work force. The meat business has made southwestern Kansas an unexpectedly diverse corner of the country.

A few hours after their arrival in the holding pens outside the factory, a plant worker will open a gate and herd No. 534 and his pen mates into an alley that makes a couple of turns before narrowing down to a single-file chute. The chute becomes a ramp that leads the animals up to a second-story platform and then disappears through a blue door.

That door is as close to the kill floor as the plant managers were prepared to let me go. I could see whatever I wanted to farther on—the cold room where carcasses are graded, the food-safety lab, the fabrication room where the carcasses are broken down into cuts—on the condition that

I didn't take pictures or talk to employees. But the stunning, bleeding and evisceration process was off limits to a journalist, even a cattleman-journalist like myself.

What I know about what happens on the far side of the blue door comes mostly from Temple Grandin, who has been on the other side and, in fact, helped to design it. Grandin, an assistant professor of animal science at Colorado State, is one of the most influential people in the United States cattle industry. She has devoted herself to making cattle slaughter less stressful and therefore more humane by designing an ingenious series of cattle restraints, chutes, ramps and stunning systems. Grandin is autistic, a condition she says has allowed her to see the world from the cow's point of view. The industry has embraced Grandin's work because animals under stress are not only more difficult to handle but also less valuable: panicked cows produce a surge of adrenaline that turns their meat dark and unappetizing. "Dark cutters," as they're called, sell at a deep discount.

Grandin designed the double-rail conveyor system in use at the National Beef plant; she has also audited the plant's killing process for McDonald's. Stories about cattle "waking up" after stunning only to be skinned alive prompted McDonald's to audit its suppliers in a program that is credited with substantial improvements since its inception in 1999. Grandin says that in cattle slaughter "there is the pre-McDonald's era and the post-McDonald's era—it's night and day."

Grandin recently described to me what will happen to No. 534 after he passes through the blue door. "The animal goes into the chute single file," she began. "The sides are high enough so all he sees is the butt of the animal in front of him. As he walks through the chute, he passes over a metal bar, with his feet on either side. While he's straddling the bar, the ramp begins to decline at a 25-degree angle, and before he knows it, his feet are off the ground and he's being carried along on a conveyor belt. We put in a false floor so he can't look down and see he's off the ground. That would panic him."

Listening to Grandin's rather clinical account, I couldn't help wondering what No. 534 would be feeling as he approached his end. Would he have any inkling—a scent of blood, a sound of terror from up the line—that this was no ordinary day?

Grandin anticipated my question: "Does the animal know it's going to get slaughtered? I used to wonder that. So I watched them, going into the squeeze chute on the feedlot, getting their shots and going up the ramp at a slaughter plant. No difference. If they knew they were going to die, you'd see much more agitated behavior."

"Anyway, the conveyor is moving along at roughly the speed of a moving sidewalk. On a catwalk above stands the stunner. The stunner has a pneumatic-powered 'gun' that fires a steel bolt about seven inches long and the diameter of a fat pencil. He leans over and puts it smack in the middle of the forehead. When it's done correctly, it will kill the animal on the first shot."

For a plant to pass a McDonald's audit, the stunner needs to render animals "insensible" on the first shot 95 percent of the time. A second shot is allowed, but should

that one fail, the plant flunks. At the line speeds at which meatpacking plants in the United States operate—390 animals are slaughtered every hour at National, which is not unusual—mistakes would seem inevitable, but Grandin insists that only rarely does the process break down.

"After the animal is shot while he's riding along, a worker wraps a chain around his foot and hooks it to an overhead trolley. Hanging upside down by one leg, he's carried by the trolley into the bleeding area, where the bleeder cuts his throat. Animal rights people say they're cutting live animals, but that's because there's a lot of reflex kicking." This is one of the reasons a job at a slaughter plant is the most dangerous in America. "What I look for is, Is the head dead? It should be flopping like a rag, with the tongue hanging out. He'd better not be trying to hold it up—then you've got a live one on the rail." Just in case, Grandin said, "they have another hand stunner in the bleed area."

Much of what happens next—the de-hiding of the animal, the tying off of its rectum before evisceration—is designed to keep the animal's feces from coming into contact with its meat. This is by no means easy to do, not when the animals enter the kill floor smeared with manure and 390 of them are eviscerated every hour. (Partly for this reason, European plants operate at much slower line speeds.) But since that manure is apt to contain lethal pathogens like E. coli 0157, and since the process of grinding together hamburger from hundreds of different carcasses can easily spread those pathogens across millions of burgers, packing plants now spend millions on "food safety"—which is to say, on the problem of manure in meat.

Most of these efforts are reactive: it's accepted that the animals will enter the kill floor caked with feedlot manure that has been rendered lethal by the feedlot diet. Rather than try to alter that diet or keep the animals from living in their waste or slow the line speed—all changes regarded as impractical—the industry focuses on disinfecting the manure that will inevitably find its way into the meat. This is the purpose of irradiation (which the industry prefers to call "cold pasteurization"). It is also the reason that carcasses pass through a hot steam cabinet and get sprayed with an antimicrobial solution before being hung in the cooler at the National Beef plant.

It wasn't until after the carcasses emerged from the cooler, 36 hours later, that I was allowed to catch up with them, in the grading room. I entered a huge arctic space resembling a monstrous dry cleaner's, with a seemingly endless overhead track conveying thousands of red-and-white carcasses. I quickly learned that you had to move smartly through this room or else be tackled by a 350-pound side of beef. The carcasses felt cool to the touch, no longer animals but meat.

Two by two, the sides of beef traveled swiftly down the rails, six pairs every minute, to a station where two workers—one wielding a small power saw, the other a long knife—made a single six-inch cut between the 12th and 13th ribs, opening a window on the meat inside. The carcasses continued on to another station, where a USDA inspector holding a round blue stamp glanced at the exposed rib eye and stamped the carcass's creamy white fat once, twice or—very rarely—three times: select, choice, prime.

For the Blair brothers, and for me, this is the moment of truth, for that stamp will determine exactly how much the packing plant will pay for each animal and whether the 14 months of effort and expense will yield a profit.

Unless the cattle market collapses between now and June (always a worry these days), I stand to make a modest profit on No. 534. In February, the feedlot took a sonogram of his rib eye and ran the data through a computer program. The projections are encouraging: a live slaughter weight of 1,250, a carcass weight of 787 pounds and a grade at the upper end of choice, making him eligible to be sold at a premium as Certified Angus Beef. Based on the June futures price, No. 534 should be worth $944. (Should he grade prime, that would add another $75.)

I paid $598 for No. 534 in November; his living expenses since then come to $61 on the ranch and $258 for 160 days at the feedlot (including implant), for a total investment of $917, leaving a profit of $27. It's a razor-thin margin, and it could easily vanish should the price of corn rise or No. 534 fail to make the predicted weight or grade—say, if he gets sick and goes off his feed. Without the corn, without the antibiotics, without the hormone implant, my brief career as a cattleman would end in failure.

The Blairs and I are doing better than most. According to Cattle-Fax, a market-research firm, the return on an animal coming out of a feedlot has averaged just $3 per head over the last 20 years.

"Some pens you make money, some pens you lose," Rich Blair said when I called to commiserate. "You try to average it out over time, limit the losses and hopefully make a little profit." He reminded me that a lot of ranchers are in the business "for emotional reasons—you can't be in it just for the money."

Now you tell me.

The manager of the packing plant has offered to pull a box of steaks from No. 534 before his carcass disappears into the trackless stream of commodity beef fanning out to America's supermarkets and restaurants this June. From what I can see, the Blair brothers, with the help of Poky Feeders, are producing meat as good as any you can find in an American supermarket. And yet there's no reason to think this steak will taste any different from the other high-end industrial meat I've ever eaten.

While waiting for my box of meat to arrive from Kansas, I've explored some alternatives to the industrial product. Nowadays you can find hormone- and antibiotic-free beef as well as organic beef, fed only grain grown without chemicals. This meat, which is often quite good, is typically produced using more grass and less grain (and so makes for healthier animals). Yet it doesn't fundamentally challenge the corn-feedlot system, and I'm not sure that an "organic feedlot" isn't, ecologically speaking, an oxymoron. What I really wanted to taste is the sort of preindustrial beef my grandparents ate—from animals that have lived most of their full-length lives on grass.

Eventually I found a farmer in the Hudson Valley who sold me a quarter of a grass-fed Angus steer that is now occupying most of my freezer. I also found ranchers selling grass-fed beef on the Web; Eatwild.com is a clearinghouse of information on grass-fed livestock, which is emerging as one of the livelier movements in sustainable agriculture.

I discovered that grass-fed meat is more expensive than supermarket beef. Whatever else you can say about industrial beef, it is remarkably cheap, and any argument for changing the system runs smack into the industry's populist arguments. Put the animals back on grass, it is said, and prices will soar; it takes too long to raise beef on grass, and there's not enough grass to raise them on, since the Western range lands aren't big enough to sustain America's 100 million head of cattle. And besides, Americans have learned to love cornfed beef. Feedlot meat is also more consistent in both taste and supply and can be harvested 12 months a year. (Grass-fed cattle tend to be harvested in the fall, since they stop gaining weight over the winter, when the grasses go dormant.)

All of this is true. The economic logic behind the feedlot system is hard to refute. And yet so is the ecological logic behind a ruminant grazing on grass. Think what would happen if we restored a portion of the Corn Belt to the tall grass prairie it once was and grazed cattle on it. No more petrochemical fertilizer, no more herbicide, no more nitrogen runoff. Yes, beef would probably be more expensive than it is now, but would that necessarily be a bad thing? Eating beef every day might not be such a smart idea anyway—for our health, for the environment. And how cheap, really, is cheap feedlot beef? Not cheap at all, when you add in the invisible costs: of antibiotic resistance, environmental degradation, heart disease, E. coli poisoning, corn subsidies, imported oil and so on. All these are costs that grass-fed beef does not incur.

So how does grass-fed beef taste? Uneven, just as you might expect the meat of a nonindustrial animal to taste. One grass-fed tenderloin from Argentina that I sampled turned out to be the best steak I've ever eaten. But unless the meat is carefully aged, grass-fed beef can be tougher than feedlot beef—not surprisingly, since a grazing animal, which moves around in search of its food, develops more muscle and less fat. Yet even when the meat was tougher, its flavor, to my mind, was much more interesting. And specific, for the taste of every grass-fed animal is inflected by the place where it lived. Maybe it's just my imagination, but nowadays when I eat a feedlot steak, I can taste the corn and the fat, and I can see the view from No. 534's pen. I can't taste the oil, obviously, or the drugs, yet now I know they're there.

A considerably different picture comes to mind while chewing (and, O.K., chewing) a grass-fed steak: a picture of a cow outside in a pasture eating the grass that has eaten the sunlight. Meat-eating may have become an act riddled with moral and ethical ambiguities, but eating a steak at the end of a short, primordial food chain comprising nothing more than ruminants and grass and light is something I'm happy to do and defend. We are what we eat, it is often said, but of course that's only part of the story. We are what what we eat eats too.

CHAPTER 17

Anthropological Perspectives on the Global Food Crisis

David A. Himmelgreen, Nancy Romero-Daza, and Charlotte A. Noble
(2012)

Like other metropolitan cities in Latin America, Bogotá, Colombia, is a city of great contrasts. On one hand, new buildings are sprouting up throughout the city sporting contemporary designs and spiraling to the sky in the backdrop of the magnanimous Andes Mountains. The *Transmilenio*, a rapid transit bus system, shuttles 1.4 million "Bogotanos" along its 84 km (54 miles) of four-lane arteries throughout the expansive city, reducing travel time by nearly one-third. Meanwhile, cars and taxies clog up the streets and avenues that cross-cut the nearly 500-year-old city. Gargantuan malls, box stores, global fast food chains, and mega-supermarkets are interspersed between bodegas, bakeries, and shoe repair shops. Sustained economic growth in Colombia even during the global recession (World Fact Book 2010) has resulted in increasing economic prosperity among a growing middle class. On the other hand, poverty and hunger are ever present in Colombia's capital city where multitudes of homeless and working poor struggle to survive on a daily basis. Throughout the city homeless people abound, picking through trash for food or scrap-metal to sell or begging for money for food, and even perhaps for drugs and alcohol. They weave in and out of traffic putting life and limb at risk and sometimes resort to mugging and vandalism. In some neighborhoods graffiti is strewn throughout the run-down buildings; political statements calling for revolution and vulgar messages share public space and add color to the often bleak settings. As in many other places, there is a widening gap between rich and poor in Colombia.

While in Colombia recently, two of the authors (Himmelgreen and Romero-Daza) volunteered to help distribute food to displaced families on the outskirts of Bogotá. More than 40 years of political instability and simmering civil war have resulted in the displacement of millions of Colombians from the countryside to the cities to escape the violence of the leftist rebels, drug cartels, and the rightist paramilitaries. Even though the violence has subsided in recent years and the economy has improved, the number of internally displaced people (IDP) has grown. Actual figures vary depending on the reporting source; while the Colombian government estimates that about 3.4 million people had been displaced by 2010, a non-governmental source places those numbers at 4.9 million, with gradual increases over the years (IDMC and NRC 2010).

In addition to the civil strife, one notable factor that is fueling this continued displacement of people as of late has been *La Niña*, a climatic event in which there is a cyclical cooling of ocean surface temperatures throughout the tropical Pacific (Nature News 2010). As result, there has been a significant increase in rainfall and extended rainy season in several countries including Colombia, Venezuela, Brazil, and Australia. In Colombia, hundreds of people have died in mudslides and flooding and over 1.5 million have become homeless because of *La Niña*-related weather (Reuters 2010). Himmelgreen and Romero-Daza volunteered with the Colombian Family Welfare Institute (ICBF) and the World Food Program (WFP) to distribute rice, oil, salt, *panela* (block of brown sugar), and *Bienestarina* (a high nutritional–value cereal for infants, pregnant women, and the elderly) to families who had been displaced by recent mudslides. As in most cases, these families, who had limited resources before losing their homes in the mudslides, saw their situation deteriorate drastically because of the inclement weather. The Colombian government estimates the rates of food security (i.e., access to food of adequate quantity and quality obtained through socially acceptable means) among IDP to be about 50%. However, considerably lower figures of about 30% are reported by non-government bodies (IDMC and NRC 2010). Thus, while in the short term, this food assistance serves to protect against malnutrition, it is only a temporary fix to the much larger problem of global poverty and food insecurity.

AIMS

Many neo-liberal economists and policy makers (Begovic et al. 2007, Bhagwati 2004, Sapsford and Garikipati 2006) have argued that a free-market economy will alleviate poverty worldwide. Unfortunately, this has not been the case as was evidenced by the Great Recession and Global Food Crisis (GFC) that began in 2008. The aims of this article are to discuss the GFC in the context of other recent global events, examine the causes and consequences of the GFC, and more importantly, explore the ways in which anthropology can be used to find solutions to the pressing problem through examples of anthropological case studies and approaches.

THE GREAT RECESSION AND THE GLOBAL FOOD CRISIS OF 2008

The global economic recession of 2008 was the worst since the Great Depression of the 1930s. Many countries including the United States were teetering on financial disaster; banks went out of business, financial markets spiraled downward like crashing airplanes, and millions of people were laid off from their jobs. It was during the early part of this Great Recession that global food prices skyrocketed and the World Food Program (WFP) declared that the increase was the biggest challenge in its 45-year history, calling the impact a "silent tsunami" that threatened to plunge millions into hunger (WFP 2008). For example, during the second quarter of 2008, the world prices for wheat and maize were three times as high as they were just five years before, and the price of rice rose five times in the same period of time. Significant price increases were found for dairy products, beef, and poultry (von Braun 2008). The United Nations Food and Agricultural Office (FAO) price index (based on changes on wholesale cost of food commodities) increased by 9% in 2006, 24% in 2007, and 51% in 2008 (Darnton-Hill and Cogill 2010). For many people, particularly those living in poverty who earn less than $2 a day and spend up to 70% of their income on food (Clemmitt 2008), these increases on the cost of food have the potential to cause much pain and suffering.

Before the current GFC, the FAO estimated that 923 million people were undernourished worldwide (FAO 2008). In 2009 it was estimated that more than one billion people were undernourished, reflecting an increase of nearly 75 million since the beginning of the GFC (FAO 2009). This is astounding considering that this represents more than 1/7th of the world's population (U.S. Census Bureau 2011).

Although the impact of the GFC is felt more strongly in poorer countries, it has also been felt in wealthier countries such as the United States. Food insecurity, which is a measure of inadequate physical, social, or economic access to food (FAO 2006), has recently risen to its highest levels since nationally representative surveys were begun in 1995. Food insecurity takes place when there is difficulty in feeding one or more household members at some point in time during the previous year. In 2007, 11.1% of households were observed to be food insecure (Nord et al. 2008). The rate increased to 14.6% in 2008 and 14.7% in 2009 (Nord et al. 2009, 2010). This translates into over 49 million people (Nord et al. 2010) or about 16% of the entire U.S. population. Seventeen million children live in food insecure households (Nord et al. 2009). Single parents, African Americans, and Hispanics are much more likely to live in food insecure households than whites. Food insecurity is not only associated with undernutrition, but also with overweight and obesity, which are more prevalent in wealthier countries.

Increasing global food insecurity and economic inflation have resulted in riots in more than 20 countries and non-violent demonstrations in at least 30 more (Messer 2009; Benson et al. 2008). This was especially so in developing countries where there is a heavy dependence on foreign food imports such as rice, wheat, corn, and soybeans. The anger and civil strife were evidenced in countries like Haiti (Mazzeo 2009) and, more recently, in Tunisia and Egypt, where rising food and fuel prices in addition to anti-government sentiment led to the ousting of the President and the fall of the entire government in the former (Ridgwell 2011) and the ousting of President Hosni Mubarak after three decades in power in the latter.

Although food prices stabilized for a period of time after the worst of the Great Recession was over, they began to climb again by the end of 2010. In fact, they hit a record high in late December 2010, according to the United Nation's FAO (CNN 2011). Fortunately, the price of some food staples such as rice has remained stable, but there is a serious concern about the rising price of wheat in the face of poor harvests in Australia where weather-related flooding has taken a dramatic toll on agriculture. Other increases in the price of sugar, oil, seeds, and meat (CNN 2011) are of concern not only in developing countries but also in industrialized ones where these commodities are extensively used in the fast-food industry and production of processed foods. Along with increased food prices there has been a significant increase in the use of food assistance programs, for instance in the United States, especially among people who are out of work or who do not earn enough money to buy food and pay for other living expenses such as housing, utilities, and prescription medications.

CAUSES AND CONSEQUENCES

In general, there has been a relative decline in global food prices since 1870 (Von Braun et al. 2008). However, there have been three major spikes in food prices over that time: the period following World War II as Europe and Japan recovered from the devastation; in the early 1970s after the Arab Oil Embargo, when oil prices skyrocketed and gas rationing was initiated; and most recently in 2008 at the beginning of the Great Recession. While the factors associated with these stratospheric increases in food prices are complex and interrelated, there are several other key ones that can be discussed in order to understand the current GFC.

BIO FUEL PRODUCTION AND TRADE

With growing concern over the dependence on oil, there has been a push to increase the production of bio fuels in countries like the United States. As a result, American farmers have reduced the amount of land used for soybean production and have increased agricultural acreage for maize, which is used to produce ethanol (Von Braun et al. 2008). In 2006, for example, the United States diverted 20% of its maize crop (14 million tons) for ethanol (Vidal 2007). This trend continues and has contributed to a reduction of maize and soybeans, as well as other cereals available for trade on global markets, thereby resulting in significant increases in food prices. Although people from poorer countries have been disproportionately affected by these increases, there is the potential for food prices to soar in wealthier countries, where unemployment remains high and wages are stagnant. The ability of families and individuals to be food secure will be further challenged if something is not done to reverse this trend.

CLIMATE CHANGE

While the public debate over climate change still rages, there is growing evidence of its impact on food systems and livelihoods (that is, the ways people support themselves and subsist). Droughts in some regions and flooding in other areas have contributed to unstable grain production; for instance, the decline in wheat production and availability of edible oils (Darnton-Hill and Cogill 2010). Dry weather in North America and in parts of Asia affected wheat production in major producers such as the United States and the Ukraine. As supplies tightened and demand grew, the cost of these food commodities increased, making it very difficult for poorer people to purchase them because their food dollars were already stretched to the limit. Crop- and specific-regions forecasts suggest that climate change will adversely impact the production of some food crops in food insecure regions around the world in the coming years (Conceição and Mendoza 2010). Also, with changing weather patterns and the encroachment of land, it is becoming increasingly difficult for nomadic peoples to raise livestock for meat and milk consumption and to use for trade for other food commodities (Clemmitt 2008).

MIGRATION, DECLINES IN AGRICULTURAL SUPPORT, AND GLOBAL MARKETS

As people find it more difficult to produce enough food to meet their needs they are increasingly moving to urban centers in search of work for survival. As a result, the production of food is falling into the hands of fewer and fewer people. At the same time, agricultural multi-national companies are displacing small-scale farmers in order to meet the food demands of a growing global population and modernizing economies. These large-scale producers rely more on fertilizer and irrigation for higher yields than their small-scale counterparts. This not only pushes the price of food higher, but also poses significant environmental hazards. Moreover, as demand for meat products increase, more agricultural commodities are being diverted for animal feed, thereby further contributing to the rise in food prices (Bloem et al. 2010). Although there have been efforts to increase small-scale, sustainable agriculture, assistance for farming has

been halved in developing countries between 1984 and 2004 (Mittal 2009). Finally, while the removal and reduction of trade tariffs have stimulated global economic growth in recent decades, such growth has come at the expense of the small-scale farmer who no longer can compete with these multi-national companies (Mittal 2010).

IMPACT OF THE FOOD CRISIS ON HEALTH AND WELL-BEING

The GFC has resulted in inadequate access to food for a great number of individuals and families all over the world. As food prices rise, and buying capacity diminishes, malnutrition becomes more and more common. Malnutrition can manifest itself as undernutrition, with the obvious signs of extreme weight-loss among children and adults and stunted or arrested growth among babies and children. However, even when there is adequate intake of calories, malnutrition can occur in the form of overweight and obesity when there is over-reliance on inexpensive foods such as pasta, white bread, rice, and other non-fortified cereal grains, and a decrease in the consumption of fruits and vegetables. While these carbohydrate-laden foods provide enough, and often excessive, amounts of calories, they tend to be void of essential minerals and vitamins. As a result, people may experience a paradoxical combination of excessive weight and inadequate nutritional status.

Inadequate nutritional status is associated with many negative health outcomes. At the most general level, there is a clear relationship between malnutrition and infection. This association, termed the malnutrition-infection cycle, was first postulated by Scrimshaw and colleagues (1968), to describe the mechanisms by which nutritional deficiencies lead to the weakening of the immune system, thus making individuals more susceptible to infectious diseases. This creates a vicious cycle, as infections further deplete the organism of needed nutrients, thus resulting in worse health outcomes. A clear example of this cyclic interaction can be seen in the context of HIV in resource-poor countries. Individuals who are malnourished are more likely to have compromised immune systems, which make them more vulnerable to HIV infection. The virus further depletes the nutritional reserves of those infected and, in the absence of adequate nutrition and medical treatment, quickly results in muscle wasting and extreme weight loss. The cycle of malnutrition and infection also hastens the progression of the disease and may lead to premature death (Suttmann et al. 1995; Tang 2003). Alarmingly, lack of access to basic food resources also increases the risk for HIV/AIDS as individuals who are food insecure and have no other means of obtaining food may involve themselves in behaviors such as transactional sex (Bryceson and Fonseca 2006, Shah et al. 2002, Weiser et al. 2007).

Malnutrition during the prenatal period may result in low-birth weight and, in severe cases, in intra-uterine growth restriction (IUGR). It can also lead to compromised immune systems and lowered immune response among newborns. Research also indicates a possible association between nutritional deficiencies and fetal abnormalities such as spina bifida and anencephaly (Carmichel et al. 2007). Babies whose immune systems are not strong are more prone to chronic and acute infections, which lead to increase morbidity and mortality. In fact, malnutrition-related conditions such as diarrheal infection are the number one cause of death among neonates and young children around the world. Diarrheal infection, in turn, further compromises the child's nutritional status by causing a lack of appetite and anorexia, decreasing absorption of essential nutrients, and contributing to the direct loss of much needed minerals and vitamins. For pregnant women, malnutrition may result in serious depletion of stored fat, compromised immune system, and pregnancy loss.

During childhood conditions such as marasmus and kwashiorkor, both of them the result of Protein Energy Malnutrition (PEM), as well as micronutrient deficiencies, such as Vitamin A, iron, and zinc deficiencies, are especially common. During the first two years of life, when most of the brain development occurs in humans, malnutrition can have serious negative consequences for children. The actual rate of brain growth can be slowed and cognitive development may be compromised, potentially leading to long-term effects. Malnourished children may also exhibit developmental delays (both in social and motor skills), and may become lethargic and unresponsive. For older children, malnutrition may lead to anxiety, apathy, delays in the development of social skills, and difficulties in concentration, thus affecting school performance (Levitsky, David and Strupp 1995, Glewwe and King 2001, Scrimshaw 1998).

While the health and well-being of adults of all ages can be compromised by lack of access to nutritious food, elderly people are at heightened risk under conditions of food insecurity. Malnutrition may significantly decrease elderly people's physical and cognitive abilities, and may magnify the deleterious effects of other conditions such as diabetes, high blood pressure, or cardiovascular disease. Among the elderly, especially those that are home-bound or institutionalized, malnutrition can result in delays in healing of existing wounds, higher susceptibility to infections, functional decline, and delays in recovering from acute health conditions (Hajjar et al. 2004).

While the links between the Global Food Crisis, malnutrition, and compromised nutritional health are patently obvious, the GFC also has important implications for mental health. As described previously, one of the effects of the food crisis has been the increase in the number of people who are "food insecure," that is, people who do not have access to food of enough quantity and quality obtained in socially acceptable ways. The inability to obtain food for themselves and for their dependents often leads people to experience increased levels of anxiety, irritability, overall stress, depression, and social isolation (Collins 2009, Hamlin et al. 2002; Heflin et al. 2005; Whitaker et al. 2006). For example, studies in Africa demonstrated an association between food insecurity and anxiety disorder (Sorsdahl et al. 2010), and

even with more serious depression (Hadley and Patil 2006). Most of these mental conditions are found among the adults (especially mothers) who face food insecurity. However, a domino effect is created as caregivers' ability to function and to relate effectively to their children is impaired. This results in increased levels of anxiety and stress among other household members. Thus, as economic conditions continue to deteriorate and more and more people experience the ravaging effects of the GFC, we are bound to see further deterioration of the physical, mental, and social health and well-being of millions and millions of individuals in all corners of the world.

ROLE OF ANTHROPOLOGY IN FINDING SOLUTIONS TO THE GFC

Given the tremendous impact of the GFC on the physical, mental, social, and economic well-being of populations around the world, there has been a call to "bring clarity and understanding to the forces underlying the food crisis to enable policymakers to establish a sustainable, food secure future" (Katz 2008:4). In response to this call, we would like to touch on some of the ways that anthropologists can contribute to understanding the complexities of the global food crisis and to informing strategies to address related outcomes. One important task for anthropologists is to highlight the ways in which political and economic contexts of food insecurity and inequities are felt locally, in communities and in households, or even reflected in the body itself. Often, the descriptions of such events as the "global food crisis" report larger, global trends, without paying due attention to the ways in which such overall patterns translate into actual consequences for households and individuals. By eliciting and highlighting the lived-experience of those most drastically affected by economic and food insecurity, anthropology can contribute much to a grounded understanding of such events.

It has been noted that within anthropology, the study of nutrition—and we would argue, food security—is fundamentally a bio-cultural endeavor (Dufour 2010). Elsewhere, the authors have posited that one way anthropologists can contribute to illustrating the connections between macro level processes and individual-level experience is through the systematic assessment of nutritional status and food insecurity among individuals and households (Romero-Daza et al. 2009). Using a combination of qualitative and quantitative methodologies, such as anthropometric measurements and dietary intake surveys (e.g., food recalls and food frequency questionnaires), important information about the growth and nutritional status of children and adults can be obtained. Further, food insecurity can be measured through surveys (such as the Household Food Insecurity Access Scale [see Coates, Swindale, and Bilinsky 2007]) and in-depth interviews. This systematic assessment can provide very important insights into the different ways in which the impact of the GFC is manifested among and even within populations.

Importantly, such analyses can lead to recognition that some groups are more vulnerable to the impacts of food crises than others. Darton-Hill and Cogill (2009) point out those segments of the population already considered vulnerable, such as women, children, refugees, internally displaced populations, and minorities, often bear the brunt of food and financial crises. While this is undoubtedly true, the GFC has also brought to the fore the vulnerability of groups that had, for the most part, been considered much less susceptible to the vagaries of food scarcity. For example, Hadley and colleagues (2009) draw attention to the experiences of youth in urban and rural Ethiopia. Through the use of household questionnaires and interviews with adolescents, these researchers examined changing levels of food insecurity during the course of the food crisis, and identified predictors of vulnerability. Results showed not only that there were high levels of food insecurity among youth, but that there was an increase in such levels through the food crisis, especially among youth from the poorest households and those in rural areas. Thus, as this study suggests, anthropologists can contribute to the assessment of changes in food security levels within single populations through time, by means of carefully constructed and rigorous longitudinal research.

The fact that urban and rural households are often differentially affected by various food and financial crises has increasingly been recognized. Darton-Hill and Cogill (2009) note that while the poor are most affected and rural areas have disproportionate numbers of the impoverished, the urban poor experience the ravages of the food crisis in a somewhat different, and often more drastic, ways. Both rural and urban poor may have to purchase much of their food; however, the rural poor may in fact have more options to access food, such as the ability to produce their own foods. The impact of the food crisis on urban populations was demonstrated in a vulnerability study of households in Lesotho in 2008. It was noted that while the majority of the ultra-poor population lived in rural areas, households in urban areas were found to have the highest level of food insecurity (Lesotho Disaster Management Authority [DMA], Lesotho Vulnerability Assessment Committee [LVAC] and the UN World Food Programme [WFP] 2008). It is estimated that poor households spend between 75 percent and 80 percent of their income on food purchases alone (IRIN 2009). In urban areas 15,000 people faced a "critical food deficit," defined as the inability to meet their food needs through production, purchases or other means of acquisition (DMA, LVAC, and WFP 2008). Over half of urban households admitted to borrowing food to get by, and more than 40 percent reduced the number of meals consumed per day (DMA, LVAC, and WFP 2008). Declining maize production and increasing prices were indicated as affecting access to food; maize prices increased 300% since 2004/2005, and the price of cooking oil rose 100% between May 2007 and May 2008 (LVAC 2008). These increases affected most households; however, the prices of commodities in urban areas increased at higher rates than prices in rural areas (DMA, LVAC, and WFP 2008). Because of the increase in food prices, a 41% expenditure deficit for urban households was expected over the next year, taking into account the costs of staple and minimum non-staple items, such as soap, paraffin for heating, matches, cooking oil, beans, salt and other household necessities (LVAC 2008). The deficit did not account for expenses such as education, medical costs, farm inputs, or other expenses such as rent, water, or electricity (LVAC 2008).

Another area to which anthropologists can contribute is through the examination of trade and food provisioning policies, with special emphasis on how global policies are localized. In the essay "Practicing Anthropology in a Time of Crisis," Brondo (2010) highlights the need for anthropologists to document the effects of resource scarcity and increasing power of transnational corporations on marginalized peoples. Such work can serve to situate globalization into local contexts. Additionally, in an examination of changes experienced by residents of southern Belize, Zarger emphasizes the importance of including the "political and historical ecologies of land use and food production when considering the local impacts of global food crises" (2009:130). Zarger underscores the role of structural adjustment and related trade policies in contributing to shifts in food production practices, yet points out that such shifts in food production are not necessarily new to Mayan livelihoods.

While initially addressing the ways economic policies have affected Haiti's vulnerability to the food crisis, Mazzeo (2009) also explored variations in rural livelihoods as contributing to differences in how communities experience food crises. He notes that lack of access to food in Haiti is "not a problem of supply; it's because of the high cost of living" (Mazzeo 2009:115). Further, he argues that the country's burgeoning dependence on staple food imports contributed significantly to its vulnerability to the food crisis and continues to present problems in terms of food security. While such broad analyses are useful to provide context, Mazzeo also explores several case studies of rural livelihoods in varying areas of Haiti. By recognizing the differences between multiple rural communities, anthropologies can contribute to tailoring solutions which are both appropriate and sustainable.

Although it is important to understand not only the larger social, political and economic context in which such crises occur as well as the local realities in which they are felt, it is also of vital importance for anthropologists to follow Lois Stanford's (2008) call for an analysis of the linkages between global and local food systems. Rosing (2009) suggests a method for studying these linkages, with the goal of teasing out the ways household and individual decisions about food are constrained and how they cope. In a study in the Dominican Republic he urges researchers to follow food from table to source rather than confining themselves to the typical examination of consumption as an outcome of production. Starting from an ethnographically grounded examination at the household level, Rosing traces factors related to food acquisition, taking us from the home to neighborhood stores, work place, the availability of staples in local markets, and to the politics of food imports. Anthropologists can further contribute to these examinations by coupling such analyses with systematic nutrition assessment to determine the impact of such factors at different levels.

Whether it is in Colombia, Lesotho, Haiti, Ethiopia, or anywhere else in the world, the Global Food Crisis has had clear detrimental effects for the health and well-being of millions of individuals and families, including many in the United States. Unfortunately, it is very likely that such effects will continue to be felt, especially in light of the very unpredictable changes brought about by global climate change. For example, while the IDP populations with whom the authors had contact in Bogotá experienced a little respite when the torrential rains stopped for a few weeks, this was short lived. As the weather deteriorated again, severe mudslides, road blockages, and ruined crops were once again daily occurrences. The increasing levels of food insecurity and ill-health among men, women, and children from the poorest areas of the country were further fueled by rises in the price of oil, which further increased the price of basic food staples. While food distribution efforts are very valuable and certainly alleviate the dire situation in which the most vulnerable people find themselves, they are a temporary—and often unsustainable—solution. A concerted effort to address the multiplicity of factors (social, economic, political, and environmental) that put people at risk is needed to design and implement long-lasting programs that respond to the needs of local communities. It is precisely in this area that anthropologists and other social scientists can best contribute their skills and expertise.

References

Begovic B, Matkovic G, Mijatovic B, Popovic D. 2007. From Poverty to Prosperity: Free Market Based Solutions. Belgrade, Serbia: Center for Liberal-Democratic Studies (CLDS).

Benson T, Minot N, Pender J, Robles M, Von Braun J. 2008. Global Food Crises. Monitoring and Assessing Impact to Inform Policy Responses. Washington, DC : IFPRI Food Policy Report, September.

Bhagwati J. 2004. In Defense of Globalization. Oxford: Oxford University Press.

Bloem M, Semba RD, Kraemer K. 2010. Castel Gandolfo Workshop: An Introduction to the Impact of Climate Change, the Economic Crisis, and the Increase in the Food Prices on Malnutrition. J Nutr 140:132S–135S.

Brondo KV. 2010. Practicing Anthropology in a Time of Crisis: 2009 Year in Review. Am Anthropol 112(2):208–218.

Bryceson DF, Fonseca J. 2006. Risking Death for Survival: Peasant Responses to Hunger and HIV/AIDS in Malawi. World Dev 34(8):1666–2006.

Carmichael SL, Yang W, Herring A, Abrams B, Shaw GM. 2007. Maternal Food Insecurity Is Associated with Increased Risk of Certain Birth Defects. Am Soc Nutr J of Nutr 137:2087–2092.

Clemmitt M. 2008. Global Food Crisis: What's Causing the Rising Prices? CQ Res 18(24):555–576. http://www.cqpress.com/product/Researcher-Global-Food-Crisis-v18–24.html (accessed January 12, 2011).

Coates J, Swindale A, Bilinsky P. 2007. Household Food Insecurity Access Scale (HFIAS) for Measurement of Food Access: Indicator Guide. Version 3. Washington, DC: Food and Nutrition Technical Assistance Project (FANTA). http://www.fantaproject.org/downloads/pdfs/HFIAS_v3_Aug07.pdf (accessed December 19, 2010 .

CNN. 2011. Global Food Prices Hit Record High. January 7. http://www.cnn.com/2011/BUSINESS/01/05/food.prices.ft/index.html (accessed January 11, 2011).

Collins L. 2009. The Impact of Food Insecurity on Women's Mental Health How it Negatively Affects Children's Health and Development. http://pi.library.yorku.ca/ojs/index.php/jarm/article/viewFile/22523/21003 (accessed January 5, 2011).

Conceição P, Mendoza RU. 2009. Anatomy of the Global Food Crisis. Third World Q 30(6):1159–1182.

Darnton-Hill I, Cogill B. 2010. Maternal and Young Child Nutrition Adversely Affected by External Shocks Such As Increasing Global Food Prices. J Nutr 140:162S–169S.

Dufour DL. 2010. Nutrition, Health, and Function. In: Larsen CS, ed. A Companion to Biological Anthropology. Malden, MA: Wiley-Blackwell, pp. 194–206.

Food and Agriculture Organization of the United Nations (FAO). 2009. Number of Hungry People Rises to 963 Million. http://www.fao.org/news/story/en/item/8836/ (accessed May 1, 2009).

Food and Agriculture Organization of the United Nations (FAO). 2008. The State of Food Insecurity in the World. Rome: Food and Agriculture Organization. http://www.fao.org/docrep/011/i0291e/i0291e00.htm (accessed December 10, 2010).

Food and Agriculture Organization of the United Nations (FAO). 2006. Trade Reforms and Food Security: Conceptualizing the Linkages. http://www.fao.org/docrep/005/y4671e/y4671e00.htm (accessed January 25, 2011).

Glewwe P, King EM. 2001. The Impact of Early Childhood Nutritional Status on Cognitive Development: Does the Timing of Malnutrition Matter? World Bank Econ Rev 15(1):81–113.

Hadley C, Belachew T, Lindstrom D, Tessema F. 2009. The Forgotten Population? Youth, Food Insecurity, and Rising Prices: Implications for the Global Food Crisis. NAPA Bull 3 (1):77–91.

Hadley C, Patil C. 2006. Food insecurity in rural Tanzania is associated with Maternal Anxiety and Depression. Am J Hum Biol 18:359–368.

Hajjar RR, Kamel HK, Denson K. 2004. Malnutrition in Aging. Internet J Geriatr Gerontology 1(1). http://www.ispub.com/ostia/index.php?xmlFilePath=journals/ijgg/vol1n1/malnutrition.xml#h1-2 (accessed January 19, 2011).

Hamelin A-M, Beaudry M, Habicht J-P. 2002. Characterization of Household Food Insecurity in Quebec: Food and Feelings. Soc Sci Med 54:119–132.

Heflin CM, Siefert K, Williams DR. 2005. Food Insufficiency and Women's Mental Health: Findings from a 3-year Panel of Welfare Recipients. Soc Sci Med 61(9):1971–1982.

Internal Displacement Monitoring Center (IDMC) and Norwegian Refugee Council (NRC). 2010. Colombia Government response improves but still fails to meet needs of growing IDP population. http://www.internal-displacement.org/8025708F004BE3B1/(httpInfoFiles)/4BCA7DF31521CC16C12577F5002CED98/$file/Colombia (accessed January 19, 2011).

Katz SH. 2008. The World Food Crisis: An Overview of the Causes and Consequences. Anthropol News 49(7):4–5.

Levitsky DA, Strupp BJ. 1995. Malnutrition and the Brain: Changing Concepts, Changing Concerns. J Nutr 125 (8S sup):2212–2220.

Lesotho Disaster Management Authority (DMA), Lesotho Vulnerability Assessment Committee (LVAC) and the UN World Food Programme (WFP). 2008. Vulnerability and Food Insecurity in Urban Areas of Lesotho: An Assessment of the Impact of High Prices on Vulnerable Households in Ten Major Cities.

Livelihood Vulnerability Assessment Committee (LVAC). 2008. Food Security and Vulnerability in Lesotho 2008. Disaster Management Authority, Office of the Prime Minister.

Mazzeo J. 2009. Lavichè: Haiti's Vulnerability to the Global Food Crisis. NAPA Bull 32 (1):115–129.

Messer E. 2009. Rising Food Prices, Social Mobilizations, and Violence: Conceptual Issues in Understanding and Responding to the Connections Linking Hunger and Conflict. NAPA Bull 32(1):12–22.

Mittal A. 2009. The Blame Game: Understanding Structural Causes of the Food Crisis. In: Clapp J, Cohen MC, eds. The Global Food Crisis: Governance Challenges and Opportunities. Waterloo, ON: Centre for International Governance Innovation (CIGI) and Wilfrid Laurier University Press, pp. 13–28.

Nature News. 2010. Return of La Niña. September 16, 2010. http://www.nature.com/news/2010/100916/full/news.2010.477.html (accessed January 24, 2011).

Nord M, Andrews M, Carlson S. 2009. Household Food Security in the United States, 2008. ERR-83, U.S. Dept. of Agriculture, Economic Research Service. November 2009.

Nord M, Andrews M, Carlson S. 2008. Household Food Security in the United States, 2007. ERR-66, U.S. Dept. of Agriculture, Economic Research Service. November 2008.

Nord M, Coleman-Jensen A, Andrews M, Carlson S. 2010. Household Food Security in the United States, 2009. ERR-108, U.S. Dept. of Agriculture, Economic Research Service. November 2010.

Reuters. 2010. Columbia Seeks Aid as Rescuers Dig Out Mudslide Victims. December 7. http://www.reuters.com/article/2010/12/08/us-colombia-disaster-idUSTRE6B70J920101208 (accessed January 10, 2011).

Ridgwell H. 2011. Rising Prices Fuel Anti-Government Sentiments across Middle East. January 20. Voice of America. http://www.voanews.com/english/news/africa/Rising-Prices-Fuel-Anti-Government-Sentiments-Across-Middle-East-114291989.html (accessed January 26, 2011).

Romero-Daza N, Himmelgreen DA, Noble CA, Turkon D. 2009. Dealing with the Global Food Crisis in Local Settings: Nonintensive Agriculture in Lesotho, Southern Africa. NAPA Bull 32(1):23–41.

Rosing H. 2009. Economic Restructuring and Urban Food Access in the Dominican Republic. NAPA Bull 32(1):55–76.

Sapsford D, Garikipati S. 2006. Trade Liberalisation, Economic Development and Poverty Alleviation. World Economy 29:1571–1579.

Scrimshaw NS, Taylor CE, Gordon JE. 1968. Interactions of Nutrition and Infection. Geneva: WHO. World Health Organ Mon Ser No. 57, p. 1–329.

Scrimshaw N. 1998. Malnutrition, Brain Development, Learning, and Behavior. Nutr Res 18(2):351–379.

Shah M, Osborne N, Mbilizi T, Vilili G. 2002. Impact of HIV/AIDS on Agricultural Productivity and Rural Livelihoods in the Central Region of Malawi. Lilongwe, Malawi: CARE Int.

Sorsdahl K, Slopen N, Siefert K, Seedat S, Stein DJ, Williams DR. 2010. Household Food Insufficiency and Mental Health in South Africa. J Epidemiol Community Health jech.2009.091462. http://jech.bmj.com/content/early/2010/04/28/jech.2009.091462.full.pdf (accessed January 19, 2011).

Stanford L. 2008. Globalized Food Systems: The View from Below. Anthropol News 49(7):7–10.

Suttmann U, Ockenga J, Selberg O, Hoogestraat L, Deicher H, Müller MJ. 1995. Incidence and Prognostic Value of Malnutrition and Wasting in Human Immunodeficiency Virus-Infected Outpatients. JAIDS and HR 8(3):239–246.

Tang AM. 2003. Weight loss, Wasting, and Survival in HIV-Positive Patients: Current Strategies. AIDS Reader 13(supp. 12):S23–S27.

U.S. Census Bureau. 2011. U.S. & World Population Clocks. http://www.census.gov/main/www/popclock.html (accessed January 21, 2011)

Vidal J. 2007. Global Food Crisis Looms as Climate Change and Fuel Shortages Bite; Soaring Crop Prices and Demand For Biofuels Raise Fears of Political Instability. The Guardian, November 3. http://www.guardian.co.uk/environment/2007/nov/03/food.climatechange (accessed January 5, 2011).

World Fact Book. 2010. Columbia. Washington, DC: Central Intelligence Agency. https://www.cia.gov/library/publications/the-world-factbook/geos/co.html (accessed January 24, 2011).

von Braun J. 2008a. Food and Financial Crises: Implications for Agriculture and the Poor. Food Policy Report No. 20. Washington, DC: International Food Policy Research Institute. http://www.ifpri.org/publication/food-and-financial-crises (accessed January 25, 2011).

von Braun J, Sheeran J, Ngongi N. 2008. Responding to the Global Food Crisis: Three Perspectives. Washington DC: International Food Policy Research Institute (IFPRI). http://www.ifpri.org/publication/responding-global-food-crisis-three-perspectives (accessed January 25, 2011).

Weiser SD, Leiter K, Bangsberg DR, Butler LM, Percy-de Korte F, Hlanze Z, Phaladze N, Iacopino V, Heisler M. 2007. Food Insufficiency is Associated with High-Risk Sexual Behavior among Women in Botswana and Swaziland. PLoS Med 4(10):e260.

World Food Program (WFP). 2008. WFP says High Food Prices a Silent Tsunami, Affecting Every Continent. http://www.wfp.org/news/news-release/wfp-says-high-food-prices-silent-tsunami-affecting-every-continent (accessed January 25, 2011).

Whitaker RC, Phillips SM, Orzol SM. 2006. Food Insecurity and the Risks of Depression and Anxiety in Mothers and Behavior Problems in their Preschool-aged Children. Pediatrics 118(3):e859–e868.

Zarger R. 2009. Mosaics of Maya Livelihoods: Readjusting To Global and Local Food Crises. NAPA Bull 32(1):130–151.

PART III

Why Do We Eat What We Eat?

UNIT IV

EXPLAINING FOODWAYS #1: MATERIALIST APPROACHES

Why do we eat what we eat? Are the means by which foods are chosen, processed, and combined simply a matter of what tastes good, or of cultural idiosyncrasy, or are they somehow related to nutritional or other biological needs? How these questions are answered provides insight into theoretical approaches used in anthropology.

Food is rich with social and ideological meaning, and food systems reflect larger systems of thought, power, and control. As omnivores, there are many things we could eat, but every human group defines a limited number of items as food, and makes even more choices at each meal. How do we choose the meal from a menu of possibilities? Is the logic of choice based somehow on an evolved wisdom of biological or ecological need? If so, what is the process by which the needs of the body are expressed as desires? Moreover, what needs are fulfilled?

The writings of cultural anthropologist Marvin Harris coalesced into a perspective that he calls *cultural materialism,* in which cultural systems and behaviors are viewed as evolved adaptations to material needs (Harris 1979 and 1985). Extending the argument to food, Harris hypothesized that food systems evolved to efficiently meet nutritional needs and to be sustainable within particular ecological limits. Simply put, we do the things we do, including growing, preparing, and eating specific foods, because they meet inescapable material needs. Harris considers purely ideological or religious explanations of food taboos to be circular: they do not lead to a deeper understanding of the taboo. His objective is to understand what is *behind* the ideology and religion. For Harris, what is dismissed by some as mere ideology or religious belief had, and may still have, an evolved logic. What culture and religion prescribe may have an ecological or biological advantage that is not readily seen.

In a well-known example in his book *Good to Eat* (1985), Harris considers the Jewish and Muslim prohibition against eating pig. He feels certain that the prohibition against eating pig, which for Jews is from the book of Leviticus, circa 450 B.C., is a law that makes some materialist sense. The challenge is to discover why eating pig is materially, as well as morally, wrong.

Moses Maimonides, a physician to the Islamic emperor Saladin, provided one explanation in the twelfth century. He wrote that the filthy and loathsome pig was forbidden because it was unwholesome. Seven centuries later, an association was discovered between trichinosis and undercooked pork, thus providing scientific support for Maimonides' idea.

Harris considers Maimonides to be on the right track, but wrong in the particulars of his argument. He points out that had Maimonides been correct, the decree should have been against undercooked pork rather than all pig products. Harris offers a more ecological explanation. He notes that pigs do not efficiently gain weight on a diet of grasses. Thus, the prohibition is basically a way of saying that pigs do not make good ecological and economic sense.

In another well-known materialist reconstruction of a past foodway, Michael Harner (1975) presented a style of argument similar to Harris for an even more controversial subject: Aztec cannibalism. Cannibalism is considered to be one of the most widespread of taboos (Arens 1979). Harner, nonetheless, clearly argues that the Aztecs practiced cannibalism and that they did so to meet nutritional needs. He makes two related points that can be viewed as hypotheses to consider.

- The Aztecs of central Mexico frequently practiced human sacrifice and cannibalism in the fifteenth century.
- Aztecs consumed human flesh to obtain a high-quality source of much-needed protein.

Harner's materialist explanation is one that is particularly interesting because it hits upon a number of key issues having to do with the quality of anthropological data and explanation. While he vigorously portrays Aztecs as cannibals, think about the perspective of the European chroniclers. What are the potential biases of his sources? (It is interesting to note that at this time Africans sometimes thought that European explorers were cannibals.) On the other hand, just because they might be biased, does this mean that the observations were incorrect? Finally, might our inability to accept cannibalism say more about us and our taboo than it does about the Aztecs?

The potential answers to the "Why cannibalism?" question are particularly interesting. As a matter of religion, sacrifice and cannibalism might be seen as a way to "appease the gods." A frequent political explanation is that sacrifice is an extreme form of social control. Having the ultimate power, the power to kill, is something that would keep the masses in line. Other explanations might be more ecological. Sacrifice is a form of killing, and this might help to limit population growth. And, finally, eating victims might provide a key source of sustenance. How can one choose among these explanations?

We may never know the truth of the extent of cannibalism and the needs it fulfilled. What would you like to know to judge whether Harner's hypothesis might be correct? Is the needed information knowable? In the face of incomplete data, what would convince you? What other types of information would provide support for the argument, and what might weaken it?

In "India's Sacred Cow," the first chapter of this section, Harris notes that many have been struck by the seeming contradiction between starving Hindus and cows that seem to run free throughout India. Why is this food source not eaten? If cows were considered food, wouldn't this help to meet important nutritional needs?

Harris wishes to demolish the stereotype that Hindu law is irrational and that Hindus would rather starve to death than eat their sacred cows. He shows how a live Indian cow contributes in a number of useful ways to the local economy. Cows are used for plowing and hauling, their milk is drunk, their dung is used for fertilizer, and when they die their leather is put to a variety of uses, while non-Hindus consume the meat. Harris concludes that, by comparison, the U.S. system of cattle production is inefficient and perhaps a bit irrational. How satisfying is Harris's explanation? Does it have the ring of a deeper explanation? Can you think of another explanation?

The work of Harris and Harner is interesting and speculative. In some cases the data are simply unavailable, and in other cases it would require an inordinate amount of time to put together a stronger test. They are great food for thought.

A more systematic analysis of a widespread practice is provided by Sera Young and colleagues in "Why on Earth?: Evaluating Hypotheses about the Physiological Functions of Human Geophagy." Geophagy, if you have not guessed by now, is the "intentional consumption of the earth." Young and colleagues report on an incredibly systematic study of the existing published literature on geophagy. Geophagy has frequently been observed and reported including in the Pemba Island, Xanzibar, Tanzania, where Young does fieldwork. There, she received only the most basic answers such as it is an addiction, the type of answer that Harris would call a circularity. A non-answer. Why an addiction?

Young and colleagues carefully review the geographic and cultural distribution in humans as well as information from other primates. They evaluate different explanations for geophagy including detoxification of parasites, increasing mineral bioavailability, and the need for a particular micronutrient. Their conclusions are far more open-ended than Harner and Harris's. Their study points towards patterns but not definite answers. Indeed, the reasons for geophagy may be as varied as the reasons for most any widespread behavior. One behavior may solve different problems depending on context. Like many questions about food, the answers are complicated...but still very interesting. What do you think?

We live in a world of insects. Insects or, more specifically, insect parts, are in pasta and on our cabbage. Individuals in North America and Europe generally do not consciously eat whole insects, but they are in a minority. Insect eating has recently gained some notoriety as an ecological alternative to the consumption of large animals and fish. Insects are tasty and ecological.

Amazonian Indians are among the many groups that regularly practice entomorphagy, the consumption of insects. Darna Dufour reports on the volume and variety of this practice in a Tukanoan village in "Insects as Food: A Case Study from the Northwest Amazon." Not unlike Richard Lee, who observed regularly what the San were eating, as part of her study of the energy flow in the village of Yapú on the upper Papurí River, Dufour sampled the insects included in the diets of the Tukanoans. She counts over twenty species that are consumed and quantified their contribution to individuals' diets. Although small in size, she finds that insects are a very important part of the diet, especially that of women.

Should we follow suit? Rather than a strange behavior, the Tukanoans, as well as the many other world cultures that eat insects, may have stumbled on something that we have not. Insects can certainly taste good and their nutritional and ecological advantages are hard to ignore.

The chapters in this section argue that diets are based on more than just what is ecologically available and also more than just what is culturally appropriate and prescribed. Diets evolve to meet nutritional and other biological needs. In different ways the authors in this section maintain that diets have an evolved logic. Might we someday follow along and begin to see the logic of eating insects? Has our diet lost its logic when cheap calories are so abundant? Has our diet lost its logic when what we eat is so readily controlled by advertisements to adults and children as well?

SUGGESTIONS FOR THINKING AND DOING NUTRITIONAL ANTHROPOLOGY

1. Reexamine the evidence for Aztec cannibalism. Identify the availability of other protein sources (including unusual sources such as algae and insects). Locate reference sources on Aztec population, ecology and food production, and human protein requirements. Does cannibalism still make sense as a protein source?

2. Explanations have consequences for action. Imagine that the fictitious project VACA has assigned you to India to solve the problem of endemic undernutrition in that country. You have read Harris and you agree with him. How would this understanding guide your actions? Conversely, what different actions might be suggested if you are not convinced by Harris?

3. Food cravings are commonly thought to reflect biological needs. A desire for salt reflects a need for sodium, and a desire for ice cream might

reflect a deficiency in calcium. Think of an example of a food craving, and investigate current understanding of whether or not it reflects physiological need.

References

Arens W. 1979. The Man-eating Myth: Anthropology and Anthropophagy. Oxford University Press: Oxford

Harris M. 1979. Cultural Materialism: The Struggle for a Science of Culture. New York: Random House.

Harris M. 1985. Good to Eat: Riddles of Food and Culture. New York: Simon and Schuster.

Harner M. 1977. The Enigma of Aztec Sacrifice. Natural History. April.

Suggested Further Reading

Arens W. 1979. The Man-eating Myth: Anthropology and Anthropophagy. Oxford University Press: Oxford. Easy reading on the quality of ethnographic data, especially as it pertains to rumors of cannibalism.

Durham WH. 1991. Coevolution: Genes, Culture, and Human Diversity. Stanford, CA: Stanford University Press. Durham presents theory and examples of "memes," or how cultural traits may be selected and evolved.

Etkin NL, ed. 1994. The Pharmacologic, Ecologic, and Social Implications of Using Noncultigens. Tucson: University of Arizona Press. An excellent compilation of cross-cultural data on plants as medicines.

Johns T. 1996. The Origins of Human Diet and Medicine. Tucson: University of Arizona Press. A wealth of interesting examples about how foods are detoxified and used for medicinal purposes.

Moffat T, Prowse T, ed. 2010. Human Diet and Nutrition in Biocultural Perspective. Berghahn Books: New York. A professionally written set of chapters all exploring human diets as intersections of biology and culture.

CHAPTER 18

India's Sacred Cow

Marvin Harris

(1978)

News photographs that came out of India during the famine of the late 1960s showed starving people stretching out bony hands to beg for food while sacred cattle strolled behind them undisturbed. The Hindu, it seems, would rather starve to death than eat his cow or even deprive it of food. The cattle appear to browse unhindered through urban markets eating an orange here, a mango there, competing with people for meager supplies of food.

By Western standards, spiritual values seem more important to Indians than life itself. Specialists in food habits around the world like Fred Simoons at the University of California at Davis consider Hinduism an irrational ideology that compels people to overlook abundant, nutritious foods for scarcer, less healthful foods.

What seems to be an absurd devotion to the mother cow pervades Indian life. Indian wall calendars portray beautiful young women with bodies of fat white cows, often with milk jetting from their teats into sacred shrines.

Cow worship even carries over into politics. In 1966 a crowd of 120,000 people, led by holy men, demonstrated in front of the Indian House of Parliament in support of the All-Party Cow Protection Campaign Committee. In Nepal, the only contemporary Hindu kingdom, cow slaughter is severely punished. As one story goes, the car driven by an official of a United States agency struck and killed a cow. In order to avoid the international incident that would have occurred when the official was arrested for murder, the Nepalese magistrate concluded that the cow had committed suicide.

Many Indians agree with Western assessments of the Hindu reverence for their cattle, the zebu, or *Bos indicus*, a large-humped species prevalent in Asia and Africa. M. N. Srinivas, an Indian anthropologist, states: "Orthodox Hindu opinion regards the killing of cattle with abhorrence, even though the refusal to kill the vast number of useless cattle which exists in India today is detrimental to the nation." Even the Indian Ministry of Information formerly maintained that "the large animal population is more a liability than an asset in view of our land resources." Accounts from

many different sources point to the same conclusion: India, one of the world's great civilizations, is being strangled by its love for the cow.

The easy explanation for India's devotion to the cow, the one most Westerners and Indians would offer, is that cow worship is an integral part of Hinduism. Religion is somehow good for the soul, even if it sometimes fails the body. Religion orders the cosmos and explains our place in the universe. Religious beliefs, many would claim, have existed for thousands of years and have a life of their own. They are not understandable in scientific terms.

But all this ignores history. There is more to be said for cow worship than is immediately apparent. The earliest Vedas, the Hindu sacred texts from the Second Millennium B.C., do not prohibit the slaughter of cattle. Instead, they ordain it as a part of sacrificial rites. The early Hindus did not avoid the flesh of cows and bulls; they ate it at ceremonial feasts presided over by Brahman priests. Cow worship is a relatively recent development in India; it evolved as the Hindu religion developed and changed.

This evolution is recorded in royal edicts and religious texts written during the last 3,000 years of Indian history. The Vedas from the First Millennium B.C. contain contradictory passages, some referring to ritual slaughter and others to a strict taboo on beef consumption. A. N. Bose, in *Social and Rural Economy of Northern India, 600 B.C.–200 A.D.*, concludes that many of the sacred-cow passages were incorporated into the texts by priests of a later period.

By 200 A.D. the status of Indian cattle had undergone a spiritual transformation. The Brahman priesthood exhorted the population to venerate the cow and forbade them to abuse it or to feed on it. Religious feasts involving the ritual slaughter and consumption of livestock were eliminated and meat eating was restricted to the nobility.

By 1000 A.D., all Hindus were forbidden to eat beef. Ahimsa, the Hindu belief in the unity of all life, was the spiritual justification for this restriction. But it is difficult to ascertain exactly when this change occurred. An important event that helped to shape the modern complex was the Islamic invasion, which took place in the Eighth Century. All Hindus may have found it politically expedient to set themselves off from the invaders, who were

Marvin Harris, "India's Sacred Cow." *Human Nature*, February 1978: 28–36. Figures have been omitted. Reprinted with permission.

beefeaters, by emphasizing the need to prevent the slaughter of their sacred animals. Thereafter, the cow taboo assumed its modern form and began to function much as it does today.

The place of the cow in modern India is every place—on posters, in the movies, in brass figures, in stone and wood carvings, on the streets, in the fields. The cow is a symbol of health and abundance. It provides the milk that Indians consume in the form of yogurt and ghee (clarified butter), which contribute subtle flavors to much spicy Indian food.

This, perhaps, is the practical role of the cow, but cows provide less than half the milk produced in India. Most cows in India are not dairy breeds. In most regions, when an Indian farmer wants a steady, high-quality source of milk he usually invests in a female water buffalo. In India the water buffalo is the specialized dairy breed because its milk has a higher butterfat content than zebu milk. Although the farmer milks his zebu cows, the milk is merely a by-product.

More vital than zebu milk to South Asian farmers are zebu calves. Male calves are especially valued because from bulls come oxen, which are the mainstay of the Indian agricultural system.

Small, fast oxen drag wooden plows through late-spring fields when monsoons have dampened the dry, cracked earth. After harvest, the oxen break the grain from the stalk by stomping through mounds of cut wheat and rice. For rice cultivation in irrigated fields, the male water buffalo is preferred (it pulls better in deep mud), but for most other crops, including rainfall rice, wheat, sorghum, and millet, and for transporting goods and people to and from town, a team of oxen is preferred. The ox is the Indian peasant's tractor, thresher and family car combined; the cow is the factory that produces the ox.

If draft animals instead of cows are wanted, India appears to have too few domesticated ruminants, not too many. Since each of the 70 million farms in India requires a draft team, it follows that Indian peasants should use 140 million animals in the fields. But there are only 40 million oxen and male water buffalo in the subcontinent, a shortage of 30 million draft teams.

In other regions of the world, joint ownership of draft animals might overcome a shortage, but Indian agriculture is closely tied to the monsoon rains of late spring and summer. Field preparation and planting must coincide with the rain, and a farmer must have his animals ready to plow when the weather is right. When the farmer without a draft team needs bullocks most, his neighbors are all using theirs. Any delay in turning the soil drastically lowers production.

Because of this dependence on draft animals, loss of the family oxen is devastating. If a beast dies, the farmer must borrow money to buy or rent an ox at interest rates so high that he ultimately loses his land. Every year foreclosures force thousands of poverty-stricken peasants to abandon the countryside for the overcrowded cities.

If a family is fortunate enough to own a fertile cow, it will be able to rear replacements for a lost team and thus survive until life returns to normal. If, as sometimes happens, famine leads a family to sell its cow and ox team, all ties to agriculture are cut. Even if the family survives, it has no way to farm the land, no oxen to work the land, and no cows to produce oxen.

The prohibition against eating meat applies to the flesh of cows, bulls, and oxen, but the cow is the most sacred because it can produce the other two. The peasant whose cow dies is not only crying over a spiritual loss but over the loss of his farm as well.

Religious laws that forbid the slaughter of cattle promote the recovery of the agricultural system from the dry Indian winter and from periods of drought. The monsoon, on which all agriculture depends, is erratic. Sometimes it arrives early, sometimes late, sometimes not at all. Drought has struck large portions of India time and again in this century, and Indian farmers and the zebus are accustomed to these natural disasters. Zebus can pass weeks on end with little or no food and water. Like camels, they store both in their humps and recuperate quickly with only a little nourishment.

During droughts the cows often stop lactating and become barren. In some cases the condition is permanent but often it is only temporary. If barren animals were summarily eliminated, as Western experts in animal husbandry have suggested, cows capable of recovery would be lost along with those entirely debilitated. By keeping alive the cows that can later produce oxen, religious laws against cow slaughter assure the recovery of the agricultural system from the greatest challenge it faces—the failure of the monsoon.

The local Indian governments aid the process of recovery by maintaining homes for barren cows. Farmers reclaim any animal that calves or begins to lactate. One police station in Madras collects strays and pastures them in a field adjacent to the station. After a small fine is paid, a cow is returned to its rightful owner when the owner thinks the cow shows signs of being able to reproduce.

During the hot, dry spring months most of India is like a desert. Indian farmers often complain they cannot feed their livestock during this period. They maintain the cattle by letting them scavenge on the sparse grass along the roads. In the cities cattle are encouraged to scavenge near food stalls to supplement their scant diet. These are the wandering cattle tourists report seeing throughout India.

Westerners expect shopkeepers to respond to these intrusions with the deference due a sacred animal; instead, their response is a string of curses and the crack of a long bamboo pole across the beast's back or a poke at its genitals. Mahatma Gandhi was well aware of the treatment sacred cows (and bulls and oxen) received in India. "How we bleed her to take the last drop of milk from her. How we starve her to emaciation, how we ill-treat the calves, how we deprive them of their portion of milk, how cruelly we treat the oxen, how we castrate them, how we beat them, how we overload them."

Oxen generally receive better treatment than cows. When food is in short supply, thrifty Indian peasants feed their working bullocks and ignore their cows, but rarely do they abandon the cows to die. When cows are sick, farmers worry over them as they would over members of the family and nurse them as if they were children. When the rains return and when the fields are harvested, the farmers again feed their cows regularly and reclaim their abandoned animals. The prohibition against beef consumption is a form of disaster insurance for all India.

Western agronomists and economists are quick to protest that all the functions of the zebu cattle can be improved with organized breeding programs, cultivated pastures, and silage. Because stronger oxen would pull the plow faster, they could work multiple plots of land, allowing farmers to share their animals. Fewer healthy, well-fed cows could provide Indians with more milk. But pastures and silage require arable land, land needed to produce wheat and rice.

A look at Western cattle farming makes plain the cost of adopting advanced technology in Indian agriculture. In a study of livestock production in the United States, David Pimentel of the College of Agriculture and Life Sciences at Cornell University found that 91 percent of the cereal, legume, and vegetable protein suitable for human consumption is consumed by livestock. Approximately three quarters of the arable land in the United States is devoted to growing food for livestock. In the production of meat and milk, American ranchers use enough fossil fuel to equal more than 82 million barrels of oil annually.

Indian cattle do not drain the system in the same way. In a 1971 study of livestock in West Bengal, Stewart Odend'hal of the University of Missouri found that Bengalese cattle ate only the inedible remains of subsistence crops—rice straw, rice hulls, the tops of sugar cane, and mustard-oil cake. Cattle graze in the fields after harvest and eat the remains of crops left on the ground; they forage for grass and weeds on the roadsides. The food for zebu cattle costs the human population virtually nothing. "Basically," Odend'hal says, "the cattle convert items of little direct human value into products of immediate utility."

In addition to plowing the fields and producing milk, the zebus produce dung, which fires the hearths and fertilizes the fields of India. Much of the estimated 800 million tons of manure produced annually is collected by the farmers' children as they follow the family cows and bullocks from place to place. And when the children see the droppings of another farmer's cattle along the road, they pick those up also. Odend'hal reports that the system operates with such high efficiency that the children of West Bengal recover nearly 100 percent of the dung produced by their livestock.

From 40 to 70 percent of all manure produced by Indian cattle is used as fuel for cooking; the rest is returned to the fields as fertilizer. Dried dung burns slowly, cleanly, and with low heat—characteristics that satisfy the household needs of Indian women. Staples like curry and rice can simmer for hours. While the meal slowly cooks over an unattended fire, the women of the household can do other chores. Cow chips, unlike firewood, do not scorch as they burn.

It is estimated that the dung used for cooking fuel provides the energy-equivalent of 43 million tons of coal. At current prices, it would cost India an extra 1.5 billion dollars in foreign exchange to replace the dung with coal. And if the 350 million tons of manure that are being used as fertilizer were replaced with commercial fertilizers, the expense would be even greater. Roger Revelle of the University of California at San Diego has calculated that 89 percent of the energy used in Indian agriculture (the equivalent of about 140 million tons of coal) is provided by local sources. Even if foreign loans were to provide the money, the capital outlay necessary to replace the Indian cow with tractors and fertilizers for the fields, coal for the fires, and transportation for the family would probably warp international financial institutions for years.

Instead of asking the Indians to learn from the American model of industrial agriculture, American farmers might learn energy conservation from the Indians. Every step in an energy cycle results in a loss of energy to the system. Like a pendulum that slows a bit with each swing, each transfer of energy from sun to plants, plants to animals, and animals to human beings involves energy losses. Some systems are more efficient than others; they provide a higher percentage of the energy inputs in a final, useful form. Seventeen percent of all energy zebus consume is returned in the form of milk, traction and dung. American cattle raised on Western range land return only 4 percent of the energy they consume.

But the American system is improving. Based on techniques pioneered by Indian scientists, at least one commercial firm in the United States is reported to be building plants that will turn manure from cattle feedlots into combustible gas. When organic matter is broken down by anaerobic bacteria, methane gas and carbon dioxide are produced. After the methane is cleansed of the carbon dioxide, it is available for the same purposes as natural gas—cooking, heating, electricity generation. The company constructing the biogasification plant plans to sell its product to a gas-supply company, to be piped through the existing distribution system. Schemes similar to this one could make cattle ranches almost independent of utility and gasoline companies, for methane can be used to run trucks, tractors, and cars as well as to supply heat and electricity. The relative energy self-sufficiency that the Indian peasant has achieved is a goal American farmers and industry are now striving for.

Studies like Odend'hal's understate the efficiency of the Indian cow, because dead cows are used for purposes that Hindus prefer not to acknowledge. When a cow dies, an Untouchable, a member of one of the lowest ranking castes in India, is summoned to haul away the carcass. Higher castes consider the body of the dead cow polluting; if they do handle it, they must go through a rite of purification.

Untouchables first skin the dead animal and either tan the skin themselves or sell it to a leather factory. In the privacy of their homes, contrary to the teachings of Hinduism, untouchable castes cook the meat and eat it. Indians of all castes rarely acknowledge the existence of these practices to non-Hindus, but most are aware that beefeating takes place. The prohibition against beefeating restricts consumption by the higher castes and helps distribute animal protein to the poorest sectors of the population that otherwise would have no source of these vital nutrients.

Untouchables are not the only Indians who consume beef. Indian Muslims and Christians are under no restriction that forbids them beef, and its consumption is legal in many places. The Indian ban on cow slaughter is state, not national, law and not all states restrict it. In many cities, such as New Delhi, Calcutta, and Bombay, legal slaughterhouses sell beef to retail customers and to the restaurants that serve steak.

If the caloric value of beef and the energy costs involved in the manufacture of synthetic leather were included in the estimates of energy, the calculated efficiency of Indian livestock would rise considerably.

As well as the system works, experts often claim that its efficiency can be further improved. Alan Heston, an economist at the University of Pennsylvania, believes that Indians suffer from an overabundance of cows simply because they refuse to slaughter the excess cattle. India could produce at least the same number of oxen and the same quantities of milk and manure with 30 million fewer cows. Heston calculates that only 40 cows are necessary to maintain a population of 100 bulls and oxen. Since India averages 70 cows for every 100 bullocks, the difference, 30 million cows, is expendable.

What Heston fails to note is that sex ratios among cattle in different regions of India vary tremendously, indicating that adjustments in the cow population do take place. Along the Ganges River, one of the holiest shrines of Hinduism, the ratio drops to 47 cows for every 100 male animals. This ratio reflects the preference for dairy buffalo in the irrigated sectors of the Gangetic Plains. In nearby Pakistan, in contrast, where cow slaughter is permitted, the sex ratio is 60 cows to 100 oxen.

Since the sex ratios among cattle differ greatly from region to region and do not even approximate the balance that would be expected if no females were killed, we can assume that some culling of herds does take place; Indians do adjust their religious restrictions to accommodate ecological realities.

They cannot kill a cow but they can tether an old or unhealthy animal until it has starved to death. They cannot slaughter a calf but they can yoke it with a large wooden triangle so that when it nurses it irritates the mother's udder and gets kicked to death. They cannot ship their animals to the slaughterhouse but they can sell them to Muslims, closing their eyes to the fact that the Muslims will take the cattle to the slaughterhouse.

These violations of the prohibition against cattle slaughter strengthen the premise that cow worship is a vital part of Indian culture. The practice arose to prevent the population from consuming the animal on which Indian agriculture depends. During the First Millennium B.C., the Ganges Valley became one of the most densely populated regions of the world.

Where previously there had been only scattered villages, many towns and cities arose and peasants farmed every available acre of land. Kingsley Davis, a population expert at the University of California at Berkeley, estimates that by 300 B.C. between 50 million and 100 million people were living in India. The forested Ganges Valley became a windswept semidesert and signs of ecological collapse appeared; droughts and floods became commonplace, erosion took away the rich topsoil, farms shrank as population increased, and domesticated animals became harder and harder to maintain.

It is probable that the elimination of meat eating came about in a slow, practical manner. The farmers who decided not to eat their cows, who saved them for procreation to produce oxen, were the ones who survived the natural disasters. Those who ate beef lost the tools with which to farm. Over a period of centuries, more and more farmers probably avoided beef until an unwritten taboo came into existence.

Only later was the practice codified by the priesthood. While Indian peasants were probably aware of the role of cattle in their society, strong sanctions were necessary to protect zebus from a population faced with starvation. To remove temptation, the flesh of cattle became taboo and the cow became sacred.

The sacredness of the cow is not just an ignorant belief that stands in the way of progress. Like all concepts of the sacred and the profane, this one affects the physical world; it defines the relationships that are important for the maintenance of Indian society.

Indians have the sacred cow; we have the "sacred" car and the "sacred" dog. It would not occur to us to propose the elimination of automobiles and dogs from our society without carefully considering the consequences, and we should not propose the elimination of zebu cattle without first understanding their place in the social order of India.

Human society is neither random nor capricious. The regularities of thought and behavior called culture are the principal mechanisms by which we human beings adapt to the world around us. Practices and beliefs can be rational or irrational, but a society that fails to adapt to its environment is doomed to extinction. Only those societies that draw the necessities of life from their surroundings, without destroying those surroundings, inherit the earth. The West has much to learn from the great antiquity of Indian civilization, and the sacred cow is an important part of that lesson.

Suggested Further Reading

Gandhi, Mohandas K. *How to Serve the Cow*. Navajivan Publishing House, 1954.

Harris. Marvin. *Cows, Pigs, Wars and Witches: The Riddles of Culture*. Random House, 1974.

Heston, Alan, et al. "An Approach to the Sacred Cow of India." *Current Anthropology*, Vol. 12, 1971, pp. 191–209.

Odend'hal, Stewart. "Gross Energetic Efficiency of Indian Cattle in Their Environment." *Journal of Human Ecology*, Vol. 1, 1972, pp. 1–27.

Raj, K. N. "Investment in Livestock in Agrarian Economies: An Analysis of Some Issues Concerning 'Sacred Cows' and 'Surplus Cattle.' " *Indian Economic Review*, Vol. 4. 1969, pp. 1–33.

CHAPTER 19

Why on Earth?: Evaluating Hypotheses About the Physiological Functions of Human Geophagy

Sera L. Young, Paul W. Sherman, Julius B. Lucks, and Gretel H. Pelto
(2011)

Geophagy is the intentional consumption of earth. It is a specific type of the more general phenomenon that is commonly referred to as "pica," the purposive consumption of non-food substances. Geophagy is widely practiced: it has been observed in hundreds of cultures on all inhabited continents (Laufer 1930; Anell and Lagercrantz 1958). Geophagy was first documented by Hippocrates (460 –380 BC) more than 2000 years ago (Hippocrates and Adams 1849). However, archeological evidence suggests that the practice of geophagy is thousands of years older and may date back to *Homo habilis* (Baudouin 1924; Clark 2001; Brady and Rissolo 2006). Earth eating continues throughout the world today (Young 2010, 2011).

Scholars from diverse fields including anthropology, behavioral ecology, biochemistry, ethology, geography, and medicine have offered a range of hypotheses for why earth is consumed. Yet, even after much investigation, geophagy remains an enigma for many reasons (Young 2010). These include the scarcity of hypothesis-driven research as well as the typically single-discipline approaches to its study. It is also due to underreporting, firstly because researchers often do not inquire about geophagy and, secondly, even if they do, fear of being judged harshly leads some geophagists to conceal their behavior (Young et al. 2008).

Because of both the prevalence of geophagy and its association with positive and negative health consequences, there is a clearly acknowledged need to understand the etiology of the behavior. Indeed, calls for elucidation of the physiological functions of this fascinating and enigmatic phenomenon are a recurring theme in the geophagy literature (e.g., Whiting 1947; Edwards et al. 1994; Geissler et al. 1997; Limpitlaw 2010).

THE HYPOTHESES

Three general physiological explanations for the etiology of human geophagy have been advanced. The first two suggest contexts in which the behavior would be adaptive, whereas the third suggests that it is not an adaptive behavior.

Hypothesis 1: Nutrient Deficiency

This hypothesis proposes that people eat earth in order to make up for dietary deficiencies of mineral micronutrients, particularly iron and zinc (Hunter 1973; Çavdar et al. 1983; Prasad 2001b) and the macromineral calcium (Wiley and Katz 1998). For brevity, these will collectively be referred to as nutrients. Because anemia (the state of insufficient red blood cells or hemoglobin) is frequently associated with geophagy (Geissler et al. 1999; Kawai et al. 2009), the most commonly reiterated of the nutrient hypotheses suggests that geophagy remedies iron deficiency. It should be noted, however, that anemia can be caused by micronutrient deficiencies other than iron, as well as infections and blood loss (Yip and Dallman 1988). Sodium deficiency has been proposed to motivate geophagy in non-human primates and other animals (Jones and Hanson 1985; Krishnamani and Mahaney 2000). However, human geophagists do not attribute their behavior to a dearth of salt (Vermeer and Frate 1979; Kraemer 2002) and with only a few exceptions (Laufer 1930), geophagic earth is not typically salty (Young et al. 2008).

Hypothesis 2: Protection

This hypothesis proposes that earth is eaten as a medicament, to reduce the short-term malaise and long-term effects of harmful chemicals and parasites and pathogens. Many human food plants produce toxic chemicals, such as tannins and glycoalkaloids to protect themselves from biotic enemies (pathogens and herbivores). Other sources of harmful chemicals in the human diet are enterotoxins secreted by food- and waterborne bacteria such as *Escherichia coli, Staphylococcus aureus, Salmonella enterica,* and *Listeria monocytogenes.* Ingestion of these toxins can cause gastrointestinal distress, dizziness, and muscle pains; in sufficient quantities, they can be mutagenic, carcinogenic, or deadly (Hui et al. 2001b). Dangerous pathogens include food- and waterborne bacteria as well as viruses and parasitic nematodes.

Sera L. Young, Paul W. Sherman, Julius B. Lucks, Gretel H. Pelto, "Why on earth? Evaluating hypotheses about the physiological functions of human geophagy." *The Quarterly Review of Biology* 86 (2011): 97–120. Reprinted with permission.

Under this hypothesis, there are two mechanisms by which geophagic earth may be protective: by *reducing the permeability* of the gut wall to toxins and pathogens and by *binding directly* to toxins and pathogens (Young 2010). The intestinal mucosal layer acts as a physical barrier between ingesta and the bloodstream by filtering out large molecules, as well as a chemical barrier by maintaining a pH gradient. Geophagic earth, especially if it is clay-rich, can bind with and thereby reinforce the protective mucosal layer and/or enhance mucosal secretion, thereby reducing permeability of the intestinal walls (González et al. 2004).

The second mechanism involves binding directly to toxins, parasites, and other pathogens. This can either render them unabsorbable by the gut or inhibit their respiration. Hladik and Gueguen (1974) first proposed that clays were protective against plant secondary compounds consumed by primates, and Profet (1992) suggested that clays could be protective against human teratogens. A number of clays found in geophagic earths are capable of binding pathogens, including viruses (Lipson and Stotzky 1983; Rey 1989; Dornai et al. 1993), fungi (Smith and Carson 1984; Lavie and Stotzky 1986a,b; Phillips et al. 2008), and bacteria (Maigetter and Pfister 1975; Said et al. 1980; Ditter et al. 1983; Gardiner et al. 1993), as well as toxins, including poisonous herbicides (Okonek et al. 1982; Lotan et al. 1983), pharmaceuticals (Tsakala et al. 1990), and plant secondary compounds (Johns 1986; Johns and Duquette 1991; Gilardi et al. 1999; Houston et al. 2001; Dominy et al. 2004). It is also possible that earth inhibits larger pathogens (e.g., geohelminths) from colonizing hosts (Krishnamani and Mahaney 2000) although the mechanism by which this occurs has not been elucidated.

Hypothesis 3: Non-Adaptive

This hypothesis proposes that there is no benefit to eating earth. Instead, people do so either because they have no food to eat or because micronutrient deficiencies have caused neurological or sensory problems. In the first case, earth is supposedly consumed to ease hunger pains when no other food is available (e.g., La Billardiére 1800; Mallory 1926; Wiley and Katz 1998). In the second case, cravings for earth are suggested to be epiphenomena of nutrient deficiencies that affect appetite-regulating brain enzymes (von Bonsdorff 1977; Youdim and Iancu 1977) or taste sensitivity (Chisholm and Martin 1981; Prasad 2001a), causing non-food substances to become appealing.

AIMS

This paper has two aims. First, we provide an updated review of the literature on geophagy in humans and, for comparison, in other vertebrates. For the human literature, our starting points were eight excellent monographs and reviews (Laufer 1930; Anell and Lagercrantz 1958; Hochstein 1968; Danford 1982; Sayetta 1986; Loveland et al. 1989; Horner et al. 1991; Reid 1992) which were then augmented by primary sources.

We compiled this information into a database that enabled us to quantitatively describe geophagy worldwide and investigate the circumstances under which it occurs. Our second aim was to use the database on human geophagy to systematically evaluate the three hypotheses for the etiology of geophagy. This paper does not directly address the cultural forces and beliefs that shape geophagy (the proximate determiners of the behavior), but rather explores the ecological triggers and physiological underpinnings of geophagy (the ultimate causes). Socioeconomic status may be an underlying cause of hunger, nutrient deficiency, or increased exposure to toxins and pathogens, but it is not a direct cause of geophagy itself. Therefore, it is not an alternative explanation for geophagy and is not tested here.

Additionally, we synthesized reports of geophagy by non-human animals to provide further insights into the distribution of the behavior and its potential physiological causes. Our starting points were several excellent reviews of geophagy in animals (Jones and Hanson 1985; Kreulen 1985; Krishnamani and Mahaney 2000; Ferrari et al. 2008). Because this information was far less detailed and comprehensive than data on humans, it was tabulated, but not analyzed statistically.

METHODOLOGY

Literature Searching

Initially, we searched online databases (Agricola, Dissertation Abstracts, Google Scholar, Human Relation Area Files, ISI Web of Science, JSTOR, Library of Congress, LexisNexis, OCLC, Proquest Historical Newspapers, PubMed, and Zoological Record) for entries containing "geophagy," "geophagia," "pica," "clay eating," "chalk eating," "cachexia Africana," "mal d'estomac," "malacia," "citta," "erde essen," "aarde eten," and "dirt eating." We sought information on geophagy in humans, non-human primates, and other vertebrates. We used the reference lists in each identified publication to locate additional primary sources. This process was iterated until no new references were found. Our search was not restricted by language, format of reference (e.g., microfiche and thesis, among others), or date of publication; the references span many languages and nearly 500 years.

Criteria and Rationale for Inclusion

We defined geophagy as the regular, purposive consumption of earth. With this definition, the mouthing behavior of young children is excluded (their earth consumption may not be intentional, but rather part of a larger behavior of environmental exploration). Instances of geophagy that were described as purely symbolic, such as the ingestion of tiny amounts during solemn occasions (oaths, mourning, tests of innocence or for religious purposes) also were excluded. Finally, if a mineral found in soil was used in the preparation of food, but was not ultimately consumed, such as during nixtamalizaton (the soaking of corn in a limestone solution before grinding), it was not considered geophagy.

The human geophagy literature can be classified into five categories: 1) individual case reports—e.g., a Turkish woman living in Paris ate chalk and clay every day (Henon et al. 1975); 2) an enumerated population—e.g., 55% of anemic Namibian women eat earth (Thomson 1997); 3) a cultural group—e.g., pregnant Otomacs regularly engage in clay-eating (von Humboldt et al. 1821); 4) soil analysis studies—e.g., montmorillonite was a major component of *ch'aqu* (Browman and Gunderson 1993:415); and 5) literature reviews in which no new data were presented— e.g., "According to La Billardiére and confirmed by the reports of Hekmeyer [clay] figures are crunched on by women and children" (Ferrand 1886: 549).

In constructing our database on human geophagy, we focused on firsthand reports of geophagy among cultural groups (category 3). If an author referred to a report of geophagy by someone else (category 5), we obtained the original document. This insured that reports were not included more than once, and that the translation was of high quality. Thus, the unit of analysis for our study is a "cultural report." We did not include reports of individual cases of geophagy (category 1) because of the likelihood of bias regarding both health consequences (people not suffering ill health are unlikely to visit a health care provider) and geographical occurrence (health care providers are not equally available worldwide). We also did not include studies of groups among whom geophagy was studied because of a biological or behavioral condition (e.g., anemia, dialysis, lead poisoning; category 2) because they were not representative of the population at large. Results from soil analyses (category 4) are drawn on throughout the paper.

In reviewing the animal literature, we focused on geophagy and excluded lithophagy (ingesting of rocks or grit). Authors referred to animal geophagy using the terms "clay licks," "mineral licks," "salt licks," and "geophagy"; all such descriptions were included in our tables and analysis. The original document was obtained whenever possible; reports citing personal communication were not included. We located 330 ethological accounts of geophagy among mammals, birds, and reptiles encompassing 297 species and 26 orders.

Constructing the Database on Human Geophagy

From each article on human geophagy we extracted information on as many of the following variables as possible: year of observation, geographic location, climate, non-food materials consumed (e.g., appearance, source, preparation), life stage of the consumer (e.g., child, adolescent, pregnant), and any associations with physiological conditions, such as gastrointestinal distress, anemia, and hunger. If several reports were made about earth eaten by the same group of people or in the same area within a 10-year span, but by different authors, these were combined into one cultural report. A custom built Web-based form was developed specifically for this project using Ruby on Rails software (http://www.rubyonrails.org/), and information from each article was entered manually. Data from biological, epidemiological, and cultural sources were included, making a biocultural analysis possible.

Our database on human geophagy included 482 publications, which contained 367 separate cultural reports of geophagy from all over the world (in supplementary material, available at *The Quarterly Review of Biology* homepage, http://journals.uchicago.edu/QRB). This database includes every obtainable, written culture-level report of human geophagy. To our knowledge, it is the most complete compilation of such information in existence. References for all sources are listed in the supplementary materials; the entire "Pica Literature Database" will be made available once all planned analyses have been completed.

Constructing a map of the frequency of occurrence of geophagy worldwide (Figure 1) presented a challenge because observations at the level of the cultural group do not "map" perfectly onto political maps, since cultures sometimes are dispersed over several countries or located in just one section of a country. To achieve a reasonable approximation, we selected the country in which the ethnic group was primarily situated at the historical time described in the original paper(s).

We used Köppen's classification system to categorize the climatic regions in which geophagy occurs (Kottek et al. 2006). The Köppen system separates climates into five categories: polar, cold, temperate, tropical, and dry (McKnight and Hess 2005). To test whether the distribution of geophagy by climate type was different from the distribution of cultural reports by climate type, we classified each of the 186 cultures in the Standard Cross-Cultural Sample (SCCS) (Murdock and White 1969) by climate type. Cultures in the SCCS were chosen because of their independence from each other, so use of the SCCS minimizes "Galton's problem" of lack of independence of cultures in close geographical proximity to each other (Naroll 1961). Additionally, we compared the geophagy distribution to the world population distribution by climate region (Staszewski 1963).

Because information on human geophagy spans 2000 years and includes reports from many fields of study, the quality and detail of observations varies widely. Accounts were written by ethnographers, colonial explorers, government officials, missionaries, medical doctors, nurses, nutritionists, and journalists. Some reports of geophagy are lengthy (e.g., more than 20 pages), and describe in detail the characteristics of individuals who practice geophagy, when in their lifetimes they do so, sources and preparation of earth, and costs, among other topics, whereas other reports are no more than brief mentions (e.g., a single phrase in a 417-page ethnographic report).

The literature on non-human geophagy was far less detailed and specific, e.g., there were few descriptions of

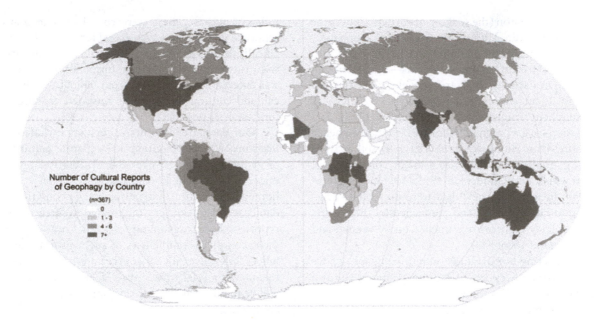

Figure 1 *Worldwide Distribution of Cultural Reports of Geophagy*

Table 1 Geophagy Scoring System Used in the Operationalization of Geophagy Frequency

Score	Terms Associated
0	Never
1	Rarely, few
2	Sometimes, occasionally
3	Frequently, common, habit, very common, quite general, many, endemic, widely, often
4	Usually, typically
5	Always

life stage, sex, or reproductive status of geophagists, nor the composition of earths consumed. The creation of an analyzable database of these reports could not yield similar insights, so we tabulated the ethological reports. Reports on geophagy in non-human primates were typically more detailed than those on geophagy in other vertebrates. A "report" was defined as a description of geophagy by a particular species in one geographic location, i.e., if there were multiple observations of the same species in the same location, they were not tallied twice.

Operationalization

To create variables in the database that could be analyzed, we first grouped the life stages of geophagists into eight categories: (1) "infants" are children younger than two years or are still breastfeeding; (2) "preadolescents" are children who have not reached puberty (3–12 years old); (3) "adolescents" are boys and girls who have reached puberty (13–18 years old); (4) "pregnant women" are adolescent

or adult women who are gestating; (5) "lactating women" are those who are breastfeeding; (6) "women" are adults whose pregnancy or lactation status is unknown; (7) "men" are adult males; and (8) "elderly" are those described in reports as being "old" or no longer bearing children. Regarding category 6, if women's reproductive status was not mentioned, we inferred that they were not pregnant or lactating, although this may have resulted in some misclassification because in many traditional societies, women of reproductive age typically were pregnant or lactating most of the time.

Data on proportions of populations or subpopulations that engaged in geophagy were rarely given in the reports we compiled. Rather, qualitative terms such as "some," "all," "frequently," and "rarely" were used instead. In an attempt to quantify these descriptive terms, we constructed a scoring system (Table 1) similar to that of Wiley and Katz (1998).

Only rarely did observers identify which subgroups within the population did not eat earth. More typically the observer would comment only on positive occurrences (e.g., "pregnant women and children eat clay"). Therefore, we standardized the frequencies by the absolute number of cultural reports made for each life stage. To do this, we divided the frequency of geophagy for each life stage by the number of cultural reports presenting information on that particular life stage (Figure 2). To reduce the geophagy frequency to a more intuitive value, we created a geophagy score, which is the mean geophagy frequency for that life stage.

When observers discussed the timing of consumption during pregnancy, terms such as "early" and "late" were used more frequently than specific months or trimesters. We classified pregnancy timing described as "early" as first trimester and grouped those described as "mid" or "late" pregnancy into a single category "second or third trimester."

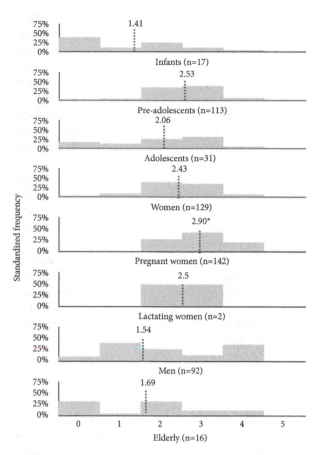

Figure 2 *Standardized Geophagy Frequencies and Mean Geophagy Score (Dotted Line) by Life Stage Based on Culture-Level Reports of Geophagy*
*Compared to pregnant women, all groups have significantly lower mean geophagy scores (p<0.0001).

"Anemia" was not a term that was in use for most of the time period encompassed by our literature review, and biomedical tests of anemia have become standard only relatively recently. Thus, associations between geophagy and mild anemia would rarely have been reported. However, we were able to identify associations with severe anemia when certain symptoms were described, e.g., pallor of skin and/or mucosal membranes and thin "watery" blood. "Chlorosis" is a term that was frequently used in the past to describe weak, pale patients; it is now considered to be synonymous with anemia (Hudson 1977). Thus, if geophagists were described as pale, having thin blood or exhibiting chlorosis, we recorded geophagy as being associated with anemia in that report.

Textures and consistencies of earths vary widely due to different proportions of the four major solid components: sand, silt, clay, and organic matter. Proportions of these components is important because each has very different effects on the body (Wilson 2003). In particular, sand is the least reactive inorganic fraction of earth, whereas clay is the most reactive (Saether and Caritat 1997). We classified geophagic earths based on qualitative descriptions in the original reports. Earth was categorized as "claylike" if the

author of the report described it in terms such as "clayey," "plastic," "moldable," "used for pottery," or as "marl."

Our database includes reports of consumption of 402 different types of earth, ranging in color from bright white to light yellow, orange, red, red-brown, purple, dark grey, black, blue, and light green. If more than one type was reported to be consumed in a culture, we used only the one that was most frequently consumed for each life stage. We chose this approach because counting more than one geophagic earth would lead to oversampling if one group ate seven types of clay, each one infrequently, whereas another group ate only one type of clay, but did so frequently. For example, if a report stated that "pregnant women rarely ate red clay but usually ate grey clay," pregnant women were classified as "usually" consumers of "grey clay."

The elemental constituents of only a few geophagic earths have been chemically analyzed; in many cases only qualitative descriptions are available. In general, it is not possible to determine the nutrient constituents of earth by visual inspection, with one exception: it can be inferred that soils contain iron if they are red in color (Jeff Wilson, personal communication). However, iron may be present if the soils are not red, because some iron-rich components result in pigmentation other than red. The calcium or zinc contents of most geophagic earths were not quantified. Even if they had been, the total elemental composition of the earth does not indicate the bioavailability of its constituents, i.e., the proportion freely available to cross an organism's cellular membranes. Bioavailability is typically much lower than total amounts (Wilson 2003).

STATISTICAL ANALYSES

All statistical analyses were performed using STATA 9.2 for Macintosh (STATA Corporation, College Station, Texas). Differences in geophagy scores among sex and life-stage categories were tested using a multilevel, mixed-effect model (to control for repeated measures within a cultural report; Figure 2). Differences between observed frequency of geophagy by circumstances of consumption and the null hypothesis were tested by using Pearson's chi-square

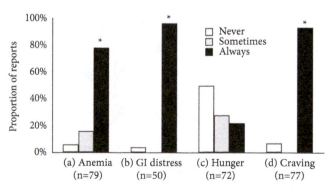

Figure 3 *Reports of the Frequency of Association of Geophagy with (A) Anemia, (B) Gi Distress, (C) Hunger, and (D) Craving*
The proportion of reports associated with anemia, GI distress, and craving was significantly higher (*) than expected under the null hypothesis (p 0.005).

analyses (see Figures 3 and 7). We tested whether nutrient requirements could predict geophagy scores (Figure 4) using Spearman's test of non-parametric correlation.

EVALUATING THE HYPOTHESES

Adaptive Hypothesis 1: Nutrient Deficiency

Association with Nutrient Deficiencies. If geophagy were a response to a nutrient deficiency, it should occur in conjunction with such a deficiency. Indeed, an association between geophagy and anemia was recognized as early as 40 AD when Cornelius Celsus, a Roman physician, wrote "those that have a bad color for a long time without jaundice, are either distrest with pains in the head, or labor under a *malacia*" (the term then used for cravings of non-food substances) (Celsus and Grieve 1756:59). The geophagy-anemia association has been confirmed repeatedly worldwide since then. For example, in Zanzibar, the Swahili term for anemia, *safura*, was mistranslated by Livingstone as "the disease of… earth eating" (Livingstone and Waller 1875:346). In 20th-century India (e.g., Hooper and Mann 1906) and on slave plantations in the Americas (e.g., Buckingham 1842), pallor was often used as a symptom of the disease of earth eating. Indeed, in our database, anemia and geophagy were associated significantly more often than would be expected under the null hypothesis (p 0.001) (Figure 3a). Available data did not permit us to test an association between geophagy and calcium or zinc deficiencies.

Frequency of Geophagy and Nutrient Requirements. If geophagy were a response to a deficiency in iron, zinc, or calcium, then we would expect people with the greatest needs to practice geophagy most often. To evaluate this corollary, we determined the daily reference intakes for each of these elements by people in each life stage (Institute of Medicine 2002; Figure 4). These values were standardized by dividing by energy requirements at each life stage to capture the relative requirements, a standard consideration in evaluating risk of nutrient deficiency.

If geophagic earth were consumed to obtain calcium, as Wiley and Katz (1998) proposed, one would expect preadolescents, adolescents, and the elderly, who have the highest calcium requirements, to engage in geophagy most frequently. If zinc deficiency were the impetus for geophagy, it should occur uniformly among all categories of adults, because they have similar zinc requirements. And, if earth were consumed to obtain iron (Hunter 1973; Abrahams 1997), we would expect infants and pregnant women to ingest earth most frequently. However, nutrient requirements were not significant predictors of geophagy scores for calcium (Spearman's rho 0.332, p 0.422), iron (Spearman's rho 0.542, p 0.165), or zinc (Spearman's rho 0.267, p 0.523). Thus, occurrences of geophagy do not parallel requirements for any of these three nutrients (Figure 4).

If geophagy were a response to nutrient deficiency, then pregnant women should consume earth most often late in gestation, when nutrient requirements are highest. Women need less iron in early pregnancy than they do when not pregnant because they are not experiencing menstrual blood loss, but later in pregnancy women's iron requirements are higher than when not pregnant because of the needs of the developing fetus (Institute of Medicine 2002). Women also need less calcium early in pregnancy compared to later, because fetal skeletal growth accelerates in mid-pregnancy; most of the calcium used by the fetus is accumulated during the third trimester (Institute of Medicine 2002). Zinc requirements do not change markedly throughout pregnancy (Institute

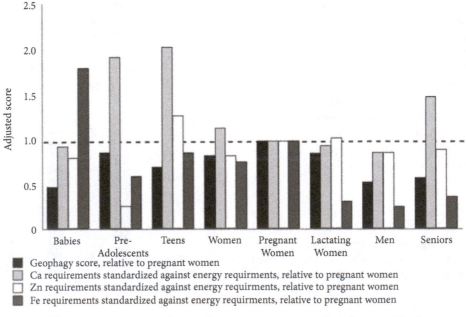

Figure 4 *Geophagy Score and Selected Nutrient Requirements, by Life Stage. All values have been standardized against those for pregnant women for ease of comparison.*

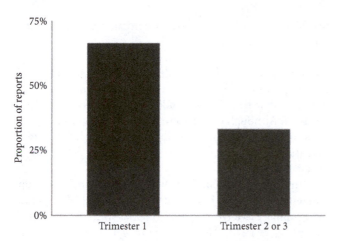

Figure 5 *Timing of Geophagy During Pregnancy (n 15)*

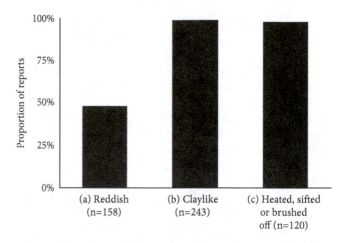

Figure 6 *Description of Geophagic Soils Showing Frequency of Reports Discussing (a) Color, (b) Texture, and (c) Preparation*

of Medicine 2002). Our data indicate that geophagy occurs nearly twice as frequently in early pregnancy as in late pregnancy (Figure 5). This pattern is not predicted by the nutrient deficiency hypothesis.

Nutrient Content of Geophagic Earth. If geophagy were an adaptive response to nutrient deficiencies, we would expect geophagic earth to contain the nutrients that are in short supply. Unfortunately, available information only enables us to evaluate this corollary for iron, and then only incompletely. Red color, indicative of the presence of iron, was reported in less than half the soils that were eaten (70 of 158; Figure 6a). Strikingly, when there was a choice between red clays and clays of other colors, the non-red clays were preferred (six of eight reports). For example, the Luo people of Kenya and Tanzania preferred the white clay sold at the market to the reddish clay that could be collected locally (Geissler 2000) and in the U.S. (Alabama), white clay was preferred over red clay (Spencer 2002). According to Vermeer (1971), the Ewe people of Ghana actually remove iron from red clay soils before consumption.

In the geophagy literature, it has been common to measure only the total elemental composition of geophagic soils (typically using acid digests). This is problematic because acid digests alone ignore much of the body's biochemistry, most critically, the pH of the intestine, the site of most elemental nutrient absorption. Because intestinal pH is much higher than the stomach, and nutrients are more soluble at low pH, equating the total elemental composition with the amount available to cross an organism's cellular membranes—i.e., its bioavailability (Semple et al. 2004)—vastly overestimates the usable nutrient content (Wilson 2003). Therefore, methods that involve only an acid digest can merely indicate if there is any element of interest present; the establishment of bioavailability requires more sophisticated techniques (Young et al. 2008).

Only five in vitro studies of geophagic samples have considered intestinal biochemistry in their analyses of

bioavailable nutrients. Two of these used the physiologically based extraction test, which includes a phase that mimics the pH and digestive enzymes in the gut, to study Ugandan (Smith et al. 2000) and Indian geophagic soils (Abrahams et al. 2006), respectively. In these studies, less than 5% of the total iron present was bioavailable. Negligible amounts of other biologically necessary minerals, including zinc, were available.

Kikouama et al. (2009) investigated trace elements released by six West African geophagic clays under conditions that mimicked the oral, gastric, or intestinal environment (samples were not passed through each stage consecutively). They found the availability of both ferric and ferrous iron to be lowest under intestinal pH, but did not calculate potential iron contribution.

A fourth in vitro study that attempted replication of intestinal conditions was conducted on two samples of South African geophagic soils (Dreyer et al. 2004). Earth was added to iron-enriched Ringer's lactate solution and the precipitation of elements at gastric and intestinal pH was measured. Black geophagic earth adsorbed sodium, potassium, and iron and liberated calcium and magnesium at pH 6.2. Iron from the Ringer solution was absorbed by the red geophagic earth at pH 6.2; no change in other elements was seen. In short, neither South African sample provided iron or zinc, but one might provide calcium.

Hooda et al. (2004) conducted the most thorough study of bioavailability because they not only examined the nutrients that geophagic materials could contribute in vitro, but their capacity to bind nutrients in suspension, thus rendering them unavailable. Results indicated that the five geophagic samples from around the world provided bioavailable calcium, magnesium, and manganese, but significantly reduced the availability of iron and zinc in suspension, suggesting that geophagic earth does not contribute these nutrients and is in fact likely to bind the iron and zinc available in ingested foods.

Most of the in vivo studies of the effects of geophagy on micronutrient absorption used outdated methods, small sample sizes, and were not adequately statistically analyzed (Young 2010). However, the limited data they do offer suggest that geophagy either decreases or does not alter micronutrient status, rather than increasing it.

Briefly, Minnich et al. (1968) demonstrated that the mean proportion of iron absorbed by people who ingested 5g of Turkish soil together with either radiolabeled iron sulfate or radio-labeled heme iron decreased by 9%. These results were subsequently replicated using other Turkish soils by members of the same research group (Çavdar and Arcasoy 1972). Talkington et al. (1970) tested the impact of two popular Texan geophagic clays on radiolabeled iron absorption and found a 1 to 3% increase in iron absorption in the presence of clay. This difference is unlikely statistically significant. Sayers et al. (1974) studied iron absorption among five habitual geophagists in South Africa. ^{55}Fe ascorbate absorption was greatly decreased when 250g of geophagic earth from participants' own supplies was eaten (mean absorption was 17.4% without earth versus 5% with earth).

In a study of 17 Turkish children, the 12 geophagists demonstrated impaired iron and zinc absorption compared to the five non-geophagists (Arcasoy et al. 1978). A second study of zinc absorption, in the presence and absence of 5g of geophagic clay, also indicated that clay impeded zinc absorption (Çavdar et al. 1983). The authors suggested that earth might bind not just with dietary zinc, but also with endogenous zinc released from the pancreas. In studies of rats, Smith and Halsted (1970) determined that modified Iranian geophagic soil could contribute dietary zinc. These results contrast with bioavailability data from in vitro analyses of unadulterated geophagic earth (Dreyer et al. 2004; Hooda et al. 2004; Abrahams et al. 2006), which indicated that little zinc was available and that some geophagic earth samples bound dietary zinc, rendering it unavailable. Finally, in the most recent in vivo study of the binding capacity of clays, pregnant rats were fed varying amounts of clay in a nutritionally complete diet (Edwards et al. 1983). The rats as well as their pups suffered skeletal and fur changes and slowed development, but exhibited no differences in hemoglobin or red blood cell count after 60 days; other nutrient indices were not evaluated. This suggests that some nutrients may have been chelated, but the data are inconclusive. Based on these few, small experimental studies, we can conclude that some geophagic clays interfere with absorption of cations, which can, in turn, result in nutrient deficiencies.

In sum, few of the available data support the hypothesis that geophagy functions to ameliorate mineral nutrient deficiencies. In fact, if clays bind dietary nutrients, this could help to explain the association between geophagy and anemia: eating certain earth might actually cause nutrient deficiencies. It is important to note, however, that presently available data on iron and zinc bioavailability are limited in quality and quantity, and information on the bioavailability of calcium and other minerals is fragmentary. More research is needed in this area.

Geophagy After the Resolution of a Deficiency. If geophagy were a response to nutrient deficiency, the resolution of that deficiency should result in cessation of the behavior. Although the literature is not extensive enough to rigorously test this corollary, there have been a few studies that assessed the effect of resolving a nutrient deficiency on pica behavior.

Three single-blinded studies suggested that iron supplementation resulted in cessation of pica behavior, including geophagy (McDonald and Marshall 1964; Mohan et al. 1968; Rogers 1972). However, there were numerous problems with the study designs, including a lack of controls, small sample sizes, and poor measurement of iron status, all of which make it impossible to attribute behavioral changes to iron supplementation alone (Reid 1992; Young 2010).

There have been two controlled double-blind studies of iron supplementation and pica. In the first (Gutelius et al. 1962), no correlation was found between changes in hemoglobin concentration and changes in pica. In the second study (Nchito et al. 2004), which focused specifically on geophagy rather than pica more generally, neither randomization to 10 months of iron supplementation nor 10 months of multivitamins significantly reduced geophagy among 402 Zambian schoolchildren. Based on multivariate logistic models, the authors concluded that neither iron supplementation nor multimicronutrient supplementation were significant predictors of geophagy (p 0.44, p 0.88, respectively). Thus, experimental data do not support the hypothesis that changes in iron status alter geophagic behavior.

There have been three studies investigating the effects of zinc supplementation on pica behavior (Bhalla et al. 1983; Chen et al. 1985; Lofts et al. 1990). Pica decreased after administration of zinc in all three, but it is not clear that this was attributable to the zinc supplementation because there was no indication of other messages given to the subjects, no controls, and no evidence of increase in zinc levels of subjects in two of the three studies (Bhalla et al. 1983; Chen et al. 1985). In sum, available data are insufficient to permit conclusions about the efficacy of zinc supplementation in causing cessation of pica (Young 2010).

In the sole study of the effects of calcium (Gutelius et al. 1963), experimental supplementation had no effect on pica behavior.

Adaptive Hypothesis 2: Protection

Association with Gastrointestinal Distress. The protection hypothesis predicts that geophagy should often be associated with gastrointestinal distress. Indeed, geophagy was associated with symptoms of gastrointestinal malaise (e.g., diarrhea, stomach pain, flatulence) in 48 of the 50 (96%) reports in which the occurrence of gastrointestinal distress was recorded (Figure 3b). This is significantly higher than would be predicted by the null hypothesis that there is no difference in geophagy by gastrointestinal malaise (p 0.001).

Clay Content of Earths. Consistent with the protection hypothesis, geophagists are highly selective about the earth they eat. In 237 of 243 cultural reports (98%) with descriptions, geophagic earth was described as clay-like (Figure 6b). Geophagists regularly expressed preferences for earth that was clay-like or smooth rather than gritty or sandy (e.g., von Humboldt et al. 1821; Beccari 1904; Vermeer and Frate 1979). Individuals sometimes went to great lengths to obtain clay-rich earth. They were willing to walk many kilometers to reach a site where a deposit of appropriate clay occurred (e.g., Forsyth and Benoit 1989). Even among clay-rich earths, there were explicit favorites. For example, one husband who dug clay for his wife from a deposit that was closer to home and less public than her preferred site; after she tasted it, she sent him back to get the *exact* clay she craved (Finger 1993).

Pathogen Content of Geophagic Earths. Under the protection hypothesis, geophagic earth should not be a vector for the transmission of parasites and other pathogens. However, parasitic infections, especially by geohelminths, have sometimes been attributed to geophagy (Hooper and Mann 1906; Anell and Lagercrantz 1958; Halsted 1968; Glickman et al. 1999). Although the parasite and pathogen contents of ingested earth were not quantified in the cultural reports in our database, there are three reasons to believe that geophagic soils typically are not vectors of geohelminth transmission.

First, geophagists typically select subsoils that are less likely to contain geohelminth eggs than earth closer to the surface, where defecation occurs (Young et al. 2007). Second, geophagists carefully prepare the earth they eat. In 118 of 120 cultural reports (98%), geophagic soils were heated, sifted, dried, or brushed off prior to consumption, rather than being excavated and immediately consumed (Figure 6c). Indeed, in Indonesia, Ghana, India, and Guatemala, an industry developed around geophagy that involved excavators, traders, and vendors (Anonymous 1881; Hooper and Mann 1906; Vermeer 1971; Hunter et al. 1989). In other places, clay preparation is handled on an individual basis, either by the consumer or someone else in the household. Whether on a large or small scale, the preparation of geophagic earth usually involves: (1) removing impurities by crushing the earth and then sifting out sand and small stones, picking off the outer crust of earth, or sometimes sieving it through cloth; and (2) baking, frying, sun drying, or smoking the earth. These preparation practices likely kill most endoparasites and other pathogens.

Third, there is little evidence to support the transmission of hookworm by geophagy (Gelfand 1945; Heymann 2004), especially since hookworms are spread transdermally. There is conflicting evidence about whether geophagy might

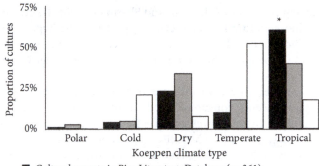

Figure 7 *Distribution of Geophagic Cultures in the Pica Literature Database (See Also Figure 1), Standard Cross-Culture Sample, and World Population Distribution by Climate Type*
The proportion of cultures in tropical areas that practice geophagy is significantly higher (*) than would be predicted by either the distribution of cultural groups in the SCCS or the worldwide population distribution by climate region (p 0.0001).

be a mechanism of transmission of whipworms (*Trichuris*) or roundworms (*Ascaris*). None of the prepared geophagic earths from Tanzania sampled by Young et al. (2007) contained live geohelminths, but in two other studies (Wong et al. 1991; Geissler et al. 1998), viable helminths were discovered in geophagic soils. This difference may be explained by the latter being conducted on soils eaten by children, who may have been more careless than adults about preparing the soil before consuming it (Young et al. 2007).

Geophagy by Climate Type. The protection hypothesis predicts that individuals who are frequently exposed to harmful foodborne microbes should frequently engage in geophagy. Foodborne pathogens multiply rapidly in hot, humid, tropical climates (Hui et al. 2001a), and species of pathogens and infectious diseases are more diverse in equatorial areas than in more northern latitudes (Guernier et al. 2004). Thus, we would expect geophagy to occur most frequently at low latitudes and altitudes. Although geophagy occurs throughout the world (Figure 1), it is especially common in tropical climate zones and exceedingly rare in polar and cold climates (Figure 7). The proportion of cultures in tropical areas that practice geophagy is much higher than would be predicted by either the distribution of cultural groups in the SCCS (p 0.0001) or the worldwide population distribution by climate region (p 0.0001).

Geophagy and Susceptibility to Toxins and Pathogens. Under the protection hypothesis, people should engage in geophagy when they are most susceptible to the harmful effects of toxins, parasites, and other pathogens. Particularly susceptible life stages are those during which rapid growth and cell division is occurring (i.e., embryogenesis and preadolescence; Bearer 1995). Furthermore, pregnant women are adaptively immunosuppressed (to avoid rejecting the embryo), so avoidance of parasites and pathogens is especially important for the woman's own health during pregnancy (Flaxman and Sherman 2000). Therefore, within a culture in which geophagy occurs, the hypothesis predicts that it should occur more frequently among pregnant women and children than among any other age or sex groups.

Indeed, the data indicate that pregnant women and preadolescents consumed earth most frequently (Figures 2 and 4). In multilevel, mixed-effect regression models of geophagy score, in which life stage is one of the independent variables and pregnant women is the reference level, the beta coefficients for all other life stages are significantly smaller. In other words, pregnant women consumed earth significantly more often than any other life stage group (p 0.0001). Thus we can reject the hypothesis that life stage cannot predict geophagy behavior.

In fact, there are more total reports of geophagy in pregnant women than reports of geophagy for all other life stages combined. Geophagy is so closely associated with pregnancy that the consumption of earth has been termed "a sign of the commencement of pregnancy" (Hooper and Mann 1906:254). In many countries, geophagy is thought of as a behavior unique to pregnancy, e.g., "It would be very surprising if pregnant women in Malawi did not eat clay. That's how you know when you are pregnant!" (Hunter 1993:75).

The protection hypothesis further predicts that geophagy should be more frequent early in pregnancy when embryonic tissues are most susceptible to damage from teratogens (Moore and Persaud 1998; Flaxman and Sherman 2000). Consistent with this, 10 of the 15 accounts that discussed the timing of geophagy during pregnancy indicated that consumption occurred during the first trimester (Figure 5).

Non-Adaptive Hypothesis 3a: Hunger

If geophagy were a non-adaptive behavior that occurs when a famished person attempts to fill an empty stomach, we would expect it to occur most often in times of food shortage or famine. We located data on hunger status of geophagists in 72 cultural reports (Figure 3c). Among these reports, geophagy was attributed solely to hunger in only 16 (22%). In contrast, hunger was explicitly not associated with geophagy in 36 reports (50%). In some of these reports, the adequacy of the food supply of geophagists was commented on directly by observers (Buckingham 1842) or indicated indirectly through discussion of the obesity of geophagists (e.g., Vermeer and Frate 1979) or the wealth of those who consumed earth (e.g., Gautier and Mc-Quoid 1853; Livingstone and Waller 1875). In the remaining 20 reports (28%), earth was sometimes eaten out of hunger while other times for "pleasure," "custom," "craving," or "habit" (e.g., von Humboldt et al. 1821). This distribution is significantly different (p 0.006) than would be expected under the null hypothesis.

The relative frequencies of geophagy by various sex and age groups (Figure 2) and its timing within pregnancy (Figure 5) also offer no support for hunger motivating

geophagy. For example, men and non-pregnant women have similar caloric requirements and so would be equally likely to engage in geophagy under this hypothesis. However, women practice geophagy much more often than men. Pregnant women require more calories (and are thus more likely to be hungry) late in pregnancy when the embryo is large and growing rapidly than early in pregnancy (Institute of Medicine 1990). Yet geophagy occurs more commonly in early than in late gestation (Figure 5). Finally, lactating women have the greatest caloric requirements of all the groups (Institute of Medicine 1990) and are therefore likely to be hungry most often. However, they are not the most frequent geophagists.

Earth Selection and Preparation. Under the non-adaptive hypothesis, if earth were being eaten simply to fill an empty stomach, any sort of earth (or any other non-toxic substance) should do. However, consumers were highly selective about the earth they ate (Figure 6). Indeed, we did not find a single report in which any type of earth was desired. Of the 77 cultural reports that mention how people felt about the earth they were eating, 72 (93%) explicitly discussed their desire for specific types of earth (Figure 3d), usually clay-rich soils. If earth was consumed as a last resort in the face of hunger, we would not expect descriptions such as "a devouring passion" (Galt 1872:403), "enjoyed" (Walker 1910: 220), and "great attachment" (Shannon 1794:375).

Quantity Consumed. Finally, if hunger motivated geophagy, we would expect that enough earth would be eaten to sate the appetite, i.e., to fill the geophagist's stomach. Although most reports did not quantify the amount of earth consumed, many described it qualitatively. The amount usually was small, for example: "a few morsels" (Maupetit 1911:179), "size of a hazelnut" (Garnier 1871:283), and "lump the size of an egg" (Whiting 1947:611). In 11 reports, the amount of earth was weighed. The modal amount that an individual consumed was approximately 30g, although in three cases more than 100g was reportedly eaten. Recently, more rigorous biomedical studies have recorded consumption of 30 – 50g of earth per individual (Geissler et al. 1997; Saathoff et al. 2002; Luoba et al. 2005; Young et al. 2010). The implication is that the usual amount of earth consumed is small, more like a medicament than a meal. Although clays can expand in volume in a moist environment, it is unlikely that the small quantities ingested would quell hunger pains, and certainly not for very long since geophagic earth provides no energy.

Non-Adaptive Hypothesis 3b: Epiphenomenon of Nutrient Deficiency

If geophagy were a non-adaptive epiphenomenon of nutrient deficiencies, we would expect the behavior to be associated with such deficiencies. In our database, anemia and geophagy are associated, but the cross-sectional nature of the data do not permit determination of temporality. If, however, a deficiency caused geophagy, the cessation of geophagy should occur upon supplementation with deficient nutrient. This is usually not the case (see the earlier section, Geophagy After the Resolution of a Deficiency). Research on the neurological and sensory consequences of nutrient deficiencies is lacking, but with current data, there is little support for this hypothesis.

GEOPHAGY IN NON-HUMAN ANIMALS

Geophagy also occurs in a wide range of non-human vertebrates (see supplementary material, Tables 2 and 3, available at http://journals.uchicago.edu/QRB). We located 79 accounts of its occurrence in 57 species of primates and 251 accounts of geophagy in 240 species of other vertebrates, including mammals (in 29 families), birds (in 13 families), and reptiles (in five families). Geophagy is likely far more common, but has gone unnoticed because detailed, long-term observations of that species' dietary habits have not been made.

Among primates, multiple hypotheses for geophagy have received empirical support. Krishnamani and Mahaney (2000:899) concluded that "mineral supplementation, adsorption of toxins, treatment of diarrhoea and pH adjustment of the gut seem the most plausible reasons why primates engage in geophagy." In our tabulation of primate geophagy, 49 of 79 accounts described geophagy as an adaptive behavior, and in the other 30 accounts, the probable function of geophagy was not specified. Among the adaptive reports, 32 (65%) attributed geophagy as probably or definitely motivated by the detoxification of plant secondary compounds or protection from parasites and pathogens (including treatment of diarrhea), and 32 (65%) attributed geophagy as probably or definitely related to obtaining nutrients. The proportions sum to more than 100% because some authors proposed multiple explanations. The vast majority of primates in which geophagy has been observed inhabit tropical areas, and detoxification was inferred most commonly in leaf- and fruit-eating primates. Ingested earth most frequently came from the forest floor and termite mounds, and often was described as having a clay-like consistency.

Among vertebrates other than primates, 176 of the 251 accounts (70%) indicated that geophagy was definitely or probably an adaptive behavior, whereas only 5 (2%) indicated that it was nonadaptive. In the other accounts the probable function of geophagy was not specified. Among the adaptive reports, 88% attributed geophagy to obtaining mineral nutrients (primarily salt and calcium) and 19% attributed geophagy to detoxification of plant secondary compounds. The proportions sum to more than 100% because some authors proposed multiple explanations.

The possibility that geophagy provides protection from parasites and pathogens was rarely considered in non-primates, and the sex and reproductive status of geophagists were infrequently mentioned. However, geophagy was described by sex and pregnancy status among 17 species of neotropical, fruit-eating bats (Bravo et al. 2008, 2010). Intriguingly, females engaged in geophagy more often than males, and pregnant females did so more often than non-pregnant females.

Studies with laboratory animals indicate that geophagy can provide relief from gastrointestinal distress. Rats cannot rid themselves of toxins through emesis, but when they are poisoned experimentally they preferentially ingest kaolin, which reduces poison-related morbidity and mortality (Mitchell et al. 1976; Burchfield et al. 1977; Watson et al. 1987; Takeda et al. 1993; Madden et al. 1999). Similar results were observed in experiments on parrots (Gilardi et al. 1999).

Animal geophagy has been observed in a wide range of climate and habitat types, although the majority of studies (especially of birds) were conducted in the tropics. Geophagy was most often detected during observations at traditionally used "clay licks," "mineral licks," and "salt licks," and need for nutrients (especially sodium and calcium) was most commonly inferred as the function of geophagy (especially in ungulates). Detoxification was inferred primarily in tropical, fruit-eating birds such as parrots and pigeons. However, the soils at many of the traditional mineral licks were described as clay-rich in composition, so detoxification and protection against pathogens may be more common than is currently recognized. Indeed, some studies attributed geophagy to both detoxification and micronutrient acquisition.

CHALLENGES TO THE INTERPRETATION OF DATA

There are several reasons for caution in interpreting our results. First is the danger of underreporting, which is inherent in any literature review. Human and animal geophagy is unquestionably underreported because it is easily missed, even by trained observers. In humans, geophagists and local informants may attempt to conceal the behavior for fear of being judged negatively or chastised, or because earth eating may be interpreted as an indication of pregnancy status (which some may want to keep private), poverty, or lack of self control (Hooper and Mann 1906; Dickins and Ford 1942; Sayetta 1986). Even when geophagists are not furtive, investigators may not know to inquire about earth eating specifically, and they "discover" geophagy only by accident (e.g., Hooper and Mann 1906; Vermeer 1966; Cooksey 1995; Rainville 1998; Grigsby et al. 1999).

Second, for human geophagy, there is considerable variability in objectivity and thoroughness among studies. Although judgmental language is stripped from our database, we wonder if the revulsion geophagy sometimes elicits has colored published reports by limiting the amount of information investigators pursued or were given in the course of fieldwork. Preconceived notions about who engages in geophagy may have also biased some of the reports. For example, if geophagy was attributed to "the weaker sex" (Maler 1692), the observer might not try to find out how often men practiced geophagy.

Third, there is an additional difficulty in studying human geophagy, and pica in general: it does not easily fit into a specific cultural conceptual category. From a cultural perspective, the people being interviewed may think of pica substances as medicines, food additives, or just cravings, and food recall questionnaires generally do not probe these issues with appropriate prompts (Young and Ali 2005). Thus, because we can only report on positive observations of geophagy, there are likely to be some false negatives (Type 2 errors), i.e., societies in which geophagy occurs, but has not been documented.

Fourth, in humans some misclassification errors probably occurred (see Methodology). However, classifying a pregnant woman as non-pregnant or an anemic person as non-anemic would only weaken the trends we discovered. And misclassification, underreporting, or false negatives would not explain the significant differences we documented among categories of geophagists within societies, including the relationships between geophagy and anemia (Figure 3a), gastrointestinal distress (Figure 3b), the predominance of the behavior among pregnant women and children (Figure 2), or the occurrence of geophagy in early pregnancy (Figure 5).

DISCUSSION

Three hypotheses have been proposed for the functional significance of human geophagy. Of these, the non-adaptive hypothesis that geophagy is an attempt to fill a hungry stomach explains few cases. Geophagy occurs when food is plentifully available. Moreover, that small quantities of earth are consumed, the age and sex biases, and the frequent association with strong cravings for specific types of earth are not consistent with the hunger hypothesis. The second non-adaptive hypothesis, that geophagy is an epiphenomenon of nutrient deficiencies that cause neurological or sensory problems, also is not supported by available data. Nutrient supplementation does not regularly cause the cessation of geophagy.

The first adaptive hypothesis is that geophagy results from nutrient deficiencies. Seemingly consistent with this hypothesis, geophagy is frequently associated with anemia. However, the timing of geophagy does not parallel the timing of changes in nutrient needs through the life span, nor within pregnancy. The irregular presence and low bioavailability of calcium, zinc, and iron in geophagic earth, the fact that iron supplementation does not reduce geophagic behavior, and the experimental data indicating that micronutrient absorption is limited after the consumption of earth cast doubt on this hypothesis.

The second adaptive hypothesis is that geophagy is a mechanism of protection against plant toxins, parasites, and other pathogens. Consistent with this hypothesis is the association of geophagy with gastrointestinal distress and with consumption of toxic substances, the high clay content of most geophagic soils (clay adsorbs dangerous chemicals and pathogens), the occurrence of geophagy in areas of the world with the highest parasite and pathogen densities (the tropics), and the sex bias and timing of geophagy during periods of greatest susceptibility to harm from parasites, pathogens, and toxins (childhood and early in pregnancy).

Use of clay in food preparation is a well-known means of neutralizing toxins (Johns and Duquette 1991; Johns 1996). In 27 reports in the Pica Literature Database, clay was used in the preparation of major food items, e.g., staple crops and fish (honey, salt, or oil were not considered major food items). In ten of these cultures (37%), clay was used in the preparation of or eaten with foods that contain harmful substances, such as Andean potatoes (which contain glycoalkaloids; Johns 1996) and Sardinian acorns (high in tannins; Wagner and Cortes 1921; Usai and Mazzarella 1969). In Western Australia, aborigines used clay in the preparation of *mene*, a tuber known to cause diarrhea when ingested raw (Grey 1841). Several of the cultural reports in our database contained explicit information about the association of geophagy with exposure to toxins. For example, people in the Northern Territory of Australia explained that they ate clay to "line the stomach" before eating fish they knew to be poisonous (Grey 1841).

The detoxifying properties of clay may even explain some of the geophagy that has been observed in times of food shortages (Figure 3c). When people are forced to eat plant parts they would normally avoid due to the secondary compounds they contain (e.g., weed stems, bark, and roots), consumption of small amounts of clay could reduce the dangers associated with ingesting these marginal foods by binding with the toxic chemicals that typically make them unpalatable (Johns 1996).

Occurrences of geophagy in non-human primates and other vertebrates also support the two adaptive hypotheses over the non-adaptive alternative. However, no conclusions can be drawn about the relative importance of micronutrient deficiencies versus protection against plant toxins in the occurrence of non-human geophagy, primarily because the possibility that geophagy provides protection against parasites and pathogens was rarely considered for non-primates. In primates, geophagy was attributed to protection from toxins and to micronutrient deficiencies with approximately equal frequencies whereas in other vertebrates geophagy was typically attributed to nutrient deficiencies. Whether this apparent difference is real is impossible to determine because many studies of primates specifically considered the protection function of geophagy, whereas most studies of other vertebrates did not. The frequency with which geophagy was reported in tropical leaf- and fruit-eating birds and mammals suggests that detoxification of plant secondary compounds is a more important function of the behavior than presently is realized.

If protection from pathogens and detoxification of plant secondary compounds are the primary functions of geophagy, what do we make of the strong and consistent associations between geophagy and anemia in humans?

There are two possibilities, both of which pertain to the complex and delicate balance between iron status and infection. Anemia can be an adaptive bodily response to infections, a nutritional adaptation whereby the sequestration of certain nutrients can protect against pathogenic agents (Prentice et al. 2007; Wander et al. 2009). Many foodborne bacteria require iron to reproduce and iron sequestration reduces bacterial growth rates. Under this hypothesis, the relationship between anemia and geophagy is correlational but not causal, that is, both the ingestive behavior and the physiological response are adaptations to minimize the severity of foodborne bacterial infections.

The second possibility is that ingestion of geophagic earth not only inhibits parasites and other pathogens but also impedes iron absorption, either by binding with dietary iron directly (Hooda et al. 2004) or with the mucin layer in the small intestine (Leonard et al. 1994) thereby making it difficult for bound iron molecules to pass through the brush border. Under this scenario, the relationship between geophagy and anemia is causal—i.e., geophagy causes anemia as a side effect of its antiparasite/pathogen benefits. Information that is presently available is insufficient to decide between these alternatives. Regardless of which is correct, the anemia-geophagy correlation could be consistent with the protection hypotheses.

Further tests of the two adaptive hypotheses would be useful. In terms of the protective hypothesis, it would be illuminating to compare the amounts and toxicities of plant secondary compounds and foodborne parasites and pathogens in the diets of geophagic and non-geophagic human societies and animal species, and among individuals within those societies or populations. Exposing laboratory animals to biotic enemies and toxins, and then feeding them geophagic earth or a placebo would also help quantify the protective effects of geophagic soils. A third test of this hypothesis would be to establish the capacity of geophagic earths to bind harmful toxins, pathogens, and endoparasites in in vivo conditions.

We hope this paper stimulates such research. More importantly, we hope readers agree that it is time to stop regarding geophagy as a bizarre, non-adaptive gustatory mistake. Our data indicate clearly that geophagy is a widespread behavior in humans and other vertebrates that occurs during both vulnerable life stages and when facing ecological conditions that require protection.

Notes

We thank Daniel Dykhuizen, Kathleen Rasmussen, Rebecca Stoltzfus, and several anonymous reviewers for their insights and useful comments on the manuscript. We would also like to acknowledge the tireless efforts of the team of library scientists and staff at the Cornell libraries, especially the Interlibrary Loan Office; they were integral to tracking down many obscure documents for the Pica Literature Database. We greatly appreciate the translations provided by Benedetta Bartali, Jen Baker, Urvashi Batra, Brian English, Tim Haupt, Jacqueline Kung'u, Helena Pachon, Rinat Ran-Ressler, Angelos Sidakalis, Owen Strijland, Vincenzo Vitelli, and Winthrop "Skip" Wetherbee. We are grateful for the following sources of financial support: the Hertz Foundation (Julius B. Lucks), the National Institutes of Health-TG #5 T32 HD007331 (Sera L. Young), The Weiss Presidential Fellowship Fund at Cornell University (Paul W. Sherman), and Wenner-Gren Foundation (Sera L. Young).

References

Abrahams P. W. 1997. Geophagy (soil consumption) and iron supplementation in Uganda. *Tropical Medicine and International Health* 2:617–623.

Abrahams P. W., Follansbee M. H., Hunt A., Smith B., Wragg J. 2006. Iron nutrition and possible lead toxicity: an appraisal of geophagy undertaken by pregnant women of UK Asian communities. *Applied Geochemistry* 21:98–108.

Anell B., Lagercrantz S. 1958. *Geophagical Customs.* Uppsala (Sweden): Studia Ethnographica Upsaliensia.

Anonymous. 1881. Land- en volkenkunde van Neerlandsch Indie: Geophagie. *Mededeelingen van wege het Nederlandsche Zendelinggenootschap* 25:293–296.

Arcasoy A., Çavdar A. O., Babacan E. 1978. Decreased iron and zinc absorption in Turkish children with iron deficiency and geophagia. *Acta Haematologica* 60:76–84.

Baudouin M. 1924. A propos de l'abrasion des dents. *La Semaine dentaire* 6:82–84.

Bearer C. F. 1995. Environmental health hazards: how children are different from adults. *The Future of Children* 5:11–26.

Beccari O. 1904. *Wanderings in the Great Forests of Borneo.* Singapore: Oxford University Press.

Bhalla J. N., Khanna P. K., Srivastava J. R., Sur B. K., Bhalla M. 1983. Serum zinc level in pica. *Indian Pediatrics* 20:667–670.

Brady J. E., Rissolo D. 2006. A reappraisal of ancient Maya cave mining. *Journal of Anthropological Research* 62:471–490.

Bravo A., Harms K. E., Emmons L. H. 2010. Puddles created by geophagous mammals are potential mineral sources for frugivorous bats (Stenodermatinae) in the Peruvian Amazon. *Journal of Tropical Ecology* 26:173–184.

Bravo A., Harms K. E., Stevens R. D., Emmons L. H. 2008. *Collpas:* activity hotspots for frugivorous bats (Phyllostomidae) in the Peruvian Amazon. *Biotropica* 40:203–210.

Browman D. L., Gundersen J. N. 1993. Altiplano comestible earths: prehistoric and historic geophagy of highland Peru and Bolivia. *Geoarchaeology* 8:413–425.

Buckingham J. S. 1842. *The Slave States of America: Volume I.* London (UK): Fisher Son and Company.

Burchfield S. R., Elich M. S., Woods S. C. 1977. Geophagia in response to stress and arthritis. *Physiology & Behavior* 19:265–267.

Çavdar A. O., Arcasoy A. 1972. Hematologic and biochemical studies of Turkish children with pica: a presumptive explanation for the syndrome of geophagia, iron deficiency anemia, hepatosplenomegaly and hypogonadism. *Clinical Pediatrics* 11: 215–227.

Çavdar A. O., Arcasoy A., Cin S., Babacan E., Gozdasoglu S. 1983. Geophagia in Turkey: iron and zinc absorption studies and response to treatment with zinc in geophagia cases. Pages 71–97 in *Zinc Deficiency in Human Subjects: Proceedings of an International Symposium held in Ankara, Turkey, April 29–30, 1982*, edited by A. S. Prasad, A. O. Çavdar, G. J. Brewer, and P. J. Aggett. New York: Alan R. Liss, Inc.

Celsus A. C., Grieve J. 1756. *Of Medicine*. London (UK): D. Wilson and T. Durham.

Chen X. C., Yin T. A., He J. S., Ma Q. Y., Han Z. M., Li L. X. 1985. Low levels of zinc in hair and blood, pica, anorexia, and poor growth in Chinese preschool children. *American Journal of Clinical Nutrition* 42:694–700.

Chisholm J. C., Jr., Martin H. I. 1981. Hypozincemia, ageusia, dysosmia, and toilet tissue pica. *Journal of the National Medical Association* 73:163–164.

Clark J. D. 2001. *Kalambo Falls Prehistoric Site: Volume III*. Cambridge (UK): Cambridge University Press.

Cooksey N. R. 1995. Pica and olfactory craving of pregnancy: how deep are the secrets? *Birth* 22:129–137.

Danford D. E. 1982. Pica and nutrition. *Annual Review of Nutrition* 2:303–322.

Dickins D., Ford R. N. 1942. Geophagy (dirt eating) among Mississippi Negro school children. *American Sociological Review* 7:59–65.

Ditter B., Urbaschek R., Urbaschek B. 1983. Ability of various adsorbents to bind endotoxins in vitro and to prevent orally induced endotoxemia in mice. *Gastroenterology* 84:1547–1552.

Dominy N. J., Davoust E., Minekus M. 2004. Adaptive function of soil consumption: an *in vitro* study modeling the human stomach and small intestine. *Journal of Experimental Biology* 207:319–324.

Dornai D., Mingelgrin U., Frenkel H., Bar-Joseph M. 1993. Direct quantification of unadsorbed viruses in suspensions of adsorbing colloids with the enzyme-linked immunosorbent assay. *Applied and Environmental Microbiology* 59:3123–3125.

Dreyer M. J., Chaushev P. G., Gledhill R. F. 2004. Biochemical investigations in geophagia. *Journal of the Royal Society of Medicine* 97:48.

Edwards A. A., Mathura C. B., Edwards C. H. 1983. Effects of maternal geophagia on infant and juvenile rats. *Journal of the National Medical Association* 75:895–902.

Edwards C. H., Johnson A. A., Knight E. M., Oyemade U. J., Cole O. J., Westney O. E., Jones S., Laryea H., Westney L. S. 1994. Pica in an urban environment. *Journal of Nutrition* 124:954S–962S.

Ferrand E. 1886. Terres comestibles de Java. *Revue d'Ethnographie* 5:548–549.

Ferrari S. F., Veiga L. M., Urbani B. 2008. Geophagy in New World Monkeys (Platyrrhini): ecological and geographic patterns. *Folia Primatologica* 79: 402–415.

Finger M. 11 December 1993. The clay eaters of Memphis. *Memphis*.

Flaxman S. M., Sherman P. W. 2000. Morning sickness: a mechanism for protecting mother and embryo. *Quarterly Review of Biology* 75:113–148.

Forsyth C. J., Benoit G. M. 1989. 'Rare, old, dirty snacks': some research notes on dirt eating. *Deviant Behavior* 10:61–68.

Galt F. 1872. Medical notes on the upper Amazon. *American Journal of Medical Sciences* 63:395–416.

Gardiner K. R., Anderson N. H., McCaigue M. D., Erwin P. J., Halliday M. I., Rowlands B. J. 1993. Adsorbents as antiendotoxin agents in experimental colitis. *Gut* 34:51–55.

Garnier J. 1871. *Voyage Autour du Monde. La Nouvelle-Calédonie (côte orientale)*. Paris (France): E. Plon.

Gautier T., McQuoid T. R. 1853. *Wanderings in Spain*. London (UK): Ingram, Cooke and Company.

Geissler P. W. 2000. The significance of earth-eating: social and cultural aspects of geophagy among Luo children. *Africa: The Journal of the International African Institute* 70:653–682.

Geissler P. W., Mwaniki D. L., Thiong'o F., Friis H. 1997. Geophagy among school children in western Kenya. *Tropical Medicine and International Health* 2:624–630.

Geissler P. W., Mwaniki D. L., Thiong'o F., Friis H. 1998. Geophagy as a risk factor for geohelminth infections: a longitudinal study of Kenyan primary schoolchildren. *Transactions of the Royal Society of Tropical Medicine and Hygiene* 92:7–11.

Geissler P. W., Prince R. J., Levene M., Poda C., Beckerleg S. E., Mutemi W., Shulman C. E. 1999. Perceptions of soil-eating and anaemia among pregnant women on the Kenyan coast. *Social Science and Medicine* 48:1069–1079.

Gelfand M. 1945. Geophagy and its relation to hookworm disease. *East African Medical Journal* 22:98–103.

Gilardi J. D., Duffey S. S., Munn C. A., Tell L. A. 1999. Biochemical functions of geophagy in parrots: detoxification of dietary toxins and cytoprotective effects. *Journal of Chemical Ecology* 25:897–922.

Glickman L. T., Camara A. O., Glickman N. W., McCabe G. P. 1999. Nematode intestinal parasites of children in rural Guinea, Africa: prevalence and relationship to geophagia. *International Journal of Epidemiology* 28:169–174.

González R., de Medina F. S., Martínez-Augustin O., Nieto A., Gálvez J., Risco S., Zarzuelo A. 2004. Anti-inflammatory effect of diosmectite in hapten-induced colitis in the rat. *British Journal of Pharmacology* 141:951–960.

Grey G. 1841. *Journals of Two Expeditions of Discovery in North-west and Western Australia, During the Years 1837, 38, and 39, Under the Authority of Her Majesty's Government: Describing Many Newly Discovered, Important, and Fertile Districts, With Observations on the Moral and Physical Condition of the Aboriginal Inhabitants.* London (UK): T. and W. Boone.

Grigsby R. K., Thyer B. A., Waller R. J., Johnston G. A., Jr. 1999. Chalk eating in middle Georgia: a culture-bound syndrome of pica? *Southern Medical Journal* 92:190–192.

Guernier V., Hochberg M. E., Guegan J.-F. 2004. Ecology drives the worldwide distribution of human diseases. *PLoS Biology* 2:e141. doi:10.1371/journal.pbio.0020141.

Gutelius M. F., Millican F. K., Layman E. M., Cohen G. J., Dublin C. C. 1962. Nutritional studies of children with pica. *Pediatrics* 29:1012–1023.

Gutelius M. F., Millican F. K., Layman E. M., Cohen G. J., Dublin C. C. 1963. Treatment of pica with a vitamin and mineral supplement. *American Journal of Clinical Nutrition* 12:388–393.

Halsted J. A. 1968. Geophagia in man: its nature and nutritional effects. *American Journal of Clinical Nutrition* 21:1384–1393.

Henon P., Gerota I., Caen J. 1975. Letter: one can remain a geophagist in Paris. *La Nouvelle Presse Médicale* 4:1431.

Heymann D. L. 2004. *Control of Communicable Diseases Manual.* Washington (DC): American Public Health Association.

Hippocrates, Adams F. 1849. *The Genuine Works of Hippocrates.* London (UK): Sydenham Society.

Hladik C. M., Gueguen L. 1974. Géophagie et nutrition minérale chez les primates sauvages. *Comptes Rendus de l'Académie des Sciences, Serie III* 279:1393–1396.

Hochstein G. 1968. Pica: a study in medical and anthropological education. Pages 88–96 in *Essays on Medical Anthropology, Southern Anthropological Society Proceedings, No. 1,* edited by T. Weaver. Athens (GA): University of Georgia Press.

Hooda P. S., Henry C. J. K., Seyoum T. A., Armstrong L. D. M., Fowler M. B. 2004. The potential impact of soil ingestion on human mineral nutrition. *Science of the Total Environment* 333:75–87.

Hooper D., Mann H. H. 1906. Earth-eating and the earth-eating habit in India. *Memoirs of the Asiatic Society of Bengal* 1:249–273.

Horner R. D., Lackey C. J., Kolasa K., Warren K. 1991. Pica practices of pregnant women. *Journal of the American Dietetic Association* 91:34–38.

Houston D. C., Gilardi J. D., Hall A. J. 2001. Soil consumption by elephants might help to minimize the toxic effects of plant secondary compounds in forest browse. *Mammal Review* 31:249–254.

Hudson R. P. 1977. The biography of disease: lessons from chlorosis. *Bulletin of the History of Medicine* 51:448–463.

Hui Y. H., Smith R. A., Spoerke D. G., Jr. 2001a. *Foodborne Disease Handbook, Volume 1: Diseases Caused by Bacteria.* Second Edition. New York: Marcel Dekker.

Hui Y. H., Smith R. A., Spoerke D. G., Jr. 2001b. *Foodborne Disease Handbook, Volume 3: Plant Toxicants.* Second Edition. New York: Marcel Dekker.

Hunter J. M. 1973. Geophagy in Africa and in the United States: a culture-nutrition hypothesis. *Geographical Review* 63:170–195.

Hunter J. M. 1993. Macroterme geophagy and pregnancy clays in southern Africa. *Journal of Cultural Geography* 14:69–92.

Hunter J. M., Horst O. H., Thomas R. N. 1989. Religious geophagy as a cottage industry: the holy clay tablet of Esquipulas, Guatemala. *National Geographic Research* 5:281–295.

Institute of Medicine. 1990. *Nutrition During Pregnancy: Part I: Weight Gain, Part II: Nutrient Supplements.* Washington (DC): National Academy Press.

Institute of Medicine. 2002. *DRI: Dietary Reference Intakes for Vitamin A, Vitamin K, Arsenic, Boron, Chromium, Copper, Iodine, Iron, Manganese, Molybdenum, Nickel, Silicon, Vanadium, and Zinc.* Washington (DC): National Academy Press.

Johns T. 1986. Detoxification function of geophagy and domestication of the potato. *Journal of Chemical Ecology* 12:635–646.

Johns T. 1996. *The Origins of Human Diet and Medicine: Chemical Ecology.* Tucson (AZ): University of Arizona Press.

Johns T., Duquette M. 1991. Traditional detoxification of acorn bread with clay. *Ecology of Food and Nutrition* 25:221–228.

Jones R. L., Hanson H. C. 1985. *Mineral Licks, Geophagy, and Biogeochemistry of North American Ungulates.* Ames (IA): Iowa State University Press.

Kawai K., Saathoff E., Antelman G., Msamanga G., Fawzi W. W. 2009. Geophagy (soil-eating) in relation to anemia and helminth infection among HIV-infected pregnant women in Tanzania. *American Journal of Tropical Medicine and Hygiene* 80: 36–43.

Kikouama J. R. O., Le Cornec F., Bouttier S., Launay A., Baldé L., Yagoubi N. 2009. Evaluation of trace elements released by edible clays in physicochemically simulated physiological media. *International Journal of Food Sciences and Nutrition* 60:130–142.

Kottek M., Grieser J., Beck C., Rudolf B., Rubel F. 2006. World map of the Köppen-Geiger climate classification updated. *Meteorologische Zeitschrift* 15: 259–263.

Kraemer S. 2002. Clay, vicks, and gold medal flour. *Southern Medical Journal* 95:1228–1229.

Kreulen D. A. 1985. Lick use by large herbivores: a review of benefits and banes of soil consumption. *Mammalian Review* 15:107–123.

Krishnamani R., Mahaney W. C. 2000. Geophagy among primates: adaptive significance and ecological consequences. *Animal Behavior* 59:899–915.

La Billardière M. 1800. *An Account of a Voyage in Search of La Pérouse, Undertaken By Order of the Constituent Assembly of France, and Performed in the Years 1791,*

1792, and 1793, in the Recherche and Espérance, Ships of War Under the Command of Rear-Admiral Bruni d'Entrecasteaux, Volume II. London (UK): J. Debrett.

Laufer B. 1930. Geophagy. Field Museum of Natural History—Anthropological Series 18:97–198.

Lavie S., Stotzky G. 1986a. Adhesion of the clay minerals montmorillonite, kaolinite, and attapulgite reduces respiration of Histoplasma capsulatum. Applied and Environmental Microbiology 51:65–73.

Lavie S., Stotzky G. 1986b. Interactions between clay minerals and siderophores affect the respiration of Histoplasma capsulatum. Applied and Environmental Microbiology 51:74–79.

Leonard A., Droy-Lefaix M. T., Allen A. 1994. Pepsin hydrolysis of the adherent mucus barrier and subsequent gastric mucosal damage in the rat: effect of diosmectite and 16,16 dimethyl prostaglandin E2. Gastroentérologie clinique et biologique 18:609–616.

Limpitlaw U. G. 2010. Ingestion of earth materials for health by humans and animals. International Geology Review 52:726–744.

Lipson S. M., Stotzky G. 1983. Adsorption of reovirus to clay minerals: effects of cation-exchange capacity, cation saturation, and surface area. Applied and Environmental Microbiology 46:673–682.

Livingstone D., Waller H. 1875. The Last Journals of David Livingstone, in Central Africa: From Eighteen Hundred and Sixty-Five to His Death. New York: Harpers and Brothers.

Lofts R. H., Schroeder S. R., Maier R. H. 1990. Effects of serum zinc supplementation on pica behavior of persons with mental retardation. American Journal of Mental Retardation 95:103–109.

Lotan N., Siderman S., Tabak A., Taitelman U., Mihich H., Lupovich S. 1983. In vivo evaluation of a composite sorbent for the treatment of paraquat intoxication by hemoperfusion. International Journal of Artificial Organs 6:207–213.

Loveland C. J., Furst T. H., Lauritzen G. C. 1989. Geophagia in human populations. Food and Foodways 3:333–356.

Luoba A. I., Geissler P. W., Estambale B., Ouma J. H., Alusala D., Ayah R., Mwaniki D., Magnussen P., Friis H. 2005. Earth-eating and reinfection with intestinal helminths among pregnant and lactating women in western Kenya. Tropical Medicine and International Health 10:220–227.

Madden L. J., Seeley R. J., Woods S. C. 1999. Intraventricular neuropeptide Y decreases need-induced sodium appetite and increases pica in rats. Behavioral Neuroscience 113:826–832.

Maigetter R. Z., Pfister R. M. 1975. A mixed bacterial population in a continuous culture with and without kaolinite. Canadian Journal of Microbiology 21:173–180.

Maler E. C. F. 1692. Disputatio Medica Inauguralis de Pica. Basel (Switzerland): Typis Johann Rudolphi Genathii.

Mallory W. H. 1926. China: Land of Famine. New York: American Geographical Society.

Maupetit. 1911. Le géophagisme au Laos Siamois. Bulletin de la Société médico-chirurgicale de l'Indochine April:176–181.

McDonald R., Marshall S. R. 1964. The value of iron therapy in pica. Pediatrics 34:558–562.

McKnight T. L., Hess D. 2005. Physical Geography: A Landscape Appreciation. Upper Saddle River (NJ): Pearson Prentice Hall.

Minnich V., Okçuoğlu A., Tarcon Y., Arcasoy A., Cin S., Yörükoğlu O., Renda F., Demirağ B. 1968. Pica in Turkey: II. Effect of clay upon iron absorption. American Journal of Clinical Nutrition 21:78–86.

Mitchell D., Wells C., Hoch N., Lind K., Woods S. C., Mitchell L. K. 1976. Poison induced pica in rats. Physiology and Behavior 17:691–697.

Mohan M., Agarwal K. N., Bhutt I., Khanduja P. C. 1968. Iron therapy in pica. Journal of the Indian Medical Association 51:16–18.

Moore K. L., Persaud T. V. N. 1998. The Developing Human: Clinically Oriented Embryology. Philadelphia (PA): Saunders.

Murdock G. P., White D. R. 1969. Standard crosscultural sample. Ethnology 8:329–369.

Naroll R. 1961. Two solutions to Galton's problem. Philosophy of Science 28:15–39.

Nchito M., Geissler P. W., Mubila L., Friis H., Olsen A. 2004. Effects of iron and multimicronutrient supplementation on geophagy: a two-by-two factorial study among Zambian schoolchildren in Lusaka. Transactions of the Royal Society of Tropical Medicine and Hygiene 98:218–227.

Okonek S., Setyadharma H., Borchert A., Krienke E. G. 1982. Activated charcoal is as effective as fuller's earth or ben   tonite in paraquat poisoning. Klinische Wochenschrift 60:207–210.

Phillips T. D., Afriyie-Gyawu E., Williams J., Huebner H., Ankrah N.-A., Ofori-Adjei D., Jolly P., Johnson N., Taylor J., Marroquin-Cardona A., Xu L., Tang L., Wang J.-S. 2008. Reducing human exposure to aflatoxin through the use of clay: a review. Food Additives and Contaminants: Part A 25:134–145.

Prasad A. S. 2001a. Discovery of human zinc deficiency: impact on human health. Nutrition 17:685–687.

Prasad A. S. 2001b. Recognition of zinc-deficiency syndrome. Nutrition 17:67–69.

Prentice A. M., Ghattas H., Cox S. E. 2007. Host-pathogen interactions: can micronutrients tip the balance? Journal of Nutrition 137:1334–1337.

Profet M. 1992. Pregnancy sickness as adaptation: a deterrent to maternal ingestion of teratogens. Pages 327–366 in The Adapted Mind: Evolutionary Psychology and the Generation of Culture, edited by J. H. Barkow, L. Cosmides, and J. Tooby. Oxford (UK): Oxford University Press.

Rainville A. J. 1998. Pica practices of pregnant women are associated with lower maternal hemoglobin level at delivery. Journal of the American Dietetic Association 98:293–296.

Reid R. M. 1992. Cultural and medical perspectives on geophagia. *Medical Anthropology* 13:337–351.

Rey C. 1989. Rotavirus viral diarrhoea: the advantages of smectite. *Annales Paediatrici* 196:1–4.

Rogers M. E. 1972. Practice of pica among iron deficient pregnant women. [MS thesis]. Auburn (AL): Auburn University.

Saathoff E., Olsen A., Kvalsvig J. D., Geissler P. W. 2002. Geophagy and its association with geohelminth infection in rural schoolchildren from northern KwaZulu-Natal, South Africa. *Transactions of the Royal Society of Tropical Medicine and Hygiene* 96:485–490.

Saether O. M., de Caritat P. 1997. *Geochemical Processes, Weathering, and Groundwater Recharge in Catchments*. Rotterdam (The Netherlands): Balkema.

Said S. A., Shibl A. M., Abdullah M. E. 1980. Influence of various agents on adsorption capacity of kaolin for *Pseudomonas aeruginosa* toxin. *Journal of Pharmaceutical Sciences* 69:1238–1239.

Sayers G., Lipschitz D. A., Sayers M., Seftel H., Bothwell T. H., Charlton R. W. 1974. Relationship between pica and iron nutrition in Johannesburg Black adults. *South African Medical Journal* 48:1655–1660.

Sayetta R. B. 1986. Pica: an overview. *American Family Physician* 33:181–185.

Semple K. T., Doick K. J., Jones K. C., Burauel P., Craven A., Harms H. 2004. Defining bioavailability and bioaccessibility of contaminated soil and sediment is complicated. *Environmental Science and Technology* 38:228A–231A.

Shannon R. 1794. *Practical Observations on the Operation and Effects of Certain Medicines in the Prevention and Cure of Diseases to which Europeans are Subject in Hot Climates, and in these Kingdoms; Particularly Those of the Liver, Flux, and Yellow Fever: Applicable Also to the Prevention and Cure of the Scurvy. Written in a Familiar Style. Recommended to the Perusal of Every Person Going to Sea, and Residing Abroad. To which are Added, Plain Directions for Private Use in the Absence of a Physician; and Observations on the Diseases and Diet of Negroes. With a Copious Explanatory Index*. London (UK): Vernor and Hood.

Smith B., Rawlins B. G., Cordeiro M. J. A. R., Hutchins M. G., Tiberindwa J. V., Sserunjogi L., Tomkins A. M. 2000. The bioaccessibility of essential and potentially toxic trace elements in tropical soils from Mukono District, Uganda. *Journal of the Geological Society* 157:885–891.

Smith J. C., Jr., Halsted J. A. 1970. Clay ingestion (geophagia) as a source of zinc for rats. *Journal of Nutrition* 100:973–980.

Smith T. K., Carson M. S. 1984. Effect of diet on T-2 toxicosis. *Advances in Experimental Medicine and Biology* 177:153–167.

Spencer T. 19 December 2002. Dirt-eating persists in rural south. *Newhouse News Service*.

Staszewski J. 1963. Population distribution according to the climate areas of W. Koppen. *The Professional Geographer* 15:12–15.

Takeda N., Hasegawa S., Morita M., Matsunaga T. 1993. Pica in rats is analogous to emesis: an animal model in emesis research. *Pharmacology, Biochemistry, and Behavior* 45:817–821.

Talkington K. M., Gant N. F., Jr., Scott D. E., Pritchard J. A. 1970. Effect of ingestion of starch and some clays on iron absorption. *American Journal of Obstetrics and Gynecology* 108:262–267.

Thomson J. 1997. Anaemia in pregnant women in eastern Caprivi, Namibia. *South African Medical Journal* 87:1544–1547.

Tsakala M., Tona L., Tamba V., Mawanda B., Vielvoye L., Dufey J., Gillard J. 1990. In vitro study of the adsorption of chloroquine by an antidiarrheal remedy traditionally used in Africa. *Journal de Pharmacie de Belgique* 45:268–273.

Usaí A., Mazzarella S. 1969. *Acorn Bread and Geophagy in Sardinia*. Cagliari (Italy): Editrice Sarda Fossataro.

Vermeer D. E. 1966. Geophagy among the Tiv of Nigeria. *Annals of the Association of American Geographers* 56:197–204.

Vermeer D. E. 1971. Geophagy among the Ewe of Ghana. *Ethnology* 10:56–72.

Vermeer D. E., Frate D. 1979. Geophagia in rural Mississippi: environmental and cultural contexts and nutritional implications. *American Journal of Clinical Nutrition* 32:2129–2135.

von Bonsdorff B. 1977. Pica: a hypothesis. *British Journal of Haematology* 35:476–477.

von Humboldt A., Bonpland A., Williams H. M. 1821. *Personal Narrative of Travels to the Equinoctial Regions of the New Continent, During the Years 1799–1804, Volume 5*. Paris (France): Longman, Hurst, Rees, Orme, and Brown.

Wagner M. L., Cortes C. W. 1921. *Das Ländliche Leben Sardiniens im Spiegel der Sprache: KulturhistorischSprachliche Untersuchungen*. Heidelberg (Germany): C. Winter.

Walker H. W. 1910. *Wanderings Among South Sea Savages and in Borneo and the Philippines*. London (UK): Witherby.

Wander K., Shell-Duncan B., McDade T. W. 2009. Evaluation of iron deficiency as a nutritional adaptation to infectious disease: an evolutionary medicine perspective. *American Journal of Human Biology* 21:172–179.

Watson P. J., Hawkins C., McKinney J., Beatey S., Bartles R. R., Rhea K. 1987. Inhibited drinking and pica in rats following 2-deoxy-D-glucose. *Physiology and Behavior* 39:745–752.

Whiting A. N. 1947. Clay, starch and soot eating among southern rural Negroes in North Carolina. *Journal of Negro Education* 16:610–612.

Wiley A. S., Katz S. H. 1998. Geophagy in pregnancy: a test of a hypothesis. *Current Anthropology* 39:532–545.

Wilson M. J. 2003. Clay mineralogical and related characteristics of geophagic materials. *Journal of Chemical Ecology* 29:1525–1547.

Wong M. S., Bundy D. A., Golden M. H. 1991. The rate of ingestion of *Ascaris lumbricoides* and *Trichuris trichiura* eggs in soil and its relationship to infection in two children's homes in Jamaica. *Transactions of the Royal Society of Tropical Medicine and Hygiene* 85: 89–91.

Yip R., Dallman P. R. 1988. The roles of inflammation and iron deficiency as causes of anemia. *American Journal of Clinical Nutrition* 48:1295–1300.

Youdim M. B. H., Iancu T. C. 1977. Pica hypothesis. *British Journal of Haematology* 36:298.

Young S. L. 2010. Pica in pregnancy: new ideas about an old condition. *Annual Review of Nutrition* 30: 403–422.

Young S. L. 2011. *Craving Earth: Understanding Pica—The Urge to Eat Clay, Starch, Ice, and Chalk.* New York: Columbia University Press.

Young S. L., Ali S. M. 2005. Linking traditional treatments of maternal anaemia to iron supplement use: an ethnographic case study from Pemba Island, Zanzibar. *Maternal and Child Nutrition* 1:51–58.

Young S. L., Goodman D., Farag T. H., Ali S. M., Khatib M. R., Khalfan S. S., Tielsch J. M., Stoltzfus R. J. 2007. Geophagia is not associated with *Trichuris* or hookworm transmission in Zanzibar, Tanzania. *Transactions of the Royal Society of Tropical Medicine and Hygiene* 101:766–772.

Young S. L., Wilson M. J., Miller D., Hillier S. 2008. Toward a comprehensive approach to the collection and analysis of pica substances, with emphasis on geophagic materials. *PLoS ONE* 3:e3147. doi: 10.1371/journal.pone.0003147.

Young S. L., Wilson M. J., Hillier S., Delbos E., Ali S. M., Stoltzfus R. J. 2010. Differences and commonalities in physical, chemical and mineralogical properties of Zanzibari geophagic soils. *Journal of Chemical Ecology* 36:129–140.

CHAPTER 20

Insects as Food: A Case Study from the Northwest Amazon

Darna L. Dufour

(1987)

Much of the recent interest in human ecology in Amazonia has centered around questions related to the amount of protein available in wild fauna on a sustained yield basis (Harris 1974; Gross 1975; Ross 1978; Chagnon and Hames 1979; Milton 1984). For the most part, wild fauna has been equated with large vertebrates. Although Beckerman (1979) pointed out that other sources of dietary protein, such as wild plants and invertebrates, need to be considered as well, the acquisition of these resources is less dramatic and has received little attention. With regard to insects this is perhaps surprising because they are a very conspicuous group and account for a large proportion of the forest's animal biomass (Fittkau and Klinge 1973:6–7). Furthermore, their use as food is very widespread and has been mentioned by a number of investigators. In his comprehensive review of the early literature, Bodenheimer (1951) cites more than 20 references. More recent work on the Yukpa (Ruddle 1973), Yanamamo (Smole 1976), Yanomami (Lizot 1977), Ache (Hurtado et al. 1985), and the Maku (Milton 1984) indicate that insect fauna continue to be included in indigenous diets.

The literature referring to the use of insects as food contains lists of edible species but little discussion of the characteristics of insects that are relevant to their selection as food resources in a tropical forest environment. Furthermore, although the suggestion that insects are an important component of indigenous diets is common (Bodenheimer 1951:11, 19; Ruddle 1973:14; Milton 1984:14), there have been no attempts to evaluate their dietary significance in terms of the frequency with which they are included in the diet, the quantities eaten, or their contribution to energy and protein intake. Lizot's (1977) work is an exception in that he estimated the percent contribution by weight of insects to Yanomami diet. His data indicate that women at Kakashiwë consumed nothing but insects during a 28-day period (1977:509).

My interest in the use of insects as food stems from fieldwork among Tatuyo-speaking Tukanoan Indians in the Northwest Amazon, and my observation that insect fauna was frequently included in the diet, sometimes in relatively large amounts. My purpose in this article is first, to define the characteristics of the insect species consumed, especially in terms of their predictability as food resources in the environment, and second, to evaluate the dietary significance of entomophagy for this population.[1] A larger goal is to provide observations and data of relevance to the question of protein availability in Amazonia. The research presented here indicates that insect fauna is frequently consumed and clearly an important food resource for Tukanoans. I thus suggest that a consideration of the role of insect fauna in the diet needs to be included in any evaluation of the adequacy of protein resources in Amazonia.

STUDY AREA

The observations reported here are based on fieldwork in the Colombian Vaupés region, primarily in the village of Yapú on the upper Papurí River between November 1976 and April 1978. The population density of the area is low, about 0.2 persons per square kilometer. The upper Papurí is a black water river draining an area of low, humid to very humid tropical rain forest broken with patches of *caatinga*, a low forest vegetation on sandy soils. Mean annual temperature is about 26°C and rainfall about 3,500 mm per year. Seasonal differences in rainfall are not well marked, but there is a long dry season of slightly less rainfall from November to February, and a short one in August. The principal rainy season begins in March, and July is usually the month of maximum rainfall. There is a second shorter rainy season from September through October.

At the time of the study, Yapú was a relatively large village settlement of over 100 persons. It was and still is considered a Tatuyo village, because the core members of the village, politically and socially, are Tatuyo, and the village is located on a site that has been occupied by Tatuyo since early in the century. The Tatuyo are one of the various linguistically defined exogamous groups of Tukanoan Indians in the Northwest Amazon (see Jackson 1983). I refer to the

Darna L. Dufour, "Insects as food: a case study from the northwest Amazon." *American Anthropologist* 89 (1987): 383–397. Reprinted with permission.

residents of Yapú as Tatuyo although members of several other groups of Tukanoans reside in the village as well.

Like other Tukanoans, the Tatuyo at Yapú are slash and burn horticulturalists. Cassava was and is the principal crop and dietary staple. During the period of field study it was supplemented with a variety of cultivated and wild vegetable foods, fish, game, and invertebrates. Neither domesticated animals nor tinned food were used. The diet has been described (Dufour 1983, 1984), and at least for adults, appears to be adequate in energy and protein.

METHODS

As part of a study of village energy flow, samples of insect material included in the diet were collected and preserved by drying (adult Coleoptera), or in 70% isopropyl alcohol (all other specimens). Almost all of the specimens were collected in the vicinity of Yapú on the Río Papurí (about 0° 31″ North and 70° 32″ West). The wasp specimens identified as *Apoica thoracica* Buysson were collected on the Caño Yi, and ants identified as *Atta laevigata* were collected at Acaricuara. Both the Caño Yi and Acaricuara sites are within 50 km of Yapú, and both species were collected for consumption while traveling with residents of Yapú. Caterpillars of the family Lacosomidae were collected at Querarimiri on the Río Cuduyari (within 80 km of Yapú) and they were reported to also occur upstream of Yapú. There are no significant differences in altitude or terrain within the region. Identifications were provided by the Insect Identification and Beneficial Insect Introduction Institute, United States Department of Agriculture (see Acknowledgments).

The proximate composition of four commonly eaten insect species was determined for representative samples preserved by traditional techniques of dry-toasting (Hymenoptera) and smoke-drying (Coleoptera larvae).[2]

The quantities of insects collected were obtained by routinely weighing all foods brought into the village for consumption. Dietary intake of insect material was ascertained using the weighed intake procedure. An observer accompanied each subject for a 24- to 72-hour period and weighed all food items prior to consumption on a 500-g dietary scale accurate to 1 g. On the occasions when it was impossible to accurately weigh food before it was consumed, weight was estimated on the basis of a duplicate portion. The protein values for animal foods were taken from the results of the proximate analyses and published food composition tables.

Weighed food intake records were kept during November through January, and May through June. In the November-January period food intakes were recorded for 72 hours for 8 men and 9 women, a total of 24 man-days and 27 woman-days. In the May-June period food intakes were recorded for 24 hours for 10 men and 13 women. November is the beginning of the long dry season and January generally the driest month of the year. May-June is the latter part of the long rainy season. The subjects were adult men and women between the ages of 18 and 55 years, all of whom appeared to be in good health, were engaged in normal activities, and were not adhering to any culturally defined food restrictions at the time.

RESULTS

Diversity of Insects Collected

The edible insects used at Yapú are listed in Table 1. These insects belong to 4 orders and include over 20 species. They are considered by order and family as this grouping defines shared characteristics of relevance to their use as food resources.

Coleoptera. A number of adult beetles, weevils, and their larvae were collected, but the most important of these were larvae of weevils, genus *Rhynchophorus*. These larvae are commonly referred to as "palm grubs" since they are found in the pith of felled palms. The Tatuyo felled palms to harvest the fruits, and often returned at a later date to harvest the larvae which subsequently developed in the pith. Palms were also cut specifically with the expectation that they would be invaded by weevils and the larvae ready to harvest in two to three months. Thus, the larvae were both a by-product of the harvesting of palm fruits and "cultivated." In the latter sense they were frequently used as a food cache by men on hunting and fishing trips away from the village.

Of the other beetles and beetle larvae collected, all were woodboring and most commonly collected from under the bark of decaying logs found in gardens, their presence detected by the sawdust tailings resulting from their woodboring activity. The larvae of these beetles were preferred over the adults, although the latter were occasionally eaten as well.

Hymenoptera. The order Hymenoptera includes ants, wasps, and bees. Ants and wasp brood were collected, but only Attine ants of the genus *Atta* were collected in quantity. *Atta* are leaf-cutting ants, conspicuous on the forest floor as they carry freshly cut leaf fragments to their subterranean nests. The genus includes two unusually large forms, the winged reproductives, or alates, and a worker with a disproportionately large head referred to as a "soldier."

Both soldiers and female alates were collected for food. Soldiers were gathered by inserting a probe, such as a palm leaf rib stripped of leaves, into a suitable nest entrance and removing those soldiers attaching themselves to it. The female alates were collected as they left the nest by the thousands in colonizing, or nuptial flights. These females, their abdomens engorged with a fatty egg mass, are very large ants and were a highly prized delicacy. The colonizing flights occurred in the early part of the principal rainy season and seemed to be triggered by a particular pattern of precipitation in which a day of very heavy rain was followed by a day of lighter rain. There was sometimes an additional flight from the nest at the beginning of the second, shorter rainy season. It was possible to predict the day of the flight very

Table 1 Summary of the Characteristics of Insects used as Food in the Northwest Amazon[a]

Species	Tatuyo name	Stage eaten	Length[b] (cm)	Weight[b] (g/ind.)	Spatial[c] dist.	Acq. rate[d] (g/h)	Temporal availability[e]
Coleoptera							
Buprestidae							
Euchroma gigantea (L.)	boopika	larva	?	?	++	?	NS
		adult	6.5	3.0d	+	?	NS
Cerambycidae							
Acrocinus longimanus (L.)	pikoroa	larva	9.0	7.7w	++	250	NS
Curculionidae							
Rhynchophorus spp.[f]	waraa	larva	5.5	3–16	+++	2,000	NS, 2–3 mos. after felling palm
		adult	?	?	+	?	NS
Passalidae							
Genus ?	yayaru	larva	4.5	1.5w	++	25	NS
		adult	4.0	1.9w	++	25	NS
Scarabacidae							
Megaceras crassum Prell	?	adult	7.0	2.2d	+	?	NS
Hymenoptera							
Formicidae[g]							
Atta cephalotes (L.)	mekaiyaa	soldier	1.0	0.1w	+++	200	NS, > 1 harvest/nest
	mekaiyaa liara	alate ♀	2.0	0.8w	+++	3200	early-mid RS, 1 flight/nest, 0430 h.
Atta laevigata (F. Smith)	ruhaa	soldier	1.0	0.1w	+++	200	NS, > 1 harvest/nest
	ruhaa liara	alate ♀	2.5	0.8w	+++	200	early-mid RS, 1 flight/nest, 1500 h.
Atta sexdens (L.)[g]	biapuna	soldier	1.0	0.1w	+++	200	NS, > 1 harvest/nest
	biapuna liara	alate ♀	2.5	0.6	+++	200	early-mid RS, 1 flight/nest, 1600 h.
Vespidae							
Apoica thoracica Buysson	utia	pupa	2.5	0.2w	+++	?	NS, 1 harvest/nest
Polybia rejecta (F.)	utia	pupa	?	0.2w	+++	?	NS, 1 harvest/nest
Stelopolybia angulata (F.)	toti utia	pupa	20	0.2w	+++	?	NS, 1 harvest/nest
Isoptera							
Termitidae; Nasutitermitinae							
Syntermes parallelus Silvestri	bupena	soldier	1.5	0.2w	+++	200	NS, > 1 harvest/nest

Continued

Table 1 *Continued*

Species	Tatuyo name	Stage eaten	Length[b] (cm)	Weight[b] (g/ind.)	Spatial[c] dist.	Acq. rate[d] (g/h)	Temporal availability[e]
		alate ♀	?	?	+++	2,000	early-mid RS, 1 harvest/nest, late afternoon
Syntermes synderi Emerson[h].	*meka bupuara*	soldier	2.0	0.2w	+++	200	NS, > 1 harvest/nest
		alate ♀	2.0	0.4w	+++	2,000	early-mid RS, 1 harvest/nest, late afternoon
Macrotermes sp.		soldier	2.2	0.3w	+++	200	NS, > 1 harvest/nest
Lepidoptera							
Hesperiidae							
Genus ?	*kiinamono*	larva	5.5	4.8w	+	<10	NS
Lacosomidae							
Genus ?	?	larva	6.0	2.8w	+++	?	long RS during 1–2 weeks
Noctuidae							
Genus ?	*batiya*	larva	6.5	4.0	+++	?	short DS—begin short RS during 1–2 weeks
Notodontidae							
Genus ?	*menehaia*	larva	4.5	0.8w	++	?	begin short RS during 1–2 weeks
Saturniidae							
Genus ?	*hutia*	larva	3.5				

[a]A number of other insects were observed being consumed but not formally identified. These included two varieties of termites (*meka rupua yabira* and *butawa*), a grub (*compiapu*), and a lemon-flavored ant (*bocorwa*).

[b]Length and weight data are average values of representative samples. Weight of specimens preserved in alcohol (w), weight of dried specimens (d), all other weights are for live insects.

[c]Spatial distribution defined as highly clumped with 50 or more individuals in close proximity in a single nest or within a single log (+++), somewhat clumped with 3–10 individuals in close proximity (++), or dispersed with individuals encountered singly (+).

[d]Acquisition rate is the maximum rate observed per attempt per person for a limited number of observations. Figures are rounded and do not include travel time to site. Search time is included in the acquisition rate for woodboring beetle larvae other than *Rhynchophorus*, but not for other insects. Acquisition time for alate ants and termites was defined by duration of swarming, which was somewhat less than one hour.

[e]Temporal availability is defined as nonseasonal (NS), i.e., available throughout the year, during the rainy season (RS) or dry season (DS). Time of the day is indicated where relevant.

[f]Larvae were collected from a variety of palms but *Mauritia flexuosa* and *Jessenia* sp. seemed to be the most important. Small and large forms of the larvae were often collected from the same palm and either represent different species or different instars of the same species. Adults were rarely used as a source of food. They are heavily sclerotized and have a very small edible portion.

[g]Two of the samples identified as *A. sexdens* were from colonizing flights that occurred between 1300 and 1400 hours. Assuming that differences in the timing of colonizing flights result in reproductive isolation, these samples may represent a subspecies of *A. sexdens*. The Tatuyo distinguish them by name, color, and taste.

[h]Tentative identification.

accurately from the weather pattern and type of activity at the nest, and the time of the flight was a recognized species specific characteristic (see Table 1). The female alates of *A. cephalotes* were particularly easy to collect since they left the nest just before dawn and could be attracted to a burning flare and caught neatly in a basket. Those of the other species of *Atta* had colonizing flights during the day, and were collected by handpicking them as they emerged from holes spread over the nest surface.[3]

Nests of several species of wasps were also collected, and the brood eaten. The species identified were all tree-dwelling social wasps. The nests of these wasps were quite large, but usually high in the trees and therefore hidden in the foliage.

Isoptera. Several species of termites were collected, but leaf-cutters of the genus *Syntermes* were the most important in the diet. The soldiers of *Syntermes* are about the same size and were collected in the same manner as the soldier ants. The female alates of *Syntermes* are smaller than alate ants of the genus *Atta*, and were collected for fishing bait as well as food. Acquisition rates were as high as those for *Atta* when leaf traps were used to channel the alates into a restricted number of exit holes.

Lepidoptera. Two species of colonial caterpillars were collected in particularly large quantities. The first, *hutia*, was a lightly haired, smallish caterpillar that nested in secondary growth and was as important for fishing bait as food. The second species, *batiya*, was a larger, brightly colored caterpillar that nested in a common primary forest tree, *Erisma Yapura*, and was collected as it descended from the canopy to pupate on the forest floor. Both species were available in only a limited portion of the range covered by their plant hosts. This patchy distribution was especially striking in the case of *batiya*. Although the host tree was very common in the area of the village, the caterpillars only appeared in a region several hours' walk to the northeast.

Two varieties of caterpillars using cultivated plants as hosts were also collected. One was found on cassava leaves, but only occasionally encountered, and the other used a cultivated tree (*Inga* sp.) as a host, but neither the tree nor the caterpillar were very common in the Yapú area. Several other varieties of edible caterpillars were named by informants, but none of these were observed being used.

Sex of the Collector

Adult men collected insect species which required felling trees (wasp brood), and splitting open felled logs (*Rhynchophorus* larvae). Men, women, and older children collected Lepidoptera and Coleoptera larvae (other than *Rhynchophorus*), and the alates of *Atta* and *Syntermes*. Women were responsible for collecting all of the ant and termite soldiers. Because this kind of collecting occurred throughout the year and was relatively time consuming, women probably devoted more time to insect collection than did men or children.

Contribution of Insects to Diet

Quantities of Insects Collected. Figure 1 shows the quantities of insects brought back to the village during a six-month period from April through June, and August through October. The Coleoptera were almost exclusively larvae of the genus *Rhynchophorus*. The quantities recorded averaged less than a kilogram per month for April, May, and June and less than 100 grams per month in August, September, and October. Coleoptera larvae seemed to be harvested throughout the year, but most were consumed away from the village by men on hunting-fishing trips, and by women in the course of gardening or other work.

Ants and termites were collected throughout the year, but collection rates showed two peaks of about 16 and 10 kg per month, respectively. The first peak was in April-May, early in the principal rainy season, when most of the nuptial flights occurred. Appreciable quantities of *Syntermes* soldiers were also collected in May because men and adolescent male initiates were adhering to ritually restricted diets in which ant and termite soldiers were the only animal food permitted. The second smaller peak in September corresponded again to nuptial flights.

The collection of caterpillars was limited to August and September, but the quantities were impressive: 26 kg of *hutia* in August and 39 kg of *batiya* in September. The value of 39 kg is the estimated fresh weight of the caterpillars calculated from the weight of smoke-dried *batiya* brought back to the village by five household groups, and an unknown proportion of what was actually harvested.

Food Value of Insects. The composition of some of the insects collected is compared to other animal foods in Table 2. The moisture content of all samples was low, and for the sake of comparison can be considered similar. The values

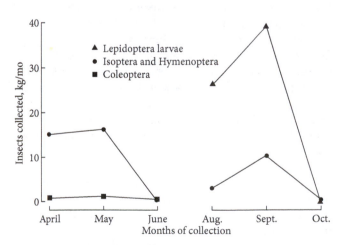

Figure 1 *Quantities of insects harvested at Yapú during two periods, April through June and August through October. Number of individuals resident in the village averaged about 108 during both periods.*

Table 2 Nutritional Value of Commonly Consumed Insects Compared With Other Animal Foods (Composition Per 100 g Edible Portion)

Food	Moisture (%)	Energy (g)	Protein (g)	Fat (g)	Ash (g)
Ants, female sexuals[a] (*Atta sexdens*)	6.1	628	39.7	34.7	1.6
Ants, female sexuals[a] (*Atta cephalotes*)	6.9	580	48.1	25.8	2.3
Termites, soldiers[a] (*Syntermes* sp.)	10.3	467	58.9	4.9	4.8
Palm grubs, smoke dried[b] (*Rhynchophorus* sp.)	13.7	661	24.3	55.0	1.0
Caterpillars, smoke dried[c] (various species)	11.6	425	52.6	15.4	4.6
River fish, smoke dried[d]	10.5	312	43.4	7.0	20.3
Tapir, smoke dried[a] (*Tapirus terrestris*)	10.3	516	75.4	11.9	3.5

[a] Proximate analyses were provided by the Instituto Agropecario de Colombia in Bogotá. Samples were prepared by dry-toasting in the field. Values are for single determinations.

[b] Proximate analyses were provided by the Instituto Colombiano de Bienestar Familiar, Bogotá, Colombia. Values are for single determinations.

[c] The values for caterpillars are from Wu Lueng, Busson, and Jardin (1968:167).

[d] Average values for two common fish, *rohe (Hoplias malabaricus)* and *wani (Aequidens latifrons)*. The fish were prepared by gutting, smoking over a slow fire until very dry, and grinding into a fine powder. This is a common method of preserving dry season surpluses of fish. The proximate analyses were provided by Dr. Gerardo Pérez G. Departamento de Química, Universidad Nacional, Bogotá, Colombia.

for river fish are the average values for two commonly used varieties, smoke-dried and ground into a powder. Since this mode of preparation includes bone and scale material, the protein value is lower than that of fileted fish.

The energy value of the insects shown is high, between 425 and 661 kcal per 100 g. The energy values for female alate ants (*Atta* sp.) and *Rhynchophorus* larvae are the highest, as both of these are rich in fat. The crude protein values for all insects are relatively high as well. The values for ants, termites, and caterpillars are higher than those for dried fish. In terms of less exotic foods the proximate composition of the ants, palm grubs, and caterpillars is comparable to that of goose liver, pork sausage, and beef liver, respectively. The composition of termite soldiers is roughly comparable to that of non-oily fish, although the latter are higher in protein.

Patterns of Insect Consumption. The frequency of insect consumption shown by the food intake records for November-January and May-June is compared to that of fish and game in Table 3. Fish was by far the most frequently consumed animal food, appearing in 88% of the diet records of males and 78% of those of females. Insects were the second, appearing in 26% of the diet records of males and 32% of those of females. Males consumed fish somewhat more frequently, and insects somewhat less frequently than did women, but these differences are not statistically significant (chi-square = 0.81, df = 1). However, insects were the only source of animal food in women's diets on 5 of the 40 days (12%) for which diet records were kept and were never the sole source in men's diets. These differences are significant.

The contributions of fish, game, and insects to the animal protein component of the diet are shown in Table 4. Most of the animal protein in the diet was from fish. Insects

provided about 4% of the animal protein in men's diets in the November-January period, and 2% in women's. Most of the insect protein in the men's diet was from palm grubs, and in the women's diet from both grubs and termites. Insects were more important in the May-June period, providing 12% of the animal protein in men's diets and 26% in women's. In both men's and women's diets most of the insect protein was from ants and termites. Animal foods provided almost 75% of the total protein in the diet in the November-January period. In May-June they provided somewhat less, about 70% of the total protein in men's diets and about 60% in women's.

Insects also contributed fat to the diet. In the November-January period the fat obtained from insects accounted for 23% and 7% of the fat provided by animal foods for men and women respectively. The corresponding figures for May-June were 18% and 20%.

DISCUSSION

Characteristics of Insect Species Included in the Diet

The species most often used for food exhibited highly clumped distributions during the part of their life cycle that was harvested. Hymenoptera (ants and wasps) and Isoptera (termites) are social insects, and therefore aggregated throughout their life cycle. Ants of the genus *Atta* form some of the largest ant colonies known (Weber 1972:1). For Coleoptera and Lepidoptera, the larval stage is, after the egg, the stage of the life cycle at which the organisms are the most numerous, and highly aggregated. The adults are more mobile and widely dispersed. Furthermore, the larval stage is often long in proportion to that of the adult (Daly 1985:426) and therefore offers a greater harvesting opportunity.

Table 3 Types of Animal Foods Consumed by Yapú Men and Women on Days Surveyed

Animal food	Man-days		Women-days	
	n	%	*n*	%
Fish only	17	50	20	50
Fish and insects	7	20	6	15
Fish and game	5	15	3	8
Fish, game, and insects	1	3	2	5
Game and insects	1	3	0	0
Game only	1	3	3	8
Insects only	0	0	5	12
No animal food	2	6	1	2
Total	34	100	40	100

Table 4 Mean Daily Animal Protein Intake of Yapú Males and Females by Source (*n* Refers to Number of Man-Days and Woman-Days; Percent Total in Parentheses)

Food source	Nov–Jan		May–June	
	M (*n* = 24)	F (*n* = 27)	M (*n* = 10)	F (*n* = 13)
Fish protein (g)	64 ± 75	56 ± 68	32 ± 30	24 ± 29
	(90)	(93)	(65)	(61)
Game protein (g)	4 ± 9	3 ± 6	11 ± 18	5 ± 13
	(6)	(5)	(23)	(13)
Insect protein (g)	3 ± 10	1 ± 3	6 ± 11	10 ± 19
	(4)	(2)	(12)	(26)
Total	70 ± 72	60 ± 66	49 ± 30	39 ± 28
	(100)	(100)	(100)	(100)

In general, the stage of the life cycle collected was the largest form and that which had the highest energy value for human consumers. For Coleoptera and Lepidoptera this is the larval stage. Larvae are devoted to feeding and exhibit a progressive increase in weight with each stage of development or instar (Chapman 1969:388). In comparison to the last instar, adult forms have a lower body mass and a hardened exoskeleton, which reduces their digestibility. In Vespidae (wasps) the pupal forms are similar to the adults in size, but softbodied and hence should be more digestible. In the case of Formicidae (ants), the female alates, with their egg mass and energy reserves in the form of fat (Weber 1972:35), have the highest energy content of any form. Of the nonreproductive forms the soldiers are the largest and have the highest edible portion. The same generalizations should be true of the termite alates and soldiers.

The insect forms collected in the largest quantities were the most predictable resources in space and time. Ants of the genus *Atta* and termites of the genus *Syntermes* inhabited nests that were irregularly distributed in the environment, but easily recognized, and the location of conveniently located nests was known. The colonies are long lived and the soldiers could be harvested repeatedly throughout the year. Alates, however, could only be collected at the time of their nuptial flights. Although of short duration, the timing of flights from particular nests was highly predictable, if both weather conditions and activity at the nest could be monitored. The latter was crucial to a successful collecting attempt, and only realistic for nest sites close to the village or near resource areas such as gardens. Attempts to predict the day of nuptial flights for nests at a distance from the village on the basis of weather patterns alone were usually unsuccessful.

Pupation of caterpillars of the families Noctuidae and Saturniidae occurred at known times of the year, on particular host plants in particular areas of forest. Although collection time was measured in days rather than hours, their temporal availability was limited, and the species collected were those occurring in areas of forest that were readily monitored. One species of caterpillar (family Lacosomidae; "outunima" in Cubeo) collected in large quantities on the Río Cuduyari occurred upstream of Yapú but was not collected during the field study, reportedly because of the uncertainty in the timing of its appearance. The patchy distribution of caterpillars is probably what makes them an important item of ceremonial exchange among Tukanoans (see Hugh-Jones 1979).

Of the Coleoptera, the distinction between those harvested in larger as opposed to smaller quantities is not as clearly defined by differences in predictability. *Rhynchophorus* larvae were essentially a managed resource, found with great regularity in the pith of felled palms. Other varieties of woodboring beetles and their larvae were also found with regularity at garden sites, but generally in smaller numbers, usually less than 20 individuals.

The other insects collected, the brood of social wasps, Hesperiid and Notodontid caterpillars, and two unidentified types of larvae, were less predictable in occurrence. Wasp nests appeared to be randomly distributed in the environment, were relatively difficult to locate, and destroyed in the harvesting process. The caterpillars appeared during recognized seasons and on known host plants, but in very small numbers. The occurrence of the two unidentified types of larvae was not easily predictable. Each appeared in the village on only one occasion, and informants claimed they were unable to locate other samples.

The insect forms collected were all relatively large insects. Soldiers and sexuals are the largest forms of *Atta* and some of the largest ants known. The soldiers and winged reproductives of *Syntermes* are the largest forms of the genus, with the exception of the queen, and fairly large insects (Araujo 1970:566). In general, beetles are considered large to medium insects. *Rhynchophorous* are among the largest of all herbivorous beetles (Crowson 1981:585), and those of the families Buprestidae, Cerambycidae, and Scarabaeidae are also large beetles (Crowson 1981:8).

Informants could name more edible insect species than were actually observed and collected during the field study. They can, for example, readily name at least 8 varieties of edible wasps, and more than 10 varieties of edible ants. There are several factors that may account for the discrepancy in number between the observed and enumerated varieties. First, the data on insect collection derived from harvest records included only the material brought back to the village and therefore underrecorded the use of insects which were typically consumed as they were collected. This was usually the case with the larvae of woodboring beetles. Furthermore, it is assumed that some of the insect material actually brought back to the village went unnoticed because it came in small packages at odd times of the day, or was effectively hidden. The latter sometimes occurred with prized foods, especially small quantities of *Rhynchophorus* larvae. The diet records provided a very accurate account of insect use, but for only a limited number of days.

Second, the period of observation may have been inadequate to record all varieties of insects that are harvested opportunistically, such as wasps, or only collected under certain social circumstances. An example of the latter was the unidentified lemon-flavored ant that was collected for use as a condiment when salt was tabooed. Third, not all varieties recognized as edible were found within the usual resource area exploited for insect fauna. Foraging for insects was usually restricted to an area within about 15 minutes' walk from the village, and in and around gardens. This was a smaller area than that exploited for fish and game resources, but essentially the same area in which most of the wild vegetable foods were collected. The only exceptions were the Noctuid caterpillars which were collected within the traditional territory of a neighboring village and in cooperation with that group, and the *Rhynchophorus* larvae "cached" near hunting/fishing camps.

Varieties of Insects Used by Other Native Amazonians

The forms of insects consumed by Tukanoans largely coincide with those reported for other traditional populations in Amazonia. The use of caterpillars and beetle larvae, especially "palm grubs," appears to be widespread and has been reported by a number of observers (Bodenheimer 1951:308; Denevan 1971:511; Lizot 1977:509; Ruddle 1973:95; Beckerman 1977:153; Milton 1984:14; Hurtado et al. 1985:17). The use of adult beetles seems to be less common, but has been reported for the Yukpa (Ruddle 1973:95) and Ache (Hurtado et al. 1985:17). The consumption of alate ants occurs in all of Amazonia (Bodenheimer 1951:305–306; Wallace 1853; Denevan 1971:511; Weber 1972:2; Ruddle 1973:95). Neither the use of soldier ants nor termites appears to be very common (Bodenheimer 1951:305), although it has been reported (Wallace 1853:243; Milton 1984:14). The consumption of wasp and bee brood has also been reported for the Yukpa (Ruddle 1973:95), but does not seem to be very common.

Dietary Significance of Insect Consumption

In terms of their proximate composition the insects consumed are comparable to other animal foods. The larval and reproductive forms are also very high in fat. The fat content of the diet is generally low (Dufour 1984), and the fat in animal foods highly valued. In terms of crude protein content the insects are generally intermediate between river fish and tapir. However, the crude protein value for whole insects with hard exoskeletons, such as ants and termites, may not be an accurate measure of the biologically available nitrogen (Redford and Dorea 1984:389). The exoskeleton of these insects is partly composed of chitin, a structural, nitrogen-containing carbohydrate. Some primates are able to digest chitin (Cornelius, Dandrifosse, and Jeuniaux 1976), but it is assumed that humans cannot (Taylor 1975:57), and therefore that the nitrogen in chitin is unavailable. A further consideration is that the crude protein value for termite soldiers is for whole insects and sometimes only the head is eaten, which has a higher proportion of muscle tissue to exoskeleton than the rest of the body.

The protein quality of the insects consumed was not determined. The amino acid composition of one species of *Atta, A. mexicana,* and four other species of insects consumed in Mexico has been reported (Elorduy de Conconi and Rodríguez 1977:168). Based on the FAO/WHO/UNU (1983) scoring pattern for the preschool child the amino acid score for *A. mexicana* is 54, which indicates that it is a food protein of intermediate value. Scores for the four other species ranged from 9 to 54. In all cases tryptophan was the limiting amino acid. This suggests that while the quality of insect protein is not as high as that of vertebrate protein, its amino acid composition is complementary to that in the dietary staple, cassava, which is limited in lysine and threonine (FAO 1970).

Insects were very frequently included in the diet, and during the May-June period contributed an appreciable proportion of the protein and fat derived from animal foods. They were less important in the diets recorded in November-January. The dietary records did not adequately sample seasonal differences in insect consumption, and it is likely that insects were also important in the diet when caterpillars were available in August and September. Over the entire year insects probably contributed 5% to 7% of all the animal protein consumed.

In general, insects were most often collected and consumed when other animal foods were available in very limited quantities, or not at all. This role of insects in damping fluctuations in the intake of animal foods reflected both seasonal variations in the availability of animal resources, and the day-to-day variability that occurred in individual households throughout the year. The high level of insect consumption recorded in May-June coincided with a seasonal peak in the abundance of alate ants and a relative low point in fish and game availability. On the other hand, the low levels of insect consumption recorded for November-January coincided with a period of average to exceptionally high fishing productivity. The actual availability of fish and game in individual households, however, was not completely dictated by seasonal factors. It depended to a large extent on the time and effort put into resource acquisition by males. Thus, even in January when fishing was the most productive, the diet records indicate that some households were consuming ants and termites collected by women.

The clearest difference between men and women in insect consumption is in the number of days insect material was the only animal food in the diet. This was 0 days for men and 5 of the 40 days for women. In all but one case in which the female declined the opportunity to eat fish, this sex difference was the result of differential access to animal foods. Such differential access frequently occurred when men were away on hunting/fishing trips and women remained in the village. It also occurred in the village because men did more visiting around mealtimes, and therefore were more likely to be served fish or game in a household other than their own. These male-female differences in diet may be an artifact of the village settlement where households occupy separate living structures, and may not have occurred in traditional longhouse settlements where communal meals were the norm.

Although insects were most often consumed on days when fish and game were in short supply, some forms, such as *Rhynchophorus* larvae and alate ants, were valued as delicacies in their own right and eaten both as snacks and with meals. Less valued insects, such as ant and termite soldiers, were most often eaten with meals at which no other animal foods were available or permitted. In some cases the quantity of insects eaten at meals was very small, not more than 10 to 15 termite soldiers' heads, or a tablespoon of dry ground ants. In these quantities the insect material functioned as a condiment. It added diversity to the meal, and thereby increased the total food energy consumed. Wild nuts and seeds were often used in a similar way. This condiment function of insects is not trivial because dietary protein is only effectively used as protein when energy intake is adequate.

The diet records were kept only for individuals not subject to food restrictions, and so they do not account for the consumption of insects during such periods. Like other Tukanoans, the Tatuyo have an elaborate system of food restrictions which forms part of their medical system (see Langdon 1975 for detailed discussion). All animal and vegetable foods fit into at least one of a series of ranked categories. The highest ranked foods, the large fish and game animals, are considered potentially the most dangerous, and the first to be removed from the diet of adults in times of illness, certain life crises, or during ritual. In general insects are ranked lower than either fish or game. The most readily available insects, ant and termite soldiers, are among the lowest ranked foods, and were sometimes the only animal foods permitted in the diet. Diets limited to water, cassava starch, and termite soldiers were adhered to by adult males during male adolescent initiation rites for as long as two weeks, by menstruating females for a day or two at a time, and in some cases of illness.

SUMMARY AND CONCLUSIONS

Given the richness of invertebrate fauna in Amazonia (Penny and Arias 1982:222), it appears that Native Amazonians include a rather limited number of species in their diet. Those insects utilized can be characterized as being relatively large, nonpoisonous, and primarily softbodied, immature forms. In terms of their overall importance in the diet they can be divided into two broad categories. The species contributing most energy and protein are those which form large, highly predictable aggregations: *Rhynchophorus* larvae, ants of the genus *Atta,* termites of the genus *Syntermes,* and Noctuid and Saturniid caterpillars. These species were sought after and could be collected in considerable quantities in any one attempt. In the second group are species that are less predictable in space and time, and/or those that occurred in smaller aggregations: woodboring beetles and their larvae, wasp brood, and some caterpillars. These insects were collected opportunistically and usually in small quantities.

The composition of the insects consumed is similar to that of other animal foods. Although they are somewhat lower in crude protein and in protein quality, their amino acid composition is complementary to that of the dietary staple. Insects were frequently included in the diet and were often used to dampen fluctuations in the availability of fish and game. The dietary data presented here suggest that insects do make a significant contribution to dietary protein intake at certain times of the year.

Insects are ubiquitous in the Amazonian ecosystem and constitute a considerable portion of the animal biomass. Their inclusion in the diets of indigenous populations should not be regarded as a mere curiosity or their importance overlooked because of their small size. They are a source of energy, animal protein and fat, and can function to add diversity to the diet. Their dietary importance will no doubt vary from group to group, but the widespread practice of entomophagy warrants further attention in any evaluation of the availability of protein resources, or the adequacy of protein intake.

Notes

The Instituto de Ciencias Naturales in Bogotá under the direction of Polidoro Pinto E. provided valuable technical support during the field study. Proximate analyses of insects were provided through the kind cooperation of Franz Pardo T. of the Instituto Colombiano de Bienestar Familiar, Bogotá, and Gerardo Pérez Gómez, Departamento de Química, Universidad Nacional in cooperation with the Instituto Agropecario de Colombia, Bogotá. I am most grateful for their assistance.

For the identification of insect material I am indebted to Lloyd Knotson, Chairman, Insect Identification and Beneficial Insect Introduction Institute of the United States Department of Agriculture, and the following specialists in his division: D. M. Anderson (Coleoptera: Curculionidae, Cerambycidae, Passalidae); W. F. Barr, Cooperating Scientist (Coleoptera: Buprestidae); R. D. Gordon (Coleoptera: Passalidae, Scarabaeidae); A. S. Menke (Hymenoptera: Vespidae); D. A. Nickle (Isoptera); D. R. Smith (Hymenoptera: Formicidae); D. M. Weisman (Lepidoptera). I am also indebted to Gary Hevel of the Smithsonian Institution for his assistance with the termite material.

Grateful acknowledgment is made to the people of Yapú whose assistance made the fieldwork possible, to Paul N. Patmore for his assistance in the field, and to Michael Little for his continuing support and encouragement.

Financial support for the fieldwork in the Vaupés was provided by a dissertation fellowship from the Social Science Research Council, a grant from the National Science Foundation to M. A. Little (No. BSN 75-20169), and a postdoctoral fellowship from the Organization of American States.

1. A paper based on a preliminary analysis of some of the data presented here was read at the 48th Annual Meeting of the American Association of Physical Anthropology in San Francisco in April 1979.

2. Analyses of moisture, nitrogen, fat, ash, and crude fiber were carried out by the Instituto Colombiano de Bienestar Familiar (Coleoptera) and by the Intituto Colombiano Agropecuario (Hymenoptera and Isoptera). Both laboratories followed the standard methods of analysis of the AOAC (1950 edition of ICBF and 1965 edition at ICA) in the determination of nitrogen, fat, ash, crude fiber, and moisture. Crude protein was calculated as nitrogen times 6.25. Carbohydrate was determined by difference (100 minus the sum of water, protein, fat, ash, and crude fiber), and the energy content was calculated as 4 kcal per gram protein, 4 kcal per gram carbohydrate, and 9 kcal per gram fat. The moisture content of fresh samples was determined by drying to a constant weight in the field using traditional methods.

3. Assuming that an *Atta sexdens* nest contains some 5,000 queens on the day of the flight (Autouri 1950 cited in Weber 1972:53) and their average weight is 0.6 g each, a nest could contain 3,000 g of queens. A total yield of 1,200 to 2,000 g for 10 collectors is then roughly one-half to two-thirds of the total biomass of alates in the colony.

References

Association of Official Agricultural Chemists. (AOAC). 1950. Official and Tentative Methods of Analysis. 7th edition. Washington, D.C.

——. 1965 Official Methods of Analysis. 10th ed. Washington, D.C.

Araujo, R. L. 1970. Termites of the Neotropical Region. *In* Biology of Termites, Vol. II. K. Krishna and F. M. Weesner, eds. Pp. 527–576. New York: Academic Press.

Autouri, M. 1950. Número de Formas Aladas e Redução dos Sauveiros Iniciais. Contribução Para o Conhecimento da Saúva *(Atta spp)*, Vol. V. Arquivos do Instituto Biológico 19:325–331. São Paulo, Brazil.

Beckerman, S. 1977. The Use of Palms by the Barí Indians of the Maracaibo Basin. Principes 22(4):143–154.

——. 1979. The Abundance of Protein in Amazonia: A Reply to Gross. American Anthropologist 81:533–560.

Bodenheimer, F. S. 1951. Insects as Human Food. The Hague: Dr. W. Junk.

Chagnon, N. A., and R. B. Hames. 1979. Protein Deficiency and Tribal Warfare in Amazonia: New Data. Science 203:910–913.

Chapman, R. F. 1969. The Insects. New York: Elsevier.

Cornelius, C., G. Dandrifosse, and C. Jeuniaux. 1976. Chitinolytic Enzymes of the Gastric Mucosa of *Perodicticus potto* (Primate Prosimian): Purification and Enzyme Specificity. International Journal of Biochemistry 7:445–448.

Crowson, R. A. 1981. The Biology of the Coleoptera. New York: Academic Press.

Daly, H. V. 1985. Insect Morphometrics. Annual Review of Entomology 30:415–438.

Denevan, W. M. 1971. Campa Subsistence in the Gran Pajonal, Eastern Peru. Geographical Review 61(4): 496–518.

Dufour, D. L. 1983. Nutrition in the Northwest Amazon: Household Dietary Intake and Time-Energy Expenditure. *In* Adaptive Responses of Native Amazonians. R. B. Hames and W. T. Vickers, eds. Pp. 329–355. New York: Academic Press.

———. 1984. Diet of Tukanoan Indians in the Northwest Amazon. Paper presented at the 83rd Annual Meeting of the American Anthropological Association, Denver.

Elorduy de Conconi, J. R., and H. B. Rodríguez. 1977. Valor Nutritivo de Ciertos Insectos Comestibles de Mexico y Lista de Algunos Insectos Comestibles del Mundo. Anales del Instituto de Biología 48:165–186. Mexico City.

Food and Agricultural Organization of the United Nations (FAO). 1970. Amino Acid Content and Biological Data on Proteins. Rome: FAO.

Food and Agricultural Organization of the United Nations, World Health Organization, and United Nations University (FAO/WHO/UNU). 1983. Energy and Protein Requirements. FAO Nutrition Report No. XX. WHO Technical Report No. XXX. Rome and Geneva: FAO.

Fittkau, E. J., and H. Klinge. 1973. On Biomass and Trophic Structure of the Central Amazonian Rain Forest Ecosytem. Biotropica 5:1–14.

Gross, D. R. 1975. Protein Capture and Cultural Development in the Amazon Basin. American Anthropologist 77:526–549.

Harris, M. 1974. Cows, Pigs, War and Witches: The Riddle of Culture. New York: Random House.

Hugh-Jones, S. 1979. The Palm and The Pleiades: Initiation and Cosmology in Northwest Amazonia. London: Cambridge University Press.

Hurtado, A. M., et al. 1985. Female Subsistence Strategies Among Ache Hunter Gatherers of Eastern Paraguay. Human Ecology 13(1):1–28.

Jackson, J. E. 1983. The Fish People: Linguistic Exogamy and Tukanoan Identity in Northwest Amazonia. New York: Cambridge University Press.

Langdon, T. A. 1975. Food Restrictions in the Medical System of the Barasana and Taiwano Indians of the Colombian Northwest Amazon. Ph.D. dissertation, Anthropology Department, Tulane University.

Lizot, J. 1977. Population, Resources and Warfare among the Yanomami. Man (n.s.) 12:497–517.

Milton, K. 1984. Protein and Carbohydrate Resources of the Maku Indians in Northwestern Amazonia. American Anthropologist 86(1):7–27.

Penny, N.D., and J. R. Arias. 1982. Insects of an Amazon Forest. New York: Columbia University Press.

Redford, K. H., and J. D. Dorea. 1984. The Nutritional Value of Invertebrates with Emphasis on Ants and Termites as Food for Animals. Journal of Zoology 203:385–395.

Ross, E. B. 1978. Food Taboos, Diet and Hunting Strategies: The Adaptation to Animals in Amazon Cultural Ecology. Current Anthropology 9:1–36.

Ruddle, K. 1973. The Human Use of Insects: Examples from the Yukpa. Biotropica 5(2):94–101.

Smole, W. 1976. The Yanomama Indians: A Cultural Geography. Austin: University of Texas Press.

Taylor, R. L. 1975. Butterflies in My Stomach. Santa Barbara: Woodbridge Press.

Wallace, A. R. 1853. On the Insects Used for Food by Indians of the Amazon. Transactions of the Royal Entomological Society of London (n.s.) 2:241–244.

Weber, N. A. 1972. Gardening Ants: The Attines. Memoirs of the American Philosophical Society, Vol. 92.

Wu Lueng, W. T., F. Busson, and C. Jardin. 1968. Food Composition Tables for Use in Africa. Bethesda: U.S. Department of Health, Education and Welfare; Health Services and Mental Health Administration; U.S. National Center for Chronic Disease Control, Nutrition Program.

UNIT V

Explaining Foodways #2: Ideology, Symbolism, and Social Power

The title to this section contains three constructs that are fundamental to anthropological research and theory in general and are central in much of the work in nutritional anthropology—*ideology, symbolism, and social power*. In our usage, as in anthropology generally, ideology is used more broadly than is typical in colloquial speech. It includes the set of explicit beliefs and values that are articulated by self-defined religious, social, and political groups, but it goes beyond that to include the full spectrum of the "ideational" or "cultural" component of the "ecological model of food and nutrition" we outlined in the first chapter. In this usage "ideology" encompasses a broad spectrum of human activities and experiences related to food.

The construct of "symbolism" is closely related to the broader construct of "ideology," but calls special attention to a particular ideological feature—namely that the object is "something that stands for or suggests something else by reason of relationship, association, convention, or accidental resemblance" (Merriam Webster Dictionary). Used in connection with food, it highlights the idea that food is not just something that tastes good or tastes bad or contains nutrients, but carries other "meanings" that go beyond its simple, outward characteristics. The construct of "social power" refers to the multiple ways in which individuals and groups of individuals exert authority over other individuals and groups, not necessarily through direct force or threat of force but by controlling access to resources, autonomy and so forth.

Food is "good to think." Food reflects identity and who we are: gender, age, social class, political persuasion, and personal style. Every social group sets limits on what constitutes food and how foods should be obtained, prepared, served, and consumed. In every culture, there are items that are edible but are not defined as food. For example, in the United States, dogs and horses are pets, and most of us would never consider consuming them, but in Europe horse meat is perfectly acceptable, and in some parts of Asia, dogs are specially bred for the table. Non-vegetarian

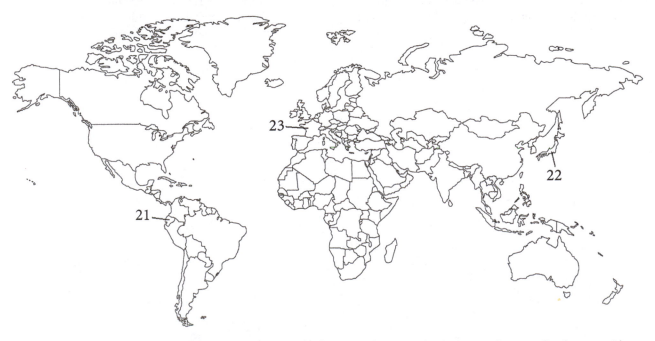

Figure 1 *Map shows the location of the groups referred to in the chapters in this section by chapter number: 21 = Zumbagua parish, highland Ecuador; 22 = Tokyo, Japan; 23 = France.*

Americans consume pigs and cows with relish, whereas the idea is abhorrent in other parts of the world. Under famine conditions, what is usually defined as nonfood may be consumed.

A useful distinction can be made between the "substance" of food—its chemical constituents—and the "circumstance" of food (Farb and Armelagos 1980). The circumstances are the social and ecological contexts in which food is embedded. For example, consider the difference between baking a cake for a friend or buying the same kind of cake at a bakery. For some people the difference (the circumstance) would be symbolically important, but for others it wouldn't matter. The different ways in which people choose to structure the menu for a celebrational dinner party could result in identical nutritional composition (substance) achieved through very different "circumstance."

Consider the many dimensions of ideational, symbolic, and social power aspects of food. Here are just a few examples:

- In North America beef was generally considered a high-status food, often associated with manliness, an association that may hark back to the rugged image of the cowboy and cattleman. Slowly, however, the widespread availability of inexpensive hamburgers and information on the relationship between red meat consumption and adult diseases has tainted beef's image. For some, beef is now symbolic of ecological destruction and personal pollution.
- Specific foods carry heavy symbolic value associated with rituals and special events. In the United States, turkey is the main dish of the Thanksgiving Day meal, and white cake is a symbol of marriage. In China, noodles symbolize longevity and are eaten on festive occasions where people want to invoke good luck.
- Food preparation techniques reflect cultural traditions, but are increasingly becoming internationalized. A few decades ago sushi was almost unknown outside of Japan or Japanese enclaves, and many people regarded consumption of raw fish negatively. Now sushi has become cosmopolitan. What will be the "in" food preparation techniques in the next 20 years?
- In most societies, a "meal" typically includes a staple food. In much of Asia, an eating event isn't a meal unless it has rice. In the United States, some individuals still feel uncomfortable with a "meal" that does not include meat, but this is decreasing. With increasing globalization, what will happen to the importance of staple foods as a defining feature of a "meal"?
- Eating etiquette is highly structured and differs from one culture to another. Eating from another's plate is accepted in many societies, whereas in ours it would be considered very poor manners. In

many societies, the male head of the household is fed first; in others this would be considered a social breach.

What are the cultural rules that define food and proper eating behaviors? Where do these rules come from, and how do they change? How universal are rules and the processes by which rules are formed? Are some of these rules meant to be resisted and broken?

Since the inception of the discipline, anthropologists have always been interested in the ideologic, symbolic, and social power aspects of food, but in ethnographic research, these topics were less salient than some other domains of ideological and symbolic activity, such as religion. However, in recent decades there has been a veritable explosion in academic research on the ideologic, symbolic, and social power aspects of food. This has occurred not just in anthropology, but in many other academic disciplines. So great is this expanding interest that many books on these topics have been produced, together with a vast number of journal articles. Consequently, trying to narrow down the choice of papers for this reader that exemplify this expansive and exciting research area was very difficult. We gave up on the idea of selecting representative papers and decided, instead, to include papers we found to be personally interesting and illustrated different approaches. We encourage readers who are interested in these subjects to continue their explorations, including looking for collections and series that are being produced by scholars in many fields.

In "The Children Cry for Bread: Hegemony and the Transformation of Consumption," Mary J. Weismantel discusses the symbolic importance of the substitution of wheat bread for barley gruel in the morning meal of indigenous families in the Ecuadorian highlands. This simple substitution is an example of "delocalization" (see chapter 38 by Pelto and Pelto for a definition and discussion of this process). In Zumbagua it is a major source of tension within families and between generations, as Weismantel demonstrates.

In the parish of Zumbagua, the morning meal is called *café*. The preparation of this meal starts with boiled water, to which is added spoonfuls of *machica*, finely ground and toasted barley meal. In recent years children have begun to ask for bread, a luxury store-bought item, instead of *machica*. Weismantel points out that in *"crying for bread,"* the children are asking for a food purchased in the market by their father, while simultaneously rejecting the home grown and processed food provided by their mother.

Beyond the symbolic expression of psychological relationships within the family, the distinction between dry bread and wet barley also represents a symbolic reflection of the indigenous social history. Bread, in contrast to barley, conjures up images of conquest, economic exploitation, and racism, while, at the same time reflecting the lure of cities, modern life, and non-indigenous culture.

Identity is also a main theme of Anne Allison's chapter, "Japanese Mothers and *Obentōs*." *Obentōs* are boxed lunches, which are prepared, in this case, for nursery school children by their mothers. They typically consist of a variety of small, individually wrapped foods, which are placed in the lunch box. There is pervasive social pressure on mothers to prepare appealing and nutritious *obentōs*, and on children to eat them quickly. Magazines and other media sources provide women with a continuous flow of information about how to prepare an *obentōs* that will be enjoyed and quickly consumed.

This chapter illustrates the methodological approach known as participant-observation as well as the application of symbolic theory in nutritional anthropology. Allison is a cultural anthropologist who lived in Japan and sent her son to nursery school there. Her study focuses on an analysis of symbolism and social power. She argues that the social pressure on mothers to prepare appealing boxed lunches reflects larger issues of mothers' roles and social position within the society. In particular the judgment that if something goes wrong the mother is to blame (in this case a child's rejection or partial rejection of the food in his or her lunch) is a symbolic means of reinforcing women's social position, regardless of whether they are also involved in income-earning work. At the same time, because of its large symbolic load, the bento box can become a vehicle for expressing an alternative view, as is illustrated by the comments that Allison shares with us from her friend Sawa.

In "Techne versus Technoscience: Divergent (and Ambiguous) Notions of Food 'Quality' in the French Debate over GM Crops," Chaia Heller explores the cultural meaning of food quality in France. As an anthropologist, Heller works with different groups within French society, including peasant farmers and scientists, in an attempt to understand their logics and divergent ideas about food quality. She suggests that what counts for quality food depends on the cultural location of the individual assessing a particular food in question.

Some in this story define food quality in terms of technoscience. For these actors, quality food is that which can be proved scientifically to be healthy to consumers. Others define food quality in terms of techne, or by the technique used in producing the food. Food quality in this case would be determined by the extent to which a food stuff has been produced by small-scale farmers in an artisanal fashion. In this way, a McDonald's hamburger is considered quality by an agent in the agro-foods industry or in a government food body. Once the burger is determined to be scientifically free of potential allergens, bacteria, or other contaminating matter, it is allowed to be called a quality food. Yet others, looking at a McDonald's hamburger through the lens of techne, rank the burger as poor in food quality. The technique would be seen as industrialized, large-scale, and lacking in cultural taste.

Heller looks closely at the French debate over genetically modified organisms (GMOs) that found their way into the French food chain beginning in 1997. In particular, she examines the ways in which a union of small family farmers, La Confederation Paysanne, asserts itself as a cultural expert on food quality. By rejecting GMO-based foods as

emerging from an industrial food system lacking "culture" and "taste," union farmers appeal to French consumers to join their cause in rejecting GMO foods. Yet as Heller illustrates, the union's attempt to define just what quality means often results in an ambiguous definition that eludes both consumers and scientists. In the French GMO controversy, we see a collision between various framings of food quality. Actors on both sides of the issue do their best to establish themselves as having the knowledge and authority in regards to food to declare GMOs as quality food or not.

In summary, the papers in this section are intended to illustrate some of the many dimensions of symbolic aspects of food. The primary focus is on the subtle and not so subtle aspects of the exercise of social power within the context of food symbolism. The exercise of symbolic power can be observed at multiple levels from the household and the community (Weismantel and Allison) to national and even international levels of discourse (Heller). What are the ways that it is expressed in your own families, communities and in your larger society?

SUGGESTIONS FOR THINKING AND DOING NUTRITIONAL ANTHROPOLOGY

The symbol aspects of food offer rich opportunities for thinking and doing nutritional anthropology.

1. In nearly all cultures, holidays are an important opportunity to express symbolic aspects of food. With your classmates, make a list of the main holidays that are celebrated in your community. Next, go out and interview five people about what foods (and menus) they use to celebrate each of the holidays. Now compare the results, first for your own interviews, then pooling the results with those of your classmates. What patterns do you see? You may find that some holidays are quite rigid with respect to the specific foods that are part of its symbolic expression and others are more flexible. What factors might help to explain that feature (of symbolic flexibility versus rigidity)?

2. The primary strategy of food advertising is to link specific products symbolically with other social values. One of the ways in ways in which you can readily observe contrasting social values (at least as perceived by the people who design advertising) is to compare the types of symbolism that are used in food ads that are directed to different types of audiences. To conduct this analysis, get several issues of different types of the following magazines: sports magazines, house-keeping/home management magazines, fashion magazines, and general interest magazines. Look through the issues to find all of the ads that relate to food and food products. For each ad, write down the values the ad is appeal-

ing to and the types of words and visuals that are used to capture the value. For example, an ad may appeal to "strength" and the picture may show barbells or a strong-looking bird in flight. Next, list all the different types of symbols you've discovered. Finally, look to see whether some symbols predominate in different types of magazines. This is another exercise that is even more interesting when you compare and pool your findings with those of classmates.

3. The concept of "comfort food" has become a part of our culture, and that phrase is now widely used in everyday speech. There are even cookbooks with "comfort food" in the title. But the specific foods that individuals consider to be "comfort foods" are highly variable from one individual to another. Explore the meaning of this cultural concept. Start by making a list of your own "comfort foods." Do you know why you regard them this way? Now find out about other people's comfort foods. Be sure to interview people of different generations, not only your own parents and grandparents, but others who come from different social and ethnic backgrounds. Can people tell you why the foods they list are comfort foods for them? What principles about food symbolism are revealed by an investigation of comfort foods?

4. To continue your exploration of symbolic aspects of foods, do a self-analysis of all of the different ways in which symbolism enters your life in relation to food. Are there foods that you give to others because they carry some special symbolic meaning? Are there foods that connect you with your ethnic background? Are there foods that you eat to rebel against authority? Remember the foods from your "comfort food analysis." How large a list can you generate of the different ways in which foods take on symbolic meaning in your life?

5. Think about the importance of food in your own life and in the lives of your friends, families, and acquaintances, apart from its role in providing nutrition and preventing you from being and feeling hungry. Make a list of all the different aspects of food symbolism that you can identify in your own life and in your social circles. How many different types of symbolic expressions were you able to identify?

Suggested Further Reading

Counihan C, Van Esterik P. 2008. Food and Culture: A Reader. Second Edition. New York: Routledge.

Douglas M, ed. 1984. Food in the Social Order: Studies of Food and Festivities in Three American Communities. New York: Russell Sage Foundation.

Anderson EN. 2005. Everyone Eats: Understanding Food and Culture. New York: NYU Press.

Goody J. 1982. Cooking, Cuisine and Class: A Study in Comparative Sociology. New York: Cambridge University Press.

Farb P, Armelagos G. 1980. Consuming Passions: The Anthropology of Eating. Boston: Houghton Mifflin.

CHAPTER 21

The Children Cry for Bread: Hegemony and the Transformation of Consumption

Mary J. Weismantel

(1989)

In this, I discuss the substitution of wheat bread for barley gruel in the early morning meal in Zumbagua, an indigenous parish of highland Ecuador. While at the macroscopic level such changes in consumption may appear to be part of an inevitable, unilinear progression from subsistence to market systems, they are experienced by households actually undergoing them as a contradictory and conflict-filled process in which ideological and cultural issues play an important part. Wheat bread for barley gruel in the early morning seems like an insignificant change, the substitution of one carbohydrate for another, but because bread enters the indigenous kitchen as part of a complex of cultural, ideological and social transformations, its significance can be greater than the effects on family nutrition or the household budget would suggest. In indigenous Andean communities today, there is a symbolic association of leavened white bread with the dominant culture; this association has historical and material aspects that relate it to general transformations in the political economy at a regional level.

Not only does purchase of breads by indigenous peasants raise social and ideological questions, but close study of this phenomenon highlights issues within the realm of economic analysis as well. As I hope to show, use of the household as an analytical unit of consumption and production can disguise very real differences between household members as economic actors. In Zumbagua, the household as a whole is involved in a combination of subsistence, commercial and wage labor activities, but the involvement of individuals in these spheres of activity is determined by their age and gender. Conflicts of interest between household members are frequently exposed and exacerbated by everyday consumption issues such as dietary innovations. These conflicts of interest between household members in turn reveal the contradictory pressures and forces at work in the nation as a whole.

Zumbagua is a rural parish of the province of Cotopaxi, in the western cordillera of the Andes. The parish today is relatively isolated and unimportant politically and economically, but this was not always the case. Zumbagua first entered the historical record as an Augustinian hacienda during the colonial period, at which time it was an important and lucrative landholding, where enormous flocks of sheep produced wool for the textile workshops of the intermontane valley. In the republican era, these Church-owned lands were taken over by the state, which used proceeds from the hacienda to fund social services in urban areas. Thus production within the parish has for several centuries been directed by national-level organizations that channelled profits from the zone into investments in the urban economy.

Because the hacienda of Zumbagua belonged to the state, it is one of the few highland areas which was directly and radically affected by the national agrarian reform law enacted in 1964. In the mid-1960s, the hacienda was dissolved and title to the land distributed among parish residents. Inequalities in land distribution quickly developed, with white[1] hacienda employees establishing themselves as an economic and social elite. However, some indigenous families have succeeded in challenging white control, although many then take on the trappings of ethnic whiteness themselves, and simply reproduce the existing system of exploitation once they attain elite status. Ethnic whiteness in Zumbagua, as in much of the Andes, is largely inseparable from integration into the cash economy. Storekeepers, busdrivers and schoolteachers are "white," even if the individuals who presently hold these jobs were "Indians" ten years ago.

At the present, most of Zumbagua's residents are both much poorer and much more ethnically indigenous in language, dress and custom than is common in Ecuador today. The population lives in widely dispersed rural households scattered over the parish's 10,000 hectares. Most of the parish is of an unusually high altitude for Ecuador, ranging from 3500–4000 meters in elevation, well above the upper limits of maize cultivation at that latitude. Residents of the parish utilize several production zones, the most important being high valley lands, used for barley, fava bean and potato cultivation, and the still higher paramo grasslands, used for

Mary J. Weismantel, "The children cry for bread: hegemony and the transformation of consumption." In *The social economy of consumption*. Monographs in Economic Anthropology, No. 6, B. Orlove and J.J. Rutz, eds. 1989. University Press of America, pp. 85–99. Reprinted with permission.

sheep and llama pastoralism and as a source of grass fuel. But although the people of Zumbagua have a strong emotional commitment to farming, it is in fact impossible for households to support themselves purely through agriculture and pastoralism. Every household is also involved in a variety of other activities, which in fact tie them to the national economy to a far greater degree than is immediately apparent. One important strategy is to send some males outside the parish as temporary wage laborers. Older workers typically find employment in small sugarcane fields and mills located in the lowlands immediately to the west of the parish, but younger men tend to go to the capital city of Quito to find work, usually in construction.

The rapid change in the relations of production of the parish in the last several decades has had a profound effect on social relations at the household level. The biggest schism is between young adults, who have come of age since the dissolution of the hacienda, and an older generation who lived under the hacienda system. The problems revealed by the issue of bread and gruel, however, do not highlight this generation gap, but rather bring to light divisions within younger families.

The proletarianization of males is creating a gender gap among young adults, which does not exist in the older generation. Males typically begin work in Quito between the ages of ten and fourteen, so that by the time a man marries at the age of twenty he has had a very different socialization than his bride. He is at home in an urban environment, speaks Spanish, listens to the radio, knows something of national sports and politics, music and slang. She, in contrast, has rarely if ever left the parish, speaks only Quichua, wears indigenous clothing, and knows the mythology, songs and elaborate Quichua riddle games of indigenous culture. She is a subsistence farmer and pastoralist, having taken over almost all the agricultural duties of the farmstead, while he is a wage laborer. Since Andean marriage does not entail a merging of financial assets and earnings, there is frequently an economic disparity between the two as well: he has money and she does not.

There is also a generation gap within these young families, between parents and children. Unlike their parents, many Zumbagua children today go to school. The children thus are becoming acculturated to national Ecuadorian society: schoolchildren understand Quichua but hardly speak it, and spend their time tearing photographs of cars, airplanes and motorcycles out of any scrap of Spanish-language magazines they can lay their hands on. The lessons they learn in the classroom, which include the rule that white, urban and professional is good and Indian, rural and peasant is bad, hardly encourage them to learn farming from their mothers and grandparents. Although their labor is very important to the family farm, most children do not look to farming as their future, regardless of whether they attend school or not.

In the above description, I have presented the roles of male and female, adult and child as fixed and predictable. In fact, however, although these descriptions are not inaccurate, they not only gloss over individual variation but also fail to reveal the conflicting attitudes individuals often feel towards the social and productive roles they play. There are few individuals, of any age or sex, who do not feel the attraction of both agricultural and proletarian lifeways, and fewer still who have not cursed the inadequate livelihood provided by both economic strategies. The fact that men who work in Quito have had to adopt more "white" cultural traits than their wives does not necessarily mean that they value "whiteness" more. The glamor of urban life and purchased goods can appeal more to women, for whom they represent an exotic and unknown world, than for their husbands, who frequently characterize the time they spend in the city as a painful exile from indigenous life.

In hacienda days, ethnic identity and productive role were determined for the people of Zumbagua by forces beyond their control. Exploitation of this work force by the national economy was then made possible by a rigid caste system in which distinctive customs preserved social boundaries. Today a new political economy prevails, and national ideologies call for the rapid assimilation of indigenous peoples. But the issue of whether such assimilation is in fact desirable is one on which the parish itself remains divided.

In Zumbagua, where ethnicity is largely a matter of socially recognized markers such as language, dress and custom, consumption choices become a major arena in which individuals and groups establish their ethnic identity. Consumption decisions thus involve a complex of issues beyond financial capacity and individual psychology. In the parish today, issues which are ultimately of a political and ideological nature, such as choices in productive strategy and cultural identity, are being argued not so much through overt debate, speechmaking and confrontations in the political arena of the parish, but rather through everyday consumption decisions being made at the household level. The pressure to assimilate does not remain at the level of abstract ideology, but pervades the textures of everyday life.

The people of Zumbagua are constantly bombarded from within and without by images of their cultural practices as being backwards and wrong. The imposition of these labels of inadequacy is part of a political and economic process which is hegemonic in nature. The erosion of the subsistence economy is inevitably occurring, an overdetermined process in which ecological degradation, overpopulation, and drastic changes in the national economy have all played a part. But the erosion of people's faith in the validity of the food and clothing, language and celebrations they grew up with is also the product of a multiplicity of forces. In an isolated rural area like Zumbagua, this message filters through in small ways, but the pressure is unrelenting. I refer to it as hegemonic because, to quote Raymond Williams, the imposition of a political order is hegemonic when it is not…"expressed in directly political forms…by direct or effective coercion…" but rather through "…a complex interlocking of political forms, and active social and cultural forms.… What is decisive is not only the conscious system of ideas and beliefs but the whole lived social process as practically organized by specific and dominant meanings and values" (Raymond Williams 1977:108–109).

The transformation of indigenous practice occurs not only when the schoolchild is taught to salute the Ecuadorian flag, but also when his mother hesitates over what foods to serve her family, fearful that there is something inadequate in a meal of homegrown foods unembellished by purchased foodstuffs or condiments. Even women who have little interaction with white outsiders, separated from them by the language barrier, learn the lessons of cultural and social inferiority. Children so young that they have scarcely ever left the farmstead have already begun to learn them too. These messages of inferiority color private consumption rituals within the household, as well as more public actions.

FOOD AND IDENTITY

My research in Zumbagua was directed towards uncovering the semiotic system that underlies the cooking of foods, a system that I refer to as cuisine. This study necessitated analysis of the relationship of Zumbagua ways of cooking to those of other Ecuadorians, the semiotic systems of people who, for the most part, are richer and whiter than those who live in the parish. For heuristic purposes, it would be possible to study Zumbagua cuisine in isolation from other cuisines that surround it, but the parish has never existed in such isolation. The cuisine of the parish has evolved as a system which, like its people, exists in a certain ethnic and class relation to other cuisines.

The people of Zumbagua are poor, rural, indigenous, and they live in the Sierra. In addition, they live above the zone of maize cultivation. All of these facts about them are reflected in their cuisine; in fact, as I discuss below, at times one food, *machica*, symbolizes all of these facts within its fan (Turner 1967) of referential meanings. Not only the diet of Zumbagua but its cuisine differs from that of the nation as a whole. Zumbagua people eat "Indian" foods in "Indian" ways: not only elements and techniques but the very syntagmatic chains by which they are combined into meals are not the same as even the stereotypical highland Ecuadorian cuisine. This difference is significant: it signifies not simply a particular way of life but one which is stigmatized.

Perhaps the quintessential *plato tipico* or traditional dish in Ecuador is the kind of dish referred to as a *seco*. In the typical *seco*, the plate holds a piece of meat (beef, chicken, goat) cooked using one of a rather limited repertoire of techniques, condiments and vegetables. At the side are perhaps some fried potatoes and another vegetable, or a relish of marinated, finely sliced onions and tomatoes with lemon and *cilantro*. The dominant element on the plate, however, is the large, unseasoned pile of white rice.

In the full midday meal or *almuerzo*, the *seco* is flanked by a preceding soup and terminal sweet *colada*, dishes that evoke a meal structure descended from pre-Hispanic patterns. But as *caldo de pata* and other Ecuadorian soups are increasingly replaced by imports like canned cream of mushroom soup, and fruit *coladas* by a soft drink or a dish of canned peaches, the earlier heritage becomes less visible even though the sequence of courses still bears its mark. The sequence of meals also continues to resist North American influences: the light, continental-style morning *cafe* is followed by the main meal, the heavy, multi-course *almuerzo* in the early afternoon, and a light meal in the evening.

To wealthy Ecuadorians whose repertoire of foods includes European and North American dishes, the *seco* and the *colada* are nostalgic reminders of the past. For most Ecuadorians, however, these dishes remain standard everyday fare. For the well-to-do, *platos tipicos* such as *seco* remain important because they symbolize the country's heritage. Unlike pizzas or sandwiches made of Wonder Bread, American cheese and bologna (*pan de miga, queso americano y pastel mexicano*), the glamorous fast foods, processed foods and snack foods that are modish among the young and the nouveaux riches, students and professional classes, *platos tipicos* are substantial, solid: bland and starchy, they reach their full flower in the traditional *almuerzo*, the heavy midday meal at which the entire family gathers. *Platos tipicos* stand for the strength of the family, that primary virtue of traditional Ecuadorian society. The ideological importance of *platos tipicos* for Ecuador is problematic, however, in a way which characterizes an Ecuadorian dilemma in seeking an autonomous identity through emphasizing the nation's heritage. For *platos tipicos* carry other messages besides "family" and "nation." They also stand for the poor, the ignorant, and the non-white: people with whom the elite, for the most part, do not wish to identify.

This opposition between the full *almuerzo* and the fast-food snack, though real, obscures a more complex hierarchy of cuisines. Shrimps *ceviches* and tropical fruits like the *grenadilla* and *chirimoya* certainly stand on the Ecuadorian side of the two rival American cuisines, North American and national, found in Quito today. But although "Ecuadorian cuisine" appears as a unified entity when opposed to sandwiches or pizzas, Ecuador in fact contains many cuisines. For example, the long-standing rivalry between highlands and coast is symbolized by potatoes vs. rice, by *locros* (stews) vs. *secos* (dry meals), by blandness vs. spiciness. This is true even though the *seco* made with rice is found throughout Ecuador, including the highlands. The *seco* dominates Ecuadorian cuisine; this dominance reflects a certain historical relationship between coast and sierra.

The *seco* also evokes the provinces rather than the capital city. In small towns and even provincial capitals, the restaurants all serve the same fare: *churrascos* and *apanados, pollo dorado, seco de chivo* (all of which are types of *secos*) appear on every menu and all are assembled on the plate in the same way. But while for Quitenos such dishes signify provincialism and a native heritage being left behind by the modern world, to the people of Zumbagua the same menu represents that outside, urban, modern world from which they feel disenfranchised.

In Zumbagua cuisine, like that of white Sierrans, there are two basic categories of dishes, *sopas* and *secos*. But in contrast to the white *almuerzo*, where *sopa* and *colada* flank a central, validating *seco*, in Zumbagua the *sopa* has a clear predominance.[2] The role of the *sopa* in Zumbagua cuisine is similar to that which Mary Douglas describes when she speaks of the power of the familiar dish to arouse in people "the flash of recognition and confidence which welcomes an ordered pattern" (Mary Douglas 1971:80). There is no doubt that the presence of the *sopa* validates most Zumbagua meals. It is the most important and most typical syntagm (dish/meal) of Zumbagua cuisine. Generally speaking, most main meals eaten in the parish consist of *sopas*. Each person sharing the meal is expected to eat at least two bowls full of soup, and more is always offered. The heavy starch content makes it a very filling meal.

The basis of these meals is boiled water. The word for "to cook," *yanuna*, itself means "to boil." Boiling is absolutely central to Zumbagua cooking practice. The essential wetness of Zumbagua dishes, which are served in bowls and eaten with spoons, contrasts sharply with the *seco*; the word *seco* itself means dry, highlighting its opposition to the water-based *sopa*. There is a strong disinclination in Zumbagua against eating any foods during a meal that have not first been immersed in hot water. Raw or dry foods are snacks meant to be eaten away from home or between mealtimes; they should not be eaten during a meal.

Beyond this underlying process of boiling in water, it is hard to write a minimal definition of a *sopa*. Unlike most peasant cuisines, everyday meals in Zumbagua may be based on any one of a variety of starches; no single complex carbohydrate predominates. It is the manner of cooking, the "ordered pattern" used, that characterizes the Zumbagua *almuirsu* (cf. Mintz 1985: 8–9).

Sopas can be divided into two basic categories, *colada* and *caldo*. The first are thick, the latter clear soups. (This distinction is not absent from our own cuisine, although it is not clearly distinguished linguistically. Cream soups, bisques, chowders and bean soups are *coladas*; consommes, broths, noodle and vegetable soups are *caldos*.) Note that potatoes, while important, do not play the role of fundamental thickener in *coladas*. While North American cuisine frequently uses potatoes as the thickening agent for a *colada*-style soup, in Zumbagua potatoes are never allowed to cook long enough to disintegrate in this fashion.[3] Other starches are used as the base of *coladas*, potatoes never. They are present in both *caldo* and *colada*, but are the validator for neither. A *colada* is validated by its thickening starch food, a *caldo* by its broth.

Whereas a *colada* must have a flour or meal of some sort used to thicken it, *caldos* may be without any starch. It is possible to make a meat broth for the sick which contains no starches at all, or only potatoes. Sick people frequently decide that they have no stomach for one or another starch, aversions which are always heeded; the extremely ill may only be able to eat pure broths. These clear broths in fact represent the quintessential *caldo*. However, neither meat broth nor its substitute, small amounts of purchased processed vegetable fat dissolved in boiling water, need to be present to make *caldo*. Hot water, noodles and salt make a perfectly acceptable *caldo*, one which cash-poor people consider somewhat desirable.

Overall, *coladas* are more common than *caldos* in everyday cuisine. A good, substantial *sopa*, the kind of meal an average family eats on a regular basis, consists of hot water thickened with home-ground barley or purchased wheat flour, cooked with a spoonful of fat, some salt, and three to five chopped onions. On most but not all days, a *sopa* also contains some extras: pieces of mutton, perhaps, or cabbage. A *sopa* should always contain enough potatoes so that each bowl served contains several, although in many households it often does not.

If potatoes are beyond many household's budget today, rice, the staple element of small-town "white" cuisine, is a rarely eaten treat. Like the sophisticated Ecuadorian confronted with emblems of popular culture from the U.S., the people of Zumbagua view dishes such as the rice-based *seco* with both hatred and desire.

Secos contrast with everyday meals in Zumbagua not only in ingredients and in their non-soup nature but in other ways as well. These include aesthetic principles about color, texture, temperature, and consistency. In the parish, it is held that to be appealing food should be liquid, thick, uniform, and barely lukewarm. This is an ideal which women strive for in their cooking. The contrast between this ideal and the norms found in "white" cuisine is clearest in the *almuerzo*, the largest and most important meal of the day, but it can be found in the lighter meals eaten in peasant households before dawn and after dusk as well.[4]

BREAD AND HEGEMONY

Throughout Ecuador, the early-morning meal is referred to as *cafe*. For most "white" Ecuadorians, *cafe* consists of a cup of hot water, served with a saucer and a spoon, into which the individual consumer mixes instant coffee and sugar. It is served with two bread rolls. This meal is familiar to indigenous residents of the parish, since it is served in the early morning in restaurants and market stalls in the "white" towns Zumbagua people frequent. In most households within Zumbagua, however, the early morning meal takes quite a different form. Although still called *cafe*, it does not contain any coffee at all. The main component is *machica*, finely ground toasted barley meal. This *cafe*, like the "white" one, involves the serving of hot water, but there are no cups or saucers in evidence. Like most other meals in Zumbagua, this one is served in deep enamel bowls.

Water is heated to boiling, and sugar is dissolved into the water. Each person is handed a bowl of this sugar-water along with a spoon. At the same time, a container filled with *machica* is placed on the ground within everyone's reach, and everyone is invited to have some: *chapuvay, chapuilla,* "go ahead and mix yourself some." There is some range in personal tastes, but most people put about an equal amount of *machica* to sugar water in their bowl. This is frequently done gradually, with leisurely actions interspersed with morning conversations. At first the hot sweet water is sipped, then bit by bit spoonfuls of *machica* are added, producing a warm sweet gruel. Sometimes a cooked gruel of sweetened, coarsely ground barley (*arroz de cebada*) is served instead of water and *machica*.

Although most households consider *machica* an absolute necessity, a substance one simply cannot live without, an alternative construction of *cafe*, familiar to everyone, substitutes bread for *machica*. Despite being a quite different form of a starch food than *machica*, in the actual consumption bread, a "dry" food which does not require immersion in water, becomes somewhat similar to other indigenous starches: as people drink spoonfuls of coffee, they break the breads into pieces and mash them into the cup, producing a sweet soupy mass not unlike a gruel.

This act of making "white" breads similar to "indigenous" gruels in the actual consumption does not negate the implied threat to indigenous identity that eating bread in the early morning contains. This threat is especially felt because of the intimate, familiar nature of *cafe*, a meal which is only shared by household members. There is a tendency in Zumbagua for special-occasion meals to be served and eaten according to rules borrowed from white cuisine, and some indigenous households self-consciously try to model even their everyday eating habits according to white forms, behavior which quickly earns them the criticism of their neighbors. But controversy over whether to adopt white forms for everyday use, such as eating *cafe* according to the white pattern where carbohydrates are eaten as dry breads, also exists within households.

Many of the early morning quarrels I witnessed in Zumbagua homes erupted over the question of bread. This conflict arises between young children and their parents. Pre-school children, especially, demand bread as their right, and refuse to accept *mishqui*, sweet gruels, or *machica* in its place. Refusal is difficult for parents, since young children, especially the youngest child, are commonly indulged a great deal. Quichua-speaking mothers mimic their children's Spanish cries for bread: "Sulu tandata munan pan, pan, pan, 'nin. Sulu wakan." They only want bread [*tanda*, Q.]. "Bread, bread, bread" they say [*pan*, Sp.]. They just cry.

In current practice, bread is definitely a member of the *wanlla* set of foods, which also includes bananas, oranges and other fruits, hard candies and cookies. It is a snack food, and is frequently given as a gift. As such, bread is a necessity in certain circumstances: it is included among the offerings to the dead on *Finados*,[5] the gifts exchanged during marriage negotiations or when asking someone to be a godparent, or as part of the redistributive flow surrounding fiesta sponsorship. Unless they are very poor, most families also buy some bread on Saturday as a treat for the children and for gift-giving in the web of *wanlla* presentations. Some of this bread is stored in the kitchen for any special occasions that might arise during the week. Many battles of will take place as mothers struggle to dole out the breads bought on Saturday as special treats, while the children demand them as daily fare. Fathers who witness these scenes seem to feel

shame at their own inadequacy, their inability to fill their children's hands with bread. They may react with anger towards the child for his unreasonable demand, or towards the mother for denying the request. Often men shout that they will buy more tomorrow, as though resenting the implication that they in fact cannot.

What seems to be taking place is a struggle on the children's part to redefine what had been a treat (*wanlla*), a luxury good which most families can afford to buy but not for every day, into a staple, a necessary part of the morning meal. This is the process which Mintz describes as intrinsic to the needs of capitalism: demand must be created, new foods must be "...transformed into the ritual of daily necessity and even into images of daily decency" (Mintz 1979:65). The children desire bread as the validation of a meal, that which seals it and marks it as satisfactory. They are pushing to redefine the role of bread in the domestic economy, not as a snack or treat but as something without which a meal would be incomplete. This redefinition implies an enlargement of the role of purchased foods in the household economy, and a preference for masculine over feminine contributions to consumption.

The change being suggested here is not the introduction of a new food into Zumbagua. Bread is already well established as a *wanlla* food, a snack or luxury food which nonetheless is a necessity in certain social interchanges. The substitution being urged by the children simply implies a change in the particular role played by bread. The significance of this change becomes clearer if we examine the meanings surrounding bread and those surrounding *machica*, the food which bread may supplant. Although other starches are important in the diet, barley, and especially *machica*, is a kind of core cultural symbol for Zumbagua. It is referred to by terms such as *bien calienticu*, food that warms you up when you eat it or *abrigaditu*, warm and comforting; people say that it is as filling as meat (although they don't mean this literally, but are using the comparison to highlight *machica*'s positive attributes). Those who have listened to the public health nurses' lectures on nutrition use the phrase *Buena alimentacion* to describe its goodness, while others simply insist that it is *alli alli mikuna* [Q.], a very good food. It is the food that is given to kittens and baby puppies, and the first solid food given to human babies. Mothers give little bags full of sweetened *machica* to their children when they send them off herding, and worry all day if a careless youngster leaves his behind.

Because it is the essential symbol of the home, *machica* is the quintessential symbol of hospitality. Some is always kept on hand to offer to visitors. It is not offered to formal guests, and certainly not to the white nurse, schoolteacher or priest, for whom, after much frantic searching, the crusty year-old jar of instant coffee is unearthed while a child is sent racing downhill to buy bread. *Machica* is for the familiar guest, for the *comadre* who always comes to help harvest or the neighbor who has come to castrate your pig. A woman loves to bring out the *machica* when her family visits from her *natal comuna*, or when sisters visit from the *comunas* into which they have married. It is as though with this single act she can recreate the disbanded family home.

The meanings attached to *machica* derive partially from the way it is made. Ideally, it is entirely produced on the farmstead. Cultural ideals demand that barley sown by a family be seed from its own stores, not purchased; the sowing, care, harvest and threshing of the crop is done by extended family members; lastly, the sifting, grinding and toasting of the grain to make *machica* is done by the women of the family. Mothers make *machica* for their children, and in-marrying women prove their allegiance to the family, and their obedience to their mother-in-law, by grinding barley in the cold hours before dawn. Where the traditional extended family is still maintained, daughters-in-law creep into their mother-in-law's kitchen at four in the morning to start making *machica*. In the newer family structure, where wage labor gives a young couple independence from parents and in-laws, couples may pay to have barley ground in the town mill. This is socially disapproved, however. Machine-ground *machica* isn't *mishqui*, sweet or tasty, people say, and older women cluck with disapproval over a house where dawn finds a cold hearth, that is, where *machica* is not being toasted in the morning. Because of this association of *machica* with female productive and social roles, women react very emotionally to their children's rejection of barley gruels. It is not only the demand for precious purchased food over abundant home-grown grains that troubles them. In demanding bread, children reject their mother's contribution to the household and reach for foods that their fathers provide.

Zumbagua adults do not feel that bread is appropriate for everyday meals because it is part of a class of food defined as *wanlla*. *Wanlla* is anything that is not part of a meal. In this sense, it could be translated as "snack," "treat," "junk food" or "dessert food," and *wanlla* can be all of these. But the second meaning of *wanlla* is "gift." All of the foods called *wanlla* are primarily purchased in order to be redistributed. The motivation is not so much altruism as the exercise of power: giving *wanlla* is a critically important social and political action in Zumbagua; no one can be a successful social actor without understanding how to give and to manipulate others into giving. Any food given as a gift can be called *wanlla*. Hence in certain contexts rice, onions, noodles, milk or any other food could be *wanlla*. Some foods, however, are always *wanlla* in nature: they do not form part of regular meals and their primary purpose, in Zumbagua eyes, is as gifts. Since eating in Zumbagua always takes the form of offering and receiving food, these goods are still *wanlla* even when bought by members of a household and consumed within that household.

Bread is the *wanlla* par excellence. It is the universally appropriate gift, the favorite treat. In Zumbagua minds, bread has none of the qualities of a staple. It is truly a *golosina*, a treat, a luxury. More so than perhaps any other food, consumption of bread is directly dependent on a family's disposable cash income. It is the one special food that everyone would like to have on hand all the time, while at the same time it is recognized that no one ever needs bread. Potatoes and barley are necessities; bread is for enjoyment.

In households where men are absent wage-workers, the relationship of husband and wife entails certain exchanges of food. Whatever the husband's job, one of the obligations of a wife is to have food ready for him when he returns home. In households where he comes home only on weekends, every other week or even only once a month, this offering on her part becomes increasingly important symbolically. She cooks the best food she has, and the form she uses is strictly indigenous, using locally produced foods like *machica* to welcome him back home. While she presents him with these boiled grain soups or gruels, he brings *wanlla*: raw foods and treats from the city. These may include noodles, flour, cookies, candies and fruit, but bread is an important component.

The relative importance of her contribution compared to his depends on the financial situation of the household. If the young couple is part of a large, landholding extended family, he may return bearing only treats and goodies. But if they are a relatively isolated, land-poor couple, she and the children may have been subsisting on nothing but *machica* and water awaiting his return, and he will then bring in a substantial supply of groceries. In treating purchased foods like bread as part of everyday meals, the children seem in some ways to be making a prediction that the latter kind of household will become more common as they grow up, a prediction that seems more likely than not. Whatever the future may be, they certainly are expressing a preference for a male-provided, purchased commodity, bread, over the female-produced complex of cooked grains. And in defining bread as part of everyday meals, they are proposing a substantial shift in the role bread plays in Zumbagua cuisine.

GRUEL AND HISTORY

This contrast between two starch food forms, one of which is produced by and represents the local economy, while the other is part of a state-level economy and so enters the local community with all the prestige and symbolic power of the state behind it, is reminiscent of the relationship between maize and potatoes described by John Murra (1975) for Inca times. According to Murra, potatoes were the humble food of humble people, while maize, the cultivation of which necessitated systems of irrigation, was associated with the imperial power of the Inca state. The ability of the Inca state to make maize into a prestige item is suggested in the fragments of myths and stories cited by Murra in which the superiority of maize over potatoes is implicitly suggested.

According to Murra, the Spanish chroniclers were blind to the competition between maize and potatoes because, coming from a grain-based economy themselves, they never considered the possibility that tubers could be a staple. I find this observation to be very pertinent to the question of breads and gruels today, since our own predisposition towards bread as a basic food, as seen in its description as the "staff of life," can prevent us from perceiving the alien nature of leavened wheat breads to household economies based on boiled foods. As Americans, we all carry with us the mythic image of home-baked bread, but in areas of the world where fuel is precious, bread baking is beyond the scope of the individual household.

Our own prejudice towards leavened bread, which can be seen in the unpleasant associations that the word "gruel" has in English, is an artifact of what Raymond Sokolov (1984:108) has called "the inexorable march of wheat." As he points out, our disdain for boiled grain dishes is not just a matter of taste but is the product of specific political and economic processes in Europe and, later, in the Americas as well. The hegemonic nature of the contrast between gruels and breads played a part in the changes in taste that accompanied the spread of the Roman Empire, for example, where Tannahill says that "Bread...was established as being more desirable than grain-pastes and porridges" (Tannahill 1973:57). According to Goody, "In Europe...the northern extension of bread from the Mediterranean was associated with its use by the conquering Romans and by the missionizing Christians, who sacralized this high-status food through its use in the Mass" (1982:180). In Zumbagua, the intonation by European priests during the Mass of "Give us this day our daily bread" has similar connotations of white validation of a high-prestige food to indigenous listeners.

Oats and barley, and the porridges and unleavened breads that are made from them, symbolized the provincialism of the Scots to the eighteenth-century writer Samuel Johnson. According to Sokolov, Johnson's jibes on the subject of Scottish culinary tradition, with its emphasis on such gruel-based dishes as haggis and flummery, are revealing of the relationship between London and the hinterlands of the British Isles. "[Johnson's]...complete insensitivity to the real situation that condemned the Celtic fringe (and the north of England) to oats and barley...is an unappealing, but, once again, typical expression of the imperial status of London" (1984:110).

In this century, Goody cites the opposition between porridges and breads as one facet of the colonized/colonizer dichotomy in Ghana, where rising black elites, who previously made much of their familiarity with European culinary habits, have only recently begun to publicly eat porridge as an affirmation of their ethnicity (Goody 1982:177, passim). Goody's comments on the production aspects of this opposition are very relevant to the Andean case. He points out that the early success of bread among European foods introduced into the area can perhaps be attributed to the possibility of producing it on a small, localized scale (1982:180). In Ecuador, bread baking and sales figure importantly among the entrepreneurial possibilities open to the lower-class "white" and cholo populations whose livelihood is based on products which appeal to and are affordable for people from the small towns and rural hinterlands of the Sierra.

As Goody points out, the contrast between leavened breads and gruels or toasted grain products is one of technology; baking bread implies use of an oven, a technology which contrasts with that of the rural household where techniques are limited to boiling and toasting (1977:180–181). Because of the high energy input required for their use, ovens in turn require some type of commercial or communal organization of production in low energy consuming economies such as that of rural Ecuador.[6]

In conclusion, then, bread in Zumbagua has for some time now been a high-status food which contrasts with local products, although its specific role in local cuisine may be changing. Family arguments over the introduction of bread into the early-morning meal involve issues larger and more complex than worries over the family budget. In addition, the roles of children and parents, men and women in these conflicts indicates the heterogeneous nature of family members both as producers and as consumers, a heterogeneity which household-level economic analysis can overlook. As to the resolution of the conflict, it remains to be seen whether the children's cries for bread and the continued erosion of the household's ability to sustain itself through subsistence agriculture will succeed in transforming everyday practice.

Notes

1. Race and ethnicity in the Ecuadorian Sierra, as in much of Latin America, is determined primarily by socioeconomic class, "Indian" and "peasant," "white" and "elite" being practically synonymous. In Zumbagua, ethnicity for permanent residents is bipolar, *blanco* (white) referring to the small local elite and *longo/a* (a derogatory term similar in connotation to the English "nigger") labeling the indigenous majority. Zumbagua "whites" would not be considered white at all by urban or upper-middle class Ecuadorians, while the metaphorical nature of these terms is demonstrated by the presence in the parish of green-eyed, fair-haired, freckled "longos," the product of the institutionalized miscegenation of hacienda days, as well as by the membership among the parish "whites" of a family of coastal blacks. Terms for people of mixed blood, such as *mestizo, cholo,* or *misti* are infrequently heard in the parish and never refer to those who were born there. The word *cholo* identifies market sellers, while professionals such as the staff of the Catholic Church or the government-sponsored clinic are referred to as *gringos,* foreigners, even when Ecuadorian. Everyone born in the parish is categorized as *blanco* or *longo,* although local gossip identifies those who are "trying to be *blanco*" or "trying to be both."

2. I use terms—*sopa* and *seco, caldo* and *colada*—which come from Ecuadorian national cuisine, but are here applied to categories used within the parish. These are not words that people of the parish themselves use. Although more acculturated and Spanish-speaking residents of the parish may use these terms to apply to Zumbagua dishes, monolingual Quichua speakers do not. Soups are commonly referred to simply as *almuirsu,* from the Spanish *almuerzo,* lunch. I have borrowed these terms to label certain implicit categories used by Zumbagua women when cooking: they refer to specific types of syntagmatic chains I discovered in their practice. I use the Ecuadorian Spanish terms because they most closely approximate native categories (not surprisingly, given the common cultural roots, European and Native American, of both cuisines) and to avoid meanings implicit in English cooking terminology.

3. Local farmers prefer varieties which retain form after boiling and consider those which break down *(deshacerse)* as inferior.

4. The Zumbagua sequence of meals is similar in concept to the typical Ecuadorian pattern, in that meals eaten after dark are light while daytime meals are heavy. As I describe elsewhere (Weismantel 1987) among current conflicts over cuisine in the parish is the issue as to whether to eat three times a day, the national pattern, or four (*cafe* {5 A.M.}, *almuirsu* {10 A.M.}, *almuirsu* {3 P.M.}, *cafe* {8 P.M.}). The latter meal structure is suited to the schedules of women who must both cook and herd sheep, but it cannot be sustained if the children attend public schools that send them home at noon for a meal.

5. Finados is the November 1–2 celebration for the dead, observed throughout the Andes. Many of the rituals of the holiday, which syncretize indigenous and Hispanic elements, suggest the symbolic significance of food and eating, and especially of starchy foods; the *colada morada* or *yana api* is in fact a gruel, made of maize in maize-producing areas, but in Zumbagua it is more frequently made of *machica*. For food symbolism in Finados, see Weismantel 1983; Hartman 1973, 1974 provides the best data on contemporary Ecuadorian practice.

6. There are communities in the Sierra that have ovens, however; these are frequently owned as money-making enterprises by certain families who undertake the roasting of pigs or the baking of quantities of breads for weddings and other special occasions.

References

Douglas, Mary. 1971. Deciphering a Meal. In *Myth, Symbol and Culture*. Clifford Geertz, ed. New York: W. W. Norton and Co., pp. 61–82.

Goody, Jack. 1982. *Cooking, Cuisine and Class: A Study of Comparative Sociology*. Cambridge: Cambridge University Press.

Mintz, Sidney. 1979. Time, Sugar and Sweetness. *Marxist Perspectives* 2:56–73.

———. 1985. *Sweetness and Power: The Place of Sugar in Modern History*. NY: Viking Press.

Sokolov, Raymond. 1984. Oat Cuisine. *Natural History* 93(4):108–111.

Tannahill, Reay. 1972. *Food in History*. NY: Stein and Day.

Turner, Victor. 1967. *The Forest of Symbols*. Ithaca: Cornell University Press.

Williams, Raymond. 1977. *Marxism and Literature*. Cambridge: Cambridge University Press.

CHAPTER 22

Japanese Mothers and *Obentōs*: The Lunch-Box as Ideological State Apparatus

Anne Allison

(1991)

Japanese nursery school children, going off to school for the first time, carry with them a boxed lunch (*obentō*) prepared by their mothers at home. Customarily these *obentōs* are highly crafted elaborations of food: a multitude of miniature portions, artistically designed and precisely arranged, in a container that is sturdy and cute. Mothers tend to expend inordinate time and attention on these *obentōs* in efforts both to please their children and to affirm that they are good mothers. Children at nursery school are taught in turn that they must consume their entire meal according to school rituals.

Food in an *obentō* is an everyday practice of Japanese life. While its adoption at the nursery school level may seem only natural to Japanese and unremarkable to outsiders, I will argue in this article that the *obentō* is invested with a gendered state ideology. Overseen by the authorities of the nursery school, an institution which is linked to, if not directly monitored by, the state, the practice of the *obentō* situates the producer as a woman and mother, and the consumer, as a child of a mother and a student of a school. Food in this context is neither casual nor arbitrary. Eaten quickly in its entirety by the student, the *obentō* must be fashioned by the mother so as to expedite this chore for the child. Both mother and child are being watched, judged, and constructed; and it is only through their joint effort that the goal can be accomplished.

I use Althusser's concept of the Ideological State Apparatus (1971) to frame my argument. I will briefly describe how food is coded as a cultural and aesthetic apparatus in Japan, and what authority the state holds over schools in Japanese society. Thus situating the parameters within which the *obentō* is regulated and structured in the nursery school setting, I will examine the practice both of making and eating *obentō* within the context of one nursery school in Tokyo. As an anthropologist and mother of a child who attended this school for fifteen months, my analysis is based on my observations, on discussions with other mothers, and on

daily conversations and an interview with my son's teacher, examination of *obentō* magazines and cookbooks, participation in school rituals, outings, and Mothers' Association meetings, and the multifarious experiences of my son and myself as we faced the *obentō* process every day.

I conclude that *obentōs* as a routine, task, and art form of nursery school culture are endowed with ideological and gendered meanings that the state indirectly manipulates. The manipulation is neither total nor totally coercive, however, and I argue that pleasure and creativity for both mother and child are also products of the *obentō*.

CULTURAL RITUAL AND STATE IDEOLOGY

As anthropologists have long understood, not only are the worlds we inhabit symbolically constructed, but also the constructions of our cultural symbols are endowed with, or have the potential for, power. How we see reality, in other words, is also how we live it. So the conventions by which we recognize our universe are also those by which each of us assumes our place and behavior within that universe. Culture is, in this sense, doubly constructive: constructing both the world for people and people for specific worlds.

The fact that culture is not necessarily innocent, and power not necessarily transparent, has been revealed by much theoretical work conducted both inside and outside the discipline of anthropology. The scholarship of the neo-Marxist Louis Althusser (1971), for example, has encouraged the conceptualization of power as a force which operates in ways that are subtle, disguised, and accepted as everyday social practice. Althusser differentiated between two major structures of power in modern capitalist societies. The first, he called, (Repressive) State Apparatus (SA), which is power that the state wields and manages primarily through the threat of force. Here the state sanctions the usage of power and repression through such legitimized mechanisms as the law and police (1971: 143–5).

Contrasted with this is a second structure of power—Ideological State Apparatus(es) (ISA). These are institutions which have some overt function other than a political and/

Anne Allison, "Japanese mothers and *obentōs*: the lunch-box as ideological state apparatus." *Anthropological Quarterly* 64 (1991): 195–208. Reprinted with permission.

or administrative one: mass media, education, health and welfare, for example. More numerous, disparate, and functionally polymorphous than the SA, the ISA exert power not primarily through repression but through ideology. Designed and accepted as practices with another purpose—to educate (the school system), entertain (film industry), inform (news media), the ISA serve not only their stated objective but also an unstated one—that of indoctrinating people into seeing the world a certain way and of accepting certain identities as their own within that world (1971: 143–7).

While both structures of power operate simultaneously and complementarily, it is the ISA, according to Althusser, which in capitalist societies is the more influential of the two. Disguised and screened by another operation, the power of ideology in ISA can be both more far-reaching and insidious than the SA's power of coercion. Hidden in the movies we watch, the music we hear, the liquor we drink, the textbooks we read, it is overlooked because it is protected and its protection—or its alibi (Barthes 1957: 109–111)—allows the terms and relations of ideology to spill into and infiltrate our everyday lives.

A world of commodities, gender inequalities, and power differentials is seen not therefore in these terms but as a naturalized environment, one that makes sense because it has become our experience to live it and accept it in precisely this way. This commonsense acceptance of a particular world is the work of ideology, and it works by concealing the coercive and repressive elements of our everyday routines but also by making those routines of the everyday familiar, desirable, and simply our own. This is the critical element of Althusser's notion of ideological power: ideology is so potent because it becomes not only ours but us—the terms and machinery by which we structure ourselves and identify who we are.

JAPANESE FOOD AS CULTURAL MYTH

An author in one *obentō* magazine, the type of medium-sized publication that, filled with glossy pictures of *obentōs* and ideas and recipes for successfully recreating them, sells in the bookstores across Japan, declares, "...the making of the *obentō* is the one most worrisome concern facing the mother of a child going off to school for the first time (*Shufunotomo* 1980: inside cover). Another *obentō* journal, this one heftier and packaged in the encyclopedic series of the prolific women's publishing firm, *Shufunotomo*, articulates the same social fact: "first-time *obentōs* are a strain on both parent and child" ("*hajimete no obentō wa, oya mo ko mo kinchōshimasu*") (*Shufunotomo* 1981: 55).

An outside observer might ask: What is the real source of worry over *obentō*? Is it the food itself or the entrance of the young child into school for the first time? Yet, as one looks at a typical child's *obentō*—a small box packaged with a five or six-course miniaturized meal whose pieces and parts are artistically arranged, perfectly cut, and neatly arranged—would immediately reveal, no food is "just" food

in Japan. What is not so immediately apparent, however, is why a small child with limited appetite and perhaps scant interest in food is the recipient of a meal as elaborate and as elaborately prepared as any made for an entire family or invited guests?

Certainly, in Japan much attention is focussed on the *obentō*, investing it with a significance far beyond that of the merely pragmatic, functional one of sustaining a child with nutritional foodstuffs. Since this investment beyond the pragmatic is true of any food prepared in Japan, it is helpful to examine culinary codes for food preparation that operate generally in the society before focussing on children's *obentōs*.

As has been remarked often about Japanese food, the key element is appearance. Food must be organized, re-organized, arranged, re-arranged, stylized, and re-stylized to appear in a design that is visually attractive. Presentation is critical: not to the extent that taste and nutrition are displaced, as has been sometimes attributed to Japanese food, but to the degree that how food looks is at least as important as how it tastes and how good and sustaining it is for one's body.

As Donald Richie has pointed out in his eloquent and informative book *A Taste of Japan* (1985), presentational style is the guiding principle by which food is prepared in Japan, and the style is conditioned by a number of codes. One code is for smallness, separation, and fragmentation. Nothing large is allowed, so portions are all cut to be bite-sized, served in small amounts on tiny individual dishes, and are arranged on a table (or on a tray, or in an *obentō* box) in an array of small, separate containers.[1] There is no one big dinner plate with three large portions of vegetable, starch, and meat as in American cuisine. Consequently the eye is pulled not toward one totalizing center but away to a multiplicity of de-centered parts.[2]

Visually, food substances are presented according to a structural principle not only of segmentation but also of opposition. Foods are broken or cut to make contrasts of color, texture, and shape. Foods are meant to oppose one another and clash: pink against green, roundish foods against angular ones, smooth substances next to rough ones. This oppositional code operates not only within and between the foodstuffs themselves, but also between the attributes of the food and those of the containers in or on which they are placed: a circular mound in a square dish, a bland colored food set against a bright plate, a translucent sweet in a heavily textured bowl (Richie 1985: 40–1).

The container is as important as what is contained in Japanese cuisine, but it is really the containment that is stressed, that is, how food has been (re)constructed and (re)arranged from nature to appear, in both beauty and freshness, perfectly natural. This stylizing of nature is a third code by which presentation is directed; the injunction is not only to retain, as much as possible, the innate naturalness of ingredients—shopping daily so food is fresh and leaving much of it either raw or only minimally cooked—but also to recreate in prepared food the promise and appearance of being "natural." As Richie writes, "...the emphasis is on presentation of the natural rather than the natural itself. It is not what nature has wrought that excites admiration but what man has wrought with what nature has wrought" (1985: 11).

This naturalization of food is rendered through two main devices. One is by constantly hinting at and appropriating the nature that comes from outside—decorating food with seasonal reminders, such as a maple leaf in the fall or a flower in the spring, serving in-season fruits and vegetables, and using season-coordinated dishes such as glassware in the summer and heavy pottery in the winter. The other device, to some degree the inverse of the first, is to accentuate and perfect the preparation process to such an extent that the food appears not only to be natural, but more nearly perfect than nature without human intervention ever could be. This is nature made artificial. Thus, by naturalization, nature is not only taken in by Japanese cuisine, but taken over.

It is this ability both to appropriate "real" nature (the maple leaf on the tray) and to stamp the human reconstruction of that nature as "natural" that lends Japanese food its potential for cultural and ideological manipulation. It is what Barthes calls a second order myth (1957: 114–7): a language which has a function people accept as only pragmatic—the sending of roses to lovers, the consumption of wine with one's dinner, the cleaning up a mother does for her child—which is taken over by some interest or agenda to serve a different end—florists who can sell roses, liquor companies who can market wine, conservative politicians who campaign for a gendered division of labor with women kept at home. The first order of language ("language-object"), thus emptied of its original meaning, is converted into an empty form by which it can assume a new, additional, second order of signification ("metalanguage" or "second-order semiological system"). As Barthes points out however, the primary meaning is never lost. Rather, it remains and stands as an alibi, the cover under which the second, politicized meaning can hide. Roses sell better, for example, when lovers view them as a vehicle to express love rather than the means by which a company stays in business.

At one level, food is just food in Japan—the medium by which humans sustain their nature and health. Yet under and through this code of pragmatics, Japanese cuisine carries other meanings that in Barthes' terms are mythological. One of these is national identity: food being appropriated as a sign of the culture. To be Japanese is to eat Japanese food, as so many Japanese confirm when they travel to other countries and cite the greatest problem they encounter to be the absence of "real" Japanese food. Stated the other way around, rice is so symbolically central to Japanese culture (meals and obentōs often being assembled with rice as the core and all other dishes, multifarious as they may be, as mere compliments or side dishes) that Japanese say they can never feel full until they have consumed their rice at a particular meal or at least once during the day.[3]

Embedded within this insistence on eating Japanese food, thereby reconfirming one as a member of the culture,

are the principles by which Japanese food is customarily prepared: perfection, labor, small distinguishable parts, opposing segments, beauty, and the stamp of nature. Overarching all these more detailed codings are two that guide the making and ideological appropriation of the nursery school obentō most directly: 1) there is an order to the food: a right way to do things, with everything in its place and each place coordinated with every other, and 2) the one who prepares the food takes on the responsibility of producing food to the standards of perfection and exactness that Japanese cuisine demands. Food may not be casual, in other words, nor the producer casual in her production. In these two rules is a message both about social order and the role gender plays in sustaining and nourishing that order.

SCHOOL, STATE, AND SUBJECTIVITY

In addition to language and second order meanings I suggest that the rituals and routines surrounding obentōs in Japanese nursery schools present, as it were, a third order, manipulation. This order is a use of a currency already established—one that has already appropriated a language of utility (food feeds hunger) to express and implant cultural behaviors. State-guided schools borrow this coded apparatus: using the natural convenience and cover of food not only to code a cultural order, but also to socialize children and mothers into the gendered roles and subjectivities they are expected to assume in a political order desired and directed by the state.

In modern capitalist societies such as Japan, it is the school, according to Althusser, which assumes the primary role of ideological state apparatus. A greater segment of the population spends longer hours and more years here than in previous historical periods. Also education has now taken over from other institutions, such as religion, the pedagogical function of being the major shaper and inculcator of knowledge for the society. Concurrently, as Althusser has pointed out for capitalist modernism (1971: 152, 156), there is the gradual replacement of repression by ideology as the prime mechanism for behavior enforcement. Influenced less by the threat of force and more by the devices that present and inform us of the world we live in and the subjectivities that world demands, knowledge and ideology become fused, and education emerges as the apparatus for pedagogical and ideological indoctrination.

In practice, as school teaches children how and what to think, it also shapes them for the roles and positions they will later assume as adult members of the society. How the social order is organized through vectors of gender, power, labor, and/or class, in other words, is not only as important a lesson as the basics of reading and writing, but is transmitted through and embedded in those classroom lessons. Knowledge thus is not only socially constructed, but also differentially acquired according to who one is or will be in the political society one will enter in later years. What precisely society requires in the way of workers, citizens, and parents will be the condition determining or influencing instruction in the schools.

This latter equation, of course, depends on two factors: 1) the convergence or divergence of different interests in what is desired as subjectivities, and 2) the power any particular interest, including that of the state, has in exerting its desires for subjects on or through the system of education. In the case of Japan, the state wields enormous control over the systematization of education. Through its Ministry of Education (Monbushō), one of the most powerful and influential ministries in the government, education is centralized and managed by a state bureaucracy that regulates almost every aspect of the educational process. On any given day, for example, what is taught in every public school follows the same curriculum, adheres to the same structure, and is informed by textbooks from the prescribed list. Teachers are nationally screened, school boards uniformly appointed (rather than elected), and students institutionally exhorted to obey teachers given their legal authority, for example, to write secret reports (*naishinsho*), that may obstruct a student's entrance into high school.[4]

The role of the state in Japanese education is not limited, however, to such extensive but codified authorities granted to the Ministry of Education. Even more powerful is the principle of the "*gakureki shakkai*" (lit. academic pedigree society) by which careers of adults are determined by the schools they attend as youth. A reflection and construction of the new economic order of post-war Japan,[5] school attendance has become the single most important determinant of who will achieve the most desirable positions in industry, government, and the professions. School attendance is itself based on a single criterion: a system of entrance exams which determines entrance selection and it is to this end—preparation for exams—that school, even at the nursery school level, is increasingly oriented. Learning to follow directions, do as one is told, and "*ganbaru*" (Asanuma 1987) are social imperatives, sanctioned by the state, and taught in the schools.

NURSERY SCHOOL AND IDEOLOGICAL APPROPRIATION OF THE OBENTŌ

The nursery school stands outside the structure of compulsory education in Japan. Most nursery schools are private; and, though not compelled by the state, a greater proportion of the three to six-year old population of Japan attends preschool than in any other industrialized nation (Tobin 1989; Hendry 1986; Boocock 1989).

Differentiated from the *hoikuen*, another preschool institution with longer hours which is more like daycare than school,[6] the *yochien* (nursery school) is widely perceived as instructional, not necessarily in a formal curriculum but more in indoctrination to attitudes and structures of Japanese schooling. Children learn less about reading and writing than they do about how to become a Japanese student, and both parts of this formula—Japanese and student—are equally stressed. As Rohlen has written, "social order is generated" in the nursery school, first and foremost, by a system of routines (1989: 10, 21). Educational routines and rituals are therefore of heightened importance in *yochien*, for whereas these routines and rituals may be the format through which subjects are taught in higher grades, they are both form and subject in the *yochien*.

While the state (through its agency, the Ministry of Education) has no direct mandate over nursery school attendance, its influence is nevertheless significant. First, authority over how the *yochien* is run is in the hands of the Ministry of Education. Second, most parents and teachers see the *yochien* as the first step to the system of compulsory education that starts in the first grade and is closely controlled by Monbushō. The principal of the *yochien* my son attended, for example, stated that he saw his main duty to be preparing children to enter more easily the rigors of public education soon to come. Third, the rules and patterns of "group living" (*shūdanseikatsu*), a Japanese social ideal that is reiterated nationwide by political leaders, corporate management, and marriage counselors, is first introduced to the child in nursery school.[7]

The entry into nursery school marks a transition both away from home and into the "real world," which is generally judged to be difficult, even traumatic, for the Japanese child (Peak 1989). The *obentō* is intended to ease a child's discomfiture and to allow a child's mother to manufacture something of herself and the home to accompany the child as s/he moves into the potentially threatening outside world. Japanese use the cultural categories of *soto* and *uchi*; *soto* connotes the outside, which in being distanced and other, is dirty and hostile; and *uchi* identifies as clean and comfortable what is inside and familiar. The school falls initially and, to some degree, perpetually, into a category of *soto*. What is ultimately the definition and location of *uchi*, by contrast, is the home, where family and mother reside.[8] By producing something from the home, a mother both girds and goads her child to face what is inevitable in the world that lies beyond. This is the mother's role and her gift; by giving of herself and the home (which she both symbolically represents and in reality manages[9]), the *soto* of the school is, if not transformed into the *uchi* of home, made more bearable by this sign of domestic and maternal hearth a child can bring to it.

The *obentō* is filled with the meaning of mother and home in a number of ways. The first is by sheer labor. Women spend what seems to be an inordinate amount of time on the production of this one item. As an experienced *obentō* maker, I can attest to the intense attention and energy devoted to this one chore. On the average, mothers spend 20–45 minutes every morning cooking, preparing, and assembling the contents of one *obentō* for one nursery school-aged child. In addition, the previous day they have planned, shopped, and often organized a supper meal with left-overs in mind for the next day's *obentō*. Frequently women[10] discuss *obentō* ideas with other mothers, scan *obentō* cookbooks or magazines for recipes, buy or make objects with which to decorate or contain (part of) the *obentō*, and perhaps make small food portions to freeze and retrieve for future *obentō*.[11]

Of course, effort alone does not necessarily produce a successful *obentō*. Casualness was never indulged, I observed, and even mothers with children who would eat anything prepared *obentō*s as elaborate as anyone else's. Such labor is intended for the child but also the mother: it is a sign of a woman's commitment as a mother and her inspiring her child to being similarly committed as a student. The *obentō* is thus a representation of what the mother is and what the child should become. A model for school is added to what is gift and reminder from home.

This equation is spelled out more precisely in a nursery school rule—all of the *obentō* must be eaten. Though on the face of it this is petty and mundane, the injunction is taken very seriously by nursery school teachers and is one not easily realized by very small children. The logic is that it is time for the child to meet certain expectations. One of the main agendas of the nursery school, after all, is to introduce and indoctrinate children into the patterns and rigors of Japanese education (Rohlen 1989; Sano 1989; Lewis 1989). And Japanese education, by all accounts, is not about fun (Duke 1986).

Learning is hard work with few choices or pleasures. Even *obentō*s from home stop once the child enters first grade.[12] The meals there are institutional: largely bland, unappealing, and prepared with only nutrition in mind. To ease a youngster into these upcoming (educational, social, disciplinary, culinary) routines, *yochien obentō*s are designed to be pleasing and personal. The *obentō* is also designed, however, as a test for the child. And the double meaning is not unintentional. A structure already filled with a signification of mother and home is then emptied to provide a new form: one now also written with the ideological demands of being a member of Japanese culture as well as a viable and successful Japanese in the realms of school and later work.

The exhortation to consume one's entire *obentō*[13] is articulated and enforced by the nursery school teacher. Making high drama out of eating by, for example, singing a song; collectively thanking Buddha (in the case of Buddhist nursery schools), one's mother for making the *obentō*, and one's father for providing the means to make the *obentō*; having two assigned class helpers pour the tea, the class eats together until everyone has finished. The teacher examines the children's *obentō*s, making sure the food is all consumed, and encouraging, sometimes scolding, children who are taking too long. Slow eaters do not fare well in this ritual, because they hold up the other students, who as a peer group also monitor a child's eating. My son often complained about a child whose slowness over food meant that the others were kept inside (rather than being allowed to play on the playground) for much of the lunch period.

Ultimately and officially, it is the teacher, however, whose role and authority it is to watch over food consumption and to judge the person consuming food. Her surveillance covers both the student and the mother, who in the matter of the *obentō*, must work together. The child's job is to eat the food and the mother's to prepare it. Hence, the responsibility and execution of one's task is not only shared but conditioned by the other. My son's teacher would talk with me daily about the progress he was making finishing his *obentō*s. Although the overt subject of discussion was my child, most of what was said was directed to me: what I could do in order to get David to consume his lunch more easily.

The intensity of these talks struck me at the time as curious. We had just settled in Japan and David, a highly verbal child, was attending a foreign school in a foreign language he had not yet mastered; he was the only non-Japanese child in the school. Many of his behaviors during this time were disruptive: for example, he went up and down the line of children during morning exercises hitting each child on the head. Hamada-sensei (the teacher), however, chose to discuss the *obentō*s. I thought surely David's survival in and adjustment to this environment depended much more on other factors, such as learning Japanese. Yet it was the *obentō* that was discussed with such recall of detail ("David ate all his peas today, but not a single carrot until I asked him to do so three times") and seriousness that I assumed her attention was being misplaced. The manifest reference was to box-lunches, but was not the latent reference to something else?[14]

Of course, there was another message, for me and my child. It was an injunction to follow directions, obey rules, and accept the authority of the school system. All of the latter were embedded in and inculcated through certain rituals: the nursery school, as any school (except such non-conventional ones as Waldorf and Montessori) and practically any social or institutional practice in Japan, was so heavily ritualized and ritualistic that the very form of ritual took on a meaning and value in and of itself (Rohlen 1989: 21, 27–8). Both the school day and school year of the nursery school were organized by these rituals. The day, apart from two free periods, for example, was broken by discrete routines—morning exercises, arts and crafts, gym instruction, singing—most of which were named and scheduled. The school year was also segmented into and marked by three annual events—sports day (*undōkai*) in the fall, winter assembly (*seikatsu happyōkai*) in December, and dance festival (*bon odori*) in the summer. Energy was galvanized by these rituals, which demanded a degree of order as well as a discipline and self-control that non-Japanese would find remarkable.

Significantly, David's teacher marked his successful integration into the school system by his mastery not of the language or other cultural skills, but of the school's daily routines—walking in line, brushing his teeth after eating, arriving at school early, eagerly participating in greeting and departure ceremonies, and completing all of his *obentō* on time. Not only had he adjusted to the school structure, but he had also become assimilated to the other children. Or restated, what once had been externally enforced now became ideologically desirable; the everyday practices had moved from being alien (*soto*) to familiar (*uchi*) to him, from, that is, being someone else's to his own. My American child had to become, in some sense, Japanese, and where his teacher recognized this Japaneseness was in the daily routines such as finishing his *obentō*. The lesson learned early, which David learned as well, is that not adhering to routines such as completing one's *obentō* on time leads to not only admonishment from the teacher, but rejection from the other students.

The nursery school system differentiates between the child who does and the child who does not manage the multifarious and constant rituals of nursery school. And for those who do not manage there is a penalty which the child learns either to avoid or wish to avoid. Seeking the acceptance of his peers, the student develops the aptitude, willingness, and in the case of my son—whose outspokenness and individuality were the characteristics most noted in this culture—even the desire to conform to the highly ordered and structured practices of nursery school life. As Althusser (1971) wrote about ideology: the mechanism works when and because ideas about the world and particular roles in that world that serve other (social, political, economic, state) agendas become familiar and one's own.

Rohlen makes a similar point: that what is taught and learned in nursery school is social order. Called *shūdanseikatsu* or group life, it means organization into a group where a person's subjectivity is determined by group membership and not "the assumption of choice and rational self-interest" (1989: 30). A child learns in nursery school to be with others, think like others, and act in tandem with others. This lesson is taught primarily through the precision and constancy of basic routines: "Order is shaped gradually by repeated practice of selected daily tasks…that socialize the children to high degrees of neatness and uniformity" (p. 21). Yet a feeling of coerciveness is rarely experienced by the child when three principles of nursery school instruction are in place: 1) school routines are made "desirable and pleasant" (p. 30), 2) the teacher disguises her authority by trying to make the group the voice and unit of authority, and 3) the regimentation of the school is administered by an attitude of "intimacy" on the part of the teachers and administrators (p. 30). In short, when the desires and routines of the school are made into the desires and routines of the child, they are made acceptable.

MOTHERING AS GENDERED IDEOLOGICAL STATE APPARATUS

The rituals surrounding the *obentō*'s consumption in the school situate what ideological meanings the *obentō* transmits to the child. The process of production within the home, by contrast, organizes its somewhat different ideological package for the mother. While the two sets of meanings are intertwined, the mother is faced with different expectations in the preparation of the *obentō* than the child is in its consumption. At a pragmatic level the child must simply eat the lunch box, whereas the mother's job is far more complicated. The onus for her is getting the child to consume what she has made, and the general attitude is that this is far more the mother's responsibility (at this nursery school,

transitional stage) than the child's. And this is no simple or easy task.

Much of what is written, advised, and discussed about the *obentō* has this aim explicitly in mind: that is making food in such a way as to facilitate the child's duty to eat it. One magazine advises:

> The first day of taking *obentō* is a worrisome thing for mother and "*boku*" (child[15]) too. Put in easy-to-eat foods that your child likes and is already used to and prepare this food in small portions (*Shufunotomo* 1980: 28).

Filled with pages of recipes, hints, pictures, and ideas, the magazine codes each page with "helpful" headings:

> First off, easy-to-eat is step one.
> Next is being able to consume the *obentō* without leaving anything behind.
> Make it in such a way for the child to become proficient in the use of chopsticks.
> Decorate and fill it with cute dreams (*kawairashi yume*).
> For older classes (*nenchō*), make *obentō* filled with variety.
> Once he's become used to it, balance foods your child likes with those he dislikes.
> For kids who hate vegetables….
> For kids who hate fish….
> For kids who hate meat…(pp. 28–53).

Laced throughout cookbooks and other magazines devoted to *obentō*, the *obentō* guidelines issued by the school and sent home in the school flier every two weeks, and the words of Japanese mothers and teachers discussing *obentō*, are a number of principles: 1) food should be made easy to eat: portions cut or made small and manipulable with fingers or chopsticks, (child-size) spoons and forks, skewers, toothpicks, muffin tins, containers, 2) portions should be kept small so the *obentō* can be consumed quickly and without any left-overs, 3) food that a child does not yet like should be eventually added so as to remove fussiness (*sukikirai*) in food habits, 4) make the *obentō* pretty, cute, and visually changeable by presenting the food attractively and by adding non-food objects such as silver paper, foil, toothpick flags, paper napkins, cute handkerchiefs, and variously shaped containers for soy sauce and ketchup, and 5) design *obentō*-related items as much as possible by the mother's own hands including the *obentō* bag (*obentōfukuro*) in which the *obentō* is carried.

The strictures propounded by publications seem to be endless. In practice I found that visual appearance and appeal were stressed by the mothers. By contrast, the directive to use *obentō* as a training process—adding new foods and getting older children to use chopsticks and learn to tie the *furoshiki*[16]—was emphasized by those judging the *obentō* at the school. Where these two sets of concerns met was, of course, in the child's success or failure completing the *obentō*. Ultimately this outcome and the mother's role in it, was how the *obentō* was judged in my experience.

The aestheticization of the *obentō* is by far its most intriguing aspect for a cultural anthropologist. Aesthetic categories and codes that operate generally for Japanese cuisine are applied, though adjusted, to the nursery school format. Substances are many but petite, kept segmented and opposed, and manipulated intensively to achieve an appearance that often changes or disguises the food. As a mother insisted to me, the creation of a bear out of miniature hamburgers and rice, or a flower from an apple or peach, is meant to sustain a child's interest in the underlying food. Yet my child, at least, rarely noticed or appreciated the art I had so laboriously contrived. As for other children, I observed that even for those who ate with no obvious "fussiness," mothers' efforts to create food as style continued all year long.

Thus much of a woman's labor over *obentō* stems from some agenda other than that of getting the child to eat an entire lunch-box. The latter is certainly a consideration and it is the rationale as well as cover for women being scrutinized by the school's authority figure—the teacher. Yet two other factors are important. One is that the *obentō* is but one aspect of the far more expansive and continuous commitment a mother is expected to make for and to her child. "*Kyōiku mama*" (education mother) is the term given to a mother who executes her responsibility to oversee and manage the education of her children with excessive vigor. And yet this excess is not only demanded by the state even at the level of the nursery school; it is conventionally given by mothers. Mothers who manage the home and children, often in virtual absence of a husband/father, are considered the factor that may make or break a child as s/he advances towards that pivotal point of the entrance examinations.[17]

In this sense, just as the *obentō* is meant as a device to assist a child in the struggles of first adjusting to school, the mother's role generally is perceived as being the support, goad, and cushion for the child. She will perform endless tasks to assist in her child's study: sharpen pencils and make midnight snacks as the child studies, attend cram schools to verse herself in subjects her child is weak in, make inquiries as to what school is most appropriate for her child, and consult with her child's teachers. If the child succeeds, a mother is complimented; if the child fails, a mother is blamed.

Thus at the nursery school level, the mother starts her own preparation for this upcoming role. Yet the jobs and energies demanded of a nursery school mother are, in themselves, surprisingly consuming. Just as the mother of an entering student is given a book listing all the pre-entry tasks she must complete, for example, making various bags and containers, affixing labels to all clothes in precisely the right place and with the size exactly right, she will be continually expected thereafter to attend Mothers' Association meetings, accompany children on fieldtrips, wash the clothes and indoor shoes of her child every week, add required items to a child's bag on a day's notice, and generally be available. Few mothers at the school my son attended could afford to work in even part-time or temporary jobs. Those women who did tended either to keep their outside work a secret or be reprimanded by a teacher for insufficient devotion to

their child. Motherhood, in other words, is institutionalized through the child's school and such routines as making the *obentō* as a full-time, kept-at-home job.[18]

The second factor in a woman's devotion to over-elaborating her child's lunch-box is that her experience doing this becomes a part of her and a statement, in some sense, of who she is. Marx writes that labor is the most "essential" aspect to our species-being and that the products we produce are the encapsulation of us and therefore our productivity (1970: 71–76). Likewise, women are what they are through the products they produce. An *obentō* therefore is not only a gift or test for a child, but a representation and product of the woman herself. Of course, the two ideologically converge, as has been stated already, but I would also suggest that there is a potential disjoining. I sensed that the women were laboring for themselves apart from the agenda the *obentō* was expected to fill at school. Or stated alternatively, in the role that females in Japan are highly pressured and encouraged to assume as domestic manager, mother, and wife, there is, besides the endless and onerous responsibilities, also an opportunity for play. Significantly, women find play and creativity not outside their social roles but within them.

Saying this is not to deny the constraints and surveillance under which Japanese women labor at their *obentō*. Like their children at school, they are watched by not only the teacher but each other, and perfect what they create, partially at least, so as to be confirmed as a good and dutiful mother in the eyes of other mothers. The enthusiasm with which they absorb this task then is like my son's acceptance and internalization of the nursery school routines; no longer enforced from outside it becomes adopted as one's own.

The making of the *obentō* is, I would thus argue, a double-edged sword for women. By relishing its creation (for all the intense labor expended, only once or twice did I hear a mother voice any complaint about this task), a woman is ensconcing herself in the ritualization and subjectivity (subjection) of being a mother in Japan. She is alienated in the sense that others will dictate, inspect, and manage her work. On the reverse side, however, it is precisely through this work that the woman expresses, identifies, and constitutes herself. As Althusser pointed out, ideology can never be totally abolished (1971: 170); the elaborations that women work on "natural" food produce an *obentō* which is creative and, to some degree, a fulfilling and personal statement of themselves.

Minami, an informant, revealed how both restrictive and pleasurable the daily rituals of motherhood can be. The mother of two children—one, aged three and one, a nursery school student, Minami had been a professional opera singer before marrying at the relatively late age of 32. Now, her daily schedule was organized by routines associated with her child's nursery school: for example, making the *obentō*, taking her daughter to school and picking her up, attending Mothers' Association meetings, arranging daily play dates, and keeping the school uniform clean. While Minami wished to return to singing, if only on a part-time basis, she said that the demands of motherhood, particularly those imposed by her child's attendance at nursery school, frustrated this desire. Secretly snatching only minutes out of any day to practice, Minami missed singing and told me that being a mother in Japan means the exclusion of almost anything else.[19]

Despite this frustration, however, Minami did not behave like a frustrated woman. Rather she devoted to her mothering an energy, creativity, and intelligence I found to be standard in the Japanese mothers I knew. She planned special outings for her children at least two or three times a week, organized games that she knew they would like and would teach them cognitive skills, created her own stories and designed costumes for afternoon play, and shopped daily for the meals she prepared with her children's favorite foods in mind. Minami told me often that she wished she could sing more, but never once did she complain about her children, the chores of child-raising, or being a mother. The attentiveness displayed otherwise in her mothering was exemplified most fully in Minami's *obentōs*. No two were ever alike, each had at least four or five parts, and she kept trying out new ideas for both new foods and new designs. She took pride as well as pleasure in her *obentō* handicraft; but while Minami's *obentō* creativity was impressive, it was not unusual.

Examples of such extraordinary *obentō* creations from an *obentō* magazine include: 1) ("donut *obentō*"): two donuts, two wieners cut to look like a worm, two cut pieces of apple, two small cheese rolls, one hard-boiled egg made to look like a rabbit with leaf ears and pickle eyes and set in an aluminum muffin tin, cute paper napkin added, 2) (wiener doll *obentō*): a bed of rice with two doll creations made out of wiener parts (each consists of eight pieces comprising hat, hair, head, arms, body, legs), a line of pink ginger, a line of green parsley, paper flag of France added, 3) (vegetable flower and tulip *obentō*): a bed of rice laced with chopped hard-boiled egg, three tulip flowers made out of cut wieners with spinach precisely arranged as stem and leaves, a fruit salad with two raisins, three cooked peaches, three pieces of cooked apple, 4) (sweetheart doll *obentō*—*abekku ningyō no obentō*): in a two-section *obentō* box there are four rice balls on one side, each with a different center, on the other side are two dolls made of quail's eggs for heads, eyes and mouth added, bodies of cucumber, arranged as if lying down with two raw carrots for the pillow, covers made of one flower—cut cooked carrot, two pieces of ham, pieces of cooked spinach, and with different colored plastic skewers holding the dolls together (*Shufunotomo* 1980: 27, 30).

The impulse to work and re-work nature in these *obentō* is most obvious perhaps in the strategies used to transform, shape, and/or disguise foods. Every mother I knew came up with her own repertoire of such techniques, and every *obentō* magazine or cookbook I examined offered a special section on these devices. It is important to keep in mind that these are treated as only flourishes: embellishments added to parts of an *obentō* composed of many parts. The following is a list from one magazine: lemon pieces made into butterflies, hard boiled eggs into *daruma* (popular Japanese legendary figure of a monk without his eyes), sausage cut into flowers, a hard-boiled egg decorated as a baby, an apple piece cut into a leaf, a radish flaked into a flower, a cucumber cut like a flower, a *mikan* (nectarine orange) piece arranged into a basket, a boat with a sail made from a cucumber, skewered sausage, radish shaped like a mushroom, a quail egg flaked into a cherry, twisted *mikan* piece, sausage cut to become a crab, a patterned cucumber, a ribboned carrot, a flowered tomato, cabbage leaf flower, a potato cut to be a worm, a carrot designed as a red shoe, an apple cut to simulate a pineapple (pp. 57–60).

Nature is not only transformed but also supplemented by store-bought or mother-made objects which are precisely arranged in the *obentō*. The former come from an entire industry and commodification of the *obentō* process: complete racks or sections in stores selling *obentō* boxes, additional small containers, *obentō* bags, cups, chopstick and utensil containers (all these with various cute characters or designs on the front), cloth and paper napkins, foil, aluminum tins, colored ribbon or string, plastic skewers, toothpicks with paper flags, and paper dividers. The latter are the objects mothers are encouraged and praised for making themselves: *obentō* bags, napkins, and handkerchiefs with appliquéd designs or the child's name embroidered. These supplements to the food, the arrangement of the food, and the *obentō* box's dividing walls (removable and adjustable) furnish the order of the *obentō*. Everything appears crisp and neat with each part kept in its own place: two tiny hamburgers set firmly atop a bed of rice; vegetables in a separate compartment in the box; fruit arranged in a muffin tin.

How the specific forms of *obentō* artistry—for example, a wiener cut to look like a worm and set within a muffin tin—are encoded symbolically is a fascinating subject. Limited here by space, however, I will only offer initial suggestions. Arranging food into a scene recognizable by the child was an ideal mentioned by many mothers and cookbooks. Why those of animals, human beings, and other food forms (making a pineapple out of an apple, for example) predominate may have no other rationale than being familiar to children and easily re-produced by mothers. Yet it is also true that this tendency to use a trope of realism—casting food into realistic figures—is most prevalent in the meals Japanese prepare for their children. Mothers I knew created animals and faces in supper meals and/or *obentōs* made for other outings, yet their impulse to do this seemed not only heightened in the *obentō* that were sent to school but also played down in food prepared for other age groups.

What is consistent in Japanese cooking generally, as stated earlier, are the dual principles of manipulation and order. Food is manipulated into some other form than it assumes either naturally or upon being cooked: lines are put into mashed potatoes, carrots are flaked, wieners are twisted and sliced. Also, food is ordered by some human rather than natural principle; everything must have neat boundaries and be placed precisely so those boundaries do not merge. These two structures are the ones most important in shaping the nursery school *obentō* as well, and the inclination to design realistic imagery is primarily a means by which these other culinary codes are learned by and made pleasurable for the child. The simulacrum of a pineapple recreated from an apple therefore is less about seeing the pineapple in an apple (a particular form) and more about reconstructing the apple into something else (the process of transformation).

The intense labor, management, commodification, and attentiveness that goes into the making of an *obentō* laces it, however, with many and various meanings. Overarching all is the potential to aestheticize a certain social order, a social order which is coded (in cultural and culinary terms) as Japanese. Not only is a mother making food more palatable to her nursery school child, but she is creating food as a more aesthetic and pleasing social structure. The *obentō*'s message is that the world is constructed very precisely and that the role of any single Japanese in that world must be carried out with the same degree of precision. Production is demanding; and the producer must both keep within the borders of her/his role and work hard.

The message is also that it is women, not men, who are not only sustaining a child through food but carrying the ideological support of the culture that this food embeds. No Japanese man I spoke with had or desired the experience of making a nursery school *obentō* even once, and few were more than peripherally engaged in their children's education. The male is assigned a position in the outside world where he labors at a job for money and is expected to be primarily identified by and committed to his place of work.[20] Helping in the management of home and raising of children has not become an obvious male concern or interest in Japan, even as more and more women enter what was previously the male domain of work. Females have remained at and as the center of home in Japan and this message too is explicitly transmitted in both the production and consumption of entirely female-produced *obentō*.

The state accrues benefits from this arrangement. With children depending on the labor women devote to their mothering to such a degree, and women being pressured as well as pleasurized in such routine maternal productions as making the *obentō*—both effects encouraged and promoted by institutional features of the educational system heavily state-run and at least ideologically guided at even the nursery school level—a gendered division of labor is firmly set in place. Labor from males, socialized to be compliant and hard-working, is more extractable when they have wives to rely on for almost all domestic and familial management. And females become a source of cheap labor, as they are increasingly forced to enter the labor market to pay domestic costs (including those vast debts incurred in educating children) yet are increasingly constrained to low-paying part-time jobs because of the domestic duties they must also bear almost totally as mothers.

Hence, not only do females, as mothers, operate within the ideological state apparatus of Japan's school system that starts semi-officially, with the nursery school, they also operate as an ideological state apparatus unto themselves. Motherhood *is* state ideology, working through children at home and at school and through such mother-imprinted labor that a child carries from home to school as with the *obentō*. Hence the post-World War II conception of Japanese education as being egalitarian, democratic, and with no

agenda of or for gender differentiation, does not in practice stand up. Concealed within such cultural practices as culinary style and child-focussed mothering is a worldview in which the position and behavior an adult will assume has everything to do with the anatomy she/he was born with.

At the end, however, I am left with one question. If motherhood is not only watched and manipulated by the state but made by it into a conduit for ideological indoctrination, could not women subvert the political order by redesigning *obentō*? Asking this question, a Japanese friend, upon reading this paper, recalled her own experiences. Though her mother had been conventional in most other respects, she made her children *obentō*s that did not conform to the prevailing conventions. Basic, simple, and rarely artistic, Sawa also noted, in this connection, that the lines of these *obentō*s resembled those by which she was generally raised: as gender-neutral, treated as a person not "just as a girl," and being allowed a margin to think for herself. Today she is an exceptionally independent woman who has created a life for herself in America, away from homeland and parents, almost entirely on her own. She loves Japanese food, but the plain *obentō*s her mother made for her as a child, she is newly appreciative of now, as an adult. The *obentō*s fed her, but did not keep her culturally or ideologically attached. For this, Sawa says today, she is glad.

Notes

The fieldwork on which this article is based was supported by a Japan Foundation Postdoctoral Fellowship. I am grateful to Charles Piot for a thoughtful reading and useful suggestions for revision and to Jennifer Robertson for inviting my contribution to this issue. I would also like to thank Sawa Kurotani for her many ethnographic stories and input, and Phyllis Chock and two anonymous readers for the valuable contributions they made to revision of the manuscript.

1. As Dorinne Kondo has pointed out, however, these cuisinal principles may be conditioned by factors of both class and circumstance. Her *shitamachi* (more traditional area of Tokyo) informants, for example, adhered only casually to this coding and other Japanese she knew followed them more carefully when preparing food for guests rather than family and when eating outside rather than inside the home (Kondo 1990: 61–2).

2. Rice is often, if not always, included in a meal; and it may substantially as well as symbolically constitute the core of the meal. When served at a table it is put in a large pot or electric rice maker and will be spooned into a bowl, still no bigger or predominant than the many other containers from which a person eats. In an *obentō* rice may be in one, perhaps the largest, section of a multi-sectioned *obentō* box, yet it will be arranged with a variety of other foods. In a sense rice provides the syntactic and substantial center to a meal yet the presentation of the food rarely emphasizes this core. The rice bowl is refilled rather than heaped as in the preformed *obentō* box, and in the *obentō* rice is often embroidered, supplemented, and/or covered with other foodstuffs.

3. Japanese will both endure a high price for rice at home and resist American attempts to export rice to Japan in order to

stay domestically self-sufficient in this national food *qua* cultural symbol. Rice is the only foodstuff in which the Japanese have retained self-sufficient production.

4. The primary sources on education used are Horio 1988; Duke 1986; Rohlen 1983; Cummings 1980.

5. Neither the state's role in overseeing education nor a system of standardized tests is a new development in post-World War II Japan. What is new is the national standardization of tests and, in this sense, the intensified role the state has thus assumed in overseeing them. See Dore (1965) and Horio (1988).

6. Boocock (1989) differs from Tobin *et al.* (1989) on this point and asserts that the institutional differences are insignificant. She describes extensively how both *yōchien* and *hoikuen* are administered (*yōchien* are under the authority of Monbushō and *hoikuen* are under the authority of the Kōseishō, the Ministry of Health and Welfare) and how both feed into the larger system of education. She emphasizes diversity; though certain trends are common amongst preschools, differences in teaching styles and philosophies are plentiful as well.

7. According to Rohlen (1989), families are incapable of indoctrinating the child into this social pattern of *shūndan-seikatsu* by their very structure and particularly by the relationship (of indulgence and dependence) between mother and child. For this reason and the importance placed on group structures in Japan, the nursery school's primary objective, argues Rohlen, is teaching children how to assimilate into groups. For further discussion of this point see also Peak 1989; Lewis 1989; Sano 1989; and the *Journal of Japanese Studies* issue [15(1)] devoted to Japanese preschool education in which these articles, including Boocock's, are published.

8. For a succinct anthropological discussion of these concepts, see Hendry (1987: 39–41). For an architectural study of Japan's management and organization of space in terms of such cultural categories as *uchi* and *soto*, see Greenbie (1988).

9. Endless studies, reports, surveys, and narratives document the close tie between women and home; domesticity and femininity in Japan. A recent international survey conducted for a Japanese housing construction firm, for example, polled couples with working wives in three cities, finding that 97% (of those polled) in Tokyo prepared breakfast for their families almost daily (compared with 43% in New York and 34% in London); 70% shopped for groceries on a daily basis (3% in New York, 14% in London), and that only 22% of them had husbands who assisted or were willing to assist with housework (62% in New York, 77% in London) (quoted in *Chicago Tribune* 1991). For a recent anthropological study of Japanese housewives in English, see Imamura (1987). Japanese sources include *Juristo zōkan sōgō tokushu* 1985; *Mirai shakan* 1979; *Ohirasōri no seifu kenkyūkai* 3.

10. My comments pertain directly, of course, to only the women I observed, interviewed, and interacted with at the one private nursery school serving middle-class families in urban Tokyo. The profusion of *obentō*-related materials in the press plus the revelations made to me by Japanese and observations made by other researchers in Japan (for example. Tobin 1989; Fallows 1990), however, substantiate this as a more general phenomenon.

11. To illustrate this preoccupation and consciousness: during the time my son was not eating all his *obentō* many fellow mothers gave me suggestions, one mother lent me a magazine, his teacher gave me a full set of *obentō* cookbooks (one per season), and another mother gave me a set of small frozen food portions she had made in advance for future *obentōs*.

12. My son's teacher, Hamada-sensei, cited this explicitly as one of the reasons why the *obentō* was such an important training device for nursery school children. "Once they become *ichinensei* (first-graders) they'll be faced with a variety of food, prepared without elaboration or much spice, and will need to eat it within a delimited time period."

13. An anonymous reviewer questioned whether such emphasis placed on consumption of food in nursery school leads to food problems and anxieties in later years. Although I have heard that anorexia is a phenomenon now in Japan, I question its connection to nursery school *obentōs*. Much of the meaning of the latter practice, as I interpret it, has to do with the interface between production and consumption, and its gender linkage comes from the production end (mothers making it) rather than the consumption end (children eating it). Hence while control is taught through food, it is not a control linked primarily to females or bodily appearance, as anorexia may tend to be in this culture.

14. Fujita argues, from her experience as a working mother of a daycare (*hoikuen*) child, that the substance of these daily talks between teacher and mother is intentionally insignificant. Her interpretation is that the mother is not to be overly involved in nor too informed about matters of the school (1989).

15. "*Boku*" is a personal pronoun that males in Japan use as a familiar reference to themselves. Those in close relationships with males—mothers and wives, for example—can use *boku* to refer to their sons or husbands. Its use in this context is telling.

16. In the upper third grade of the nursery school (*nenchō* class; children aged five to six) my son attended, children were ordered to bring their *obentō* with chopsticks and not forks and spoons (considered easier to use) and in the traditional *furoshiki* (piece of cloth which enwraps items and is double tied to close it) instead of the easier-to-manage *obentō* bags with drawstrings. Both *furoshiki* and chopsticks (*o-hashi*) are considered traditionally Japanese and their usage marks not only greater effort and skills on the part of the children but their enculturation into being Japanese.

17. For the mother's role in the education of her child, see, for example, White (1987). For an analysis, by a Japanese, of the intense dependence on the mother that is created and cultivated in a child, see Doi (1971). For Japanese sources on the mother-child relationship and the ideology (some say pathology) of Japanese motherhood, see Yamamura (1971); Kawai (1976); Kyūtoku (1981); *Sorifu seihonen taisaku honbuhen* (1981); *Kadeshobo shinsha* (1981). Fujita's account of the ideology of motherhood at the nursery school level is particularly interesting in this connection (1989).

18. Women are entering the labor market in increasing numbers yet the proportion to do so in the capacity of part-time workers (legally constituting as much as thirty-five hours per week but without the benefits accorded to full-time workers) has also increased. The choice of part-time over full-time employment has much to do with a woman's simultaneous and almost total responsibility for the domestic realm (Juristo 1985; see also Kondo 1990).

19. As Fujita (1989: 72–79) points out, working mothers are treated as a separate category of mothers, and non-working mothers are expected, by definition, to be mothers full time.

20. Nakane's much quoted text on Japanese society states this male position in structuralist terms (1970). Though dated, see also Vogel (1963) and Rohlen (1974) for descriptions of the social roles for middle-class, urban Japanese males. For a succinct recent discussion of gender roles within the family, see Lock (1990).

References

Althusser, Louis. 1971. *Ideology and ideological state apparatuses (Notes toward an investigation in Lenin and philosophy and other essays)*. New York: Monthly Review.

Asanuma, Kaoru. 1987. *"Ganbari" no kozo (Structure of "Ganbari")*. Tokyo: Kikkawa Kobunkan.

Barthes, Roland. 1957. *Mythologies*. Trans. by Annette Lavers. New York Noonday Press.

Boocock, Sarane Spence. 1989. Controlled diversity: An overview of the Japanese preschool system. *The Journal of Japanese Studies* 15(1): 41–65.

Chicago Tribune. 1991. Burdens of working wives weigh heavily in Japan. January 27, Section 6. p. 7.

Cummings, William K. 1980. *Education and equality in Japan*. Princeton NJ: Princeton University Press.

Doi, Takeo. 1971. *The anatomy of dependence: The key analysis of Japanese behavior*. Trans. by John Becker. Tokyo: Kodansha Int'l. Ltd.

Dore, Ronald P. 1965. *Education in Tokugawa Japan*. London: Routledge and Kegan Paul.

Duke, Benjamin. 1986. *The Japanese school: Lessons for industrial America*. New York: Praeger.

Fallows, Deborah. 1990. Japanese women. *National Geographic* 177(4): 52–83.

Fujita, Mariko. 1989. "It's all mother's fault": Childcare and the socialization of working mothers in Japan. *The Journal of Japanese Studies* 15(1): 67–91.

Greenbie, Barrie B. 1988. *Space and spirit in modern Japan*. New Haven CT: Yale University Press.

Hendry, Joy. 1986. *Becoming Japanese: The world of the preschool child*. Honolulu: University of Hawaii Press.

———. 1987. *Understanding Japanese society*. London: Croom Helm.

Horio, Teruhisa. 1988. *Educational thought and ideology in modern Japan: State authority and intellectual freedom*. Trans. by Steven Platzer. Tokyo: University of Tokyo Press.

Imamura. Anne E. 1987. *Urban Japanese housewives: At home and in the community*. Honolulu: University of Hawaii Press.

Juristo zōkan Sōgōtokushu. 1985. Josei no Gensai to Mirai (The present and future of women). 39.

Kadeshobo shinsha. 1981. *Hahaoya (Mother)*. Tokyo: Kadeshobo shinsha.

Kawai, Hayao. 1976. *Bosei shakai nihon no Byōri (The pathology of the mother society—Japan)*. Tokyo: Chūō koronsha.

Kondo, Dorinne K. 1990. *Crafting selves: Power, gender, and discourses of identity in a Japanese workplace*. Chicago IL: University of Chicago Press.

Kyūtoku, Shigemori. 1981. *Bogenbyō (Disease rooted in motherhood)*. Vol. II. Tokyo: Sanma Kushuppan.

Lewis, Catherine C. 1989. From indulgence to internalization: Social control in the early school years. *Journal of Japanese Studies* 15(1): 139–157.

Lock, Margaret. 1990. Restoring order to the house of Japan. *The Wilson Quarterly* 14(4): 42–49.

Marx, Karl and Frederick Engels. 1970 (1947). *Economic and philosophic manuscripts*, ed. C.J. Arthur. New York: International Publishers.

Mirai shakan. 1979. Shufu to onna (Housewives and women). Kunitachishi Komininkan Shimindaigaku Semina - no Kiroku. Tokyo: Miraisha.

Mouer, Ross and Yoshio Sugimoto. 1986. *Images of Japanese society: A study in the social construction of reality*. London: Routledge and Kegan.

Nakane, Chie. 1970. *Japanese society*. Berkeley: University of California Press.

Ohirasōri no Seifu kenkyūkai. 1980. Katei kiban no jujitsu (The fullness of family foundations). (Ohirasōri no Seifu kenkyūkai - 3). Tokyo: Okurashō Insatsukyōku.

Peak, Lois. 1989. Learning to become part of the group: The Japanese child's transition to preschool life. *The Journal of Japanese Studies* 15(1): 93–123.

Richie, Donald. 1985. *A taste of Japan: food fact and fable, customs and etiquette, what the people eat*. Tokyo: Kodansha International Ltd.

Rohlen, Thomas P. 1974. *The harmony and strength: Japanese white-collar organization in anthropological perspective*. Berkeley: University of California Press.

———. 1983. *Japan's high schools*. Berkeley: University of California Press.

———. 1989. Order in Japanese society: attachment, authority, and routine. *The Journal of Japanese Studies* 15(1): 5–40.

Sano, Toshiyuki. 1989. Methods of social control and socialization in Japanese day-care centers. *The Journal of Japanese Studies* 15(1): 125–138.

Shufunotomo Besutoserekushon shiri-zu. 1980. Obentō 500 sen. Tokyo: Shufunotomo Co., Ltd.

Shufunotomohyakka shiri-zu. 1981. 365 nichi no obentō hyakka. Tokyo: Shufunotomo Co.

Sōrifu Seihonen Taisaku Honbuhen. 1981. Nihon no kodomo to hahaoya (Japanese mothers and children): kokusaihikaku (international comparisons). Tokyo: Sōrifu Seishonen Taisaku Honbuhen.

Tobin, Joseph J., David Y.H. Wu, and Dana H. Davidson. 1989. *Preschool in three cultures: Japan, China, and the United States*. New Haven CT: Yale University Press.

Vogel, Erza. 1963. *Japan's new middle class: The salary man and his family in a Tokyo suburb*. Berkeley: University of California Press.

White, Merry. 1987. *The Japanese educational challenge: a commitment to children*. New York: Free Press.

Yamamura, Yoshiaki. 1971. *Nihonjin to haha: Bunka toshite no haha no kannen ni tsuite no kenkyu (The Japanese and mother: Research on the conceptualization of mother as culture)*. Tokyo: Toyo-shuppansha.

CHAPTER 23

Techne versus Technoscience: Divergent (and Ambiguous) Notions of Food "Quality" in the French Debate over GM Crops

Chaia Heller

(2007)

With the rise of industrial agriculture and the agrofoods industry in postwar France, there has been a gradual, steady explosion of discourse regarding food quality. Debates about food safety gained steam in the 1970s, along with discussions regarding impacts of the industrial model on the vitality of the French countryside, a zone that constitutes a cultural lifeway, an arena of artisanal production, and a profitable national tourist commodity (Mendras 1976). In turn, the rise of processed, "fast," or mass-produced foods in France sparked discussions regarding a national loss of "taste" and "culture" and a general decline in French food "quality."

Drawing from ethnographic research, I explore the ways in which the Confédération Paysanne (CP), France's second largest agricultural union of family farmers, invokes notions of French food quality as part of their campaign against genetically modified organisms (GMOs).[1] In particular, I examine the ways in which CP farmers, marginalized from industrial agriculture, are becoming key actors in reconfiguring new understandings of food quality, establishing themselves as a potent symbol of agricultural technes, or artisanal food production.

In exploring the French food quality debate, I examine a series of foundational binaries that circulate through actors' narratives about GM foods. First, the nature–culture binary—a dichotomy studied critically by a range of social theorists in recent decades (Bookchin 1982; Haraway 1991; Palsson and Rabinow 1999; Rabinow 1996b; Strathern 1980)—represents a central heuristic through which actors structure their discourses about food quality. As I illustrate, however, this nature–culture binary is shot through with broader discourses of denaturalization and deculturalization, which are associated in turn with ideas of technoscience and globalization.

For instance, actors in the global GMO debate often discuss GM food's lack of "naturalness," based on what Donna Haraway (1997) describes as a perceived transgression of natural orders or laws. In contrast, actors in the French case may discuss GM food's lack of "culturalness" or a GMO's rupture with artisanal food production. The French case then gives rise to yet another binary, that between *techne* and *technoscience*: an opposition of artisanal technes of production as compared to foods associated with technoscience-driven industrial agriculture. In this way, the GMO debate pivots around three binaries: nature versus culture, culture versus nonculture, and techne versus technoscience.

Finally, two poles of "food quality" spin out of these three binaries: techne-driven food quality and technoscience-driven food quality. Proponents of the former call for a more "cultural" definition of *food quality*: one based on adherence to traditional agricultural practices. Promoters of the latter, the technoscience-driven food quality associated with GMOs, may assume a more "technical" definition of *food quality*, a meaning more grounded in quantifiable risks to human health and the environment.

It is useful to note here, that *techne* is derived from the Greek word *technion*, which is associated with the term *craft*. For the ancient Greeks, techne represented art's practical application, as opposed to products of human invention produced through rational domains such as geometry or science. In contemporary philosophy, techne has been used by theorists ranging from Martin Heidegger (1977) to Murray Bookchin (1982) when distinguishing between technique associated with an artistic, rather than a mechanistic, episteme. Techne also echoes with James Scott's discussion of *metis*, which he defines as local "premodern" forms of knowledge and practice often marginalized by modern state and capital formations (Scott 1998).

As I illustrate in what follows, the CP's rejection of GMOs and fast food is predicated on the notion that such foods are the negation of techne-driven food quality, representing instead the embodiment of technoscience-driven food quality. As instances of "nonculture," GMOs are "junk

Chaia Heller, "Techne versus technoscience: divergent (and ambiguous) notions of food 'quality' in the French debate over GM crops." *American Anthropologist* 109 (2007): 603–615. Reprinted with permission.

food" (or what CP farmer José Bové refers to as *la malbouffe*); they are the antithesis of techne-driven food embodied in Roquefort cheese or Champagne.

In France, the natural domain (defined often as that which is "not urban") is often regarded in agricultural rather than wilderness terms; so French nature is tightly fused with notions of culture-as-agriculture. Agricultural technes of production such as Roquefort cheese are thus regarded as "natural-as-agricultural," as opposed to GMOs, which are often perceived as products of an industrially driven technoscience.

After providing a brief history of the problematization of "quality" in France during the postwar period by powerful institutions, I examine these two poles of quality drawn from techne and technoscience. In particular, I examine the prominence of the technoscience definition of *quality* among actors at National Institute of Agricultural Research (the French equivalent of the U.S. Department of Agriculture; hereafter abbreviated from the French as INRA). As I illustrate, such actors tend to invoke primarily technoscience-driven definitions of technical quality to support their claims about food quality.

In the next part of the article, I examine how the CP deploys techne-driven food quality to promote their overall agenda and their anti-GM campaign. First, I explore changes in the union's notions of quality over the past several decades: changes that move from a focus on food production to food consumption. In particular, I examine the ways in which the union struggles to link ideas of food quality with either artisanal techne or technoscience. Second, I examine the CP's anti-GMO campaign, analyzing the cultural place and meaning of the union's discourses of techne-related food quality in the French imagination. I note that, despite the union's ambiguous definition of *food quality*, they successfully designate GMOs as "la malbouffe," or bad-quality food, establishing themselves as protectors of artisanal technes of food quality.

The CP's anti-GMO campaign provides insight into the ways in which controversies over food quality are becoming key sites at which activist institutions attempt to regain power and legitimacy in an economic and agricultural milieu from which they are generally disenfranchised. The CP's story is about how marginalized groups of farmers attempt to define *food quality* in "techne terms" to promote models of agriculture that counter those favored by government and large corporate bodies.

The Problematization of "Quality" in Postwar France

The problematization of French agriculture emerges during a period known as Les Trentes Glorieuses (lit., "The Glorious Thirty"; 1945–75). Paradoxically, just at the time when France found economic prosperity and established itself as an agricultural superpower, significant discussion regarding the quality of French food emerged in tandem.

Les Trentes Glorieuses were at least in part facilitated by the Politique Agricole Commun (Common Agricultural Policy; hereafter, PAC), a European-wide agricultural policy encouraging industrial agriculture by giving greater subsidies to large-scale and intensive producers. French agricultural banks, for instance, favored large-scale and intensive enterprises, excluding small farmers from access to low-interest loans (Blanc 1977). By the early 1960s, France had morphed into a heavily subsidized, export-oriented agricultural economy that favored an intensive, chemicalized agricultural apparatus while also promoting a growing agrofoods and fast foods industry (Chavagne 1988).

After resolving its initial problems of production by providing its own "primary materials," such as grains, milk, and livestock, French government bodies and industry turned its focus to questions of consumption. During the 1970s, marketing agents and corporations began to promote "value-added" products such as processed and prepackaged foods, while also encouraging a French fast-food industry. As sociologist Rick Fantasia (1995) points out, by the early 1970s, French entrepreneurs were successfully imitating the U.S. fast-food model. By 1989, French (or European) firms or investors owned 80 percent of the 777 fast food hamburger restaurants in France, introducing chains with U.S.-sounding names such as "Crip-Crop," "Dino-Croc," or "Chicken Shop" (Fantasia 2000).

Those changes in food-production systems had been met with concerns raised by various stakeholders in French society. The growing agrofoods industry brought few economic benefits, for instance, to family farmers. For agricultural unions such as the CP, the new industrial system entailed production surpluses—and ensuing price drops—disenfranchising small farmers along the way. Small farmers that survived were often those able to establish a niche for themselves by producing artisanal products (Malassis 1997:18) or by supplementing their incomes with off-farm employment.

By the 1980s, supermarkets (which also emerged during Les Trentes Glorieuses) began to gradually replace the local direct-sale market system that had prevailed before the war. Over the decades, these *hypermarchés* have become flooded with industrially mass-produced wines, cheeses, pâtés, and chicken, not to mention a broader array of frozen, instant, and prepackaged foods. Cheaper, mass-produced versions of traditional products drew consumer attention away from artisanal equivalents as consumers bought their Christmas *pâté de foie gras* in the local hypermarché for less than half price rather than in the local direct-sale market where farmers traditionally sold their products.

As I note below, although the CP's initial concerns about the disenfranchisement of small farmers constitutes the union's main concern, it is the latter concern about an ambiguously defined and techne-driven food "quality" that ends up constituting the cornerstone of the CP's campaign against industrial agriculture and GM technologies.

The 1980s: Problematizing "Quality" by Powerful Institutions

The problematization of French food quality emerged in the 1980s as a technique of governance (Foucault 1991). As Akhil Gupta illustrates in the case of Indian farmers (1998:293), "quality discourse" can become a technology for depoliticizing and normalizing concerns of small farmers (and those of the general public) regarding the social and political consequences of industrial agriculture.

This particular technique of governance constitutes a response by powerful institutions to "consumer attitudes" regarding problems associated with industrial agriculture—problems that came to a head in the early to mid-1990s (Heller 2006). The Bovine Spongiform Encephalopathy (BSE, or "mad cow disease") scandal that began in 1994 resulted in a significant drop in French beef sales. Subsequently, French consumer magazines and advocates began to discuss an increasing public concern for "quality" products, such as "farm products" and organic agriculture (Marris 2001).

Following the BSE scandal and the subsequent controversy in 1997 surrounding GM crops, "quality" became amplified as a concern not only by consumers but also by government actors and French scientists as well. By the early 1990s, discourses about food quality and food-related risk had become a central forum in which to discuss perceived problems associated with productivist agriculture (Levidow 1997), without directly addressing questions of political and economic power, agricultural inequality, and so on (Jasanoff 2005:95).

As Raymond Williams (1976) suggests, historical processes are not merely "reflected" by language but, rather, occur within it. Williams's concept of "keywords" is useful in tracing the term *quality*, which indeed circulated through a variety of domains at this time, forming semantic clusters with terms such as *safety* or *risk* by actors operating within a technoscience idiom, while clustering with terms such as *traditional* or *artisanal* by actors defining quality in techne terms.

During this period, governmental and scientific bodies published literature that called for "quality" as the solution to problems associated with industrial agriculture. For instance, a text published by the French Academy of Agriculture, *Two Centuries of Progress in Agriculture and Food, 1789–1989* (1990), called for France to move from a "technological" or productivist model of agriculture to one concerned with "quality." In 1998, environmental minister Dominique Voynet argued for "quality" in her introduction to the Ministerial Report, *Management of the Territories and the Environment*. According to Voynet, "Food self-sufficiency, the principal goal assigned to the PAC in the fifties and sixties, has been not only achieved, but has been surpassed" (1998:14). In light of this achievement, Voynet called for farmers to protect the "vitality of the territory" by promoting ecological agricultural techniques and focusing on "products of *le terroir* and quality labels" (Voynet 1998:8). Guy Paillotin, president of INRA, echoed Voynet

in his opus, *Tais-toi et mange!* (*Shut Up and Eat!* [1999]). Paillotin posited that agriculture can find a new opportunity in "this era of over-production" by "privileging quality and diversity of products that express the particular richness of a *terroir* (or a particular agricultural zone)" (Paillotin 1999:14).

As a technology of governance, "quality" discourse draws attention away from political concerns such as the material and cultural conditions of small farmers disenfranchised from the system. Paillotin, Voynet, and other powerful actors focus instead on "quality," on establishing new agricultural zones for "controlled label status," and on endorsing the creation of new *signes de qualité* (quality labels), such as *produit fermier* (farm product) and *label rouge* (red label associated with items of superior production). Calls for small farmers to become protectors of quality products of le terroir serve as distractions from (and compensation for) the political and economic disenfranchisement of small farmers in the postwar period, normalizing their increasingly marginal status.

Techne and Technoscience: Ambiguities of Food "Quality" at INRA

Discourses of food quality are highly context specific. Indeed, for some actors, ideas of food quality derive from agricultural technoscience as the quality of a product is cast in quantitative terms—specifically, in measurable environmental or health risks associated with particular agricultural practices. For other actors, food quality implies techne-driven quality, product quality defined in relation to the scale of production or the degree to which a product has been traditionally cultivated by drawing from local savoir faire.

Technoscientific discourses about food quality often embody an instrumental rationality, one that normalizes productivist agriculture, for instance, by evaluating it in terms of "calculable" environmental and health risks alone (Heller 2001a), rather than production scale or process (see Table 1). In contrast, discourses about techne-driven food quality often reflect a systemic disenchantment with the instrumental rationality embedded in productivist agriculture itself, promoting a model scaled to support the cultural identities and artisanal practices of small farmers.

During my research stay in France, I interviewed over 50 actors at INRA–Versailles (a research station located

Table 1 Comparison of Techne Versus Technoscientific Notions of Quality.

Techne-driven food "quality"	Technoscience-driven food "quality"
cultural, qualitative rationality quality of life for producers savoir-faire embedded in production process	instrumental, calculative rationality product safety for consumers managed risk of production process

just outside of Paris) who were engaged in various aspects of producing *plants transgéniques* (transgenic plants). Interviewees ranged from postdoctoral students to high-ranking directors of research. By casting food quality in technical terms of health and environmental risk or "safety," INRA actors tended to eclipse issues of culture or quality of life associated with the agriculture production process itself. A technoscience-driven notion of food quality fails to address a productivist rationality of industrial agriculture that has historically disenfranchised small farmers, leading to problems of overproduction and price drops. Instead, INRA actors promoted environmentally friendly forms of productivist agriculture, or a GM agriculture, and new "quality" food labels that appealed to consumers' desires for techne-driven quality.

At INRA, discourses about food quality were couched within a technoscience idiom. For instance, the key INRA publication on GMOs, "Transgenic Plants in Agriculture" (Khan 1996), addresses questions of quality in terms of environmental or health risks associated with particular applications of GM technologies. In a section on "Food Quality," the publication discusses the importance of creating "quality" GM products by assessing and monitoring the potential risks by appealing to technoscience:

> An essential question concerns the consequences of genetic transformation on the quality of food destined for human consumption....In the case where products are not the equivalent of traditional products, control mechanisms used in all industrialized countries will carefully examine the potential risks. [INRA 1998:15]

Indeed, on-the-ground interviews with most INRA actors engaged in GM-related plant research revealed a profound preoccupation with the theme of technoscience-driven quality. In nearly every interview or discussion dealing with GMOs, INRA actors equated food quality with food safety, describing a French public that had recently decided that their agriculture had become industrialized and unsafe.

It is crucial to note, however, that INRA actors' narratives were far from monolithic. Instead, their "personal," "off-the-record," and "nonscientific" understandings of food quality were often identical to those of their non-scientific counterparts. For instance, when speaking as "scientists," INRA actors would often assume a technical definition of *quality*. When speaking "personally" as a "gourmand," or when simply chatting over an informal lunch, actors would often switch discursive registers. Reminding me often about U.S. citizens' "lack of food culture," actors would discuss the robustness of French food quality associated with technes of artisanal production. I refer to this discursive switching as "discursive compartmentalization" (Heller 2004), a phenomenon in which actors change discursive frames according to the specific position of cultural expertise from which they are speaking at a particular time.

Indeed, when speaking "as scientists," many INRA actors' narratives would begin with a discussion of the publics' questioning of industrial agriculture (and of GMOs), locating this problem within a context of overproduction: a context in which the public can "afford" to demand fewer food-related risks. For INRA director of science research, Roger D., the GMO debate emerges out of a postscarcity situation in which consumers no longer accept a "risky" productivist agriculture:

> And so now, consumers are demanding to know what is on their plates....Now the French consumer has had enough of the risks. They want to know what is on their plates. They want a quality product. And the issue of GMOs finds itself within this debate. [Roger D., personal communication, February 12, 1998]

In a conversation with an INRA postdoctorate researcher, Sylvie M., she shifted focus to considering how issues of quality and environmental protection can solve problems of technical quality associated with overproduction:

> We already have too much food. We have stocks and stocks of wheat. I think it should be about producing better, not more. We should be producing better quality, using less pesticides, for instance. I think it's good for researchers to be looking into environmental problems. [Sylvie M., personal communication, March 2, 1998]

In many narratives, actors discuss INRA's shift from an emphasis on "quantity" to one of "quality." For INRA research director, Edouard L., "quality" is the solution to public concern with problems of food safety, environmental pollution, and overproduction associated with intensive agriculture:

> Due to mad cow, citizens are asking where agriculture is going. They are concerned about pollution and problems of overproduction, about a loss of quality. And so now, INRA does more research and sells their findings, about how to improve quality. That's the new focus here. [Edouard L., personal communication, April 4, 1999]

Although most INRA actors discuss INRA's intention to produce better technoscience-driven quality, there were some who expressed a desire to improve the techne-driven quality of products by encouraging small farmers to produce artisanal "quality products." Yet discussions of artisanal quality tend to be highly instrumentalized, framed in terms of product profitability. Here Henri P. (an INRA environmental expert) infuses a discourse about techne-driven quality with an economistic discourse about the potential profitability of producing farm-made products with added value:

> At INRA, we're saying that there should be agriculture of quality. For instance, you make more money from producing pâté de foie gras than you do by simply raising a duck. The same goes for wine or cheese. When you eat a preprepared meal, for instance, you are paying Danone not for the basic food product, but for the packaging, the advertising, transport, etc. With foie gras, you are paying for the work of the farmer. [Henri P., personal communication, May 21, 1999]

Before concluding my discussion of INRA actors, it is worth adding that the concept of the "GMO" was at the time a relatively new cultural entity in the scientific world. Although most INRA actors had recently become accustomed to discussing GMOs and food quality with reporters and in other public forums, most reported that they had been drawn into a foreign debate with which they had nothing to do. Despite the fact that they had become cultural symbols of GMOs in the French media, INRA scientists generally felt misunderstood, wrongly accused, and generally confused by the commotion. One day over lunch, Henri P. articulated the sentiments of many:

> We had never even heard of a "GMO" until reporters started coming in here to ask us about them. The Confédération Paysanne, they think we make "GMOs." I have always worked on transgenic plants that have nothing to do with food at all. Why are they (the reporters and farmers) accusing us? All I do is work on understanding the genetic structure of a plant, understanding specific genetic mutations. They blame us because they have nowhere else to go. Why don't they ask American companies that actually produce them! [Henri P., personal communication, April 18, 1999]

Indeed, many at INRA–Versailles utilized transgenic methods in researching the plant model *Arabidopsis*, a scientifically useful plant owing to its relatively simple genetic structure. I met no one at INRA who was conducting research or development on genetically engineered food such as corn, soy, or canola (the crops on which the controversy was based) per se.

THE CONFÉDÉRATION PAYSANNE: *AGRICULTURE PAYSANNE* AND (AMBIGUOUS) NOTIONS OF FOOD QUALITY

As we have seen, problematizing food quality is a technique of governance, a means by which powerful institutions problematize, normalize, and depoliticize social and political issues associated with industrial agriculture. In what follows, I illustrate the ways in which the CP deploys discourses of food quality as a technique of resistance, a means by which the union asserts the legitimacy of small-scale agriculture within an agricultural system dominated by large-scale intensive producers.

The CP was formed in 1987 by a network of family farmers across France who had been disenfranchised from the industrial agricultural model promoted by the French and European subsidy and loan system. Reclaiming the pejorative or "backward" term *paysan*, peasant, the CP redefined the paysan as a worker-identified farmer standing in solidarity with international peasant and indigenous groups struggling to protect traditional lifeways affected by both industrial agriculture and the governmental policies that promote it (Heller 2005).

While positioning itself in relation to large-scale agricultural production on a national level, the CP also has an international scope and vision. The CP was key in founding the European Peasant Coordination and Via Campesina, two NGOs that are cornerstones of the wider international antiglobalization movement that focuses on the rights of peasants and indigenous people internationally.

Shifting from "Quality of Life" for Producers to "Quality Foods" for Consumers

The CP underwent a primary shift in recent decades regarding their discourses of food quality. Beginning in the late 1980s and early 1990s, the CP moved away from a production-centered discourse that emphasized the farmer's right to production and to a "quality of life." In this shift, they adopted a more consumer-oriented food discourse: one that emphasized the consumers' demand for "quality" food. In adopting a consumer-oriented discourse, the union adopted an increasingly ambiguous definition of *food quality*, one that equivocates between notions of agricultural techne and technoscience.

To examine this shift, I first explore the union's initial emphasis on production, and the accompanying demand for "quality of life" for small producers living in rural areas. When first founded in 1987, the Marxist-oriented CP demanded for paysans the same right to produce as other laboring societal sectors (Heller 2001a). Their ongoing focus on production scale (a demand that farm subsidies be distributed among the greatest number of small farms, rather than among fewer large farms) reflects their belief that agriculture and rural life should constitute a quality of life available to the greatest number of French citizens (Aubineau 1997). Currently, this lifeway is inaccessible to most paysan families, as over 50 percent of spouses living on family farms are obliged to work part time, off the farm, in factories, transportation, retail, and so on. In such cases, one full-time worker can "afford" to be employed on the family farm (Dufour, personal communication, October 12, 1998).

Questions of production scale and quality of life for farmers are central to CP discourse. At any CP action, demonstrators may be found singing, "Trois petites fermes, c'est mieux qu'une grande," which translates to "three little farms are better than a big one," was the CP's anthem in the late 1980s, and is still sung during CP actions addressing problems related to French and European agricultural policy. However, by the early to mid-1990s, the union began to shift from a primary emphasis on production scale and quality of life for producers toward the adoption of a more consumer-oriented discourse.

Seeking alliances with consumers' associations and government bodies intent on shaping consumer behavior amidst various food controversies, the CP was determined to establish for itself a distinctive niche within the broader productivist landscape: a niche that France's largest productivist agricultural union, the FNSEA (National Federation of Agricultural Enterprises), could not hope to occupy.

Note that this discursive shift in emphasis (from production to consumption) is implicit, rather than openly discussed within the CP. At no time during my research did actors ever discuss the union's increasing focus on consumer-related food quality. When questioned about this rhetorical shift, many key CP actors appeared perplexed or even slightly amused by the observation.

As early as the 1970s (previous to the founding of the CP), French family farmers in various movements tried to encourage consumers' associations to broaden their understanding of quality to include questions of production scale and to define quality foods as not only technically "safe" but also as promoting the livelihood of small farmers. As CP farmer Jean Caberet explains, 1970 was a pivotal year for family farmers struggling to position themselves in relation to consumer organizations and in relation to risk-oriented technoscience-driven quality:

> In 1970, the UFC did a boycott on chicken and veal (due to hormones used in the production process) and this hurt paysans a great deal. Prices fell. And so paysans became very sensitive to problems of quality. You see, since the 1960s, we were told to produce and produce, without thinking about quality. And in the end, prices fell, and consumers were not happy with the quality. And so we had to rethink productivism and quality. And we also learned that we had to work with consumers, to make sure our actions supported each other. [Jean Caberet, interview, February 9, 1999]

The CP struggles to define *quality* in a way that aligns the interests of paysans and consumers. In May of 1999, at a conference about GM-related agriculture and health sponsored by Stop! A la PAC Folle (the words *PAC Folle* is a play on the term *Vache Folle*, or "mad cow"), there was a clash between production and consumer-oriented framings of "quality." Below, Pierre-Andre Deplaude (CP national secretary) and Marie-José Nicoli (president of the Union Fédérale des Consommateurs, France's largest consumers' union) present a production versus consumer approach to quality:

DEPLAUDE: We want all paysans to be able to produce quality products, but we also want to be able to generate employment for paysans as well. We cannot forget this. You could have industrial agriculture produce quality products as well. But this is not at all what we seek.

NICOLI: We are not necessarily opposed to an intensive agriculture. We just want to have diversity and quality. The issue is health safety for everyone. Consumers shouldn't have to worry about whether they are going to be allergic to their food or whether they will become resistant to antibiotics. As consumers, we want it all!...I'm sorry, but paysan products are just too expensive, Sir! We want a diversity of choices, we want safe products, affordable products.

DEPLAUDE: You have to understand that there is a problem of unemployment among paysans. That

paysans are disappearing. No one talks about this. Agriculture loses four times as many jobs a year than any other profession. Madame Nicoli, I find your position toward GMOs to be contradictory. We must be critical of industrialized agriculture. We must be sensitive to the death of the paysan. [Field notes, May 7, 1999]

By invoking a rationality of solidarity-based production, Deplaude calls for consumers' associations such as the UFC to incorporate discourses of production scale into their notion of quality in support of small farmers. Nicoli responds by invoking a technoscience-driven notion of quality, drawing on instrumental and economistic rationality of individual choice. For Nicoli, the scale of production is irrelevant to matters of food quality. Instead, a quality product is one that prioritizes issues of product safety, rather than paysan *solidarité*.

To address these conflicts, the CP initiated in 1992 an alliance between paysans, consumers' associations, and ecology groups called "l'Alliance Paysan, Écologistes, et Consommateurs." According to CP organizer Jean-Damien Therreux, who heads up the GMO campaign, the Alliance came out of a desire to foster solidarity between groups addressing issues of food and agriculture:

> In 1992, we created the Alliance, along with other groups. We did it to try to circulate other discourses, to show that it's important to promote good quality as well as good prices. Consumers and environmentalists don't know that much about agricultural policy, they don't really understand what productivist agriculture is. They don't understand how it affects paysans as well as product quality. [Therreux, personal communication, October 11, 1999]

Defining *quality* in a consumer-driven market is not an easy proposition. For the CP to gain the support of consumers' organizations, they must convince consumers that paysans can produce affordable products comparable to those produced by heavily subsidized industrial farmers: the same farmers that have put them out of business because of their ability to produce more for less. At the same time, the CP must present itself as producing a distinctive product, one different from the one produced by FNSEA industrial farmers. In so doing, they must equate industrial food production with low food quality. Although a tempting strategy, most CP farmers are well aware, as Deplaude admits above, that industrial farmers could indeed mass-produce "quality" products—if indeed it is technoscience, rather than technes of production, that define *food quality*.

Agriculture Paysanne: CP Understandings of Food Quality

By 1999, the CP considered how best to publicly assert CP product quality within the consumer milieu. Internal discussions had emerged within the union about the possibility of establishing a French food quality label (*signe de qualité*) specifically for CP products: one that would be distinguishable from organic labels and from "sustainable agriculture" (an idea many CP actors associate with Britain and northern Europe). This reliance on *signes de qualité*—such as the *appellation d'origine controllé* ("term of controlled origin," established in 1919)—has long been a strategy by which French farmers have been able to both reify and secure agricultural products and markets by establishing an almost primordial link between product and *terroir*, a term that refers to a specialized agricultural region such as Champagne (Ulin 1997).

This CP label would be anchored in the union's central platform, Agriculture Paysanne (AP). The AP platform made its first debut in 1987 at the CP's founding meeting in Rennes. AP constituted a system of worker-identified small farmers expressing solidarity with sustaining the lifeways of small farmers. Over the next decade, the CP further refined AP, presenting in 1998 the Charter for Agriculture Paysanne That Respect the Farmer while Meeting Societal Needs to CP membership (see Bové and Dufour 2001:204). AP promotes the CP's agricultural model as a global alternative to industrial and intensive farming models within the context of PAC and policies related to the General Agreement on Terrifs and Trade (GATT).

AP thus defines the criteria associated with CP food production that, presumably, would be incorporated into a CP food label. To understand the potential meaning of such a label, it may be useful to briefly explore the ten key principles that comprise the AP platform. These principles present a distinct divergence from other anti-industrial agricultural discourses—such as sustainable or organic agriculture—that generally define *food quality* by invoking technoscientific ideas of toxicity, chemicalized artificiality, or the inverse, naturalness.

The Ten Principles of Paysan Agriculture:

1. production and distribution that allow for the greatest number of farmers to earn a viable income;
2. solidarity with farmers in Europe and the rest of the world;
3. respect for nature that will ensure its use by future generations;
4. diligent use of rare resources;
5. transparency in all relations of purchasing, production, processing, and sale of agricultural produce;
6. ensuring the good quality, taste, and safety of all produce;
7. maximum autonomy for farmers;
8. partnership with other sectors living in rural areas;
9. maintenance of the diversity of animals, plants, and land for both their historic and economic value; and
10. remaining conscious of the long-term and global context.

—BOVÉ AND DUFOUR 2001

AP departs from sustainable and organic agriculture discourses by emphasizing the idea of production scale rather than production methods: for instance, sustainable methods are generally regarded as those utilizing techniques that cause the least physical harm to present and future lands, waterways, workers, and so on. For the CP, the question of scale is a social, rather than primarily technoscientific or environmental, concept, reflecting a form of social solidarity, a collective concern to increase the overall number of farmers employable within a given region.

Significantly, the idea of "organic agriculture" is not a necessary component of AP. Once again, the CP represents a sharp departure from small farmer movements in northern Europe, Great Britain, or the United States, which tend to identify with organic agriculture as the primary alternative to industrial farming. In fact, only a minority of CP farmers utilize organic farming methods. Although many regard "organics" as too expensive and impractical, others choose to focus their energy on reinvigorating a rural world around a small-scale model.

AP also diverges from sustainable and organic agriculture discourses in its understanding of "nature." Out of the ten AP principles, only one makes explicit reference to "nature," positing it as integral to the agricultural context, rather than standing in inherent opposition to it (see principle 3). The other more indirect reference (principle 9) represents a call to maintain diversity of animal and plant species for distinctly social reasons ("historic and economic value").

Yet although "nature" is not central to AP discourse, the way CP actors portray "nature" is of tremendous political significance, as they invoke keywords such as *nature, rare resources*, and *diversity* (see principles 3, 4, and 9), terms that became increasingly salient in Europe during the 1990s. In light of new European discourses on environment and nature, CP farmers refer to the "diversification" of rural areas through European and French agricultural policy as "multifunctionality," the elaboration of paysan tasks beyond the primary activity of production.

Agricultural multifunctionality implies several things. First, it suggests technes of production, the idea of adding value to farm products such as milk or meat by producing artisanal cheeses, meats, and pâtés. Second, *multifunctionality* entails ideas of rural restoration and maintenance subsidized by the European Union. The inclusion of these environmentally oriented keywords into the ten principles of agriculture paysanne signals the CP's attempt to establish itself as a powerful conduit of national and European agricultural policy.

Protecting the French landscape (in addition to maintaining the quality of French food), then, becomes a central component of CP policy. In addition, the union takes up keywords such as *transparency* (found in principle 5), terms often found in politicized circles. By the 1990s, the term *transparency* (clustered together with other words such as *quality* and *safety*) had become a keyword in governmental, consumer, scientific, and corporate circles during the food scares associated with productivist agriculture. These crises began in the 1970s with the first hormone-treated veal affair and continue today in the furor over hormone-treated beef, mad cow disease, and GMOs. The CP incorporates transparency into their ten key principles and includes the term in their substantial consumer-oriented discourse used in general communications with the press.

Notions of multifunctionality signal the CP's move away from its initial focus on production and fair wages. In the AP charter, a section entitled "Farming to Serve Society" concludes with a telling statement:

> To respond to the needs (of society), farming produces two types of goods: commercial goods (foodstuffs) and non-commercial goods (environment, landscape). [Confédération Paysanne 1998]

Thus, among the many goals of the CP, at least three are quite apparent. In addition to seeking employment for small farmers and producing "quality" foods appealing to consumers, the CP seeks to engage in landscape preservation.

For many CP farmers, multifunctionality represents a necessary means of economic survival. CP literature thus frames multifunctionality optimistically, portraying it as a form of land-based stewardship. Other CP members, however, share a more pessimistic view of multifunctionality. Former CP national secretary Réné Riesel, in particular, spoke candidly about multifunctionality as entailing paysans beginning to "play the multifunctionality game by becoming gardeners rather than farmers... becoming little show pieces in the countryside, becoming 'museumified' " (Reisel, interview, March 3, 1999).

The CP's choice to become multifunctional in regards to food production and landscape preservation represents another shift in union discourse away from a production-centered discourse that privileged the quality of life of the small farmer who earns a fair wage by producing food exclusively. We can best observe this shift in emphasis by examining an excerpt from the 1989 version of the AP charter. Here, CP actors describe agriculture in philosophical terms (as a pleasurable lifeworld) rather than as a multitasking strategy that obliges farmers to navigate their way through supranational subsidy bodies:

> That work be pleasurable is perhaps the "most" important thing. Economics and productivity are meaningless if working conditions are physically or psychologically painful. Quality of life means choosing to value life, it's a balance between work, leisure, culture, and engagement in the world. [Confédération Paysanne 1998:9]

In the above passage, the CP articulates a particular rationality of agricultural production: that agriculture is not simply a technical means of production but a quality of life in itself. The CP's original emphasis on production scale stemmed, at least in part, from the fact that it would allow the greatest number in rural areas to enjoy a pleasurable quality of rural life.

Ambiguous "Quality": Production Scale or Method?

Of all CP discourses, those regarding quality are perhaps the most ambiguous and contradictory. Although the CP attempts to establish itself as a key expert on food quality when among powerful institutions, its notion of "quality" is not defined in technical, artisanal, or organic terms. The contradictions found in discourses about scale and method among various CP actors—and between public CP policy and private CP practice—appear to be implicit ones. I rarely, if ever, heard a CP actor point to or reflect on the ambiguity of the term *quality* and its equally ambiguous criteria based on agricultural scale or method.

CP discourse embodies an unarticulated tension between the following: (1) questions of agricultural method (i.e., utilization of chemicalized or organic methods and degree of agricultural intensity such as the number of animals being raised on a given plot of land); (2) questions of production scale (the actual size of the plot of land being used in agricultural production); and (3) the relationship between these two and the broader issue of food quality.

Although CP literature often suggests a necessary link among these elements, many CP farmers note, off the record, that the CP intentionally does not clearly define criteria regarding CP production scales or methods. Whereas some CP farmers own or rent relatively large-scale enterprises (although not comparatively as large as those held by big producers in the FNSEA), many others use chemical inputs and even farm intensively, albeit on relatively smaller plots of land.

This hesitance to determine specific standards for farm scale or method is apparent when reading the ten key AP principles. As many CP farmers suggested to me, this hesitance is because of the union's valorization of inclusivity. By avoiding clear criteria on production scale and method, the CP is able to include a diverse range of small farmers struggling to survive by utilizing a variety of farming strategies.

The union's ambiguous definition of *food* is particularly apparent in a 1998 AP pamphlet. The section entitled "Products of Quality" demonstrates the union's awareness of the word *quality* as a marketing tool, a technoscientific notion of safety, an assertion of cultural discourses surrounding taste, and even a vague assertion regarding production scale and intensity.

> The idea of quality is increasingly used as a marketing tool. Often, it conjures a simplistic idea, image, or guarantee of quality. Without strictly codifying this notion of quality, we assert that it addresses, at the very least, issues of taste and safety. The concern of agriculture paysanne is to promote production systems not on the basis of marketability, but on the basis of safety and taste. The first goal is to eliminate the agricultural causes of certain food dangers, certain food components consumed by the population. The size of the farm, as well as the level of intensity, are directly linked to the product quality. [Confédération Paysanne 1998:8]

Although critiquing marketing agents' instrumental and simplistic use of the term *quality*, the CP itself veers toward making similar assertions. Although positing that production scale and method (intensity) are "directly linked" to food quality, the authors do not determine what those links might be. In this AP charter, the authors fail to identify which scale or methods are to be associated with product safety and taste.

Establishing the value of small-scale farming in a world increasingly dominated by large-scale agribusiness is challenging, particularly when large-scale agribusiness can mimic "alternative" methods such as organic (Pollan 2006) or even artisanal agriculture. As it attempts to assert the distinctiveness of CP food quality, the CP often finds itself on shaky discursive ground.

In the spring of 1999, at a meeting at the CP headquarters in Paris, a group of paysans were discussing the CP food label idea. At one point, one of the national secretaries turned to the rest of the group and said,

> You know, eventually, the big growers and the agrofoods company will create small-scale production lines of artisanal products, or they will produce non-GMO and organic products. Big producers can produce "quality" if they want to. It's just a matter of time. [Field notes, May 20, 1999]

The rest of the group sat quietly for several seconds, shaking their heads in knowing disbelief. Finally, one of the other national secretaries summed it up when he uttered one of my favorite sayings, "N'importe quoi," which in this context meant something like "they'll do anything…anything at all."

Although CP actors use discourse on "quality" to bolster claims about France's need for paysan farmers, the union's discourse is weakest when it attempts to make technical claims about quality related to agricultural methods. As noted below, despite these manifold contradictions, the CP successfully deploys a consumer-oriented discourse on techne-driven quality after 1999, establishing itself as a necessary niche within a broader agricultural landscape dominated by technoscience-driven agribusiness.

THE CP'S ANTI-GMO CAMPAIGN: TECHNE VERSUS TECHNOSCIENCE

By becoming spokespeople for food quality, the CP hopes to establish a legitimate and economically tenable position for family farmers in French society. Toward this effort, the union began in the 1990s to establish themselves as a symbol of artisanal technes of production, presenting themselves to the public as small farmers who produce "value-added" farm-made products. The CP's anti-GMO campaign illustrates the ways in which the union appeals to often ambiguous understandings of food quality in their attempt to establish themselves as key players in international debates about GM foods.

Before exploring the CP's use of ambiguous food quality, I will briefly contextualize the CP's anti-GMO campaign.

Agricultural biotechnology represents a strategy devised by governments and corporations searching for new domains of capital accumulation during the postindustrial years of the early 1970s. Rather than seek primarily to increase agricultural productivity (the main objective of industrial agriculture), agricultural biotechnology seeks to enhance the ability of corporate and government bodies to monopolize seed production (originally the domain of public institutions such as the U.S. Department of Agriculture and small regional seed companies) and to create highly specialized seeds and chemical imputs designed for large-scale agribusiness.

Whereas agricultural biotechnology builds on and retains previous industrial models of intensive large-scale agricultural production, GM technologies are designed as well to benefit large-scale agrochemical and biotechnology industries abandoning Fordist forms of vertical integration for new globalized chains of commodity production (Heller 2001b).

Agricultural biotechnology was first largely developed in the 1980s by small start-up companies in California's Silicon Valley, which were eventually bought up by multinational agrochemical companies such as Monsanto and Novartis (Rabinow 1996a). By the fall of 1996, these multinationals began to export their first generation of GM crops to Europe in the form of GM seeds for cultivation and food products processed primarily with GM soy and corn. As the first shipments of GM products arrived on French soil, French NGOs were already plugged into an international network of anti-GMO activists located in countries including southern India, Europe, the United States, Canada, Australia, Japan, Brazil, and Mexico. Greenpeace-France greeted the first ships carrying GM seeds on shore dressed in white hazard gear, gleaning considerable national press along the way.

The CP formally launched its own anti-GMO campaign in 1997 (Confédération Paysanne 1998). Although their early campaign tended to emphasize issues of food risk, appealing to the authority of science experts (a dominant trend in the overall debate during this period), their later discourse emphasized questions of food quality, drawing from their own forms of cultural expertise (Heller 2001a).

The union's success at establishing themselves as the key spokespeople for the anti-GMO movement in France (and throughout Europe and much of the world) was tied to a series of events surrounding one of the union's key activists, a Roquefort milk supplier from southern France named José Bové. Already known in France as an anti-GMO activist, Bové was arrested in August of 1999 for "dismantling" a McDonald's in the southern town of Millau. The 300 activists that accompanied Bové in prying off signs and tiles at the building site that day were contesting the decision of the WTO to place a hefty surtax on Roquefort cheese, the mainstay of the area's income. According to the CP, this surcharge resulted from U.S. pressure on the WTO to punish Europe for banning U.S. hormone-treated beef (Heller 2001b). Bové rose to stardom when he forfeited bail, choosing instead to remain in prison for three weeks. During his imprisonment, the union stood behind Bové, organizing and galvanizing supporters, as his cause came to symbolize the fight of French food quality against industrial agriculture symbolized by McDonald's, the WTO, and U.S. multinationals such as Monsanto.

Techne-Driven Agriculture and the Rise of La Malbouffe

Bové popularized a unique anti-GMO discourse by linking issues of food quality to perceived problems of globalization. By 1999, Bové had become a key spokesperson for national and international anti-GMO and antiglobalization networks. The centerpiece of his discourse is the term *la malbouffe*, which literally means "bad quality food" and which he equates with GMOs, McDonald's, and all products of industrial and GM agriculture (Heller and Escobar 2003). La malbouffe is the antithesis of an agriculture associated with such artisanal products as Roquefort cheese.

By the end of 1999, la malbouffe constituted what Raymond Williams refers to as a keyword, a potent term found in semantic clusters with other highly salient terms that together do not merely reflect social reality but, rather, constitute new forms of cultural beliefs and practices through their usage (Williams 1976). In June of 2006, a Google search summoned up 34,200 references to *la malbouffe*. A perusal through the virtual pages of la malbouffe–related links shows a panoply of discourses about problems associated with French food quality—all of them traceable to Bové's original narratives about the crisis in French food. The first page, for instance, yields headers such as "la malbouffe dévastatrice" (la malbouffe, the devastator) that address "the link between food security and la malbouffe" and "les méfaits de la malbouffe" (the evil doings of la malbouffe). Such virtual pages often discuss problems related to the quality of French wines and associated issues of maintaining the aesthetic value of French agriculture (Heller 2006).

In addition to its tenure as a media magnet, the term *la malbouffe* has had an impressive activist career as well. In November of 1999, a few months after the McDonald's incident, the CP illegally shipped (at Bové's prodding) 300 kilos of Roquefort from the Papillon Roquefort Company over the border to the Seattle WTO meetings, circumventing Clinton's extra tariff that had raised the price of Roquefort almost threefold (Heller 2004:94).

In each media appearance that week, Bové discussed the need to counter la malbouffe with quality food such as Roquefort. As a producer of ewe's milk for Roquefort cheese, Bové is linked to a particularly potent cultural symbol. As the first French product to achieve controlled origin status (*appellation d'origine controllé*) in 1921, Roquefort embodies artisanal ideas of "le terroir," the distinctive geography of a French region, that, when combined with the traditional savoir faire of the French paysan and artisan, renders products of French high culture such as wines, cheese, or pâtés (Hervieu 1996). To receive controlled origin

status, Champagne can only be produced in Champagne, Bourgogne in Bourgogne, and Roquefort only in one particular arid zone in southern France.

Through the idea of "la malbouffe," Bové both articulates and reconfigures a set of cultural concerns about the survival of technes of agricultural production. *La malbouffe* stands for a perceived placelessness associated with industrial agriculture–associated products such as GMOs as well as "fast" and processed foods. For Bové, the antidote to la malbouffe is a food quality associated with agricultural technes of production deeply rooted in specific times, places, and traditions associated with peasant and indigenous food practice.

The Unique Place of Technes of "Food Quality" in the French Nature–Culture Configuration

To better appreciate the cultural salience of la malbouffe and its meaning within the French GMO food quality controversy, we will now examine the specific place of "culture" and "nature" within French society. In France, the GMO debate is framed in primarily agricultural terms, as paysans constitute the key spokespeople for the cause. In contrast, in countries such as the United States, Australia, and those of the United Kingdom and northern Europe, ecology groups primarily rally the cause. As I note below, the emergence of CP paysans as key symbols for the anti-GMOs movement in France is linked to local understandings of nature, culture, and their relation to food quality discourses (Heller 2006).

GMOs are uniquely located in the French imagination in relation to the nature–culture dichotomy. Although most anti-GMO activists define GMOs as examples as poor food quality, what they mean by *quality* differs in some significant ways. For most northern European (as well as British, U.S., and Australian) anti-GMO activists, GMOs represent poor food quality because they are unnatural. In contrast, for French anti-GMO activists, GMOs are examples of poor food quality (or la malbouffe) because they are noncultural.

Clearly, there is no monolithic "French" understanding of nature and culture. However, in my research with both French paysans and actors involved in a variety of governmental, scientific, consumer, and corporate forums, I uncovered among actors a unique nature–culture configuration that departs from the "classical" Western nature–culture dualism (Strathern 1980).

As Marilyn Strathern illustrates in her canonic work "No Nature, No Culture: The Hagen Case" (1980), the nature–culture dualism represents a distinctive Western way of organizing reality. Drawing from Strathern's crucial insights, I note in my own research that although the nature–culture dualism is indeed a Western construct, it tends to be organized in two primary ways: presocial and social. Whereas many in the West posit "nature" in opposition to "culture," others in the West construct "nature" in more social terms.

In the latter case, nature stands in historical continuity with culture, as the two ideas are linked together in the idea of agriculture. French nature romanticism indeed tends to portray nature as le terroir, a particular agricultural region associated with specific forms of artisanal food production. This social understanding of nature suggests what Neil Smith refers to as the social production of nature (1996:49), the socialization of nature through human activity or labor.

In my discussions with actors regarding the French anti-GMO movement, they would often appeal to a reified "French nature," in their attempts to explain why the ecology movement is less prominent in France than in "Anglo-Saxon" countries, or why French people have a particular relationship to ideas of food quality. For Pascal R., a key INRA researcher, the question of ecology is different in France because of France's lack of nature:

> You see, there is no nature in France. There are still some valleys, some ravines, and a few forests, but they are quite small, just a few hectares. The environment in France is a product of systems of human practice and so you can't treat the environmental question like you can in other countries, the Anglo-Saxon countries. [Pascal R., interview, May 12, 1999]

In the West, then, there are two primary understandings of nature: one precultural and one cultural. In addition, there are two primary understanding of culture: one based on the Germanic notion of culture as *kultur* (inherited essence) and one on the French notion of culture as *cultiver* (process; see Pandian 1985:30).

French understandings of culture-as-*cultiver* find their origins in the preclassical Latin term *cultus*, which has two meanings, one material, one semiotic. First, *cultus* refers to the cultivation of the material or biological world. *Culture* is the term for both an agricultural crop and for the microorganisms used in the fermentation process required for making cheese and wine. Second, *cultus* implies the idea of developing cultural knowledge. To be cultured, then, is to be cultivated, to have developed an understanding of cultivated things, such as French wine, cheese, literature, or philosophy.

In turn, the 18th-century French notion of "civilization," derived from the Latin *civis* or *civilitas*, is in turn linked to the idea of "cultiver": the notion of modern progress as a universal process of development. Rather than constitute a national or cultural essence, civilization represents a developmental process, a model of upward mobility constituted by stages of human development (Pandian 1985).

As we have seen, French understandings of nature and culture put a unique spin on the Western nature–culture dualism. Instead of a fundamental tension between nature and culture, the two categories are understood as two dimensions of one continuous process of development that entails the nurturing of both material and semiotic worlds. Again, instead of a binary between nature and culture, France is marked by a binary between culture and nonculture, between people and things that are cultivated and not cultivated.

In questions of French food quality, then, the primary opposition is not necessarily between natural and unnatural foods but, rather, between cultured and noncultured foods, the latter associated with technoscience-driven agribusiness. Thus, in the French nature–culture configuration, GMOs are la malbouffe not necessarily because they are unnatural but, rather, because they are perceived as noncultural. They are patented biological commodities, products of sterile laboratories, designed to fit every climate of monocropping agriculture. For Bové, GM agriculture is an "immutable mobile" (Latour 1987), wiping out small farmers everywhere, perpetuating a model of agriculture that turns rural areas into empty placeless zones, occupied mostly by tourists or agribusiness. As a noncultivated entity, GMOs, like fast food, become shorthand for globalization. They represent the opposite of culture, cultivation, and civilization.

It is useful to point out, however, that the French are not unique in their fetishization of nature-as-agriculture. In the United States, for instance, actors reify the naturalness of Vermont-based agriculture (Heller 1999), such as artisanal Vermont cheese (Paxson 2006). The difference is that the United States also counterpoises this notion of nature as agriculture against a notion of nature as pristine wilderness. And furthermore, when U.S. citizens reject foods because of a lack of wholesomeness, they tend to denounce the food as unnatural and artificial, rather than as lacking in cultural savoir faire. U.S. citizens' rejection of McDonald's is largely based on discourses of technical quality (health and obesity), rather than on the "un-Americanness" of the food.

CONCLUSION

Over the past several decades, the ambiguous term *quality* has become a keyword used by states, corporations, and other powerful institutions to normalize and depoliticize problems associated with industrial agriculture. As I have argued, just as institutions such as INRA appeal to ambiguous ideas of "quality" to promote their agricultural agendas, unions such as the CP make similar attempts.

The CP's anti-GMO campaign represents an instance in which the union successfully appealed to techne-driven food quality—despite the fact that union members do not necessarily utilize artisanal production scale or methods. Yet by asserting the cultural contrast between symbols such as Roquefort cheese and GMOs (the latter being an example of la malbouffe), the union is able to transform a technique of governance into a potent means to establish their own cultural authority regarding food, agriculture, and processes of globalization—as well as possibly constituting the basis for establishing a new food quality label, *Agriculture Paysanne*. It is the CP's ability to argue for GMO's lack of cultivation or savoir faire that finds resonance with the general French public. In an age of globalization in which technoscientific placelessness is often juxtaposed against technes of place-based production, Bové's comparison between a GMO and the McDonald's nowhere land of uniform hamburgers proves truly compelling.

Notes

I would like to thank Arturo Escobar, Rick Fantasia, Les Levidow, Alan Goodman, and Deborah Heath, whose insights greatly informed many of the thoughts articulated here. Special thanks go to the National Science Foundation who made my research in France possible. Gratitude is also owed to Bruno Latour and Michel Callon at the Centre de Sociologie de l'Innovation for an important year of intellectual support and guidance. My deepest gratitude goes to the many scientists of INRA–Versailles and members of the Confédération Paysanne who generously welcomed me into their homes and workplaces as I tried to put the pieces together.

1. During 1997–2000, I conducted ethnographic research, spending weekends with CP farm families throughout the country, attending CP meetings and conferences at the union's headquarters outside of Paris, and participating in a variety of CP demonstrations. My research, however, did not end in 2000. As is the case with many public debates about science, the French GMO debate has yet to find *closure*—truly a problematic and tenacious term within science studies generally (Nelkin 1992). As the French GMO debate continues to unfold, I have continued to study it virtually, from afar, and during short visits to the country.

References

Aubineau, Andre. 1997. De 1987 a 1997: Une autre politique agricole (From 1987 to 1997: Toward a new agricultural policy). Campagnes Solidaires 107:89.

Blanc, Michel. 1977. Les paysanneries francaises (The French peasantry). Paris: Delarge.

Bookchin, Murray. 1982. The Ecology of Freedom. Palo Alto, CA: Cheshire Books.

Bové, José, and Francois Dufour. 2001. The World Is Not for Sale: Farmers against Junk Food. London: Verso Books.

Chavagne, Yves. 1988. Bernard Lambert: 30 ans de combat paysan (Bernard Lambert: 30 years of peasant struggles). Baye: Editions La Digitale.

Confédération Paysanne. 1998. Technologies génétiques: Pour un moratoire sur la mise en culture et la commercialisation pour l'application du principe du precaution (Genetic technologies: Toward a moratorium on planting and commercialization in accordance with precaution principle). Paris: La Confédération Paysanne.

Fantasia, Rick. 1995. Fast Food in France. Theory and Society 24:201–243.

———. 2000. Restaurants rapides pour "societe sans classes" (Fast-food restaurants for a "classless society"). Le Monde Diplomatique 554:6–7.

Foucault, Michel. 1991. Governmentality. In The Foucault Effect: Studies in Governmentality. Graham Burchell, Colin Gordon, and Peter Miller, eds. Pp. 87–105. Chicago: University of Chicago Press.

French Academy of Agriculture. 1990. Deux Siecles de Progres Pour l'Agriculture et L'Alimentation, 1789–1989 (Two centuries of progress in agriculture and food, 1789–1989). Paris: Technique et Documentation Lavoisier.

Gupta, Akhil. 1998. Postcolonial Developments: Agriculture in the Making of Modern India. Durham, NC: Duke University Press.

Haraway, Donna. 1991. Simians, Cyborgs, and Women: The Reinvention of Nature. New York: Routledge.

———. 1997. Modest_Witness@Second_Millennium. FemaleMan©_Meets_OncoMouse™: Feminism and Technoscience. London: Routledge.

Heidegger, Martin. 1977. The Question Concerning Technology. In Martin Heidegger: Basic Writings. David Farrell Krell, ed. William Lovitt, trans. Pp. 73–82. New York: Harper and Row.

Heller, Chaia. 2001a. From Scientific Risk to Paysan Savoir-Faire: Peasant Expertise in the French and Global Debate over GM Crops. Science as Culture 11:5–37.

———. 2001b. McDonald's, MTV, and Monsanto: Resisting Biotechnology in the Age of Informational Capital. In Redesigning Life. B. Tokar, ed. Pp. 405–420. London: Zed Books.

———. 2004. Risky Science and Savoir-Faire: Peasant Expertise in the French Debate over Genetically Modified Crops. In The Politics of Food. Marianne Lien and Brigitte Nerlich, eds. Pp. 81–101. Oxford: Berg Press.

———. 2005. From Scientific Risk to Paysan Savoir-Faire: Divergent Rationalities of Science and Society in the French Debate over GM Crops. Ph.D. dissertation, Department of Anthropology, University of Massachusetts, Amherst.

———. 2006. Post-Industrial "Quality" Agricultural Discourse: Techniques of Governance and Resistance in the French Debate over GM Crops. Social Anthropology 14(3):319–334.

Heller, Chaia, and Arturo Escobar. 2003. From Pure Genes to GMOs: Transnationalized Gene Landscapes in the Biodiversity and Transgenic Food Networks. In Genetic Nature/Culture: Anthropology and Science beyond the Two-Culture Divide. A. Goodman, D. Heath, and M. S. Lindee, eds. Pp. 155–176. Berkeley: University of California Press.

Hervieu, Bertrand. 1996. Au bonheur des campagnes (The goodness of the countryside). Paris: Éditions de l'Aube.

Jasanoff, Sheila. 2005. Designs on Nature: Science and Democracy in Europe and the U.S. Princeton: Princeton University Press.

Khan, Axel. 1996. Transgenic Plants in Agriculture. L'Institute De Recherche Agriculturel. P. 63. Montrouge: John Libbey Eurotext.

Latour, Bruno. 1987. Science in Action. Cambridge, MA: Harvard University Press.

Levidow, Les. 1997. European Biotechnology Regulation: Framing the Risk Assessment of a Herbicide-Tolerant Crop. Science, Technology, and Human Values 22(4):472–505.

Malassis, Louis. 1997. Les Trois Ages De L'Alimentaire (Three eras of food production). In Les Industries Agro-Alimentaires En France (The French agro-food industry). Jacques Marseille, ed. Pp. 9–18. Paris: Le Monde-Editions.

Marris, Claire. 2001. Public Views on GMOs: Deconstructing the Myths. EMBO Reports 21(7):545–548.

Mendras, Henri. 1984. La fin des paysans (The last of the peasantry). Arles: Actes Sud.

National Institute of Agricultural Research (INRA). 1998. Introduction. *In* Organismes Genetiquement Modifies A l'INRA: Environment, Agriculture, Alimentation. Paris: Athena Arts Graphiques.

Nelkin, Dorothy. 1992. Controversies: Politics of Technical Decisions. 3rd edition. Newbury Park, CA: Sage.

Paillotin, George. 1999. Tais-toi et mange! L'agriculture, le scientifique, et le consommateur (Be quite and eat! Farmers, scientists, consumers). Paris: Bayard Editions.

Palsson, Gisli, and Paul Rabinow. 1999. Iceland: The Case of a National Human Genome Project. Anthropology Today 15(5):14–18.

Pandian, Jacob. 1985. Anthropology and the Western Tradition: Toward an Authentic Anthropology. Chicago: Waveland Press.

Paxson, Heather. 2006. Artisanal Cheese and Economies of Sentiment in New England. *In* Fast Food/Slow Food: The Cultural Economy of the Global Food System. Richard Wilk, ed. Pp. 201–218. London: Berg Press.

Pollan, Michael. 2006. The Omnivore's Dilemma: A Natural History of Four Meals. New York: Penguin Press.

Rabinow, Paul. 1996a. Artificiality and Enlightenment: From Sociobiology to Biosociality. *In* Essays on the Anthropology of Reason. pp. 91–111. Princeton: Princeton University Press.

———. 1996b. Making PCR: A Story of Biotechnology. Chicago: University of Chicago Press.

Scott, James. 1998. Seeing Like a State: How Certain Schemes to Improve the Human Condition Have Failed. New Haven, CT: Yale University Press.

Smith, Neil. 1996. The Production of Nature. *In* Future Natural: Nature, Science, Culture. George Robertson, Melinda Mash, Lisa Tickner, Jon Bird, Barry Curtis, and Tim Putnam, eds. pp. 35–54. London: Routledge.

Strathern, Marilyn. 1980. No Nature, No Culture: The Hagen Case. *In* Nature, Culture and Gender. Carol MacCormack and Marilyn Strathern, eds. Pp. 174–223. Cambridge: Cambridge University Press.

Ulin, Robert. 1997. Vintages and Traditions: An Ethnohistory of Southwest French Wine Cooperatives. American Anthropologist 99(3):664–665.

Voynet, Dominique. 1998. Preface to Agriculture, monde rural et environment: Qualite oblige (Preface to agriculture, the rural world, and the environment: quality oblige). Paris: La Documentation Francaise.

Williams, Raymond. 1976. Keywords: A Vocabulary of Culture and Society. New York: Oxford University Press.

UNIT VI

ADAPTING FOODS TO PEOPLE AND PEOPLE TO FOODS

Not only do people eat different kinds of foods, but foods themselves contain many different sorts of chemical compounds and elements, only some of which are nutrients. How a particular food is prepared for consumption affects the presence, and even the availability, of some compounds, elements and nutrients. For example, the amount of vitamin C (a compound) is greater in raw foods than in cooked foods because vitamin C is heat sensitive and damaged by cooking. How people process and prepare foods is especially important for staple foods, those foods that are consumed in greatest quantities and thereby provide most of the energy in the diet. Some groups process and prepare foods in ways that have amazingly significant consequences for the quality of their diets. Two classic examples are discussed in the chapters in this section: (1) the food processing techniques used by Amazonian Indians to eliminate cyanide, a toxic compound; (2) the alkaline processing of maize (corn in U.S. English) that alters the biological availability of the vitamin niacin.

The cyanide story is developed by Darna Dufour in the chapter "A Closer Look at the Nutritional Implications of Bitter Cassava Use." Dufour, a biological anthropologist, lived for almost 2 years with Tukanoan Indians in the Amazon (Figure 1) and became fascinated by the fact that these people consumed cassava, a cyanide-containing root, that they themselves considered highly toxic in a raw state. Cassava was probably domesticated thousands of years ago somewhere in South America and has been the dietary staple of native Amazonians for a very long time. What is the cyanide doing there in the root in the first place? Who knows, but cyanide is a compound found in many wild plants, and we hypothesize that it is produced by the plant as a protection against predation—a kind of natural insecticide. It is not found in many domesticated plants, or at least not in the parts of the plant normally eaten. Humans can tolerate small amounts of cyanide in the foods they eat and the air they breathe (cigarette smoke contains cyanide) because they can detoxify it

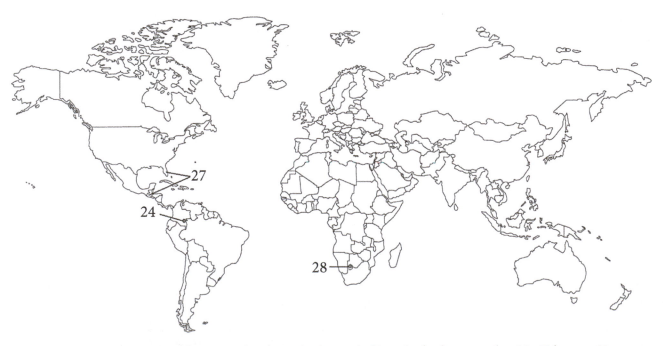

Figure 1 *Map shows the location of the groups referred to in the chapters in this section by chapter number: 24 = Tukanoans, Vaupes region, Colombia; 27 = Maya, rural Guatemala and Indiantown, Florida, United States; 28 = !Kung Bushmen of the Dobe area of Botswana.*

metabolically. Large amounts of cyanide, however, can overpower the detoxification process and lead to illness, and sometimes death. The amount of cyanide present in the cassava cultivated by Tukanoan Indians is large enough to cause illness and death. So how can they use cassava as a dietary staple? This is the question Dufour attempts to answer.

The processing of maize is another example of a strategy that improves the nutritional value of a plant food. Maize does not contain a toxin; it is an ordinary grain in terms of its chemical composition. But curiously enough, the niacin (a B vitamin) in maize is not as biologically available to humans as one would assume looking at the chemical composition of the raw grain itself. As Barrett Brenton notes in his chapter, "Pellegra, Sex and Gender: Biocultural Perspectives on Differential Diets and Health," the maize processing technique developed by native peoples in the Americas increases the biological availability (bioavailability) of niacin to human consumers. It is a technique that relies on soaking maize kernels in an alkaline solution before cooking, as strange as that might sound.

Does alkaline processing make a difference nutritionally? Yes, it certainly appears to because there is no evidence that native peoples on maize-based diets ever suffered from pellagra, the disease of niacin deficiency. On the other hand, there is ample evidence of pellagra in individuals who eat a maize-based diet that does not use alkaline processing. A good example is the outbreak of pellagra among sharecroppers in the southern United States in the early twentieth century who lived on a diet of maize, pork fat, and molasses. Interestingly, Brenton also notes that in this population, the prevalence of pellagra was much higher in females than males and asks if this could be due to social factors (women having more restricted diets than men), or perhaps to biological differences between males and females.

Not only does the way people process and prepare foods alter foods' chemical composition, but humans also vary in how they digest and metabolize some of the compounds and elements in foods. How could that be? Food is taken into the mouth, where it is chopped, mashed, and mixed with saliva. It goes to the stomach, where it is mixed with acid to further its breakdown into small particles, and then into the small intestine, where enzymes complete the breakdown of food particles into compounds and elements that can be absorbed through the wall of the intestine. We call this enzymatic breakdown digestion, and it is here where problems can occur because one needs a particular enzyme for each type of compound. Peptidase works on the chemical bonds in proteins (peptide bonds), sucrase works on the chemical bonds of sucrose (plant sugar), lactase works on the chemical bonds of lactose (milk sugar), and so on. The production of enzymes is a function of one's genetic code and normal diet.

Most people produce sufficient quantities and types of enzymes to digest the foods in their normal diet, but there are some interesting exceptions. Some Inuit do not produce the sucrase to digest sucrose. We assume this is because plants have become a significant part of their diet only in the past

50 years or so. The classic exception is that of lactase. Not all people, as adults, produce sufficient lactase to digest lactose (milk sugar). Why that might be? Who are these people? What social meanings are attached to milk drinking? These are some of the questions addressed in Andrea Wiley's chapter, "'Drink Milk for Fitness': The Cultural Politics of Human Biological Variation and Milk Consumption in the United States."

The last two papers in this section look at the relationship between food and people in a slightly different way. They consider nutritional status as a measure of the adequacy of the whole diet. Nutritional status refers to the biological condition (status) of the organism. Common measures are the growth rate of children and the body size and fatness of adults. These measures reflect disease history as well as some other environmental factors, but diet is usually considered a primary determining factor.

The first of the two chapters by Barry Bogin is "Maya in Disneyland: Child Growth as a Marker of Nutritional, Economic and Political Ecology." Bogin, a biological anthropologist, spent many years studying the growth of Mayan children in Guatemala, and later when some Mayan families immigrated to the United States, the growth of Mayan children in the United States (Figure 1). The migration set up a classical natural experiment: members of a single biological (genetic) population living in two very different environments. Bogin found that the Mayan children in the United States grew faster and taller than those in Guatemala, a clear demonstration that the small body size of the Maya in Guatemala was not genetic. Bogin also argues that we can think about the relationship between body size and environment in another way: the shortness of the Maya in Central America is an indicator that the Central American environment is less optimal for human growth than the U.S. environment. Growth is also used as an indicator of environmental conditions in other chapters in this volume including chapter 33 by Adolfo Chávez and colleagues, "The Effect of Malnutrition on Human Development," and chapter 34 by Reynaldo Martorell, "Body Size, Adaptation, and Function."

The second of the two chapters in this section, "!Kung Nutritional Status and the Original 'Affluent Society'—A New Analysis," is also by Barry Bogin (Figure 1). In this chapter he analyzes the nutritional status of !Kung hunter-gatherers in the 1960s, and comes to the conclusion that they were not as well-nourished as we have generally assumed. Rather, he argues, they were in an environment where food resources were "scarce" and as a result adults showed evidence of undernutrition. Bogin's analysis and conclusion are particularly important as the !Kung have become the quintessential example of hunter-gatherers, and few had ever questioned the adequacy of their nutritional status. The !Kung are described in two other chapters (chapters 2 and 7), both written by Richard Lee: "Eating Christmas in the Kalahari," and "What Hunters Do for a Living, or, How To Make Out on Scarce Resources."

What have we learned from the chapters in this section? People can adapt or manipulate the chemical composition of foods in ways that make them more nutritious. People have also adapted to food, in the sense that they have evolved the genetic capacity to digest compounds in foods that comprise their usual diets. Lastly, we learned from Bogin that the growth of children and the body size of adults are plastic characteristics in that they are influenced by the environment, especially the nutritional environment. And given that, we can think of nutritional status as a measure of the quality of the nutritional environment.

SUGGESTIONS FOR THINKING AND DOING NUTRITIONAL ANTHROPOLOGY

1. Make a list of all the foods you consume today that contain maize (corn) or some product derived from maize. Read labels and look for ingredients such as corn oil, hydrogenated corn oil, cornstarch, corn syrup, high-fructose corn syrup (HFCS), cornmeal, corn flour, hominy, grits. What percentage of all the foods you ate contained some form of maize?

2. What kinds of special foods and food products are available at your local supermarket for lactose-intolerant people? Find out what kinds of dairy foods lactose-intolerant people can *usually* tolerate. The key here is *usually*, because we know that lactase production depends to some extent on usual diet.

3. Find out why artificial sweeteners, such as NutraSweet and Equal, and "sugar-free" products, such as Diet Pepsi, contain a warning: PHENYLKETONURICS: CONTAINS PHENYLALANINE. What is phenylalanine? Who are phenylketonurics, and why do they need to avoid phenylalanine?

4. Make a list of all the "wild" foods you have ever eaten. Consider "wild" plant foods those plants that are not cultivated, e.g., the dandelions in the front lawn. Consider "wild" animals to be those that are not farmed or managed by humans in any way. Some fish are caught wild, some are farmed. Some animals that you might think of as wild, like elk and deer, are often farmed. Describe your list. Is it mostly plant foods or animal foods? How many foods does it contain compared to the number of different foods you usually eat?

Suggested Further Reading

Coe M. 2011. The Maya. 8th edition. London: Thames & Hudson, Ltd. Synthesis of our current understanding of Mayan civilization in pre-Columbian times.

Gibbons A. 2006. There's More than One Way to Have Your Milk and Drink It, too. Science 314:1672. Brief account of recent identification of genetic variants in Africans that allow adults to digest lactose (milk sugar).

Katz SH, Hediger ML, Valleroy LA. 1975. Traditional Maize Processing Techniques in the New World. Science 184:765–773. Classic description and analysis of the effects of traditional maize processing on the bioavailability of niacin.

Roe D. 1973. A Plague of Corn: The Social History of Pellagra. Ithaca, NY: Cornell University Press. Description and analysis of the social conditions and diets associated with outbreaks of the nutritional deficiency disease known as pellegra.

Sostak M. 1983. Nisa: The Life and Words of a !Kung Woman. New York: Vintage Books. An engrossing account of !Kung life as hunter-gatherers as told by one woman.

Wiley AS. 201. Re-Imaging Milk. New York: Routledge. Highly readable biocultural approach to animal milk as a food for humans.

CHAPTER 24

A Closer Look at the Nutritional Implications of Bitter Cassava Use

Darna L. Dufour

(1995)

Cassava, or manioc (*Manihot esculenta* Crantz), is the traditional dietary staple of many native Amazonians. Although it is very productive on the *tierra firme* soils of Amazonia, it is one of the few food crops in which the content of cyanide can create problems of toxicity, and therefore its use is a potential source of nutritional stress.

In the last 20 years there has been a tremendous increase in the research on cassava (for reviews, see Cock 1985; Okezie and Kosikowski 1982). This research has been stimulated by the growing importance of cassava in both human and animal diets. Cassava is now the fourth most important source of food energy in the tropics worldwide (Cock 1982), and its use is expected to double before the year 2000 (Okezie and Kosikowski 1982). The potential toxicity of cassava is considered one of the major limiting factors in its use for both culinary purposes and animal feed (Okezie and Kosikowski 1982), and some researchers consider the "bitter," or high-cyanide, cultivars unsuitable for human food (Gomez et al. 1984). Cyanide toxicity associated with cassava consumption has been linked to a number of health problems in Africa (Nestel and MacIntyre 1973; Ermans et al. 1980; Osuntokun 1981; Rosling 1987).

Among indigenous peoples in Amazonia, the high-cyanide, or so-called "bitter," cassava appears to have been the staple crop in the Amazon basin, northeastern South America, and the Antilles (Nordenskiold 1924; Steward and Faron 1959). Low-cyanide, or "sweet," cassava was more widely distributed (Nordenskiold 1924) but tended to be part of a crop complex dominated by either maize or bitter cassava (Renvoize 1972). The exception to this is on the eastern slopes of the Andes where sweet cassava was the staple crop (Steward 1959). The elaborate processing systems associated with "bitter" varieties have long attracted the attention of anthropologists and other observers, but their actual effectiveness in reducing toxicity has received little attention. Other important questions regarding the toxicity of the cultivars used, the distribution of bitter and sweet cultivars, and the roles of bitter and sweet cassava in the adaptation of native peoples have gone unanswered.

The purpose of this [article] is to report the results of recent research on the use of bitter cassava by Tukanoan Indians in northwest Amazonia, and in doing so to focus attention on the use of cassava by native Amazonians. In addition I would like to reconsider some of the commonly cited disadvantages of cassava use. These disadvantages are, first, that it is a crop with low nutrient density and hence is a relatively poor source of dietary protein and minerals. Second, the "bitter" varieties of cassava require extensive processing, which further reduces protein and mineral content. The third disadvantage, proposed by Spath (1981), is that the residual toxicity, i.e., cyanide, in a cassava-based diet increases the need for the amino acids methionine and cystine, which are generally more abundant in animal than in plant proteins. This last disadvantage is part of the broader question of the toxicity of cassava.

The fieldwork reported here was done in 1984–86 with Tukanoan Indians in the Colombian Vaupés, primarily in the village of Yapú on the Papurí River.[1] The characteristics of this group have been discussed previously (Dufour 1983). Ecologically the Vaupés is an area of low elevation covered with dense tropical rain forest broken with patches of *caatinga* (a type of low forest occurring on white sand) and drained by black-water rivers. In climatic terms the area is humid to very humid. Precipitation averages 3,500 mm a year, and temperatures average 26°C. During the long "dry" season from about November to February, precipitation averages between 150 and 200 mm per month (PRORADAM 1979:13).

Yapú is a village settlement of Tatuyo-speaking Tukanoan Indians. Like other traditional Tukanoans, those at Yapú are swidden horticulturalists whose principal crop is cassava. Secondary crops include plants such as taro (*Colocasia* spp.), sweet potato (*Ipomoea* sp.), arrowroot (*Maranta ruiziana*), bananas, plantains, and a number of fruits. Animal foods are obtained from fishing, hunting, and gathering (Dufour 1983).

Darna L. Dufour, "A closer look at the nutritional implications of bitter cassava use." In *Indigenous peoples and the future of Amazonia: an ecological anthropology of the endangered world*, L. Sponsel, ed. University of Arizona Press, 1995, pp. 149–165. Reprinted with permission.

CASSAVA

Cassava is a perennial woody shrub belonging to the family Euphorbiaceae. It is native to the Neotropics and well adapted to the low fertility, highly acid soils that are common in Amazonia (Rogers 1965; Moran 1973; Cock 1985; Howeler 1985). It is tolerant of drought as well as high rainfall, so long as drainage is good (Cock 1985:18). It is grown primarily for its starchy storage roots, but the leaves are also used as food.

The plant and the edible roots are referred to as both cassava and manioc. Cassava is now the more widely used term in English, and it is the one I will use here. It is probably derived from *casabe, cazabe,* or *kasabi,* the Taino (Arawak) word for cassava bread (Carrizales 1984; Jones 1959:29). Manioc is from the Tupí-Guaraní *mandioca* (Sauer 1950), and is also the word for the plant in French.[2]

The toxicity of cassava results from the presence of cyanogenic glucosides that break down into glucose and hydrogen cyanide (prussic acid) upon hydrolysis. Hydrolysis results from contact between the glucosides and the endogenous enzyme linamarase; it occurs when plant tissues lose their physiological integrity or are damaged by processes such as harvesting, peeling, or grating. All cassava cultivars contain cyanogenic glucosides, but the concentrations vary greatly between cultivars and with season, climate, and edaphic conditions (Coursey 1973; Bourdoux et al. 1980). The distinction between sweet and bitter cassava is common throughout Amazonia, and indeed throughout the world. In general it refers to roots that can simply be peeled, boiled, and eaten, as opposed to those that are considered bitter or toxic and require additional processing before being consumed. In a more precise way, *sweet* is used to refer to cassava roots with cyanide concentrations of less than 100 ppm, and *bitter* is used for those with concentrations of greater than 100 ppm fresh weight (FW). This is the sense in which the terms are used here.

CASSAVA IN NORTHWEST AMAZONIA

Tukanoans at Yapú maintain about 100 named cassava cultivars, all but two of which they classify as *kii* and consider "bitter." These are the dietary staples. The remaining two are referred to by the Geral term *makasera* and are considered "sweet." A sample of common kii cultivars from Yapú had cyanide concentrations ranging from 280 to 531 ppm FW, with a mean of 454 ppm FW. Hence, they are properly considered "very bitter," or high-cyanide containing (Dufour 1988a). There is no information on the cyanide content of the cultivars used by other native Amazonians, but in comparison to those of other areas of the world, the average cyanide concentration of the Yapú cultivars is the highest of any reported.

In the northwest Amazon, cassava appears in the diet in a number of forms, the most important of which are *casabe,* a bread, and *fariña,* a toasted meal. Casabe is a uniquely Amazonian use of cassava and traditionally was the most widespread mode of preparation (Schwerin 1971:12). Among Tukanoans, casabe is a thick, soft bread made fresh daily from white-fleshed roots. It is the preferred accompaniment to fish, game, and insects, and when those are not available, it is eaten after being dipped in a "pepper pot." Fariña is the basis of meals when people are traveling or working away from the village, and it is most commonly consumed as a drink—a small amount swirled in water.

The Tukanoan processing technique for casabe is elaborate and has been described previously (Dufour 1985, 1989; Hugh-Jones 1979). It is shown schematically in Figure 1. First, the roots are rasped to remove the outermost layer of peel, and then they are washed and grated. Grating reduces the roots to a fine, watery mash, which is then separated into three fractions: liquids, starch, and fiber. The separation is accomplished by washing (with water and extracted juices) and squeezing the mash in a basketry strainer to remove the starch and liquids from the more fibrous portion, and then allowing the starch to settle out of the wash water. Once the starch has settled, the supernatant is decanted off and boiled immediately to make the beverage *manicuera.* The other two products, starch and fiber, are stored at least overnight but preferably for 48 hours, and then are recombined and baked as a casabe. To prepare casabe, the fiber is dewatered in a *tipiti* (basketry sleeve press), lightly toasted, and then mixed with the starch. The starch is also used to thicken beverages (*mingao*) and fish porridges (*puné*).

Casabe can also be prepared by simply dewatering and baking the freshly grated mash. This type of casabe is not very commonly consumed in Yapú and is referred to here as "fresh casabe." It is a denser bread and lacks the fermented taste of ordinary casabe. When baked as a cracker-thin cake it is used as an ingredient in beer. Other types of casabe include those made from plain starch, in either a thick or a thin form, and those made from the raw, fermented mash destined for fariña.

Fariña is prepared from yellow-fleshed roots that are trimmed off the stem end and soaked in stream water until softened (two to four days), then peeled, grated, allowed to ferment for a minimum of three days, dewatered with a tipiti, sifted to produce an even texture, and toasted (see Fig. 1). The type of fariña prepared by Tukanoans is called *farinha d'agua* in Brazil.

EFFECTIVENESS OF PROCESSING TECHNIQUES

The effectiveness of the processing techniques used to prepare casabe and fariña in detoxifying roots was assessed in a series of experiments conducted at the Centro Internacional de Agricultura Tropical (CIAT) in Cali, Colombia, and is discussed in detail in Dufour (1989). In these experiments we measured the loss of free cyanide, or HCN, and total cyanide, which includes both HCN and cyanogenic glucosides. Cyanide in the form of cyanogenic glucosides is also referred to as bound cyanide, i.e., cyanide bound to glucose.

The changes in total and free cyanide that occurred during processing for casabe are shown in Table 1. There was only a modest reduction in total cyanide with rasping and grating.

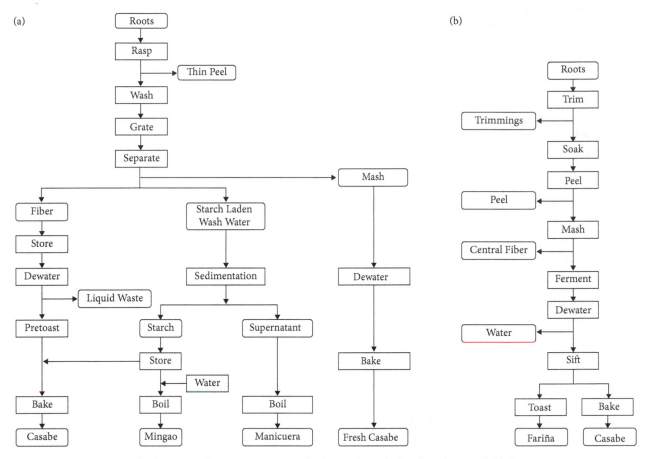

Figure 1 *Flow diagram of Tukanoan-style cassava processing for (a) casabe and related products and (b) fariña.*

The grated mash, however, showed a dramatic increase in free cyanide, indicating that the grating resulted in the conversion of cyanogenic glucosides to the free form. Since free cyanide is water soluble, most of the remainder was concentrated in the wash water and then volatilized with cooking. The boiled juice, manicuera, contained only 0.8 percent (FW basis) of the initial concentration of total cyanide.

The cyanide levels in the starch and fiber continued to decline slowly during storage and with cooking. The casabes made with starch and fiber that had been stored for 48 hours contained less than 4 percent of the initial total cyanide. Those made with starch and fiber stored 24 hours contained more than twice as much, as did the fresh casabes.

The effectiveness of the Tukanoan technique in reducing cyanide levels in cassava is due to several factors. First, grating causes extensive disintegration of the plant tissues, and the subsequent mixing ensures maximal contact between the enzyme and the glucosides, a process that maximizes the conversion of bound to free cyanide. Second, the inner peel is grated along with the pulp. This facilitates hydrolysis because enzymatic activity in the peel is higher than in the pulp (Bruijn 1973; Nambisan and Sundaresan 1985). This practice of including the inner peel has been reported only for Tukanoans and Karinya (Karl Schwerin, personal communication). Third, the washing of the mash concentrates most of the free cyanide in the wash water, where it can be effectively volatilized by boiling.

Cyanide losses during the processing of fariña are shown in Table 2. The roots showed a gradual decline in total cyanide with trimming and soaking, and when softened (day 6), contained only 21 percent of the initial total cyanide. The loss of cyanide can be attributed to enzyme hydrolysis and volatilization of HCN, as well as to fermentation (Ayernor 1985:94). The roots showed additional small decreases in cyanide content with peeling and mashing, and in the first days of fermentation. The fermented mash on day 10 contained only 2.4 percent of the initial total cyanide. Total and free cyanide content was further reduced by toasting (see values on a dry matter basis).

The values for total and free cyanide obtained in the processing experiment are comparable to those found in fariña samples collected in the Colombian Vaupés region. These had concentrations of 8.3 ± 2.59 ppm total cyanide and 6.2 ± 0.48 ppm free cyanide on a fresh weight basis (n = 24).

ROLE OF PROCESSING STEPS IN DETOXIFICATION

The results of these processing experiments challenge some of the assumptions held by anthropologists regarding the role of Amazonian processing techniques in detoxification. Three common assumptions are that the peeling, the use of the tipiti, and the application of heat are the important

Table 1 Changes in Total and Free Cyanide in Cassava Roots Processed for Casabe. Values Are the Average of Three Processing Runs with MCOL 1684 and Three with MVEN 25 on a Fresh Weight Basis (FW). Dry Matter Values in Parentheses

| Day | Process Stage | Moisture % | Cyanide, ppm FW | | F/T % | Total Cyanide % Initial |
			Total	Free		
Day 1	Whole roots	64	528 (1,441)	76 (211)	14	100.0
	Rasped roots	65	411 (1,158)	72 (227)	18	77.8
	Mash (grated roots)	64	416 (1,136)	289 (789)	69	78.8
	Fiber, fresh	74	103 (396)	54 (215)	52	19.5
	Starch, fresh	49	91 (182)	75 (148)	82	17.2
	Wash water[a]	92	153 (3,229)	130 (3,138)	85	29.0
	Manicuera	82	4 (19)	3 (10)	75	0.8
	Mash, dewatered	50	236 (451)	173 (330)	73	44.7
	Casabe, fresh	29	40 (58)	10 (15)	25	7.6
Day 2	Fiber, sour	73	80 (290)	56 (206)	70	15.1
	Fiber, sour, dewatered	56	68 (153)	44 (96)	65	12.9
	Starch, sour	48	62 (120)	50 (99)	81	11.7
	Casabe, ordinary	26	39 (55)	25 (35)	64	7.4
Day 3	Fiber, sour	72	60 (209)	37 (129)	62	11.4
	Fiber, sour, dewatered	58	40 (96)	28 (68)	70	7.6
	Starch, sour	45	39 (72)	35 (64)	90	7.4
	Casabe, ordinary	25	17 (22)	7 (10)	41	3.2

[a]Dry matter values are for a single processing run.

Table 2 Changes in Total and Free Cyanide in Cassava Roots Processed for Fariña. Values Are for One Processing Run with MCOL 1684 on a Fresh Weight Basis (FW). Dry Matter Values in Parentheses

| Day | Stage | Moisture % | Cyanide, ppm FW | | F/T % | Total Cyanide % Initial |
			Total	Free		
Day 1	Whole roots	67	328 (972)	42 (124)	13	100.0
Day 2	Soaked roots	67	247 (758)	18 (56)	7	75.3
Day 3	Soaked roots	70	222 (744)	34 (113)	15	67.7
Day 4	Soaked roots	73	175 (642)	63 (232)	36	53.3
Day 5	Soaked roots	73	104 (338)	40 (149)	38	31.7
Day 6	Soaked roots	69	68 (251)	36 (116)	53	20.7
	Peeled-grated	68	35 (109)	18 (55)	51	10.6
Day 7	Fermented mash	66	11 (32)	10 (29)	92	3.4
Day 8	Fermented mash	66	10 (30)	8 (23)	80	3.0
Day 9	Fermented mash	66	8 (22)	7 (20)	75	2.4
Day 10	Fermented mash	66	6 (16)	4 (11)	67	1.8
	Fariña	3	8 (8)	4 (4)	50	2.4

steps in detoxification. A fourth assumption is that processing significantly reduces the nutritional value of cassava (Sponsel 1986).

First, peeling, which was assumed to remove a large portion of the cyanide (Dole 1978), does not really achieve that in the "bitter" varieties, although it certainly does in the "sweet." Rather, when very bitter cultivars are used, leaving the inner peel intact when the roots are grated facilitates hydrolysis.

Second, the tipiti, that famous and unique basketry sleeve press, has been assumed to play a key role in detoxification (Carrizales 1984). However, as Dole (1978) pointed out, the tipiti's principal function is dewatering. It can function in detoxification because both the glucosides and free cyanide are water soluble, but its role depends on when in the processing sequence it is used. In the Tukanoan processing sequence used for casabe, dewatering is done after there has been adequate time for hydrolysis and volatilization of free cyanide; hence it plays a very minimal role in detoxification. The use of the tipiti would be most important when freshly grated roots were used for casabe and when cooking was done shortly after grating. This method of preparing casabe, however, does not appear to be very common. Other groups that make casabe without extracting the starch typically let the mash set overnight before baking it (Lancaster et al. 1982; Seigler and Pereira 1981). This should allow adequate time for both hydrolysis and volatilization of HCN, even if the mash is dewatered before it is stored.

The key tool in detoxification is the one that precedes the tipiti in the processing sequence—the grating board. This instrument macerates the plant material and in doing so allows hydrolysis to proceed rapidly. In the preparation of fariña, the long period of soaking is the most effective part of the process in detoxifying the roots. Again the tipiti is not very important because the total cyanide content has already been reduced more than 98 percent before it is used.

A third assumption is that because heat volatilizes free cyanide, the application of heat results in detoxification (Schwerin 1985). A corollary of this is that simple methods of processing, such as boiling and baking, are adequate for detoxification (Roosevelt 1980:129). But in elaborate processing systems such as that of the Tukanoans, the application of heat is of only minimal importance because most of the glucosides have been converted to free cyanide and released before heat is applied. The application of heat in this type of processing system is probably most important in gelatinizing the starches and producing the desired texture in foods. Further, although the application of heat will volatilize HCN, it usually stops hydrolysis because the enzyme linamarase is deactivated at 72°C. Therefore, if heat is applied before hydrolysis has been completed, the food can retain significant amounts of bound cyanide, which is thermally stable up to 150°C (Nambisan and Sundaresan 1985).

It follows that simple cooking techniques such as boiling and roasting can eliminate free cyanide but will not be as effective in removing cyanogenic glucosides (Cooke and Maduagwu 1978). In boiling, free cyanide is lost to the air through volatilization, but bound cyanide goes into solution and can be found in the cooking water. Thus, cooked dishes, such as stews, in which the cooking water is consumed retain as much as 88 percent of the total cyanide (Bruijn 1971, cited in Cooke and Maduagwu 1978; Cooke and Maduagwu 1978). In areas such as India, where bitter cultivars are boiled, the cooking water is not consumed and is actually changed two or three times during cooking (Nambisan and Sundaresan 1985). This practice of changing the cooking water has not been reported for indigenous groups in Amazonia.

The roasting of whole cassava roots by burying them in hot ashes is done in the northwest Amazon with sweet cultivars and has been reported for a number of groups in Amazonia (Schwerin 1971). Cyanide loss under these kinds of conditions has not been studied, but it is probably similar to that observed during the baking of cassava chips in ovens, which has been shown to be a relatively ineffective method of reducing cyanide levels, again because the enzyme linamarase is inactivated at 72°C and linamarin is heat stable to 150°C (Cooke and Maduagwu 1978). It is doubtful that in normal roasting, as done by indigenous peoples, the root tissues reach 150°C, since they are thoroughly cooked at less than 100°C. Thus the roasting of whole tubers in ashes would probably remove little of the total cyanide.

In summary, the simpler methods of processing such as boiling and roasting are not very effective in reducing cyanide concentration and are only suitable for use with low-cyanide roots. This finding suggests that the exclusive use of these techniques will be confined to populations using low-cyanide cultivars. It does not follow, however, that groups using more complex processing techniques are necessarily using high-cyanide cultivars.

The fourth common assumption is that processing significantly reduces the nutritional value of cassava (Sponsel 1986). This is not a valid generalization; nutritional loss depends on the type of processing done. In some processing systems the loss of minerals in soaking, washing, and dewatering can be as high as 40 to 70 percent, and the loss of soluble proteins as high as 50 percent (Meuser and Smolnik 1980). The processing technique used for casabe, however, is nutritionally conservative. Waste is limited to the outer peel (<2 percent fresh weight), and the consumption of manicuera makes available the minerals and soluble proteins that would otherwise be lost. This advantage can only be gained if processing is done in small batches and the liquids boiled and consumed shortly afterward, because they deteriorate rapidly in both raw and cooked states. Retention of the peel also increases the nutritional value of cassava products because the peel fraction is higher in both minerals and protein than the pulp.

CYANIDE EXPOSURE AND THE INCREASED NEED FOR AMINO ACIDS

To estimate the exposure to dietary, cassava-borne cyanide in Yapú we determined food intake for 24 adults (12 males and 12 females) using the 3-day weighed intake method during

Table 3 Sources of Energy and Protein in the Diets of 24 Yapú Adults (means ± SD)

	Energy, % Total	Protein, % Total
Cultigens: Manioc	79.8 ± 9.00	20.9 ± 13.41
Other	9.0 ± 7.91	14.6 ± 16.28
Wild vegetable products	1.4 ± 4.04	0.8 ± 2.39
Wild animal products	8.5 ± 7.05	61.4 ± 28.73
Store foods	2.1 ± 4.46	2.4 ± 9.63

Table 4 Mean Daily Energy, Protein, and Cyanide Intakes of 24 Yapú Adults

	Mean ± SD
Energy, kcal	2272 ± 746.4
kcal/kg	42.9 ± 12.7
Protein, g	43.3 ± 23.12
g/kg	0.82 ± 0.43
Total Cyanide, mg	20.0 ± 8.29
mg/kg	0.4 ± 0.11
Free Cyanide, mg	9.1 ± 3.24
mg/kg	0.2 ± 0.04

Table 5 Yapú Diet Compared to FAO/WHO/UNU Suggested Pattern (Preschoolers) for Critical Amino Acids

Amino Acid	FAO	Yapú Diet
Lysine	58	70
Methionine + Cystine	25	34
Threonine	34	40
Tryptophan	11	11

November 1986. Energy and protein values for Tukanoan foods were taken from food composition tables, principally those of Wu Leung and Flores (1961) and Dufour (1988b). Cyanide values for cassava-based foods were taken from the processing done in the present study and samples collected in Yapú.

Results of the food intake study are shown in Tables 3 and 4. The overall composition of the diet is similar to that reported previously for this population (Dufour 1983). Total cyanide intakes were on the order of 20 mg/day (0.4 mg/kg/day), and free cyanide intakes were approximately half that value, 9 mg/day (0.18 mg/kg/day).

The metabolic detoxification of dietary cyanide occurs principally via the conversion of cyanide to thiocyanate, which is then excreted in urine. The key enzyme in this reaction contains sulphur, which is derived from sulphur-containing amino acids, methionine and cystine. Reliance on this metabolic pathway increases the need for these two amino acids. For the Yapú diet, cyanide detoxification would require about 2 mg/kg/day of methionine. This estimate may be high, however, as the toxicity of intact cyanogenic glucosides has not been established. If only free cyanide, which definitely requires detoxification, is considered, the methionine requirement would be about 1 mg/kg/day.

What does this imply in terms of the adequacy of the current Yapú diet? The dietary data indicate that adults' crude protein intakes average 0.85 grams per kilogram of body weight per day. This is 96 to 102 percent of the FAO/WHO/UNU Safe Level (1985), depending on how the digestibility of the diet is estimated. Energy intake is 45 kilocalories per kilogram of body weight and appears to be adequate, so we can assume that dietary protein is probably not being used to supply energy. The amino acid pattern of the Yapú diet is compared to the FAO/WHO/UNU suggested pattern requirement for preschool children in Table 5. The FAO/WHO/UNU requirement for methionine and cystine is 25 mg/kg/day, and the Yapú diet provides approximately 34 mg/kg/day. Thus, even if the additional requirements for detoxification of 2 mg/kg/day are considered, sulphur-containing amino acids do not appear to be limiting in this diet. This is noteworthy inasmuch as Yapú protein intakes are barely adequate by FAO/WHO/UNU (1985) standards.

Spath's (1981) contention that the reliance on cassava as a dietary staple increases the minimum daily requirement for methionine is valid, but the Yapú data indicate that this increase in need is quite small. I think that given this small increase in need and the limited nature of our understanding of human amino acid requirements, it would be difficult to support Spath's (1971) argument that methionine alone may be acting as a limiting factor in Amazonia.

CONCLUSIONS AND IMPLICATIONS FOR FUTURE RESEARCH

The results presented here indicate that cassava may not be quite so poor a source of protein and minerals as we have assumed, but as is true of other staple foods, its nutritional value is a function of processing. Although Tukanoans cultivate very bitter varieties of cassava, their processing system is effective in detoxifying the roots. The residual cyanide in food products is low, and the current diet of adults appears to provide adequate quantities of the sulfur-containing amino acids used in the metabolic detoxification of dietary cyanide.

What are the implications of these results for future research? I would like to make two suggestions. First, a number of the health problems associated with cassava use in Africa are the direct result of inadequate processing. Given the preference for high-cyanide cassava varieties in Amazonia, the potential for these same sorts of problems is clearly present if less efficient processing techniques are adopted in the future. Presently, in the more traditional villages like Yapú, cassava processing is highly constrained culturally and there is almost no variation between women or over time in how products are prepared. Cassava processing is, however, an extremely time-consuming activity. As women's expectations change with acculturation, cassava processing techniques may also change. In more acculturated areas like Mitu, there has been a shift to fariña and a virtual abandonment of casabe and associated products. The quality of the fariña for sale suggests that the traditional long fermentation period is being shortened.

Further, since metabolic detoxification of cassava-borne cyanide is dependent on sulfur-containing amino acids, a decrease in the quantity or quality of protein in the current high-cassava diet would increase the risk of cyanide-related health problems. The general assumption is that dietary quality, including animal protein consumption, decreases with acculturation, but there are few empirical data available.

I believe that the strong cultural preference for bitter cassava varieties by at least some native Amazonians deserves more attention. To my knowledge, it is the only example of selection for the more toxic varieties of a given crop. In the Yapú area this selection does not appear to be related to productivity differences between the bitter and sweet cultivars, but it does appear to be related to qualitative differences in the food products made from bitter and sweet cultivars (Dufour 1993).

Notes

1. This research was supported by NSF grant number BNS-8519490, a Fulbright research grant, and an Early Career Development Award from the University of Colorado. I thank Felipa and Cándido Muñoz of Yapú, Vaupés, Colombia, for the processing work at CIAT; T. Salcedo of CIAT for the laboratory analyses; and the Instituto Colombiano de Antropología for its collaboration. I also thank Paul N. Patmore and Richard Wilshusen for their assistance with the fieldwork, and J. Cock, R. Best, and C. Wheatley of CIAT for their support.

2. In Central America and northern parts of South America the plant is referred to as *yuca*, also a Taino word (Carrizales 1984). In Brazil, Paraguay, and Argentina it is referred to as *mandioca* (Albuquerque 1969), and in parts of Colombia, as *mañoco*.

References

Albuquerque, M. de. 1969. *A mandioca na Amazonia*. Belém, Brazil: Superintendencia do Desenvolvimento da Amazonia.

Ayernor, G. S. 1985. Effects of the Retting of Cassava on Product Yield and Cyanide Detoxification. *Journal of Food Technology* 20:89–96.

Bourdoux, P., A. Mafuta, A. Hanson, and A. M. Ermans 1980. Cassava Toxicity: The Role of Linamarian. In *Role of Cassava in the Etiology of Endemic Goitre and Cretinism*, edited by A. M. Ermans, N. M. Mbulamoko, F. Delange, and R. Ahluwalia, pp. 15–28. Ottawa: International Development Research Centre Monograph IDRC-136e.

Bruijn, G. H. de 1973. The Cyanogenic Character of Cassava (*Manihot esculenta*). In *Chronic Cassava Toxicity*, edited by B. Nestle and R. MacIntyre, pp. 43–48. Ottawa: International Development Research Centre Monograph IDRC-010e.

Carrizales, V. 1984. Evolución histórica de la tecnología del cazabe. *Interciencia* 9(4):206–13.

Cock, J. H. 1982. Cassava: A Basic Energy Source in the Tropics. *Science* 218:755–62.

———. 1985. *Cassava: New Potential for a Neglected Crop*. Boulder, Colo.: Westview Press.

Cooke, R. D., and E. N. Maduagwu 1978 The Effects of Simple Processing on the Cyanide Content of Cassava Chips. *Journal of Food Technology* 13:299–306.

Coursey, D. G. 1973 Cassava as Food: Toxicity and Technology. In *Chronic Cassava Toxicity*, edited by B. Nestel and R. MacIntyre, pp. 27–36. Ottawa: International Development Research Centre Monograph IDRC-010e.

Dole, G. E. 1978. The Use of Manioc Among the Kuikuru: Some Interpretations. In *The Nature and Status of*

Ethnobotany, edited by R. I. Ford, pp. 217–49. Ann Arbor: Museum of Anthropology, University of Michigan.

Dufour, D. L. 1983. Nutrition in the Northwest Amazon: Household Dietary Intake and Time-Energy Expenditure. In *Adaptive Responses of Native Amazonians*, edited by R. Hames and W. Vickers, pp. 329–55. New York: Academic Press.

———. 1985. Manioc as a Dietary Staple: Implications for the Budgeting of Time and Energy in the Northwest Amazon. In *Food Energy in Tropical Ecosystems*, edited by D. J. Cattle and K. H. Schwerin, pp. 1–20. New York: Gordon and Breach.

———. 1988a. Cyanide Content of Cassava (*Manihot esculenta*, Euphorbiacae) Cultivars Used by Tukanoan Indians in Northwest Amazonia. *Economic Botany* 42 (2):255–66.

———. 1988b. The Composition of Some Foods Used in Northwest Amazonia. *Interciencia* 13(2):83–86.

———. 1989. Effectiveness of Cassava Detoxification Techniques Used by Indigenous Peoples in Northwest Amazonia. *Interciencia* 14(2):88–91.

———. 1993. The Bitter Is Sweet: A Case Study of Bitter Cassava (*Manihot esculenta*) Use in Amazonia. In *Tropical Forests, People and Food: Biocultural Interactions and Applications to Development*, edited by C. M. Hladik, A. Hladik, O. F. Linares, H. Pagezy, A. Semple, and M. Haldey, pp. 575–88. Paris: UNESCO/Parthenon.

Ermans, A. M., N. M. Mbulamoko, F. Delange, and R. Ahluwalia, eds. 1980. *Role of Cassava in the Etiology of Endemic Goitre and Cretinism*. Ottawa: International Development Research Centre Monograph IDRC-136e.

FAO/WHO/UNU. 1985. *Energy and Protein Requirements*. Geneva: World Health Organization.

Gomez, G., et al. 1984. Effect of Variety and Plant Age on the Cyanide Content of Whole-root Cassava Chips and Its Reduction by Sun-drying. *Animal Feed Science and Technology* 11:57–65.

Howeler, R. H. 1985. Mineral Nutrition and Fertilization of Cassava: A Review of Recent Research. In *Cassava Research, Production and Utilization*, edited by J. H. Cock and J. A. Reyes, pp. 249–320. Cali, Colombia: CIAT.

Hugh-Jones, C. 1979. *From the Milk River*. Cambridge: Cambridge University Press.

Jones, W. O. 19590 *Manioc in Africa*. Stanford, Calif.: Stanford University Press.

Lancaster, P. A., J. S. Ingram, M. Y. Lim, and D. G. Coursey 1982 Traditional Cassava-based Foods: Survey of Processing Techniques. *Economic Botany* 36:12–45.

Meuser, F., and H. D. Smolnik. 1980. Processing of Cassava to Gari and Other Foodstuffs. *Starch/Starke* 32:116–22.

Moran, E. F. 1973. Energy Flow Analysis and the Study of *Manihot esculenta* Crantz. *Acta Amazonica* 3(3):29–39.

Nambisan, B., and S. Sundaresan. 1985. Effect of Processing on the Cyanoglucoside Content of Cassava. *Journal of Science of Food and Agriculture* 36:1197–1203.

Nestel, B., and R. MacIntyre, eds. 1973. *Chronic Cassava Toxicity*. Ottawa: International Development Research Centre Monograph IDRC-010e.

Nordenskiold, E. 1924. *The Ethnography of South America Seen from Mojos in Brazil*. Goteborg: Erlanders Boktryckeri Aktiebolag.

Okezie, B. O., and F. V. Kosikowski. 1982. Cassava as Food. *Critical Reviews in Food Science and Nutrition* 17(3):259–75.

Osuntokun, B. O. 1981. Cassava Diet, Chronic Cyanide Intoxification and Neuropathy in Nigerian Africans. *World Review of Nutrition and Dietetics* 36:141–73.

PRORADAM (Proyecto Radargrametrico del Amazonas) 1979 *La Amazonia y sus recursos*. Bogotá: Republica de Colombia.

Renvoize, B. S. 1972. The Area of Origin of *Manihot esculenta* as a Crop Plant: A Review of the Evidence. *Economic Botany* 26:352–60.

Rogers, D. J. 1965. Some Botanical and Ethnological Considerations of *Manihot esculenta*. *Economic Botany* 19(4):369–77.

Roosevelt, A. C. 1980. *Parmana: Prehistoric Maize and Manioc Subsistence Along the Amazon and Orinoco*. New York: Academic Press.

Rosling, H. 1987. *Cassava Toxicity and Food Security*. Uppsala, Sweden: Tryck kontakt.

Sauer, C. O. 1950. Cultivated Plants of Central and South America. In *Handbook of South American Indians*, edited by J. H. Steward, pp. 507–33. Washington, D.C.: United States Government Printing Office.

Schwerin, K. H. 1971. The Bitter and the Sweet: Some Implications of the Traditional Techniques for Preparing Manioc. Paper presented at the annual meeting of the American Anthropological Association.

———. 1985. Food Crops in the Tropics. In *Food Energy in Tropical Ecosystems*, edited by D. J. Cattle and K. H. Schwerin. New York: Gordon and Breach.

Seigler, D. S., and J. F. Pereira. 1981. Modernized Preparation of Casave in the Llanos Orientales of Venezuela. *Economic Botany* 35(3): 356–62.

Spath, C. D. 1981. Getting to the Meat of the Problem: Some Comments on Protein as a Limiting Factor in Amazonia. *American Anthropologist* 83(2):377–79.

Sponsel, L. E. 1986. Amazon Ecology and Adaptation. *Annual Review of Anthropology* 15:67–97.

Steward, J. H., and L. C. Faron. 1959. *Native Peoples of South America*. New York: McGrawHill.

Wu Leung, W. T., and M. Flores. 1961. *Food Composition Table for Use in Latin America*. Bethesda, Md.: Interdepartmental Committee on Nutrition for National Defense, National Institutes of Health.

CHAPTER 25

Pellagra, Sex and Gender: Biocultural Perspectives on Differential Diets and Health

Barrett P. Brenton

(2000)

BACKGROUND

Pellagra's social history contains a complex story of dietary, socioeconomic, ethnic, and gender inequality. None of the work to date on this disease has focused on the fact that both mortality and morbidity rates for women have been more than double that of men. This calls for a biocultural approach and hypothesis that investigates the clear difference and synergism of pellagra rates related to sex *and* gender. I will argue below that to do so, one must begin to integrate the age-dependent role of estrogen during the female lifecycle (from menarche to menopause) with differential gender-based food consumption patterns. This short research report draws from U.S. mortality statistics covering the period 1900–1950, a time during which pellagra was most prevalent. My objective here is to highlight how clear the evidence is for differential mortality rates between males and females based on diet and digestion.

Put plainly, pellagra is a disease of poverty and social inequality (Brenton 1998). It has severely affected far more women than men. The disease results primarily from deficiencies in the B-vitamin niacin and the amino acid tryptophan. Both of these nutrients are limiting factors in diets of maize eaters. Pellagra has been generally correlated to high-maize and low-protein diets over the past three centuries. Indigenous New World peoples are believed to have been protected from this disease by the use of alkali processing techniques. With the addition of culinary ash or lime this process increases the bioavailability of both niacin and tryptophan (Katz et al. 1974). Consequently, the first descriptions of pellagra were in the Old World during the 18th century as maize was becoming more common as a staple food. This "plague of corn" was rampant in some marginalized European peasant populations for centuries and prevalent among poor U.S. Southerners in the early decades of the twentieth century (Etheridge 1972; Roe 1973). Without the benefit of an alkali cooking tradition scores of impoverished peoples consumed primarily maize-based diets and suffered its consequences. This ranged from the polenta eaters of Italy to the consumption of grits in southern U.S. cuisine. Pellagra continues to be a problem in refugee populations and is still endemic in some South African communities (Brenton 1998).

Pellagra is one of the great detective stories in the history of nutrition (see Carpenter 1981; Etheridge 1972; Roe 1973; Terris 1964). Early on, an association was made between a high-maize diet and poverty among those with the greatest affliction, but for over two centuries many other theories were put forth to explain this malady. This included: 1) a high maize diet with little or no milk, meat or fresh vegetable supplements; 2) spoiled or rotten grain; 3) a disease spread by insects; 4) bad heredity, a question of eugenics, and 5) an overall consequence of poverty.

One thing that was fairly consistent was the description of this malady. Pellagra literally translated as "rough or angry skin" became popularly known as the affliction of the four "D's." Each "D" characterized one of the classic symptoms of the debilitating sequence of the disease: Dermatitis, Diarrhea, Dementia, with the fourth and final "D," Death. It affects children, men, and women, but again differentially. What follows is a brief history of pellagra in the U.S. during the first half of this century.

A BRIEF HISTORY OF PELLAGRA IN THE U.S. 1900–1950

Although first described in the U.S. during the 19th century, by 1910 the U.S. Public Health Service recognized a rapid increase in pellagra mortality. Efforts were then put forth to make physicians aware of the disease and its diagnosis. Interestingly enough, an industrial milling and degerming processes of corn and wheat, which completely removed most of the niacin, became common around 1905 when pellagra rates began to rise. In addition, for southern states where pellagra rates were the highest, grits were no longer being made as "hominy grits," which involved the alkali processing of maize into hominy, but were only grits as a process of this new milling process. Unfortunately, these grits were still being sold as hominy grits.

Barrett P. Brenton, "Pellagra, sex and gender: biocultural perspectives on differential diets and health." *Nutritional Anthropology* 22 (2000): 20–24. Reprinted with permission.

From 1914 onward, studies by Dr. Joseph Goldberger, a U.S. Public Health Service officer, came to the conclusion that pellagra was related to a poor diet lacking good sources of protein, which was in part a consequence of poverty (Goldberger 1918; Terris 1964). Yet his ideas did not receive widespread acceptance for almost 20 years. For a brief time period after 1917 pellagra mortality actually dropped related to WWI. This was due to increased wages at cotton mills in the south and because of an increased interest in victory gardens, with access to fresh vegetables. Soon after the war however economic depression returned and pellagra morbidity soared to epidemic proportions.

Pellagra mortality rates quickly subsided during the mid 1930s to early 1940s in part from "New Deal" programs and later WWII which provided employment, higher wages, and again incentives for victory gardens. In addition, niacin was isolated as a B complex vitamin that served as a pellagra-preventative (PP) factor which could be provided to patients in the form of yeast. By 1943 corn and wheat flours were being fortified with niacin. This was probably the greatest contributor to a sustained decrease in pellagra.

PELLAGRA SEX AND GENDER

One of the most striking characteristics of pellagra mortality is that in the U.S. from 1900–1950 rates for women were consistently *double* that of men (Miller 1978). Even more alarming is the fact that pellagra morbidity rates (those diagnosed with the disease) could be up to 20 times greater for women, with a common two to three fold difference being prevalent. Why? I propose that pellagra morbidity and mortality rates for females eating high maize and low protein diets are greater than males due to a complex biocultural interaction and synergism of:

(a) Unequal access to nutrient quality foods and therefore inadequate intakes of niacin and tryptophan by women due to both poverty and gender inequality, and

(b) Estrogen's demonstrated inhibitory effect on converting the amino acid tryptophan to niacin, a major pathway for meeting our daily niacin requirements.

Putting a theoretical debate on the conflation of sex and gender aside, this proposal operates on the condition of distinguishing between: gender (a category of sexual identity as women, men, etc.), *and* sex (a category of being biologically male or female).

A few brief gendered explanations for why women suffered from pellagra much more than men in the U.S. south during the first half of this century are focused on differential and unequal access to quality foods within the household. This difference has been noted by both researchers of the time (Carpenter 1981; Terris 1964) and social historians (Etheridge 1972). For example:

(a) As primary wage earners, men were given consideration and preference at the dinner table, they also had pocket money to spend on foods outside of the home;

(b) Women as wage earners made less than men, thus decreasing their spending power for food items;

(c) Women would give protein quality foods, especially milk, to their children first;

(d) Women would generally eat last after everyone else in the family had a chance to eat;

(e) Women, especially in southern states, strongly upheld the culinary triad of maize (in the form of grits), molasses, and fat-back pork; a combination that clearly contributed to pellagra..

Understandably these examples cannot encompass an enormous amount of household variation. Yet, they begin to add up as a formidable set of risk factors in the etiology of pellagra. In addition, it forces us to take a serious look at the gender-specific historical consequences of food accessibility, inequality and the biology of poverty. Following through with a biocultural approach we also need to incorporate the impact of biological sex.

PELLAGRA AND SEX

Although the conversion rate of tryptophan to niacin is only 60:1 (Henderson 1983), our dietary requirements of niacin are usually met in this way. This pathway is especially important in diets which are low in niacin, as in the case of intensive maize eaters. The diets of pellagrins would have further exacerbated their condition with low tryptophan/protein diets. From a biological/physiological/biochemical perspective, it has been shown that estrogen can block or inhibit the biochemical conversion of the essential amino acid tryptophan to the B-vitamin niacin when diets are minimally adequate for tryptophan (Bender and Totoe 1984; Shibata and Toda 1997). In short, it seems that the Kynurenine pathway responsible for the tryptophan to niacin conversion is inhibited by estrogen.

However, at the same time pregnancy and lactation can actually increase the conversion of tryptophan to niacin by enhancing that biochemical pathway (National Research Council 1989; Wolf 1971). This would only be to a limited degree or not at all in diets low in both tryptophan and niacin.

A 1990 survey of a pellagra outbreak among Mozambican refugees in Malawi showed that the morbidity rate was almost 8 times higher among women than men (Malfait et al. 1993). Pregnant and lactating females had lower rates, although not significantly different, than other women. There are other, although inconsistent, reports in the historical literature that pregnant females have lower rates of pellagra, but the rates soon rose after they had given birth (Saunders 1911). Unfortunately it is not clear whether or not these women were breastfeeding with prolonged periods of lactation.

A strong argument for the impact of estrogen can also be found when one notes that in the U.S. during some of the worst outbreaks of pellagra, the maximum number of pellagra deaths for females occurred at a mean age category of 30–34 years of age, when females are well into maximum estrogen production during reproductive years. Reports consistently stress that females between 20 and 40 are at the highest risk for developing pellagra. This can also be clearly seen in the age-dependent role of estrogen during the female lifecycle (from menarche to menopause). The onset of pellagra shows a dramatic increase in pellagra around the age of menarche and drops off sharply by age 50 and the onset of menopause. For males, pellagra rates begin to rise after age 35 peaking at around age 60. These observations are consistently noted in both mortality and morbidity rates for the U.S. and in other countries as well. In sum, mortality rates for females closely follow an age-related curve from menarche to menopause linked to life history levels of estrogen.

CONCLUSIONS

The physiology and social history of pellagra combined provide a biocultural case study for understanding the etiology of a disease and its socio-cultural implications. Although thousands of people died during the height of the pellagra era, we must remember that hundreds of thousands of people were inflicted. The U.S. history of pellagra shows us how the scientific community and policy makers had to come to the realization that nutrition and disease are related, and the role that poverty plays in that relationship (Bollet 1992; Kunitz 1988). I argue that we must also incorporate the biocultural dimensions of gender and sex into these discussions.

With the synergism of sex and gender in action, it is tempting to question the role of Native American females/ women in the biocultural evolution of maize culinary traditions that stressed the use of alkali processing techniques to prevent the onset of pellagra and allow higher maize consumption. Although beyond the scope of this presentation and reserved for future publications, issues of race and ethnicity also figure heavily into differential pellagra morbidity and mortality. Black females had by far the highest morbidity and mortality rates for pellagra. White males had the lowest.

This integrative research is instrumental in determining dietary recommendations and establishing international food policy and public health intervention programs regarding differential female and male physiology and nutrition, and gender differences in access to foods, both today and in past societies.

Periodic episodes and outbreaks of pellagra around the world are a testament to the biology of poverty. As anthropologists we often feel helpless to intervene in the political-economic conditions under which poverty is accepted and promoted. We can however continue to be critical of those conditions under which political and economic exploitation occurs and remind the public that poverty has both a very real and usually deleterious biological effect on the human condition.

References

Bender, D. A. and L. Totoe, 1984, Inhibition of Tryptophan Metabolism by Oestrogens in the Rat: a Factor in the Aetiology of Pellagra. British Journal of Nutrition 51:219–224.

Bollet, A.J., 1992, Politics and Pellagra: The Epidemic of Pellagra in the U.S. in the Early Twentieth Century. The Yale Journal of Biology and Medicine 65:211–221.

Brenton, B. P., 1998, Pellagra and Nutrition Policy: Lessons from the Great Irish Famine to the New South Africa. Nutritional Anthropology 22(1):1–11.

Carpenter, K. J. (ed.), 1981, Pellagra. Stroudsburg, PA: Hutchinson Ross.

Etheridge, E.W., 1972, The Butterfly Caste: A Social History of Pellagra in The South. Westport, CT: Greenwood.

Goldberger, J., 1918, Pellagra: Its Nature and Prevention. Public Health Reports 33:481–488.

Henderson, L.M., 1983, Niacin. Annual Review of Nutrition 3:289–307.

Katz, S. H., M.L. Hediger, and L.A. Valleroy, 1974, Traditional Maize Processing Techniques in the New World. Science 184:765–773.

Kunitz, S. J., 1988, Hookworm and Pellagra: Exemplary Diseases in the New South. Journal of Health and Social Behavior 29: 139–148.

Malfait, P. et al., 1993, An Outbreak of Pellagra Related to Changes in Dietary Niacin among Mozambican Refugees in Malawi. International Journal of Epidemiology 22: 504–511.

Miller, D. F., 1978, Pellagra Deaths in the United States. American Journal of Clinical Nutrition 31:558–559.

National Research Council, 1989, Recommended Dietary Allowances. 10th Revised Edition. Washington D.C.: National Academy Press.

Roe, D.A., 1973, A Plague of Corn: The Social History of Pellagra. Ithaca, NY: Cornell University Press.

Saunders, E.B., 1911, The Gynecological, Obstetrical and Surgical Aspects of Pellagra. American Journal of Insanity 68: 541–551.

Shibata, K. and Satoko, T., 1997, Effects on sex hormones on the metabolism of tryptophan and niacin and to serotonin in male rats. Bioscience, Biotechnology, and Biochemistry 61(7):1200–1202.

Terris, M. (ed.), 1964, Goldberger on Pellagra. Baton Rouge, LA: Louisiana State University Press.

Wolf, H., 1971, Hormonal Alteration of Efficiency of Conversion of Tryptophan to Urinary Metabolites of Niacin in Man. The American Journal of Clinical Nutrition 24:792–799.

CHAPTER 26

"Drink Milk for Fitness": The Cultural Politics of Human Biological Variation and Milk Consumption in the United States

Andrea S. Wiley

(2004)

That populations vary with respect to their capacity to digest milk in adulthood is well known among biological anthropologists and organizations in the United States involved in the formulation and enactment of food and nutrition policies. This variation in response to milk derives from genetic regulation of lactase, the enzyme that breaks down the milk sugar lactose. In most populations, lactase activity declines during childhood; in relatively few does lactase activity remain high throughout adulthood. Cross-culturally, persistence of lactase activity into adulthood correlates with (1) fresh milk consumption; (2) a central role for milk production in the domestic economy; (3) positive evaluation of milk and other dairy products; and (4) physiological capacity to digest and, hence, tolerate lactose. This article is primarily concerned with how the anthropological interpretation of lactase persistence compares to those offered by institutions in the United States that have an impact on dietary recommendations for consumption of cow's milk, an important agricultural commodity. Because polices often reflect the biases and agendas of their authors, the portrayal of lactase persistence by the dominant ethnic group—U.S. citizens derived from northern Europe, who are largely lactase persistent—is likely to indicate ethno- or biocentric bias, insofar as it promotes milk consumption and downplays the significance of other biologies.

First, I outline the state of knowledge about the biology of lactase persistence, especially its genetic foundations, and what is known about population variation in these genotypes. The anthropological discussion builds on this genetic information and seeks to understand the evolutionary causes of population variation. Next, describe the stories told by various U.S. institutions—the United States

Department of Agriculture (USDA) and the dairy industry, professional medical associations, nutritionists and dieticians, and antimilk coalitions. Despite widespread acknowledgement that a substantial minority of people in the United States—and the majority in the world—are lactase impersistent as adults, it appears that the strong cultural value placed on cow's milk and governmental support of the dairy industry inhibit policies that put the anthropological understanding of lactase persistence into practice. Thus, while the latter emphasizes biological variation in milk digestive physiology and the unique historical processes that produced it, this perspective has been subsumed into subtly disguised normalizing discourses that downplay the significance of this diversity and promote a modal biological response to milk that should facilitate its consumption by all U.S. citizens throughout life.

Given the interconnections between discourses of biological variation, dietary recommendations, and political economic forces supporting the U.S. dairy industry, a biocultural perspective is particularly relevant to this analysis. In using the biocultural label, I consider not only how cultural factors influenced biological evolution (as is surely the case in the evolution of lactase persistence) but also how understandings of human biological variation are constructed and elaborated within a cultural context.

THE BIOLOGICAL FOUNDATION OF LACTASE PERSISTENCE

Lactase (more technically, lactase-phlorizin hydrolase [LPH]) is an enzyme found in the brush border of the jejunum of the mammalian small intestine. It functions to break down lactose, a sugar found only in mammalian milks, into its component sugars, glucose and galactose. Because lactose cannot be absorbed directly, lactase is necessary for the digestion and metabolic utilization of milk sugar. In most mammalian species, lactase production is high at birth and begins to decline around the time of weaning. As a result,

Andrea S. Wiley, "'Drink milk for fitness': the cultural politics of human biological variation and milk consumption in the United States." *American Anthropologist* 106(2004): 506–517. Reprinted with permission.

adult mammals produce only residual quantities of lactase. Up through the latter part of the 20th century, researchers debated whether lactase activity could be maintained or induced by a diet containing lactose. Although a few studies suggested that it could be, most concluded that the decline of lactase production occurred independently of lactose in the diet (Sahi 1994b). Human studies from the 1960s indicated that contrary to earlier beliefs, most humans followed the basic mammalian pattern (Bayless and Rosensweig 1966, 1967), and that lactase activity in adults could not be increased by providing lactose.

It is now well understood that the age-related decline in lactase production is regulated genetically, and that there is both individual and population variation in this trait. While frequencies of adult lactase activity are somewhat continuously distributed across populations, two patterns are easily distinguished: (1) populations in which high frequencies of adults continue to produce high levels of lactase in adulthood and (2) populations in which lactase production declines to low levels by adulthood (Sahi 1994a). Several thorough reviews describe population frequencies of lactase persistence (cf. Durham 1991; Flatz 1987; Sahi 1994a; Scrimshaw and Murray 1988; Simoons 1978). While studies of individual populations vary tremendously in their methodology and sample populations, it is clear that high rates of lactase persistence are found only among northern Europeans; South Asians; herding populations of the Middle East, Arabian Peninsula, and sub-Saharan Africa; and descendents of these populations.

Populations also vary in the age at which lactase activity declines, from one to two years to 20 years. Those groups with high rates of persistence exhibit later average ages of onset among members who are impersistent (Sahi 1994a). Neither the mechanism underlying this age variation nor its significance is well understood.

TERMINOLOGY

A number of terms are employed to describe the biological phenomenon of lactase activity in adults, and their usage provides insights into how various authors or institutions view variation in this phenotype. The terms *lactose tolerance/intolerance* are most common in vernacular usage. These refer to the subjective experience of gastrointestinal symptoms after lactose consumption (bloating, diarrhea, cramps), which vary considerably across individuals. It is quite possible to have high lactase activity but report intolerance or, more frequently, to have biologically assayed low lactase activity but report no symptoms of intolerance. Other terms are thus preferred, although there is no consensus on which are best. In recognition that low levels of lactase activity are modal for the human species, many authors prefer *lactase persistence/nonpersistence, lactase restriction*, or *high/low lactose digestion capacity*.

The term *adult-type hypolactasia* has gained currency as a way to describe low levels of lactase activity among adults, although Timo Sahi (1994b), a leading proponent of

this terminology, dismisses the possibility of using *hyperlactasia* as its counterpart. However, given that hypolactasia is the norm for the species, individuals with higher lactase activity in adulthood could properly be described as having *hyperlactasia. Lactase deficiency* implies pathology, as do the descriptors *lactose maldigestion* and *malabsorption*. Furthermore, terminology that includes the word *lactose* implies that lactose is part of the diet; *lactose maldigestion* or *malabsporption* would never manifest if lactose was not being consumed.[1] Changes in lactase activity or the digestion of lactose among adults can also stem from nutritional factors (e.g., protein malnutrition), pathologies of the small intestine, and gastrointestinal infections. When any of these result in low levels of lactose digestion, *secondary hypolactasia, malabsorption*, or *maldigestion* is the diagnostic label. Adult-type hypolactasia that derives exclusively from age-related declines in lactase activity is considered primary.

Throughout this article I will use the terms *lactase persistence/impersistence*. These are preferred because they are relatively value free, implying neither pathology nor having *too much* or *too little* or *high* or *low* lactase activity.

THE ANTHROPOLOGICAL STORY OF LACTASE PERSISTENCE

Variation in adult lactase production appears to be under strong genetic control, and genealogical studies have found a pattern that is consistent with a dominant mode of expression for the alleles associated with lactase persistence (Kretchmer 1972; Sahi 1994a). The gene for the lactase enzyme is found on chromosome 2 and is not variable across populations in ways that correlate with differences in lactase persistence. Regulation of the lactase gene is variable, however, and there are four common variants of the lactase haplotype (A, B, C, and U). A is most common in northern Europe, with declines in frequency across southern Europe and India, where B and C are more common. U is notably absent among Indo-European populations but is found in most others. Haplotype diversity is greatest in sub-Saharan African populations (Hollox et al. 2000). Lactase persistence is most frequently associated with the A form but is found occasionally with the other forms (Harvey et al. 1998; Hollox et al. 2000).

Recently a noncoding segment of DNA upstream from the lactase gene has been identified as a site of variation in adult lactase activity (Enattah et al. 2002). Individuals with the C nucleotide at a locus in the 13th intron or a G in the 9th intron (these two introns being eight kilobases apart) within a neighboring gene about 14 kilobases upstream from the lactase gene were lactase impersistent, while those with T or A at these same loci were lactase persistent. Although the exact mechanism by which these loci regulate lactase production remains unclear, current evidence points to their action at the level of gene transcription, as most studies demonstrate variation in mRNA levels between those who are lactase persistent or impersistent, a pattern that becomes evident during childhood (Wang et al. 1998).

It is widely accepted that the origins of animal domestication set the stage for selection favoring the ability to digest lactose in adulthood—for without exposure to mammalian milk in adulthood, presumably no advantage would derive from continued production of lactase. Indeed, all populations with high rates of lactase persistence have long histories of dairying. Given that milk is rich in several nutrients (protein, fat, calcium, sugar), Frederick Simoons (1978, 2001) proposed that individuals with a mutation allowing them to consume the milk of domesticated mammals throughout life would have been healthier and better nourished than those without it. Researchers have suggested that a three to seven percent fitness advantage would have been sufficient to generate the high frequencies of lactase persistence found in dairy-dependent populations (Flatz 1987; McCracken 1971). However, as William Durham (1991) pointed out, there are many populations with long histories of domesticating dairy animals that also have low rates of lactase persistence. These groups often make use of fermented milk products (e.g., yogurt, kefir) or cheese. Bacterial fermentation results in dairy products that are low in lactose, while the process of cheese making involves draining off the lactose-rich whey from milk solids. Thus, having a history of dairying is necessary but not sufficient for explaining global variation in lactase persistence, and only populations drinking substantial amounts of *fresh* milk would have benefited from the ability to digest lactose.

Noting that lactase persistence and fresh milk consumption correlated with latitude, Durham (1991) proposed that the low levels of UV light found at high latitudes would have selected for lactase persistence among dairying populations living there. This hypothesis was based on the observation by Gebhard Flatz and Hans Rotthauwe (1973) that the presence of lactose in the small intestine enhances calcium absorption. Vitamin D is synthesized in skin cells in the presence of UV light and facilitates calcium uptake, but when exposure to UV light is reduced—and Vitamin D synthesis is, thus, likewise diminished—lactose, which is found only in fresh milk, can increase calcium absorption. The calcium absorption hypothesis was recently subjected to critical review by Simoons (2001), who concluded that there is scant osteoarchaeological, historical, or biomedical evidence to support it. Further, while this may help explain the very high frequencies of lactase persistence found among northern Europeans, it has little relevance for understanding lactase persistence in populations at lower latitudes. There, other nutritional advantages to adult milk consumption, such as hydration or the use of lactose as a carbohydrate, a nutrient rare in the diets of exclusive pastoralists, may have accrued to those able to digest fresh milk.

Another hypothesis that has received relatively little attention is that since the genetic markers associated with lactase persistence are known in geographically diverse areas, lactase persistence could have spread prior to the rise of dairying cultures. B. Anderson and C. Vullo (1994) proposed that lactase *im*persistence was selected for as a defense against falciparum malaria, the most deadly form of the parasitic disease. Milk is a very rich source of the B-vitamin riboflavin, and malarial parasites require riboflavin to multiply in red blood cells. In the context of riboflavin deficiency at a level tolerated by a human host, malarial reproduction is significantly inhibited (Dutta et al. 1985). Thus, early reduction in lactase production would lead to earlier termination of breastfeeding; this in turn would generate riboflavin deficiency (from decreased milk intake) sufficient to reduce malarial infection without being overly deleterious to the child. Because populations vary in the age at which lactase activity may decline, later age of onset of lactase impersistence would have been tolerated in populations not exposed to deadly forms of malaria (e.g., northern Europeans, who have both high rates of lactase persistence and later ages of onset of impersistence among those with that genotype). However, a study in Sardinia showed that three villages with varying exposure to malaria did have different frequencies of other known adaptations to malaria (e.g., G-6PD deficiency and β-thalassemia) but did not vary in their rates of lactase persistence (Meloni et al. 1998). This hypothesis also fails to explain why some populations would remain lactase persistent throughout life, given that this is the derived (i.e., evolutionarily recent) condition for mammals.

While selection probably played a key role in the spread of lactase persistence among some dairying populations, other evolutionary forces have also contributed to global diversity in adult lactase activity. Genetic drift may have been important in reducing diversity in genes associated with lactase activity in non-African populations, given that there is greater variation within contemporary African populations (Hollox et al. 2000). Clearly, gene flow has also played an enormous role among historical and contemporary populations, especially in areas colonized by northern European populations (Flatz 1987). Collectively, these forces have generated the more-or-less continuous distribution in population frequencies of lactase persistence.

OTHER STORIES: LACTASE PERSISTENCE AND HEALTH POLICY IN THE UNITED STATES

The anthropological story of lactase persistence is a story of human variation: Lactase impersistence is the norm for the species and persistence is the unusual condition. Individuals in most populations experience declines in lactase production during childhood and, hence, have little of the enzyme required to fully digest milk in adulthood. As expected, these are also populations that historically have made little use of fresh milk. Conversely, populations with high rates of lactase persistence have included dairy farming as an intrinsic part of the food economy and extensive use of dairy products in their cuisines (Durham 1991). These practices have become entrenched in many areas permanently colonized by Europeans in particular (e.g., United States, Canada, New Zealand, Australia). While the extent to which fresh milk was a large part of traditional European diets is unclear, it is now widely consumed in European-derived populations in the United States. Milk is especially recommended for children, teenagers, and adult women; it is considered necessary to support the needs of fetal growth during pregnancy and milk production during lactation, to build and maintain a strong skeleton, and to ward off osteoporosis at older ages. Whether these recommendations are well supported by evidence is a matter of some contention, especially given that other populations maintain adequate fetal and child growth and bone density in the absence of milk consumption (cf. Bertron et al. 1999; Feskanich et al. 1997; Heaney 2000; Specker and Wosje 2001; Weinsier and Krumdieck 2000). While I have reviewed this topic elsewhere (Wiley 2004), here the question is whether the anthropological story of variation in lactase activity has any currency in policies promoted by U.S. policy-making institutions dealing with food, nutrition, or health, given the hegemony of European culinary traditions and agricultural practices. What other discourses about this aspect of human biological variation are constructed by such institutions?

USDA and the National Dairy Council (NDC)

The USDA has a dual mandate within the U.S. government: to promote U.S. agricultural interests and to issue food and nutrition guidelines that promote the health of U.S. citizens. That these two missions might be at odds with one another was apparently not considered when the USDA was created. At the time, undernutrition was a considerable problem; however, in the current dietary environment of hyperabundance of relatively cheap agricultural commodities (e.g., corn, wheat, milk) and dietary guidelines that encourage consumption of calorie dense foods, conflict between these goals is becoming more visible as rates of obesity and its concomitant health problems continue to rise (Nestle 2002).

Dairy products make up about 11 percent of U.S. agricultural commodities (U.S. Department of Commerce 2002). In the Dairy Production Stabilization Act of 1983, the U.S. government authorized the USDA to oversee national programs for "dairy product promotion, research, and nutrition education as part of a comprehensive strategy to increase human consumption of milk and dairy products" (USDA 2002:5). In 1990, the Fluid Milk Promotion Act specifically targeted fluid (fresh) milk. In justifying this act, Congress stated that

> (1) fluid milk products are basic foods and a primary source of required nutrients such as calcium, and otherwise are a valuable part of the human diet; and (2) fluid milk products must be readily available and marketed efficiently to ensure that the people of the United States receive adequate nourishment; and (3) the dairy industry plays a significant role in the economy of the United States. [USDA 1990]

These programs are run by groups such as the Fluid Milk Board, the National Dairy Council (NDC), and the National Dairy Promotion and Research Board (NDPRB), among other state and regional organizations. Under a check-off system, local dairy farmers pay a mandatory fee per unit of milk produced to support the activities of these groups, the vast majority of which focus on advertising (USDA 2002).

The USDA is also responsible for developing and promoting dietary guidelines for U.S. citizens. The food pyramid, the most widely disseminated guide to eating in the United States, includes a separate category for dairy products and recommends two to three servings of dairy products per day (www.nal.usda.gov/fnic/Fpyr/pmap.htm). The primary (though not exclusive) justification for such a recommendation is based on milk products as rich sources of calcium. Moreover, even though there are some "alternative" nonofficial food pyramids designed for minority populations accessible through the USDA site, all of them also contain dairy products (www.nal.usda.gov/fnic/etext/000023.html#xtocid2381818). As Marion Nestle (2002) noted in her careful study of links between government diet and nutrition policy and food industries, several representatives of the dairy industry including the NDC and NDPRB were on the advisory committee charged to develop the 2000 Dietary Guidelines for Americans. Not surprisingly, they opposed any suggestion to include alternatives to dairy foods, especially as sources of calcium (such as fortified soy "milk") in the dairy section.[2] Among other blatant conflations of government policy and the dairy industry was the 1998 appearance of then-secretary of health and human services Donna Shalala in one of the popular "got milk?" advertisements.

Thus, in both of its roles the USDA is involved in promoting the consumption of dairy products—especially fresh milk—among all U.S. citizens. However, the agency has been forced to recognize that substantial numbers of ethnic minorities may have low levels of the enzyme lactase or consider themselves lactose intolerant. With the increasing presence of peoples of Asian, Latin American, or African descent in the United States, up to 25 percent of the adult population may be lactase impersistent. The NDC recognizes that approximately 100 percent of all Native Americans, 90 percent of all Asian Americans, 80 percent of all African Americans, 53 percent of all Hispanic Americans, and 15 percent of all Caucasians are "lactose maldigesters" (NDC 2003b).

In their publications, the USDA and the various dairy promotion organizations first make a clear distinction between their preferred term *lactose maldigestion* and *lactose intolerance*. Lactose intolerance refers to the "gastrointestinal symptoms experienced by some individuals who have low levels of lactase, the enzyme necessary to digest lactose" (NDC 2003b). These symptoms include nausea, vomiting, bloating, cramps, and excess flatulence. However, they argue that this condition is relatively rare, and that *lactose maldigestion* is more common. Importantly, individuals with lactose maldigestion may have low levels of lactase but do not experience gastrointestinal symptoms following consumption of lactose-containing dairy products so long as their physiological capacity to digest lactose is not exceeded. Thus, according to the NDC, such people can—and should—consume milk.

The NDC contends that rates of reported lactose maldigestion are likely to overestimate those who actually suffer negative symptoms after milk consumption, also in part because these symptoms may mimic those of other gastrointestinal illnesses. Individuals who suspect they are lactose intolerant should be objectively tested by a physician using the breath hydrogen test, which measures the amount of hydrogen expelled in a person's breath following digestion of lactose. The NDC is, however, careful to note that those tests may generate false positives (again inflating the rate of "true" intolerance) because the lactose challenge is much greater than that found in a glass of milk. Furthermore, many individuals may claim to be lactose intolerant not because they have physiological symptoms but, rather, because of negative "culturally based attitudes towards milk learned at a young age" (NDC 2003b). Such persons may never acquire a taste for milk if they live in a family that does not make milk a part of their regular diet.

The USDA and dairy promotion agencies recommend "several easy steps to overcome lactose intolerance." The first and most vital step is to see a physician immediately in order to be correctly diagnosed. If a low level of lactase activity is verified, an individual must *not* conclude that he or she should avoid dairy products but, rather, find creative ways to include dairy products in the diet. The NDC warns that "avoiding dairy foods can cause inadequate intakes of calcium and many other essential nutrients. A deficiency of calcium increases the risk of developing osteoporosis, hypertension, and possibly some types of cancer," but "fortunately, tolerance to lactose can be improved by adjusting the amounts and types of dairy foods consumed" (NDC 2003a). These modifications include drinking small amounts of milk with meals to slow the process of absorption, starting with small servings and slowly working up to larger quantities in a process that suggests the building of a tolerance to lactose. Other solutions to intolerance include consuming aged, hard cheeses, yogurt with active bacterial cultures, lactose-free milk, or taking over-the-counter lactase enzyme tablets or drops prior to the consumption of lactose-containing dairy products. Nondairy sources of calcium are denigrated as having much less calcium than milk, or it is suggested that their calcium is much less bioavailable than that in milk.[3]

Nutrition and Dietetics Perspectives

The reach of the U.S. government's nutrition policy is extensive. Its impact is clear in the nutritional recommendations made by practicing nutritionists and dieticians, as well as in the food assistance programs that the USDA supports. Organizations such as the American Dietetics Association (ADA), the professional unit to which registered dietitians belong; the American School Food Service Association (ASFSA); and nutrition textbooks tend to take the approach of the USDA and NDC. Given that nutritionists and dieticians are those who provide dietary advice to individuals in clinical, public health, food assistance program-related, and other settings, their interpretation of lactase impersistence is likely to have practical significance.

A popular nutrition text has a separate "nutrition focus" section on lactose intolerance in which there is discussion of population variation in the ability to digest lactose, although reduction in lactase activity is described as a "primary *disease*" (Wardlaw and Insel 1996). Individuals suspecting lactose intolerance should find out by trial and error how much lactose they can comfortably tolerate and

> easily adjust the amount of dairy products in their diet. Such people need not avoid all milk and milk products; nor is this recommended because these foods are very good sources of calcium, riboflavin, potassium, and magnesium. Although these four nutrients are present in other food groups, many people don't eat much of these alternative sources. [Wardlaw and Insel 1996:75–76]

The ADA presents a "fact sheet" on lactose intolerance, which was supported by a grant from McNeil Consumer Products, makers of Lactaid°. The fact sheet reviews population variation in lactase production—and, in an interesting departure from NDC statements—suggests that lactose intolerance is very common. It does, though, go on to recommend that individuals adopt the various strategies outlined by the NDC—for example, consuming smaller amounts of dairy more frequently or choosing lower lactose-containing dairy products, but, not surprisingly, two of its six suggestions include taking exogenous lactase. Nestle (2002) has noted that among professional nutrition associations, the ADA is more likely to promote food industry interests in its publications, and it is one of the links (the other being the NDC) listed at www.whymilk.com, the interactive website of the popular "got milk?" campaign.

The ASFSA, a nonprofit organization of professionals in school nutrition programs, also vigorously promotes milk consumption in part through its close association with the National School Lunch Program. Since the 1946 inception of the National School Lunch Act, the government has required that fluid milk be offered as part of meals that are eligible for federal reimbursement. Note that the National School Lunch program, like the USDA, has a dual purpose, as outlined in the Act of 1946:

> It is hereby declared to be the policy of Congress, as a measure of national security, to safeguard the health and well-being of the Nation's children and to encourage the domestic consumption of nutritious agricultural commodities and other food, by assisting the States, through grants-in aid and other means, in providing an adequate supply of food and other facilities for the establishment, maintenance, operation and expansion of nonprofit school lunch programs. [USDA 2003]

Twenty years later, private institutions devoted to the care and education of children were also made eligible for these federal milk reimbursements. And, in 1968, an amendment to the Child Nutrition Act was approved that read: "Minimum nutritional requirements shall not be construed to prohibit substitution of foods to accommodate the medical or other special dietary needs of individual students" (USDA 2003). Presumably, this covered those with lactose intolerance. Of note is a presentation from the ASFSA website that celebrates Boston schools' success at promoting lactose-free milk in their food programs, which resulted in increases in milk sales (Focus on Children: Boston Public Schools 2003); also educational materials from the NDC are easily accessed though the ASFSA site (www.asfsa. org).[4]

The Special Supplemental Nutritional Assistance Program for Women, Infants, and Children (WIC) was authorized in 1974 to provide subsidies for specific nutrient-rich foods for pregnant or breastfeeding women and infants and children up to five years of age. Fluid milk and cheese are featured among the foods that are allowed (others are infant formula, cereal, eggs, dried beans, peanut butter, tuna fish, and carrots). The majority (over 60 percent) of WIC recipients (which numbered over eight million in 2002) are minorities—the largest percentage of which are Hispanics, African Americans, Asian Americans, and Native Americans, all populations with high frequencies of lactase impersistence (www.ers.usda.gov/publications/fanrr27/fanrr27d.pdf). In recognition of individuals with "special" dietary needs, WIC allows lactose-reduced or lactose-free milk, or the substitution of more cheese for milk in its food packages, but no nondairy substitutes.

Professional Medical Associations

Given that government nutrition policy explicitly targets milk for consumption by U.S. citizens to maintain optimal health, how do medical institutions, whose members are involved in clinical practice, assess the issue of milk consumption and lactase impersistence? Publicly available materials from three relevant medical organizations (American Academy of Pediatrics [AAP]; American Academy of Family Practitioners [AAFP]; and American College of Gastroenterology [ACG]) provide insight into this issue. These groups all make the crucial distinction between *lactose intolerance* and *lactase impersistence* but tend to focus on *lactose intolerance*. This makes sense in that from their perspective, lactose intolerance is the relevant clinical condition; individuals experiencing uncomfortable or painful symptoms because of underlying lactase impersistence would be those most likely to seek medical help.

While medical organizations appear to consider lactase impersistence as "normal" for the human species, citing the usual surveys of its frequency in different populations, their language nonetheless tends to medicalize it and treat it as the deviant condition. For example, the AAP uses the language *lactose maldigestion*, but in the discussion of global variation, it refers to *lactase deficiency*:

late-onset lactase *deficiency* (adult hypolactasia) is a common *disorder*. Approximately 90% of adult Ameri-

can blacks and 60% to 80% of Mexican-Americans, native American Indians, Asians, and most middle-Eastern and Mediterranean populations have *abnormal* findings on lactose tolerance tests. [AAP 1985, emphasis added][5]

Likewise, lactase impersistence is described by the ACG as: "a shortage of the enzyme lactase, which is *normally* produced by the cells that line the small intestine" (www.acg.gi.org/patientinfo/cgp/cgpvol3.html#food, emphasis added). Note that these are descriptions of lactase impersistence, not specifically the clinical symptoms associated with lactose intolerance.

Unlike the NDC, which recommends an objective lactose-challenge test by a clinician, medical organizations tend to favor self-diagnosis of lactose intolerance. In their educational materials, both the AAFP and ACG recommend that individuals diagnose themselves by eliminating all dairy products from their diet for several weeks to ascertain whether this eases their symptoms. This is followed by a dairy challenge to see if symptoms reappear. If they do, the "treatment" is simple: Avoid dairy products. However, they also suggest that by trial and error individuals should figure out how much of which dairy products they can tolerate without negative symptoms. Those who find themselves reacting to most dairy products are advised to take exogenous lactase before they consume them.

Again, the concern for those who avoid milk products is that they would not meet their calcium needs. Most medical organizations recommend dairy products such as yogurt, cheese, or lactose-reduced milk, especially for children, who are seen as particularly in need of not only the calcium in dairy products but also the protein, Vitamin D (which is not an intrinsic part of milk; milk is *fortified* with Vitamins A and D), and, in the case of fresh milk, water for hydration. Other fortified foods, such as orange juice, or dark green leafy vegetables, legumes, and fish are recommended, and calcium supplementation is advised for those who "significantly limit their dietary intake of milk products" (www.acg.gi.org/patientinfo/cgp/pdf/food_I%7E1.pdf).

While the AAP expresses concern that children with lactase impersistence obtain sufficient calcium, their statement also outlines the potential problems associated with milk consumption among such children. The nutrients in milk may not be fully absorbed; if diarrhea results, nutrients are lost and there is a risk of dehydration. Furthermore, the AAP and others express concern about the use of lactose in medicines such as birth control pills, antacids, and other prescription and over-the-counter drugs (AAP 1985). Lactose is used as a filler, an anticaking agent, and a flavor to make pills more palatable. While only a very few individuals with severe intolerance are likely to be sensitive to these small amounts, including lactose among the inactive ingredients in medicines (estimated at up to 20 percent of prescription drugs and six percent of over-the-counter medicines; www.gastro.org/public/brochures/lactose.html) indicates a lack of appreciation for population diversity in physiological responses to lactose.

Antimilk Groups

Despite overt sponsorship of milk consumption by state and federal governments, there is vigorous—if not well-coordinated—antimilk sentiment, suggesting that milk's merits are not entirely uncontested within the United States. Two primers for this "movement" with intentionally sensationalist titles are *Milk: The Deadly Poison* by Robert Cohen (1997), the self-proclaimed "notmilkman" who also maintains a website www.notmilk.com, and *Don't Drink Your Milk! The Frightening New Medical Facts about the World's Most Overrated Nutrient* by Frank Oski (1977). The Physician's Committee for Responsible Medicine (PCRM) and People for the Ethical Treatment of Animals (PETA) are two organizations actively promoting the message that milk is neither an ideal nor necessary food.[6] Both groups cite studies implicating milk consumption as a contributing factor to numerous health problems (from prostate and breast cancer to osteoporosis; see www.pcrm.org or www.milksucks.com). Lactose intolerance is on the list of potential problems associated with milk consumption; as with clinicians, antimilk groups are more concerned with negative physiological outcomes and less interested in lactase impersistence per se. The latter is folded into *lactose intolerance* in this description:

> LACTOSE INTOLERANCE: Fifty million Americans experience intestinal discomfort after consuming milk, cheese, or ice cream (*Postgraduate Medicine* 1994:95). Symptoms include stomach pain, gas, and diarrhea.
>
> Lactose, a milk sugar, is made up of two other sugars, glucose and galactose. Galactose has been identified as a causative factor in heart disease, cataracts, and glaucoma. Most adults "lack" the enzyme, lactase, to break down lactose. Instead, lactose is broken down by bacteria in the lower intestines. Their own body wastes combine with those sugars to ferment into toxins causing bloating and cramps.
>
> Once a correct diagnosis is established, there is a simple cure: NOTMILK!
>
> In April of 1999, the *Journal of Clinical Gastroenterology* (volume 28:3) reported: "Introduction of a lactose-free dietary regime relieves symptoms in most patients…who remain largely unaware of the relationship between food intake and symptoms." [Cohen 1998]

Unlike the dairy industry, which claims that the prevalence of lactose intolerance is *over*estimated, Cohen suggests that it is *under*diagnosed as a source of gastrointestinal complaints. And, instead of following the "simple steps" that the dairy industry outlines for individuals with symptoms of intolerance, the solution is straightforward: Avoid dairy products. Because the antimilk contingent considers there to be sufficient evidence that milk may cause rather than prevent various health problems, this avoidance is not deleterious but, in fact, beneficial to one's health.

A related resource, accessible from www.nomilk.com, is the website of Steve Carper, author of *Milk: Not for Every Body* (1995; the site can also be accessed at http://ourworld. compuserve.com/homepages/stevecarper/). On Carper's "lactose planet," the lactose intolerance clearinghouse has an extensive array of information, much of which reads like the discussion in an introductory biological anthropology textbook. Again a clear distinction is made between *lactose intolerance* and *lactase impersistence*, and the evolutionary explanation for lactase persistence is presented (i.e., pastoralist or Vitamin D–deficient populations gained some advantage by drinking milk). Carper is not opposed to milk consumption per se but wants to alert the public about the myriad potential problems associated with milk consumption and provide information on alternatives.

The clash between the antimilk platform of the PCRM and the promilk agenda of USDA and NDC came to a head in two articles in the *Journal of the National Medical Association*, a journal devoted to health issues that concern peoples of African descent (www.nmanet.org). At the heart of the debate was the policy significance of biological variation in adult lactase production. Authors from the PCRM alleged that the *Dietary Guidelines for Americans* are biased against minorities insofar as dairy products are recommended for all U.S. citizens (Bertron et al. 1999). They concluded that the *Guidelines*

> encourage dairy products for daily consumption by all Americans, despite differences in tolerances for dairy products, preferences for other calcium-rich foods and susceptibilities to osteoporosis, as well as the lack of scientific evidence of benefit from dairy products for members of racial minorities. In this regard, federal nutrition policies do not yet address the needs of all Americans. [Bertron et al. 1999:156]

In this case, recognition of significant population variation in lactase persistence and relatively high frequencies of impersistence among minorities in the U.S. warrants rethinking the explicit national policy of encouraging—indeed, mandating—dairy product consumption by all. Those with different digestive biologies are being forced to conform to European-derived norms of dietary behavior, which the authors contend are associated with increased risk for various diseases such as osteoporosis and ovarian cancer, among others. This charge echoed a 1979 lawsuit in which the Federal Trade Commission sued the California Milk Producers Advisory Board for its advertising campaign "Everybody needs milk." However, the judge ruled that there was insufficient evidence that milk was a significant threat to individuals with lactose intolerance, arguing further that

> Milk is one of the most nutritious foods in the nation's diet, and from the standpoint of the population as a whole, or even significant population groups, is literally "essential, necessary and needed." The withdrawl of milk

from any major population group would amount to a nutritional disaster. [Katz 1981:267]

A response to PCRM appeared in the same journal three years later in an article titled "Overcoming the Barrier of Lactose Intolerance to Reduce Health Disparities," authored by NDC researchers (Jarvis and Miller 2002). In this counterclaim, the authors argued that the relatively high rates of lactose maldigestion and the concomitant low milk intake among minority populations are significant contributors to their higher rates of several chronic diseases (osteoporosis, hypertension, stroke, colon cancer). The basis of the claim is evidence suggesting that calcium and "other dairy related nutrients" may reduce the risk of these diseases, although at present most studies presenting such results have relied on correlations and retrospective data, rather than demonstrating a direct causal link between milk consumption and lower risk of these diseases. Thus, to reduce disparities between the relative health advantages enjoyed by whites, "Physicians can help reduce the disease burden and health care costs in minority populations by committing themselves to helping their clients overcome the barrier of lactose intolerance" (Jarvis and Miller 2002:64). This is to be accomplished by providing such clients with "several simple strategies that allow those with low lactase activity to consume dairy products," as outlined previously. Furthermore, in a separate publication, the NDC argues that although "Many minorities have low levels of lactase...stereotyping all minorities as lactose intolerant is inappropriate" (NDC 2003b). Thus, the claim of bias against minorities evident in recommendations to consume milk is turned on its head to suggest that individuals who fail to consume milk because of fears of symptoms (often misplaced, the NDC researchers claim) from lactose maldigestion are at risk of major chronic diseases and well-known health deficits because of their dietary choices, as well as to accuse the authors from the PCRM of racial stereotyping. The NDC materials explicitly confirm that the Dietary Guidelines are for *all* U.S. citizens, that dairy foods are required to provide nutrients not found in other types of foods, and that minorities are especially at risk of calcium-deficiency diseases as a function of lower dairy consumption (NDC 2003b).

DISCUSSION

At the heart of these various stories about lactase persistence/impersistence are two key issues. One is the nature and significance of biological diversity in lactase production in adulthood and its relationship to milk consumption. The second, and related, issue is the appropriateness of milk in the diet of contemporary U.S. citizens, which should be reflected in food and nutrition policies. All of the stories contain some appreciation for biological diversity of adult lactase production. They acknowledge that lactase impersistence is very common in the world and that there are substantial minorities within the U.S. who are lactase impersistent. Some go further in describing the evolutionary

scenarios that might have generated differences in lactase activity, focusing on the nutritional benefits that might have accrued to populations that were able to exploit fresh milk. Thus, the older advertising slogan "Drink Milk for Fitness" had an unintentional (?) link to evolutionary explanations, but, of course, it went further by making this a blanket statement that suggested that everyone's physical and, perhaps, Darwinian fitness might be enhanced by milk consumption. While it makes sense that the dairy industry would want to endorse this concept, with the exception of the antimilk contingents, milk continues to be recommended by diverse institutions, albeit in forms and quantities that individuals find physiologically acceptable.

This suggests the entrenched nature of milk in U.S. culinary culture, national identity, and agricultural economy. As Melanie DuPuis (2002) has shown, even in the 19th century when milk consumption was more often than not associated with infectious disease from the unsanitary conditions of its production and distribution, it had already achieved the status of "nature's perfect food." Milk's positive symbolism is overdetermined: its white color, association with things pastoral and maternal and the innocence of babies, and its biblical references (several being odes to a "land that floweth with milk and honey"), among others. In the 20th century, with improvements in sanitation (pasteurization, refrigeration) and discoveries in nutrition, one nutrient in particular—calcium—has come to symbolize the inherent goodness of milk. The current justification for promoting milk rests almost exclusively on this mineral, and the United States, it is proclaimed, is facing a "calcium crisis" (NDC 2003b). This crisis—whether real or imagined—correlates with a decline in milk consumption and evidence that most U.S. citizens, milk drinkers included, consume less than the Recommended Daily Allowance (RDA) for calcium (the average is 801 milligrams, while the RDA is at least 1,000 milligrams; USDA 1998).[7] Whether the RDA for calcium is too high or too low is a matter of some contention (Anderson 2001; Matkovic and Ilich 1993), but suffice it to say here that the solution to the calcium "crisis," at least according to the USDA and NDC, is to consume more milk rather than consume other foods rich in calcium—such as fish bones, dark green leafy vegetables, nuts, or legumes. The USDA notes that milk and dairy products make up 73 percent of the calcium available in the U.S. food supply and, hence, dairy is the best and most readily available source of calcium (NDC 2003b). It should be noted that hunter-gatherers living on wild foods are able to consume ample quantities of calcium (above the U.S. RDA) from nondairy sources (Eaton et al. 1999). On the other hand, it appears that much of the world's population consumes well below the U.S. RDA for calcium without apparent detriment (Food and Agriculture Organization 2002).

By and large, aside from the allegations of the antimilk groups, the NDC and the USDA constitute the main voice in shaping the dominant rhetoric about biological diversity in lactase production. Their story is constructed around the inherent goodness of milk and the benefits of a biological make-up that allows for daily consumption of abundant quantities. As DuPuis noted, the apparent superiority achieved by European dairying cultures during the colonial period was in part attributed to their dairy-based diet. She quotes the famous nutritionist E. V. McCollum in National Dairy Council advertisements from the 1920s:

> The people who have achieved, who have become large, strong, vigorous people, who have reduced their infant mortality, who have the best trades in the world, who have an appreciation for art, literature and music, who are progressive in science and every activity of the human intellect are the people who have used liberal amounts of milk and its products. [DuPuis 2002:117]

Not only was drinking milk and consuming other dairy products seen as superior, it was also viewed as normal and normative. This perspective endured through the 1960s when studies began to demonstrate population variation in lactase persistence, with the modal global form being lactase impersistence. However, despite widespread recognition of this distribution, lactase impersistence remains implicitly pathological, as evidenced in widely used terminologies and definitions. Such medicalizing of non-Western, particularly African biologies appears in the colonial period and remains evident in the example of lactase impersistence (cf. Comaroff and Comaroff 1992; Gould 1981; see Tapper 1995 for discussion of the analogous example of sickle-cell anemia). To be fair, lactose intolerance, which may result from lactase impersistence, is a cluster of uncomfortable physiological symptoms for which a person might seek medical help, but it is important to acknowledge that these only manifest in the context of milk consumption.

The significance of biological variation in lactase persistence is downplayed by the USDA and dairy industry. First, they consider it to be an "overblown" issue, citing evidence that lactase impersistence is not always associated with symptoms of lactose intolerance. Although they acknowledge that a large portion of adults—particularly in minority populations in the United States—are likely to have low levels of lactase, this should not prevent them from consuming milk. Much research sponsored by the NDC has been focused on determining just how much milk people who self- or medically diagnose lactose maldigestion can consume; their published studies show that up to two or even three cups of milk can be consumed by individuals testing positive for lactose maldigestion, as long as these are spread throughout the day (Suarez et al. 1997, 1998). Anthropological studies have also noted discordance between lactase status and symptoms of intolerance. For example, Susan Cheer and John Allen (1997) found that Tokelau islanders in New Zealand had high frequencies of lactase impersistence, as diagnosed in breath hydrogen tests, but lactase status was not highly correlated with either consumption of dairy products or perceived symptoms of lactose intolerance.

From the USDA and NDC's perspective, avoidance of milk is not an acceptable strategy, regardless of one's lactase status. To consume milk in the United States is to be healthy;

to avoid milk is to put oneself at risk of a variety of long-term ailments. Thus, diversity in adult lactase production is essentially meaningless for most individuals who, they suggest, can happily consume milk and be healthier for it. At the same time, the NDC retains a vision of lactase impersistence as problematic, not so much because it may provoke gastrointestinal symptoms but, rather, because it may result in reduced milk consumption. The very term *maldigestion* suggests a malady, and the following passage describes the deviant nature of this condition: "Data from most studies suggest that individuals with primary lactose *deficiency* consume less milk than those who digest milk *normally*" (Jarvis and Miller 2002:58, emphasis added). So while they acknowledge underlying biological variation, it is of no practical significance; it should not be a barrier to consuming milk and enjoying the health benefits it confers to those who have a history of drinking milk and continue to do so regularly. One can and should "overcome" this biological deficit to achieve full participation in U.S. culinary culture and its self-evident salutary consequences.

Because biological variation is discounted, the NDC suggests that it is negative cultural attitudes about milk that reduce its consumption by minority groups. Arthur Whaley noted this same trend in epidemiological studies: "Ethnic/racial groups are often seen as having misperceptions and unhealthy behaviors learned through cultural socialization that increase their risk for adverse health outcomes" (2003:738). Hence, individuals in such groups should be educated about the value of milk in their diets and enact behavioral changes; the source, value, or integrity of diverse "cultural attitudes" are dismissed. Drinking milk is no less than full enculturation into U.S. life. Yet the increasing diversity of the U.S. public must be acknowledged and celebrated to some extent, especially if the goal is to sell more milk and reverse the decades-old downward trend in milk consumption. Thus, efforts to embrace that diversity while simultaneously unifying it into a common milk-drinking experience have escalated.[8] It is impossible to avoid the images in popular culture from the wildly successful "got milk?" advertising campaign, which feature famous role models of various ethnic backgrounds sporting milk mustaches.[9] This campaign has both increased milk sales and reached iconic status. This practice is not lost on antimilk groups, who complain that it is misleading because of the relatively high frequency of lactase impersistence/lactose intolerance among groups of African, Asian, or Latin American descent (and who have also subverted the "got milk?" slogan in various ways; see www.milksucks.com). Given the rapid growth of this demographic group, the NDC explicitly targets Hispanics in its current advertising strategy (USDA 2002); by using minority role models, it hopes to instill a positive association with milk and encourage milk consumption among minority children. Given that food preferences are established in childhood (Rozin 1983, 1990), this strategy should pay off for the dairy industry in the short and long term.

So how do we construct reasonable food policy based on our current understanding of population variation in adult lactase production? Both the NDC and PCRM have valid claims—that to characterize minorities as *lactase impersistent* (or *lactose intolerant*) is to engage in racial stereotyping and that to mandate milk consumption for all U.S. citizens is discriminatory against those with lactase impersistence (and especially those with lactose intolerance). To some extent the claims and counterclaims about the healthiness of milk are irrelevant to this discussion, although it is a travesty to attribute health deficits among minorities to their "failure" to drink milk. Milk is neither the elixir of life, whose consumption will surely prevent chronic disease, nor is biology destiny—drinking moderate amounts of milk is not likely to be seriously problematic for most people with lactase impersistence. Various lactose-reduced options exist for those who wish to consume dairy, but at the same time, an increasingly diverse U.S. public is being led to believe that they must consume milk to be healthy, and traditional cuisines and alternate sources of calcium are largely discredited.

CONCLUSION

It is heartening to see widespread acknowledgment of human biological variation in adult lactase activity among policy-making institutions in the United States. The evolutionary stories that go along with it have received less attention, except insofar as they acknowledge that some benefit accrued to certain populations that were able to exploit milk throughout life. These benefits are hailed and emphasized by those institutions promoting milk; they are less evident in the stories told by those who question milk's cultural and biological supremacy. The biology that facilitates ongoing milk consumption is likewise celebrated; other digestive physiologies are seen as abnormal or deficient in some way and need to be "overcome."

However, in achieving such broad acceptance, the anthropological context for appreciating biological and cultural diversity is easily lost, especially when it threatens to thwart marketing goals or undermine accepted wisdom, in this case, about the inherent goodness of milk for "every body." When it comes to describing biological variation, the axiom that biological variation within populations is greater than variation between populations is rarely appreciated, as *populations* are labeled as *lactose intolerant* or *lactase persistent*. Yet in the quest for examples of patterned genetic variation among human populations, work in biological anthropology may promote this interpretation, reifying population differences while downplaying the tremendous amount of individual variation in response to lactose. This is where the evolutionary perspective is most useful, in the sense that it describes the *process* by which genetic change comes about and the important social and natural environmental factors that generate such change without reference to discrete population groupings.

This example further illustrates the utility of a biocultural perspective in anthropology, and one that attempts to understand how human biology, especially human biological variation, is constructed and elaborated within a cultural

context. Here, biological variation in lactase production in adulthood runs up against a dietary culture characterized by extensive use of dairy products and a political economic context in which the USDA and dairy industry ally to increase milk consumption among a U.S. public of increasing biological, ethnic, and dietary diversity. The story that they tell about lactase persistence has become the dominant story; challenges to it are trivialized or described as subversive. This axis of biological variation, so celebrated by biological anthropologists, is relegated to a somewhat interesting yet, ultimately, meaningless fact, except insofar as it threatens to impede full enculturation into a dairy-consuming culture.

Notes

I gratefully acknowledge the help of a group of excellent anthropology students at James Madison University, most especially Adam Southall, for his careful research and comments on this manuscript. Likewise, Angel Shockley, Naheed Ahmed, Haley Thrift, and Jessica Fowler contributed useful insights. Kim Butler's thesis work on milk advertising was particularly helpful. Ric Thompson, Alex Brewis, and Richard Lippke all provided valuable feedback on earlier drafts of this article. The editors of *AA* were very helpful in recasting the article for the broadest anthropological audience.

1. A lack of consistency in terminology is evident in introductory biological anthropology textbooks. In a sample of four textbooks, two referred to *lactase impersistence* simply as *lactose intolerance* (Jurmain et al. 2000; Relethford 2003); one referred to it as *lactase deficiency* (Stein and Rowe 2000); and another referred to it as *low digestive capacity* (Boyd and Silk 2003).

2. In a preliminary proposal for new revised Dietary Guidelines, calcium-enriched soy products are added as an alternative in the dairy category (see www.usda.gov/cnpp/pyramid-update/FGP%20docs/TABLE%201.pdf). It remains to be seen whether this will be kept in the final version, although Dean Foods, one of the largest dairy corporations, also owns Morningstar, which makes Sun Soy, a soymilk brand.

3. Robert Heaney and Connie Weaver (1990) found that the calcium available in kale was higher than that in milk. Other sources disparage the calcium density and bioavailability of vegetable foods: "A person would need to consume 8 cups of spinach, nearly 5 cups of red beans, or 2 cups of broccoli to get the same amount of calcium absorbed from 1 cup of milk" (NDC 2003b).

4. It should also be noted that many schools have "pouring rights" contracts with soft drink corporations, and students often choose soft drinks over milk at school. Given the high sugar content of soda and its potential contribution to the current epidemic of childhood obesity, this issue is a key concern of ASFSA members.

5. These population groupings are regularly used in descriptions of variation in lactase activity in the United States. That these are diverse kinds of groups, which reflect commonly used national, regional, "racial," or ethnic identities is not considered.

6. These groups have been described as "the most immediately dangerous," because of their sometimes terrorist tactics (Heaney 2001:160). Further, their influence is decried:

We confront a recent, very modern efflorescence of militant groups that oppose all use of animal products and aim to effect a nutritional policy outcome similar to that of the creationists with regard to evolution. Those who care about nutrition, those who think nutrition important for the public health general, need to realize that the present-day skirmishes may be only the first wave of a growing battle. [Heaney 2001:163]

7. This decline in milk consumption is usually traced to the rise in the consumption of soda, bottled water, juice, and sports drinks. Also, while U.S. citizens widely acknowledge that milk "does a body good," this earlier advertising slogan had little positive impact on milk consumption. Only after the initiation of the "got milk?" campaign did milk consumption rebound somewhat (Manning 1999).

8. Promilk attitudes and governmental policies are increasingly evident on a global scale. Thus, immigrants to the United States may already come with attitudes shaped by these policies from their home countries.

9. Recently, some have started wearing lactose-reduced milk mustaches.

References

American Academy of Pediatrics. 1985. "Inactive" Ingredients in Pharmaceutical Products. Pediatrics 76(4):635–643.

Anderson, B., and C. Vullo. 1994. Did Malaria Select for Primary Adult Lactase Deficiency? Gut 35:1487–1489.

Anderson, John J. B. 2001. Calcium Requirements during Adolescence to Maximize Bone Health. Journal of the American College of Nutrition 20(2):186S–191S.

Bayless, Theodore M., and N. S. Rosensweig. 1966. A Racial Difference in Incidence of Lactase Deficiency: A Survey of Milk Intolerance and Lactase Deficiency in Healthy Adult Males. Journal of the American Medical Association 197:968–972.

———. 1967. Incidence and Implications of Lactase Deficiency and Milk Intolerance in White and Negro Populations. Johns Hopkins Medical Journal 121:54–64.

Bertron, Patricia, Neal D. Barnard, and Milton Mills. 1999. Racial Bias in Federal Nutrition Policy, part 1: The Public Health Implications of Variations in Lactase Persistence. Journal of the National Medical Association 91(3):151–157.

Boyd, Robert, and Joan B. Silk. 2003. How Humans Evolved. New York: W. W. Norton and Co.

Carper, Steve. 1995. Milk Is Not for Every Body: Living with Lactose Intolerance. New York: Facts on File.

Cheer, Susan M., and John S. Allen. 1997. Lactose Digestion Capacity and Perceived Symptomatic Response after Dairy Product Consumption in Tokelau Island Migrants. American Journal of Human Biology 9(2):233–246.

Cohen, Robert. 1997. Milk: The Deadly Poison. Englewood Cliffs, NJ: Argus Publishing.

———. 1998 Lactose Intolerance. Electronic document, www.notmilk.com/forum/988.html, accessed October 2, 2003.

Comaroff, John, and Jean Comaroff. 1992. Ethnography and the Historical Imagination. Boulder: Westview Press.

DuPuis, E. Melanie. 2002. Nature's Perfect Food: How Milk Became America's Drink. New York: New York University Press.

Durham, William. 1991. Coevolution: Genes, Culture and Human Diversity. Stanford: Stanford University Press.

Dutta, P., J. Pinto, and R. Rivlin. 1985. Antimalarial Effects of Riboflavin Deficiency. Lancet 2(8463):1040–1043.

Eaton, S. Boyd, S. B. Eaton III, and Melvin J. Konner. 1999. Paleolithic Nutrition Revisited. In Evolutionary Medicine. W. R. Trevathan, E. O. Smith, and J. J. McKenna, eds. pp. 313–332. New York: Oxford University Press.

Enattah, Nabil Sabri, Timo Sahi, Erkki Savilahti, Joseph D. Terwilliger, Leena Peltonen, and Irma Varvela. 2002. Identification of a Variant Associated with Adult-Type Hypolactasia. Nature Genetics 30:233–237.

Feskanich, Diane, Walter C. Willett, Meir J. Stampfer, and Graham A. Colditz. 1997. Milk, Dietary Calcium, and Bone Fractures in Women: A 12-Year Prospective Study. American Journal of Public Health 87:992–997.

Flatz, Gebhard. 1987. Genetics of Lactose Digestion in Humans. Advances in Human Genetics 16:1–77.

Flatz, Gebhard, and Hans W. Rotthauwe. 1973. Lactose Nutrition and Natural Selection. Lancet 2:76–77.

Focus on Children: Boston Public Schools. 2003. Marketing—Best Practice. Boston Public Schools Lactose-Free Milk Public Awareness and Education Campaign. Electronic document, www.asfsa.org/meetingsandevents/archive/mc2003/marketing_boston.ppt, accessed October 2.

Food and Agriculture Organization. 2002. Human Vitamin and Mineral Requirements. Rome: Food and Nutrition Division, FAO.

Gould, Stephen Jay. 1981. The Mismeasure of Man. New York: W. W. Norton and Co.

Harvey, C. B., Edward J. Hollox, Mark Poulter, Yangxi Wang, M. Rossi, S. Auricchio, T. H. Iqbal, B. T. Cooper, R. Barton, M. Sarner, R. Korpela, and Dallas M. Swallow. 1998. Lactase Haplotype Frequencies in Caucasians: Association with the Lactase Persistence/Nonpersistence Polymorphism. Annals of Human Genetics 62:215–223.

Heaney, Robert P. 2000. Calcium, Dairy Products and Osteoporosis. Journal of the American College of Nutrition 19(2):83S–99S.

———. 2001 The Dairy Controversy: Facts, Questions, and Polemics. In Nutritional Aspects of Osteoporosis. P. Burckhardt, B. Dawson-Hughes, and R. P. Heaney, eds. Pp. 155–164. New York: Academic Press.

Heaney, Robert P., and Connie M. Weaver. 1990. Calcium Absorption from Kale. American Journal of Clinical Nutrition 51:656–657.

Hollox, Edward J., Mark Poulter, Marek Zvarik, Vladimir Ferak, Amanda Krause, Trefor Jenkins, Nilmani Saha, Andrew I. Kozlov, and Dallas M. Swallow. 2000. Lactase Haploytpe Diversity in the Old World. American Journal of Human Genetics 68:160–172.

Jarvis, Judith K., and Gregory D. Miller. 2002. Overcoming the Barrier of Lactose Intolerance to Reduce Health Disparities. Journal of the National Medical Association 94(2):55–66.

Jurmain, Robert, Harry Nelson, Lynn Kilgore, and Wenda Trevathan. 2000. Introduction to Physical Anthropology. Belmont, CA: Wadsworth/Thomson Learning.

Katz, Robert S. 1981. Dairy Council Perspective on Lactose Intolerance. In Lactose Digestion: Clinical and Nutritional Implications. David M. Paige and Theodore M. Bayless, eds. P. 267. Baltimore, MD: Johns Hopkins University Press.

Kretchmer, Norman. 1972. Lactose and Lactase. Scientific American 227(4):70–78.

Manning, Jeff. 1999. Got Milk? The Book. Rocklin, CA: Prima.

Matkovic, Velimir, and Jazminka Z. Ilich. 1993. Calcium Requirements for Growth: Are Current Recommendations Adequate? Nutrition Reviews 51(6):171–180.

McCracken, Robert D. 1971. Lactase Deficiency: An Example of Dietary Evolution. Current Anthropology 12:479–517.

Meloni, T., C. Colombo, G. Ruggiu, M. Denena, and G. F. Meloni. 1998. Primary Lactase Deficiency and Past Malarial Endemicity in Sardinia. Italian Journal of Gastroenterology and Hepatology 30:490–493.

National Dairy Council. 2003a. Dairy Food Sensitivities: Facts and Fallacies. Electronic document, www.nationaldairycouncil.org/lvl04/nutrilib/digest/dairydigest_683b.htm, accessed May 30.

———. 2003b Lactose Intolerance and Minorities: The Real Story. Electronic document, www.nationaldairycouncil.org/lv104/nutrilib/relresearch/lactose_int_1.html, accessed August 7.

Nestle, Marion. 2002. Food Politics: How the Food Industry Influences Nutrition and Health. Berkeley: University of California Press.

Oski, Frank A. 1977. Don't Drink Your Milk! The Frightening New Medical Facts about the World's Most Overrated Nutrient. Chicago: Wyden Books.

Relethford, John H. 2003. The Human Species. New York: McGraw Hill.

Rozin, Paul. 1983. Human Food Selection: The Interaction of Biology, Culture and Individual Experience. In The Psychobiology of Human Food Selection. L. M. Barker, ed. pp. 225–254. Westport, CT: AVI Publishing Co.

———. 1990 Acquisition of Stable Food Preferences. Nutrition Reviews 48:106–113.

Sahi, Timo. 1994a. Genetics and Epidemiology of Adult-Type Hypolactasia. Scandinavian Journal of Gastroenterology 29(suppl. 202):7–20.

———. 1994b Hypolactasia and Lactase Persistence: Historical Review and the Terminology. Scandinavian Journal of Gastroenterology 29(suppl. 202):1–6.

Scrimshaw, Nevin S., and E. B. Murray. 1988. The Acceptability of Milk and Milk Products in Populations with a High Prevalence of Lactose Tolerance. American Journal of Clinical Nutrition 48(4):1083–1159.

Simoons, Frederick J. 1978. The Geographic Hypothesis and Lactose Malabsorption. American Journal of Digestive Diseases 23:963–980.

———. 2001 Persistence of Lactase Activity among Northern Europeans: A Weighing of Evidence for the Calcium Absorption Hypothesis. Ecology of Food and Nutrition 40(5):397–469.

Specker, Bonnie, and Karen Wosje. 2001. A Critical Appraisal of the Evidence Relating Calcium and Dairy Intake to Bone Health Early in Life. In Nutritional Aspects of Osteoporosis. P. Burckhardt, B. Dawson-Hughes, and R. P. Heaney, eds. Pp. 107–123. New York: Academic Press.

Stein, Philip L., and Bruce M. Rowe. 2000. Physical Anthropology. New York: McGraw Hill.

Suarez, Fabrizis L., Jacqueline Adshead, Julie K. Furne, and Michael D. Levitt. 1998. Lactose Maldigestion Is Not an Impediment to the Intake of 1,500 mg. Calcium Daily as Dairy Products. American Journal of Clinical Nutrition 68:1118–1122.

Suarez, Fabrizis L., Dennis A. Savaiano, Paul A. Arbisi, and Michael D. Levitt. 1997. Tolerance to the Daily Ingestion of Two Cups of Milk by Individuals Claiming Lactose Intolerance. American Journal of Clinical Nutrition 65:1502–1506.

Tapper, Melbourne. 1995. Interrogating Bodies: Medico-Racial Knowledge, Politics, and the Study of a Disease. Comparative Studies in Society and History 37:76–93.

U.S. Department of Agriculture. 1990. Fluid Milk Promotion Act of 1990. Electronic document, www.ams.usda.gov/dairy/fldact.htm, accessed August 7, 2003.

———. 1998 Data Tables: Food and Nutrient Intakes 1994–1996. Electronic document, www.barc.usda.gov/bhnrc/foodsurvey/ home.htm, accessed October 15, 2003.

———. 2002 Report to Congress on the National Dairy Promotion and Research Program and the National Fluid Milk Processor Promotion Program. Washington, DC: USDA.

———. 2003 The National School Lunch Program: History and Development. Electronic document, www.fns.usda.gov/cnd/INCLUDES/NSLPBackgroundandDevelopment.htm#NATIONAL%20SCHOOL%20LUNCH%20ACT%20APPROVED, accessed October 2, 2003.

U.S. Department of Commerce. 2002. Statistical Abstract of the United States: 2002. Washington, DC: U. S. Census.

Wang, Yangxi, Clare B. Harvey, Edward J. Hollox, Alan D. Phillips, Mark Poulter, Peter Clay, John A. Walker-Smith, and Dallas M. Swallow. 1998. The Genetically Programmed Down-Regulation of Lactase in Children. Gastroenterology 114:1230–1236.

Wardlaw, Gordon M., and Paul M. Insel. 1996. Perspectives in Nutrition. Baltimore, MD: Mosby.

Weinsier, Roland L., and Carlos L. Krumdieck. 2000. Dairy Foods and Bone Health: Examination of the Evidence. American Journal of Clinical Nutrition 72:681–689.

Whaley, Arthur L. 2003. Ethnicity/Race, Ethics, and Epidemiology. Journal of the National Medical Association 95(8):736–742.

Wiley, Andrea S. 2004. Does Milk Make Children Grow? Poster presented at the Human Biology Association Meetings, Tampa, FL, April 14.

CHAPTER 27

Maya in Disneyland: Child Growth as a Marker of Nutritional, Economic, and Political Ecology

Barry Bogin

(2012)

First, let me explain the title of this essay. "Maya in Disneyland" refers to two groups of Maya people from Guatemala who immigrated to Los Angeles, California, and Indiantown, Florida. Astute readers will make the connection to the two Disney Corporation properties located in these same regions of the United States of America. My use goes further than the geographical propinquity of the Maya immigrants to these theme parks. I follow the meaning of "Disneyland" as given by geographer Robert D. Sack (1992) whose focus is "… basically on the symbolism of American places and American mythological history" (Fraim n.d.). The act of migration to the United States places the Maya families within the social and physical context of North American symbolism, history, and behavior. The Maya bring their own cultural history and values, which are thousands of years older than the American symbolism of Disneyland, and the confrontation of the old and the new play out in terms of a syncretism and synergism between beliefs and practice relating to diet, behavior, and health.

We will return to the two Maya immigrant groups a bit later in this essay. Before doing so, we move to the second part of the title. The measurement of height, weight, and other dimensions of the human body has a long history in Anthropology. Working in the late 19th and early 20th Centuries, Franz Boas used studies of human growth to show the economic and social effects of migration from Europe to the United States (Bogin 1999, pp.34–36). The United States–born offspring of immigrants from southern and eastern Europe averaged 4–5 centimeters (2") taller, and often had longer heads, than their parents. Boas used these findings to dismiss the idea that Greeks, Neapolitans, Bohemians, Jews, and other ethnic groups from impoverished areas of Europe belonged to distinct biological "races." Instead, Boas showed that improved living conditions changed the body size and body shape of new Americans.

Today, the physical growth and development of human beings are used by anthropologists, economists, historians, epidemiologists, physicians, and others as sensitive indicators of the quality of the social, economic, and political environment in which they live (Tanner 1981, Komlos 1994, Fogel 1986, Schell 1986, Bogin 1999, Steckel 2008). The journal *Economics and Human Biology* is devoted to these topics and the *American Journal of Human Biology* and *Annals of Human Biology* publish many related articles. James Tanner (1986) said it best when he wrote that growth is a mirror for society. By this he meant that, "The growth amongst the various groups which make up a contemporary society reflects rather accurately the material and moral condition of that society."

Anthropologists use the growth of infants, children, juveniles and adolescents, in terms of height, weight, and body composition (e.g., fatness and muscularity), to assess nutritional status and health status for both individuals and the community. The reason that anthropometry (body measurement) serves this purpose is that the development of the human phenotype is highly plastic. *Plasticity* refers to the ability of many organisms to change their biology or behavior during ontogeny to respond to changes in the environment, particularly when these are stressful. Plasticity is one of the three types of biological adaptations defined by Gabriel Lasker (1969). The first and second types are "those genetically entrenched in the population by repeated natural selection and those dependent on a capacity to acclimatize in the short run" (Lasker 1969:1484). Lasker characterizes the third type of adaptation as "modification of an individual during his growth and development…the process is essentially irreversible after adulthood…and may be separately designated as plasticity" (Lasker 1969: 1484). Due to a long developmental period before adulthood, human beings are, perhaps, one of the most plastic of all species and hence one of the most variable in terms of physical form and behavior.

The remainder of this essay investigates how plasticity in body growth reflects the nutritional, economic, and political ecology of Maya children and juveniles living in Guatemala and the United States.

WHO ARE THE MAYA?

There are an estimated 7–8 million Maya living in Guatemala, the Yucatan Peninsula of southern Mexico, Belize, El

Salvador, and western Honduras (Lovell 2000). The majority, about 6.5 million, live in the highlands of Guatemala (Tovar Gomez 1998, The World Bank 2004, WHO 2010). This makes the Maya the largest Native American ethnic group.

Common features of rural lifestyle, economic activities, kinship and marriage systems, religion, philosophy, and a brutal history since the Conquest of the Americas binds all Maya together into a shared cultural identity. There are, however, 22 or so Maya languages, each associated with a specific Maya group such as the Yucatec Maya of southern Mexico and the K'iche (Quiche), Mam, Q'eqchi (Qekchi), and Q'anjob'al (Kanjobal) of Guatemala. Maya orthography has changed over time. I will use current spellings of Maya group names. The living Maya are the biological and cultural descendants of the people inhabiting the same culture area prior to European contact in the year 1500 CE[1]. Archaeology of the region indicates that hunter-gatherers and small scale farmers existed in the region for thousands of years. It is not certain which of these groups became the Maya. By about 250 CE a Maya cultural identity was well established and the people were organized in several state-level societies, ruled by priest-kings and an elite class of political-religious leaders. Each Maya state group maintained armies and a workforce of peasants that produced food using a mosaic system of "...agricultural fields, raised wetland fields, kitchen gardens, terraced hills, and. managed forests" (McNeil et al. 2010). Maya plant and animal husbandry cultivated a diversity of species to provide food; medicinal plants; and wild animals for protein food and honey, firewood, and building materials. The peasants also supplied labor to build monumental architecture, such as the sites of Tikal, Palenque, and Calakmul. These city-states, located in tropical forest lowlands, were sites of economic, social, political, and religious power. The Maya left us records of these activities, carved in stone monuments and written on paper books. There were hundreds of such books, each called a codex. All but a few of these books were burned by the Spanish in their zeal to subdue, Christianize, and control the Maya.

Sometime after 900 CE, and after centuries of warfare and environmental change, most of those Maya kingdoms were disbanded, although centers such as Uxmal in the Yucatan peninsula remained vibrant until about 1200 CE. The lowland urban centers located in today's Guatemala were abandoned. Most of the people migrated to the highlands located in Western Guatemala. There they lived in sophisticated chiefdomship societies and continued to construct adobe and stone buildings and temples, but on a much smaller scale than previously.

This is how the Spanish and Portuguese Conquistadors encountered the Maya. The Europeans took advantage of existing competition between chiefdomships to foment greater civil discord, and then turned on their Maya allies. New infectious diseases introduced by the Conquistadors, such as smallpox, bubonic plague, and measles, spread rapidly among the Maya, and without any biological or social resistance whole villages of Maya were decimated. "Between 1519 and 1632 eight epidemics lashed Guatemala, with more localized episodes occurring over the same period" (Lovell 2000, p. 115). Maya from both royal and commoner families died by the tens of thousands. The political, economic, and religious leadership was decimated. War and disease destroyed the basis of Maya livelihood and social cohesion. Within a century the Maya were conquered and forced to labor for their new masters. It is estimated that there were about two million Maya people living in what is today Guatemala in the year 1500. By 1625, this Maya population declined to a nadir 128,000 people (Lovell & Lutz 1996).

In the past 200 years or so, Maya culture has been characterized by subsistence and market-oriented agriculture, small-scale animal holdings (sheep, chickens, a cow, or burro) augmented by craft specialization. An example of a Maya woman wearing traditional woven and embroidered clothing is given in Figure 1. Other characteristics of traditional Maya culture are social behavior relating to household economy, endogamy (marriage within the

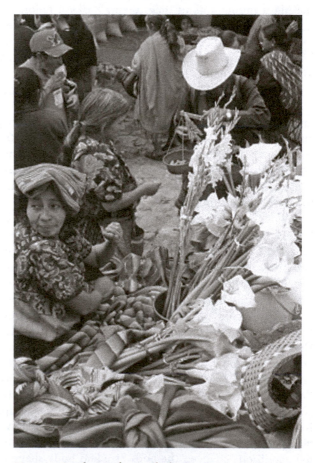

Figure 1 *Sunday market in Chichicastenango, Guatemala. The women selling flowers wear traditional Maya clothing. The embroidery on the blouse (called a huipil) is typical to this village. The men wear European-style clothing, which is typical for many Maya men in Guatemalan society. The mixture of clothing styles is another example of cultural syncretism in Maya life.*

community), collective religious practice, use of the Maya calendar, and communication in a Maya language. Some aspects of modern-day traditional Maya culture predate the Conquest; others are postcolonial syncretic blends between various Maya and Spanish social-religious practices.

Many Maya believe that they have *sangre de la raza*, meaning blood of the pre-Conquest Maya, running in their veins. Genetic and dental studies do show that the Maya form a definable biological population (Gomez-Casado et al. 2003, Cucina and Tiesler 2004, Scherer 2007). Maya differ in these traits from the Mestizo and Ladino ethnic groups of Mexico and Central America, who show greater biological and social affinities with their Spanish, Portuguese, and other European ancestors. It is very important to emphasize that the Maya are not a distinct "race." The genetic and dental traits of the Maya are shared to some extent with all human beings, but are expressed in a statistically higher frequency within the Maya population. This reflects the Maya preference to marry other Maya.

More than biology, it is Maya cultural traits that continue to distinguish them from the other major ethnic group in Guatemala, the Ladinos. In contrast to the Maya, Ladinos usually wear Western clothing, claim Spanish or other European ancestry, and practice social behavior derived largely from Spain or elsewhere in Europe. As of 2010, Guatemala's total population was about 13 million, divided about evenly between Maya and Ladino (WHO 2010). After independence from Spain in 1821, Ladinos assumed political power and they continued to socially and economically dominate the Maya (Lovell 2000, 2010). Forced labor recruitment persisted well into the twentieth century, and to this day indigenous lands continue to be confiscated. Ladino peasants and the urban poor of Guatemala also suffered under both postcolonial and state regimes. Any resistance by either Maya or the Ladino poor has been met with harsh military repression.

During the late 1970s and early 1980s the social, economic, and political fates of Guatemala's Maya and poor Ladino population deteriorated further. One observer explains that during this time Guatemala experienced a particularly bloody decade of civil war that has severely changed life there, especially for the Maya. The guerrilla insurgency and the overwhelming response by the military in Guatemala resulted in the destruction of hundreds of Maya towns and villages. The Maya of the mountainous area where the guerrilla forces found refuge were caught in an uprising that left them most vulnerable: they could not quickly leave their lands and villages like the insurgents and could not defend themselves against the weaponry of the state. As Beatriz Manz (1988) has documented, the destruction of the villages and societal structures in the area has been thorough (Burns 1989:21–22).

Tens of thousands of Maya were killed during the civil war, and more than 250,000 fled across the border into Mexico. Among the most numerous of those fleeing the country were Q'anjob'al-speaking Maya from northwest Guatemala. The Mexican government disbanded many of the refugee camps in the late 1980s. Some refuges returned to Guatemala, some assimilated into Mexican society, and some journeyed to "*El Norte*"—the United States. It is estimated that since the onset of civil war in Guatemala in 1978, as many as half a million Guatemalan Maya have come to the US (Loucky and Moors, 2000).

In my own research, I study the growth and nutritional status of several groups of Mayan children and juveniles between the ages of 5 and 12 years old. One group lives in their homeland of Guatemala, and another lives in the United States. The Maya in Guatemala live in rural villages to the northwest of Guatemala City. These villages have no safe source of drinking water. Townspeople depended on an unreliable supply of water from rain swollen streams, or from shallow wells. Water from these sources is contaminated with fertilizers and pesticides used on nearby agricultural fields and by human and farm animal wastes. Recently, some villages have dug deep wells, but the water taken from these is often contaminated by the time people drink it because water is stored in unhygienic containers. Adding to this, most homes lack running water and have only pit toilets. Farm animals, dogs and cats have free access within homes and there are limited food storage facilities. All of this is caused by the poverty of the rural population. Guatemala has the second largest proportion of population living in poverty of any nation in the Americas—the first is Haiti with 72% of the total population living in poverty. The World Bank (2003) estimates that about 87% of the Maya in Guatemala live in poverty, meaning that these Maya families live on less than US$2.00 per day. This compares with the estimate of 56% of all Guatemalans, Maya and Ladino, living in poverty. Economists for the World Bank define poverty in terms of the ability to purchase a minimum "food basket" equaling 2172 kilocalories (kcals) of food consumption per day. This energy intake value is the minimum average daily caloric requirement for a 'typical' Guatemalan person, based on a weighted average of the population taking into account the age and sex distribution and the assumption of moderate physical activity (The World Bank, 2003). Added to the cost of this minimum "food basket" is an allowance for essential non-food items. The total cost of the "food basket" plus other essential purchases comes to US$560.90 per year in 2000 dollars. To put this in perspective, it is quite easy to spend this amount on one dinner for a party of six people at a "nice" restaurant in New York, London, Paris, or Moscow.

Using this estimate of the cost for the required kcals/day provides a stark picture of nutritional status for Maya in Guatemala. The situation is even worse when we consider the composition of the diet. Most of the kcals consumed by the poor are from corn and corn-based foods, such as tortillas. These basic carbohydrates are supplemented with black beans, other vegetables, and occasionally eaten small portions of meat and fruit (see Box 27–1). A "meal" of two tortillas with a pinch of salt is commonly reported by anthropologists who have lived with Maya families (for example, Glittenberg 1994). The result on nutritional status

BOX 1   THE TRADITIONAL MAYA DIET IN GUATEMALA

The diet of any human social group must provide sufficient energy and adequate quantities of each of the 45–50 essential nutrients required by human beings. Failure of the diet to meet these needs results in poor growth and development, illness, or death. A popular misconception is that the Maya diet is based on only three foods—corn, black beans, and squash (Box 1, Figure 1). If that were the case, then there would be no Mayan people because these three foods do not supply all needed nutrients. In fact, the traditional Maya diet of the mid-20th Century was composed of at least 108 different food items. The Institute of Nutrition of Central America and Panama (INCAP) conducted food surveys in several Guatemalan villages between 1950 and 1969. The original data were recorded in the form of INCAP internal reports, in Spanish. Dr. Odelia I. Bermudez and colleagues (2008) accessed these archival data and published the basic findings, along with new analyses of the nutritional content of some foods. These surveys "...document the intake of foods and beverages in households from rural and semirural communities across Guatemala"..."To collect dietary data, INCAP used a mixed methodology that included a food record with weighing of the foods prepared the day of the first visit, followed by 24-hour recalls over the next 7 days. Dietary analysis of the data was based on the Food Composition Table for Central America and Panama; data on a few items originating from the United States were analyzed with the use of the US Department of Agriculture (USDA) Handbook No. 8" (Bermudez et al. 2008, p. 279).

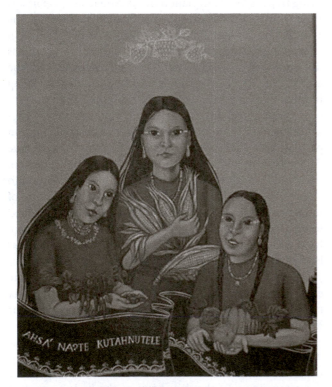

Figure 1 *The 3 sisters—corn, beans, and squash by Mary Lee Prescott. This painting depicts the Iroquois people. Corn, beans, and squash are important foods for many Native American peoples, ranging from parts of South America, throughout Central America and Mexico, and north into the Southwest and Mississippi Valley and its tributaries within the United states. With permission of the Bear Paw Gallery. http://www.bearpawartgallery.com.*

Table 1 Number of Foods Consumed by Traditional Rural Maya Families According to Food Group (from Bermudez et al. 2008)

Food Groups	INCAP studies (1950–60)
Corn, corn tortilla, and corn atole	3
Corn tamales	2
Beans	3
Rice	1
Bread	3
Breakfast cereals	1
Other cereals (e.g., pasta)	2
Milk, dairy products, and egg	8
Meat, beef, and pork	11
Game meat[a]	3
Chicken and turkey	2
Fish and shellfish	5
Green leafy vegetables	11
Green and yellow vegetables	4
Other vegetables	17
Potatoes, root crops, and plantain	4
Fruit[b]	13
Fats and oils	2
Sugar	2
Beverages[c]	4
Snacks[d]	0
Desserts[e]	3
Soups	0
Other mixed dishes with meat	0
Miscellaneous[f]	4
Total number of foods	108

[a] Meat from wild animals hunted for food.
[b] Fruits include fresh, dried (raisins), and canned fruit and 100% fruit juices.
[c] Beverages include soft drinks, fruit-flavored sweetened drinks, tap water, bottled water, tea, coffee, and alcoholic beverages.
[d] Snacks include salty appetizers, including potato and corn chips and popcorn.
[e] Desserts include pastry, cakes, ice cream, sweetened gelatin, and pudding.
[f] Miscellaneous includes salt, spices, and seasonings.

As shown in Box 1, Table 1, Bermudez and colleagues identified 22 food groups and a total of 108 foods from the nine INCAP studies of rural Maya families. "Vegetables" is the most diverse food group, with 36 items, including green leafy vegetables, green and yellow vegetables, other vegetables, potatoes, root crops, and plantains. Some of these vegetables are wild plants native to rural Guatemala, for example a leafy plant called *busnay*. "Fruit" is the next most diverse group with 13 items, then "milk, dairy products and eggs" with 8 items. All other food groups have 5 or fewer items. Wild animals, listed as "game meat," were hunted for food, and "fish and shellfish," mainly those caught in rivers such as small fish, shrimps, and crabs, were important sources of animal protein. Some of these riverine foods were home-processed by drying and salting for long-term storage. Meat, from beef, pork, chicken, and turkey, along with eggs, milk and dairy were eaten, but rarely and in relatively small quantities. Although the number of corn-based products and "beans" seems small, in fact these food groups did comprise the bulk of the food eaten. "Desserts" comprised "...traditional dishes such as *rellenitos de platano* (sweetened plantain fritters) and rice pudding..." (Bermudez et al. 2008, p. 281).

Processed foods totalled only 12 (11%) of the 108 total food items. These processed foods included two kinds of sugar (highly refined white sugar and a less refined brown sugar called *panella*), two types of beverages, including coffee and alcohol, ice cream (very rarely), and cooking oil.

The daily intake of energy, macronutrients (carbohydrates, fats, protein), and several micronutrients (vitamins and minerals) are listed in Box 1, Table 2. In their analysis, Bermudez and colleagues estimated the daily energy intake of the rural Maya of the INCAP studies at 2044 kcal. Based on their reported intakes of macronutrients (carbohydrates, fats, proteins) the total energy intake is only 1795 kcals per day. The difference is 249 kcals, but it is not stated where these other kcals come from. One possibility is alcohol, and if this is the case these are "empty" kcals as alcohol has virtually no other essential nutrients.

To make better sense of the data in Box 1, Table 2, I compare the values with the percent of the Daily Recommended Intake (DRI) of the Food and Nutrition Board, National Academy of Sciences, United States (http://iom.edu/en/Global/News%20Announcements/~/media/Files/Activity%20Files/Nutrition/DRIs/DRISummaryListing2.ashx). These values are based on the recommended DRI for physically active adult women ages 19–30 years old with a height of 150 cm, the average height of Maya women, and a 'thin' BMI of 18.5. Women of this age range are in their prime reproductive years. Indeed, during pregnancy and lactation the nutritional requirements of these women increase, but for the purposes of this analysis it is sufficient to use DRIs for non-pregnant, non-lactating Maya women. Adult men need more of most nutrients, except iron, due to their larger body size.

The value of 1795 kcals per day of energy intake is only 87% of the recommended daily intake for adult women. If these Maya women had a 'normal' BMI of 24.9, they would be consuming only 71% of required kcals. It would be virtually impossible to maintain normal weight for height on that kcal deficit. Calcium, iron, and thiamine are consumed in sufficient amounts. Foods such as corn tortillas and black beans are good sources of those nutrients. Riboflavin, niacin, and especially vitamin C are deficient in the diet.

The contribution of carbohydrates to total energy intake was 74%, and that of fats and protein, respectively, 11% and 15%. This breakdown is not, in itself, unhealthy and, indeed, is recommended by some nutritional consultants (Willet and Skerett 2005). The

Table 2 Average Estimated Daily Intake of Energy, Macronutrients, of the Traditional Rural Maya Diet[a] and Percent of the Daily Recommended Intake (DRI) of the Food and Nutrition Board, National Academy of Sciences, United States[b]

Nutrient	INCAP studies (1950–1960)[c]	Percent of DRI or total kcals
Energy (kcal)	1795	87
Carbohydrates g (kcal)	334 (1336)	74
Total fat g (kcal)	21.1 (189.9)	11
Protein g (kcal)	67.3 (269.2)	15
Micronutrients		Percent of DRI
Calcium (g)	1.1	100
Iron (mg)	19.8	110
Thiamin (mg)	1.2	100
Riboflavin (mg)	0.7	64
Niacin (mg)	11.3	81
Vitamin C (mg)	37.5	50

[a] From Bermudez et al. 2008.

[b] http://iom.edu/en/Global/News%20Announcements/~/media/Files/Activity%20Files/Nutrition/DRIs/DRISummaryListing2.ashx. The values are based on the recommended DRI for physically active adult women ages 19–30 years old with a height of 150 cm, the average height of Maya women, and a BMI of 18.5; adult men need more of most nutrients, except iron.

[c] Bermudez et al. (2008) report a total energy value of 2044 kcals. The value of 1795 reported here is based on the contribution of carbohydrates, fats, and proteins as given by Bermudez et al. It is likely that alcohol consumption makes up the difference in kcals, but alcohol contributes no other nutrients and alcohol is consumed rarely by traditional adult Maya women and never by their children.

problem for the rural Maya is they do not have enough food to eat to meet energy and nutrient requirements.

The DRIs recommended by the Food and Nutrition Board of the United States are 45–65% carbohydrate, 20–35% fat, and 10–35% protein. The typical United States diet tends to be at the upper DRI intake for fat and the lower range of intake for carbohydrates and protein. Maya-Americans likely consume a diet closer to that typical for the United States, and they certainly consume more total kcals per day than the Maya of rural Guatemala. The shift from the traditional rural Maya diet in Guatemala may be one of the reasons for the increased stature, and especially body weight, of the Maya-Americans.

is a dismal. The percentage of infants under one year of age meeting recommended nutritional requirements is presented in Table 1.

By 5 years of age, 44% of all Guatemalan children are stunted, meaning they have a height-for-age falling below the third percentile of height expected for their age based on international references for growth. Nutritional deficiencies plague adults as well as infants and children. More than 35% of all adult Guatemalan women are anemic

(low iron). Guatemalans also have the lowest levels of iodine and folic acid of all peoples in Central America and Panama (Marini and Gragnolati 2003). Nutritional deficiencies in the young compromise adult health, including intellectual skills and capabilities, and in turn the nutritional deficiencies of women compromise the growth and development of their fetuses. It is a vicious cycle, one which recycles poverty and poor health, low birth weight, and risks for stunting from generation

Table 1 Percentage of Guatemalan Infants Younger than 1 Year Old Fulfilling Nutrient Requirements

Fulfillment of Requirements	Energy (Kcal)	Proteins	Vitamin A*	Iron
>100%	16%	35%	66%	2%
75–100%	8%	38%	29%	0%
50–75%	57%	15%	3%	3%
<50%	18%	12%	2%	95%
<25%	–	–	–	34%
Sample size = 352				

* Taking into account fortified sugar.
Source: Marini and Gragnolati 2003.

to generation (Garn et al. 1984, Bogin 1988: 148–159, Varela-Silva et al 2007).

STUDIES OF MAYA GROWTH IN GUATEMALA AND THE UNITED STATES

Along with colleagues from the Universidad del Valle de Guatemala in Guatemala City, I began working with the schoolchildren of one Maya village in 1979. We measured Maya children attending the state-run primary and middle school in the village. This village is only 15 miles (25 km) from Guatemala City. The parents of the children in this village worked mostly at clothing factories and in the business of growing ornamental flowers for export to North America and Europe. I thought that these activities might raise the standard of living for the families of the village, at least compared with more deeply rural Maya farming villages. I hoped to see improvements in nutritional status of the children as reflected in better growth. Our research in the new village did not support my expectations.

Parents working in the clothing factories and the flower export business are laborers and are treated and paid poorly. Many work on a piecemeal basis, for instance being paid about US$0.25 per shirt completed (this was the wage in the late 1980–1990s period). At this rate, an adult can earn only a few dollars a day. The nutritional status of the villagers is typical of the poor in Guatemala (Table 1), with Maya youngsters eating less than 75% of the food they need. Surveys by a group of foreign health workers in the village find that almost 30 percent of the girls and 20 percent of the boys are deficient in iodine, that most of the children suffer from intestinal parasites, and that many have persistent ear and eye infections. As a consequence, their health is poor and their height reflects it: they average about 7.5 cm (3 inches) shorter than better-fed Guatemalan children and juveniles.

As mentioned at the start of this essay, the Maya I work with in the United States live in Los Angeles, California and in the rural agriculture community of Indiantown in central Florida. In this research I have partnered with Dr. James Loucky, a social anthropologist with many years' experience in Guatemala and in Maya communities in the United States. Other academic colleagues are Prof. Patricia Smith, an economist at University of Michigan-Dearborn, Dr. Ines Varela-Silva, a specialist in energy expenditure at Loughborough University, and Dr. Luis Rios, a biological anthropologist from Spain. I also have support of Maya community leaders, especially Mr. Antonio Silvestre in Florida. Working with Dr. Loucky, my other academic colleagues, and Mr. Silvestre has proven to be immensely valuable to develop biocultural perspectives and better understandings of Maya nutritional status and health.

The findings reported here come from studies we conducted between 1992 and 2000, although I have visited the Maya communities in Florida several times since then. The Maya families belong to the Q'anjob'al language group. Q'anjob'al speakers come from a relatively small region in the northwest Guatemala highlands. Indeed, most of the families in our sample come from one town and several smaller hamlets surrounding this town. Thus, the Florida and California Maya we measured are from the same ethnic and geographic origin in Guatemala. They are compared with Kaqchikel-speaking Maya living in Guatemala from the village where I worked and from other villages nearby. Biological and social differences between these language groups are minor and there are no known genetic explanations for differences in physical growth that we find between the Guatemala and USA Maya.

At the time of our research the political status of the Maya in the United States was heterogeneous and included many who applied for (and in some cases won) political asylum, others who gained legal rights to work and residency, and many who remained undocumented. Without legal residence people live in fear of arrest and deportation. During my visit to Indiantown in 2008, a Maya mother was arrested by immigration authorities and then taken away from her children, who were born in the United States and are therefore U.S. citizens. Hard work by Sister Mary Dooley, the Director of the Hope Rural School in Indiantown, and Mr. Silvestre secured the mother's release and return to her children.

In Florida, adult Maya worked as day laborers in agriculture, landscaping, construction, child care, and other informal sector jobs. In Los Angeles, most Maya over the age of 15 toiled for 50 or more hours a week doing low-wage manual sewing work in the sweatshops of the garment district (Loucky, 1993, 1996). A few Maya established their own sewing contracting shops (*fábricas*) with five to 25 employees, including other Maya. A few were beginning to work as paraprofessionals (nurses' aides) or as semiskilled workers (hairdresser, electronic technician). In both Indiantown and Los Angeles the Q'anjob'al Maya organized voluntary support organizations that helped with resettlement, employment, and housing and also sponsored community religious and cultural events designed to promote Maya values and ethnic identity.

OUR SAMPLES OF CHILDREN

In Indiantown, children of all ethnicities attending the two elementary schools were measured during February of 1992 and again in March of 2000. Four ethnic groups—Maya, Mexican, white, black—provided large enough samples for statistical analysis in the age range of 5 to 12 years. Chronological age was ascertained from birth certificates, official school records, or other proof of date of birth such as asking parents twice for the birth date. The place of birth of the parents and the child and the length of the child's residence in the United States were also collected. Several members of the Maya community assisted with the gathering of this information. The names of the ethnic groups used here reflect the self-reported names provided by the children of Indiantown or by their school teachers. The Los Angeles Maya children were measured at Christmas parties sponsored by a Maya cultural organization in December 1992 and 1999. A few children were measured in their homes. As in Florida, children were asked to self-identify their ethnicity, or, in the case of the young children, adults familiar with the child were asked.

We measured the youngsters for height, weight, sitting height, arm circumference, and triceps skinfold. The rationale for each of these measurements is as follows. Since height increases over time, it is an indicator of the history of nutritional status and health of a child. In contrast, weight can both increase and decrease over time and, therefore, relates more to recent nutrition and health status. Sitting height is a measurement of the length of the upper body (head, neck, and trunk). Subtracting sitting height from total height provides an estimate of leg length. Leg length is a sensitive indicator of the quality of early life because the legs grow relatively faster than the trunk of the body during the first 7 years after birth (Bogin and Varela-Silva 2010). Circumferences and skinfolds are generally accepted measures for body composition (i.e., lean body mass and fat mass). Body composition is often used as a proxy for nutritional status. Lean body mass is an indicator for the body's reserves of protein, and fat mass is an indicator of the body's reserves of energy.

Most Maya families arrived in the 1980s as refugees escaping a civil war as well as a political system that threatened them and their children. In the United States they

found security and started new lives, and before long their children began growing faster and bigger. Our data show that the average increase in height among the first generation of these immigrants was 5.6 cm (2.2 inches), which is one of the largest single-generation increases in height ever recorded. When people migrated from the poverty of rural life in Eastern Europe to the cities of the United States just after World War I, such as my own grandparents did, the increase in height of the next generation was only about 2.54 cm (1 inch).

One reason for the rapid increase in stature is that in the United States the Maya have access to treated drinking water and to a reliable supply of food. Especially critical are school breakfast and lunch programs for children from low-income families, as well as public assistance programs such as the federal Women, Infants, and Children (WIC) program and food stamps. That these programs improve health and growth is no secret. What is surprising is how fast they work. Mayan mothers in the United States tell me that even their babies are born bigger and healthier than the babies they raised in Guatemala, and hospital statistics bear them out. These women must be enjoying a level of health so much improved from that of their lives in Guatemala that their babies are growing faster in the womb.

Of course, plasticity means that such changes are dependent on external conditions, and unfortunately the rising height—and health—of the Maya is in danger from political forces that are attempting to cut funding for food stamps and the WIC program for immigrants. In fact, Congress cut the WIC program's budget by about 30 percent for 2012. By one estimate, this means some 300,000 families will lose benefits (http://zesterdaily.com/zester-soapbox-articles/1345-mitt-romneys-safety-net-is-not-working). It is likely that the negative impact on the lives of poor Americans, including the Mayan refugees, will be as dramatic as were the former positive effects.

The improvements in height continued with our measurements in 1999–2000. We show this in Figure 2. The measurements for boys and girls are combined, as there are no meaningful differences between them. The data for Maya in the United States combine the groups measured in Los Angeles and Indiantown. In 1992 (labeled Maya-USA1992) we measured 211 Maya boys and girls. In 1999–2000 (labeled Maya-USA2000) we measured 431 Maya boys and girls. These groups are compared with a sample of 1348 Maya boys and girls measured in Guatemala in 1998 and the National Health and Nutrition Examination Survey (NHANES) of the United States. The NHANES surveys are national random, stratified sampling of all non-institutionalized persons in the United States and include the ethnic groups 'White', 'Black', 'Mexican-American', and 'other Hispanic'. For this analysis we use the combined NHANES I and II references data for 'White' and 'Black' boys and girls published by Frisancho (1990). Reference data for Hispanics (mostly Mexican-Americans) were not part of the NHANES I and II.

The Maya-USA2000 sample is, on average, 11.4 cm (4.5") taller across the ages of 5 to 12 years than the Maya of the same ages in Guatemala. As shown in Figure 3, Maya-Americans have a significantly smaller sitting height ratio, meaning relatively longer legs, than Maya of the same age in Guatemala. This change in body proportions is due to the fact that 6.9 cm (2.7") of the increase in height is due to longer legs. The increase in leg length amounts to 61% of the increase of total stature. Sitting height ratio was once thought to be a fairly unalterable characteristic, one that defined so-called racial groups. But, it is now known that changes in leg length relative to total height is a sensitive indicator of the quality of the environment for human growth during the first 7 years of life (Bogin and Varela-Silva 2010).

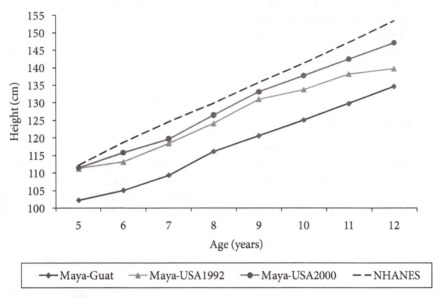

Figure 2 *Mean height of Maya boys and girls in Guatemala (Maya-Guat) and in the United States (Maya-USA) compared with the median height of boys and girls in the United States (NHANES, from Bogin and Loucky 1997).*

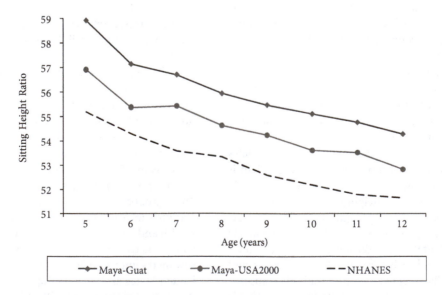

Figure 3 *Mean sitting height ratio (SHR) of Maya boys and girls in Guatemala (Maya-Guat) and in the United States (Maya-USA) compared with the Median SHR of United States boys and girls (NHANES). SHR is defined as [(sitting height/height)*100]. A smaller SHR indicates relatively longer legs for a given height. The mean difference in leg length=7.02 which is the average difference in estimated leg length between the Maya-Guat group and the Maya-USA2000 group (from Bogin and Loucky 1997).*

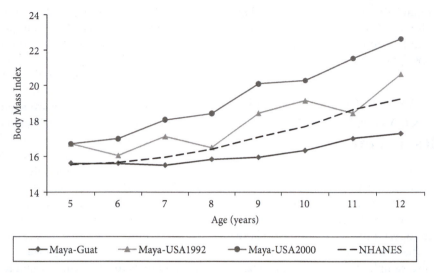

Figure 4 *Mean body mass index (BMI) of Maya boys and girls in Guatemala (Maya-Guat) and in the United States (Maya-USA) compared with the median BMI of United States boys and girls (from Bogin and Loucky 1997). BMI is defined as [weight in kg / height in m²].*

Not all bodes well for the Maya-American children and juveniles. They are taller and longer-legged, but they are also showing more overweight and obesity. In Figure 4 the body mass index (BMI) is shown. BMI is widely used to estimate fatness—a higher BMI value indicating more body fatness. BMI is an imperfect estimate of fatness in children, especially those children with short legs. A relatively large trunk and head will raise BMI even when body fatness is not high. This may be seen in Figure 4 for the lines representing BMI for Maya in Guatemala and the NHANES median. These two lines are quite close until age 8 years, but the Maya in Guatemala aged 5–8 years are known to be both short and very thin (low body fatness). The Maya-Americans have higher BMIs than the average American boy or girl in the NHANES I and II samples. Part of this difference is due to the Maya-American having relatively shorter legs than the NHANES sample, but our measurements of skinfolds and arm circumference show that the Maya-Americans are much fatter than Maya-Guatemalans.

The nutritional status of 6 to 12 years olds living in Indiantown, Florida, in the year 2000 is summarized in Table 2. The Maya-Americans show more stunting, overweight and obesity than any other ethnic groups living in Indiantown (stunting is height < 3rd percentile of the United States CDC growth reference; overweight is BMI > 85th percentile on the CDC reference; obesity is BMI > 90th percentile on the CDC reference; Kuczmarski 2000).

What explains the incidence of stunting, overweight, and obesity among the Maya of Indiantown? We interviewed 290 of the Maya children and juveniles we measured regarding their diets and patterns of physical activity. We were able to survey parents of only 42 of the private school children regarding their family's socioeconomic status,

Table 2 Prevalence of Stunting, Overweight and Obesity: Indiantown 2000

	Stunted	Overweight	Obese	n
Maya	11.5%	48.6%	25.3%	296
Mexican	3.8	35.0	28.0	157
Haitian	7.7	30.8	23.1	13
Euro. Amer.	0.0	24.5	18.4	49
African Amer.	0.7	31.7	25.9	139
Others	0.0	41.7	38.9	36
TOTAL	6.1	39.7	33.5	690

including income, number of offspring in the family, and remittances sent back to Guatemala. We offered the survey in both Spanish and English and noted which version the parent chose. The choice of language proxies the degree of assimilation to the United States.

Our analysis of these data (Smith et al. 2002) finds statistically significant evidence that children who report that watching TV or playing computer games as a favorite pastime face a higher risk of overweight. This is hardly surprising as these sedentary activities are associated with greater fatness in many studies. Maya children and juveniles with more siblings face a higher probability of overweight and obesity. This was unexpected, as more mouths to feed might lead to less food intake per person. Perhaps the number of children in a family is correlated with some other factor positively related to BMI, such as type of food served or amount of physical activity. Finally, children whose parents answered the questionnaire in Spanish face a lower risk of weight problems. If indeed these families are less assimilated to United States culture and lifestyles, then perhaps they retain more of their traditional Maya traditions in terms of diet, physical activity, and leisure time pursuits which are less likely to lead to overweight in their offspring.

THE INTERGENERATIONAL INFLUENCES HYPOTHESIS AND OUR CONTINUING RESEARCH

The 11.5% of stunted Maya-American children and juveniles in our total sample is unexpected, given the very high rates of overweight and obesity in this same group. Positive energy balance, via more food intake, less energy expenditure, or both, is expected to result in greater growth in both height and body mass. There were only five stunted children in our questionnaire sample, too few for any meaningful analysis of the causes of stunting. But, other studies also report the combination of stunting and overweight in groups similar to the Maya-Americans, that is, traditional cultural groups undergoing a rapid transition in lifestyle due to migration to developed nations such as the United States. In developing nations, obesity has increased dramatically in the last decade, but a high prevalence of stunting still coexists (reviewed in Varela-Silva et al. 2007, 2009). This combination of stunting and overweight in the same population is called the "short-plump syndrome" and, more recently, the nutritional dual-burden.

The intergenerational influences hypothesis (IIH) is one explanation for this. The IIH was proposed by Irving Emanuel (1986) as "…those factors, conditions, exposures and environments experienced by one generation that relate to the health, growth and development of the next generation." The IIH includes "fetal programming," "perinatal adaptive responses," "life history trade-offs," "developmental adaptations," and related concepts in the literature (Varela-Silva et al 2009). The original IIH was proposed to account for the persistence of low birth weight across generations. In the context of our research with the Maya, the IIH relates to the existence of a non-genetic mechanism in which malnutrition of the mother during her own fetal and early postnatal development will have negative health consequences for her offspring, especially risks for low birth weight and overweight/obesity later in life.

How do these non-genetic mechanisms work across generations? The change in height of American and Dutch people over the past few generations provide an example. Consider these statistics: in 1850 Americans were the tallest people in the world, with young adult American men averaging 167.6 cm (5'6"). In the years 2003–2006 European-American men averaged 178 cm (5'10"), but have fallen in the standings and are now only the 7th tallest people in the world. In first place are the Dutch at 183 cm (6') and then men from Sweden, Germany, Finland, Czech Republic, and Denmark (in all of these groups, and just about everywhere else, women average about 13–15 cm [5.5"] less than men at all times). Americans are about 2 cm shorter, on average,

than all these European populations. Remember, 2 cm is the average increase in stature of European immigrants to the United States in the late 19th and early 20th Centuries (it is a myth that African groups, such as the Tutsi, are or have ever been the tallest people in the world; Tutsi men average 170.2 cm or 5'7").

Back in 1850 Dutch men averaged only 5'4"—the shortest men in Europe. So what happened? Did all the short Dutch move over to the United States? Did the Dutch back in Europe get an infusion of "tall genes"? Neither. In both America and the Netherlands life got better, but more so for the Dutch, and height increased as a result. After the turn of the century both the United States and the Netherlands began to protect the health of their citizens by purifying drinking water, installing sewer systems, regulating the safety of food, and, most important, providing better health care and diets to children. The children responded to their changed environment by growing taller. After World War II, the Dutch decided to provide public health benefits to all of the public, including the poor. In the United States, meanwhile, improved health is enjoyed most by those who can afford it. The poor often lack adequate housing, sanitation, and health care. The difference in our two societies can be seen at birth: in 1990 only 4% of Dutch babies were born at low birth weight (LBW <2500 grams, or 5.5 lbs), compared with 7% in the United States. For white Americans the LBW rate was 5.7%, and for black Americans the rate was a whopping 13.3%. The difference in LBW between whites and blacks reflects the history of slavery and inequality as well as continuing disparities in socioeconomic status (Jasienska 2008). These disparities between rich and poor in the United States carry through to adulthood: high income black and white Americans are taller than low income blacks and whites by about 1.5 cm (0.6"), but do not differ within same socioeconomic category. The height gradient according to education differences is even greater—white and black men with a university education average about 3 cm taller than men with no formal education and 2 cm taller than men with only an elementary school education (Komlos and Baur 2004).

The increase of stature in the Netherlands, the United States, and the other nations took place over 160 years, or 6–7 generations. The intergenerational influences hypothesis explains the trend in height in the following way. If a girl is undernourished and suffers poor health during infancy and childhood then the growth of her body, including her reproductive system, is usually reduced. With a shortage of energy and raw materials, she can't build more cells to construct a bigger body; at the same time, she has to invest what materials she can get into repairing already existing cells and tissues from the damage caused by disease. She also must allocate energy and body materials to basic metabolism to maintain her body, essential physical labor, and, if possible, play and other social behavior. Her shorter stature as an adult is the result of all the compromises her body makes between these demands while growing up.

Such a woman can pass on her short stature to her child, but genes may have nothing to do with it. If she becomes pregnant, her small reproductive system probably won't be able to supply a normal level of nutrients and oxygen to her fetus. The functioning of other organs in her body, including the kidneys and pancreas, may also be deranged. The harsh maternal environment reprograms the fetus to grow more slowly than it would if the woman was healthier, so she is more likely to give birth to a smaller baby. Low-birth-weight babies tend to continue their prenatal program of slow growth through childhood. By the time they are teenagers, they are usually significantly shorter than people of normal birth weight. Some particularly striking evidence of this reprogramming comes from studies on monozygotic twins, which develop from a single fertilized egg cell and are therefore identical genetically. But in certain cases, monozygotic twins end up being nourished by unequal portions of the placenta. The twin with the smaller fraction of the placenta is often born with low birth weight, while the other one is normal. Follow-up studies show that this difference between the twins can last throughout their lives.

Our current studies of Maya growth and nutritional status focus on intergenerational influences on the risk for stunting and overweight of 7- to 9-year-old boys and girls. We are now working in Merida, Mexico. Merida is the largest city in the Yucatan peninsula, which is part of the Maya culture area. The Yucatecan Maya share with Guatemala Maya the same long history of social, economic, and political repression at the hands of European colonists and, more recently, from the political regimes of Mexico and Central America (Montejo, 1999). In addition, the Maya population, especially those who migrated recently from rural areas to slums of Merida, is confronting the effects of the nutrition transition, shifting from the consumption of traditional foods to westernized fast foods that are high in energy but nutritionally poor (Leatherman and Goodman 2005). This nutritional transition, along with the legacy of poverty and low social conditions, increases the risk for overweight and associated diseases, stunting, and overall impaired growth (Fernald 2007; Gurri et al. 2001).

So far we find that the Maya mothers are short, with 69.4% of the 206 women measured below 150 cm (59") height. Stunting is detected in 21% of their children and overweight in 33%, with 2.4% both stunted and overweight. In principle it should be virtually impossible for a 7–9 year old to be simultaneously stunted and overweight. Mother's height below 150 cm and the child's birth weight below 3000 grams (6.6 lbs) both are statistically significant predictors of stunting in the child (Varela-Silva et al. 2009). These results support the IIH. Mother's whose own growth was compromised pass on similar risks to their offspring and a lower birth weight indicates that the intergenerational influences are at work before birth. We found no clear effects on the risk for overweight that support the IIH.

In 2010 we collected more data from 58 Maya families in Merida. This research is in cooperation with Dr. Federico Dickinson and colleagues of the *Centro de Investigación y de Estudios Avanzados* (Cinvestav) in Merida. We expanded our theoretical perspective to consider not only the IIH, but also current nutritional and behavioral risks for child overweight/obesity. Our original plan for data collection is shown in Figure 5. Working down the boxes on the left side of Figure 5, we estimate the mother's nutrition and health when she was a girl by measuring both her adult stature and knee height, which is the length measured from the heel of the foot to the top of the knee cap. As explained above, undernutrition, disease, and heavy workloads in the first 7 years of life stunt the legs more than the rest of the body, and the lower leg is most affected. We weigh the mothers

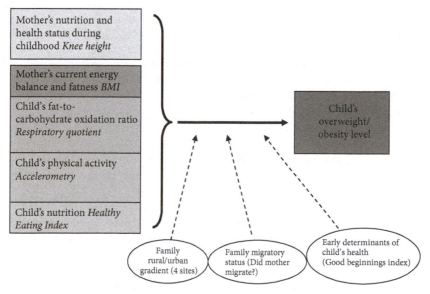

Figure 5 *The next step in our research—intergenerational, nutritional, and behavioral risks for Maya child obesity.*

and calculate their BMI to provide a single measurement of current energy balance and fatness. We were not able to measure the child's fat-to-carbohydrate oxidation ratio due to insufficient funds. The ratio will tell us something about the child's metabolic use of different kinds of energy containing nutrients. Based on other research, we predict that due to the intergenerational history of undernutrition Maya children will tend to use energy from carbohydrate foods and store energy from the fat in foods as fat on their body. In Merida, where fat is more plentiful in processed foods, this type of metabolism places the Maya children at risk for overweight. We did use the Actiheart, a combined heart rate monitor and accelerometer, to measure physical activity over a one week period. Accelerometers record body movement of any type, while the heart rate monitor tells us the physical intensity of the movement. The final box indicates that we interviewed mothers about the eating habits of their children.

The ellipses at the bottom of the figure indicate that we planned to work at four sites, three in the Yucatan as well as Indiantown, Florida. Again, lack of funding limited us to the one site in Merida. We did collect family migration history and other demographic variables, such as fertility history of the mother, family size, and household composition. Finally, we collected information of the child's early life, including place of birth (hospital or home), birth weight, record of immunizations, and history of serious illness. Most of these data were copied from medical clinic visit health cards maintained by the families.

We are using all of these data to build statistical and biocultural models of risks for overweight/obesity and risks for stunting. Some of our findings are published in scientific journals (Wilson et al. 2011a; 2011b). New field-work to collect more data on three generations—grand-mothers, their daughters and grandchildren—is currently underway.

SUMMARY

The decisions of Maya parents to migrate to the United States or from rural to urban Mexico are best viewed as rational responses to the nutritional, economic, and political ecology for child development. From a biocultural perspective, there are significant implications from our Maya research.

Human phenotypes, represented in this essay as growth in height, weight, body proportions, and body composition, are sensitive indicators of the physical, economic, and political environment. Much of the 20th Century research on the factors influencing plasticity in human phenotypes focused on only the physical environment—for instance, the hypoxia of high altitude, the cold and heat of latitude extremes, or the nutritional stress experienced in traditional agricultural communities. Often, little can be done to alter the physical environment, and we ascribe variation in human physical and behavioral phenotypes to inevitable accommodations to them.

However, all people live within social, economic, and political environments that also have powerful effects on human phenotypes. A newer wave of anthropological research is concentrating on biocultural interactions between these social, economic, and political environments. Our studies of "Maya in Disneyland" are part of this new wave. In their physical growth the Maya-American children show some of the symbolism of the United States—"...the symbolism of American places and American mythological history." People with bigger bodies are a major part of United States mythological history. Think of George Washington, Abraham Lincoln and Paul Bunyon. Maya-Americans gain American bigness in both height and fatness. The former seems "good" and the later seems "bad." The juxtaposition of "good and bad" are also part of United States symbolism and mythology—think "cowboys and Indians." The growth changes experienced by the Maya are likely due to the abundance of food ("good") and the abundance of low physical activity leisure time ("bad") that symbolically characterize the United States today. Future generations of Maya-Americans, indeed all Americans, will need to come to terms with the reality and the symbolism of the United States if they wish to maintain a good nutritional balance and good health.

Notes

1. "CE stands for "Common Era." It is a relatively old term that is experiencing rapidly increased usage in recent years. It is expected to eventually replace AD. The latter is an abbreviation for "Anno Domini" in Latin or "the year of the Lord" in English. The latter refers to the approximate birth year of Yeshua of Nazareth (a.k.a. Jesus Christ). CE and AD have the same value; 2004 CE = 2004 AD. The word "common" simply means that it is based on the most frequently used calendar system: the Gregorian Calendar. BCE stands for "Before the common era." It is expected to eventually replace BC, which means "Before Christ," or "Before the Messiah." Years in the BC and BCE notation are also identical in value" (quoted from http://www.religioustolerance.org/ce.htm, accessed 01 December 2010).

References

Aragón CJ. 2001. La Quinceañera. In: Girlhood in America: an encyclopedia, Volume 1. Forman-Brunell M, ed. ABC-Clio/Greenwood: Santa Barbara, California, pp. 535–539.

Bermudez OI, Hernandez L, Mazariegos M, Solomons NW. 2008. Secular Trends in Food Patterns of Guatemalan Consumers: New Foods for Old. Food and Nutrition Bulletin 29:278–287.

Bogin B. 1988. Patterns of Human Growth. Cambridge: Cambridge University Press.

Bogin B. 1999. Patterns of Human Growth, 2nd edition. Cambridge: Cambridge University Press.

Bogin B, Loucky J. 1997. Plasticity, Political Economy, and Physical Growth Status of Guatemala Maya Children Living in the United States. Am J Phys Anthropol 102:17–32.

Bogin B, Varela-Silva MI. 2010. Leg Length, Body Proportion, and Health: A Review with a Note on Beauty. Int J Environ Res Public Health 7:1047–1075.

Burns A. 1989. The Maya of Florida. Migration World 27(3/4):20–26.

Cucina T. 2004. Dental Morphometry and Biological Affinity in Pre-Contact and Contact Maya Populations from the Peninsula of Yucatan. Mexicon 26(1):14–19.

Emanuel I. 1986. Maternal Health During Childhood and Later Reproductive Performance. Ann N Y Acad Sci 477:27–39.

Fernald L. 2007. Socio-Economic Status and Body Mass Index in Low-Income Mexican Adults. Soc Sci Med 64:2030–2042.

Fogel R. 1986. "Physical Growth as a Measure of the Economic Well Being of Populations: The Eighteenth and Nineteenth Centuries." In Falkner F, Tanner J, eds. Human Growth, 2nd ed, vol. 3. New York: Plenum, pp. 263–281.

Fraim J. The Symbolism of Place. http://www.symbolism.org/writing/books/sp/3/page4.html (accessed November 4, 2010).

Frisancho AR. 1990. Anthropometric Standards for the Assessment of Growth and Nutritional Status. Ann Arbor: University of Michigan Press.

Garn SM, Pesick SD, Pilkington JJ. 1984. The interaction between prenatal and socioeconomic effects on growth and development in childhood. In Borms J, Hauspie R, Sand C, Susanne C, and Hebbelinck M, eds. Human Growth and Development. New York: Plenum, pp. 59–70.

Glittenberg J. 1994. To the Mountain and Back: The Mysteries of Guatemalan Highland Family Life. Waveland Press: Long Grove, Illinois.

Gómez-Casado E, Martínez-Laso J, Moscoso J, Zamora J, Martin-Villa M, Perez-Blas M, Lopez-Santalla M, Lucas Gramajo P, Silvera C, Lowy E, Arnaiz-Villena A. 2003. Origin of Mayans According to HLA Genes and the Uniqueness of Amerindians. Tissue Antigens. 61:425–436.

Gurri F, Balam Pereira G, Moran E. 2001. Well-Being Changes in Response to 30 Years of Regional Integration in Maya Populations From Yucatan, Mexico. Am J Hum Biol 13:590–602.

Jasienska G. 2009. Low Birth Weight of Contemporary African Americans: An Intergenerational Effect of Slavery? Amer J Hum Biol 21:16–24.

Komlos J, ed. 1994. Stature, Living Standards, and Economic Development. Chicago: University of Chicago Press.

Komlos J, Baur M. 2004. From The Tallest to (One of) the Fattest: The Enigmatic Fate of the American Population in the 20th Century. Econ Hum Biol 2:57–74.

Kuczmarski RJ. 2000. CDC Growth Charts: United States. Advance Data from Vital and Health Statistics. No. 314. Hyattsville, MD: National Center for Health Statistics.

Lasker GW. 1969. Human Biological Adaptability. Science 166:1480–1486.

Leatherman T, Goodman A. 2005. Coca-Colonization of Diets in the Yucatan. Soc Sci Med 61:833–846.

Loucky J. 1993. Central American refugees: Learning new skills in the U.S.A. In Howard MC, ed. Contemporary Anthropology, 4th ed. New York: HarperCollins, pp. 228–230.

Loucky J. 1996. Maya Americans: The emergence of a transnational community. In Hamilton N, Chinchilla N, eds. Central Americans in California. Los Angeles: Center for Multiethnic Studies and Transnational Studies, University of Southern California, pp. 30–34.

Loucky J, Moors MM. 2000. The Maya Diaspora: Guatemalan Roots, New American Lives. Philadelphia: Temple University Press.

Lovell WG. 2000. A Beauty That Hurts: Life and Death in Guatemala. Austin: University of Texas Press.

Lovell WG. 2010. A Beauty That Hurts: Life and Death in Guatemala, 2nd edition. Austin: University of Texas Press.

Lovell WG, Lutz CH. 1996. A Dark Obverse: Maya Survival in Guatemala, 1520–1994. The Geographical Review 86: 398–407.

Manz B. 1988. Refugees of a Hidden War: The Aftermath of Counterinsurgency in Guatemala. Albany: State University of New York Press.

Marini A, Gragnolati M. 2003. Malnutrition and Poverty in Guatemala. World Bank Policy Research Working Paper 2967, http://econ.worldbank.org/external/default/main?pagePK=64165259&theSitePK=469372&piPK=64165421&menuPK=64166093&entityID=000094946_03020804020125

McNeil CL, Burney DA, Burney LP. 2010. Evidence disputing deforestation as the cause for the collapse of the ancient Maya polity of Copan, Honduras. Proc Natl Acad Sci U S A 107:1017–1022.

Montejo V. 1999. Voices from Exile: Violence and Survival in Modern Maya History. Norman, OK: University of Oklahoma Press.

Sack RD. 1992. Place, Modernity, and the Consumer's World: A Relational Framework for Geographical Analysis. Baltimore: The Johns Hopkins University Press. Schell LM. 1986. Community health assessment through physical anthropology: Auxological epidemiology. Hum Org 45:321–327.

Scherer AK. 2007. Population structure of the Classic period Maya. Am J Phys Anthropol. 132: 367–380.

Smith P, Bogin B, Varela-Silva M, Orden B, Loucky J. 2002. Does Immigration Help or Harm Children's Health? The Mayan Case. Soc Sci Q 83:994–1002.

Steckel RH. 2008. Biological Measures of the Standard of Living. J Econ Perspect 22: 129–152.

Tanner JM. 1981. A History of the Study of Human Growth. Cambridge: Cambridge University Press.

Tanner JM. 1986. Growth as a mirror of the conditions of the society: secular trends and class distinctions. In Demirjian A, ed. Human Growth, a Multidisciplinary Review. London: Taylor & Francis Ltd, pp. 3–34.

The World Bank. 2004. Poverty in Guatemala. Washington, DC: World Bank.

Tovar Gómez M. 1998. Perfil de los Pueblos Indígenas de Guatemala. Un acercamiento a la problemática, procesos y cultura milenaria de los pueblos indígenas de Guatemala. Informe para el Banco Mundial; Guatemala.

Varela-Silva M, Frisancho A, Bogin B, Chatkoff D, Smith P, Dickinson F, Winham D. 2007. Behavioral, Environmental, Metabolic and Intergenerational Components of Early Life Undernutrition Leading to Later Obesity in Developing Nations and in Minority Groups in the USA. Coll Antropol 31:39–46.

Varela-Silva MI, Azcorra H, Dickinson F, Bogin B, Frisancho AR. 2009. Influence of Maternal Stature, Pregnancy Age, and Infant Birth Weight on Growth During Childhood in Yucatan, Mexico: A Test of the Intergenerational Effects Hypothesis. Am J Hum Biol. 21:657–663.

Willett WC, Skerrett PJ. 2005. Eat, Drink, and Be Healthy. Free Press/Simon & Schuster: New York.

Wilson H, Dickinson F, Griffiths P, Bogin B, Varela-Silva MI. 2011a. Logistics of using the Actiheart physical activity monitors in urban Mexico among 7- to 9-year-old children. Am J Hum Biol. 23:426–428.

Wilson HJ, Dickinson F, Griffiths PL, Azcorra H, Bogin B, Varela-Silva MI. 2011b. How useful is BMI in predicting adiposity indicators in a sample of Maya children and women with high levels of stunting? Am J Hum Biol. 23:780–789.

WHO. 2010. World Health Organization, Country Cooperation Strategy at a Glance, Guatemala. http://www.who.int/countries/gtm/en/ (accessed November 6, 2010).

CHAPTER 28

!Kung Nutritional Status and the Original "Affluent Society"—A New Analysis

Barry Bogin

(2012)

The 1960s were heady times for Planet Earth. The pace of change increased for the independence of former Colonies from the European powers, for the Civil Rights movement in the United States, for United States hegemony in world affairs—including the Cuban missile crisis, the Vietnam War, and CIA activity in Latin America—for the Women's Rights and Feminism movements, for the introduction of "the Pill" (pharmacological contraception) and the sexual revolution, for the continuing Cold War with the Soviet Union, including Soviet and United States space programs culminating in the moon landing of 1969. A few key events of that decade include the assassinations of John Kennedy, Robert Kennedy, and Martin Luther King Jr., the anti-war movement, and the Beatles, which was a portent of a new power of "youth culture" in music, clothing, and other arenas (think of "hippies," the Woodstock music festival, and "swinging London").

Academia in general, and anthropology in particular, were caught up in the "Sixties."

Richard Lee, the author of the chapter in this reader "What hunters do for a living, or, how to make out on scarce resources" (originally published in 1968), recalls the impact:

> In the early 1960s, the anthropological world was excited by the new data pouring in from field studies on nonhuman primates and from the Leakeys' discoveries of ancient living floors associated with fossil man. The ethnographic study of a contemporary hunter-gatherer group seemed to be the next logical step. Irven DeVore and I chose to work in Africa rather than in Australia because we wanted to be close to the actual faunal and floral environment occupied by early man.

—Lee 1979a, pp. 303–304

The few remaining human hunting-gathering people alive in the 1960s were estimated to be less than 1% of the total human population (Lee and Devore 1968). They were viewed as a precious and dwindling resource for study by anthropologists. The above quote expresses the two prevailing anthropological reasons for the value of research on the Dobe !Kung people of the Kalahari Desert in Botswana: 1) Africa is the continent of origin for the human species, and 2) living hunter-gatherers such as the Dobe !Kung provide a window to view the human past when all people lived by foraging. The purpose of the Kalahari Research Project initiated in 1963 by Lee and DeVore was to document and understand the, "...basic adaptive strategies of the hunting and gathering way of life" (ibid, p. 304). The fundamental conclusion at the time of the field research (the mid-1960s), is that "The Dobe-area Bushmen live well today on wild plants and meat, in spite of the fact that they are confined to the least productive portion of the range in which Bushman peoples were formally found" (Lee 1968, p. 43). That conclusion is repeated in many of the publications of members of the Kalahari Research team, and as recently as 2010 by team member Nancy Howell who succinctly states, "...most of [the Dobe !Kung] seem to be healthy and vigorous" (p. 49).

The conclusions of the Kalahari Research Project are that the !Kung were well nourished, "live well" on their foraged diet, and were vigorous in terms of a high level of physical activity. These conclusions have been questioned in the past by researchers from a variety of disciplines (Panter-Brick et al 2001, see especially chapters by Froment, Jenike, Pennington, and Rowley-Conwy, Stillitoe 2002, De Souza 2006, Bogin 2009). Recent research shows that many living foragers and traditional horticulturalists and pastoralists live within adverse nutritional and infectious disease ecologies, often exacerbated by social instability and warfare (Gray et al. 2008, Gurven et al. 2008, McDade et al. 2008). Froment (2001, p. 259) finds that, "Coping with hazards and a heavy burden of diseases, hunter-gatherers do not live—and have never lived—in the Garden of Eden; they are not affluent, but poor, with limited needs and limited satisfaction, and little access to any facility."

From these perspectives, the living foragers are not representative of optimal, favorable, or even normative human biological conditions. Rather, the living foragers are remnants of the past. They have suffered from exploitation by more powerful pastoral and agriculture-based societies in the historical past, by Colonial-era powers in the recent past, and by the nation-states in which the foragers now reside (Bodley, 1999; Trigger, 1999).

The new analysis presented in this chapter provides additional evidence that the !Kung of the 1960s were neither well nourished, healthy, or especially vigorous. These findings are based on the original data for nutritional intake, energy expenditure, and anthropometry (height, weight, and body composition) collected by the Kalahari Research Project team. The new analysis makes use of estimates of food composition and human energy requirements that became available after 1980, that is, after the original publications by the Kalahari Research Project team. The goal of the new analysis is not to criticize or disparage the original research. In fact, the fieldwork and data collection of the Kalahari Research Project represent some of the finest anthropological, nutritional, and ecological work ever done. The purpose of the new analysis is to help refine understanding of the nutritional anthropology of the !Kung—a people and culture that occupies a central, almost intellectually sacred, place in the biocultural study of the human species.

THE ORIGINAL AFFLUENT SOCIETY?

The findings of the Kalahari Research Project regarding !Kung nutritional status were welcomed and adopted by several influential academics into a revised view of the nature of the hunting and gathering lifestyle. The old view was that foragers lived precariously, always on the brink of hunger, ill health, and death. This is a view that extends back in time to at least the year 1651 when Thomas Hobbes' book *Leviathan* was published. In that book Hobbes described the natural state of humankind before the creation of centralized state political systems—such as rule by kings, pharaohs, emperors, and the like—as one with,

> no Knowledge of the face of the Earth; no account of Time; no Arts; no Letters; no Society; and which is worst of all, continuall feare, and danger of violent death; And the life of man, solitary, poore, nasty, brutish, and short.

One of the major contributions of Anthropology was to show how Hobbes' view was both ethnocentric and incorrect. Every student of introductory anthropology now learns of the socially rich and philosophically complex nature of human culture in all human societies, past and present, including the traditional anthropological groupings of bands, tribes, chiefdoms, and states. The archeological and skeletal evidence from the Paleolithic (> 10,000 BP—years before present), long before the advent of human dependence on animal and plant domestication, shows people living in social groups, some relatively large in population size, and enjoying a relatively good standard of living as evidenced by good physical growth, successful reproduction, sophisticated technology, and complex ideological systems (Cohen and Armelagos 1984,

Formicola and Giannecchini 1999, Gage 1998, Mathers and Henneberg 1995, Ruff et al. 1993, Wood 1994, Steckel and Rose 2002). Longevity in the past was not "short," for as long ago as 50,000 BP many people lived to be 50 to 70 years old (Caspari and Lee 2006, Koningsberg and Herman 2006, Paine and Boldsen 2006).

The Hobbesian view was, however, common in anthropological writings and textbooks through the 1950s. These notions of "Paleolithic poverty" and the alleged dire circumstances of living foragers were challenged by Marshall Sahlins (1972) in his book *Stone-age Economics*, especially the first chapter titled "The original affluent society." The premise of this chapter is that the hunting and gathering lifestyle provides sufficient food, adequate material means for housing, clothing, and other goods, and abundant leisure time. "A good case can be made that hunters and gatherers work less than we do; and, rather than a continuous travail, the food quest is intermittent, leisure abundant, and there is a greater amount of sleep in the daytime per capita per year than in any other condition of society" (Sahlins, 1972, p. 14).

Sahlins' "The original affluent society" provided the post-1960 perspective of the hunting and gathering lifestyle that is still common in anthropological and popular scientific opinion today. Sahlins' chapter is worth reading by anyone interested in foragers, in economics, and in the nature of anthropology in the late 1960s and 1970s. Sahlins' views are firmly situated within Marxian anthropology, an anti-capitalist attitude, and anti-progress ideology—which are all to the good! The capitalistic, pro-progress ideology of the previous 100 years held that farming was better than foraging, and that industrialization was superior to both. Sahlins' conclusions about the affluence of hunters and gathers was firmly documented and supported by ethnographic studies of foraging societies including the Arunta and other Arnham Land peoples of Australia, the Mbuti Pygmies of Central Africa, the Yahgan of Tierra del Fuego, the !Kung of Botswana and the Hadza of Tanzania (citations in Sahlins 1972). The !Kung play an especially important role in Sahlins' analysis due to the detailed quantitative and qualitative data collected by the Kalahari Research Project team. Sahlins' chapter "The original affluent society" helped to elevate the writings of Richard Lee to a central place in nutritional anthropology.

The !Kung diet of low, but adequate energy intake, a wide variety of foods, greater intake of fruits and vegetables than meat, little or no or dairy foods, coupled with moderate to vigorous physical activity is the basis of a health advice book written by some members of the Kalahari research project team (Eaton et al. 1989). Much current medical and academic health advice follows on from that book and others like it (for example, Willet 2005, Lindeberg 2005, Cordain 2010, but see Nestle 2000 for a critique). All sorts of diet and health pundits extol the benefits of the hunting and gathering lifestyle of peoples such as the !Kung—search the Web with terms such as "Stone-age diet," Paleolithic diet," "hunter-gather diet," and "evolution diet."

But, what if newer data from nutritional science and newer interpretations of human nutritional biology show that the !Kung forager diet was not adequate and that the !Kung hunter-gatherers of the 1960s were not healthy? If this is the case, then how might the anthropological and nutritional view of the !Kung's "affluence" be altered?

"You Can Never Be Too Rich or Too Thin" – Wallis Simpson, Duchess of Windsor

Is it possible for a group of people to be well-nourished and at the same time very thin? Is it possible for a group of people to be well-nourished and relatively short? The !Kung of the 1960s were one of the thinnest human groups ever measured. By the word "thin" I mean that the !Kung had one of the smallest reserves of body fat and arm muscle mass measured for any non-institutionalized human group (that is, excluding concentration camp victims and prisoners of any type, as well as hospitalized persons). The !Kung were also relatively short in stature.

Nancy Howell, who was part of the original Kalahari Research project team, writes that, "One of the most distinctive features of the !Kung people is their small body size. They are short and slender and fine-boned. Many people are so thin that bones and muscles are readily seen through the skin, even though most of them seem to be healthy and vigorous" (2010, p. 49).

Just how short and thin are the !Kung? Here I use the data for height, weight, skinfold, and arm circumference measurements of the Dobe area !Kung taken by Richard Lee, Nancy Howell, and other members of the Kalahari Research Project between August 1967 and May 1969. The data are publically available online at the University of Toronto Research Repository https://tspace.library.utoronto.ca/handle/1807/10395. Once at this site click on "view all…" located in the right side column. Another means of access is the site https://tspace.library.utoronto.ca/. I used the internal search engine to find "Nancy Howell," which provided a list of data files. Searching for "Richard Lee" will produce lists including many photographs of the !Kung and many articles.

Analysis of the data finds that, on average, !Kung children follow the 3rd percentile of stature and weight of the United States National Center for Health Statistics (NCHS 2000) references. This means that the average !Kung child is shorter and lighter than 97% of all children in the United States. !Kung adult height and weight median values are 160.7 cm and 48.6 kg for men and 149.9 cm and 42.1 kg for women (ages 20–84 years old). From a statistical perspective, median values are better than mean values to represent the average, or central tendency, of growth measurements used to assess nutritional status (Bates et al. 2011). In terms of median percentiles of height, !Kung men fall at 3.4 and !Kung women at 3.8 of the NCHS references. In terms of median weight percentiles !Kung men fall at 1.4 and !Kung women at 3.5 of the NCHS references.

If we consider the entire distribution of measurements, then these median values indicate that nearly 50% of all children and adults have heights and weights that lie below the 3rd percentile value. Public health professionals, including medical doctors, epidemiologists, and human growth specialists, consider that any individual with such small height or weight warrants investigation for a disease, a growth disorder (such as a genetic or hormonal problem), or severe undernutrition. When an entire population is found to have 50% of all heights and weight below the 3rd percentile it is a strong indication of severe disease, undernutrition, or both (World Health Organization 1995, Bogin et al. 2007). There is no evidence that the !Kung have a genetic or hormonal disorder that might explain their small body size. This means that disease and/or undernutrition are the likely cause.

To help understand the small body size of the !Kung I compared the weight-for-age of !Kung with that for Maya refugee infants and children. The Maya data were collected by Dr. Faith Warner in 1995. These Maya families were originally from the Ixcán region of western highlands in Guatemala. They fled Guatemala in the 1970s and early 1980s due to the violence of the Civil War and were settled in a refugee camp in Campeche, Mexico, in 1984 (Warner et al. 2005, Warner 2007). The name of this camp is Maya Tecún. The anthropometric data for these refugee children have not been published previously and the data were kindly provided by Dr. Warner.

The measured weights of both !Kung and Maya were transformed to z-scores (standardized values). Z-score transformation allows comparison of boys and girls, different ages, and different ethnic groups all to the same standard, or a reference, for growth. The z-scores presented here were calculated using the comprehensive references for growth developed by Frisancho (2008). These growth references are based on the National Health and Nutrition Survey (NHANES III) of the United States, conducted from 1988–1994. This was a national sampling of all non-institutionalized persons in the United States, based on a random, stratified sampling protocol. A total of 31,311 persons were measured, including the ethnic groups "white," "black," "Mexican-American," and "other Hispanic." The Frisancho comprehensive growth references were produced by statistically smoothing the original NHANES III data to remove skewness and construct normally distributed percentiles for each growth variable. The Frisancho comprehensive growth references provide percentiles for many anthropometric measurements used in nutritional analysis for males and females from 2 months to 90 years of age. Because these comprehensive "…references were developed using a large sample size and statistical methods applicable to all populations they provide a uniform baseline useful for evaluating growth and nutritional status of individuals and populations, irrespective of ethnicity" (Frisancho 2008, p. 115).

The weight z-scores for individuals are plotted in Figure 1, which also includes a "best-fitting average line" of the weight-for-age z-scores as estimated by least squares regression. A z-score of "0" corresponds to the 50th percentile of the reference, in this case meaning the median, or average, weight of healthy, well-nourished infants and children at any given age. A z-score of "+2" or greater corresponds to the 97th percentile and above (the heaviest for their age) and a z-score of "-2" or smaller corresponds to the 3rd percentile (the lightest for their age).

Between birth and 4 months of age, the distribution of !Kung weights is "normal" in relation to the median of the comprehensive references. Eight of the !Kung infants have weights at or above +2 z-scores, which is quite heavy. I asked Dr. Nancy Howell about the methods for weighing infants and she explained that some infants were measured in clothing or bundled in a blanket. The extra weight of these items is the likely reason for measurements above +2 z-scores. It seems that the Kalahari Research Project team members were not carefully trained in the methods of anthropometry. Standard methods of weighing newborns is to measure them nude or in minimal clothing, such as a diaper. If it is necessary to measure infants with clothing, then examples of the clothing or blanket must be weighed separately and that weight must be subtracted from the gross weight of the clothed infant to more accurately estimate the true weight of the newborn. In contrast to the !Kung measurements, the Maya infants and children, at all ages, were weighed in the nude or with only a diaper (Warner et al 2005). The Maya infants begin life at the '0' line, meaning their birth weights are at about the median weight of the reference. Immediately after birth the Maya infants' weight declines relative to the reference and continues to decline until about age 42 months.

After one month or so, the !Kung infants were weighed with less clothing and their weights relative to the reference seem to drop very fast. The removal of blankets and clothing explains part of this decline, but a real slowing of growth relative to the references also occurred. This is evident by the fact that by age 6 months, when infants were likely to be measured in minimal or no clothing, the !Kung z-scores are about equal to those of the Maya. The !Kung weights stabilize at about 24 months and then drop again after 30 months. !Kung infants are weaned, meaning that the mother stops all lactation between 24–48 months of age (Konner 1978), with an average weaning age of 42 months (Sellen 2001). Complimentary foods (non-breast milk foods) are introduced as early as 3 months of age. Complementary feeding is not a problem, so long as the foods are safe and nutritionally adequate. Indeed, after the age of 6 months breast-milk alone cannot meet the energy and nutrient requirements of human infants for healthy growth. The complementary foods provided to !Kung infants are not sufficient in quality, in quantity, or both to meet growth needs, as the z-scores decline throughout the first 24 months. An increased rate of weaning of !Kung infants after age 30 months may explain the decline in z-scores from that age onward. Once weaned, the infants and children must eat foods prepared for them by older people. Those foods are clearly not meeting growth requirements. Please notice in Figure 1 that the !Kung children's z-scores continue to decline up to age 60 months, and probably continue to decline for several more years. Note also that the !Kung fall farther below the references than do the Maya, who seem to stabilize by 54 months.

The growth in weight of the Maya refugee infants and children living in a Mexican camp is similar to the growth

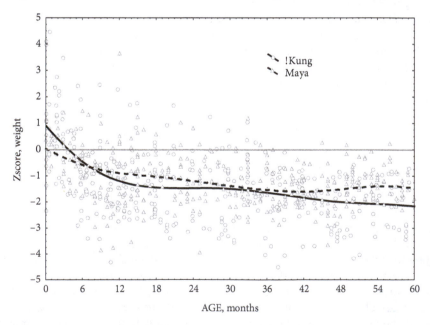

Figure 1 *Comparison of z scores for weight of !Kung (open circles) and Maya refugee (open triangles) infants and children aged 0–60 months. The solid horizontal line lies at the "0" z-score, that is, the median value of weight-for-age of the Comprehensive References for growth (Frisancho 2008). The curved solid line is the average weight-for-age z-score of the !Kung sample as estimated by least squares regression. The broken curved line is the average weight-for-age z-score of the Maya sample as estimated by least squares regression.*

of rural Guatemala Maya discussed in my chapter "Maya in Disneyland" in this book. Those rural Guatemalan Maya are unquestionably suffering from undernutrition, infectious disease, and for children and juveniles over age 6 years the demands from physical labor, such as carrying firewood, tending to animals, and care for younger siblings. These conditions also existed in the refugee camp: "Life was seen as extremely difficult in Maya Tecún, with men and women identifying a lack of water, poor land, extreme heat, illness, and insufficient food, household goods, and clothing as major problems that they faced on a daily basis" (Warner 2007, p.197). In addition the Maya refugees suffered from "…war-induced trauma, isolation, lack of social support, and the restrictions of encampment…" (Warner 2007, p.195). An unpublished report by Faith Warner and Jennifer Soika ("Child Anthropometry and Cultural Variation in Four Mayan Refugee Communities," Bloomsburg University) finds that between 60–70% of the Maya refugee infants and children are undernourished based on weight-for-age. Warner and Soika used Mexican growth references as the basis of comparison to assess the data (Ramos Galvan 1975). If the Frisancho comprehensive references were utilized the rates of undernutrition would be greater, because the Mexican references are based on a sample that is, overall, smaller in height and weight than the NHANES III sample.

Given the adverse conditions of life in the Mexican refugee camp, and the similar pattern of growth of the Maya and !Kung, the most reasonable interpretation of the growth of the !Kung infants and children is that it is due to inadequate food intake, disease, or a combination of both. Small size of !Kung infants and children sets the pattern of growth for older ages, as !Kung adults remain relatively short and light throughout their lives.

Another method of nutritional assessment is the body mass index, or BMI, which is a ratio of weight-for-height. BMI is calculated as [(weight in kilograms) / (height in meters)^2 x 100]. BMI is often used to estimate fatness, as greater amounts of body fat for a given height will increase the BMI value. Indeed, BMI works well as an estimate of fatness for adults of the industrialized nations, which are characterized by high levels of food intake and low levels of physical activity. There are problems in the interpretation of BMI when it is applied to human groups practicing more traditional lifestyles, such

as foraging, farming and animal husbandry. People engaged in physical labor may have greater amounts of muscle for a given height, and this will also increase BMI.

Even so, a comparison of adult BMI values for 21 societies practicing traditional methods of subsistence, including foraging, pastoralism, and non-mechanized farming finds that !Kung BMI is the 4th lowest for both men and women (Walker et al. 2006; data kindly provided by Dr. Robert Walker). !Kung men have an average BMI of 19.5 and !Kung women average 18.8. Ranking below the !Kung are the Aeta of the Philippine Islands who practice a mixed economy of foraging, farming and animal husbandry, several peoples of Arnham Land, Australia, who are foragers and farmers (these are the same Arnham Land people of Sahlins' "original affluent society"), the Turkana of Kenya who are pastoralists, and the Walbiri who are Australian foragers. These groups have average BMI values from 17–19.4. International references for BMI (World Health Organization 1995) specify that a BMI value less than 18.5 indicates "thinness" and is a risk for health. BMI values between 18.5 and 24.9 are considered "normal" and the least risk for adverse health. BMI above 25 indicates "overweight." In the Kalahari Research Project database there are 194 men and 202 women with BMI values. They range from 18–84 years old with a mean age = 41.3 years and 87% are less than 60 years old. In total, 44% of these !Kung have BMI values less than 18.5. Only one man, age 39 years, has a BMI above 25 and his value is 25.8.

A more direct estimate of fatness is the measurement of skinfolds and arm circumference (Bates et al. 2011). Skinfolds estimate the amount of fat stored between the skin and the underlying muscle. Arm circumference, in conjunction with the triceps skinfold, provides an estimate of muscle tissue on the arm. Body fat accumulates when energy intake exceeds the body's energy requirements for basal metabolism, physical activity, combating disease, reproduction, and other needs. Body fat is lost when these needs exceed energy intake.

The Kalahari Research Project team measured triceps and subscapular skinfolds and mid-upper arm circumference on !Kung children and adults. Here I report the findings for adults between the ages of 18–84 years old. Individual !Kung men and women were measured on more than one occasion during the period August 1967 to May 1969. This was done to

Table 1 Descriptive Statistics for Triceps and Subscapular (SSCAP) Skinfolds and Mid-Upper Arm Circumference of !Kung Men and Women 18-84 Years Old*

	Men					Women				
	N	Median	Z-score	Range	Comp Ref M	N	Median	Z-score	Range	Comp Ref M
Triceps, mm	286	5.1	-1.6	3.0-12.0	10.7	312	9.5	-2.5	3.6-24.9	21.7
SSCAP, mm	282	6.2	-2.9	3.7-12.6	17.6	301	7.2	-2.6	3.8-19.5	20.2
ARM CIRC, cm	100	23.3	-3.1	16.2-29.5	31.3	94	20.6	-2.2	16.8-27.4	29.3

*The !Kung data are compared with the median values from the comprehensive reference (Comp Ref M) of Frisancho (2008).

assess body fatness in the rainy vs. dry seasons. At each occasion, three skinfold measurements were usually taken on each person. Here I present all of the data collected, as the average of the measurements taken on each occasion for each person. This means that some individual !Kung contribute multiple measurements, but it also ignores seasonal variation for these same people and, therefore, the results provide an overall assessment of !Kung fatness and nutritional status.

A summary of the findings is given in Table 1, along with comparisons to the comprehensive references of Frisancho (2008). Men and women are shown separately because women usually have greater body fat and larger skinfolds than men. !Kung women do have larger skinfolds than !Kung men, and the sex differences are of about the same relative magnitude as the sex difference between reference men and women. However, compared with the reference data the !Kung are very thin, meaning low fat reserves on their bodies. The references are based on the United States population of 1988–1994, admittedly a population with high levels of overweight and obesity. Even so, there is no way to interpret the !Kung values as "healthy." The median z-score values for the two skinfolds are between -2.9 and -1.6 of the reference. In terms of only the triceps skinfold, 36% of adults have a z-score less than -2.0 and 64% less than -1.5. These values are considered as below average to very low by Frisancho (2008) and the World Health Organization (1995).

The !Kung arm circumference z-score values average -3.1 for men and -2.2 for women, both very small values. As described in Lee's 1968 essay (see chapter 7), the !Kung do a good deal of physically demanding labor, which places a premium on muscle health. Small arm circumference means the !Kung are laboring with less muscle than may be needed for optimal work outputs, which for the !Kung means insufficient production of food. Taken together, the low fat reserves of the !Kung, their small arm muscle mass, and the demands of their physical labor mean that they are living very close to the limits of survival and that they are highly susceptible to starvation during times of food shortage.

!KUNG NUTRITIONAL BALANCE: ANOTHER INPUT-OUPUT ANALYSIS

The "affluence" of the hunter-gatherer lifestyle, as described by Sahlins (1972), is in large part based on a very careful input-output analysis of !Kung work carried out by Richard Lee and other members of the Kalahari Research Project team. The essay by Lee (1968; chapter 7 in this book) summarizes the meticulous collection of hours of work per person, as well as the total amount of food collected (see Lee 1969 for the detailed analysis). Based on methods of analysis available in the late 1960s, Lee writes (1968, p. 39), "One can tentatively conclude that even a modest subsistence effort of two or three days work per week is enough to provide an adequate diet for the !Kung Bushmen." Compared to the five to six day work week of many people involved in industry, business, intensive agriculture, and even academia, the !Kung do seem to enjoy an affluence of leisure time.

A decade later, Lee (1979b) revised his input-output analysis, recalculating and increasing in the contribution of "Other vegetable" foods in the diet. The numbers of both the 1969 and 1979 energy input-output analyses are given here in Table 2. In addition, I provide a "new analysis" of the data based on estimates of the energy value of foods in the !Kung diet that were published after 1979.

My new analysis helps to explain the poor nutritional status of the !Kung, as estimated from the anthropometric data. Using the best methods and data available at the time, Lee (1969) reported that the !Kung produce an average of

Table 2 Input-Output Analyses of the Dobearea !Kung Diet*

Class of food	Per capita consumption					New analysis	Lee 1969	Lee 1979
	Percent contribution by weight	Weight in grams	Protein grams	Fat	Carbs	Kcals per day[2]	Kcals per day[3]	Kcals per day[3]
Meat	37/**31**	230	48.3[1]	7.8	0	264	690	690
Mongongo nut	33/**28**	210	60.5	120.3	5.0	1345	1260	1365
Other vegetable	30/**41**	190/**300**[5]	1.9			133[4]/**210**	190	300
Total	100	630/**740**				1742/**1819**	2140	2355

* Numbers in bold typeface indicate the revisions made by Lee (1979b).

[1] Based on 21 g/100g carcass (Ntiamoa-Baidu 1997/ FAO), Lee 1979b gives 15g/100g carcass and only 10% shrinkage due to water content, but Ntiamoa-Baidu 1997/FAO gives 70% moisture in raw meat. Lee estimates 300kcal/100g raw meat. Ntiamoa-Baidu (1997/FAO) wild game average is 114.6kcal/100g).

[2] Based on 4kcal/g for protein and carbohydrate, 9kcal/g for fat;

[3] Based on 3.4kcal/g for protein, 8.37kcal/g for fat

[4] Nutrient content of these "other vegetable" foods is not given by Lee (1969) and is not known. Lee estimates 1kcal/gram of collected vegetable. I compiled a list of 19 fruits and vegetables, including corn, white potatoes, avocado, peas, beans, apples and oranges, totaling 3,185 grams and providing 2,230 kcal, or 0.7 kcal/gram.

[5] Lee 1979b increased vegetable to 300g/day, which includes mongongo fruit and some other vegetables.

2140 kcals per person per day. In 1979b that value increased to 2355 kcals per person per day. Lee estimated that the average per capita energy expenditure of the !Kung is 1975 kcals/day, based on the Dobe area population of 336 people, with 30% men, 35% women, and 35% people under 15 years old. The difference between energy input and output is a profit of 165 kcals for the 1969 estimate and 380 kcals for the 1979b revision.

For my new analysis I use the same contribution by weight of the collected and hunted food that Lee carefully measured. The energy value of that food is re-estimated using data for the nutritional value of meat from wild animals published in a report from the Food and Agricultural Organization (FAO) of the United Nations (Ntiamoa-Baidu 1997). The FAO report lists the nutritional value of 19 species of African mammals, many of which are part of the !Kung diet, such as porcupine, duiker, wild pig, and bushbuck. The seed and fruit of the mongongo tree (*Ricinodendron rautaneii*) are mainstays of the !Kung diet, comprising about 30% of all energy intake. I use the mongongo nutritional analysis by Graz (2007) to estimate the kcal value of the mongongo fruit and nut. The energy value of vegetable foods eaten by the !Kung, other than the mongongo, is difficult to estimate because most of those plants have not been analyzed in the laboratory. Lee (1969) provided an estimate of 1.0 kcal per gram from these "Other vegetables." I compiled a list of 19 vegetable foods for which energy values per gram are known (see Table 2, footnote 4). These are all domesticated plants and as such are likely to provide more edible material and more energy than wild plants as they are bred for human food use. The average energy value of these 19 domesticated plant foods is 0.7 kcal/gram.

Based on these more recent data for the energy value of the !Kung diet I find that the average intake is 1742 kcals per person per day using Lee's 1969 values for the weight of the food and 1819 kcals per person per day using Lee's 1979 revision. The energy value from mondongo nuts and fruits increases a bit from Lee's 1969 analysis and is very close to his 1979 estimate. The energy value of other vegetables falls by a small amount. It is the energy value of meat that falls the most, to less than half that estimated by Lee. The major reason for this is that Lee suggested a 10% 'shrinkage' in the weight of meat when cooked. The reason for 'shrinkage' is not specified by Lee in any of his publications that I have read.

The weight of a portion of meat can shrink when cooked due to loss of fat or water. Wild game meat is generally of low fat. The FAO reports that wild game has a median weight of 3.4 grams of fat per 100 grams of meat. More important is the amount of water and other fluids, as the median moisture by weight of wild game is 70 grams per 100 grams of meat (Ntiamoa-Baidu 1997). The value is 73g/100g for meats from domesticated ox, sheep, and pig (Ntiamoa-Baidu 1997).

Due to the low fat and high moisture content of wild animals the energy value of cooked game meat is considerably lower than the 300 kcal per 100 grams that Lee estimated. Indeed, the FAO analysis of African wild mammals reports a median value of 114.6 kcal/100grams of cooked meat. The two African mammal species on the FAO list with highest energy content are the South African porcupine (*Hystrix africae-australis*),which is 46 grams of fat and provides 549 kcal per 100 grams, and the Greater Cane rat (*Thryonomys swinderianus*), which is 16.8 grams of fat and provides 263 kcal per 100 grams. No species of rat is listed as consumed by the !Kung and the amount of porcupine consumed amounts to only 4% of the total weight of meat brought to the camp (Lee 1979b, p. 206). Warthogs contribute 65% of the total weight of meat consumed, and warthogs average 1.6 grams of fat and provide 110 kcal per 100 grams. Even the energy value of domesticated animals, such as chicken, beef and pork, averages 194 kcals/100 grams, and these animals have a median fat content of 13% (Ntiamoa-Baidu 1997, http://www.ars.usda.gov/Services/docs.htm?docid=18877).

Lee (1968, 1969, 1979b) does not appear to mention the consumption of offal, but it is likely that the !Kung consume the internal organs, bone marrow, and other parts of the animals they hunt in addition to skeletal muscle meat. The FAO report on the nutritional value of wild African animals does not mention offal. I was able to find nutritional analysis of domestic beef and lamb offal from The English Beef & Lamb Executive website (http://www.simplybeefandlamb.co.uk/download-booklet). Liver, kidney, tongue, and oxtail are listed, with a range of energy values from 88–171 kcals per 100 grams. Domestic animals have more fat and therefore more kcals/100grams than most wild animals. So, even with the consumption of all edible parts of their animal prey the !Kung could not ingest 300 kcal/100 grams.

The new values for energy input fall short of Lee's estimate of !Kung energy expenditure, by either -233 kcal or -156 kcal per person per day. Moreover, the energy imbalance becomes even worse if newer formulae for estimating energy expenditure are used. These newer formulae are published by the FAO (Food and Agriculture Organization et al. 1985; 2004). Using the FAO methods, Nancy Howell (2010) estimates that the Dobe area !Kung population requires 2069.4 kcal/day/person. This makes the energy deficit grow to between -250.4 and -327.4 kcal/person/day.

If the !Kung were in true energy deficit, then they would have all been dead. A deficit of 3500 kcal results in the loss, on average, of one pound (0.454 kg) of body weight. At a daily deficit of -250 kcals/day a !Kung adult would lose 2.1 pounds every 30 days, or 26 pounds (11.8 kg) in a year. Clearly this is impossible to sustain and survive. It is likely that some errors in the observation or estimation of the food consumed occurred. All anthropological fieldwork is susceptible to these types of errors, even a project as careful and well controlled as the Kalahari Research Project. It is also likely that !Kung people "snack" by eating food items found while foraging for the larger types of food that are carried back to camp. Such snacking may add enough kcals to bring the !Kung just into positive energy balance. It is very clear, however, that by any input-output analysis !Kung energy intake is maintained at a level close to the minimum required for life and that their energy balance is precarious. The small, stature, low body weight, "thin" BMIs, and very small skinfolds and arm circumferences of the !Kung of all ages make sense in light of their minimally positive energy intake, coupled with periods of moderate to vigorous energy expenditures in food production.

Affluence or Economy of Effort?

The "affluence" of !Kung lifestyle is tied to their leisure time. Lee (1968, 1969, 1979b) points out the work required by the !Kung for food production amounts to 2.4 days per week. Sahlins (1972) used this number to describe the !Kung, and other living foragers as having abundant leisure time with more daytime sleep than in agricultural and industrial societies. Given the new energy input-output analysis provided here, there is another interpretation of the leisure and daytime sleep of foragers such as the !Kung. They may be conserving the limited energy available to them for survival.

The !Kung may be practicing a strategy for success made famous by Winston Churchill. In 1946, at the age of 18 years old, the historian Paul Johnson met Churchill and he writes of the encounter that Churchill, "…gave me one of his giant matches he used for lighting cigars. I was emboldened by that into saying, 'Mr. Winston Churchill, sir, to what do you attribute your success in life?' and he said without hesitating: 'Economy of effort. Never stand up when you can sit down, and never sit down when you can lie down.' And he then got into his limo" (Johnson 2009).

People with energy deficiency, or living at a delicate energy balance, do practice an economy of effort. One example are studies by Gerald B. Spurr and colleagues of marginally undernourished boys and girls, ages 6–16 years old, in the city of Cali, Colombia. These boys and girls adjust their energy expenditure according to energy intake. In one quasi-experiment (Spurr and Reina 1988), normal and undernourished boys were observed at a summer day camp. They were encouraged to increase their physical activity by playing sports and other games. The undernourished boys were not able to keep up with the normally nourished boys during the morning session. At mid-day both groups received a meal and the undernourished boys received an extra 760 Kcals of food, all of which was consumed. During the afternoon play session the undernourished boys were able to keep up with the normal group for about 2 hours, which is about the time they expended the extra 760 kcals eaten at lunch.

The Zapotec people live in the region of Oaxaca, Mexico. Like the Maya, the Zapotecs are the descendants of native peoples who occupied the Americas before the year 1492. Also like the Maya, the Zapotecs have lived under social, economic, and nutritional adversity for the past 500+ years. Biocultural research with the Zapotecs has been carried out by Robert M. Malina and colleagues for several decades. In one study (Malina and Buschang 1985), height, weight, hand

grip strength, running speed, standing long jump, and ball throw for distance were measured in a sample of Zapotec boys and girls aged 6 to 15 years old. Compared to a sample of healthy, well-nourished boys and girls from schools in Philadelphia, the Zapotecs are significantly shorter and lighter—about the same body size as Maya of the same ages. Malina and Buschang adjusted the data statistically for the differences in body size—smaller people are less strong and run, jump, and throw less than taller people—and found that the Zapotec grip strength was still less than expected. The same was true for running speed and the long jump. In contrast, Zapotec throwing distance was greater than that of the Philadelphia sample. Overall, Malina and Buschang report that the reduced stature of the Zapotecs negatively affects their running and jumping, and their reduced weight results in less muscle strength – meaning, less muscle mass on the body. Zapotec children and adolescents are clearly less healthy and vigorous than better nourished people.

From his research with Colombian boys and girls, combined with research from Zapotecs of Mexico and other peoples with chronic energy deficiency (CED), Spurr concluded that, "In pre-school children, CED results in decreased activity as a first line of defense against decreased rate of growth" (1990, p. 139). If the CED continues, then growth is reduced and by the time these CED children are of school age they have reduced physical activity as a result of their small size (Spurr 1990). Two clear cases of the growth of infants and children suffering from CED, Maya and !Kung, are shown in Figure 1. The leisure of !Kung children, who tend to stay near camp and not expend energy in food production (Lee 1968, 1979), may be a result of their poor nutritional status. It may also be a social strategy by adults to protect the fragile health of the children.

Evidence of fragile health comes from Nancy Howell's path breaking books on !Kung demography (1979, revised edition 2000) and her more recent book on !Kung life history and health (2010). Howell (2010, p.15) writes that 20% of !Kung newborns died before age one year and "…about 45% died by age 15…." The !Kung have one of the highest pre-adult mortality rates of any human society. This seems prima facie evidence that infant and child health is quite fragile, most likely due to undernutrition. I know of a few Guatemala Maya villages, with gross undernutrition and high levels of infectious disease, that ever experienced a nearly 50% mortality for under 5 year olds, and that is only for pre-term or low birth weight infants (Mata et al. 1976).

The physical activity of !Kung adults is also dictated by nutritional status. In studies of malnourished Colombian adults engaged in physical labor, such as cutting sugar cane, Spurr found that taller men with greater muscle mass could do more work per day and earn more money (Spurr, 1983). Indeed, studies of human physical work capacity from around the world find that smaller bodied adults cannot maintain the higher work capacity levels, and work productivity, of larger bodied adults (Ulijaszek 2000). Spurr succinctly summarized this relationship by writing that, "…malnutrition is accompanied by a reduced PWC [physical work capacity] … and the degree of depression is related to the severity of the depressed nutritional status and to the loss of muscle mass" (Spurr, 1983, p. 21). !Kung adults have small body size and very small arm circumference, both indicating low amounts of muscle mass. It seems most parsimonious to explain the so-called "leisure time" of the !Kung—the many hours or days of rest between bouts of physical activity in food production, socializing, and trance dancing—as a physiological limitation of their marginal nutritional status. Trance dancing is an important part of !Kung ritual life, and men may expend considerable energy by dancing all night. The dancing comes with a productivity cost, because "…those who have entered trances the night before rarely go out hunting the following day" (Lee 1968, p. 37). Periods of daytime rest after hunting or trance dancing may be a biocultural strategy to maximize their "economy of effort." The !Kung are not lazy, but they do have to pace out their work episodes to stay within nutritional and physiological limitations.

THE PACE OF KNOWLEDGE

The Kalahari Research Project (KRP) was one of the first of a new type of anthropological fieldwork with a biocultural perspective. It was one of the first studies with a truly interdisciplinary team of social, medical, and biological scientists. Many members of the KRP team are currently eminent academics. Richard Lee is today one of the world leaders of hunter-gather studies and the rights of indigenous peoples. Lee started the Kalahari Peoples Fund, a non-profit source of support for educational, economic, and social development of the !Kung and related peoples. This was another "first" in applied anthropology. Given this distinguished history, the new analysis of !Kung nutrition presented here is in no way a criticism of the work of Lee or any member of the KRP team. Like any academic field, nutritional anthropology develops by building on existing research, refining its methods, and re-analyzing prior interpretations.

The question of forager nutritional status is important because for about 99% of human evolutionary history all people lived by hunting and gathering foods from their local environments. The domestication of plants and animals is a recent event. It is possible that dogs were domesticated, or semi-domesticated more than 100,000 years BP, but more likely less than 40,000 years BP (Verginelli et al. 2006). Dogs may have assisted people while hunting, eaten wastes around human camps, and been eaten (but a cuisine based on dogs is not likely). Rice may be the earliest of the major plant foods to be domesticated, at about 14,000 BP (Fuller 2007, Hirst, 2010). Mass production of domesticated foods is less than 10,000 years old and the human dependence on agriculture less than 6000 years old. In the broad timescales of human evolution and archaeology, domestication and agriculture occurred "just yesterday."

It is quite correct to state that the foraging, "…way of life has been the most successful and persistent adaptation [people] have ever achieved" (Lee and DeVore, 1968, p. 3). Writing in 1968, Lee and DeVore state that of the 150 billion people who have ever lived, more than 60% lived as foragers, about 35% lived since the advent of agriculture, and less than 5% lived within industrial societies. But, to place these statistics in context, it is vital to state that less than 1/1000th of the people alive today make any part of their living by hunting and gathering. People in these societies are mostly part-time foragers, as they acquire many foods and other items via trade or purchase. It is likely that in this year of 2012, there is no human society that lives by full-time foraging.

Even so, in some ways all people alive today retain some of the biological, sociological, economic, and psychological constitution of our foraging ancestors. This makes the biocultural study of the forager way of life important as possible window on "human nature" (Lee and Devore, 1968; Lee and Daly 1999; Panter-Brick et al. 2001). Viewed another way, ancient foragers possessed genomic, behavioral, and emotional elements that are common to living people. In this perspective our biological and cultural "line of sight" on foragers works in both directions—foragers are as much like us, the agro-industrialists, as we are like them. Deprive us of our nutritional, social, and emotional needs and we suffer from poor physical growth and adverse health. Hunter-gatherers, such as the !Kung, are no different.

Sahlins (1972, p.40) clearly understood the facts of forager nutritional anthropology when he wrote, "Hunter-gatherers consume less energy per capita per year than any other group of human beings." Despite this paucity of energy intake, Sahlins continues by adding, "Yet when you come to examine it the original affluent society was none other than the hunter's—in which all the people's material wants were easily satisfied." Were the !Kung ever an "affluent society"? Possibly, but they were not affluent in the 1960s. In fact they were suffering from high rates of infant and child mortality, poor physical growth, and limitations on work capacity.

References

Bates CJ et al. 2011. Nutritional assessment methods. In: Geissler C and Powers H, editors. Human Nutrition with CD-ROM, 2nd edition. Burlington, MA: Elsevier.

Bodley JH. 1999. Hunter-gatherers and the colonial encounter. In: Lee RB and Daly R, editors. The Cambridge encyclopedia of hunters and gatherers. Cambridge: Cambridge University Press. p 465–472.

Bogin B. 1999. Patterns of human growth, 2nd edition. Cambridge University Press: Cambridge.

Bogin B et al. 2007. Life history trade-offs in human growth: adaptation or pathology? Am J Hum Biol 19:631–42.

Bogin B. 2009. Childhood, adolescence, and longevity: A multilevel model of the evolution of reserve capacity in human life history. Am J Hum Biol 21:567–77.

Caspari R and Lee SH. 2006. Is human longevity a consequence of cultural change or modern biology? Am J Phys Anthropol 129:512–517.

Cohen MN and Armelagos GJ, editors. 1984. Paleopathology at the origins of agriculture. Orlando, FL: Academic Press.

Fuller DQ. 2007. Contrasting patterns in crop domestication and domestication rates: recent archaeobotanical insights from the Old World. Ann Bot 100:903–24.

Cordain L. 2010. The Paleo Diet: Lose Weight and Get Healthy by Eating the Foods You Were Designed to Eat. Wiley: New York.

De Souza RG. 2006. Body size and growth: the significance of chronic malnutrition among the Casiguran Agta. Ann Hum Biol 33:604–619.

Eaton SB et al. 1988. The Paleolithic prescription: a program of diet & exercise and a design for living. New York: Harper & Row.

Food and Agriculture Organization, World Health Organization, and United Nations University (FAO/WHO/UNU). 1985. Energy and Protein Requirements (Report of joint FAO/WHO/UNU expert consultation; WHO technical report series no. 724). Geneva: World Health Organization.

Food and Agriculture Organization, World Health Organization, and United Nations University (FAO/WHO/UNU). 2004. Human Energy Requirements. Report of a Joint FAO/WHO/UNU Expert Consultation. Geneva, World Health Organization.

Formicola V and Giannecchini M. 1999. Evolutionary trends of stature in upper Paleolithic and Mesolithic Europe. J Hum Evol 36:319–333.

Frisancho A. 2008. Anthropometric standards. an interactive nutritional reference of body size and body composition for children and adults. Ann Arbor, MI: The University of Michigan Press.

Froment A. 2001. Evolutionary biology and the health of hunter-gather populations. In: Panter-Brick C et al. editors. Hunter-gatherers: an interdisciplinary perspective. Cambridge: Cambridge University Press. p 239–266.

Gage TB. 1998. The comparative demography of primates: with some comments on the evolution of life histories. Ann Rev Anthropol 27:197–221.

Graz FP. 2007. *Schinziophyton rautanenii* (Schinz) Radcl.-Sm. In: van der Vossen HAM and Mkamilo GS, editors. PROTA 14: Vegetable oils/Oléagineux [CD-Rom]. Wageningen, Netherlands: PROTA.

Gray S et al. 2009. Mixed-longitudinal growth of Karimojong girls and boys in Moroto District, Uganda. Am J Hum Biol 21:65–76.

Gurven M et al. 2008. Aging and inflammation in two epidemiological worlds. J Gerontol 63A:196–199.

Habicht J-P et al. 1974. Height and weight standards for preschool children. How relevant are ethnic differences in growth potential? The Lancet 1:611–15.

Hirst KK. 2010. History of rice: archaeological evidence for the history of rice. http://archaeology.about.com/od/domestications/a/rice.htm (accessed 27 Novemeber 2010).

Howell N. 1979, 2nd edition 2000. Demography of the Dobe !Kung. New York: Aldine de Gruyter.

Howell N. 2010. Life Histories of the Dobe !Kung: Food, Fatness, and Well-Being Over the Lifespan. Berkeley, CA: University of California Press.

Jenike M. 2001. Nutritional ecology: diet, physical activity and body size. In: Panter-Brick C, Layton RH and Rowley-Conwy P, editors. Hunter-gatherers: an interdisciplinary perspective. Cambridge: Cambridge University Press. p 205–238.

Johnson P. 2009. Churchill. New York: Viking.

Koningsberg LW and Herrmann NP. 2006. The osteological evidence for human longevity in the recent past. In: Hawkes K and Paine RR, editors. The evolution of Human life history. Santa Fe, NM: School of American Research. p 267–306.

Konner M. 1978. Nursing frequency and birth spacing in !Kung hunter-gatherers. IPPF Med Bull 15:1–3.

Lee RB. 1968. What hunters do for a living, or how to make out on scarce resources. In: Lee RB and DeVore I, editors. Man the hunter. New York: Aldine. p 30–48.

Lee RB. 1969. !Kung bushman subsistence: an input-output analysis. In: Vayda AP. (ed): Environment and cultural behavior. University of Texas Press, Austin. p 47–79.

Lee RB. 1979a. Hunter-gatherers in process: the Kalahari Research Project, 1963–1976. In: Foster GM et al., editors. Long-term field research in social anthropology. New York: Academic Press. p 303–21.

Lee RB. 1979b. Men, women, and work. In: The !Kung San: Men, women, and work in a foraging society. Cambridge University Press, p 250–80.

Lee RB and Daly R. 1999. The Cambridge Encyclopedia of Hunters and Gatherers. Cambridge University Press.

Lee RB and DeVore I, editors. 1968. Man the hunter. New York: Aldine.

Lindeberg S. 2005. "Palaeolithic diet ("stone age" diet)". Scandinavian Journal of Food & Nutrition 49:75–7.

Malina RM and Buschang PH. 1985. Growth, strength, and motor performance of Zapotec children, Oaxaca, Mexico. Human Biology 57:163–181.

Mata LJ et al. 1976. Antenatal events and postnatal growth and survival of children in a rural Guatemalan village. Ann Hum Biol 3:303–15.

Mathers K and Henneberg M. 1995. Were we ever that big? Gradual increase in hominid body size over time. Homo 46:141–173.

McDade TW. 2008. Maintenance versus growth: investigating the costs of immune activation among children in lowland Bolivia. Am J Phys Anthropol 136:478–84.

Nestle M. 2000. Paleolithic diets: a skeptical view. Nutrition Bulletin 25:43–47.

Ntiamoa-Baidu Y. 1997. Wildlife and food security in Africa. FAO Conservation Guide 33. Food and Agriculture Organization of the United Nations. FAO, Rome (Italy). Forest Resources Division. http://www.fao.org/docrep/w7540e/w7540e00.htm

Paine R and Boldsen J. 2006. Paleodemographic data and why understanding Holocene demography is essential to understanding human life history evolution in the Pleistocene. In: Hawkes K and Paine R, editors. The evolution of Human life history. Santa Fe, NM: School of American Research. p 307–330.

Panter-Brick C et al., editors. 2001. Hunter-gatherers: an interdisciplinary perspective. Cambridge: Cambridge University Press.

Pennington R. 2001. Hunter-gatherer demography. In: Panter-Brick C et al., editors. Hunter-gatherers: an interdisciplinary perspective. Cambridge: Cambridge University Press. p 170–204.

Ramos Galván R. 1975. Somatometría Pediátrica en Niños en la Ciudad de México. Archivos de Investigación Médica 6, Supp.1:83–396.

Rowley-Conwy P. 2001. Time, change and the archaeology of hunter-gatherers: how original is the 'Original Affluent Society'? In: Panter-Brick C et al., editors. Hunter-gatherers: an interdisciplinary perspective. Cambridge: Cambridge University Press. p 39–72.

Ruff CB et al. 1993. Postcranial robusticity in *Homo*. I: Temporal trends and mechanical interpretation. American Journal of Physical Anthropology 91:21–53.

Sahlins M. 1972. Stone-age economics. Aldine: Hawthorne, New York.

Sellen DW. 2001. Comparison of infant feeding patterns reported for nonindustrial populations with current recommendations. J. Nutr 131: 2707–15.

Spurr GB. 1983. Nutritional status and physical work capacity. Yearbook of Physical Anthropology 26:1–35.

Spurr GB. 1990. Physical activity and energy expenditure in undernutrition. Prog Food Nutr Sci. 14:139–92.

Spurr GB and Reina JC. 1988. Influence of dietary intervention on artificially increased activity in marginally undernourished Colombian boys. Eur J Clin Nutr 42:835–46.

Steckel RH and Rose JC, editors. 2002. The backbone of history. Cambridge: Cambridge University Press.

Stillitoe P. 2002. After the 'affluent society': cost of living in the Papua New Guinea highlands according to time and energy expenditure-income. J Biosoc Sci. 34:433–61.

Trigger DS. 1999. Hunter-gather peoples and nation-states. In: Lee RB and Daly R, editors. The Cambridge encyclopedia of hunters and gatherers. Cambridge: Cambridge University Press. p 473–479.

Ulijaszek SJ. 2000. Work and energetics. In: Stinson S et al., editors. Human Biology: An Evolutionary and Biocultural Perspective. New York: Wiley. p 345–376.

Verginelli F et al. 2006. The origins of dogs: archaeozoology, genetics, and ancient DNA [article in Italian]. Med Secoli 18:741–54.

Walker R et al. 2006. Growth rates and life histories in twenty-two small scale societies. Am J Hum Biol 18:295–311.

Warner F et al. 2005. Child anthropometry and cultural variation in four Mayan refugee communities. Paper presented at the American Association of Physical Anthropologists 74th Annual Meeting, Milwaukee, Wisconsin, April 2005.

Warner F. 2007. Social Support and Distress among Q'eqchi' Refugee Women in Maya Tecún, Mexico. Medical Anthropology Quarterly 21:193–217.

Willet W. 2005. Eat, drink and be healthy: the Harvard Medical School guide to healthy eating. New York: Simon and Schuster.

Wood JW. 1994. Dynamics of human reproduction: biology, biometry, demography. Hawthorne, NY: Aldine.

World Health Organization. 1995. Physical status: the use and interpretation of anthropometry. WHO technical report series: 854. Geneva, Switzerland: World Health Organization. http://helid.desastres.net/en/d/Jh0211e/

UNIT VII

Foods as Medicine

At first glance the distinction between food and medicine may seem clear enough when you inventory your medicine cabinet and your refrigerator. The items in your medicine cabinet are probably tablets of various shapes, colors, and sizes, and bottles of moderately foul-tasting liquids, all of which have specific instructions about how often and how much to consume them, as well as why you should consume them; that is, a description of the symptoms they promise to alleviate. In the refrigerator, on the other hand, there may be items like bottles of fruit juice, cartons of milk, eggs, carrots, jams, condiments, and other things you might eat straight away or prepare to eat later. The packaging of items in the refrigerator or cupboard may have a great deal of printing, but no specific directions as to how often or in what amounts the foods should be consumed, and usually no specific instructions as to why they should be consumed. Consume as desired!

The distinction between substances that are "food" and substances that are "medicine" is a very fine line and is culturally determined. Consider these two definitions from the New Oxford American Dictionary: medicine is "a compound or preparation used for the treatment or prevention of disease, esp. a drug or drugs taken by mouth" and food is "any nutritious substance that people or animals eat or drink, or that plants absorb, in order to maintain life and growth." So when is a substance a food and when is it a medicine? Moreover what is a medicine in one cultural context might be a food in another.

The distinction is even less clear when we look at the effect of specific foods in relation to prevention and curing of disease. A classic Western culture example is scurvy, a severe disease characterized by joint pain, muscle weakness, bleeding gums, and, ultimately, death. Today we know that scurvy is a result of an inadequate intake of vitamin C (ascorbic acid) and the symptoms can be rapidly reversed with vitamin C supplements. In the eighteenth century, when scurvy was devastating the crews of British sailing ships on their voyages of exploration around the globe, no one knew that ascorbic acid is an essential nutrient that cannot be synthesized by humans but must be obtained from external sources. However, the British knew that the symptoms could be cured by eating fresh vegetables. Captain James Cook, the famous explorer, reported that outbreaks of scurvy in his crew caused him to make a number of unscheduled stops to get the edible "green stuff" that would cure it (Watt 1981). The problem on these sailing ships was that the diet was limited to food that was easily preserved and transported, such as "biscuits," oatmeal, dried peas, butter, cheese, and beer. Eventually the British discovered that carrying lemons on board could eliminate the need to go ashore for edible green stuff. In essence, British sailors, soon called "limeys," first used particular foods to cure a disease and then learned to use another food to prevent that same disease.

A more current example is the use of diet to treat the problem of high serum (blood) cholesterol levels, not a disease per se, but a well-known risk factor for developing cardiovascular disease. In the case of high serum cholesterol, two types of diet therapy are recommended: (1) reduce the amount of animal foods in the diet, and hence the amount of cholesterol coming from dietary sources (the human body also produces cholesterol from other compounds); and (2) to increase high-fiber foods, such as oat bran, fruits, and legumes, that act to limit the amount of cholesterol absorbed in the small intestine.

This section explores relationships of food and medicine from biocultural and sociocultural perspectives. Two papers in this section, the contributions of Nina Etkin and Lauren Blum and colleagues, illustrate multiple features of nutritional anthropological approaches to the study of foods, including analyses that draw out the relationships between foods and medicine, and between cultural concepts of illness and curing. They both ground their research in a firm, elaborated scholarship of historical background in which they examine specific foods (chili in the case of Etkin and liver and greens in the Blum et al. study) in relation to their cross-cultural and historical uses. They both use ethnography in a specific culture (the Hausa) so that the reader understands the rich cultural elaborations and interpretations of the specific foods within their broader cultural context. It is chance that these two highly sophisticated and methodologically sound studies were conducted in the same cultural group, although in different specific geographic settings. For us, the readers of the papers, this happy coincidence helps to fill in the larger picture of the ways in which these foods function within the culture. In both of these studies we see the adaptive nature of cultural practices.

There are many books and articles about spices that people who are interested in this varied and endlessly fascinating topic can read. Nina Elkin's paper, and the book from which it was drawn (Elkin 2006), is an excellent way to begin your studies of spices. The first part of the paper presents the botanical classification of species and their chemical properties. She continues with a succinct, but thorough, review of the cultural history of spices, concluding with a short review of chili. The paper then shifts ground to examine the many dimensions of chili in Hausa culture, with an emphasis on its role in prevention and healing of disease. That description and interpretation reflects Elkin's in-depth ethnographic research of the type that characterizes anthropological approaches to food and nutrition studies.

The paper by Lauren Blum and colleagues begins with a nutritional issue—the problem of vitamin A deficiency. Vitamin A deficiency is one of the most serious and pervasive nutritional problems in poor countries around the world. It is responsible for untold life-long suffering from blindness, and is implicated in child mortality through its effects on immune system functioning. It has been, and continues to be, a primary focus for nutrition intervention programs. Like the study by Elkin, this paper sets the research squarely within an anthropological theoretical and methodological framework. You should note the use of an ethnographic technique that is often used by medical anthropologists: the presentation of scenarios that describe specific biomedical conditions and permit the investigator to ask a series of questions about how the respondent understands, interprets, and deals with the issue. By describing the symptoms of different levels of vitamin A deficiency, this technique permitted the investigators to obtain a nuanced and differentiated view of Hausa perceptions and practices. One of the most interesting findings from this study was the discovery that, apparently, the cultures in this part of the world, where vitamin A deficiency has been present for a long time, have independently discovered the role of vitamin A-rich foods as a treatment for this significant disease.

Chocolate! It's widely loved, sometimes addictive, fraught with symbolic value, subject of scholarship, art, commerce, and scientific research, a "drug" that we give to children without a second thought, and a food that plays a role in prevention and healing of disease in many cultures around the world. In his fascinating paper, "From Aphrodisiac to Health Food: A Cultural History of Chocolate," Louis Grivetti provides an overview of chocolate's history, from its roots in pre-Hispanic Mexico to the present day. In the Aztec (Mexican) medical system, the stimulant aspects of chocolate were recognized to such an extent that it was forbidden for women and children for fear their more sensitive bodies would be harmed by the strong drug. As a medicine it was used to treat a variety of ailments. This paper provides a small window, almost a peephole, into a very complex subject, one that has drawn scholars from a variety of fields, not to mention all the chefs and food writers who have described culinary aspects of chocolate. To expand your knowledge about the breadth and depth of the topic, readers should consult the massive and scholarly collection of papers that Grivetti and his colleagues have put together (see suggested readings below).

Jill Dubisch, in "You Are What You Eat: Religious Aspects of the Health Food Movement," steps us back in time to the emerging health food movement in the United States in the 1970s. She describes the structure of some of the health foods movement's core beliefs, and sets them in an historical context. Most importantly, she shows how characteristics of the movement conform to some aspects of theoretical models of religions and how they function. This paper, appropriately, does not attempt to assess the status of the beliefs in relation to scientifically derived knowledge. Analyses of contemporary biomedical systems from a sociocultural perspective would similarly reveal many features it shares with religious systems. It is very important that you, as a reader, do not fall into the trap of thinking that because the analysis examines the movement for its symbolic and religious aspects, the content of the beliefs is necessarily incompatible with scientific understanding. On the contrary, many of the beliefs that are central tenets of the health food movement have demonstrated scientific validity. In fact, rigorous, contemporary research on the preventive and curative properties of foods continues to reveal the capacity of many different foods to contribute to physical and mental health, as well as the importance of consuming healthful diets.

In summary, the chapters in this section invite us to take a closer look at two conceptual categories, food and medicine, that are so much a part of daily life that we don't usually spend time thinking about what they mean. These examples underscore the general observation that all human societies classify foods into a limited set of categories, use these categories to define their diet, and relate diet to health.

SUGGESTIONS FOR THINKING AND DOING NUTRITIONAL ANTHROPOLOGY

1. Go to a bookstore or browse the Internet for books on diet. How many of them are directly related to health (not just to weight loss)? What are the different kinds of health themes and diseases that books on diet cover? What areas of health are not represented in the publications on diet?
2. Explore the ways in which ideas about the healing role of foods enter into your own personal or family culture. What kinds of foods were you given as a child to help you when you were sick? Were there any foods that were used to prevent illness? Which of these foods are parts of your personal health management today? Then talk with family members of an older generation to find out if there are any foods

that they used as medicine that are no longer part of their current medical management. Compare the results of your informal self and family evaluation with friends and classmates, particularly those who belong to different ethnic groups.

References

Watt J. 1981. Some consequences of nutritional disorders in eighteenth century British circumnavigations. In Watt J, Freeman RJ, Bynum WF, eds. Starving Sailors: The Influence of Nutrition Upon Naval and Maritime history. Bristol, UK: National Maritime Museum, pp. 51–72.

Suggested Further Reading

Etkin NL. 2006. Edible Medicines: an Ethnopharmacology of Food. Tucson: University of Arizona Press.

Johns T. 1996. The Origins of Human Diet and Medicine: Chemical Ecology. Tucson: University of Arizona Press.

Grevetti L, Shapiro H-Y, eds. 2009. Chocolate: History, Culture and Heritage. New York: Wiley.

CHAPTER 29

Spices:
The Pharmacology of the Exotic

Nina Etkin
(2006)

In the dreams of all who pushed back the limits of the unknown world there is the same glitter of gold and precious stones, the same odor of far-fetched spices.

—Sir Walter Raleigh

For much of the history of biomedicine, the boundary between medicines and foods was blurred. Spices in particular moved fluidly from one category to the other, sold not only by grocers and spice merchants but also by apothecaries and physicians. Interchangeable use of the terms *spicer*, *pepperer*, and *apothecary* and their European-language counterparts reflected commercial and public, as well as medical professionals', perceptions of overlap.

Western science has paid more attention to the healthful potential of spices relative to other food categories. One reason is the assumption that, because spices played a prominent role in the early history of Western medicine, these items are more likely to have significant pharmacologic action. This rationale is faulty, in view of the fact that much of biomedical practice was based in a succession of iterations on the paradigm of humors and was ineffective well through the nineteenth century. As it turns out, the premise that spices are an especially pharmocodynamic group of plants does have an empirical foundation but one that has been only relatively recently substantiated according to bioscientific standards of evidence.

Spices differ from other domesticated and commercialized plant species in at least one pharmacologically significant way: the marked organoleptic qualities that signal the presence of allelochemicals, which have been bred out of many cultivated food plants, have been retained in the domesticated spices that are valued specifically for those flavors, scents, and other redolences. In recent decades this, as well as an expanded pharmacologic potential, has been corroborated for many spices through the characterization of specific functional compounds with discrete activities. Further, I suggest that bioscience finds spices compelling because, like pharmaceuticals, they are specific (have unique

and distinguishing tastes), small (in volume), and powerful (in the stimuli they emit and, in many cases, physiologic action). In this way, spices fit an allopathic model of healing: indeed, by virtue of these features, we might say that spices embody the quintessence of biomedicine.

This chapter treats spices generally, through definition and historical review, highlights chile pepper in a case study of a transglobal spice, and offers a novel approach that emphasizes evolution and context to explore the pharmacological potential of spices.

DEFINITIONS

If carbohydrate-rich superfoods anchor a cuisine (see chapter 1), spices are its sails. These botanically diverse items serve many functions. In all the world's cuisines they flavor, color, and preserve foods. Throughout history spices have served as gifts or obligations to the ruling class and as currency in commercial transactions; they are medicines (spice of life) and were included among grave goods and in embalming fluids (spice of death). As perfumes and cosmetics, spices disguise the taste and smell of unpalatable foods[1] and body odor. They mediate life-cycle ceremonies by marking individuals (e.g., monks, brides) through scent and color. Commonly they are the medium of transaction for witchcraft and sorcery and are burned as incense and fumigants for religious and funerary rites. Culturally, spices are signatures (flavor or signal prints) that distinguish the cuisines of ethnically diverse peoples and, within groups, mark social asymmetries through varied applications, combinations, and frequency and volume of consumption.

The food industry defines spices as "the dry parts of a plant, such as roots, leaves, and seeds, [that] impart to food a certain flavor and pungent stimuli" (Hirasa and Takemasa 1998: 1). Generally, the term *spice* has been used to refer to dry parts of plants of tropical or semitropical origin, whereas *culinary herb* has designated the aromatic leaves or seeds of nonwoody temperate plants. *Condiments*, which by some definitions are multicomponent and added to already-prepared foods, may be spices as well. These even semifixed definitions do not serve, however: the origin of some flavoring plants is not known (or of interest) outside of botany

Nina L. Etkin, "Spices: the pharmacology of the exotic." In *Edible Medicines: An Ethnopharmacology of Food*. N. Etkin. Tucson: University of Arizona Press, 2006, pp. 83–106. Figures have been omitted. Reprinted with permission.

or food-science circles; places of origin do not necessarily correspond to contemporary places of production and consumption; and more than one plant part of a spice or herb may be used to flavor foods. Substantively, then, these categories overlap; the distinctions are Eurocentric, based in how people who write about food flavors came to know and use these plants. Further, these are functional definitions, not botanical ones which might, for example, highlight the clustering of spice genera in certain families, such as Labiatae, Piperaceae, Umbelliferae, and Zingiberaceae (Table 1).

In this chapter I use the term *spice* inclusively, to designate all varieties of food flavorings, fragrances, flavor enhancers, colorings, appetite stimulants, and other stimuli from the tropics of Africa, Asia, and the Americas; the composite Mediterranean/Middle East/North Africa area; and the colder regions of northern Europe and Asia (Appendix).[2] Further, I entertain other definitions of spices that resonate simultaneously their phytochemistry, roles in traditional and transformed cuisines, and medicinal properties.

TASTE

The flavor of a spice is imparted by volatile essential oils, which are primarily constituted by terpenes (carbon-oxygen-hydrogen compounds; see Table 2). Monoterpenes (ten-carbon compounds) typically are strongly aromatic and very volatile. Essential oils are complex compounds that vary in the relative proportions of individual chemicals of which they are comprised. The flavor characteristics of individual plants of the same spice species can vary with growth conditions (soil, hydration, temperature), collection (time of harvest, duration of drying), and the circumstances of storage and transport. The pungency of a spice, like its taste, depends on the concentration and composition of essential oils. Pungent compounds are classified with reference to the structural characteristics summarized in Table 2, where, in descending order of presentation, they range along a continuum of perception from hot, which diffuses through the mouth, to sharp, which stimulates the oral and

Table 1 Botanical Classification of Spices[a]

Monocotyledonae

Liliiflorae	Liliaceae	chives, garlic, onion
	Iridaceae	saffron
Scitaminae	Zingiberaceae	cardamom, galangal, ginger, melegueta pepper, mioga, turmeric
Orchidales	Orchidaceae	vanilla

Dicotyledonae

Sympetale

Tubiflorae	Labiatae	basil, lavender, marjoram, mint, oregano, perilla, rosemary, sage, savory, thyme
	Solanaceae	chile, paprika
	Pedaliaceae	sesame
Campanulatae	Asteraceae	chicory, tarragon

Archichlamydeae

Piperales	Piperaceae	African cubebs, Benin pepper, black pepper, cubebs, long pepper
Ranales	Myristicaceae	mace, nutmeg
	Lauraceae	bay, cinnamon
	Illiciaceae	star anise
Rhoeadales	Brassicaceae	cress, horseradish, mustard
Rosales	Fabaceae	fenugreek, licorice, tamarind
Geraniales	Rutaceae	flower pepper, Japanese pepper
Myrtiflorae	Myrtaceae	allspice, clove
Umbelliflorae	Umbelliferae	ajwain, aniseed, caraway, celery, coriander, cumin, dill, fennel, parsley

[a] Angiospermae (flowering plants); Hirasa and Takemasa (1998).

Table 2 Pungent Compounds in Spices

Basic structure	Spice	Pungent constituents[a]	Sensation
Acid amide group R-CO-N-R-R	chile black pepper, white pepper	capsaicin piperine, chavicine	hot
Carbonyl group R-CO-R	ginger	zingerol*, shogaol*	
Thioether group R-S-R	onion	diallyl sulfide*	
Isothiocyanate group R-N-C-S	horseradish mustard	allyl-thiocyanate* allyl-thiocyanate* p-hydroxybenzyl isothiocyanate	sharp

Modified from Hirasa and Takemasa (1998).
[a]Volatile compounds are identified by an asterisk.

nasal mucous membranes. Most sharp compounds are volatile and are identical to the flavor compounds of that spice; most hot compounds are nonvolatile, thus distinct from the flavor principles (Hirasa and Takemasa 1998).

A CULTURAL HISTORY OF SPICES

The geopolitical significance of spices is revealed in their cultural history. Aromatic and pungent plants have been used in food preparation for thousands of years. For example, as early as the third century BCE, black pepper (*Piper nigrum*) from India was an item of commerce in the Middle East, and Malukan cloves (*Syzygium aromaticum* [L.] Merr. & Perry, Myrtaceae) were traded to China. Some eastern Asian origin myths center on spices, underscoring their prominence in consolidating political power. As Arabian Muslim cultural influences moved through North Africa into the Iberian Peninsula, small quantities of rare and valuable commodities were transported, including cloves, cinnamon (*Cinnamomum zeylanicum* Blume, Lauraceae), pepper, and nutmeg (*Myristica fragrans*), as well as the more affordable saffron (*Crocus sativus*), cumin (*Cuminum cyminum* L., Umbelliferae), and coriander (*Coriandrum sativum* L., Umbelliferae). These spices were transported for consumption and trade, with care to carry seeds as well to begin production in new lands. In the West it was not until the first century CE that there was a sizeable increase in the use of spices to flavor food. Until recent times, spices were expensive and their exchange value overlapped that of precious metals and gemstones. In the early years of the spice trade, merchants generated mystery about the origin of spices, which contributed to their appeal and, as a corollary, market value. The accelerated regional circulation and eventual globalization of spices is intimately linked to European discovery of indigenous cultures and foods, colonialism, and mercantile capitalism.

Spices, especially those endemic to the tropics, have a history of substantial geopolitical significance. Mesopotamia and India were centers of spice origins and trade in the first century BCE, and ancient overland spice trade routes (e.g., the Incense Route) peppered the terrain that linked the eastern Mediterranean to Asia and Southeast Asia. Late in the first century CE, the Romans learned how to harness the wind systems (monsoons) of the Indian Ocean (which the Arabs might already have known and concealed) and built ships on a greatly increased scale, which ended the Arab monopoly of trade with India.

Much of the European voyaging of later centuries involved the search for direct trade routes to the spice-producing regions in the East. The exploration of Asia by Marco Polo (1254–1324) established Italy, specifically Venice, as the Medieval center of the European spice and drug trade. In the early 1400s Portugal initiated a systematic program of exploration and became the leader among European navigating countries. Later in that century Portuguese ships first crossed the equator, Bartholomew Díaz rounded the Cape of Good Hope (1486), Christopher Columbus reached the Americas (1492), and Vasco da Gama found a route to India's west coast (1498). In the late 1400s, Pedro Alvarez Cabral, commander of Portugal's first merchant voyage to India (1500), established two trading posts on the west coast, thus shifting the centers of commerce from Italy and Egypt to the ports of Portugal and Spain.

By the mid-1500s overland spice trade with the East had been reestablished, including the shipment of as much as a million pounds of black pepper over traditional routes through the eastern Mediterranean. But even that was less than 20 percent of the volume of spices that reached Europe via Spanish and Portuguese ports. Over the next few centuries, competition for control of spice-producing regions was the cause of much of the military conflict among European nations and great suffering among indigenous populations forced into plantation spice production for export to

Europe. By the end of the 1600s the Dutch colonizers had virtually driven the Portuguese and English out of the Spice Islands (Maluku) of eastern Indonesia (the East Indies) and established monopolies not only in nutmeg, mace (*Myristica fragrans*), cloves, and cinnamon but also in pepper, ginger (*Zingiber officinale* Roscoe, Zingiberaceae), and turmeric (*Curcuma longa* L., Zingiberaceae). A century later, England was in the ascendancy, and the United States had become a major player in world spice trade. Compared with other tropical products such as sugar and tea, spices had a minor role in the economy of the British colonial empire, and the Dutch were the leading spice traders in the nineteenth and early twentieth centuries. It is safe to generalize that spice commerce was critical to many national economies, as evidenced by repeated and costly expeditions to spice-growing regions and the extension of struggles for control to political rivalries and military conflict (Toussaint-Samat 1992; Andaya 1993; Dalby 2000).

Today spice production and commerce are far less centralized than in earlier times, having expanded to include many countries in the tropics and a few in the temperate zones: for example, Brazil is a major source of black pepper, Jamaica produces allspice (*Pimenta dioica* [L.] Merr., Myrtaceae) and ginger, and the United States, Canada, and Europe are significant sources of sesame seed (*Sesamum indicum* L., Pedaliaceae), basil, parsley (*Petroselinum crispum* [Miller] A. W. Hill, Umbelliferae), and other herbs. In recent years, the United States has been the world's main spice buyer, followed by Germany, Japan, and France (Davidson 1999).

UNIQUE TASTES BECOME TRANSCULTURAL FLAVORS: THE CASE OF CHILE

New World Roots of Popular Fruits

This section highlights chile, arguably the most commonly consumed spice worldwide. *Capsicum* is the botanical and in some sectors the popular name for a plant genus that includes diverse species and cultivars: chile, pimento, pimiento, paprika, and bell (or sweet/green) peppers. A genus of the family Solanaceae, capsicums are related to the New World tomato (*L. esculentum*) and potato (*S. tuberosum*) and to the Old World eggplant (*Solanum melongena* L.) and the toxic black nightshade (*Solanum nigrum* L.).

All capsicums are New World natives. Wild chile peppers originated in present-day Bolivia to southwestern Brazil and spread throughout South and Central America via seed dispersal by birds (if nonpungent taxa are included in the genus, a second center of diversity is Mesoamerica). For 8000 years or so, wild chiles were an integral element in the diets of peoples of the Yucatan Peninsula and southern Mexico, where they served also as currency. Chiles featured prominently in the spiritual life of the Aztec, Maya, and Inca,

who called them "bird peppers" and identified particular avian taxa as conveyors of knowledge about and propagators of the fruit (Nabhan 1997, 2004). Chiles were forbidden during fasts intended to appease the gods, and the Inca venerated the chile as a holy plant, one of the four brothers of their creation myth. Chiles were domesticated by 3000 BCE, and were cultivated in as many as thirty varieties by 500 CE, when the Aztec Empire flourished.

In 1493 Christopher Columbus returned from his quest for a western route to the East carrying a pungent spice that he found on the Caribbean island Española (Haiti/Dominican Republic). Believing he had reached the East, Columbus created some confusion by identifying the natives as Indians and calling the pungent spice *pimiento* after the Asian Indian black pepper (*pimienta*), which he so desperately sought. The indigenous Arawak of Española called the fruit *axí*, which was transliterated to the Spanish *ají*, still used today in the Dominican Republic, other parts of the Caribbean, and much of South America. Some Amerindian groups in the Andean region retain the ancient terms *uchu* and *huayca*. The Nahuatl Mexican term *chilli* was transliterated to the Spanish *chile*, both of which are regarded as variants of the *Oxford English Dictionary's* primary spelling *chilli* (Andrews 1995, 2003).

In contrast to the stammeringly slow adoption of the New World tomato, potato, and other "discovered" foods, the pungent capsicums spread east with marked speed. From Europe chile peppers rapidly diffused along established spice trade routes to Africa and Asia, where the plants adapted to the geoclimatic conditions of the tropical Old World. Even in the face of opposition from the real (black) pepper traders in Europe, chiles spread from the New World to Europe and Asia in about fifty years. On India's Malabar (southwest) Coast, three varieties of chile were developed for export along ancient trade routes to Europe through the Middle East and along the new Portuguese route around Africa to Europe. Portuguese traders introduced chiles to Japan and Southeast Asia; from there, seed dispersal by birds established chiles throughout humanly inaccessible inland areas and insular Southeast Asia. Caravan routes linking the Middle East, India, Burma, and China introduced New World foods, one artifact of which is the more prominent role of chile in the cuisines of southwestern Hunan and Szechuan, compared with other regions of China.

At the end of the fifteenth century, the Mediterranean was characterized by two discrete trading arenas: the Spanish-dominated western Mediterranean and the Ottoman Empire to the east. At the center of the European spice trade, Venice depended on goods from Asia via the Ottomans, who received commodities from Portuguese ports on the Malabar Coast and Persian Gulf. Products that reached central Europe were disseminated to other parts of Europe. Supplies from Asia and Portuguese sources in Africa, India, and Lisbon also reached Antwerp, the primary European port. Along these routes, between 1535 and 1585, chiles were introduced into the markets of Italy,

Germany, England, the Balkans, and Moravia but became prominent in the cuisines only of Turkey and the Balkans. When the Napoleonic Wars interrupted European spice supplies, Balkan paprika substituted for the original American cultivars.

After chile trade and consumption had become established in the Middle East, Asia, and Europe, Spain played a more prominent role in circulating New World plants: an Acapulco-Manila trade route operated for 250 years to transfer goods between Mexico and eastern Asia. Spanish colonies in what are now New Mexico and Florida traded with the Caribbean and Mexico, receiving chiles and other goods, forty years before the introduction of the first chiles to a British colony (Virginia) in 1621 (Dewitt and Bosland 1995; Ho 1995; Dewitt 1999; Andrews 2003).

Although taxonomists and historians are clear in designating chile as native to tropical America, many contemporary world cultures understand it to be intrinsic to their own traditional cuisines and culinary identities. The apparent enthusiasm, or at least ease, with which diverse cultures embraced chiles reflects not so much an invention of tradition as it testifies to how well chiles conform to established palates. Through a syncretization of flavors, chiles were readily adopted into cuisines already marked by pungent spices such as cloves, ginger, and long (*Piper longum* L. Piperaceae), black (*P. nigrum*), flower (*Zanthoxylum zanthoxyloides* Lam., Rutaceae), and African melegueta (*Aframomum melegueta* Schumann, Zingiberaceae) peppers. They thrived in the new environments and in many areas became a spontaneous crop, growing and reseeding itself without human agency. Historians further speculate that the ready adoption of capsicums marks their confusion with black pepper, affordable then only by the wealthy. Indeed in many areas chile overshadowed or replaced the original pungents as a less expensive spice. Today India, China, and Pakistan lead the world in chile production. Familiarity with chile-flavored Szechuan dishes, Indian curries, and West African soups makes it difficult to conjure the short history of chiles in those regions.

Chile Embellishes Cuisines and Pharmacopoeias Around the World

Chile pepper was widely embraced not only as a food flavoring but also as medicine. In its region of origin, Aztec peoples relieved toothache with chile juice and mixed chile with maize flour to treat sore throat, asthma, and cough; the Maya also treated respiratory disorders with chile fruit and applied its juice to infected wounds. These applications were diffused and embellished and other uses were discovered, as chile was introduced around the world. The apprehension of these medicinal uses in the context of pharmacologic actions listed in the Appendix rationalizes many indigenous pharmacopoeias (although not all preventive and therapeutic objectives overlap pharmacologic action). In contemporary Western societies, chiles are among the more commonly used botanical supplements and phytoceuticals.

Hausa Cultural Construction of *Barkono*/Chile

The relatively recent introduction of chile into West Africa stands in stark contrast to its importance for populations of the region, including Hausa in northern Nigeria. In Hurumi, at least one of the three daily meals centers on a dense, bland grain porridge, *tuwo*, made from guineacorn or millet or less commonly from rice or maize. The chief ingredients of several varieties of *miya* (the companion, piquant soup) are tomato (*tumatir*), various cultivated and wild leaves (*ganye*), okra (*kubewa*), garden egg (*yalo, Solanum melongena* L., Solanaceae), pumpkin (*kabewa, Cucurbita pepo*) and/or melon (*agusi, Citrullus lanatus* [Thunb.] Mansf., Cucurbitaceae), peanut (*Arachis hypogaea*) or palm oil (*man ja, Elaeis guineensis* Jacq., Palmae) and/or butter (*man shanu*), and ideally meat or fish. The varied flavors of miya are imparted by combinations of the fermented soup base daddawa with salt, chile pepper, and the compound spice *yaji* (discussed below). Other dishes provide appropriate, if less esteemed, substitutes for tuwo da miya for the morning and midday meals. These include gruels and vegetable-leaf mixtures supplemented by peanuts, beans, rice, spices, and oils. Between-meal foods include various traditional calorie-, fat-, and/or protein-dense snacks and seasonal fruits. For contemporary villagers, the substance of cuisine, but less so its rhythm (meal and food-type sequencing), has been impacted on all levels by Hurumi's increased participation in the global economy.

Among singlet spices, *barkono*/chile is the signature of Hausa cuisine in northern Nigeria. Hausa themselves characterize their flavor repertoire as narrow and identify barkono as their primary flavor principle; outsiders (e.g., from other regions of Africa and Europe) typically characterize Hausa cuisine as remarkably hot. Hurumi residents use barkono to refer generally to chile peppers, but they further differentiate among cultivars with reference to taste, shape/size, and suitability for medicine. *Tsiduhu* is the smallest and hottest of local chiles; barkono fruit is small, and it and tsiduhu are favored medicinally because they are more powerful. The fruit of *bunsurun barkono* (goat's chile) is somewhat larger and not very hot. *Ataruhu* has a round and lobed shape; *dan kadana* is a larger, long and thin variety; and *tattasai*, the largest local chile, is drupe-shaped. These last three, milder chiles are indicated for children's medicines.

The most common Hausa medicinal uses of barkono are for intestinal disorders, including worms; abrasions and wounds; fevers; and *sabara*, a complex spirit-caused disorder, a strong disease requiring strong medicine, with internal and external phases that include one or more of these symptoms: swellings that can develop into pustular sores that may itch and fuse, fever, sloughing. For example, barkono is snorted to induce sneezing, which helps to externalize the internal phase of rash diseases such as measles and chickenpox, while medicines taken later in the therapeutic process are directed at symptom resolution. Barkono is a powerful deterrent against sorcery. For *ciwon gindi*, a type of lower back pain, chile promotes the egress of accumulated *majina* (phlegm) at the locus of soreness. In another medicinal domain, barkono is featured among proscribed foods for certain conditions, for example, *fara*, a symptom complex marked chiefly by anemia, a weakened state of health for which powerful foods and medicines risk exacerbation and complications leading to *shawara*, an overlapping symptom complex that intersects hepatitis.

The cultural significance of barkono is reflected among compositional elements of *Bori*, the indigenous, pre-Islamic Hausa religion that centers on the mediation of *iskoki*/spirits who reside in the invisible city of Jangare, one of whose twelve houses is headed by Barkono.[3] In other words, ancient Hausa religious traditions were transformed some time after 1493, so that the New World barkono was added to or replaced something in the existing foundational structure of Bori. The cultural significance of chile in Hausaland is further evidenced by the metaphoric uses of barkono, as is apparent in these proverbs:

> *Namiji barkono ne. Sai a tauna shi a san yajinsa.*
> A husband is like a pepper. Not until you chew do you know how hot he is. [Experience reveals a man's character.]
> *Audu barkono ne (barkonam mutane ne).*
> Audu is a chile (a chile person). [Audu is irascible.]
> *Ta sha barkono.*
> She ate a chile. [She is angry.]

Political Economy, Globalization, Commodification

The transposition of the American chile to cuisines and pharmacopoeias around the world provides an interesting, and in some ways unique, example of the confluence of food traditions, geopolitics, and the cultural construction and social negotiation of foods and medicines. From the perspective of political economy, chile peppers were not simply an introduced commodity; in large part they took the place of black pepper, an item that carried high social and cultural salience in many parts of the world. Black pepper itself, as well as chile and other spices, and cash crops such as tobacco (*Nicotiniana tabacum* L., Solanaceae) and coffee all are integral to an extended history of European imperial expansion that included colonization and the appropriation of local peoples and their products. Like other globalized commodities, chile peppers were more than simple introductions and substitutions; they were further transformed in their cultures of destination, where they have become key elements of highly diverse cuisines, pharmacopoeias, and languages.

PHYSIOLOGIC EFFECTS OF SPICES

The scientific literature on spices is vast and has been expanding rapidly in recent years. As evidence, over an arbitrarily selected recent two-year span (2004–2005),

virtually every issue of the following journals included one or more articles on the medicinal uses and pharmacology of one or more spices: *Pharmaceutical Biology*, *Journal of Ethnopharmacology*, and *Planta Medica*. These figures from PubMed searches also reveal scientific interest: garlic was the subject of 1984 articles, onion of 1616, capsicum of 875, cinnamon of 513, ginger of 454, and turmeric of 360. Spices that in the last several hundred years have been incorporated into Western cuisines, as well as spices that Western scientists identify as the signature of non-Western cuisines (e.g., capsicum, ginger), are overrepresented in these scientific studies.

Because the phytochemistry of spices has been better characterized than that of any other functional or taxonomic group, more is known about their potential interactions with pharmaceuticals, foods, and other botanicals. Still, this knowledge is only emergent. Some interactions can be predicted intuitively. For example, in theory, plants that contain eugenol and other platelet inhibitors may potentiate anticoagulant drugs. However, we must seriously question whether this is clinically significant, as it applies to almost all the plants in the Appendix, whose use is widespread; also, interactions depend strongly on whether the plant and drug are consumed at or near the same time, as well as on how the plant is prepared, combined with other foods and drugs, and consumed.

Although the category spices embraces considerable botanical and phytochemical diversity, subgroups of spices can be linked through similar physiologic effects. For example, pungent compounds stimulate body heat production, influence blood pressure in the peripheral circulation, promote lipid metabolism, and affect metabolic regulation through nervous system and hormonal influences. They enhance digestion by promoting peristalsis and the secretion of digestive enzymes, stimulating the liver to produce acid-rich bile, and increasing absorption into the blood from the intestines. Antioxidant activity characterizes many spices, especially those in the Labiatae: phenolic glucosides, caffeic acid, protocatechuic acid, rosmarinic acid, and phenylpropionic acid in oregano (*Origanum vulgare* L.), and carnosol, rosmanol, epirosmanol, and isorosmanol in rosemary (*Rosmarinus officinalis* L.); combinations of antioxidant and other spices have synergistic effects (Beckstrom-Sternberg and Duke 1994; Hirasa and Takemasa 1998; Platel and Srinivasan 2004).

By way of illustration, the Appendix lists some of the constituents and isolated physiologic effects of thirty-three spices selected to represent a variety of organoleptic qualities, places of origin, botanical growth form (habit), plant parts, and phytochemical spectra. This compilation resonates the bioscientific research paradigm in which natural products are reduced to their constituents and/or extracts and studied through controlled laboratory protocols that range across in vitro assays, animal studies, and human clinical contexts. The challenge is to connect these disembodied observations in an analytic framework that represents real people's experiences with spices in both medicinal and dietary contexts.

The remainder of this chapter moves beyond catalogues of constituents and activities to suggest novel approaches to the ethnopharmacology of spices. This is accomplished by considering one class of activity, antimicrobial action, and addressing that from both an evolutionary and a contextualized perspective that focuses on composite spices.

NOVEL APPROACHES TO SPICE PHARMACOLOGY

Antimicrobial Action

Because the germ theory of disease has been the predominant paradigm in the West for the last hundred years, the antimicrobial action of spices has been a special subject of attention. Spices are prominently represented in the pharmacopoeias of contemporary indigenous groups who use these plants to treat wounds, abscesses, and systemic infections; in childbirth and early postpartum; and to improve the healthful qualities of foods. Thousands of years ago in China and India spices were used medicinally and to preserve foods. Similarly, in the West people have taken advantage of the antimicrobial attributes of spices for centuries. Ancient texts record systematic use of spices in places of their endemicity. The ancient Egyptians embalmed the dead with spices such as thyme (*Thymus vulgaris* L., Labiatae), cinnamon, and cumin. In early Greece and Rome mint was used to prevent milk from spoiling and coriander extended the shelf life of meats. Spices were consumed in such high volume in the Middle Ages that one might regard them more as foods, although they also played a specific role in treating infectious diseases such as typhus and cholera.

Starting in the 1880s and at an increasing pace through the twentieth century, biomedical research concentrated on the antimicrobial action of spices. Today, the growing problem posed by drug-resistant microorganisms accelerates bioscientific search for more effective preventions and treatments, including (again) a special interest in spices. Volatiles and pungent spices tend to have strong antimicrobial activity, as do constituents that include aldehyde (–CHO) or hydroxyl (–OH) groups. Especially when one employs the expanded definition of spice, literally tens of thousands of studies establish antimicrobial action against a taxonomically diverse range of organisms, including some of the most important pathogenic bacteria and toxin-producing microorganisms that affect humans, such as cholera, tuberculosis, dysentery, and staphylococcal infection. It is not possible to determine how important a role knowledge of such activity factors into the decisions that shape cuisines, but it would surely be wrong to suppose that it was not at all significant.

Evolutionary Implications of Spiced Cuisines. A recurrent theme in the literature on antimicrobial spices is the role they may play in food safety. Some authors invoke an evolutionary trajectory of adaptive responses, noting the antiquity and ubiquity of spice use, including during times and in places in which food preservation could not be supported by refrigeration or cognate technologies. For example, Sherman and colleagues advanced these four predictions (Billing and Sherman 1998: 4; Sherman and Flaxman 2001: 145): spices kill or inhibit food-spoilage microorganisms; spice use should be heaviest in hot climates, where (unrefrigerated) foods spoil most rapidly; spices with the most potent antimicrobial properties should be favored in areas where foods spoil most quickly; and, within a country, meat recipes should be more heavily spiced than vegetable recipes.

Their correlational study inferred (but did not measure directly) how spices affect people's health by quantifying the frequency of spice use across a range of cultures and geographies. Inclusion criteria limited the research to meat-inclusive[4] cuisines and minimally 50 (preferably more than 100) recipes from at least two traditional cookbooks. The researchers analyzed 4578 recipes from 107 cookbooks representing thirty-six countries, sixteen of the nineteen major language groups, and every continent. Additional data were compiled on the antimicrobial activities of individual spices, their botanical characterization, and temperature ranges for each country. The forty-three spices include groups that cohere around one or a small number of shared constituents, for example, "capsicum" includes all members of that genus that produce capsaicin and "onion" groups onion, garlic, leek, and other *Allium* spp.

Sherman and colleagues' findings bear out their predictions.[5] Their literature review, like the one I conducted, uncovered substantial antimicrobial activity for many spices; and all spices in their study were used medicinally in diverse indigenous therapeutic systems. Whereas the medicinal use of spices is episodic (in response to the diagnosis of specific and general symptoms) and includes consumption in relatively large volume, in cooking spices are used in small quantities and added routinely. This suggests that spiced foods may prevent food spoilage and remedy chronic problems such as micronutrient deficiencies and persistent enteric infection.

In general, the cuisines of hot-climate countries include numerous spices, which are used frequently (in more than 40 percent of recipes); cold-climate country cuisines use fewer spices and less often (in fewer than 5 percent of recipes). Significant positive correlations hold between mean annual temperature and the number of recipes that include at least one spice, mean number of spices per recipe, the proportion of frequently used spices in each country, and the mean proportion of recipes that call for each strongly inhibitory spice used in each country (at least 75 percent microbial inhibition). There is also a positive (but not significant) correlation between the proportion of microorganisms inhibited by each spice and the percentage of countries that use that spice, that is, antimicrobially more potent spices are used more broadly. Whereas there is no correspondence between mean annual temperature and the number of spice plants growing in a country, positive correlations exist between the number of countries in which each spice grows and the number that use it. Further, mean annual temperature and the proportion of spices used in the countries in which they grow are positively correlated. In other words, although people in hot countries do not have a larger selection of locally growing spices, they use a higher percentage of those that are available, especially the more potent antimicrobials. Finally, meat-based recipes from all thirty-six countries designate a significantly larger number of spices than vegetable-based recipes, an average of 3.9 and 2.4 spices, respectively; and the proportions of dishes that include more than one spice and more than one strongly antimicrobial spice are significantly higher for meat, compared to vegetable, dishes (Sherman and Hash 2001).

The methodology of these studies can be criticized on several counts. For example, only the United States and China are regarded to have regional cuisines (an artifact of the cookbooks located by the authors), and then only "northern" and "southern"; from isolated recipes one cannot know how often that dish is consumed. Still, the argument is compelling that cuisines are shaped in part by the antimicrobial action of spices.

In Sherman and colleagues' explanation, enhancing the palatability of foods is only a proximate explanation of spicing, while the ultimate reason is that spices inhibit or kill food-spoiling microorganisms. We are not served by deciding between proximate and ultimate explanations and should instead consider the multiplex and complementary nature of a suite of objectives that underlie food choice and preparation: pharmacologic action *and* aesthetics, learned tastes, and the cultural construction of cuisines.

Spices in the Context of Complex Cuisines

As described above, many spices are synergists that enhance the bioavailability and potency of companion phytochemicals. Thus, we may apply a biocultural perspective that explores spice complexes in which a number of discrete flavors are blended. I selected three region-specific composite spices, with overlapping constituents, to explore the intersection of cultural constructions of cuisine and pharmacologic potential.

Ayurvedic Trikatu. The Sanskrit term for three acrids, *trikatu*, is a traditional Ayurvedic formulation that combines the fruits of long and black peppers and ginger rhizome in equal portions. Although not technically a culinary spice, trikatu has a long history as a digestive and is marketed today as a food supplement. In this way, trikatu provides a pharmacologically and culturally interesting contrast for Chinese five-spice and Hausa yaji, discussed below. Trikatu is an essential element of many, even more complex botanical mixtures that are used in the treatment of a wide variety of disorders. While some contemporary Ayurvedic practitioners dismiss the addition of trikatu as a prescription that "lacks reason" and is employed "only for the sake of rhyme," others invoke the traditional explanation that these acrids help to restore balance among the *doshas* (dynamic forces) *kapha*, *pitta*, and *vata*.

Occasional citations in the scientific literature note that trikatu increases the potency of medicines already clinically judged effective in their own right, as when added to the leaves of Malabar nut/*vasaka* (*Justicia adhatoda* L., Acanthaceae) in the treatment of asthma (Atal et al. 1981). More recent studies have determined that trikatu affects the pharmacokinetic profile of drugs; specifically, it promotes bioavailability of some (e.g., vasicine, sparteine, phenytoin, propranolol, theophylline, sulfadiazine, and tetracycline) and reduces the bioavailability of others (e.g., the antituberculosis drugs isoniazid and rifampicin) (Johri and Zutshi 1992; Karan et al. 1999). Once it had been determined that the primary compound responsible for these effects is piperine, a major alkaloid in peppers (but not in ginger), investigations have concentrated on this phytoconstituent, rather than on the conventional three-part crude drug preparation. This approach is consistent with a biomedical research protocol that narrows inquiry to discrete, isolatable units. This course of study both clarifies, by identifying known or characterizable phytoconstituents, and oversimplifies, by taking out of the mix the effects of other constituents and by fragmenting the cultural integrity of this traditional spice complex. The constituents and activities of these three spices are summarized in the Appendix and suggest significant pharmacologic potential beyond synergisms.

Still, these findings have implications for polypharmacy, dose and timing of medications, and the redesign of drug administration. For example, the cost and difficulty of parenteral administration of some drugs may be mitigated by changing to oral administration accompanied by trikatu or other drug potentiators. Further, because trikatu is comprised of three culinary spices, exploration of its pharmacologic profile reinforces how consumption outside of clinical contexts may influence health.

Chinese Five-Spice. The highly aromatic Chinese five-spice is pungent, fragrant, hot, and slightly sweet all at once. It is comprised of equal amounts of star anise (*Illicium verum* Hook f., Illiciaceae), clove, cinnamon, fennel, and flower pepper. Regionally variable optional ingredients include ginger, galangal (*Alpinia officinarum* Hance, Zingiberaceae), and licorice. Although one could argue that increasing the number of components erodes the integrity of the five, this offers an example of how rules are created to break rules, in this case normative cuisine prescriptions. In some sectors it is referred to as the "five-spice family," underscoring both its compound nature and its structural symmetry in Chinese cosmology, which is characterized by five-part domains: the universe is composed by earth, wood, fire, metal, and water, five phases that are associated with virtually everything else, so that human circumstances are understood through the integration of five colors, five large body organs, and so on. In the context of food and medicine, the five tastes include sour, salt, bitter, sweet, and piquant, and the five smells are fragrant, scorched, rancid, rotten, and putrid. Elements of the five-part domains must be carefully balanced among themselves and with parallel domains, so that the universe is harmonized by the integration of social life, cooking, medicine, and other activities. Scholars agree that throughout history the distinction between Chinese food and medicine has been especially porous (Anderson 1988).

Individually and in various permutations, these five plants figure prominently in the medical traditions of China: all are used as digestive tonics and for gastrointestinal disorders; star anise and flower pepper are diuretic, flower pepper also is carminative, cinnamon is analgesic and antiemetic and is used during the postpartum and to slow aging, and fennel is used in pain management (Simoons 1991).

This complex perspective on health and healing invites us to speculate about the pharmacologic potential of the five spices (Appendix), for example, how the phytochemical characteristics of individual components are interpreted in the light of overarching principles of balance, judgments about the efficacy of complex versus singlet preparations for disease prevention and therapy, and how the individual as diner engages the last stage of preparation of medicinal foods by using sauces and other table items to create order out of disparate elements.

Yaji in Northern Nigeria. Based on my intimate knowledge of its cultural constructions in Hausa diet and medicine, I can speculate more productively about the pharmacologic potential of the composite spice *yaji*. As barkono is the singlet signature flavor of Hausa cuisine, yaji is its composite counterpart, offering nuances of taste and a complex texture. It contains barkono, as well as *citta maikwaya* (melegueta pepper), *cittar aho* (ginger), *fasakwari* (flower pepper), *kanumfari* (clove), *kimba* (guinea pepper), *kulla* (thonningia), and *masoro* (Benin pepper) (see Appendix). Of these, only barkono is cultivated locally. Hurumi residents purchase prepared yaji or individual constituents at markets. Some women prepare yaji in volume, powdering the ingredients together with mortar and pestle (accompanied by much sneezing throughout the compound), in anticipation of their own needs as well as for sale throughout the village.

The plants that comprise yaji all are pharmacologically dynamic. Singly and together they represent significant antimicrobial, anti-inflammatory, antioxidant, and carminative potential and are vitamin rich (Appendix). These activities take on more meaning in the context of the specific culinary and medicinal uses of yaji, such as in the early postpartum and for male circumcision.

Haihuwa/Childbirth. Like most traditional cultures, Hausa regard pregnancy as a predominantly healthful phase for the duration of which concerns center on good nutrition, and virtually none of the circumstances of pregnancy is treated with medicines. Certainly, the potential for complications is widely understood. Gestational age, for example, can influence the baby's viability. Hausa say that a child born prematurely in the seventh month will survive, because the body lacks form, but a child born during the eighth month surely will die (see below, *kaciyar maza*). Conversely, the first forty days postpartum are regarded as a period of risk for both the new mother (*mai jego*), who risks infection and other complications of childbirth, and

the baby (*jinjiri*) for whom the primary concerns are *fara* (see above) and *mayankwaniya*, another symptom complex that overlaps marasmus (protein-calorie malnutrition) and can incorporate or eventuate from *fara*.

A complex suite of medicines and behaviors address health concerns, as well as assure progress in the child's development and the mother's ability to breastfeed. Mai jego should avoid both literal and figurative exposure to *dauda*/pollution, which extends to not having sexual relations with her husband for the forty-day period. After birth the mother's body is raw and must be "cooked."[6] Medicines and foods are structured around restoring to the body the heat and blood lost during childbirth, especially to the reproductive organs. The room and bed are warmed with glowing embers; aromatic medicines are burned to repel spirits, such as the gum of *maje* (*Daniellia oliveri* Hutch and Dalz, Fabaceae) and *tazargade* (*Artemisia* spp., Asteraceae), which may be embellished by adding spices. Large volumes of water are boiled to wash the mother and baby twice per day (*wankan jego, wankan jinjiri*), the water cooking their bodies, with plants (yaji and other antimicrobial species) added to the water to prevent complications and to treat any symptoms that develop. Other leafy branches are the vehicles that deliver (splash) the water, such as *darbejiya* (neem, *Azadirachta indica* A. Juss., Meliaceae) and *tsamiya* (tamarind, *Tamarindus indica* L., Fabaceae). Mai jego is encouraged to eat well: all her food must be cooked; her meals should include meat, eggs, and other nutrient-dense foods and, especially, should be liberally flavored with yaji.

In anticipation of the birth, mai jego's husband purchases (or commissions relatives' preparation of) large quantities of yaji, which she not only consumes with each meal but also gifts in small amounts to female relatives and friends who visit. Yaji also figures prominently among the visitors' gifts for the new mother. This both assures the physical health of mai jego and jinjiri and, symbolically and in fact, redistributes healthful food/medicine among a larger population. The aromatic and pungent flavor of yaji assures that the womb is properly heated and cleansed. Concern in the postpartum with the restoration of heat through fire, medicine, and food—featuring yaji—finds parallels in the rules that govern Hausa male circumcision.

Kaciyar Maza/Male Circumcision. In a structural analogue to childbirth, the Hausa barber-surgeon (*wanzami*) can circumcise boys when they are seven or nine years of age but not eight years old. An age cohort of boys may be circumcised at the same time, in a public ceremony marked by discrete stages (cutting, bleeding, washing, applying medicines) that culminate in the *dan shayi* (circumcised boys) eating a special gruel, flavored with yaji. In addition to the "seven and nine but not eight" principle and yaji that marks both haihuwa and kaciya, other structural analogues are embodied in the rules that govern cold, food, and pollution for a fifteen-day phase of partial seclusion and rest for dan shayi. Care must be taken so that *sanyi* (cold) does not penetrate the vulnerable body of the boy: fires warm the sleeping hut for the recovery period, and dan shayi eat foods similar to those for mai jego: warm foods, meat and other calorie- and fat-dense foods, all generously flavored with yaji.[7] Medicines are administered to prevent dauda, dirt or infection, also a metaphor for pollution. Menstruating women, who are *karni* (religiously polluted), should not care for or visit dan shayi, other (sexually mature) adults should stay away as well, and the boy's parents do not have sexual relations during the recovery phase.

Healthful Qualities of Yaji for Liminal Phases.   The foregoing discussion briefly introduces symbolic symmetries that link the postpartum and circumcision recovery in Hausa society. Not only are these liminal phases marked in much the same way as other life-cycle transitions that have high social salience, but they also constitute periods of heightened health risk that share concerns for infection, inflammation, *kumbura* (edema), and blood/heat loss. The aromatic constituents and pungent tastes of yaji impart a physical sensation of heat, and the individual spices embody significant pharmacologic potential.

———

This chapter began with a comprehensive definition for a biodynamic class of botanicals that serve diverse functions, especially as foods and medicines. The overview of the cultural history of spices overlaps issues of political economy, globalization, and commodification, as expanded in the case study of chile pepper. The general treatment of the physiologic effects of spices suggests their broad-based biopotential and connects to the next section, which offered a novel approach to the pharmacology of spices: extending conventional catalogues of activities and constituents, attention was directed to one activity class, antimicrobials, which was explored from both an evolutionary and a contextualized perspective that examined the cultural constructions and pharmacologic potential of composite spices. This chapter has focused on spices as a discrete category of culinary and medicinal products, whereas plants discussed in the next chapter cohere around a means of preparation. The fermentation of foods and medicines has important health implications from the perspectives of nutrient content and the prevention and mediation of pathologic processes.

Notes

1. There is some debate about the widely held belief that spices are/have been used to mask the taste of already spoiled foods. While this seems to rest on a conventional wisdom that food supplies are unsafe in the absence of modern technology, we have ample evidence for food preservation and other safety measures in both contemporary and historical populations. Further, this ignores both the health risks of ingesting spoiled food, as well as the fact that spices not only add flavor but also bring out existing flavors including, presumably, the taste of putrefaction.

2. The seasonings salt and sugar seem obvious inclusions but are not treated in this chapter because each has an extensive literature of its own documenting complex social, medicinal, and culinary

histories (e.g., Mintz 1985, 1996; Lovejoy 1986; Attwood 1992; Montanari 1994; Laszlo 2001; Kurlansky 2002; Woloson 2002). These ubiquitous and low-cost seasonings of the modern era were expensive commodities in their early histories, salt itself (and to a lesser extent sugar) serving as currency at various times and places. Like the other spices discussed in this chapter, salt and sugar have interesting clinical applications, and their global patterns of production and consumption offer insight into the political economy of food sourcing, globalization, and commodification.

3. Although formerly condemned by Islamic clerics in the jihad of the early nineteenth century, Bori continues to exist in regionally variable, attenuated forms (in part because the iskoki find parallels in the Islamic *jinn*/spirits). It follows an idiom of affliction to which people are drawn to resolve physical, psychological, and social problems. Integral to Bori are musicians, noninitiates who preserve the oral traditions through song; *yam Bori*, the adepts ("horses"); and divine spirits who reside in the invisible city Jangare and deliver to their victims, in turn, illness and misfortune then resolution. Cure is effected as the adepts are first drawn into trance and dancing then "mounted" by the spirit; in the end, they serve as a medium for that spirit's voice through mimetic representation of its appearance and actions. Jangare social organization finds parallels in Hausa society: it is governed by *Sarkan Aljan* (Chief of Spirits), with or without a royal court; authority is further divided among twelve *zauruka* (houses, sing, *zaure*) that are distinguished by ethnicity, occupation, and descent: for example, *Zauren Turawa*, house of North African spirits, whose head is *Barkono*/chile pepper; *Zauren Kutare*, house of the lepers, headed by *Kuturu* the leper (Besmer 1983).

4. The authors focused on meat-inclusive recipes because the spoilage rate of animal products is greater and associated with more instances of food-borne illness than are vegetables: dead plants, compared to animal flesh, are better protected from microorganisms due to the presence of antimicrobial phytochemicals, difficult-to-digest lignin and cellulose, pH lower than what supports most bacteria, and low fat content. A recipe is qualified as "meat-based . . . [if] at least one-third of its total weight or volume consists of red meat, poultry, pork, veal or seafood" (Billing and Sherman 1998: 6).

5. The examples of lemon, lime, and black and white peppers at first seem to contradict the hypothesis. Although they number among the "five most commonly used spices and appear in the meat-based cuisine of every country in [the] sample, they are among the least effective" antimicrobials, and their use does not correlate with temperatures (Billing and Sherman 1998: 17). However, these spices act synergistically with other spices and foods and could, arguably, play an adjuvant role in the collective antimicrobial action. The issue of spice blends is treated in the section Spices in the Context of Complex Cuisines.

6. One of the most instructive of Hausa symbolic representations links human reproduction and alimentation. The fundamental metaphor of this allegory likens eating with intercourse, both expressed in the homonym verb *ci*. Elaborations of the *ci* allegory include the homonym *sanwa* for both semen and cooking water; describing the vagina as the locus of consumption; surgical excision during the naming ceremony of the *beli* (uvula) and the *tantani* (hymen), appendages that are understood to block consumption; and in rude vernacular reference to divorced women as *bazawara* (leftover, partially consumed food). Further elaborations are apparent in the rules that govern birth and the early postpartum, as well as in songs, proverbs, and epithets. Corollary

symbolic expressions that link gestation to food production include the representation of the penis and vagina as, respectively, the pestle and mortar (based on structure/function) and the penis and testicles as the *murhu* (three-stoned cooking hearth). Similarly, the developing fetus rests on a murhu while developing in the *mahaifa* (womb). Reproductive development finds an analogue in the fire that is alimentation: the cooking, forming, and transforming from raw to cooked (see also Darrah 1980).

7. Hausa food rules for circumcision are developed in more detail in chapter 1, Food in Celebration.

References

Andaya, Leonard Y. 1993. *The World of Maluku: Eastern Indonesia in the Early Modern Period.* University of Hawai'i Press, Honolulu.

Anderson, E. N. 1988. *The Food of China.* Yale University Press, New Haven, Conn.

Anderson, Jennifer L. 1991. *An Introduction to Japanese Tea Ritual.* State University of New York Press, Albany.

Andrews, Jean. 1995. *Peppers: The Domesticated Capsicums.* Rev. ed. University of Texas Press, Austin.

Andrews, Jean. 2003. Chili peppers. In *Encyclopedia of Food and Culture.* S. H. Katz, ed. Pp. 368–378. Charles Scribner, New York.

Atal, C. K., U. Zutshi, and P. G. Rao. 1981. Scientific evidence on the role of Ayurvedic herbals in bioavailability of drugs. *Journal of Ethnopharmacology* 4(2): 229–232.

Attwood, Donald A. 1992. *Raising Cane: The Political Economy of Sugar in Western India.* Westview Press, Boulder, Colo.

Beckstrom-Sternberg, S. M., and James A. Duke. 1994. Potential for synergistic action of phytochemicals in spices. In *Spices, Herbs, and Edible Fungi.* G. Charalambous, ed. Pp. 201–223. Elsevier, Amsterdam.

Besmer, Fremont E. 1983. *Horses, Musicians, and Gods: The Hausa Cult of Possession-Trance.* Bergin and Garvey, South Hadley, Mass.

Billing, Jennifer, and Paul W. Sherman. 1998. Antimicrobial functions of spices: why some like it hot. *Quarterly Review of Biology* 73(1): 3–49.

Chaaib, F., E. F. Queiroz, K. Ndjoko, D. Diallo, and K. Hostettmann. 2003. Antifungal and antioxidant compounds from the root bark of *Fagara zanthoxyloides.* *Planta Medica* 69(4): 316–20.

Dalby, Andrew. 2000. *Dangerous Tastes: The Story of Spices.* University of California Press, Berkeley.

Darrah, Alan C. 1980. A Hermeneutic Approach to Hausa Therapeutics: The Allegory of the Living Fire. Ph.D. diss., Department of Anthropology, Northwestern University.

Davidson, Alan. 1999. *The Oxford Companion to Food.* Oxford University Press, Oxford.

Dewitt, Dave. 1999. *The Chile Pepper Encyclopedia.* William Morrow, New York.

Dewitt, Dave, and Paul W. Bosland. 1995. *The Pepper Garden.* Ten Speed Press, Berkeley, Calif.

Duke, James A. 1985. *Handbook of Medicinal Herbs.* CRC Press, Boca Raton, Fla.

Galal, Ahmed M. 1996. Antimicrobial activity of 6-paradol and related compounds. *International Journal of Pharmacognosy* 34(1): 64–69.

Gyamfi, M. A., N. Hokama, K. Oppong-Boachie, and Y. Aniya. 2000. Inhibitory effects of the medicinal herb, *Thonningia sanguinea,* on liver drug metabolizing enzymes of rats. *Human Experimental Toxicology* 19(11): 623–631.

Hirasa, Kenji, and Mitsuo Takemasa. 1998. *Spice Science and Technology.* Marcel Dekker, New York.

Hladik, C. M., and B. Simmen. 1996. Taste perception and feeding behavior in nonhuman primates and human populations. *Evolutionary Anthropology* 5: 58–71.

Ho, P. T. 1995. The introduction of American food plants into China. *American Anthropologist* 55: 191–201.

Johri, R. K., and U. Zutshi. 1992. An Ayurvedic formulation: 'trikatu' and its constituents. *Journal of Ethnopharmacology* 37: 85–91.

Karan, R. S., V. K. Bhargava, and S. K. Carg. 1999. Effect of trikatu, an Ayurvedic prescription, on the pharmacokinetic profile of rifampicin in rabbits. *Journal of Ethnopharmacology* 64: 259–264.

Kiba, A., H. Saitoh, M. Nishihara, K. Omiya, and S. Yamamura. 2003. C-terminal domain of a hevein-like protein from *Wasabia japonica* has potent antimicrobial activity. *Plant and Cell Physiology* 44(3): 296–303.

Kurlansky, Mark. 2002. *Salt: A World History.* Walker and Company, New York.

Kurzer, Mindy S. 2000. Hormonal effects of soy isoflavones: studies in premenopausal and postmenopausal women. *Journal of Nutrition* 130: 660S–661S.

Kwon, Y. S., W. G. Choi, W. J. Kim, W. K. Kim, M. J. Kim, W. H. Kang, and C. M. Kim. 2002. Antimicrobial constituents of *Foeniculum vulgare.* *Archives of Pharmacal Research* 25(2): 154–157.

Laszlo, Pierre (Mary Beth Mader, trans.). 2001. *Salt: Grain of Life.* Columbia University Press, New York.

Lovejoy, Paul E. 1986. *Salt of the Desert Sun: A History of Salt Production and Trade in the Central Sudan.* Cambridge University Press, Cambridge.

Mintz, Sidney W. 1985. *Sweetness and Power: The Place of Sugar in Modern History.* Penguin Books, New York.

Mintz, Sidney W. 1996. *Tasting Food, Tasting Freedom: Excursions into Eating, Culture, and the Past.* Beacon Press, Boston.

Nabhan, Gary. 1997. *Cultures of Habitat: On Nature, Culture, and Story.* Counterpoint Press, Washington, D.C.

Nabhan, Gary. 2004. *Why Some Like It Hot.* Island Press, Washington, D.C.

Newall, Carol A., Linda A. Anderson, and J. David Phillipson. 1996. *Herbal Medicines: A Guide for Health Care Professionals.* Pharmaceutical Press, London.

Ohtani, I. N. Gotoh, J. Tanaka, T. Higa, M. A. Gyamfi, and Y. Aniya. 2000. Thonningianins A and B, new antioxidants from the African medicinal herb *Thonningia sanguinea*. *Journal of Natural Products* 63(5): 676–679.

Platel, Kalpana, and K. Srinivasan. 2004. Digestive stimulant action of spices: A myth or reality? *Indian Journal of Medical Research* 119: 167–179.

Research and Editorial Staff of the Pharmacists' Letter and Prescribers' Letter. 2003. *Natural Medicines Comprehensive Database*. 5th ed. Therapeutic Research Faculty, Stockton, Calif.

Sherman, Paul W., and Samuel M. Flaxman. 2001. Protecting ourselves from food. *American Scientist* 89: 142–151.

Sherman, Paul W., and Geoffrey A. Hash. 2001. Why vegetable recipes are not very spicy. *Evolution and Human Behavior* 22(3): 147–163.

Simoons, Frederick J. 1991. *Food in China: A Cultural and Historical Inquiry*. CRC Press, Boca Raton, Fla.

Toussaint-Samat, Maguelonne (Anthea Bell, trans.). 1992. *History of Food*. Blackwell, Oxford.

Walton, Nicholas J., Melinda J. Mayer, and Arjan Narbad. 2003. Vanillin. *Phytochemistry* 63(5): 505–515.

Woloson, Wendy A. 2002. *Refined Tastes: Sugar, Confectionery, and Consumers in Nineteenth-Century America*. Johns Hopkins University Press, Baltimore, Md.

APPENDIX: SOME COMMON SPICES

English name[a]	Genus species	Family	Origin[b]	Constituents and activities[c]
Allspice tree/fruit	*Pimento dioica* (L.) Meer.	Myrtaceae	TAm	carene, caryophyllene, curcumene, cymene, eugenol, limonene, phellandrene, pinene, thujene, thymol relieves pain, carminative, inhibits blood clots, expectorant, bactericide, fungicide
Aniseed herb/seed	*Pimpinella anisum* L.	Umbelliferae	Med	anethole, anise ketone, bergapten, methyl chavicol, estragole, flavonol, limonene, linalool, myristicin, α-pinene, rutin, scopoletin, umbelliferone antifungal, carminative, expectorant, anticonvulsant, estrogenic, lactagogue, relieves psoriasis, stimulates hepatic regeneration
Annatto shrub/fruit pulp	*Bixa orellana* L.	Bixaceae	TAm	anethole, apigenin, bixin, borneol, camphor, carotenoids, estragol, eucalyptol, eugenol, gallic acid, linalool, luteolin, pyrogallol, maslinic acid antibacterial, inhibits blood clots, estrogenic
Basil herb/leaf	*Ocimum basilicum* L.	Labiatae	TAs	anethole, borneol, cineole, methyl chavicol, methyl cinnamate, estragol, eucalyptol, eugenol, linalool, ocimeme, safrole anticancer, antibacterial, inhibits blood clots, lowers blood sugar, expectorant, carminative
Benin pepper vine/fruit	*Piper guineense* Schnm. & Thonn.	Piperaceae	TAf	β-caryophyllene, cubebeme, germacrene, limonene, piperine antitumor, antifungal, analgesic, carminative, anti-inflammatory, antioxidant
Black pepper, white pepper vine/fruit	*Piper nigrum* L.	Piperaceae	TAs	β-bisabolene, camphene, myristicin, phellandrene, pinene, piperidine, piperine, safrol antibacterial, antifungal, expectorant, lowers blood pressure, diuretic, carminative, anti-inflammatory, antioxidant
Caraway herb/seed	*Carum carvi* L.	Umbelliferae	NEA	carvone, carveol, limonene antibacterial, antifungal, carminative, antispasmodic, anticancer
Celery seed herb/seed	*Apium graveolens* L.	Umbelliferae	Med	apiogenin, apiin, bergapten, celereodise, delerin, glycolic acid, limonene, phthalides, β-selinene, umbelliferone bacteriostatic, antifungal, inhibits blood clots, anti-inflammatory, lowers blood pressure, carminative, antispasmodic, lowers serum glucose, diuretic, antitumor
Chile	*Capsicum annuum* L.	Solanaceae	TAm	capsaicin, capsanthin, capsicidin, capxanthin, carotene, ferredoxin, solanine, scopoletin antibacterial; lowers serum triglycerides, stimulates lipid mobilization from fat tissue; carminative; increases blood flow to skin; antiulcer; diminishes cluster headache; counter-irritant for rheumatism, arthritis, neuralgia, and lumbago; antioxidant, anti-inflammatory
Cinnamon tree/bark	*Cinnamomum zeylanicum* Blume	Lauraceae	TAs	cinnamaldehyde, eugenol, methylhydroxy chalcone, pinene, safrole, linalool, tannins antibacterial, antiviral, antifungal, antiseptic, antihelminthic, carminative, antispasmodic, anti-diarrheal, inhibits blood clots, antipyretic

(Continued)

Appendix (Continued)

English name[a]	Genus species	Family	Origin[b]	Constituents and activities[c]
Clove tree/flower bud	*Syzygium aromaticum* (L.) Merr. & Perry	Myrtaceae	TAs	campestrol, eugenol, eugenin, pinene, sitosterol, stigmasterol, vanillin antibacterial, antiviral, fungistatic, antihelminthic, carminative, anti-inflammatory, inhibits blood clots, antispasmodic, anticancer, anti-emetic, trypsin potentiating, lowers blood sugar, analgesic
Fennel herb/leaf, seed	*Foeniculum vulgare* Miller	Umbelliferae	NEA	anethole, camphone, dillapianol, estragole, fenchone, limonene, pinene antimicrobial, carminative, antispasmodic, estrogenic, expectorant
Fenugreek herb/leaf, seed	*Trigonella foenum-graecum* L.	Fabaceae	Med	coumarin, disogenin, fenugreekine, tigogenin, trigonelline antiviral, lowers serum cholesterol, lowers blood pressure, anticancer, lowers blood sugar
Flower pepper shrub, tree/fruit	*Zanthoxylum zanthoxyloides* Lam., Z. spp.	Rutaceae	TAf	phenylethanoid derivative, fagaramide, fagaronine, hesperidin, zanthoxylol antisickling, antioxidant, antifungal, tumor inhibition, antibacterial
Galangal herb/rhizome	*Alpinia officinarum* Hance	Zingiberaceae	TAs	cineole, linalool, galangol, galangin, α-pinene antibacterial, antifungal, carminative, antitumor, antiulcer
Garlic herb/bulb	*Allium sativum* L.	Liliaceae	NFA	ajoene, allicin, alliin, alliinase, s-allylmercaptocysteine, citral, diallyl sulfide, geraniol, linalool, α- and β-phellandrene, prostaglandins, scordinins antibacterial, antifungal, antiviral; lowers serum cholesterol, serum triglycerides, and low density lipoproteins; increases high-density lipoproteins; blocks aortic lipid deposition; lowers blood pressure; antihepatotoxic; antineoplastic; stimulates immune system; decreases blood sugar; inhibits blood clots
Ginger herb/rhizome	*Zingiber officinale* Roscoe	Zingiberaceae	TAs	β-bisabolene, galanolactone, geraniol, gingerol, gingerdione, shogaol, zingerone, zingiberine antimicrobial, antihelminthic, carminative, antinausea, stomachic, lowers blood sugar, antiulcer, decreases serum cholesterol, inhibits blood clots, antioxidant, anti-inflammatory
Guinea pepper tree/fruit	*Xylopia aethiopica* (Dunal) A. Rich	Annonaceae	TAf	carene, linalool, imonene, myrcene, phellandrene, pinene, thujene, xylopic acid antibacterial, antimalarial
Horseradish herb/root	*Armoracia rusticana* P. Gaertner, Meyer & Scherb.	Brassicaceae	NFA	ally-thiocyanate, asparagine, gluconasturtiin, glucosinolates, peroxidase enzymes, scopoletin, sinigrin antibacterial, antispasmodic, lowers blood pressure, carcinostatic
Lemongrass herb/leaf	*Cymbopogon citratus* (Nees) Stapf.	Poaceae	TAs	citral, geraniol, limolene, pinene, perpineole antibacterial, analgesic, antipyretic, antioxidant, uterine stimulant
Licorice shrub/ rhizome, root	*Glycyrrhiza glabra* L.	Fabaceae	Med	asparagin, eugenol, glycyrin, glabrin, glabridin, glabrol, glycyrrhizin, indole, licoricone, linalool, umbelliferone antibacterial, antiviral, anti-inflammatory, antihepatotoxic, inhibits blood clots, antiulcer, antispasmodic, expectorant, laxative
Long pepper vine/fruit	*Piper longum* L.	Piperaceae	TAs	β-caryophyllene, β-bisabolene, pentadecane, piperine amoebicidal, bactericidal, antifungal, carminative, anti-inflammatory, antioxidant
Mace, nutmeg tree/fruit	*Myristica fragrans* Houtt.	Myristicaceae	TAs	camphene, dipentene, elincin, eugenol, geraniol, linalool, myristicin, α- and β-pinenes, safrole antimicrobial, antioxidant, antitumor, carminative, reduces cholesterol, diuretic, inhibits blood clots
Melegueta pepper herb/fruit	*Aframomum melegueta* Schumann	Zingiberaceae	TAf	caryophyllene, gingerol, humulene, paradols, shogaol, zingerone antibacterial, antifungal, anti-schistosomal
Oregano herb/leaf	*Origanum vulgare* L.	Labiatae	NEA	β-bisabolene, cavracrol, p-cymene, linalool, rosamarinic acid, thymol antibacterial, antifungal, anticancer, antioxidant, antihepatotoxic

(Continued)

Appendix *(Continued)*

English name[a]	Genus species	Family	Origin[b]	Constituents and activities[c]
Star anise tree/fruit	*Illicium verum* Hook f.	Illiciaceae	TAs	anethole, anisic acid, methyl chavicol, cineole, estragole, nerolidol, perpineol, phellandrene, safrole, salicylic acid antimicrobial, neurotropic, carminative, relieves respiratory inflammation, expectorant, estrogenic
Tamarind tree/fruit pulp	*Tamarindus indica* L.	Fabaceae	TAf	geranial, geraniol, limonene, methyl salicylate, safrole, tamarindienal, tartaric acid antioxidant, carminative, laxative, antischistosomal, antifungal, antibacterial
Thonningia parasitic herb/ flower	*Thonningia sanguinea* Vahl.	Balanophoraceae	TAf	thonningianins a and b antioxidant, antibacterial, anti-anaphylactic, antihepatotoxic
Turmeric herb/rhizome	*Curcuma longa* L.	Zingiberaceae	TAs	curcumin, turmerin, turmerone, ukonan c, zingiberen antibacterial, antifungal, anti-inflammatory, antihepatotoxic, antioxidant, antitumor, estrogenic, lowers cholesterol, anti-venom, lowers blood sugar, stimulates immune system
Vanilla liane/seed pod	*Vanilla planifolia* Jackson	Orchidaceae	TAm	anisic acid, caffeic acid, catechin, guaiacol, vanillin anticariogenic, antioxidant, antibacterial, antiyeast, antimutagenic, liver protective
Wasabi herb/root, stem	*Wasabia japonica* (Miq) Matsum.	Brassicaceae	NEA	chitinase, hevein, isothicyanate antibacterial, antifungal, anticancer, inhibits blood clots
Wormseed herb/leaf	*Chenopodium ambrosioides* L.	Chenopodiaceae	TAm	ascaridole, p-cymene, geraniol, hydroperoxides, limonene, myrcene, methyl salicylate, pinene, spinasterol, urease antihelminthic, antifungal, trypanocidal, amoebicidal, diuretic

a. Growth form, habit/plant part is shown after the name.

b. TAs, tropical Asia; TAm, American tropics; Med, Mediterranean/Middle East/North Africa: NEA. northern/temperate Europe and Asia: TAf, tropical West Africa.

c. Information is complied from Duke (1985). Galal (1996), Newall et al. (1996). Hirasa and Takemasa (1998), Gyamfi et al. (2000), Morimitsu et al. (2000), Kwon et al. (2002), Chaaib et al. (2003), Kiba et al. (2003), Research and Editorial Staff (2003), Walton et al. (2003).

CHAPTER 30

Coping with a Nutrient Deficiency: Cultural Models of Vitamin A Deficiency in Northern Niger

Lauren S. Blum, Gretel H. Pelto, and Pertti J. Pelto

(2004)

The importance of vitamin A deficiency as a public health problem in developing countries has become increasingly evident. Thirty years ago it was recognized as a cause of permanent blindness, which affected a small proportion of children (the most malnourished) in all developing countries. Then it was found to be responsible for up to 50 percent of child deaths in some communities (Beaton et al. 1993). Recent evidence documents the negative consequences of nightblindness in pregnancy, which is a sign of an early stage of the deficiency (Christian 2000; Christian et al. 2000). This paper presents the results of an ethnographic study of vitamin A deficiency in a Hausa community in northern Niger, in which we sought to understand local people's explanations of the signs and symptoms of vitamin A deficiencies, their beliefs about the etiology of these problems, and their management strategies for dealing with them. From a theoretical perspective we were particularly interested in how local knowledge of the stages of the deficiency is organized. From a practical perspective we wanted to understand how the cultural "explanatory models" affected household management strategies, including utilization of alternative care resources in the community.

We set out to examine the Hausa peoples' cultural belief systems (explanatory models) concerning the signs and symptoms of vitamin A deficiency in order to relate these models to the Sahelian ecological setting of West Africa. The physical environment and economic marginality of the Hausa make them highly vulnerable to periodic nutritional deficiencies as there is a continuing degradation of food production in the area in addition to sharp seasonal changes in food availability. Also, their cultural models concerning biomedically defined "vitamin A deficiency symptoms" are of both practical and theoretical importance. This is because the various manifestations of vitamin A deficiency,

especially as they affect the eyes, constitute a connected system of causality in the biomedical and nutritional sciences, yet these ocular manifestations would seem to be difficult to place within a single theoretical model on the basis of direct experience alone. Thus, understanding the make-up of cultural model(s) concerning the range of these visual/ocular problems can provide clues as to how cultural knowledge concerning health and illness problems is constructed from peoples' direct experiences within ecological settings of food scarcity.

The term "explanatory model" was introduced by Kleinman (1980:105–106) to refer to individuals' culturally constructed ideas about the etiology, symptom patterns, expected or appropriate treatments, and expectations of outcomes, of specific illness events. As pointed out by Kleinman and other medical anthropologists, individual explanatory models draw on various elements of "cultural models" currently available in given communities. Mattingly and Garro (1994; cf. Rubel and Hass 1990) have pointed out that individuals' explanations of illness episodes (i.e., individual explanatory models) tend to be highly congruent with the main lines of illness concepts and ideas indigenous to their local communities. On the other hand, due to differences in specific illness experiences, differential access to local knowledge, and other factors there are local intracommunity variations.

Many researchers (e.g., Beine 2003; Mattingly and Garro 1994; Ross et al. 2002) have used the concepts of "cultural models" and "explanatory models" interchangeably, as do we. This linking of individual cognitive processes and products with group cultural knowledge underscores our theoretical assumption that individuals' problem-solving, as it relates to illnesses and other matters, is generally a social, interactional process that draws on elements of cultural information and understandings currently available within their respective social networks. This model coincides with that of Strauss and Quinn (1997), who state, with regard to explanatory processes (assigning meaning to things and events), that these "states [meanings] are produced through the interaction of two sorts of relatively stable structures: intrapersonal, mental structures (which we will also call "schemas" or "understandings" or "assumptions") and

Lauren S. Blum, Gretel H. Pelto, and Pertti J. Pelto, "Coping with nutrient deficiency: cultural models of vitamin A deficiency in northern Niger." *Medical Anthropology* 23 (2004):195–227. Reprinted with permission.

extrapersonal, world structures. The relative stability of the world and our schemas has the effect that both in a given person and in a group of people who share a way of life, more or less the same meanings arise over and over" (6). Beine (2003) has recently used the same conceptual framework for examining cultural models of HIV/AIDS in Nepal.

In this conceptual framework it is useful to identify the individual components, or "building blocks," for cultural models. Above, Strauss and Quinn refer to those components as "schemas" ("schemata" in Beine's usage). Specific schemas concerning illnesses would include the various individual explanations of causality, categorizations of signs/symptoms, varieties of alternative treatments and healers, and many other broad or narrow concepts. All or most of the schemas, or understandings, about illness are likely to be "common cultural property" in small communities sharing similar life experiences. On the other hand, intragroup variation in explanatory models comes about from unique individual experiences as well as from the use of differing processes when combining and constructing explanations of individual events and circumstances.

For example, in the case of experiences of nightblindness due to vitamin A deficiency, some individuals may have lighter workloads and very little inconvenience, while others (e.g., pregnant women caring for small children or living in poorer households) may have to deal with demanding family obligations and inadequate lighting, causing serious disturbance. Such differences can lead to different constructions of "severity" and other elements of explanatory models. Also, due to physiological (including genetic) differences, in practically all types of illness there is considerable variation in the severity of individual symptoms.

In our theory of illness and treatment-seeking behavior we do not, of course, assume that ideational cultural models are the sole, or even the main, causes of individual actions. Many researchers have pointed out that, for example, treatment-seeking behaviors depend very much on economic resources, attitudes, and cooperative family members as well as on another very important variable—the accessibility of various health care facilities.

Returning to the schemas, or components, of cultural models of illness, many of the crucially important strands of information are simply not available to societies that lack the technology, or transmitted knowledge, to deal with bacteria, viruses, micronutrients, and other significant agents involved in pathologies. People who have no apparatus for "seeing" micro-organisms might stumble on effective treatment through some sort of trial and error, but not because they have schemas for constructing a notion of germ theory with regard to specific illnesses. As pointed out by Alland (1970:117) in his presentation of an ecological approach to the study of human health and illness, some pathological conditions are more amenable than are others to empirical, pragmatic analysis. Allard stated, "where symptoms are clear-cut and diseases fairly common, many societies have developed a consistent set of treatments specific to the symptoms themselves." In such cases the treatments are more likely to be effective, and decisions about remedial actions somewhat easier to take, provided the medicines or other remedies are locally available and affordable.

Schemas involved in human health and illness come in various sizes and levels of generality. Concepts of "hot" and "cold" are widespread throughout Latin America (Rubel and Hass 1990) as well as many other parts of the world (Leslie 1998). Individual symptoms, illnesses, medications, foods, and other things are classified to varying extent as "hot/heaty" or the opposite. Thus the "hot-cold" schema provides an explanatory component for a very wide range of human illnesses and conditions. At a much more specific level, certain individual foods and bodily symptoms may be considered as "heaty" or "cold," depending on localized experiences and usages.

In some societies various forms of witchcraft, "ill winds," "evil eye," and other "supernatural" schemas play a very large role in cultural models of illness (Blanchet 1984; Dillon-Malone 1988; Lepowsky 1990; Stone 1988). Alland (1970) pointed out that, where such broad schemas are pervasive and where diagnosis of illness is very feebly related to specific signs and symptoms, people are unlikely to develop truly effective empirical treatments of illnesses.

The analysis of cultural models of HIV/AIDS in recent literature is important because it illustrates an oft-neglected phenomenon—the social connotations and stigmatization attached to specific illnesses. As Beine and others have pointed out, stigmatization can have direct consequences for individual treatment-seeking as well as for preventive behaviors. The dynamics of stigmatizing schemas in the case of HIV/AIDS corresponds to what Nichter (1994) has referred to as "connotative aspects of illness." The more recent studies of cultural models have therefore expanded the scope and definition of "explanatory models" of illnesses beyond the denotative meanings upon which a biomedical perspective usually focuses.

We include a discussion of explanatory models of HIV/AIDS here because its extreme contrast with our discussion of vitamin A deficiency highlights some important features of explanatory models. The case of HIV/AIDS is perhaps the most extreme example of a pathology for which the direct experiences of individuals provide scant clues about the causes or sources. The time from initial infection to the first signs of illness is usually several years. Therefore, throughout the world, people have been introduced to a social and cultural construction of HIV/AIDS that is very largely imposed from the outside—that is, through mass media news and HIV/AIDS intervention campaigns. Programs designed to raise awareness of HIV/AIDS began by introducing the name of the illness, explaining the pathways of transmission, and then emphasizing ways of preventing the spread of HIV.

When a specific local population receives such "awareness information" from the outside world, local cultural schemas are invoked to integrate the new information into existing explanatory models. In the United States, the first explanatory models led to the label "gay disease," while in

Haiti, HIV/AIDS came to be attached to the concept of voo-doo (Farmer 1994). Beine (2003) states that, in the context of Nepal, the cultural model of HIV/AIDS was constructed from a combination of traditionally available cultural elements (schemas) concerning serious illnesses plus strong inputs from externally directed mass media campaigns. He points out that, in Nepal, "the strong association of AIDS with sex has activated the traditional randi (promiscuity) schema" (281). Beine believes that the randi schema, as part of the explanatory model, is a major factor in the stigmatizing of individuals infected (or believed to be infected) with HIV. He examined the ways in which several main elements from traditional explanatory schemas developed into the full-blown cultural model of HIV/AIDS in Nepal.

The construction of HIV/AIDS cultural models in different societies is an extreme example of a very widespread phenomenon. In all social groups today the construction of understandings about illnesses involves a combination of local cultural ideas and new kinds of information from the wider world. In the case of the Hausa of Niger, all cultural models of health problems include some reflection of the availability of Western cosmopolitan medical services. Practically everywhere in the world, health care involves pluralistic systems, with the result that explanatory models nearly always include schemas concerning treatment-seeking at government clinics or hospitals, or with private allopathic practitioners, as well as criteria for turning to traditional healers or home remedies.

Our study of cultural models of the signs/symptoms of vitamin A deficiency is therefore related to macro influences at two levels: (1) the broader economic and ecological environments that strongly influence food availability and periodic shortages, and (2) the complex interactions of local traditional health care with externally developed cosmopolitan medical concepts and treatment.

VITAMIN A DEFICIENCY

Vitamin A deficiency produces diverse health problems, including visual difficulties of progressive severity, from nightblindness to the ulceration of the eye and permanent blindness. It also increases the severity of infectious disease episodes and the risk of child mortality (Sommer and West 1996). These effects on the progress of infections have only been recognized in recent years and have been much more difficult to isolate than have the more directly observable effects on the eyes.

The only dietary sources of preformed vitamin A are found in animal sources (e.g., eggs, milk, liver, fish oils), with the highest concentrations in animal livers. Many plant foods contain carotenoids, some of which are precursors that are converted into vitamin A in the body (Parker 1996). In the rest of this article, both foods with preformed vitamin A and those with high levels of vitamin A precursors are referred to as vitamin A-rich foods.

In this study we focused on the following signs and symptoms of vitamin A deficiency: nightblindness and

corneal lesions referred to as Bitot's spots. As background for interpreting the cultural management of vitamin A deficiency, it is important to differentiate between moderate vitamin A deficiency and the stages of xerophthalmia that represent more severe deficiencies. Generally, the first ocular symptom is maladaptation to dim light, commonly known as nightblindness (Sommer and West 1996). This affliction most often occurs among poorly nourished women during pregnancy and in young children, among whom physiological demands are particularly high. As the deficiency progresses, more severe forms of eye damage, which are less common, appear in the form of corneal lesions, the first stage of which is referred to as Bitot's spots. The progression from corneal lesions to irreversible corneal destruction (including extrusion of the eyeball) can occur very rapidly, particularly when a severe infectious disease, such as measles, results in rapid depletion of marginal vitamin A stores (Sommer and West 1996).

Although severe xerophthalmia is irreversible, the milder ocular symptoms can be reversed very rapidly (in as little as four hours) when individuals ingest preformed vitamin A (Sommer and West 1996). The action of vitamin A in reversing, as well as in preventing, nightblindness and eye lesions, occurs in the gut, where retinol is bound to a retinol-binding protein, which permits its transport to cells.

A high prevalence of ocular manifestations of vitamin A deficiency in a population is an indicator of severe environmental constraints and economic deprivation, and it is associated with high rates of childhood malnutrition and mortality. In areas of chronic low dietary intakes of vitamin A-rich foods, prevalence rates of deficiency are expected to be high, especially among women of reproductive age and young children. For example, studies conducted in rural Nepal found that nightblindness affected 10 to 20 percent of pregnant and lactating women and up to 13 percent of preschool children (Katz et al. 1995; WHO/UNICEF 1995). Xerophthalmia, the condition produced by severe vitamin A deficiency, tends to cluster within the poorest regions and districts in developing countries, and it is the poorest segments of populations that have the highest risks of severe deficiencies (Beaton 1993; Katz et al. 1993).

Vitamin A deficiencies can also show marked seasonal variations, corresponding to periods of food shortages, epidemics of childhood illnesses, and outbreaks of warfare (which bring about scarcity of foods). When food sources of vitamin A are inadequate body reserves are subsequently depleted, and insufficient stores can be further compromised by illness. In Mali, where clinical vitamin A deficiency is a significant problem, epidemiological studies have shown that seasonal variation in the magnitude and degree of vitamin A deficiency is associated with cyclical changes in vitamin A intake in the diet and disease trends (Resnikoff 1996). In northern regions there is a significant correlation between the length of the dry season and the prevalence of xerophthalmia (Resnikoff, personal communication, October 1997).

Plotting the geographical distribution of xerophthalmia shows that clinical vitamin A deficiency is most prevalent in Southeast Asia and Sub-Saharan Africa, accounting for approximately 90 percent of global subclinical and clinical vitamin A deficiency (Underwood 1997). In Africa, the combination of measles with depleted vitamin A stores is reported to be responsible for as high as 40 percent of childhood blindness, and it constitutes a clinical public health problem in all of the countries spanning the Sahelian strip of Africa (Hussey and Klein 1990; Foster and Yorston 1992). Since 1987 Niger, where our study was conducted, has been on a list of countries in which vitamin A deficiency represents a public health problem (WHO/IVACG/UNICEF 1988).

THE RESEARCH SITE

The research was carried out in the land-locked country of Niger, located in the Sahelian region of West Africa. At the time the study was conducted, approximately 85 percent of the population of Niger was living in rural areas. Rural populations in the north are primarily nomadic herders, while the southern portion of the country is comprised of more sedentary, crop-growing communities. In many parts of Niger cyclical droughts, rapid desertification, and general ecological degradation, accelerated by demographic pressures, are forcing agricultural activities into low rainfall zones. Agricultural communities in the marginal areas are particularly vulnerable to unpredictable harvests and periodic food deficits. In addition, a sharp decline in world uranium prices—which in the past provided significant revenue for Niger—has had deleterious effects on the national economy. These factors, along with recent political instability, contribute to Niger's present ranking among the poorest nations in the world.

The study site, Filili[1] is a Hausa-speaking, predominantly Islamic community that borders the Sahelian ecological zone. This is a northern pastoral region where annual rainfall averages 200 to 300 millimeters. Historical records give evidence of a complex framework of social relations and economic interactions among the Fulani pastoralists, Tuarag nomadic traders, and the Hausa farming populations living in this agro-pastoral zone (Fuglestad 1983). Exceptional harvests in the first half of the 20th century earned Filili a designation as one of the millet granaries of the country. However, there are also records suggesting that the area has been subjected to cyclical droughts that periodically resulted in widespread famine. During the lean periods the inhabitants suffered serious health problems, and many people migrated, at least temporarily, to the more southerly regions, out of the famine-stricken area. Today, village elders make frequent references to the dramatic changes in the local ecology that have transpired over the past three decades as desert conditions gradually encroach on the land.

Filili is located 185 kilometers north of the capital city and is the county seat and the home of a number of government offices. At the time the study was conducted (1993–94) the community consisted of 17 quartiers (neighborhoods) and four adjoining villages, with a total population of 19,525. The residential area, which is transected by a paved road, is bounded by government buildings to the south and a market and commercial district located at the northernmost part of the town. Local leadership falls under the traditional chief, or Sarki, who is accountable to regional and national officials. The Sarki's role includes the collection of taxes, resolution of disputes, and participation in ritual ceremonies. Each neighborhood is comprised of clusters of household compounds characterized by similarities in ethnic background, occupation group, and socioeconomic status. The neighborhoods have a traditional political structure ruled by a berama (neighborhood chief) who reports to the Sarki.

The gida, which is translated as "household," or "compound," is the central unit of social organization in Hausa culture (Wall 1988). The gida refers to the housing structure as well as the patrilineal kinsmen who reside in the dwelling. Following traditional Hausa practices, residential complexes in Filili are often comprised of a central courtyard with small adobe houses or adjoining rooms on the periphery, and the compound is surrounded by a mud wall. Interspersed among the larger compounds are families living in one-room, straw-roofed, round huts—an indication of poor economic conditions. Quarters located on the outskirts of town consist mainly of these one-room huts and frequently are not protected by the traditional Hausa wall that separates households and affords a level of privacy.

The Food System and Health Care Resources in Filili

Filili is primarily a farming community, although some local people are employed in government offices. The harsh economic environment precludes self-sufficient grain production as a realistic aim for the poorer farmers in the community. Seasonal variability in precipitation and low frequency of rainfall prevents farmers from attaining the production levels necessary even for subsistence, and periodic drought causes further deterioration of the land and decreases the potential for food production. As a result, a large percentage of farming families are forced each year to migrate to the neighboring bush areas for six or seven months to cultivate the land and harvest crops. Paradoxically, as the ecological situation has progressively eroded over the past few decades, impoverishment has prevented farmers from extricating themselves from farming as their primary means of producing food and income. Increases in migration rates to coastal countries and to Burkina Faso during the off-season is particularly prevalent among the most vulnerable economic groups, who have less capital and fewer cash-earning opportunities (Sutter 1982).

In this northern zone, where Fulani pastoralists spend most of the year grazing herds, the Hausa farmers also invest in domestic animals. The wealthier families own cows, but poorer families can only afford to maintain small ruminants such as sheep and goats to minimize risks of food scarcity. Over recent years, the region reports large losses of both small and large livestock, which is concomitant with the end of the hot season and the onset of the rains. Apparently, when grazing becomes restricted and foliage is meager, animals reach a low nutritional state and the most vulnerable of them cannot support the dramatic drop in temperature that comes with the first rains.

Both economic and environmental factors limit food availability and the consumption of a variety of foods in Filili, where chronic dietary deficiency exists and general nutrition is poor. Although historically dairy products and meat were central to the diet, the majority of residents are unable to afford the regular consumption of these highly valued foods (the exception is the skimmed milk used in hura, a millet-based drink that comprises an essential component of the daily diet). Most residents must rely heavily on cereals and tubers during the summer months, when millet stores are depleted and market costs are high. Fresh fruits and vegetables are imported from southern regions in small quantities, but these items are costly and only available seasonally, so they play only a small role in local diets. In addition to the food produced through farming, most families must purchase staples in the weekly market and from vendors and shops. People also rely on a range of edible wild plants, which women collect in the surrounding bush.

The best sources of vitamin A-rich foods are expensive and are viewed as luxury foods. On market days the male household head may purchase grilled meat, including pieces of liver, which are distributed among family members. Foods that make up a larger percentage of vitamin A in the local diet include essential sauce ingredients such as indigenous green leaves and pumpkin and maize (which is commonly consumed as an alternative to the staple millet). While small quantities of drumstick tree, baobab, or red sorrel leaves are added to the sauce on a daily basis, women and children also eat the snack food kupto, a popular mixture made of green leafy vegetables, ground peanuts, oil, onion, and spices. When in season, mangoes, which are eaten as a special snack, provide an important source of vitamin A.

A pronounced feature of the diet is seasonal variation. The soudure, or hungry months, when both food supplies and money are scarce, occur during the most physically demanding time of year. This is between June and September, when people are preparing for the harvest. During this period of privation many people must reduce food intake and resort to a more monotonous dietary regime, consisting of less valued foods and often dominated by dried cassava and a diluted version of the traditional millet drink.

Health Resources

The Hausa medical system in Niger is characterized by medical pluralism. This system encompasses a range of resources, from biomedically trained personnel working at the government medical center, marabouts, bokas, and wazami, to self-treatment, and it can involve the use of two or more health care options concurrently. At the time of this study, two physicians were attached to the government health center in Filili. The rest of the staff working in the health facility included trained midwives, registered nurses, nurse assistants, and social workers.

Marabouts, who are holy men and Koranic teachers, are also recognized as health providers. They are solicited to restore relationships between humans and the supernatural by treating illnesses perceived as potentially inflicted by Allah. To administer treatment, the marabouts typically consult the Koran for guidance. They locate appropriate passages from the Koran, which they write on wooden slates with black ink. The wood is then cleansed with water and the individual seeking care consumes the prayer water. In all cases, treatment can only be successful with Allah's approval.

Bokas, who work primarily as herbalists, are known to treat inexplicable health conditions, such as convulsions or mental and physical handicaps, that are attributed to iska, spirits believed to possess mystical powers. In Filili, the title of boka also refers to someone who practices sorcery. In order to remedy these conditions, the boka must exorcise the spirits.

Wazami (barbers) work from their homes, or roam the streets offering services. They may also be summoned to family compounds. In addition to cutting hair and shaving beards, their repertoire of services includes bloodletting, male circumcision, scarification, uvulectomy, and the removal of a hypertrophied hymen. Wazami are considered to be experts in determining blood status and in identifying illness associated with "bad" or "old" blood.

In general, home treatments for illness draw on a range of alternatives, including dietary or herbal remedies or the use of local goods or resources known to counteract the principal cause of the illness. In markets and stores a diverse range of inexpensive pharmaceuticals can be purchased, including so-called "panaceas" from Nigeria and medicines from Europe and the United States, often with expired "use-by" dates. These are touted as all-purpose remedies for a wide range of symptoms and ailments, including malaria, colds, diarrhea and dysentery, general fatigue, various aches and pains, and sexual dysfunction.

RESEARCH METHODS

This research was part of a larger cross-cultural study carried out in six different countries (Blum et al. 1997; Kuhnlein and Pelto 1997). The fieldwork took place in a series of five two-month sessions over a 14-month period in 1993–94. The research schedule permitted us to capture seasonal food variation that might affect vitamin A deficiency as well as household economic fluctuations reflecting work schedules and influencing food intake.

The research strategy included a mix of qualitative and quantitative methods. The first step of data gathering involved interviewing key informants in order to explore the topical domain of vitamin-rich foods and to collect local terminology related to vitamin A deficiency. Key informants were interviewed throughout the duration of the research process, providing primary data on cultural interpretations of vitamin A deficiency. Interviews were conducted with experienced mothers who had raised several children, with other primary caretakers (including grandmothers), and with fathers of preschool children. A variety of health providers were also interviewed to ascertain their views on illness categories, illness causation, and treatment practices.

Hypothetical case scenarios were used as a technique to elicit local knowledge and attitudes about ocular signs associated with vitamin A deficiency and to identify perspectives about treatment alternatives and preferred sources of care. The case scenarios were constructed from information provided by key informants and were pilot tested several times to ensure relevance and appropriateness in the local context.

Case scenarios were employed to obtain the following data: (1) terminology and concepts related to signs and symptoms of clinical vitamin A deficiency and the illnesses with which they are associated; (2) beliefs surrounding the etiology of symptoms and expectations concerning their progression; (3) home remedies used to prevent or treat the range of ocular manifestations; (4) health resources available in the community for treatment of vitamin A deficiency and the anticipated treatment for nightblindness as well as a more advanced sign of xerophthalmia; (5) expected recovery time and evidence of improvement following treatment; (6) patterns of care-seeking for varying signs and symptoms; and (7) relevant considerations that influence choice and punctuality of treatment action. A limitation of the case scenario method is that the information provided in response to the scenario is likely to reflect perceptions of appropriate treatment rather than actual behavior. Ongoing interviews with key informants permitted us to validate data related to the connection between cultural knowledge and actual health-seeking actions. Additional supporting information came from case histories of individuals with past experiences of the symptoms of vitamin A deficiency.

The data gathering using hypothetical scenarios was carried out in a sample of 100 households. The sample was identified by designating every sixth household unit in a community map until the desired number of households with children between six months and six years of age was obtained. The full interview protocol was completed with 92 mothers. Mothers were selected as the designated respondents because they have the primary responsibility for meeting the basic needs of members of the household, including caring for sick children and selecting among therapeutic options. All of the interviews were carried out in Hausa by the senior author, usually with an accompanying local assistant.

During the structured interviews respondents were verbally presented with three scenarios, which were accompanied by visual aids prepared by a local artist to depict the storyline. Interviews lasted approximately one hour, and respondents were encouraged to give open-ended answers to questions. Concerning treatment options, they were asked which treatment they would use first and then what they would do if that failed to produce the desired results. If mothers felt that two different treatment strategies needed to occur concurrently, then this was noted in their response. The results presented below are based on the following scenarios: one each for nightblindness in a child and a pregnant woman, and one for a more severe form of vitamin A deficiency, which involves the development of a white spot in the conjunctiva (Bitot's spot) of a child.

The nightblindness scenario for a child is as follows:

> Adamou is three years old. He is a very active little boy who has many friends with whom he plays in the neighborhood. However, for the past week, as the day ends and the sun sets, Adamou chooses to quit playing with his friends. He just sits alone. He seems frustrated and sad and is afraid to move around. His mother, Amina, has noticed his recent inactivity at nightfall and wonders what should be done. What do you advise?

The scenario for a pregnant woman is as follows:

> Fati is seven months pregnant. She is more tired than she was during her first pregnancy and is finding it difficult to keep up with her 15-month-old son, Hamissou. Furthermore, as her pregnancy progresses, she has noticed that it has become impossible to see at night. As the sun sets, Fati is no longer able to continue the household chores, particularly preparation of the evening meal. Fati's husband, Abdou, expects the evening meal to be ready for him when he returns home from a long day of work. What is wrong with Fati? Do you have any advice for her?

The scenario for a more severe ocular sign of xerophthalmia in a child is:

> Ousmane is small for a five-year-old. He has had a very difficult childhood, suffering from continual bouts of diarrhea and malnutrition. Ousmane was sick with a fever and rash but he is now better. Yesterday, Ousmane's mother Saratou noticed a white foamy patch on the white part of his eye. This afternoon the white part of Ousmane's eye appears to be dry and the white foamy area has gotten bigger. Saratou recognizes that this is unusual but doesn't know what to do. What do you suggest?

FINDINGS

The interviews reveal that both nightblindness and more severe manifestations of vitamin A deficiency are known conditions in Filili. In the full sample of 92 households, approximately one-fourth of the respondents (26 of 92) reported experiences of past episodes of nightblindness, generally in pregnancy. Two of the young children in the study households had recently gone through episodes of nightblindness. One woman had lost sight in one eye at the age of five years, during a bout with measles, but none of the children in the current study households had suffered permanent loss of sight.

The biomedical sign that is glossed in English as "nightblindness" is widely referred to in Filili as dundumi. Table 1 presents the scenario results on the etiology of dundumi. Typical of the responses for the scenario on nightblindness in a young child was that of a woman who said that Adamou was suffering from dundumi, an affliction that she attributed to a diet deficient in essential foods. There was strong cultural consensus for food-related causes of dundumi in both children and women, and for the most part causation was formulated as a lack of "good foods." The missing dietary items included liver, red meat, dairy products, and dark green leafy vegetables. Within the context of nightblindness, these foods are known as magani dundumi (medicine for nightblindness). Dundumi is associated with chronic hunger and poverty. As a male informant explained, "People get this when they don't eat meat or when they don't drink milk. If people have animals they don't get this. If they have animals, they receive milk and this isn't a problem. But if they don't have animals and they don't have money, this can be a common problem." One woman suggested that nightblindness is also related to anago (a drastic change in the diet), which could be precipitated by a move to the bush or the abrupt removal of a critical component of the diet (such as breastmilk). She pointed out that "anango can give you eye problems." Another key informant stated, "If you don't feel hunger you don't get dundumi. Hunger gives dundumi."

The scenario of a pregnant woman with nightblindness elicited similar responses to those elicited for the young boy. Table 1 shows that 65 percent of respondents associated the condition with a deficient diet. Some respondents viewed the etiology of dundumi in pregnancy as directly related to the demands placed on the body during pregnancy, which

Table 1 Mothers' Perceptions of Causes of Nightblindness from Case Scenarios

Cause (a)	Nightblindness (%)	
	Three-year-old child (n=51)	Pregnant woman (n=57)
Food-related		
Lack of good food	71	65
Hunger	12	–
Insufficient blood-rich foods	4	–
Salt intake (b)	4	2
Insufficient vitamin-rich foods	2	–
Pregnancy-related		
Demands of pregnancy	–	20
Hard work in pregnancy (c)	–	8
Poor birth spacing	–	4
Other physical		
Over exposure to sun	10	4
Comes with rainy season	–	2
Blood fell into the eyes	5	2
Poor blood	4	2
Tiredness	2	–
Non-physical		
Evil spirit	2	2
Allah's will	2	–
Don't know	2	2

(a) Multiple responses were permitted.

(b) For a child, this was too little salt; for a pregnant woman, it was too much salt.

(c) Includes two responses for accumulated hardship of pregnancies.

can exacerbate the internal imbalance caused by a poor diet or hunger. In contrast to childhood, nightblindness in pregnancy is commonly perceived as a normal condition in the last trimester, and it is thought to be caused by the additional nutritional requirements of pregnancy combined with the strenuous physical rigors of women's daily work-loads. Although women viewed dundumi as a condition of pregnancy and believed it would disappear with deliv-ery, they stressed the importance of undertaking treatment quickly because the problem could interfere with their work responsibilities. They pointed out that male household heads would not be understanding if nightblindness—considered an innocuous condition—interfered with household duties, especially the evening food preparation. As the data in Table 1 demonstrate, spiritual or non-physical causes of dundumi are virtually absent from the etiological explanation for either children or pregnant women.

Respondents' answers concerning the etiology of the corneal lesions depicted in the scenario of a child with xerophthalmia are shown in Table 2. Respondents referred to the white spots of the corneal lesions with a descriptive phrase: furin cikin ido (white in the eye).

As seen in Table 2, 63 percent of the women attrib-uted furin cikin ido to duca (measles), which is associated with a high temperature and corashi (lesions). These lesions are thought to develop inside the body, from where they then enter the eye. One woman stated, "Duca gives this to children, it makes their eyes white." Twenty percent of the mother-respondents indicated that the child's condition was wahala tamoa, a phrase that draws attention to the hardship of malnutrition. Many respondents explained that poorly nourished children are more susceptible than are well nour-ished children to complications of duca, including eye signs. Moreover, women depicted a vicious cycle in which chil-dren suffering from measles refuse to eat, thus exacerbating their already weak state and inducing additional weight loss, which would often be accompanied by diarrhea.

In general, respondents linked furin cikin ido to "heat-producing" illnesses such as measles, diarrhea, and chickenpox. Older informants mentioned smallpox as a precursor to the eye conditions presented in the scenario. Heat-producing illnesses are believed to induce lesions inside the body, which can attack and "eat" away at the eye and potentially "ruin" one or both eyes. According to

Table 2 Mothers' Perceptions of Causes of a White Spot in the Child's Eye from Case Scenarios

Cause (a)	White spot in a young child's eye (%) (n=51)
Related to heat-producing and other childhood illnesses	
Measles	63
Malnutrition	20
Diarrhea	8
Diarrhea with malnutrition	6
Heat in the body	6
Chickenpox	2
Breastmilk-related	
Bad breastmilk	4
Mother lacked adequate breastmilk	2
Abrupt weaning from breastmilk	2
Child weaned early	2
Care-related	
Mother failed to care for child	2
Lack of cleanliness	2
Failed to get medicine quickly	2
Non-physical	
Allah's will	6
Evil spirit	2
General hardship	2
Don't know	2

(a) Multiple responses were permitted.

one informant, "Those children with lesions, with karambo (chickenpox) or duca, this can ruin their eyes. The lesions can go into the eyes and destroy them." Measles is considered the most lethal of these childhood illnesses and is widely recognized for its ability to create extreme heat, causing one or both eyes to close and leading to blindness. As a respondent explained, "We say that if a child gets duca, it is important to look into the eyes. We don't allow the eyes to close because if they close they will be ruined." A shut eye signals the degree to which the heat has engulfed the child and indicates potential deadly consequences. Signs of deterioration or closure of the eye are also an indication that the child's life is at risk. One respondent stated, "These problems can destroy the eyes and enter the body, killing the child."

Table 3 provides the results on first treatment recommendations. In the case of nightblindness, a majority of respondents recommended a food-related home remedy, often consisting of consuming grilled liver, dripping blood from the liver into the eyes, eating beef or goat meat, or eating green leaves, particularly baobab and red sorrel leaves. Eighty-one percent of mother-respondents recommended an indigenous food remedy for a child, while 64 percent gave this as their first recommendation for a pregnant woman. The most common recommendation with regard to a food remedy involved the ingestion of grilled liver. For example, one respondent explained, "When we have dundumi, we buy grilled liver that has not been cooked long. We take a piece of liver and bite into it. This transmits the goodness in the blood of the liver to the eyes. We next take two pieces of liver and place them on the eye—the juice or blood goes into the eyes, dissipating bad blood that has collected. We then eat the remaining liver."

Because the blood in the liver is considered critical to treatment, respondents insisted that the liver should not be overcooked. Women specified that the liver is to be consumed only by the individual suffering from the affliction (which is highly unusual in this culture, where sharing is essential to survival). Five respondents proposed that grilled liver simply be placed on the eye so that it could absorb the bad blood, and a few specified that blood from the liver should be consumed. Other recommended dietary remedies included beef, mutton, or intestines. Some respondents suggested that, if the family could not afford meat, then leaves of baobab, red sorrel, bean, or horseradish could be given. Women referred to dark green leaves as magani talaka—medicine for poor people who, in this instance, were suffering from nightblindness.

While most respondents simply recommended the consumption of mounds of boiled leaves mixed with oil and onions, others provided more elaborate advice concerning ritual components. For example, one informant described the following remedy: "Here we cook surre [red sorrel], put it in a dish and put the dish in a room at prayer hour when the sun is setting and there is little light. We allow the person with dundumi to seek out the dish in the dark. When she finds the dish she puts it near her eyes so that the wind from the leaves gets into the eyes. Afterwards that person is supposed to eat the leaves." She indicated that the procedure should be repeated one or two times and that the container should hold the equivalent of about six cups of leaves. She also emphasized that the leaves are not to be shared. She continued, "All of this is from lame [a deficient intake of 'good' foods] or rishin ci nama [not eating meat]. They don't eat good foods like meat and oil, and this leads to rishin ganiwa [not being able to see]. Lame comes with wahala [hardship]. When we don't have millet we get wahala. When we are full we don't have wahala."

Respondents who recommended a food-related home remedy expected the treatment to reverse the symptoms. Women have such confidence in the therapeutic properties of food remedies that, if a dietary therapy does not cure the nightblindness within a few days, then they presume that the affliction has been misdiagnosed. It is also noteworthy

Table 3 Mothers' Suggestions for Initial Treatment from Case Scenarios

Treatment	Nightblindness in a three-year-old child (%) (n=57)	Nightblindness in a pregnant woman (%) (n=58)	White spot in the eye of a young child (%) (n=54)
Home food remedy	81	64	–
Dispensary	11	29	52
Concurrent home remedy/dispensary	5	3	2
Mother should eat better	2	–	–
Capsule from store	–	2	–
Boka	–	2	4
Marabout	–	–	5
Home non-food remedy	–	–	37
Nothing to do	1	–	2

that older people and younger women who had moved into Filili from the bush (where there is less food variety) had a greater appreciation for and knowledge of the therapeutic properties of indigenous foods and exhibited a more profound understanding of the deficiency than did those who had not lived in the bush.

As is also apparent from Table 3, while, for the majority of women we interviewed, food-based remedies are clearly the first treatment choice for dundumi (nightblindness), some respondents said they would turn to the dispensary for help. The dispensary was a more attractive first option for the pregnant woman with dundumi than for the child with dundumi. No respondent recommended a traditional healer for a child, and only two respondents felt that a boka should be the first recourse for the pregnant woman.

In contrast, for the case scenario featuring a child with furin cikin ido (a white spot in the eye), half of the respondents recommended that the boy be taken for biomedical care, while 37 percent indicated that his condition required a non-food based home treatment. Those women who advised that care be sought at the dispensary based their advice on the seriousness of the problem, the superiority of eye medication available through the government health structure, and the ability of health personnel to diagnose eye problems. On the other hand, the mothers who elected to administer therapy at home prioritized treating measles and its accompanying fever with one of many indigenous remedies, none of which involved the ingestion of food. Specific treatment for the eye problem was viewed primarily as an important strategy to save the eye, secondary to curing the underlying illness. A protective measure involves placing freshly sliced onions around the eyes or on the eyelids of a child with measles: the stinging sensation prevents the eye from closing, forcing exposure to colder air and thus saving the eye. As an informant explained, "People say that if there is no water in the eye, if it dries up, the eye will close and the eye will be lost. Because of this, when the eye has problems, they try to keep the eye open."

To elicit information on what to do if the first treatment failed to bring about a satisfactory solution, another set of questions was asked, following the procedure utilized by Young (1980). As shown in Table 4, when responding to questions on dundumi, the most popular second choice if the first strategy failed was the dispensary. It is only after food remedies or the dispensary have not produced results that some respondents suggested that the help of a traditional healer should be sought. For a child with furin cikin ido the dispensary is the most popular choice when the first strategy fails to bring about an improvement. As is the case with less severe illness, with severe illnesses traditional healers become a much more attractive option when neither home remedies nor clinic have been successful. In all cases, a small minority of respondents suggest that the sick child should be brought to the hospital.

Despite the fact that women recognize the rapid sequential progression of clinical manifestations of vitamin A deficiency and associate these signs with dangerous health complications, patterns of care-seeking suggest that mothers would be less apt to explore consecutive treatment options for furin cikin ido than for dundumi. Apparently, the local understanding of the gravity of the condition leads women to believe that the appearance of corneal lesions means that loss of eyesight is almost inevitable, hence the decision not to take further action. As one woman explained, "Blindness can occur very, very quickly, before we know what is happening."

Table 4 Mothers' Suggestions for Subsequent Treatments if the First Treatment Fails

Treatment options	Nightblindness in a three-year-old child	Nightblindness in a pregnant woman	White spot in the eye of a young child
Second treatment			
Dispensary	40	37	30
Home remedy (a)	10	14	13
Traditional healer (b)	4	3	6
Total	54	54	49
Third treatment			
Dispensary	9	13	4
Home remedy	5	9	6
Traditional healer	14	13	9
Hospital	2	1	5
Total	30	36	24

(a) For nightblindness, food remedies were recommended; for xerophthalmia, nonfood remedies were recommended.

(b) Includes boka and marabout.

CASE HISTORIES OF NIGHTBLINDNESS

In addition to the scenario results, further insights about community responses to nightblindness were provided through case histories. Two examples follow.

A Family with Dundumi

Aichatou, who is the second of three wives, had experienced dundumi during all four of her pregnancies. She and her family live on the periphery of town in three straw huts: one wife occupies each hut, and the children sleep with their biological mother. A few days prior to the first interview, all of the women and children in the compound were suffering from dundumi. According to Aichatou, "When the sun set we couldn't see anything, we were like blind people." She explained that they grilled liver. After the liver was cooked, the "juice" was dripped into their eyes and the liver was subsequently consumed. Although the co-wives laughed when they recounted the story, they lamented, "This is a big ciwo [hurt]. It's awful: one minute you can see and the next your sight goes away." In this home dundumi has occurred with such regularity that it has become a normal affliction. The consumption of liver as an effective treatment is known by all family members, even the youngest, who is just three years old.

A Woman with Dundumi

Four years ago, when Mariama was six months pregnant, she developed dundumi. She attributed this to lame (lack of good foods), which she explained was caused by inadequate funds due to her husband's absence from Filili. When her husband returned to Filili she was once again able to include meat in her diet, and the dundumi went away. However, immediately following the birth of her baby, they moved to the bush, where they spent the entire farming season. Two months later she again had dundumi. She explained, "In Filili there is a variety of foods available, but in the bush the diet is very monotonous. Sai anago [an abrupt change in the diet]. There is no wild game and, furthermore, during the rainy season there is no money to purchase foods. Sai wahala [hardship]." An old woman living in the bush told her to cook liver briefly, place it in a pot when it was still hot, and lean over the pot with her eyes open so that the "new blood" from the liver would go into her eyes. Mariama stated that, although she followed this treatment, she was still having difficulty seeing at night. She decided to try red sorrel leaves, and she explained that red sorrel is also a remedy for dundumi but a less costly one. She first cooked the leaves in a sauce and then made kupto (the green leafy dish mixed with peanuts). After she consumed these concoctions, the dundumi disappeared.

DISCUSSION

In biomedical theory nightblindness and Bitot's spots are manifestations of the same underlying problem—a deficiency of vitamin A. Our data show that, in the local belief system in Filili, these two problems are the results of very different constructs, each of which is attributed to a different etiology and requires a different treatment than does the other. An outstanding feature of the causal explanations associated with nightblindness involves diet. In view of the strong role of diet in the local etiology, it is not surprising to find that dietary measures figure importantly in its management. On the other hand, the manifestation of a white spot in the eye is believed to be caused by the "hot" diseases with which it is often associated. For this condition the primary thrust of management is treatment directed to the dangerous condition of excess heat.

There is a strong cultural consensus in Filili regarding both the etiology and treatment strategies for nightblindness. Most people believe that it is appropriately handled at home, and management knowledge is widespread so that most respondents know the most biomedically efficacious remedies. There is also a consensus on the causes of a white spot in the eye (associated with xerophthalmia), but there is ambiguity about the best response. Half of the respondents felt that seeking biomedical treatment from the health clinic was the best choice, whereas others had greater faith in the power of traditional home treatments to deal with heat-producing illnesses and the lesions they cause. The local understanding of the gravity of the condition may also engender a belief that little can be done to prevent the loss of the eye. Although we do not have direct measures of respondents' perceptions of the self-efficacy of their management strategies for Bitot's spots, the evidence from the scenarios and case histories suggests that families have high expectations concerning their ability to cure nightblindness and low expectations concerning their ability to treat white spots in the eyes.

The widely shared confidence in using home remedies to treat nightblindness rather than seeking care outside the household is likely associated with differences in the efficacy of treatment. A unique feature of nightblindness compared to other manifestations of the same underlying problem is that it can be reversed with the ingestion of vitamin A-rich foods. The response to dietary treatment can be dramatic, reversing a condition that involves blindness and resulting in normal vision within a few hours. In contrast, more severe signs do not generally respond to food or other treatment. Conversely, clinical manifestations commonly result in permanent scarring or damage to the eye.

What is striking about the etiological explanations and management of nightblindness is how closely they correspond to contemporary biomedical knowledge and treatment. This high level of correspondence raises questions about how the two different models—the biomedical and the Filili—have come to be so similar. Has the Filili model been recently introduced through nutrition education and biomedical practice? If not, then is this a case of independent discovery? Or does it represent diffusion from another, non-biomedical explanatory system?

If their explanatory model for nightblindness were a product of diffusion from modern, Western biomedical concepts, then we would expect that younger, educated people would be more knowledgeable and more accepting of the dietary strategies for treating the problem than would older, uneducated people. However this is not the case. We found that it was the older people, including those living in more isolated areas, who were most knowledgeable about the food remedies for nightblindness. Also, the ritualistic components in the remedies point to a "non-modern" source of the belief system. We would also expect that, if the sources of the knowledge were to be found in Western biomedicine, then explanations of nightblindness and Bitot's spots would be closely linked.

To explore other possible sources for these cultural models we reviewed research related to nightblindness in other parts of West Africa. In her study in the Sahelian zone of Mali, Dettwyler (1989) found that nightblindness is widely known. Traditional cures for this problem most commonly involved the consumption of liver and entailed elaborate descriptions of food rituals. Dettwyler reports a common dietetic remedy, which villagers indicated is very effective if repeated two or three days in a row: "You take a piece of goat liver and cook it directly over the flame of the fire. Next you rub the liquid from the liver in your eyes and then throw the piece of liver into your house at night. You go into the house and try to find the liver in the dark. When you have found it, you come outside and eat it" (32).

Data that Campbell (1993) collected in Burkina Faso show that nightblindness is recognized in diverse ethnic groups. Liver is also commonly reported as a cure for nightblindness. Once again treatment is often ritualistic, involving throwing a piece of cooked liver into a dark room. The individual with the condition is required to search for and immediately consume the liver. In northern Ghana, where local languages have specific terms for nightblindness, research on ethnographic aspects of vitamin A uncovered widespread use of therapy for this condition— therapy that generally entailed consuming large portions of meat or liver. Accounts of the treatment once again illuminated traditional rituals imbued with folk explanations (P. Arthur, personal communication, March 1995). For instance, informants explained that a child who is suffering from nightblindness is placed in a corner of a dark room. A piece of chicken liver (the choice of chicken liver seems to be significant because it is considered a delicacy) is put in another corner, and the child is then asked to find it. If the child is able to locate the liver and consume it, then her/his nightblindness is cured.

Keith's (1991) data from Niger show that nightblindness is believed to occur in humans and animals, particularly during pregnancy, and in both cases it is widely attributed to a lack of good foods. Male respondents explained that, in humans, nightblindness signifies poverty, particularly an inability to purchase meat. A study of the folk etiology of nightblindness and local remedies conducted by Muderhwa, Adamou, and Maman (1993) in the northern pastoral zone of Niger found that people commonly associate nightblindness with inadequate consumption of meat or liver, and, more generally, with poor nutrition. A large majority of the 239 people interviewed in that study mentioned liver as the best therapeutic food source.

It is evident that Filili residents and people living in other regions of West Africa maintain remarkably similar cultural interpretations of and treatment responses to nightblindness. All of these sites share common environmental and economic features, including periodic food shortages— particularly with regard to foods rich in vitamin A—thus leading to high rates of nightblindness. If food insufficiency is the cause of a physiological problem, then it is not difficult to understand why the treatment would consist of supplying certain foods. But what kind of foods? How did the hypothetical "health specialists" fix on liver as the appropriate remedy? The answer might be found in the high cultural value placed on meat, particularly liver, as a "powerful" food.

In Filili liver is widely esteemed, particularly for its high blood content. Residents believe that the consumption of "blood-rich" food is critical to the maintenance of good health. People of all ages are in need of these foods on a regular basis but particularly during times of sickness, when blood-rich foods are necessary to restore health.

Respondents indicated that the levels of blood in the body can change dramatically through time because blood has a definite lifespan. Therefore, blood should be replenished on a regular basis. Strenuous work, over-exposure to the sun, and/or illness can ruin the blood, causing it to age quickly, stopping circulation, and/or "killing the blood," thus leading to death. Symptoms associated with "old blood" include fatigue and generally poor health. These indicators signal that the person needs to be bled. Following this process, an intake of blood-rich foods returns new blood to the body, increasing circulation and restoring health.

With regard to Filili concepts of foods, liver is the food item that is richest in blood. Other foods with elevated blood content include red meats, which also have a high cultural value, as well as beans, milk, and cow's butter. To a lesser degree, green leafy vegetables, which are often consumed as a substitute for more expensive blood sources, are also believed to contain blood. Therefore, in the case of nightblindness, the use of green leafy vegetables would have been a readily available and logical treatment, particularly for families who could not afford meat.

The Filili interpretation of the more serious and less common vitamin A deficiency sign—Bitot's spots—is also based on naturalistic observations. The people rightly associate the condition with serious illness, particularly measles. However, at that point their general "theory of physiology and bodily conditions," referring to "heat" and "heatiness," provides a ready explanation of the illness. Thus we can suggest that the humoral theory interferes with the possibility of developing cultural explanations based on nutritional deficiency. The possibility of developing a food-based remedy is further lessened by the fact that the signs and symptoms of xerophthalmia, unlike those of nightblindness, are not readily affected by food supplementation.

SUMMARY AND CONCLUSIONS

Residents of Filili are enmeshed in a vicious cycle of low food production and poverty, and this has a direct effect on food acquisition and consumption patterns. As a result, most inhabitants must rely on a monotonous diet dominated by bulky foods and less costly items. They must also contend with extreme seasonal variations in food availability. This is particularly true of fruits and vegetables, which are available on a limited basis only during short spans of the year. The combination of economic and ecological factors limiting food production and acquisition predisposes Filili residents to nutritional deficiencies, including vitamin A.

The specific illness symptoms we selected for study were derived from an etic, biomedical perspective, in which they "belong together" because they constitute a set of conditions on a continuum of nutritional status. While these signs share one common feature—they affect eyesight—there is no reason to assume that they constitute a unitary illness domain in explanatory systems other than biomedicine. In the cultural understandings of nightblindness and Bitot's spots among people in Filili, these two illness symptoms have different etiologies and, therefore, require different treatment strategies.

There are strong similarities between the cultural models of nightblindness in Filili and other communities in West Africa where vitamin A deficiency is prevalent. The similarities in the explanatory models, taken together with the strong resemblances in their ecological and economic circumstances, suggest that diffusion of the nutritional explanation was powerfully reinforced by the peoples' common experiences regarding the effects of periodic food deprivations.

The West African cultural model for nightblindness is an example of a very large class of folk models around the world in which illness etiology is attributed to a dietary problem. The problems may be variously constructed as a deficiency of specific foods, a dietary imbalance, consumption of inappropriate foods, or, in some cases, over-consumption of "dangerous foods." The local explanation for a white spot in the eye is not associated with diet, although some respondents indicated that poor nutrition may contribute to the child's illness. As our focus in this article is primarily on perceptions related to a nutrient deficiency, we have not pursued broader questions concerning the distribution of beliefs and practices related to heat-producing illnesses, which is the larger context to which xerophthalmia relates.

Thirty years ago, Alland (1970) developed a series of hypotheses concerning the effects of particular attributes of diseases on the development of cultural models of explanation and management. One of the factors he identified as potentially important is time—the amount of time from exposure to the illness-causing agent to manifestation of the disease as well as the amount of time it takes for a treatment to have some observable effects on the ailment. He suggested that the shorter the interval, the more likely it was that an efficacious model would be developed and maintained. The contrasts among the signs and symptoms of nightblindness, Bitot's spots, and HIV/AIDS point to the importance of the variations in time-links to causal mechanisms and time-sequences in treatment effects. For nightblindness, a dramatic improvement in eyesight occurs following the ingestion of liver. Therefore, the connections are relatively direct and time links are very short, thus maximizing the possibilities for rational, empirical responses. In the case of Bitot's spots, the link between cause and effect is more difficult; and HIV/AIDS pose enormous time-gaps, which, in Alland's terms, makes rational cause and effect analysis extremely difficult except in a highly technological society. Thus, it seems probable that the widespread similarities in this form of treatment for nightblindness throughout West Africa are explained by a basic process in the generation of indigenous cultural knowledge for coping with illness.

The theoretical approach proposed by Alland, which we are applying to the effects (symptoms) of vitamin A deficiency in northern Niger, emphasizes the rationality of peoples' cultural coping strategies in dealing with health threats. Unfortunately, with regard to most illnesses, particularly those brought about by viruses, bacteria, and other microorganisms, causal mechanisms are invisible, thus precluding rational cause-and-effect problem solving. In societies that do not have microscopes and other forms of modern technology, the construction of explanatory models for various human illnesses has led to the use of various magical, religious, and other non-natural systems. In the case of health problems that arise from temporary food deficiencies, the pathways to naturalistic explanations are somewhat more clear.

Following Alland, we suggest that the ecological conditions in West Africa have exposed people to conditions in which sharp fluctuations in food availability resulted in nightblindness being a common experience. Those conditions also made the recognition of causal linkages more likely, thus leading to the use of efficacious therapeutic approaches.

Note

1. A pseudonym has been used to protect the identity of the research community.

References

Alland, A. 1970 Adaptation in Cultural Evolution: An Approach to Medical Anthropology. New York: Columbia University Press.

Blanchet, T. 1984 Meanings and Rituals of Childbirth in Bangladesh. Dhaka: University Press.

Beaton, G. H., R. Martorell, K. J. Aronsen, B. Edmonston, G. McCabe, A. C. Ross, and B. Harvey 1993 Effectiveness of Vitamin A Supplementation in the Control of Young Child Morbidity and Mortality in Developing Countries. Toronto: University of Toronto International Nutrition Program.

Beine, D. K. 2003 Ensnared by AIDS: Cultural Contexts of HIV/AIDS in Nepal. Kathmandu: Mandala Book Point.

Blum, L. S., P. J. Pelto, G. H. Pelto, and H. V. Kuhnlein 1997 Community Assessment of Natural Food Sources of Vitamin A. Boston: International Nutrition Foundation.

Campbell, J. 1993 Vitamin A Consumption in Burkina Faso: A Qualitative Study. Washington, D.C.: Academy for Educational Development.

Christian, P. 2000 Night Blindness during Pregnancy and Subsequent Mortality among Women in Nepal: Effects of Vitamin A and β-Carotene Supplementation. American Journal of Epidemiology 152(6):542–547.

Christian, P., K. P. West, S. K. Khatry, J. Katz, S. C. LeClerg, E. Kimbrough-Pradhan, S. M. Dali, and S. R. Shrestha 2000 Vitamin A or Beta-Carotene Supplementation Reduces Symptoms of Illness in Pregnant and Lactating Nepali Women. Journal of Nutrition 130(11):2675–2682.

Dettwyler, K. A. 1989 Communication for Vitamin A: Field Study in Macina. Washington, D.C.: Academy for Educational Development.

Dillon-Malone, C. 1988 Mutumwa Nchimi Healers and Wizardry Beliefs in Zambia. Social Science and Medicine 26(11):1159–1172.

Farmer, P. 1994 AIDS Talk and the Constitution of Cultural Models. Social Science and Medicine 38(6):801–809.

Foster, A. and D. Yorston 1992 Corneal Ulceration in Tanzanian Children: Relationship between Measles and Vitamin A Deficiency. Transaction of the Royal Society of Tropical Medicine and Hygiene 86(4):454–455.

Fuglestad, F. 1983 A History of Niger, 1850–1960. Cambridge: Cambridge University Press.

Hussey, G. D. and M. Klein 1990 A Randomized, Controlled Trial of Vitamin A in Children with Severe Measles. New England Journal of Medicine 323:160–164.

Katz, J., S. L. Zeger, K. P. West, J. M. Tielsch, A. Sommer 1993 Clustering of Xerophthalmia within Households and Villages. International Journal of Epidemiology 22:709–715.

Katz, J., S. K. Khatry, K. P. West, J. H. Humphrey, S. C. LeClerq, E. K. Pradhan, R. P. Pokhrel, A. Sommer 1995 Night Blindness during Pregnancy and Lactation in Rural Nepal. Journal of Nutrition 125:2122–2127.

Keith, N. J. 1991 Field Research in Birni'n Konni: Vitamin A Communication Project. Washington, D.C.: Academy of Educational Development.

Kleinman, A. M. 1980 Patient and Healers in the Context of Culture: An Exploration of the Borderland between Anthropology, Medicine and Psychiatry. Berkeley: University of California Press.

Kuhnlein, H. V. and G. H. Pelto, eds. 1997 Culture, Environment and Food to Prevent Vitamin A Deficiency. Boston: International Nutrition Foundation.

Lepowsky, M. 1990 Sorcery and Penicillin: Treating Illness on a Papua New Guinea Island. Social Science and Medicine 30(10):1049–1063.

Leslie, C., ed. 1998 Asian Medical Systems: A Comparative Study. New Delhi: Motilal Banarsidass Publishers.

Mattingly, C. and L. G. Garro. 1994 Narrative Representations of Illness and Healing. Introduction. Social Science and Medicine 38(6):771–774.

Muderhwa, N. D., D. Adamou, and M. L. Maman 1993 Promotion de la Production et de la Consummation des Aliments Riches en Vitamine A. Bouza, Niger: FAO.

Nichter, M. 1994 Anthropological Approaches to the Study of Ethnomedicine. Yverdon, Switzerland: Gordon and Breach Publishers.

Parker, R. S. 1996 Absorption, Metabolism and Transport of Carotenoids. FASEB Journal 10(5):542–551.

Resnikoff, S. 1996 Primary Eye Care and Prevention of Nutritional Blindness in West Africa. In Nutritional Blindness in Developing Countries, Interdisciplinary Symposium. C. A. Ribaux and M. Frigg, eds. Pp. 70–82. Basel, Switzerland: Sight and Life.

Ross, J. L., S. L. Laston, P. J. Pelto, and L. Muna 2002 Exploring Explanatory Models of Women's Reproductive Health in Rural Bangladesh. Culture, Health and Sexuality 4(2):173–190.

Rubel, A. J. and M. R. Hass 1990 Ethnomedicine. In Medical Anthropology: Contemporary Theory and Method. T. M. Johnson and C. Sargent, eds. Pp. 115–131. New York: Praeger Publishers.

Sommer, A. and K. P. West 1996 Vitamin A Deficiency: Health, Survival and Vision. New York: Oxford University Press.

Stone, L. 1988 Illness Beliefs and Feeding the Dead in Hindu Nepal: An Ethnographic Analysis. Ceredigion, Wales: Edward Mellin Press.

Strauss, C. and N. Quinn 1997 A Cognitive Theory of Cultural Meaning. Cambridge: Cambridge University Press.

Sutter, J. 1982 Peasants, Merchant Capital and Rural Differentiation: A Nigerian Hausa Case Study. Ph.D. dissertation, Cornell University.

Underwood, B. 1983 Paper presented at the Cornell International Lecture Series, Department of Nutrition, Cornell University, Ithaca, NY.

Wall, L. 1988 Hausa Medicine: Illness and Well-Being in a West African Culture. Durham, NC: Duke University Press.

WHO/UNICEF 1995 Global Prevalence of Vitamin A Deficiency. MDIS Working Paper No. 2, Geneva: World Health Organization.

WHO/IVACG/UNICEF Task Force 1988 Vitamin A Supplements: A Guide to Their Use in the Treatment and Prevention of Vitamin A Deficiency and Xerophthalmia. Geneva: World Health Organization.

Young, J. C. 1980 A Model of Illness Treatment Decisions in a Tarascan Town. American Ethnologist 7(1):106–131.

CHAPTER 31

From Aphrodisiac to Health Food: A Cultural History of Chocolate

Louis E. Grivetti

(2005)

Chocolate is more than a confection, more than a dessert, more than a delightful pleasure. When drunk as cocoa or eaten as a solid bar of chocolate, consumers share a common connection through a vast spectrum of time. *Theobroma cacao*, the tree that bears the pods and beans that are ultimately made into chocolate, was probably domesticated initially in the western regions of the Amazon basin about 4000 years ago. Another suggestion is that domestication and human use of cacao first took place within a geographical area that today encompasses the modern states of Tabasco, Oaxaca, and Chiapas in southern Mexico, northern Guatemala, and Belize.

The story of cacao and chocolate begins with the early Olmecs who lived in Mesoamerica more than 3000 years ago. The story extends through the 16th-century Spanish conquest and colonization of Central America, when frothy cacao beverages prepared at the court of King Montezuma were served to Cortés and his troops. Chocolate facts and myths are linked with the spread of this beverage into Europe and North America during the late 16th and early 17th centuries. Today, in the 21st century, consumers welcome chocolate in a variety of ways, whether as a primary meal item or as a dessert, but always as a delightful pleasure.

Linguistic specialists, among them Martha Macri and her students at the University of California, Davis, have suggested that chocolate-related terms probably originated with the early Olmec civilization, passed to the Mayans, and then to the Mexica/Aztecs. Beans from cacao trees were differentiated by the ancients into two primary types: the term *quauhcacahuatl* represented the best-quality beans that were used as a form of currency, while the word *tlacacahuatl* applied to lower-quality beans used to prepare beverages. The English word cacao is derived linguistically from the Nahuatl (Aztec language) words *cacahuatl* or *xoxocatl*, generally translated as "a beverage prepared from cacao and water."

How Cacao Came to Humans

In ancient Mayan texts cacao has a divine origin—it is truly a gift from the gods. Xmucane, one of the creation gods, invented nine beverages, and from these, humans were formed who were able to feed themselves. Of these nine beverages, three were made with cacao and corn. Then came a time when historical events shifted geographically from the Mayan lowlands and southern regions of modern Mexico as new immigrants arrived from the north and poured into the central valley of Mexico. These immigrants, the Toltecs, built the astonishing pyramids located at Teotihuacan. According to Toltec religious texts, the god Quetzalcóatl planted the first earthly cacao tree in a field at the site of Tula to honor good, hard-working humans who lived and toiled there.

The Toltecs, themselves, experienced cultural upheaval in the 14th century as their world was disrupted by the arrival of people known as the Mexica (Aztecs). Mexica warriors subdued the indigenous tribes that had flourished in the valley and constructed their capital, Tenochtitlan, on two islands in Lake Texcoco. By the 16th century, the Aztecs had installed a strong economic, military, and political presence within the valley. Tenochtitlan at this time was an extraordinary architectural achievement, with a population variously estimated by scholars as between 250–350,000, making the capital one of the largest cities in the world.

The Mexica/Aztecs loved chocolate. More correctly, the Mexica nobility and male soldiers loved chocolate. Cacao/chocolate was not available to all the Mexica and others living in the central valley. It was served as a beverage only to adult males, specifically priests, government officials, military officers, distinguished warriors, and sometimes to the bravest enemy captives before sacrifice. The Mexica held that cacao/chocolate beverages were intoxicating and stimulating and, therefore, not suitable for women and children.

Arrival of the Spanish

Just as the Mexica had replaced the Toltecs, a new invading force changed the culture of the New World. Spanish expeditionary forces arrived on the eastern shore of what is now modern Mexico in 1519, an event that initiated revolutionary

Louis E. Grivetti, "From aphrodisiac to health food: a cultural history of chocolate." *Karger Gazette* 68 (2005):1–3. Reprinted with permission.

regional changes and new chapters in the complex history of chocolate. Hernando Cortés landed near modern Vera Cruz. After burning his ships he led his troops inland toward the Mexica capital where his army was received by King Montezuma. Cortés, himself, and several of his literate officers wrote accounts of their march and documented events of the Mexica conquest. Several passages reflect direct observation of cacao-sellers in Tenochtitlan, while others describe behavior at dinners hosted by Montezuma where chocolate was served: *From time to time the men of Montezuma's guard brought him, in cups of pure gold, a drink made from the cocoa-plant, which they said he took before visiting his wives... I saw them bring in fifty large jugs of chocolate, all frothed up, of which he would drink a little (Bernal Díaz del Castillo: 1560).*

This passage by Bernal Díaz is the first documentation in a European language to associate chocolate drinking with sexual activity (but would not be the last). Missing from the earliest Spanish documentation, however, is any suggestion that chocolate was consumed both as a food and as a medicine—two roles that ultimately dominated later European descriptions of this interesting food.

MEDICAL USES OF CHOCOLATE IN MEXICA TEXTS

While the earliest Spanish accounts do not report medicinal uses for chocolate, the written record is not silent. Indigenous Mexica medical views of cacao/chocolate are recorded in several documents, among them the *Codex Barberini*, Latin 241, commonly known as the *Badianus Manuscript* (1552) and the *Florentine Codex* (1590). While both manuscripts postdate Spanish colonial contact, they were compiled by Spanish priests who obtained the information from Mexica respondents, so the views probably reflect earlier, pre-European-contact behavior.

The *Badianus Manuscript*, written in both Nahuatl/Aztec and Latin, is a Mexica herbal that identifies more than 100 medical conditions common to the central valley, and their treatments. The manuscript contains a striking color painting of a cacao tree among the healing plants identified in the text. There is also a passage describing how cacao flowers were strewn in perfumed baths to reduce the fatigue experienced by Mexica government administrators.

The *Florentine Codex* was compiled by the priest Bernardino de Sahagún who arrived in New Spain in 1529. While many priests associated with the early decades of Spanish colonial rule in Mexico (or New Spain) viewed local inhabitants as savages, and their customs, traditions, and literary documents as "ungodly," Sahagún did not. He was curious about Mexica medical knowledge and sought to learn as much as he could about their social traditions and history. Sahagún's Mexica informants reported a vast array of knowledge that he dutifully recorded and preserved for posterity. Without his labor and efforts to preserve this information, 21st-century scholars would have relatively few documents to work with and interpret when attempting to understand and reconstruct the precolonial era.

The information within the Florentine Codex is critical to understanding the early medical-related history of chocolate. The document reports that Mexica respondents warned against excessive drinking of cacao prepared from unroasted beans, but praised it if used in moderation. They reported that drinking large quantities of green cacao made consumers confused and deranged, but if used reasonably, the beverage both invigorated and refreshed. Another passage from the *Florentine Codex* reveals that cacao was mixed with various medicinal products and used to offset or mask the flavor of ill-tasting drugs. Sahagún's informants also reported that a local product known as *quinametli* (identified as "bones of ancient people called giants") was blended with chocolate and used to treat bloody dysentery.

CHOCOLATE ARRIVES IN EUROPE

While many recent texts and websites provide readers with a precise year and a specific event whereby chocolate was first introduced to Europe, food historians always debate "firsts" and the so-called "first" arrival of chocolate in Europe is a subject of conjecture to say nothing of myth. Chocolate may have been introduced to Europe via the Spanish court in 1544, when Dominican friars are said to have brought Mayan nobles to meet Prince Philip. I suspect, though, that this oft-cited statement is probably more allegorical than precise. It is correct to say, however, that within a century of the arrival of the Spanish in Mexico, both culinary and medicinal uses of chocolate had spread from Mexico to Spain, France, England, and elsewhere within Western Europe (entering through Spain and Portugal) and probably North America as well (entering through the Spanish settlement at St. Augustine, Florida). Throughout Europe, chocolate was considered an "exotic" beverage—in competition with coffee and tea—and consumers readily developed their passion and desire for this dark, strangely "exciting" drink. In England chocolate houses emerged as the "rage of the day," where wealthy, powerful Englishmen debated politics and global affairs over steaming cups of hot chocolate. Indeed, the so-called "Queen's Lane Coffee House on High Street," Oxford, began serving both coffee and chocolate in 1650 and still serves both beverages today in the 21st century.

CHOCOLATE AS FOOD—CHOCOLATE AS MEDICINE

From the 16th through early 19th century, numerous European travel accounts and medical texts documented the presumed merits and medicinal value of chocolate. Using library holdings of the Library of Congress, Washington, DC, the British Museum, and the University of California, as well as translations of original hand-written documents located at various archives in Mexico, Spain, and elsewhere, my research team has identified more than 100 medical uses for chocolate prescribed by physicians during the past 475 years[1].

Presented here is a brief "taste" of these rich chocolate-related passages from selected historical monographs. On inspection, these samples reveal that chocolate products were used to treat a myriad of human disorders:

Francisco Hernández (1577) wrote that pure cacao paste prepared as a beverage treated fever and liver disease. He also mentioned that toasted, ground cacao beans mixed with resin were effective against dysentery and that chocolate beverages were commonly prescribed to thin patients in order for them to gain "flesh."

Agustin Farfan (1592) recorded that chili peppers, rhubarb, and vanilla were used by the Mexica as purgatives and that chocolate beverages served hot doubled as powerful laxatives.

José de Acosta (1604) wrote that chili was sometimes added to chocolate beverages and that eating chocolate paste was good for stomach disorders.

Santiago de Valverde Turices (1624) concluded that chocolate drunk in great quantities was beneficial for treatment of chest ailments, but if drunk in small quantities was a satisfactory medicine for stomach disorders.

Colmenero de Ledesma (1631) reported that cacao preserved consumers' health, made them corpulent, improved their complexions, and made their dispositions more agreeable. He wrote that drinking chocolate incited love-making, led to conception in women, and facilitated delivery. He also claimed that chocolate aided digestion and cured tuberculosis.

Thomas Gage (1648) described a medicinal chocolate prepared with black pepper used to treat "cold liver." Gage wrote that chocolate mixed with cinnamon increased urine flow and was an effective way to treat kidney disorders.

Henry Stubbe (1662) wrote that consumers should drink chocolate beverages once or twice each day to relieve tiredness caused by strenuous business activities. He reported that ingesting cacao oil was an effective treatment for the Fire of St. Anthony (i.e., ergot poisoning). Stubbe also described chocolate-based concoctions mixed with Jamaica pepper used to treat menstrual disorders, and other chocolate preparations blended with vanilla to strengthen the heart and to promote digestion.

William Hughes (1672) reported that cough could be treated by drinking chocolate blended with cinnamon or nutmeg. He wrote that chocolate nourished the body, induced sleep, and cured the "pustules, tumors, and swellings commonly experienced by hardy sea-men who had long been kept from a diet of fresh foods," symptoms akin to scurvy.

Sylvestre Dufour (1685) wrote that medicinal chocolate commonly contained anise-seed as an ingredient, and that such mixtures were used to treat bladder and kidney disorders. He described a type of medical chocolate blended with achiote (Bixa orellana) that produced a product of a blood-red color, used to reduce the "fever of love."

Nicolas de Blégny (1687) reported that chocolate mixed with vanilla syrup soothed lung inflammations and lessened the "ferocity of cough." He identified medicinal chocolates that contained as ingredients "syrup of coins," "drops of gold tincture," and "oil of amber" that treated indigestion and heart palpitations.

De Quélus (1718) wrote that drinking chocolate was nourishing and essential to good health. He said that drinking chocolate "repaired exhausted spirits," preserved health, and prolonged the lives of old men. Further, he claimed that an ounce of chocolate contained as much nourishment as a pound of beef.

Antonio Lavedan (1796) claimed that chocolate was beneficial but only if drunk in the morning, and he strongly cautioned against afternoon use of this beverage. He wrote that chocolate alone—with no other food—could keep consumers robust and healthy for many years, and remarked that drinking chocolate prolonged life.

Brillat-Savarin (1825) wrote that chocolate was a "wholesome, agreeable food, nourishing, easily digested, and an antidote to the inconveniences ascribed to coffee." He claimed that chocolate was best suited to those who exercised their brains, especially clergymen, lawyers, and travelers, and he recommended a concoction of cacao mixed with amber dust as a treatment for the ill-effects of hangover.

Auguste Saint-Arroman (1846) reported that chocolate—while suited to both the aged and weak—was dangerous if drunk by the young. He identified a recipe for medical chocolate that included iron filings, used to treat chlorosis in women.

Saint-Arroman's monograph on chocolate is intriguing for other reasons. He provided a recipe whereby chocolate was prepared from roasted cacao, sugar, and aromatic substances, such as ginger, pimento, and cloves, and sometimes vanilla and cinnamon. He also wrote that a common form of Spanish chocolate included the bulb of the root of arachis or "earth pistachio," better known in English as the peanut (*Arachis hypogaea*). Peanuts, domesticated initially in the Americas (perhaps Brazil), were taken to Europe and initiated there as a field crop. The Saint-Arroman account represents one of the earliest reports to document the blending of chocolate and peanuts, whether as medicine or as food, a blend that today in the 21st century represents a favorite combination for millions of consumers globally.

While chocolate has been prescribed in past centuries to patients suffering from "alpha to omega" (from anemia, angina, and asthma to wasting, weakness, and worms), its long history in medical treatment has been a controversial one. While 21st-century physicians would not claim that chocolate cured cancer, gout, jaundice, rheumatism, scurvy, snake bite, or syphilis (as claimed in the past), examination of the historical medical accounts reveals five consistent, reasonable, medical-related uses:

1. For emaciated patients in order to restore weight—certainly an important treatment for patients with wasting diseases such as tuberculosis.
2. To stimulate the nervous systems of feeble patients, especially those suffering from apathy, exhaustion, or lassitude—an action which we might now attribute to the theobromine and caffeine in chocolate.
3. To calm, soothe, and tranquilize patients identified as "over-stimulated," especially those suffering from strenuous labor or "serious mental activity"—here, it is the pleasurable taste and flavor sensations, coupled with a relaxing effect, which would produce the mellow mood.
4. To improve digestion and elimination. Chocolate was said to strengthen, calm, or soothe "stagnant stomachs," stimulate the kidneys and hasten urine flow, improve bowel function, soften stools, and even cure or reduce hemorrhoids.
5. To bind medicinal ingredients and to mask the flavors of ill-tasting drugs, uses which are reflected in the modern view that "a little bit of chocolate makes the medicine go down."

Although not consistent through time, there are also intriguing historical accounts that suggest eating or drinking chocolate could/would have had a positive effect on patients beyond merely the placebo effect and pleasure of consuming this food. Hughes wrote in 1672 that drinking chocolate alleviated asthma spasms; Stubbe wrote in 1662 that drinking chocolate increased breast milk production; and Colmenero de Ledesma suggested in 1631 that drinking chocolate could expel kidney stones. Modern science has identified the vasodilatation and diuretic effects that follow chocolate consumption, and with chocolate's high energy value, the concept that chocolate could be a galactagogue (milk producer) can at least be considered.

But chocolate, of course, is not a panacea for all of life's ills. Countering the well-documented positive and potentially positive medical effects of chocolate consumption identified in historical documents, these same texts offer other claims that may be discounted: effective against ergot poisoning (claimed by Stubbe in 1662); effective in delaying the growth of white hair in men (claimed by Lavedan in 1796); effective in reducing tumors/pustules (claimed by Hughes in 1672).

RECENT CHOCOLATE-RELATED FIELDWORK

Throughout the centuries chocolate has been used as both a food and medicine in many regions of the world. Since 2000, our team has conducted fieldwork in selected countries of Central America and the Caribbean where we have sought information on culinary, health, and medical uses as reported by traditional populations.

Mexico

In the geographical region of the Mixtec Alta in the Central Valley of Oaxaca, Mexico, *curanderos* (traditional healers) informed us that chocolate beverages were prescribed to cure bronchitis. In this region *curanderos* use cacao beans to treat the medical condition known as *espanto* or *susto*, an illness thought to result when persons have been startled or frightened. The treatment for *espanto/susto* reflects the high importance played by cacao in Mixtec society and the value placed upon cacao beans. Both patient and healer return to the exact location where the fright occurred: the *curandero* brings quantities of tobacco, bowls of fermented beverages, herbs, and cacao beans. The healer feeds the earth by planting cacao beans as a form of payment to the forces that caused the disease. The explanation given us was that by restoring wealth to the earth (in pre-Spanish times, cacao beans served as a type of money), the evil that caused the fright would become distracted, whereupon the person suffering from *espanto/susto* could be treated and returned to health. Elsewhere in the El Istmo region of eastern Oaxaca, residents told us that chocolate beverages were commonly served to children at the morning meal as a type of talisman that protected children against the stings of scorpions, bees, or wasps.

The most intriguing uses of chocolate in Mexico are ancient cultural rituals blended with a veneer of Christianity. The celebration called *Dia de la Muertos* (Day of the Dead) lasts from October 31 through November 2. At this time chocolate plays a central role in the cultural/social life of Mexican families. During *Dia de la Muertos*, the living must fulfill their obligations to the deceased, a responsibility known as *guelaguetza* (reciprocity). Chocolate is prepared locally as balls, tablets, and as hot beverages that are exchanged among friends and relatives. Foods, beverages, and especially chocolate products are placed on *ofrendas* (offering tables/altars) erected at homes and local cemeteries. Chocolate in either solid or liquid form is offered to the memory of dead children on the night of October 31, the day specifically known as *Dia de los Angelitos* (Day of the Little Angels). Deceased adults are honored with chocolate offerings on November 1 or *Todos Santos* (All Saints' Day). Families visit the cemeteries at night where they gather in a family atmosphere to think about and remember the deceased. During the evening "watch," family members drink hot chocolate.

The Christian faithful at Oaxaca use chocolate in other religious celebrations as well. December 25 initiates the Twelve Days of Christmas, a period that extends through the New Year and ends on January 6 (Epiphany: the traditional date for the arrival of the Magi at Bethlehem). During the day and evening of January 5, homes of relatives and friends are visited and guests are served a festival food called *La Rosca de Reys* (The Three Kings Bread). This bread is eaten with hot chocolate, prepared using water or milk. A tiny figure of the infant Jesus is baked inside the bread. Whoever receives the doll in their slice is obligated to organize the next chocolate-related festival—February 2 or *Dia de la Calendaria* (Candlemas)—when tamales and hot chocolate are prepared as festive dishes.

Dominican Republic

Chocolate beverages continue to be widely used in the Dominican Republic as traditional medicine, whether to improve kidney function, reduce anemia, or to halt diarrhea. Chocolate is prescribed by healers to treat sore throat, to ease "over-exerted brains" (among persons engaged in heavy thinking), and to soothe stomach ache. Other respondents stated that chocolate beverages blended with coconut milk and onion reduced symptoms of the common cold. Still others said that chocolate beverages strengthened the lungs and energized consumers.

California, USA

Our team members have also worked among the Mixtec Indian community located at Madera, a small town in the San Joaquin Valley of California, with cultural roots in the state of Oaxaca in southern Mexico. We were interested in the maintenance or abandonment of chocolate-related customs and traditions after immigration to the United States. Mixtec residents we interviewed reported that chocolate was consumed in three ways in Madera: (1) as *Champurado*, a mixture of chocolate, maize flour, and boiling water, (2) as a basic beverage prepared with water or milk, or (3) as *Mole*, a chocolate sauce commonly served with festive turkey dishes.

Favorite Oaxaca recipes that normally blended cacao, sugar, cinnamon, and almonds were widely desired and missed—so much so that individuals returning to Oaxaca for short-term visits were given "wish lists" to fulfill and bring back to Madera, items that included Oaxaca-style chocolate. American-style chocolates, widely available throughout the community, were eaten but not considered as "real" chocolate, or types widely desired by respondents.

The Mixtec we studied in California were a community in transition and individuals were undergoing various levels of acculturation. Still, interviews we conducted related a strong, sustained use of chocolate in a medicinal context. Respondents reported that regular drinking of chocolate was healthy; that chocolate blended with fresh beaten eggs combated fatigue; that chocolate mixed with a *manzanilla*-based herbal tea alleviated pain; and chocolate mixed with cinnamon and *ruda* (rue) eased stomach ache. The Mixtec living at Madera reported that eating and drinking chocolate also had two additional effects. We were told that some individuals drank chocolate to lower their high blood pressure. Alternatively, "lethargic" individuals who drank chocolate would experience elevated blood pressure and no longer feel tired. Many in the community reported that drinking chocolate eased symptoms of the common cold.

THE GLOBALIZATION OF CHOCOLATE

We have written elsewhere that chocolate is more than a beverage, more than a confection, that chocolate is more than the sum of its interesting phytochemicals [1]. To taste chocolate is to share a common connection through history—from the early Olmecs more than three thousand years past, to the period of frothy cacao beverages prepared at the court of King Montezuma, into the 20th- and 21st-century era of the contemporary chocolate bar. A number of books have been published recently on chocolate-related botany, economics, history, lore, and medical/nutritional properties [2–5]. These books are good places to begin. Further, those interested in chocolate history and lore should be encouraged to go online: a search with the key words "chocolate" and "cacao," and various spelling variants, will reveal thousands of book titles and nearly 23 million websites (as of July 1, 2005). Hundreds of these sites claim to host "real" chocolate "facts" and "correct chocolate-related timelines." Some of these are generally correct; others, however, fit more within the realm of fiction, while the majority merely copy chocolate-related dates and events from one site onto another without critical scrutiny regarding the information source and whether or not the information is correct. It is more interesting, instead, to search the web for specific chocolate-related or sociocultural aspects of chocolate: search for chocolate-related advertisements from magazines, newspapers, and signs; chocolate-related collectibles, whether boxes and tins, candy molds, posters, chocolate pots/cups/saucers, even chocolate-related toys. What one encounters during such searches is exposure to how chocolate fits into many aspects of cultures throughout the world, how it links peoples and cultures through time and geographical space—from Austria to Zambia, from precolonial Central and South America to the 21st century of the Common Era: chocolate has become part of the "social gloss" of millions throughout the world today.

Our chocolate-related research has revealed a consistent, global fascination with this wonderful food. Eating chocolate may alter the mind and be pleasing to consumers because of its theobromine content. But chocolate is more. Chocolate alters the mind through a myriad of pleasurable sensations as the flavor and taste sensations flood the mouth, stimulating memories of the consumer's childhood, youth, and adult years. It is not the same with other foods: memories of broccoli, liver, and turnips hold no such places in the pantheon of great food-related experiences, but memories of chocolate allow consumers to recall wonderful days and pleasurable events. If there is a "true history of chocolate," it will remain forever elusive, the threads too long, too tangled to ever fully unravel. The traces extend through most of the fields in the humanities (art, literature, music, poetry, theater), the social sciences (anthropology, economics, geography, history, psychology, sociology), as well as the agricultural and biological, medical, even physical sciences (too many to identify). But maybe that very mystery—tempting our research—together with the endless human inventiveness in its use, will ensure that chocolate remains one of the most intriguing foods on this planet.

ACKNOWLEDGMENTS

I would like to thank the following colleagues and students who contributed to the research and field studies that are mentioned in this article: Dr. Martha Macri and her student Diane Barker who summarized Mayan language cacao/chocolate-related terminology; Dr. Sylvia Escarcega who provided the information on Day of the Dead and medicinal practices among the Mixtec-speaking community of Oaxaca; Rebecca Schacker who provided the fieldwork information on cacao/chocolate-related healing practices in the Dominican Republic; Dr. Jim Grieshop and Timateo Mendoze who undertook fieldwork on cacao/chocolate-related healing practices among the Mixtec-speaking community of Madera, California. This research was funded, in part, through a generous grant from Mars Incorporated.

References, Numbered

1. Dillinger TL, Barriga P, Escarcega S, Jimenez M, Salazar Lowe D, Grivetti LE: Food of the gods: cure for humanity? A cultural history of the medicinal and ritual use of chocolate. J Nutr 2000;130 (Suppl): 2057S–2072S.
2. Coe SD, Coe MD: The True History of Chocolate. Thames and Hudson, London, 1996
3. Knight I: Chocolate and Cocoa: Health and Nutrition. Blackwell, Oxford, 1999
4. Rosenblum M: Chocolate: A Bittersweet Saga of Dark and Light. North Point, New York, 2005
5. Young AM: The Chocolate Tree: A Natural History of Cacao. Smithsonian Institution Press, Washington, DC, 1994.

References, Other

Brillat-Savarin JA: The Physiology of Taste. New York, Houghton Mifflin, 1825(?).

Colmenero de Ledesma A: Curioso Tratado de la Naturaleza y Calidad del Chocolate. Madrid, Francisco Martinez, 1631.

de Acosta J: The Naturall and Morall Historie of the East and West Indies. Intreating of the Remarkable Things of Heaven, of the Elements, Metals, Plants and Beasts. London, Val. Sims for Edward Blount and William Aspley, 1604.

de Blégny N: Le bon usage du thé, du caffé et du chocolat pour la préservation et pour la guérison des maladies. Paris, Michallet, 1687.

De la Cruz M: The Badianus Manuscript, Codex Barberini, Latin 241, Vatican Library; an Aztec Herbal of 1552. Baltimore, Johns Hopkins University Press, 1940.

de Valverde Turices S: Un Discurso del Chocolate. Seville, J. Cabrera, 1624.

Diaz del Castillo B: The Conquest of New Spain. New York, Penguin, 1983.

Dufour PS: The Manner of Making of Coffee, Tea, and Chocolate as it Is Used in Most Parts of Europe, Asia, Africa and America, with Their Vertues [sic.]. London, William Crook, 1685.

Farfan A: Tractado Breve de Medicina [1592]. Madrid, Ediciones Cultura Hispanica, 1944.

Gage T: The English American: His Travail by Sea; or a New Survey of the West Indies Containing a Journall [sic.] of Three Thousand Three Hundred Miles within the Main Land of America. London, Cotes, 1648.

Hernández F: Historia de las Plantas de la Neuva Espana. Mexico City, Imprenta Universitaria, 1577.

Hughes W: The American Physitian [sic], or A Treatise of the Roots, Plants, Trees, Shrubs, Fruit, Herbs etc. Growing in the English Plantations in America: Describing the Place, Time. Names, Kindes, Temperature, Vertues and Uses of Them, either for Diet, Physick, etc. whereunto Is Added a Discourse of the Cacao-Nut-Tree, and the Use of its Fruit; with All the Ways of Making of Chocolate. The Like Never Extant Before 1672. London, J. C. for William Crook the Green Dragon without Temple-Bar, 1672.

Lavedan A: Tratado de Los Usos, Abusos, Propiendades y Virtudes del Tabaco, Café, Te y Chocolate. Madrid, Imprenta Real, 1796.

Quélus D: The Natural History of Chocolate: Being a Distinct and Particular Account of the Cocoa-Tree Its Growth and Culture, and the Preparation, Excellent Properties, and Medicinal Vertues of Its Fruit. Wherein the Errors of Those Who have Wrote upon this Subject Are Discovered; the Best Way of Making Chocolate is Explain'd; and Several Uncommon Medicines Drawn from It, Are Communicated. London, J. Roberts, 1718.

Sahagun B: General History of the Things of New Spain [Florentine Codex, 1590]. Santa Fe, The School of American Research and the University of Utah Monographs of The School of American Research and The Museum of New Mexico, 1981.

Saint-Arroman A: Coffee, Tea and Chocolate: Their Influence upon the Health, the Intellect, and the Moral Nature of Man. Philadelphia, Townsend Ward, 1846.

Stubbe H: The Indian Nectar, or, a Discourse Concerning Chocolata [sic.]: The Nature of the Cacao-Nut and the Other Ingredients of that Composition Is Examined and Stated According to the Judgment and Experience of Indian and Spanish Writers. London, J. C. for Andrew Crook, 1662.

CHAPTER 32

You Are What You Eat: Religious Aspects of the Health Food Movement

Jill Dubisch
(1981)

Dr. Robbins was thinking how it might be interesting to make a film from Adelle Davis' perennial best seller, *Let's Eat Right to Keep Fit*. Representing a classic confrontation between good and evil—in this case nutrition versus unhealthy diet—the story had definite box office appeal. The role of the hero, Protein, probably should be filled by Jim Brown, although Burt Reynolds undoubtedly would pull strings to get the part. Sunny Doris Day would be a clear choice to play the heroine, Vitamin C, and Orson Welles, oozing saturated fatty acids from the pits of his flesh, could win an Oscar for his interpretation of the villainous Cholesterol. The film might begin on a stormy night in the central nervous system....

—Tom Robbins, *Even Cowgirls Get the Blues*

I intend to examine a certain way of eating; that which is characteristic of the health food movement, and try to determine what people are communicating when they choose to eat in ways which run counter to the dominant patterns of food consumption in our society. This requires looking at health foods as a system of symbols and the adherence to a health food way of life as being, in part, the expression of belief in a particular world view. Analysis of these symbols and the underlying world view reveals that, as a system of beliefs and practices, the health food movement has some of the characteristics of a religion.

Such an interpretation might at first seem strange since we usually think of religion in terms of a belief in a deity or other supernatural beings. These notions, for the most part, are lacking in the health food movement. However, anthropologists do not always consider such beliefs to be a necessary part of a religion. Clifford Geertz, for example, suggests the following broad definition:

A *religion* is (1) a system of symbols which acts to (2) establish powerful, pervasive, and long-lasting moods and motivations in men by (3) formulating conceptions

of a general-order of existence and (4) clothing these conceptions with such an aura of factuality that (5) the moods and motivations seem uniquely realistic. (Geertz 1965: 4)

Let us examine the health food movement in the light of Geertz's definition.

HISTORY OF THE HEALTH FOOD MOVEMENT

The concept of "health foods" can be traced back to the 1830s and the Popular Health movement, which combined a reaction against professional medicine and an emphasis on lay knowledge and health care with broader social concerns such as feminism and the class struggle (see Ehrenreich and English 1979). The Popular Health movement emphasized self-healing and the dissemination of knowledge about the body and health to laymen. One of the early founders of the movement, Sylvester Graham (who gave us the graham cracker), preached that good health was to be found in temperate living. This included abstinence from alcohol, a vegetarian diet, consumption of whole wheat products, and regular exercise. The writings and preachings of these early "hygienists" (as they called themselves) often had moral overtones, depicting physiological and spiritual reform as going hand in hand (Shryock 1966).

The idea that proper diet can contribute to good health has continued into the twentieth century. The discovery of vitamins provided for many health food people a further "natural" means of healing which could be utilized instead of drugs. Vitamins were promoted as health-giving substances by various writers, including nutritionist Adelle Davis, who has been perhaps the most important "guru" of health foods in this century. Davis preached good diet as well as the use of vitamins to restore and maintain health, and her books have become the best sellers of the movement. (The titles of her books, *Let's Cook It Right, Let's Get Well, Let's Have Healthy Children*, give some sense of her approach.) The health food movement took on its present form, however, during the late 1960s, when it became part of the "counterculture."

Jill Dubisch, "You are what you eat: religious aspects of the health food movement." In *The American Dimension: Cultural Myths and Social Realities*. W. Arens and S. P. Montague, eds. Mayfield Publishing Company, 1981, pp. 115–127. Reprinted with permission.

Health foods were "in," and their consumption became part of the general protest against the "establishment" and the "straight" life-style. They were associated with other movements centering around social concerns, such as ecology and consumerism (Kandel and Pelto 1980: 328). In contrast to the Popular Health movement, health food advocates of the sixties saw the establishment as not only the medical profession but also the food industry and the society it represented. Food had become highly processed and laden with colorings, preservatives, and other additives so that purity of food became a new issue. Chemicals had also become part of the food-growing process, and in reaction terms such as "organic" and "natural" became watchwords of the movement. Health food consumption received a further impetus from revelations about the high sugar content of many popular breakfast cereals which Americans had been taught since childhood to think of as a nutritious way to start the day. (Kellogg, an early advocate of the Popular Health movement, would have been mortified, since his cereals were originally designed to be part of a hygienic regimen.)

Although some health food users are members of formal groups (such as the Natural Hygiene Society, which claims direct descent from Sylvester Graham), the movement exists primarily as a set of principles and practices rather than as an organization. For those not part of organized groups, these principles and practices are disseminated, and contact is made with other members of the movement, through several means. The most important of these are health food stores, restaurants, and publications. The two most prominent journals in the movement are *Prevention* and *Let's Live*, begun in 1920 and 1932 respectively (Hongladarom 1976).

These journals tell people what foods to eat and how to prepare them. They offer advice about the use of vitamins, the importance of exercise, and the danger of pollutants. They also present testimonials from faithful practitioners. Such testimonials take the form of articles that recount how the author overcame a physical problem through a health food approach, or letters from readers who tell how they have cured their ailments by following methods advocated by the journal or suggested by friends in the movement. In this manner, such magazines not only educate, they also articulate a world view and provide evidence and support for it. They have become the "sacred writings" of the movement. They are a way of "reciting the code"—the cosmology and moral injunctions—which anthropologist Anthony F. C. Wallace describes as one of the important categories of religious behavior (1966: 57).

IDEOLOGICAL CONTENT OF THE HEALTH FOOD MOVEMENT

What exactly is the health food system? First, and most obviously, it centers around certain beliefs regarding the relationship of diet to health. Health foods are seen as an "alternative" healing system, one which people turn to out of their dissatisfaction with conventional medicine (see, for example, Hongladarom 1976). The emphasis is on "wellness" and prevention rather than on illness and curing. Judging from letters and articles found in health food publications, many individuals' initial adherence to the movement is a type of conversion. A specific medical problem, or a general dissatisfaction with the state of their health, leads these converts to an eventual realization of the "truth" as represented by the health food approach, and to a subsequent change in life-style to reflect the principles of that approach. "Why This Psychiatrist 'Switched,'" published in *Prevention* (September 1976), carries the following heading: "Dr. H. L. Newbold is a great advocate of better nutrition and a livelier life style. But it took a personal illness to make him see the light." For those who have experienced such conversion, and for others who become convinced by reading about such experiences, health food publications serve an important function by reinforcing the conversion and encouraging a change of life-style. For example, an article entitled "How to Convert Your Kitchen for the New Age of Nutrition" (*Prevention*, February 1975) tells the housewife how to make her kitchen a source of health for her family. The article suggests ways of reorganizing kitchen supplies and reforming cooking by substituting health foods for substances detrimental to health, and also offers ideas on the preparation of nutritious and delicious meals which will convert the family to this new way of eating without "alienating" them. The pamphlet *The Junk Food Withdrawal Manual* (Kline 1978) details how an individual can, step by step, quit eating junk foods and adopt more healthful eating habits. Publications also urge the readers to convert others by letting them know how much better health foods are than junk foods. Proselytizing may take the form of giving a "natural" birthday party for one's children and their friends, encouraging schools to substitute fruit and nuts for junk food snacks, and even selling one's own baking.

Undergoing the conversion process means learning and accepting the general features of the health food world view. To begin with, there is great concern, as there is in many religions, with purity, in this case, the purity of food, of water, of air. In fact, there are some striking similarities between keeping a "health food kitchen" and the Jewish practice of keeping kosher. Both make distinctions between proper and improper foods, and both involve excluding certain impure foods (whether unhealthful or non-kosher) from the kitchen and table. In addition, a person concerned with maintaining a high degree of purity in food may engage in similar behavior in either case—reading labels carefully to check for impermissible ingredients and even purchasing food from special establishments to guarantee ritual purity.

In the health food movement, the basis of purity is healthfulness and "naturalness." Some foods are considered to be natural and therefore healthier; this concept applies not only to foods but to other aspects of life as well. It is part of the large idea that people should work in harmony with nature and not against it. In this respect, the health food cosmology sets up an opposition of nature (beneficial) versus culture (destructive), or, in particular, the health food movement against our highly technological society. As products of our industrialized way of life, certain foods are unnatural; they produce illness by working against the body. Consistent with this view is the idea that healing, like eating, should proceed in harmony with nature. The assumption is that the body, if allowed to function naturally, will tend to heal itself. Orthodox medicine, on the other hand, with its drugs and surgery and its non-holistic approach to health, works against the body. Physicians are frequently criticized in the literature of the movement for their narrow approach to medical problems, reliance on drugs and surgery, lack of knowledge of nutrition, and unwillingness to accept the validity of the patient's own experience in healing himself. It is believed that doctors may actually cause further health problems rather than effecting a cure. A short item in *Prevention*, "The Delivery Is Normal—But the Baby Isn't," recounts an incident in which drug-induced labor in childbirth resulted in a mentally retarded baby. The conclusion is "nature does a good job—and we should not, without compelling reasons, try to take over" (*Prevention*, May 1979: 38).

The healing process is hastened by natural substances, such as healthful food, and by other "natural" therapeutic measures such as exercise. Vitamins are also very important to many health food people, both for maintaining health and for healing. They are seen as components of food which work with the body and are believed to offer a more natural mode of healing than drugs. Vitamins, often one of the most prominent products offered in many health food stores, provide the greatest source of profit (Hongladarom 1976).

A basic assumption of the movement is that certain foods are good for you while others are not. The practitioner of a health food way of life must learn to distinguish between two kinds of food: those which promote well-being ("health foods") and those which are believed to be detrimental to health ("junk foods"). The former are the only kind of food a person should consume, while the latter are the antithesis of all that food should be and must be avoided. The qualities of these foods may be described by two anthropological concepts, *mana* and *taboo*. Mana is a type of beneficial or valuable power which can pass to individuals from sacred objects through touch (or, in the case of health foods, by ingestion). Taboo, on the other hand, refers to power that is dangerous; objects which are taboo can injure those who touch them (Wallace 1966: 60–61). Not all foods fall clearly into one category or the other. However, those foods which are seen as having health-giving qualities, which contain *mana*, symbolize life, while *taboo* foods symbolize death. ("Junk food is…dead.…Dead food produces death," proclaims one health food manual [Kline 1978: 2–4].) Much of the space in health food publications is devoted to telling the reader why to consume certain foods and avoid others ("Frozen, Creamed Spinach: Nutritional Disaster," *Prevention*, May 1979; "Let's Sprout Some Seeds," *Better Nutrition*, September 1979).

Those foods in the health food category which are deemed to possess an especially high level of *mana* have come to symbolize the movement as a whole. Foods such as honey, wheat germ, yogurt, and sprouts are seen as

representative of the general way of life which health food adherents advocate, and Kandel and Pelto found that certain health food followers attribute mystical powers to the foods they consume. Raw food eaters speak of the "life energy" in uncooked foods. Sprout eaters speak of their food's "growth force" (1980: 336).

Qualities such as color and texture are also important in determining health foods and may acquire symbolic value. "Wholeness" and "whole grain" have come to stand for healthfulness and have entered the jargon of the advertising industry. Raw, coarse, dark, crunchy, and cloudy foods are preferred over those which are cooked, refined, white, soft, and clear. (See Table 1.)

Thus dark bread is preferred over white, raw milk over pasteurized, brown rice over white. The convert must learn to eat foods which at first seem strange and even exotic and to reject many foods which are components of the Standard American diet. A McDonald's hamburger, for example, which is an important symbol of America itself (Kottack 1978), falls into the category of "junk food" and must be rejected.

Just as the magazines and books which articulate the principles of the health food movement and serve as a guide to the convert can be said to comprise the sacred writings of the movement, so the health food store or health food restaurant is the temple where the purity of the movement is guarded and maintained. There individuals find for sale the types of food and other substances advocated by the movement. One does not expect to find items of questionable purity, that is, substances which are not natural or which may be detrimental to health. Within the precincts of the temple adherents can feel safe from the contaminating forces of the larger society, can meet fellow devotees, and can be instructed by the guardians of the sacred area (see, for example, Hongladarom 1976). Health food stores may vary in their degree of purity. Some sell items such as coffee, raw sugar, or "natural" ice cream which are considered questionable by others of the faith. (One health food store I visited had a sign explaining that it did not sell vitamin supplements, which it considered to be "unnatural," i.e., impure.)

People in other places are often viewed as living more "naturally" and healthfully than contemporary Americans. Observation of such peoples may be used to confirm practices of the movement and to acquire ideas about food. Healthy and long-lived people like the Hunza of the Himalayas are studied to determine the secrets of their strength and longevity. Cultures as yet untainted by the food systems of industrialized nations are seen as examples of what better diet can do. In addition, certain foods from other cultures—foods such as humus, falafel, and tofu—have been adopted into the health food repertoire because of their presumed healthful qualities.

Peoples of other times can also serve as models for a more healthful way of life. There is in the health food movement a concept of a "golden age," a past which provides an authority for a better way of living. This past may be scrutinized for clues about how to improve contemporary American society. An archaeologist, writing for *Prevention* magazine, recounts how "I Put Myself on a Caveman Diet—Permanently" (*Prevention*, September 1979). His article explains how he improved his health by utilizing the regular exercise and simpler foods which he had concluded from his research were probably characteristic of our prehistoric ancestors. A general nostalgia about the past seems to exist in the health food movement, along with the feeling that we have departed from a more natural pattern of eating practiced by earlier generations of Americans (see, for example, Hongladarom 1976). (Sylvester Graham, however, presumably did not find the eating habits of his contemporaries to be very admirable.)

The health food movement is concerned with more than the achievement of bodily health. Nutritional problems are often seen as being at the root of emotional, spiritual, and even social problems. An article entitled "Sugar Neurosis" states "Hypoglycemia (low blood sugar) is a medical reality that can trigger wife-beating, divorce, even suicide"

Table 1 Health Food World View

	Health Foods	**Junk Foods**	
cosmic	LIFE	DEATH	
oppositions	NATURE	CULTURE	
	holistic, organic	fragmented, mechanistic	
basic	harmony with body	working against body	
values	and nature	and nature	undesirable
and	natural and real	manufactured and	attributes
desirable	harmony, self-	artificial disharmony,	
attributes	sufficiency, independence	dependence	
	homemade, small scale	mass-produced	
	layman competence	professional esoteric	
	and understanding	knowledge and jargon	
	whole	processed	
	coarse	refined	
beneficial	dark	white	harmful
qualities	crunchy	soft	qualities
of food	raw	cooked	
	cloudy	clear	
	yogurt*	ice cream, candy	
	honey*	sugar*	
	carob	chocolate	
specific	soybeans*	beef	specific
foods with	sprouts*	overcooked vegetables	taboo
mana	fruit juices	soft drinks*	foods
	herb teas	coffee,* tea	
	foods from other cultures:	"all-American" foods: hot dogs,	
	humus, falafel, kefir, tofu,	McDonald's hamburgers,*	
	stir-fried vegetables,	potato chips,	
	pita bread	Coke	
	return to early American	corruption of this original	
	values, "real" American	and better way of life	
	way of life	and values	

*Denotes foods with especially potent mana or taboo.

(*Prevention*, April 1979: 110). Articles and books claim to show the reader how to overcome depression through vitamins and nutrition and the movement promises happiness and psychological well-being as well as physical health. Social problems, too, may respond to the health food approach. For example, a probation officer recounts how she tried changing offenders' diets in order to change their behavior. Testimonials from two of the individuals helped tell "what it was like to find that good nutrition was their bridge from the wrong side of the law and a frustrated, unhappy life to a vibrant and useful one" (*Prevention*, May 1978: 56). Thus, through more healthful eating and a more natural life-style, the health food movement offers its followers what many religions offer: salvation—in this case salvation for the body, for the psyche, and for society.

Individual effort is the keystone of the health food movement. An individual can take responsibility for his or her own health and does not need to rely on professional medical practitioners. The corollary of this is that it is a person's own behavior which may be the cause of ill health. By sinning, by not listening to our bodies, and by not following a natural way of life, we bring our ailments upon ourselves.

The health food movement also affirms the validity of each individual's experience. No two individuals are alike: needs for different vitamins vary widely; some people are more sensitive to food additives than others; each person has his or her best method of achieving happiness. Therefore, the generalized expertise of professionals and the scientifically verifiable findings of the experts may not be adequate guides for you, the individual, in the search of health. Each person's experience has meaning; if something works for you, then it works. If it works for others also, so much the better, but if it does not, that does not invalidate your own experience. While the movement does not by any means disdain all scientific findings (and indeed they are used extensively when they bolster health food positions), such findings are not seen as the only source of confirmation for the way of life which the health food movement advocates, and the scientific establishment itself tends to be suspect.

In line with its emphasis on individual responsibility for health, the movement seeks to deprofessionalize knowledge and place in every individual's hands the information and means to heal. Drugs used by doctors are usually available only through prescription, but foods and vitamins can be obtained by anyone. Books, magazines, and health food store personnel seek to educate their clientele in ways of healing themselves and maintaining their own health. Articles explain bodily processes, the effects of various substances on health, and the properties of foods and vitamins.

The focus on individual responsibility is frequently tied to a wider concern for self-sufficiency and self-reliance. Growing your own organic garden, grinding your own flour, or even, as one pamphlet suggests, raising your own cow are not simply ways that one can be assured of obtaining healthful food; they are also expressions of independence and self-reliance. Furthermore, such practices are seen as characteristic of an earlier "golden age" when people lived

natural lives. For example, an advertisement for vitamins appearing in a digest distributed in health food stores shows a mother and daughter kneading bread together. The heading reads "America's discovering basics." The copy goes on, "Baking bread at home has been a basic family practice throughout history. The past several decades, however, have seen a shift in the American diet to factory-produced breads.... Fortunately, today there are signs that more and more Americans are discovering the advantage of baking bread themselves." Homemade bread, home-canned produce, sprouts growing on the window sill symbolize what are felt to be basic American values, values supposedly predominant in earlier times when people not only lived on self-sufficient farms and produced their own fresh and more natural food, but also stood firmly on their own two feet and took charge of their own lives. A reader writing to *Prevention* praises an article about a man who found "new life at ninety without lawyers or doctors," saying "If that isn't the optimum in the American way of living, I can't imagine what is!" (*Prevention*, May 1978: 16). Thus although it criticizes the contemporary American way of life (and although some vegetarians turn to Eastern religions for guidance—see Kandel and Pelto 1980), the health food movement in general claims to be the true faith, the proponent of basic Americanness, a faith from which the society as a whole has strayed.

SOCIAL SIGNIFICANCE OF THE HEALTH FOOD MOVEMENT FOR AMERICAN ACTORS

Being a "health food person" involves more than simply changing one's diet or utilizing an alternative medical system. Kandel and Pelto suggest that the health food movement derives much of its popularity from the fact that "food may be used simultaneously to cure or prevent illness, as a religious symbol and to forge social bonds. Frequently health food users are trying to improve their health, their lives, and sometimes the world as well" (1980: 332). Use of health foods becomes an affirmation of certain values and a commitment to a certain world view. A person who becomes involved in the health food movement might be said to experience what anthropologist Anthony F. C. Wallace has called "mazeway resynthesis." The "mazeway" is the mental "map" or image of the world which each individual holds. It includes values, the environment and the objects in it, the image of the self and of others, the techniques one uses to manipulate the environment to achieve desired end states (Wallace 1966: 237). Resynthesis of this mazeway—that is, the creation of new "maps," values, and techniques—commonly occurs in times of religious revitalization, when new religious movements are begun and converts to them are made. As individuals, these converts learn to view the world in a new manner and to act accordingly. In the case of the health food movement, those involved learn to see their health problems and other dissatisfactions with their lives as stemming from improper diet and living in disharmony with nature. They are provided with new values, new ways of viewing their environment, and new techniques for achieving their goals. For such individuals, health food use can come to imply "a major redefinition of self-image, role, and one's relationship to others" (Kandel and Pelto 1980: 359). The world comes to "make sense" in the light of this new world view. Achievement of the desired end states of better health and an improved outlook on life through following the precepts of the movement gives further validation.

It is this process which gives the health food movement some of the overtones of a religion. As does any new faith, the movement criticizes the prevailing social values and institutions, in this case the health-threatening features of modern industrial society. While an individual's initial dissatisfaction with prevailing beliefs and practices may stem from experiences with the conventional medical system (for example, failure to find a solution to a health problem through visits to a physician), this dissatisfaction often comes to encompass other facets of the American way of life. This further differentiates the "health food person" from mainstream American society (even when the difference is justified as a return to "real" American values).

In everyday life the consumption of such substances as honey, yogurt, and wheat germ, which have come to symbolize the health food movement, does more than contribute to health. It also serves to represent commitment to the health food world view. Likewise, avoiding those substances, such as sugar and white bread, which are considered "evil" is also a mark of a health food person. Ridding the kitchen of such items—a move often advocated by articles advising readers on how to "convert" successfully to health foods—is an act of ritual as well as practical significance. The symbolic nature of such foods is confirmed by the reactions of outsiders to those who are perceived as being inside the movement. An individual who is perceived as being a health food person is often automatically assumed to use honey instead of sugar, for example. Conversely, if one is noticed using or not using certain foods (e.g., adding wheat germ to food, not eating white sugar), this can lead to questions from the observer as to whether or not that individual is a health food person (or a health food "nut," depending upon the questioner's own orientation).

The symbolic nature of such foods is especially important for the health food neophyte. The adoption of a certain way of eating and the renunciation of mainstream cultural food habits can constitute "bridge-burning acts of commitment" (Kandel and Pelto 1980: 395), which function to cut the individual off from previous patterns of behavior. However, the symbolic activity which indicates this cutting off need not be as radical as a total change of eating habits. In an interview in *Prevention*, a man who runs a health-oriented television program recounted an incident in which a viewer called up after a show and announced excitedly that he had changed his whole life-style—he had started using honey in his coffee! (*Prevention*, February 1979: 89). While recognizing the absurdity of the action on a practical level,

the program's host acknowledged the symbolic importance of this action to the person involved. He also saw it as a step in the right direction since one change can lead to another. Those who sprinkle wheat germ on cereal, toss alfalfa sprouts with a salad, or pass up an ice cream cone for yogurt are not only demonstrating a concern for health but also affirming their commitment to a particular life-style and symbolizing adherence to a set of values and a world view.

CONCLUSION

As this analysis has shown, health foods are more than simply a way of eating and more than an alternative healing system. If we return to Clifford Geertz's definition of religion as a "system of symbols" which produces "powerful, pervasive, and long-lasting moods and motivations" by "formulating conceptions of a general order of existence" and making them appear "uniquely realistic," we see that the health food movement definitely has a religious dimension. There is, first, a system of symbols, in this case based on certain kinds and qualities of food. While the foods are believed to have health-giving properties in themselves, they also symbolize a world view which is concerned with the right way to live one's life and the right way to construct a society. This "right way" is based on an approach to life which stresses harmony with nature and the holistic nature of the body. Consumption of those substances designated as "health foods," as well as participation in other activities associated with the movement which also symbolize its world view (such as exercising or growing an organic garden), can serve to establish the "moods and motivations" of which Geertz speaks. The committed health food follower may come to experience a sense of spiritual as well as physical well-being when he or she adheres to the health food way of life. Followers are thus motivated to persist in this way of life, and they come to see the world view of this movement as correct and "realistic."

In addition to its possession of sacred symbols and its "convincing" world view, the health food movement also has other elements which we usually associate with a religion. Concepts of mana and taboo guide the choice of foods. There is a distinction between the pure and impure and a concern for the maintenance of purity. There are "temples" (health food stores and other such establishments) which are expected to maintain purity within their confines. There are "rabbis," or experts in the "theology" of the movement and its application to everyday life. There are sacred and instructional writings which set out the principles of the movement and teach followers how to utilize them. In addition, like many religious movements, the health food movement harkens back to a "golden age" which it seeks to recreate and assumes that many of the ills of the contemporary world are caused by society's departure from this ideal state.

Individuals entering the movement, like individuals entering any religious movement, may undergo a process of conversion. This can be dramatic, resulting from the cure of an illness or the reversal of a previous state of poor health, or it can be gradual, a step-by-step changing of eating and other habits through exposure to health food doctrine. Individuals who have undergone conversion and mazeway resynthesis, as well as those who have tested and confirmed various aspects of the movement's prescriptions for better health and a better life, may give testimonials to the faith. For those who have adopted, in full or in part, the health food world view, it provides, as do all religions, explanations for existing conditions, answers to specific problems, and a means of gaining control over one's existence. Followers of the movement are also promised "salvation," not in the form of afterlife, but in terms of enhanced physical well-being, greater energy, longer life-span, freedom from illness, and increased peace of mind. However, although the focus is this-worldly, there is a spiritual dimension to the health food movement. And although it does not center its world view around belief in supernatural beings, it does posit a higher authority—the wisdom of nature—as the source of ultimate legitimacy for its views.

Health food people are often dismissed as "nuts" or "food faddists" by those outside the movement. Such a designation fails to recognize the systematic nature of the health food world view, the symbolic significance of health foods, and the important functions which the movement performs for its followers. Health foods offer an alternative or supplement to conventional medical treatment, and a meaningful and effective way for individuals to bring about changes in lives which are perceived as unsatisfactory because of poor physical and emotional health. It can also provide for its followers a framework of meaning which transcends individual problems. In opposing itself to the predominant American life-style, the health food movement sets up a symbolic system which opposes harmony to disharmony, purity to pollution, nature to culture, and ultimately, as in many religions, life to death. Thus while foods are the beginning point and the most important symbols of the health food movement, food is not the ultimate focus but rather a means to an end: the organization of a meaningful world view and the construction of a satisfying life.

References

Ehrenreich, Barbara, and Deidre English. 1979. *For Her Own Good: 150 Years of the Experts' Advice to Women.* Garden City, N.Y.: Anchor Press/Doubleday.

Geertz, Clifford. 1965. "Religion as a Cultural System." In Michael Banton, ed., *Anthropological Approaches to the Study of Religion.* A.S.A. Monograph No. 3. London: Tavistock Publications Ltd.

Hongladarom, Gail Chapman. 1976. "Health Seeking Within the Health Food Movement." Ph.D. Dissertation: University of Washington.

Kandel, Randy F., and Gretel H. Pelto. 1980. "The Health Food Movement: Social Revitalization or Alternative Health Maintenance System." In Norge W. Jerome, Randy F. Kandel, and Gretel H. Pelto, eds., *Nutritional Anthropology.* Pleasantville, N.Y.: Redgrave Publishing Co.

Kline, Monte. 1978. *The Junk Food Withdrawal Manual.* Total Life, Inc.

Kottak, Conrad. 1978. "McDonald's as Myth, Symbol, and Ritual." In *Anthropology: The Study of Human Diversity.* New York: Random House.

Shryock, Richard Harrison. 1966. *Medicine in America: Historical Essays.* Baltimore: Johns Hopkins University Press.

Wallace, Anthony F. C. 1966. *Religion: An Anthropological View.* New York: Random House.

PART IV

Too Little and Too Much: Nutrition in the Contemporary World

UNIT VIII

Undernutrition and Its Discontents

We are in the midst of a shift in language from "malnutrition" to "undernutrition." Today we use the term "undernutrition" when we are referring to conditions of inadequate intake of the essential nutrients that everyone needs in order to survive and thrive. This shift in language is necessary because we are now much more aware of the existence of other forms of malnutrition, even in conditions where people can get enough to eat, or even more than enough to eat. In fact, obesity is also a serious malnutrition problem, so we need a way of distinguishing the malnutrition that comes from not having enough to eat from other forms of nutrition-related pathology.

Under the heading of undernutrition, it is disheartening to find a wide continuum of conditions from outright starvation to more subtle, but nonetheless pernicious effects of inadequate intake of both macronutrients (protein and energy) and micronutrients (vitamins and minerals). What are the causes of undernutrition? What are its consequences? Many of the papers throughout this volume are directly or indirectly concerned with the causes of undernutrition. They take up various aspects of the complex determinants of food systems and examine how those determinants result in diets that are sometimes inadequate to meet the macronutrient and micronutrient needs of particular populations and subgroups within populations. For example, in the section on the cultural ecology of infant and young child feeding, the papers describe and analyze the ways in which multiple determinants lead to patterns of infant feeding that do not always optimize children's nutritional intake and nutritional status. In contrast to papers in other sections of the book that examine nutrition as the "endpoint" or "outcome" of analysis, in this section undernutrition is the starting point. We focus first on its consequences for individuals, and, by extension, the societies in which they live (the papers by Adolfo Chávez and colleagues, Reynaldo Martorell, and Richard Bender and Darna Dufour). In the papers by Alex de Waal and Alan Whiteside and by Catherine Panter-Brick and colleagues, we turn attention to larger system consequences, including the societal responses for ameliorating and treating undernutrition.

In the spectrum of consequences of undernutrition, death is the direst. Death from undernutrition is not only caused by starvation. Outright starvation is rare, except under exceptional circumstances of war and famine. The vast majorities of deaths from undernutrition occur in infants and young children and are the result of its effects on various biological functions, particularly its effects on the immune system. In 1993 Pelletier, Frongillo, and Habicht showed that undernutrition kills by increasing the severity of common childhood infections. Across the world, in different ecological, economic, and socio-cultural conditions, at every level of undernutrition, undernourished children are more likely to die than are children in the same communities and countries who are not undernourished. Well-nourished children survive childhood diseases, such as diarrhea, pneumonia and measles, but undernourished children are much more likely to die when they get sick. In epidemiological terms we can say that the "case fatality rate" of infectious diseases is higher when a child is undernourished. In 2008 a group of epidemiological investigators concluded that 35% of deaths in infants and children birth to 5 years in the world today are due to undernutrition. When neonatal deaths are excluded an even higher proportion of deaths involve nutrition. Thus, as a public health problem, the various forms of undernutrition, including deficiencies of micronutrients, play a very large role in child deaths in the contemporary world.

When, in the 1960s, Dr. Adolfo Chávez and his colleagues at the National Institute of Nutrition in Mexico undertook a study to demonstrate that mild to moderate undernutrition had major consequences for child health and development their hypothesis was quite radical. Within the nutrition and public health community there was general agreement that serious nutrient deficiencies were a cause for concern. But some individuals doubted whether a smaller degree of growth stunting due to inadequate nutrition, the type Chávez and colleagues witnessed every day in Mexican peasant communities, was affecting anything other than child size. Chávez decided to conduct a long-term experiment in which he gave nutrition supplements to women during pregnancy and then their children, and compared the supplemented children to their older siblings, who did not receive the supplements. All children, both supplemented and unsupplemented had access to free health care at the clinic the researchers set up in the community.

The paper in this reader (chapter 33) is a comprehensive report on the long-term study. It summarizes many aspects of growth and development resulting from supplementation, sequentially as the children got older and more outcomes could be examined. Among the many findings that demonstrate the pernicious effects of undernutrition are growth stunting, increased percent of time that children are sick, decreased levels of activity, decreased interest in exploring their environments, and other effects on personality and intellectual development. Viewed across the years of the study, the breadth of the negative consequences is stunning.

A primary consequence of undernutrition is that children fail to grow well. In the absence of adequate food to meet needs for growth and other functions, one of the primary biological adaptations the body makes is to slow down or even stop growing. Consequently growth faltering during the period when a child should be showing measurable increases in height and weight is an important indicator that the child is experiencing the process of becoming undernourished. Although adult size within a population is also influenced by genetics, short stature in adulthood generally indicates that the individual experienced undernutrition in childhood.

Is the reduction in growth that occurs with undernutrition a "no cost" adaptation, as some people have argued? Reynaldo Martorell takes up the question in his paper on "Body Size, Adaptation, and Function." This paper was originally published as part of a larger symposium, "Small but Healthy," which was published in 1989 in the journal *Human Organization.* The symposium was designed to examine multiple aspects of the so-called "small but healthy hypothesis." Each of the chapters in the symposium dealt with different aspects of the fallacy of the concept of a "no cost adaptation" to undernutrition. Today, very few people subscribe to the idea that children can be small, but healthy. The reason for including this paper in the reader today is that Martorell makes four basic points in his paper that everyone should be aware of: 1) adults in developing countries have small body sizes largely as a result of poor diets and infection during childhood; 2) monitoring growth in children is widely accepted as an excellent tool for detecting health problems; 3) the conditions that give rise to stunting affect other aspects, such as cognitive development; and 4) girls who are stunted in childhood are, in adulthood, at greater risk of giving birth to stunted infants who, in turn, are at greater risk of dying in infancy. In this short paper, which draws on data from many parts of the world, we find a clear argument for regarding growth stunting as an important indicator of undernutrition, with all of its short-term and long-term functional consequences.

Richard Bender and Darna Dufour continue the examination of the consequences of undernutrition in their paper, "Hungry But Not Starving: Functional Consequences of Undernutrition in Adults." They take us from its effects in childhood to the continuation of those effects on adults. They present the concept of work capacity as a biological phenomenon, explaining how it is measured and how it relates to undernutrition. The effect of a specific micronutrient deficiency, iron, is then discussed. In addition to the negative effects of anemia on work capacity, anemia has many other negative consequences, including its potential role in maternal mortality during childbirth. It is important to remember that iron deficiency, with all of its negative consequences, is very widespread in the world today. Together with the chapters by Chávez and colleagues and Martorell, the paper by Bender and Dufour shows us that undernutrition is never benign. Even relatively low levels of deficiencies during critical periods of life have serious, lifelong consequences.

The paper on famine in Southern Africa by Alex de Waal and Alan Whiteside was published in the midst of a food crisis. As the authors point out, "Droughts and famines have afflicted large parts of Africa throughout history." These have been well publicized, to such an extent that many people in more affluent countries have become inured to the pictures of suffering and death that occur during food crisis situations. The fact that serious perturbations in food systems lead to hunger and ultimately to starvation is well known and well documented. There is also strong evidence to show that food system perturbations are directly linked to climatic conditions and climate change, which in turn reflect the influences of socio-political and economic forces and geopolitics. While a secondary reason for including this chapter in the book is to remind our readers that famines continue to happen with devastating consequences, our primary motivation is the important insights underlying the authors' hypothesis. In this paper DeWaal and Whiteside call attention to another critical feature in the fragility of food systems, another factor that links directly to undernutrition—the physical health of the people who have responsibility for producing food and sustaining local food systems. Their dramatic hypothesis is that HIV/AIDS has become so prevalent in Southern Africa that it not only affects the individual families who are living with the disease, but the capacity of the entire society to produce food. Their hypothesis draws attention to the consequences of disease on nutritional well being, not just at the individual and family level, but also on the societal level.

Catherine Panter-Brick and colleagues take up an additional critical aspect of undernutrition—namely contemporary responses to the societal challenges presented by severe food shortages and the ensuing undernutrition. They examine the responses at multiple levels, from the international agencies to local communities. Panter-Brick and colleagues begin their analysis by questioning the appropriateness of the term "crisis" for the situation in the Sahel. Crisis implies a short-term problem that is amenable to short-term solutions. However, they point out that "In some localities...the 'food crisis' of 2004–6 was not necessarily *qualitatively* different from other years. Seasonal hunger and food crises are part and parcel of habitual, 'normal' experience." To underscore this point she notes that "Indeed, in 2007 after the food crisis was ostensibly over, Niger's children still suffered a 50% chronic and 10% acute malnutrition rate...A new crisis emerged in 2010, following floods in the north in late 2009 and a season of unpredictable rains, and then compounded by further flooding in August 2010."

A primary feature of this chapter, which is often missing from analyses of nutrition interventions undertaken by non-anthropologists, is the emic perspective, the views of the families who needed help. Panter-Brick and colleagues skillfully contrast the rationales and assumptions of the people who set up and run programs with those of people in the communities. In particular they identify sources of "disjunction" between the two sets of players. Of particular importance are differences in understandings of "vulnerability." They suggest "some parental views of vulnerability prevented some malnourished children from having access to emergency nutrition programmes." Closely related to vulnerability are the problems that occur because of "targeting." Most nutrition programs, including those that are put in place during emergencies, "target" their resources to subject sub-groups and exclude others. Often targeting is by age, so that children below and above particular ages are excluded because biological and epidemiological research shows that they are not likely to benefit from a particular intervention. This feature creates many tensions at the interface between intervention programs and families, not just in emergency situations, but also in usual, onoing public health and nutrition programs. However, it can be particularly acute in emergency situations. As articulated by Panter-Brick and colleagues, "The explicit goal of emergency feeding and therapeutic programmes is to save the lives of the most vulnerable individuals. By contrast, parents seek to address the vulnerability of *all* of their children and the long-term livelihoods of the whole household.... There is a strong local ethos of non-discrimination between children within a household. A widely expressed sentiment was that 'all children are the same.'" Moreover, excluding other children in the household, and even those of neighbors, is seen as violating fundamental social values. In concluding their chapter, Panter-Brick and colleagues take up the very difficult issues of moving families and communities out of aid, and the challenges of sustaining support when international agencies can no longer do so.

In conclusion, the chapters we have selected for this section provide a picture of holistic, anthropological approaches to the critical and pervasive issue of undernutrition in the contemporary world. Some of the authors are anthropologists by training; all of them use a biocultural perspective to describe and analyze the complex interactions between biology and behavior that produce the negative functional consequences of living in social systems that fail to provide all of their members with sufficient food to meet their nutritional needs. The papers include a range from a focus on individuals to international socio-cultural and political dynamics in order to illustrate the breadth of research on one of the most serious problems of humanity.

Suggestions for Thinking and Doing Nutritional Anthropology

1. Many tools have been developed to help people learn how to understand the nature of undernutrition, food insecurity, and how to measure it. When it comes to learning new skills, there is no substitute for first-hand experience, but learning the basics is excellent preparation. Whether you plan to work on issues related to undernutrition or over-nutrition or just want to be an informed person, knowing the basics about how to conduct anthropometric measurements is a skill that will stand you in good stead. The Food and Agricultural Organization (FAO), which is a UN agency based in Rome, has made it possible for people everywhere to do this through a free on-line course. Here is the link: http://www.foodsecinfoaction.org/dl.

   To learn how to do anthropometry, follow the link to "Nutritional status assessment and analysis" in the Learning Center: Courses on Food Insecurity. You will need to register on the website to get access to the courses. Registration is simple, with clear instructions.

   There are many other courses you may be interested in, including courses on policies related to food security, program issues, such as targeting, communicating about food insecurity, and so on. This ambitious and extensive site is supported by the European Union.

2. The World Health Organization has recently created a public access website where you can obtain a great deal of information about nutrition, both undernutrition and over-nutrition. To learn about the site and how to use it, pick a specific nutrient and follow the links to the information about your nutrient. You can start your search here: http://www.who.int/nutrition/en/ and then follow the links to the e-LENA website. (The WHO Nutrition website in general and the e-LENA website are both excellent sources of information on many aspects of nutrition.)

References

Black RE, Allen LH, Bhutta ZA, Caulfield LE, de Onis M, Ezzati M, Mathers C, Rivera JR. 2008. Maternal and child undernutrition: global and regional exposures and health consequences. The Lancet 371(9608): 243–260.

Pelletier DL, Frongillo Jr. EA, Habicht J-P. 1993. Epidemiologic evidence for a potentiating effect of malnutrition on child mortality. American Journal of Public Health 83(8):1130–1133.

Pelto GH, ed. 1989. Small but Healthy. Symposium Human Organization, 48(1): 11–52.

Suggested Further Reading

Hadley C. Three Pillars of Food Insecurity: Getting to the Guts of Utilization. http://foodanthro.wordpress.com/2011/05/24/the-three-pillars-of-food-insecurity-getting-to-the-guts-of-utilization/. This article by Craig Hadley for the Society for the Anthropology of Food and Nutrition. In addition to this article the website of

SAFN is a veritable gold mine of information on many topics in nutritional anthropology.

Victora CG, Adair L, Fall C, Hallal PC, Martorell R, Richter L, Sachdev HS. Maternal and child undernutrition: consequences for adult health and human capital. The Lancet 371(9609): 340–357. This important paper is a follow-up on the topic of long-term consequences of undernutrition during pregnancy and early childhood. If you cannot get it through your library you can also access it directly at the Lancet journal website. This is one of a number of papers that the journal makes available free of charge to the public, and you can read it by signing up on their website.

Bodley J. 2008. The Price of Progress. In Victims of Progress, Fifth edition. Lanham, MD: Altamira Press. Available at http://www.wcc.hawaii.edu/facstaff/dagrossa-p/articles/PriceOfProgress.pdf. This article, although not focused exclusively on undernutrition, includes discussions about what happens to diet quality in small-scale societies when their social and dietary systems are distorted by confrontations with external socio-political systems.

CHAPTER 33

The Effect of Malnutrition on Human Development: A 24-Year Study of Well-Nourished and Malnourished Children Living in a Poor Mexican Village

Adolfo Chávez, Celia Martínez, and Beatriz Soberanes

(1995)

CHRONIC MALNUTRITION

It was recognized in the 1950s that the severe forms of protein-energy malnutrition, kwashiorkor and marasmus, were associated with marked cognitive effects (Scrimshaw et al., 1968) although the lasting effects on survivors were unknown. The predominant type of malnutrition in Latin America has changed dramatically during the second half of this century. On the one hand, the prevalence of acute and severe forms of malnutrition that bring death to children has steadily declined. On the other hand, chronic malnutrition, which causes physical and intellectual impairments in the affected populations, has increased substantially.

Marginal or chronic malnutrition is a consequence of early malnutrition that is more noticeable between 8 and 20 months of age. Many individuals who experience childhood malnutrition survive and reach adult age. However, these individuals are "vulnerable survivors" with very specific developmental deficiencies that are the result of chronic malnutrition experienced during early childhood.

This study reports on an 18-year follow-up that gives us the opportunity to describe the natural history of two exceedingly important problems in developing countries: poverty and malnutrition. These data contribute to our understanding of the consequences of early childhood poverty and malnutrition for the individual's performance at birth, during the school-age period, and during adolescence and young adulthood.

Adolfo Chávez, Celia Martínez, and Beatriz Soberanes, "The effect of malnutrition on human development: a 24-year study of well-nourished and malnourished children living in a poor Mexican village." In *Community-based longitudinal nutrition and health studies: classic examples from Guatemala, Haiti, and Mexico.* N. S. Scrimshaw, ed. Boston: International Nutrition Foundation for Developing Countries, 1995, pp. 79–124. Amended and reprinted with permission.

The worldwide problem of malnutrition is related to the consumption of deficient and monotonous diets that are based on roots and cereals. Cross-sectional studies conducted in developing countries have shown that few children have the symptoms and clinical signs of severe protein-energy or micronutrient malnutrition. Furthermore, the majority of these children seemed to tolerate well their chronic exposure to suboptimal diets. However, pioneering studies in Mexico (Ramos-Galván, 1949; Cravioto et al., 1966; Cravioto and DeLicardie, 1968) showed that subclinical malnutrition, manifested only by impaired growth, significantly impaired intersensory perception. Concurrently Mönckeberg (1967) showed a significant relationship between growth retardation and reduced cognitive performance in low socioeconomic groups in Chile.

In this period, Federico Gómez, the Director of the Hospital Infantil de Mexico, proposed a classification of malnutrition based on weight-for-age that has been widely adopted. First degree malnutrition was identified as 10 to 25% below normal weight-for-age, second degree as 25 to 40% below and third degree as greater than 40% below standards for well-nourished children for whom the normal range was plus or minus 10%. First and second degree malnutrition correspond to what is now called *marginal nutrition* (Gómez, 1946; Canosa et al., 1968).

The longitudinal study described in this [article] was carried out to understand the consequences of moderate malnutrition. Emphasis was on determining the relationship between chronic malnutrition and the physical, mental, and behavioral development of the individuals. To understand this relationship, the research design must control for nonnutritional factors that also affect human developmental needs by including longitudinal observations of both malnourished and well-nourished children living under the same social and ecological conditions.

By 1967, the year in which this study was planned, it was recognized that subclinical malnutrition associated with growth retardation was associated with deficits in learning and behavior. However, there was no agreement as to the extent with which these associations were due to malnutrition or to concurrent genetic, cultural or other environmental factors. As a result of this debate, this study was designed as an intervention in which it was possible to control for nonnutritional factors.

We decided to follow a small number of subjects prospectively in great detail, for two reasons. The data collection, which included measurements of milk volumes, interviews, and direct observations of child behavior, required field workers to live with the families for at least three consecutive days every two months. The ethics of observing a control group of subjects without nutritional supplementation during the study has been questioned. The researchers considered the study to be ethical because its results would help to motivate decision-makers to invest in and support efforts to improve the nutritional status of the poor in Mexico and throughout the world, an expectation amply realized. Moreover, the control group benefited from the same enhanced medical care and stimulation as the supplemented group. Without a control group no children would have received a supplement.

Several of the social goals of the project were achieved. In 1973, a few months after the first report of the project was presented, the Mexican government launched a major program called Orientación Familiar, which taught women how to improve their infant feeding practices. The program promoted partial breast-feeding at three months of age, which meant the inclusion of clean foods available at home in addition to breast milk (Muñoz de Chávez and Chávez, 1986). This program was delivered to more than two million households by a large number of rural women who were trained in the use of educational materials. This was the largest public health effort that resulted from the study in Tezonteopan, which together with other smaller studies, was instrumental in decreasing the severity of malnutrition in Mexico.

Most of the original observations in Tezonteopan were made by the resident researcher Celia Martínez between 1968 and 1973. She still lives in the village 24 years after the initiation of the study and has also conducted, at times with few resources and little support, follow-up studies during adolescence and young adulthood. It is to her that we owe the accumulation of knowledge from this extraordinarily detailed study that illustrates how the functioning of poor Mexican infants is damaged by malnutrition and how it can be improved with better primary health care and nutrition.

A POOR VILLAGE: ITS REALITY AND PROBLEMS

Tezonteopan had 1,495 inhabitants when the study was initiated in 1968. The village was very isolated, even though it was only 9 km from a paved road to Mexico City, only 2.5 hours away.

Tezonteopan covers 200 ha of agricultural land and was founded in 1884 by 18 families that ran away from a neighboring hacienda. In 1938 the government provided the village with an additional 552 ha of agricultural land. Agriculture is the main source of income for the villagers, who grow corn, beans, and squash for subsistence and peanuts as a cash crop.

The vast majority of the families are poor and have access to only 2 or 3 ha of land. Income received from crops is just enough to pay for the loans that are provided in kind or as cash by the local shop owners. These loans are usually used to acquire consumption and production goods and to cover expenses related to social events and health care.

In 1968 most of the dwellings were built of reeds or adobe and had only one room. The quality of life, including the level of hygiene, was very poor and the village lacked basic infrastructure such as electricity and potable water. At the beginning of the study, the average family income was 1 US$ per day.

In the two years prior to the initiation of the study, overall mortality was 18.5/1,000, infant mortality was 126/1,000 births, and the preschool mortality was 16.9/1,000 inhabitants. The annual birth rate was 58.8/1,000, which in part can be explained by the predominantly young population living in the village. Despite the high mortality, the birth rate was still high and the population increased. The secular trends (1966–1990) of fertility and mortality are presented in Table 1.

The period of fertility was short because the onset of menarche usually was late, at about 15.5 years of age, and the women reached menopause at the relatively young age of 40.5 years (A Chávez and Martínez, 1973). The period of postpartum amenorrhea was very long and lasted for 13.5 months. Therefore the birth intervals were long, with a mean duration of 27 months. The fecundity rates were high because the women had nine children in their short reproductive lives, only five of whom survived until adolescence or early adulthood.

The diet in the village was deficient in nutrients because meat products were hardly ever consumed. Corn provided two-thirds of the daily energy intake, and the remaining calories were provided by beans, sugar (in coffee and tea), and sometimes pasta, bread, and wild vegetables. The infant feeding patterns were very consistent in the village. Infants were given only breast milk up to 8 to 10 months of age. At this

Table 1 Demographic Data on the Community (Mean of 5 Years Around the Annual Rate)

Demographic Data	1966	1972	1978	1984	1990
Total population	1355	1779	2195	2577	2918
Birth rate	58.8	50.4	45.1	40.0	33.2
General mortality rate	18.5	12.5	9.6	9.7	6.9
Demographic growth rate	38.3	40.3	35.5	30.3	26.3
Preschooler mortality rate	16.9	7.5	11.9	6.3	2.6
Infant mortality rate	126	108	77	78	62

age other foods—*atole* (corn gruel), soups, and tortillas—were gradually introduced into the diet.

Since the project was designed around a nutritional intervention, it was decided to minimize the inclusion of other types of interventions such as health care and community development. For this reason, only basic health care was provided, and community events were supported only when this was specifically requested by the villagers.

Important changes took place in the community during the study. This was undoubtedly the result of the presence of the research team and the interest of the Mexican government in the community development of rural areas. At the beginning, these changes were slow; electricity and potable water were not requested by the villagers until the third and fifth year of the study, respectively. After this period the villagers wanted to experience a faster rate of community development, and by 1980 several projects were planned. These included the introduction of irrigation pumps, more profitable crops such as tomatoes, machines for removing peanut husks, and trucks for transporting agricultural products. The research center fully supported and communicated all these requests to the authorities in charge of making these decisions.

The process of change in the village was interrupted in 1982 as a result of a national economic crisis. The sharp increment in outmigration by young villagers that took place around this time probably reflected the fear and anguish caused by this crisis. In 1982, the first peasants went to work in a neighboring community, and now, 10 years after the first migrations, there are 150 villagers working in the United States and Canada.

In spite of the several changes that have taken place since 1975 as a result of social and economic openness, many aspects of basic life in the village have not changed. For example, in the 1990s almost all families have television and video sets. However, the villagers still sleep on a mat on the floor, and the houses still have the same appearance and size, even though they now use more brick and concrete. Most of the houses still lack windows and are as contaminated as before. The food habits and environmental conditions of the people are still the same, even though they now have higher incomes and water taps inside the households.

Infant feeding habits have changed: infants are now given more foods in addition to breast milk and are introduced to these foods at earlier ages. The families are now more likely to give cows' milk as a complement to breast milk. These changes in infant feeding practices are due to the fact that the families have seen the superior development of the children who were supplemented in the study.

There have been important improvements in health in the village. It is paradoxical that small changes could bring about such large effects. The community is still trying to produce more agricultural products, in spite of the national economic crisis of the last 10 years. However, the villagers are also obtaining resources by more diversified strategies that include migration. These recent migration patterns have brought about the most important changes that have benefited the village. In spite of the scarcity of credit and the decline in the prices of agricultural products, the community is now less isolated and more likely to seek external resources. Chronic or moderate malnutrition still persists today at about the same level as before, but there has been a decline in the number of cases of severe malnutrition. Regretfully, these changes have not been enough to promote the healthy development of the survivors.

THE LONGITUDINAL INTERVENTION STUDY: DESIGN AND IMPLEMENTATION

The study was planned as an intervention in which one group of mother-infant dyads received food supplementation while a second group remained untreated. Whereas the treated group would tell us if an adequate nutritional status could be attained even under adverse socioeconomic conditions, the untreated group would provide important information about the natural course and consequences of chronic malnutrition (Madrigal and Avila, 1990).

This project was conceived as a study of cases and not as an epidemiological survey. At that time there were data suggesting that the problem of marginal malnutrition was related to breast-feeding (Martinez and Chávez, 1967). For this reason it was decided to devote a substantial amount of effort to measuring the quantity of breast milk produced and ingested. A great deal of effort also went into making behavioral observations of the children. This component was included because the research team believed that suboptimal child behavior was one of the main consequences of malnutrition. Because behavioral studies can only be done by direct observation in the households, the sample size could not be large. Based on a statistical procedure for taking into account the possibility of dropouts from the study, it was estimated that 20 dyads would be enough to test the behavioral hypotheses.

The supplemented and unsupplemented groups did not enter the study at the same time, because the people in the villages could have questioned the provision of food to some but not to other children. For this reason, during the first year of the study, only the non-supplemented women and their newborns were recruited into the study. During the second and third year of the study, all the women who became pregnant received food supplementation. At the time of birth of the children, dyads with similar physical and socioeconomic characteristics to the unsupplemented group were recruited for continued supplementation.

The United States National Institutes of Health (NIH) initially funded the study for four years and later extended this period to seven years. The Mexican Council for Science and Technology (CONACYT) funded the project for another seven years. The project has continued to be funded by smaller grants, one of which was provided by the United Nations University (UNU).

The study was initiated in February 1968, and the first three months were devoted to a general study of the community and to establishing a close relationship with the families. Following this period, all the pregnant women in the village were studied. By the end of the first year, in June 1969, a group of 41 mother-infant dyads had been recruited. Twenty of these 41 women were selected for the measurements of milk production and intake and behavioral observations. The selection was based on socioeconomic status and maternal health, age, and anthropometry. The growth of the children of the remaining 21 dyads was followed longitudinally into the adolescent period.

The women and their children born in 1968 and 1969 were not given supplemental food and did not receive any type of intervention except in emergency situations. These children grew up with the support of their families under the usual conditions of the village. They were breast-fed for a prolonged period of time, and weaning foods were usually introduced with hesitation and at a very late age in an unsanitary environment that constantly led to constant infections.

These children were born with low birth weight. They grew well in the first three months but then their growth velocity declined and therefore they began to suffer malnutrition. Of the 20 children who were selected for the full study, two were treated and dropped from the study because they developed severe malnutrition, one with edema and the other with marasmus. One of them was replaced by another child. Another child died of an infection under very difficult circumstances and one child emigrated. Therefore this group had a final sample size for the full study of 17 children. The total number of newborns of that year was later further reduced from 41 to 36 due to two additional migrations. This group has been analyzed and included in several reports dealing with preschoolers and teenagers.

The following year a second group of pregnant women was recruited and supplemented twice per day with a nutritious drink immediately following the first report of amenorrhea. The drink was made by mixing milk with fruits and was designed to provide 400 kcal per day and appropriate amounts of iron, niacin, riboflavin, and vitamins A and C. The intake of the food supplement was monitored, and it was shown that it provided 325 kcal per day. Supplemented women had similar socioeconomic and physical characteristics as the women in the nonsupplemented group that was recruited the previous year.

Supplemented subjects were matched at birth with their counterparts in the unsupplemented group, according to the physical and social characteristics of the mother-infant dyad. In addition to the 20 supplemented women who were included in the full study, another 20 women were also given food supplements and studied in some aspects of their development. The fact that the experimental and the control groups entered the study at different times was necessary, not only for interactions with the community but for logistic reasons.

The children in the experimental group began to receive supplementary food as soon as they showed the first signs of growth faltering, at about 12 weeks of age. First, the children were offered a bottle with milk during the night. When the children started to request to be breast-fed more often, even though they were being offered the bottle with milk, they were also given fruits and vegetables. Afterwards the infants were fed ad libitum with milk and a variety of strained foods. The research team always advised the women to continue breast-feeding during this time.

When the children were four years old, they were supplemented twice per day with a sandwich and a glass of milk. When the children began attending school, they sometimes missed one of the daily episodes of supplementation because they preferred to remain playing at school during recess instead of going out to receive their supplement. However, the children always received the supplementation after school hours. The supplementation intervention ended when the children were 10 years of age.

Throughout the study, special care was taken to ensure that the only between-group difference was the nutritional supplementation. Measures were taken to balance the amount of contact with research workers and any other procedure that could have been considered a nonnutritional intervention.

Throughout the 24 years of existence of the Centro Rural de Tezonteopan, a variety of nutrition and child development parameters have been studied. The unsupplemented children are, as this report is being written, 22 years old and therefore have become young adults. The children in the supplemented group are now between 17 and 20 years of age. The range of ages in the latter group is explained by the fact that the large amount of effort needed for planning and implementing the project caused a slowdown in the rate of recruitment of subjects during the last years of the intervention phase.

The different types of studies are presented in the Results. The special methodologies that were employed are presented and discussed below.

(a) All the women were included in longitudinal follow-ups of anthropometry and in a special study on fertility and reproduction.

(b) The studies on food intake during early infancy included measurements of milk volume using a 72-hour test-weighing procedure at 2, 8, 16, 24, 36, 56, and 78 weeks of age.

(c) The behavioral follow-up looking at mother-child interactions was the most significant component of the study. These observations were made between breast-feeding episodes while the observer was seated in a corner of the house pretending to read a book. Every 40 seconds the investigator looked over the book to make a "visual photograph" of the mother-child interaction (e.g., holding, feeding, kissing, verbalizing, degree of physical activity, etc.). Seventeen parameters were captured and written down every time a "visual photograph" was created. This procedure was carried out for 1.5 hours during the morning after the child woke up and for another 1.5 hours in the afternoon. This methodology is derived from that used for ethological observations of primates and is the one that captured the most important differences between the supplemented and unsupplemented children.

(d) A similar methodology was used during the school period. The researchers made a hole in the wall of the classroom so that they could make behavioral observations of the children (e.g., standing, sleeping, attention span) while attending class. Each observation period lasted 1.5 hours and yielded information that discriminated between supplemented and unsupplemented children. Several national and international knowledge and problem-solving tests were also administered during the school period.

(e) The physical activity of the infants was evaluated by observing the number of contacts that the heel made with the bed. Afterwards physical activity was measured as the number of steps taken in a specified period of time (10 minutes per hour for 10 consecutive hours).

(f) The longitudinal assessments involving neurological, psychological, and cognitive measurements were done following traditional methods (A Chávez and Martínez, 1982).

(g) Morbidity was recorded daily and the study also included a microbiological assessment of fecal contamination of household objects and members.

The experimental design was selected to test the hypothesis that nutrition during early childhood is an environmental factor that has a strong negative impact on long-term human development and function. The design of the study also contributed to a better understanding of the development of children in a deprived environment. It was also possible to study the life cycle in the families, since it included the follow-up of subjects from the time that they were in their mother's womb until they became pregnant.

The final objective of the project was to identify the critical point at which interventions that will achieve an optimal development in socioeconomically disadvantaged populations are most cost-effective.

THE FIRST EIGHT MONTHS OF LIFE

The first impact of the supplementation interventions was on the mothers themselves. By the eighth month of pregnancy, the supplemented women consumed 20% more food (2,410 cal and 70.7 g protein vs 2,055 cal and 53.3 g protein) and had a higher pregnancy weight gain (+3.4 kg) than unsupplemented women. Among supplemented women, menstruation returned by 7.5+2.6 months postpartum, 6.2 months earlier than among unsupplemented women. An important consequence of this delayed return of menstruation was that the birth interval decreased from an average

of 27 months to 19 months (A Chávez and Martínez, 1973). This effect cannot be attributed to decreased rates of breast-feeding, because *all* the supplemented women were breast-feeding an average of 7.3 times per day by the time that menses returned.

In this community, infants can be considered as extra-uterine fetuses who depend on their mothers for survival during their first months of life. Then infants are fed almost exclusively on breast milk. Solid foods usually begin to make a critical nutritional contribution when the infant is beyond six to eight months of age.

The placenta is a very efficient organ for the transfer of nutrients from the mother to the fetus even when she is poorly nourished. However, this study demonstrates that maternal supplementation under these circumstances can improve birth weight. The newborns of supplemented mothers weighed 2,970 g at birth and were 180 g heavier than their counterparts in the unsupplemented group (A Chávez and Martinez, 1979c). This 6.5% increase in birth weight, as trivial as it might seem, is important for several reasons. First, this was the beginning of the anthropometric differences that persisted throughout life. Second, 39% (14/39) of the newborns in the unsupplemented group, but only 7.5% (3/40) of those in the supplemented group, were low birth weight (<2.5 kg) infants. Third, food supplementation was also associated with increased total length, leg length, thorax circumference, ratio of head to thorax circumference, and ratio of leg to total length (A Chávez, 1978).

An important question is whether the decline in breast milk production even in the supplemented mothers is due to maternal malnutrition or is a natural phenomenon in the human species. The latter is a possibility, because all mammals follow a parabolic pattern of milk production, with a short incremental period and a long and progressive decremental stage. There is no reason for the human species to follow a different pattern of lactation. To respond to this question, the women who were supplemented during pregnancy continued to be supplemented during lactation. The

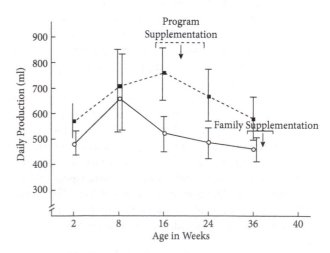

Figure 1 *Milk consumption by the infants of supplemented (---) and unsupplemented (—) mothers.*

total milk volumes plotted in Figure 1 show remarkable between-group differences. As with other mammals, breast milk production among supplemented women followed a parabolic pattern, peaking at four months, followed by a gentle decline.

The literature indicates that in developing countries, children begin to slow their growth at about three months of age. Therefore, it is important to consider the role of breast-feeding in the future of the child. A key finding from this study is that intake or production of breast milk in the unsupplemented group increased during the first eight weeks of lactation and fell thereafter (Martínez and Chávez, 1971). In the supplemented group it increased at least to 16 weeks. Unfortunately, milk volume measurements were not taken within the 8- to 16-week interval. However, by 16 weeks the milk volume had already decreased.

At eight weeks, the infants of unsupplemented mothers were consuming 32 ml per nursing episode, and by 16 weeks this figure decreased to 41 ml per episode. In Figure 2 a comparison of the breast milk intake per kilogram of body weight between the village children and Japanese children fed breast milk ad libitum with bottles indicates that the decrease in milk volume observed in the village after eight weeks is abnormal. This decline in breast milk production occurred despite the fact that children were breast-feeding about 13 times every 24 hours. Therefore, it is important to underscore that the decline in breast milk production is due to maternal supply and not infant demand. This decrease in breast milk production has important nutritional and developmental consequences for the child.

Chemical analysis of the milk samples indicated that the breast milk of unsupplemented women was not diluted according to the progressive pattern typical of other mammals. Unsupplemented women continued producing concentrated milk after their infants were eight weeks of age.

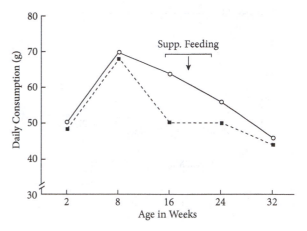

Figure 3 *Milk solids consumed by the infants of supplemented (—) and unsupplemented (---) mothers.*

By contrast, the milk of supplemented women was diluted beyond the expected range. Figure 3 includes the consumption of breast milk solids and shows that both groups of women secreted the nutrients following a pyramid-type pattern, although the peak is sharper among supplemented women. The peak for supplemented women was followed by a more gradual decline in the concentration of nutrients in breast milk after the infants were 3 months of age.

> The between-group difference in the nutrient content of breast milk was 16% less in the supplemented group during the first eight months of life of the child. Although this difference does not seem large, it is important to underscore that it was greatest between 8 and 24 weeks. During this short period of time, the unsupplemented children ceased to be able to obtain all the breast milk that they demanded. To a certain extent, this also happened with the supplemented children, although in this case this phenomenon was observed at an older age and with a more gradual onset.

The decline in breast milk consumption by the children of poorly nourished mothers that begins at two to three months of age is the first insult that leads to malnutrition during early childhood. This situation could be easily corrected by introducing complementary foods available in the household by three months of age as required to maintain weight gain.

Figure 4 shows the between-group differences in energy intake. The deficiency in energy intake in the unsupplemented group begins at 12 weeks and is not corrected later. By eight months of age, the between-group differences in nutritional status are not readily apparent to the observer, i.e., the unsupplemented children were not obviously malnourished. However, more detailed analysis of their nutritional status shows some impairments. Photographs confirmed that supplemented and unsupplemented mother-child pairs had different attitudes and different characteristics of the skin, adipose and muscular tissues (Chávez and Martínez, 1982).

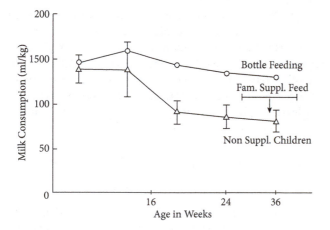

Figure 2 *Milk consumption per kg of weight by age during the first nine months by infants receiving breast milk alone without complementary cow's milk feeding, cow's milk by bottle to complement breast milk, and children given complementary cow's milk and whose family was given additional food from 27 to 41 weeks that was partially shared with the infant.*

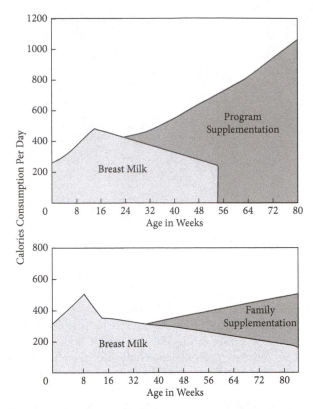

Figure 4 *Mean caloric consumption per day by age during the first two years after birth by infants whose mothers received food supplementation during pregnancy and who were given complementary feeding when growth began to falter (upper diagram) compared with the caloric intake of infants whose mothers were unsupplemented and who received only the complementary food spontaneously provided by the family (lower diagram).*

By eight months, the unsupplemented children had already been exposed to two nutritional insults. The first occurred in utero due to a deficient transfer of nutrients across the placenta. The second occurred at about three months of age due to a decrease in maternal breast milk production. In view of these insults, why were there so few clinical manifestations? First, breast-feeding allows infants to recover partially from the in utero insult. During the first three months of life, the infant has access to an abundant supply of milk and grows at a very fast rate. Second, biological mechanisms protect the child against nutritional insults. This is illustrated by the fact that the child can maintain lean tissue at the expense of his fat reserves. Another coping mechanism is a reduction in physical activity. This hidden malnutrition is likely to have negative long-term consequences for the future development of the child, even though dramatic effects are not evident by eight months of age.

As shown in Figure 5, the between-group difference in weight is small at eight months. Furthermore, it is still not possible to detect significant differences in the infants' utilization of nutrients, physical activity, or behavior. However, some indicators show consistent differences. Perhaps the most pronounced differences can be seen in neurological

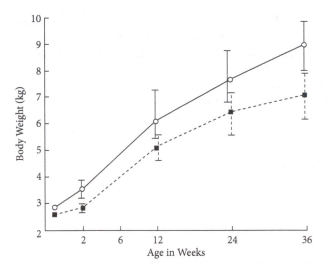

Figure 5 *Weight increase in the first 36 weeks of children in the maternal supplementation and complementary feeding group (—) compared with children breast-fed by unsupplemented mothers who received no complementary food from the program (---).*

development both at birth and during early infancy (Rodríguez et al., 1979). By eight months, the unsupplemented child had less reflex control and poorer psychomotor development (A Chávez et al., 1975). There were also some behavioral differences. Unsupplemented children cried more, played less, and had less than optimal family interaction (A Chávez and Martínez, 1975).

The fact that there were no obvious clinical manifestations of malnutrition up to eight months of age has led some people to recommend exclusive breast-feeding for a minimum of six months. However, this study does not support this argument, since the breast milk supply begins to decline by three months, and small developmental, biological, and behavioral deficits begin to appear. These deficits become larger as the child grows older in a socioeconomically deprived environment.

In short, on the one hand, children who reach eight months of age with acceptable growth, such as weighing more than 8 kg, will be more likely to crawl, to demand attention, and to have better immunological defenses. On the other hand, a child who reaches eight months under adverse conditions grows less well, has a poor appetite and low levels of physical activity and social interaction and is likely to become more malnourished.

THE "VALLEY OF DEATH" BETWEEN 8 AND 20 MONTHS

Even though breast-fed, socioeconomically disadvantaged children living in developing countries go through a period of particularly high health risks between 8 and 20 months of age. The most vulnerable children die during this period that can be characterized as the "valley of death." The vast majority of those individuals who survive this period are the "vulnerable survivors."

The child needs to have adequate reserves to survive the passage through this period. The valley of death represents both a biological and a cultural reality. It is a biological phenomenon because it is linked with nutrition and infections. It is also related to culture because it is in part determined by child-rearing practices. Both adverse cultural and biological factors are present simultaneously during weaning and illness. In the valley of death, there are three situations in which feeding practices and health interact with each other.

The *first* is related to the finding that by eight months, the mothers, both supplemented and unsupplemented, cannot produce enough milk to meet the nutritional demand of their infants. At around this age, the volume of milk produced plateaus at about 450 ml per day. It is likely that this is a common situation among poor people, since similar findings were obtained in an urban area (Pérez-Hidalgo, 1970). This amount of breast milk is valuable for the nutrition of the infant. Therefore, prolonged breast-feeding is recommended for those women who do not have enough resources to obtain and safely handle cow's milk or a combination of foods. Although breast milk should be a major component of the infant's diet during the valley of death, it is also important to feed clean digestible foods as soon as possible.

The *second* feeding problem that occurs during this period is the tendency of children of this age to develop anorexia when the organism is exposed to an insult, particularly an infection. The anorexia during the passage through the valley of death contrasts with the good appetite of children younger than eight months who demand to be breast-fed even during episodes of severe diarrhea. This is desirable, because the infant replenishes nutrients that are being lost because of diarrhea. Some of this anorexia could be due to malnutrition, or perhaps it is normal at this age since the same phenomenon is observed among well-nourished children.

The *third* issue that needs to be considered is that during this period many children are weaned from the breast. Earlier it was believed that this was the cause of malnutrition, because the children were abruptly weaned without being offered foods of adequate protein quality and content. There is no doubt that weaning from the breast is an important event; however, it is often done at an age when the child is already malnourished. In fact, it is possible that women decide to stop breast-feeding because they notice an insufficient milk supply long before weaning. In the case of Tezonteopan, weaning from the breast during this period was not an issue, since only three of the unsupplemented women stopped breast-feeding before 20 months, and this did not pose a health risk to their children at this time.

A second period of decline in breast milk production was observed when the children were about 13 months of age. This is often associated with a new pregnancy. According to common wisdom, when a mother becomes pregnant during the period encompassing the valley of death, the child becomes jealous and changes his personality. What happens in reality is that the malnourished child becomes sad and irritated, and cries frequently. These signs could be interpreted as indicators of an increase in the severity of malnutrition related to the low milk supply produced by the mother.

The other biological phenomenon characteristic of the valley of death is related to infections, since this is the period when the child loses the passive immunity received from his mother and has acquired only limited active immunity. It is also the time when the child moves around in unsanitary areas and foods contaminated with pathogens are introduced. While not all immunity is lost by eight months, the epidemiological observations, however, show clearly that the supplemented and unsupplemented children had different patterns of frequency, duration, and severity of infectious diseases (Figure 6).

The role played by culture is similar to what has been reported for other socioeconomically disadvantaged groups. For this reason, it is possible to talk about a culture of poverty during the valley of death. In Tezonteopan weaning foods are introduced very late and in small quantities at about eight months of age. These foods are often withdrawn from the infant's diet with illness, particularly fevers and diarrhea, without taking into account the nutritional needs of the child. Another example is the practice of giving the child a corn tortilla to lick. Every time the tortilla falls down, the caretaker picks it up and gives it back to the child, even though it has dirt on it. The child is not able to ingest the tortilla and for this reason it obtains a minimum nutritional benefit from it. The same could be said of other foods that were given to the unsupplemented group, such as *atoles* and soups. Very frequently these foods contain fewer nutrients and are contaminated.

The differences in energy consumption after eight months between the supplemented and unsupplemented groups can be seen in Figure 4. In the supplemented group, the energy intake increases gradually, following the children's

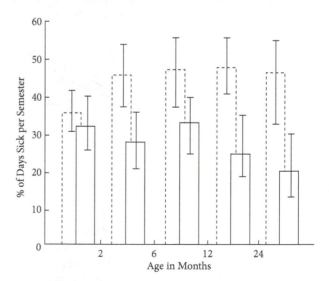

Figure 6 *Percentage of days sick per semester in the first 30 weeks of children in the maternal supplementation and complementary feeding group (—) compared with children, breast-fed by unsupplemented mothers, who received no complementary food from the program (---).*

requirements. In the unsupplemented group, on the other hand, energy intake declines and reaches a nadir at about 10 to 11 months of age, unfortunately. At this point, the intake of non-breast-milk foods is still very small. Given the low nutrient intakes observed among the unsupplemented group in the valley of death, it is surprising that children survive and even show a small advance in their development. At two months of age, when the child weighs about 4 kg, he obtains almost 500 kcal from breast milk. Afterwards the energy intake declines from breast milk.

The growth curve shown in Figure 7 corresponds to the increments in body surface (Wetzel plot) and shows that by the third month, the growth of the unsupplemented child begins to falter in relation to that of the supplemented child. This difference becomes more pronounced between four and eight months of age. The figure represents the averages of 17 cases that were followed closely. However, if individual cases were plotted, a zigzag pattern with arrested, accelerated, or decelerated periods of growth would appear. This is due to episodes of illness that have negative growth effects through direct biological mechanisms (i.e., altered metabolism, anorexia, reduced absorption) and exogenous cultural mechanisms (i.e., withdrawal of solid food).

The growth patterns of supplemented and unsupplemented children differ not so much in the number and severity of infections as in the speed of recuperation from infections. Supplemented children had frequent episodes of infections during this period, and their growth and appetite were also affected. However, they recovered sooner from illness and ate very well while recovering from infections. Their anthropometry was better than that of the unsupplemented children. Between 6 and 18 months, the supplemented children grew less than normal, but they returned rapidly to their expected growth pattern between 18 and 24 months. The unsupplemented children recover very slowly,

and before they can catch up fully, another episode of infection commonly occurs.

With the findings from this study, it is possible to clarify the relative importance of malnutrition and infection as determinants of child health in developing countries. Several researchers insist that infectious diseases are the main determinants, but this study shows that supplemented children are able to recover from infections sooner. This observation allows us to ascertain that nutrition is a more important determinant of child health than disease, because a well-nourished child is able to recuperate and return to his normal growth pattern in spite of suffering frequent episodes of infectious diseases.

It is not clear how the unsupplemented children can survive the valley of death while consuming less than 500 kcal/day and facing so many illnesses. However, the two principal factors are their reduced body size and less physical activity (A Chávez et al., 1972). Figure 8 shows clear between-group differences in physical activity.

There was no apparent between-group difference in physical activity at eight months of age. It is possible that the method of measurement of physical activity (i.e., the number of times that the feet touched the side of the crib) was not sensitive enough to pick up differences, because it is common to wrap the infants with blankets in the study village. After 10 months of age, however, the differences were remarkable, showing that as they grew older, the supplemented children increased their physical activity whereas the unsupplemented children did not.

As in other underdeveloped communities, almost all the children developed clinical signs of malnutrition at some point during the study. However, their symptoms were transient and improved even without medical care. Cross-sectional studies conducted in underdeveloped villages have reported similar nutritional findings to those encountered

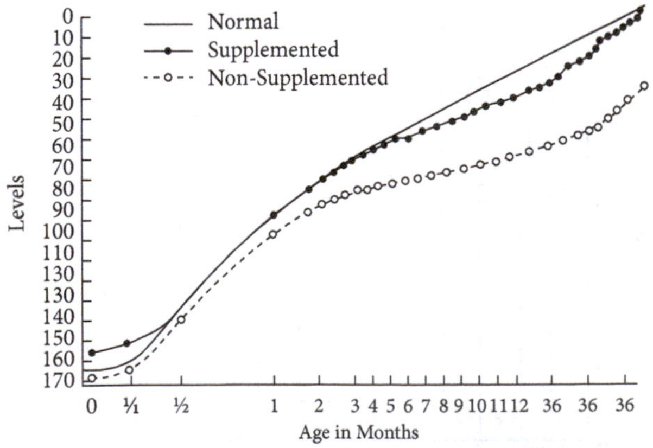

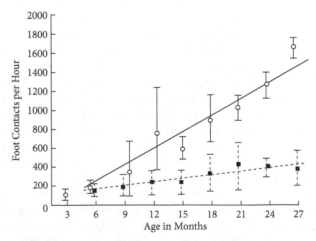

Figure 7 *Levels of growth in the first 36 weeks of children in the maternal supplementation and complementary feeding group (--•--) compared with children breast-fed by unsupplemented mothers and who received no complementary food from the program (--○--). Children in the supplemented group of children match levels of growth for well-nourished children (—) during the first four months of infancy.*

Figure 8 *Number of foot contacts per hour in the first 27 weeks of children in the maternal supplementation and complementary feeding group (—) compared with children breast-fed by unsupplemented mothers and who received no complementary food from the program (---).*

in Tezonteopan. Only 26.3% of the children under five years of age can be classified as having type II or type III malnutrition (i.e., moderate to severe malnutrition). This would suggest that the nutritional status of the population is heterogeneous. This is misleading, however, because the studies have examined children of different ages and at different stages of nutritional stress.

A frequency distribution of the nutritional status of the 41 unsupplemented children indicated that 14.6% were severely malnourished (i.e., type III malnutrition) when they were experiencing their worst nutritional status, 78.1% had type II malnutrition at worst, and only 7.3% had no worse than type I malnutrition at some point during the study. This is the real distribution of malnutrition in the community and is different from the prevalence estimates. With a cross-sectional study, it would have not been possible to detect these high levels of severe malnutrition, because all the children do not become malnourished at the same point in time and several of them could have already been dead when the study was conducted. Therefore severely malnourished children in the sample did not die in the Tezonteopan study, because they received medical care as soon as they began to become severely malnourished if they were not recovering spontaneously.

The previous data show that underdeveloped regions can have only a moderate prevalence but a high incidence of moderate to severe malnutrition. Therefore malnutrition can be the underlying cause of mortality during the critical period of human development studied in Tezonteopan. Furthermore, prenatal malnutrition associated with low birth weight, immaturity at birth, and low breast milk output after two to three months increases the relevance of nutrition for public health.

There is no doubt that malnutrition between 8 and 20 months adversely affects neurological function and other phenomena that have social repercussions. The low energy intake in the unsupplemented children and their reduced levels of physical activity are directly related to behavioral outcomes such as longer sleep periods and desire to remain in the crib for longer periods of time. It is also possible that malnourished children are carried for longer periods of time on their mothers' backs because they do not move and remain quiet. It is also possible that the low levels of physical activity have an indirect relationship with the suboptimal level of stimulation and interaction between the fathers and siblings and the malnourished child (A Chávez et al., 1975; A Chávez and Martínez, 1975).

In sharp contrast with the unsupplemented group, the supplemented children were more active, slept less, and did not want to remain in the crib or to be carried by their mothers for a long period of time. Fathers were often involved with the care of the supplemented children and smiled at and played with their offspring. The siblings also had to participate sooner and more intensely in the care of the child. All these events brought relatively more stimulation and interaction to the supplemented children.

Although the differences in physical activity explain part of the differences in behavior, stimulation, and degree of interaction, there might be other factors that also contribute to explaining these outcomes.

It is possible that malnutrition by itself is related directly to several personality traits. The unsupplemented children were withdrawn and insecure, and they cried frequently. The crying can be attributed to hunger and to the request to be breast-fed. However, the facts that even after eight months of age these children still cried frequently and with anguish during periods of anorexia and had low levels of physical activity (Figure 9) indicate different personality traits of supplemented and unsupplemented children.

Between 8 and 20 months, the unsupplemented children did not smile at their fathers, played less by themselves or with other individuals, and felt secure only if they were close to their mothers. The need to be in direct physical contact was so strong that several of them held to their mothers with great force for prolonged periods of time (Figure 10).

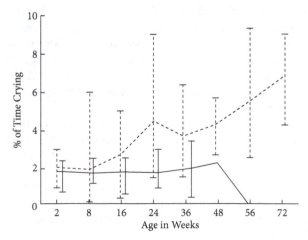

Figure 9 *Percentage of time crying in the first 27 weeks by children in the maternal supplementation and complementary feeding group (—) compared with children breast-fed by unsupplemented mothers and who received no complementary food from the program (---).*

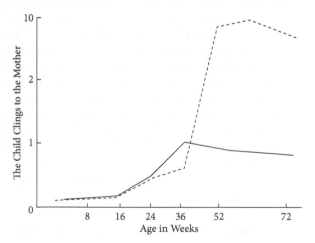

Figure 10 *Children observed clinging to the mother in the first 72 weeks in the maternal supplementation and complementary feeding group (—) compared with children breast-fed by unsupplemented mothers, who received no complementary food from the program (---).*

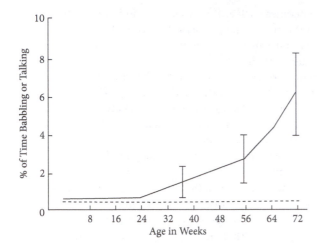

Figure 11 *Babbling in the first 72 weeks by children in the maternal supplementation and complementary feeding group (—) compared with children breast-fed by unsupplemented mothers, who received no complementary food from the program (---).*

Several of the unsupplemented children were afraid of their fathers and siblings and did not like to be cleaned. They hardly ever vocalized and only communicated by crying (Figure 11).

In general, the results show that the malnourished child is very insecure, and this leads to a passive and dependent personality. These characteristics of infant behavior become even worse as a result of several cultural practices that are frequently found in under-developed communities. In general, the mothers do not take the initiative to stimulate their offspring. As a result, there is a poor maternal-child interaction, which is limited to breast-feeding when the child cries or simply swinging the child in the crib or carrying him on her back.

In the case of the supplemented group, it is clear that the children stimulated responses from other people, demonstrating that supplementary feeding can break the passivity and apathy in the family. The children initiated interactions not only with their mothers but also with their fathers, siblings, neighbors, and animals. The behavior of the supplemented children changed traditional cultural patterns, since the fathers became involved with the care of young children. This was possible because the supplemented children were too active and difficult to be taken care of by their mothers alone, and also had happy personalities that attracted the fathers.

The developmental delays of the unsupplemented children stabilize at the end of the valley of death at 20 months of age. Afterwards their developmental curves run parallel to and always below those of the supplemented and reference children. As a result, the unsupplemented child leaves the valley of death as a vulnerable survivor.

The Preschool Survivor and the Nutritional Crisis at School Entrance

The nutritional status of the children who grow up in Tezonteopan stabilizes at about 20 months of age, and their rate of weight growth becomes similar to that observed in well-nourished populations. The increments in linear growth are of a smaller magnitude than those in weight, and as a result, the children from the village experience a progressive increment in weight relative to height. Ramos Galván (1969) refers to this phenomenon as homeorrhexis.

All the study children were still being breast-fed at 20 months, and their breast milk intake was about 400 ml/day (i.e., 35 ml/kg of body weight). The consumption of non-breast-milk foods, such as tortillas, corn *atole*, and beans, was low, and these foods were of poor quality. The total daily energy and protein consumption were 526 kcal and 11.2 g, respectively (A Chávez and Martínez, 1982).

How is it possible that the 20-month-old children from Tezonteopan can stabilize their nutritional status if they are surviving on such a low food intake? It almost seems impossible that the unsupplemented children could gain weight as fast as the supplemented or well-nourished children who consumed at least twice the amount of food. At this age the physiological needs of the child decrease and there is also a large adaptive reduction in physical activity; however, the child may still be unhealthy. The findings that by 20 months the unsupplemented child has a stable food consumption and energy expenditure, and that his activity level decreases in relation to the supplemented child, support this hypothesis.

The pattern of changes in body proportions is interesting. The malnourished children are born with shorter legs, and during the first eight months the size of the legs substantially catches up with that of the rest of the body. Between 8 and 20 months, the legs and the trunk of malnourished and well-nourished children grow at the same rate. However, after 20 months the growth rate of the legs of malnourished children again declines in relation to the well-nourished children.

The rate of increase in head circumference is analogous to the growth rate of the legs. This rate is the same in supplemented and unsupplemented children until 20 months of age, after which the rate declines among the unsupplemented children. Given this finding, why do the unsupplemented children who experience homeorrhexis seem to have large heads? The reason is that the small circumference of the thorax, coupled with a relatively large waist circumference, gives the child the appearance of being younger with a normal head size.

It is possible that the ratio between head and thorax circumference, rather than weight-for-age or weight-for-height, is the best indicator of nutritional status between 20 months and six years. This ratio is always <1 for malnourished and >1 for well-nourished children. Other indicators that might be sensitive to the nutritional status at this age are the ratios of upper to lower body length and of thorax to head circumference.

The severity and frequency of infections decrease beginning at 20 months. The duration per episode of diseases such as respiratory infections and diarrhea declines among the well-nourished relative to the malnourished.

At this age there is also some degree of stabilization in neurological function and mental performance. Beginning at 20 months of age, the unsupplemented children increase their performance at the same rate as the supplemented children, although the latter maintain a constant 10% to 15% advantage. By three years of age, the unsupplemented children almost reach the level of the supplemented children in language development and social behavior. However, after a short time their curves separate again, and later the unsupplemented show similar improvement rates as the supplemented children.

The differences in physical activity that can be attributed to the food supplementation are remarkable, and between 20 and 36 months there is a sevenfold difference in favor of the supplemented children.

Between 20 and 40 months, the household time-sampling methodology that was previously used to assess behavior was switched to a method based on placing the child in an open-field square area that had toys on one side and the mother on the other. This method allowed behavior to be studied at a predetermined time and place. The differences in behavior between supplemented and unsupplemented children remained constant. The unsupplemented children did not move around the square area, did not play with the toys, and did not move from their mothers' sides, where they remained crying and requesting to be held in their arms. By contrast, the supplemented children played with the toys, showed them to their mothers, and moved around the square area without fear or insecurity.

These results show that the malnourished children do not experience complete compensatory adaptations beginning at 20 months of age. These children are shorter, more ill, and heavily dependent on their mothers because they have a withdrawn personality. It is difficult to understand the basis for the insecurity experienced by malnourished children. It could be caused by a general feeling of weakness or lack of control of the environment, and/or by their immature personalities. These characteristics of insecurity and fear are responsible for the crisis faced by the malnourished child when he enters school for the first time.

At around six or seven years of age, the homeorrhetic mechanism observed among malnourished children (i.e., to

spare weight at the expense of height) is reversed. At this age the children increase their linear growth rate at the expense of weight, and several symptoms of malnutrition begin to appear. Table 2 shows the difference in weight and height between the well-nourished and the malnourished children at the end of the preschool and at the beginning of the school period.

Beginning at five years, the unsupplemented children begin to catch up in linear growth, and by eight years they have reduced their deficit with respect to the supplemented children by about 4 cm. By contrast, the deficit in weight of the unsupplemented children increases during this period of time.

When applying the Jenss reference growth model to the children of Tezonteopan, it was found that the unsupplemented children experience their maximum deviation in growth rates at five to seven years of age (A Chávez and Martínez, 1982).

The morbidity data indicated that at six and seven years of age the malnourished children experience a small and statistically nonsignificant increase in the number of episodes and duration per episode of illness when compared with the supplemented group. This finding might be explained by the exposure to new microbes in school.

In the school, the children were observed every 45 seconds for 1.5 hours at arrival and before leaving the school for the day. Twelve behavioral items were recorded, and the children were unaware that they were being observed (Schlaefper, 1986). There were large between-group differences in school behavior and performance. Table 3 summarizes 3,240 behavioral observations per year per child. Statistics are not presented, due to the large sample size and the large between-group differences. The first column shows the results of the second daily observations and the second column shows the results that include both daily observations. These two columns are presented because the unsupplemented children performed even worse at the end of the day, perhaps because of fatigue. This is likely to have occurred because by the end of the day these children reduced their level of activity and increased the time spent sleeping. Unsupplemented children participated less in class, were more distracted, slept more, played less, and cried more on arrival at school than their supplemented counterparts.

There were also substantial between-group differences, which are difficult to interpret, at six and seven years of age in a series of written tests. The unsupplemented children had an average grade of 6.5 ± 1.9 out of 10, and 38.3% failed to pass the school year. By contrast, none of the supplemented children had to repeat the school year, and their average grade was 8.1 ± 0.5.

Several teachers, who were unaware of which group the children belonged to, were trained to apply several tests of knowledge to the study children. Table 4 shows the results of these tests. It indicates that there were between-group differences in favor of the supplemented children, even at the beginning of the school period (see Detroit-Engel test). This

Table 2 Differences in Average Weight and Height Between Supplemented and Unsupplemented Children

Age (yrs)	Weight (kgs)	Height (cms)
5.0	3,989	9.5
5.5	4,109	9.0
6.0	4,387	8.2
6.5	4,629	7.4
7.0	5,030	7.0
7.5	4,845	5.4
8.0	4,869	5.6

Table 3 Classroom Activities of Children (Percentage of Time in Activity in 3,240 Observations During 3 Hours in the First School Year)

Behavior	End of Day Observations		Total Observations	
	Not Supplemented	Supplemented	Not Supplemented	Supplemented
Active participation[a]	1.9%	11.7%	4.3%	13.9%
Passive participation[b]	11.3%	19.3%	10.1%	18.1%
Classroom movement	4.8%	23.1%	7.7%	24.5%
Distracted	52.6%	31.6%	54.4%	30.2%
Sleepy	8.5%	0.0%	4.5%	0.7%
Crying	3.0%	1.4%	4.7%	0.6%
Fighting	0.8%	1.3%	0.4%	1.0%
Out of classroom/other behavior	17.1%	11.6%	13.9%	11.0%

[a]Obey instructions, participate or interact with the teacher.
[b]Look at the teacher, read or look at the book or answer in chorus.

Table 4 Results of Tests in the First School Year

Test	Not Supplemented	Supplemented
Beginning of year Detroit-Engel	6.5 ± 1.9	8.1 ± 0.5
Middle of year L. Filho	8.8 ± 1.4	13.3 ± 0.9
End of year Detroit-Engel	19.4 ± 2.5	36.1 ± 3.1
End of year International	6.2 ± 1.0	7.9 ± 0.7
End of year National	6.3 ± 1.2	8.6 ± 0.9

result is interesting, because none of the children received preschool education. By the end of the school year, the between-group differences in the knowledge tests were even larger, perhaps as a result of the school learning experience.

The knowledge of the children was also measured during the second year. However, the between-group comparisons are invalid, because the large proportion of unsupplemented children who repeated the school year had been previously exposed to these tests. In addition, two unsupplemented children were taken out of school by their parents.

COMMENTS: NUTRITION IN THE LIFE CYCLE AND SOCIAL DEVELOPMENT

The results of this study show that malnutrition is tightly linked to health, well-being, and educational opportunities in the community. Malnutrition is both the cause and the effect of the limited opportunities for socioeconomic development of the study population.

Malnutrition begins at birth, as illustrated by the finding that newborns of unsupplemented mothers were 180 g lighter. Almost 40% of these children were born with low birth weight (<2.5 kg). During the first two to three months of life, the unsupplemented children experienced only a partial recovery from in utero malnutrition. This is because they had

access to adequate nutrition after birth, since their mothers had an initially adequate milk supply until this age. However, the maternal milk supply was soon no longer sufficient, and the children's nutritional status deteriorated. However, because this deterioration took place slowly it was not obvious to the parents or even the physicians. This is unfortunate, because this is the period when the functional deficits associated with malnutrition begin to appear (Chávez and Martínez, 1979a). It can be detected by periodic weighing.

From three to eight months the children were hungry, as evidenced by their demand to be breast-fed 20 or more times per day, and they began to change their morphology and general appearance, as illustrated by changes in skin texture and adipose tissue. During this period the children began to be insecure and unhappy. However, the mothers and the physicians were unable to interpret these signs correctly, as illustrated by the practice of prolonged exclusive breast-feeding.

The period between 8 and 20 months of age is the valley of death, when malnutrition becomes apparent. During this period, when the transfer of maternal immunity decreases, there is a synergism between malnutrition and infection, resulting from the unsanitary environment in which the child lives, and lower resistance due to malnutrition. The valley of death is also characterized by many behavioral deficiencies, some of which may be triggered by lower levels of physical activity and a more timid and apprehensive personality, both traits that lead to reduced interaction between the child and his mother, family, and environment (Allen et al., 1992).

The interaction between malnutrition and poverty is apparent throughout the life cycle. Maternal malnutrition, as reflected by low weight gain during pregnancy, and poor health are related to low birth weight (Allen et al., 1992). Afterwards, the mother influences the nutritional status of her child through her breast-feeding practices. The consequences of an inadequate maternal milk supply in this population, for satisfactory development after the infant reaches about three months of age, are far more serious than is currently accepted.

Breast milk is the first "push" for the development of the child, but among malnourished women this push is short-lived and not as strong as it should be. The maternal production of breast milk in Tezonteopan is enough to meet the nutritional requirements of the infant only for the first two to three months of life. During this period, the mother increases her milk supply, but it suddenly drops to a level of 500 to 600 ml and remains at this lower level. It is likely that this is a common phenomenon throughout the disadvantaged areas of the world. The decreased milk supply is not enough to continue "pushing" the child in his development and is responsible for a deterioration of his nutritional status. By eight months of age, the milk deficit, together with inadequate complementary feeding and the increased nutritional needs for physical activity and recovery from infection, worsens the situation of the child. The survivors in communities like Tezonteopan grow less, spend less energy, and interact less with their environment than well-nourished children (A Chávez and Martínez, 1979b).

The sudden stabilization in nutritional status and reactivation of growth and development that takes place at 20 months of age is surprising. However, this reactivation takes place at a pace adequate for the chronological, but not for the biological or functional, age of the child. Therefore, there is no catch-up in the developmental processes in this period. Between 20 months and six to seven years of age, the unsupplemented child's appearance and behavior are those of a younger individual. Character and personality are withdrawn, but nutrition problems are not apparent. At the beginning of the school period, the linear growth of the supplemented children is similar to that of the unsupplemented children, but the latter exhibit deficits in weight and in mental and behavioral development. Moreover, the unsupplemented children did not do well in school. More than one-third failed to pass the first year of school, and the remaining perhaps should have also failed because their grades were very low. The poor school performance of these children can be attributed to malnutrition, since the supplemented children passed their first year of school without problems.

Adolescence is usually considered a period of nutritional crisis. In this study, however, the between-group differences tended to narrow during this period. This is related to adaptation mechanisms of the unsupplemented children, including delayed onset and longer duration of puberty, which allowed them to partially recover from their deficits. In addition, cultural factors that limit the opportunities for progress slowed down the development of supplemented children during adolescence. However, it is important to note that unsupplemented subjects did not reach the levels of performance of the supplemented children during adolescence. Their physical, mental, and behavioral performance was also worse.

From these results it seems likely that certain behavioral and cultural characteristics that have been considered as typical of poor agricultural societies are due to malnutrition. Among them are passivity, lack of motivation for change, and limited decision-making abilities, which together explain the tendencies for the limited progress and development in these communities. It is possible to break the vicious cycle of malnutrition and social development in several ways. The approach adopted has almost always been to promote investment in increased production and create the conditions for savings and reinvestment. This has not worked in the poor rural environment, where it is difficult to save and reinvest. Nutrition is an area that deserves special attention because, as this study shows, it improves the quality of human resources, an essential factor for development. A society with more capable individuals not only can produce more but can improve its technological competence. Improved nutrition is both an instrument for development and an end in itself. Better nutrition improves health and physical and mental capabilities, the instruments and outcomes of development.

This study shows that it is not difficult to improve the nutritional status of individuals. While more material and human resources were expended in this study due to the research nature of the project than would be required, it shows that much can be achieved with relatively little investment. Applied nutrition programs are needed because they can maximize the benefits per unit of investment. The data from this study show that the target age for nutritional interventions should be three to eight months to prepare the child for a healthy entrance into the valley of death. Children should weigh 8 kg by eight months of age. The second priority of these programs should be the valley of death, because this is the period when the nutritional problem becomes worse. At this age, programs are curative rather than preventive, since the children are already malnourished (VA Chávez et al., 1988).

An important programmatic priority is the care of the pregnant woman. Gestation is an extremely important period because, as this study shows, the deficits in physical development observed in the unsupplemented group at the end of the study are proportional to those present at birth. The issue of how best to improve the nutritional status of pregnant women has not been resolved. Suboptimal nutrition during pregnancy is related to social conditions, the treatment of women in society, employment, age at marriage, birth interval, and many other factors that currently cannot be addressed with cost-effective programs.

Programmatic actions need to address the malnutrition-infection complex with simple measures. These should be driven by a primary health approach involving food and hygiene, sometimes called the "bread and soap" approach. With political commitment, this is a feasible strategy. The implementation of primary health care measures in the communities involving essential nutrition and health interventions at the household level is within the reach of most Latin American countries. These measures should include immunization, provision of essential micronutrients, elimination of parasites, and educational messages regarding the need for complementary feeding beginning at three months of age. Measures that will improve nutrition during pregnancy are also needed.

These and other studies have documented the nature of the malnutrition problem and its consequences. Furthermore, the technology to combat the problem of malnutrition is available. It is hoped that the findings of this study will help to mobilize the sociopolitical will to solve the problem that is still lacking in many developing countries.

References

Allen LH, Backstrand JR, Chávez, A, Pelto GH. 1992. *Functional implications of malnutrition. People cannot live by tortillas alone: the results of Mexico CRSP. Final Report of Mexico Project.* Human Nutrition Collaborative Research Program, USAID, Washington, DC, June 1992.

Canosa C, Salomón, JB, Klein R. 1968. "Nutrition growth and mental development." In: *Proceedings of the International Congress of Pediatrics*, Mexico.

Chávez A. 1978. "Effects of mother's nutrition on infant body morphology." In: *Birth-Weight Distribution as an Indicator of Social Development.* SAREL/WHO Report R:2, Sweden.

Chávez A, Martínez C. 1973. "Nutrition and development of infants from poor rural areas III. Maternal nutrition and its consequences on fertility." *Nutr Rep Intern* 7:1.

Chávez A, Martínez C. 1975. "Nutrition and development of children from poor rural areas. V. Nutrition and behavioral development." *Nutr Rep Intern* 11:466.

Chávez A, Martínez C. 1979a. "Effects of maternal undernutrition and dietary supplementation on milk production." In: Aebi H, Whitehead, RG, eds. *Maternal Nutrition During Pregnancy and Lactation.* Bern: Hans Huber Publ.

Chávez A, Martínez C. 1979b. *Nutrición y Desarrollo Infantil.* Nueva Editorial Interamericana, México.

Chávez A, Martínez C. 1979c. "The effect of maternal supplementation on infant development." In: Effects of maternal nutrition on infant health. Arch Latinoamer Nutr Supplement 1, Dec 1979.

Chávez A, Martínez C. 1982. *Growing Up in a Developing Community.* INCAP-UNU Publ.

Chávez A, Martínez C, Bourges H. 1972. "Nutrition and development of infants from poor rural areas. II. Nutritional level and physical activity." *Nutr Rep Intern* 5:139.

Chávez A, Martínez C, Soberanes B. 1991. "Effects of early malnutrition on the physical, mental and social condition of rural adolescents." Symposium of the IX Meeting of the L.S. Nutrition Society, San Juan, PR.

Chávez A, Martínez C, Yashine T. 1975. "Nutrition, behavioral development and mother-child interaction in young rural children." *Fed Proc* 34:1574.

Chávez VA, González-Richmond A, Cifuentes E, Batrouni L, Madrigal H, Martínez C, Mata A. 1988. "Alcances del sistema de paquetes selectivos en los programas de atención primaria." *Rev Sal Pub Méx* 30:446.

Cravioto J, DeLicardie ER. 1968. "Intersensory development of school aged children." In: Scrimshaw NS, Gordon JE, eds. *Malnutrition, Learning and Behavior.* Cambridge, MIT Press: 252–69.

Cravioto J, DeLicardie ER, Birch HG. 1966. "Nutrition, growth and neurointegrative development: an experimental and ecologic study." *Pediatrics* 38(suppl. 2, Pt. 2):319–72.

Gómez F. 1946. "Desnutrición." *Bol Med Hosp Inf Méx* 3:543.

Jelliffe DB. 1966. *The Assessment of Nutritional Status of the Community (with Special Reference to Field Surveys in Developing Regions of the World).* Geneva: WHO.

Madrigal H, Avila CA. 1990. *Encuesta Nacional de Alimentación del Medio Rural.* Publ División de Nutrición L-89, Tlalpan, D.F., México.

Martínez C, Chávez A. 1967. "La lactancia y los hábitos de alimentación infantil en una comunidad indígena." *Rev Méx Social* 29:223.

Martínez C, Chávez A. 1971. "Nutrition and development of children from poor rural areas. I. Consumption of mothers' milk by infants." *Nutr Rep Intern* 4:139.

Mönckeberg F. 1978. "Effect of early marasmic malnutrition on subsequent physical and psychological development." In: Scrimshaw NS, Gordon JE, eds. *Malnutrition, learning and behavior.* Cambridge, MA: MIT Press: 269–77.

Muñoz de Chávez M, Chávez A. 1986. "Evaluación de un programa de educación masiva para mejorar la alimentación infantil rural." *Rev Inv Clín Méx* 38(Suppl: La Nutrición en México 1980–1985):153.

Pérez-Hidalgo C. 1970. "Valor nutritivo de la leche materna procedente de madres Méxicanas urbanas." *Salud Publ Méx* 12:236.

Ramos-Galván R. 1949. "La desnutrición infantil en México: sus aspectos estadísticos, clínicos, dietéticos y sociales." *Bol Med Hosp Inf Méx* 5:84.

Ramos-Galván R. 1969. "El significado de las edades pediátricas." *Acta Pediatr Latinoamer* 1:65.

Rodríguez R, Rubio F, Martínez C, Chávez A. 1979. "Nutrition and development of children from poor rural areas. VIII. The effect of mild malnutrition on children's neurological development." *Nutr Rep Intern* 19:315.

Schlaepfer LVA. 1986. "A longitudinal study in a rural Mexican community: analysis of the growth, health and nutrition aspects (0–10 years of age)." Doctoral thesis, University of Maryland, College Park, MD.

Scrimshaw NS, Taylor CE, Gordon J. 1968. *Interactions of Nutrition and Infection.* Geneva: WHO.

Seckler D. 1982. "Small but healthy. A basic hypothesis in the theory, measurement and policy of malnutrition." In: Sukhatme PV, ed. *New Concepts in Nutrition and Their Implications for Policy.* Pune, India: Maharasthra Assoc Sc Res Institute.

CHAPTER 34

Body Size, Adaptation, and Function

Reynaldo Martorell

(1989)

An economist by the name of David Seckler proposed the "small but healthy" hypothesis a few years ago (Seckler 1980, 1982). This hypothesis has generated a lively literature (Messer 1986), including heated debates and thoughtful but sometimes emotionally charged rebuttals from nutritionists such as Gopalan (1983) and Latham (1984). Seckler's views have sparked a great deal of interest because they result in policy and programmatic implications which differ markedly from the conventional. The "small but healthy" hypothesis implies a world in which the problem of malnutrition is no longer of massive proportions since most of the world is "small but healthy." In Seckler's world, the only individuals who are "truly" malnourished are those showing clinical signs of malnutrition. The latter, Seckler tells us, should be the first priority of nutrition policy, and nutritional resources should not be squandered on the "small but healthy population." My presentation is not a comprehensive critique of Seckler's ideas nor of the resulting policy implications, but rather it is a selective discussion of issues that seem to have been ignored by Seckler. First allow me to briefly describe some of the principal elements of the "small but healthy" hypothesis.

SECKLER'S "SMALL BUT HEALTHY" HYPOTHESIS

Seckler's "small but healthy" child is the child who is short but not thin. In the Waterlow classification, this refers to children whose heights are two standard deviations below the median of the reference population but whose weight for heights are above this criterion (see Table 1). In the jargon of the day, these children are said to be "stunted but not wasted." This group of children makes up a significant proportion of the population in many Third World countries and is the majority in India, Bangladesh, and some African nations (Martorell 1985). Children who are wasted, on the other hand, are far less common, and rarely exceed 10% of the population, even in areas where nutritional problems are a serious concern (Martorell 1985). Wasting is synonymous with marasmus and Seckler has no objection to classifying

these children as unhealthy. To repeat, it is the stunted but not wasted child who Seckler calls "small but healthy."

According to Seckler (1980, 1982), most nutritional scientists believe in what he calls the "Deprivation Theory." This view holds that an individual is healthy and well nourished if he grows along his genetically determined growth curve. On the other hand, growth significantly below this curve indicates that the individual is malnourished and in poor health. Seckler believes that this view is incorrect and instead proposes the "Homeostatic Theory of Growth." In this theory, the single potential growth curve is replaced by the concept of a broad array of potential growth curves. Within the bounds of this potential growth space, the child may move through various paths of size and shape without suffering any functional implications. Seckler tells us that while the *deprivation* theory of nutritionists postulates a continuous functional relationship between small size and impairments, his *homeostatic* theory postulates a threshold relationship. Seckler (1982:129) goes on to tell us that "smallness may not be associated with functional impairments over a rather large range of variation; but the system explodes into a high incidence of functional impairments at the lower bound of size." The stunted but not wasted child is within this safe zone, or to use his words, "small but healthy."

I am certain that the vast majority of researchers do not agree with the "deprivation theory" as formulated by Seckler. Growth retardation is widely recognized as a response to a limited nutrient supply at the cellular level. The maintenance of basic metabolic functions takes precedence and resources are diverted away from growth and physical activity. The concurrence of growth retardation and functional impairments is the rationale for the use of

Reynaldo Martorell, "Body size, adaptation and function." *Human Organization* 48(1989): 15–20. Reprinted with permission.

Table 1 Waterlow's Classification

		Height	
		<2 SD	≥2 SD
Weight for height	<2 SD	Stunted and wasted	Not stunted but wasted
	≥2 SD	Stunted but not wasted	Normal

anthropometric indicators as risk indicators of poor health and as predictors of mortality. It is incorrect to claim that nutritional scientists uniformly hold that growth retardation and functional impairments are linearly related. In fact, much of the research shows curvilinear relationships (see Martorell and Ho 1984 for a review of the literature). Minor and brief interruptions in growth are not likely to be a cause of concern, whereas chronic patterns of growth retardation leading to stunting invariably are.

My remarks are limited to a discussion of four issues. The first issue is that the causes of stunting are unhealthy. Second, I will emphasize that linear growth retardation is a danger signal and not an innocuous adjustment to environmental stimuli. Third, I will discuss the fact that the factors that affect linear growth also affect other functional domains. Finally, I will refer to the fact that stunted adults suffer certain disadvantages.

THE PROCESS OF STUNTING IS UNHEALTHY

First, I would like to underscore that the *process* of stunting is unhealthy. Seckler implies that the child is healthy while he is becoming stunted so long as he avoids wasting, and that stunting has no functional implications once it has occurred. Throughout his writings we are presented with the image of the child who "indifferently" adjusts his growth trajectory in response to environmental stimuli while enjoying perfect health. Moreover, he seems to ascribe only a small role to

nutrition and infection factors in causing smallness. Seckler proposes that there are two kinds of smallness. The first, he says, is "smallness due to poverty, and to poor physical and socio-economic environments" (Seckler 1982:134). The second is "smallness due to malnutrition, a pathological state of deficiency entailing functional impairment of individuals" (Seckler 1982:134).

There are no known mechanisms through which poverty can affect growth which do not involve nutrition and infection. Examples of mechanisms through which socio-economic factors influence growth in children are shown in Figure 1. The relative importance of the components of poverty will vary from place to place, but these will always lead to low dietary intakes and/or infection which result in decreased nutrient availability at the cellular level and which then gives rise to growth retardation (Chen 1983). The diets of poor children are generally deficient in both quantity and quality and these characteristics are the result of several factors: limited food availability *per se*, inappropriate infant feeding practices and the influence of infections on appetite. Infections will also have direct effects on nutrient metabolism and thus lead to poor nutrient utilization. In short, there are not two kinds of smallness. Rather, the basic cause of stunting is poverty and the effects on size are mediated through poor diets and infection.

We know a great deal about the timing of stunting (see Martorell and Habicht 1986 for a detailed discussion of this subject). One of the best available illustrations of the development of stunting is a figure published in Waterlow and Rutishauser (1974; see Figure 2). By expressing mean growth rates in length in populations of preschool children from developing countries as a percentage of the average velocity in the reference population, one will obtain curves which are similar to the ones shown in Figure 2 for Jamaica, Gambia, and Uganda. The choice of reference population, as noted below, matters little if at all. Growth in length in the first few months of life is generally as fast in Third World children as in reference populations. Growth retardation begins anywhere from the second to the sixth month and

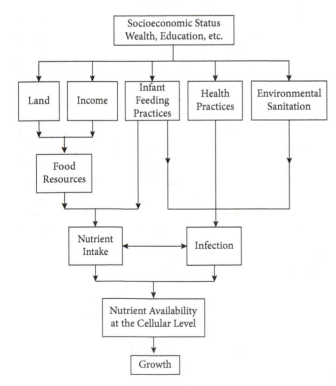

Figure 1 *Examples of mechanisms through which poverty influences growth in children*

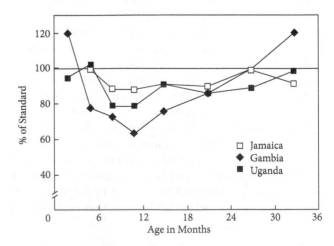

Figure 2 *Relative velocity curves for length for young children from three countries (from Waterlow and Rutishauser 1974).*

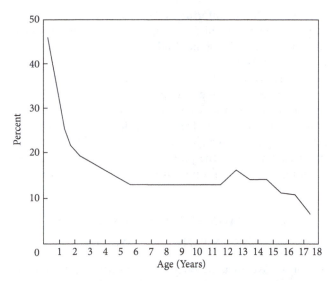

Figure 3 *Proportion of protein requirement due to growth needs at various ages in boys* (from data in FAO/WHO/UNU 1985).

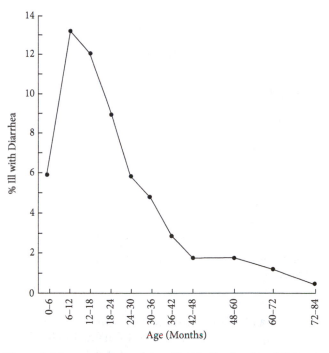

Figure 4 *Mean percentage of time ill with diarrhea from birth to seven years of age in Guatemalan children* (from Martorell and Habicht 1986).

continues till about three years of age. Growth rates generally equal those in reference populations after about three years of age.

The period from three months to as long as three years is the period of weaning in traditional societies, which I define as the transition from total dependence on mother's milk to complete reliance on the local diet. Stunting is a phenomenon intimately associated with the perils of this period. Numerous factors play a role in determining nutrient intake and infectious disease patterns, including infant feeding practices, the nature of the local diet and the foods offered to children, environmental sanitation, and the degree of contamination of foods and liquids.

Weaning brings together powerful factors which lead to stunting. The first two years of life is a time when growth is very rapid and therefore a time when adverse factors are going to have a significant and lasting effect. Also, infancy and the second year of life are when nutritional requirements, expressed as energy or as nutrients per kg per day, are greater than at any other subsequent time of life. As shown in Figure 3, a greater proportion of the requirement for protein is due to growth during this critical phase of human development than is the case later. Thus, growth rates are not only fastest during the weaning period, but also account for a greater share of the total nutrient demand than is the case later on in life.

Another feature is that infections, particularly diarrheal diseases, occur most frequently during the first two to three years of life. This is illustrated in Figure 4 which shows the percent of time Guatemalan children are ill with diarrhea from birth to seven years of age. The first two years or so of life is a time when children's immunological systems are maturing rapidly and when they are first coming into contact with disease pathogens. If children survive to four or five years of age, they will be healthier than they were earlier in life.

There is now considerable evidence from a variety of settings showing that almost all of the growth retardation observed in Third World populations has its origin in this stormy period of weaning (Billewicz and McGregor 1982; Hauspie et al. 1980; Dahlmann and Petersen 1977; Satyanarayana et al. 1980, 1981). By the time children in developing countries are three to four years of age, many are already destined to be stunted adults.

Ethnicity or race plays a minor role in determining population differences in length during the weaning period. In fact, it has been rather difficult to show that there are ethnic differences in growth potential in prepubescent children. Differences associated with poverty, on the other hand, are easy to demonstrate (Victora et al. 1986) and far overshadow those which might be ascribed to race or ethnicity (see Martorell 1985 for a review of the literature).

GROWTH RETARDATION IS A RISK INDICATOR

The second issue I want to address is that linear growth is our best indicator of child health. *Good growth means good health.* Seckler, you will recall, claims that linear growth retardation has no functional implications. Only wasting implies an impaired state and therefore only wasting represents a nutritional and public health problem. This is a very narrow and out-dated clinical view of the problem of malnutrition.

Seckler's views ignore that there is a continuum of responses as children face nutritional deficits. As indicated in Figure 5, at severe levels of deficiency, linear growth ceases

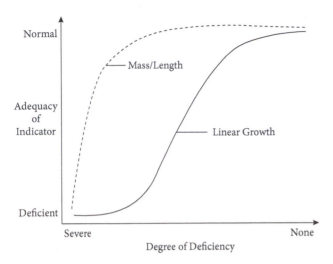

Figure 5 *Response of anthropometric indicators to varying degrees of deficiency.*

altogether and it becomes necessary to use tissue reserves as an energy and nutrient source to maintain vital functions. However, at less severe stages, normal mass to length dimensions will be maintained as it may be possible to cope with dietary deficits simply by slowing down in growth and by decreasing physical activity. This seems to be the situation in Latin America where moderate linear growth retardation occurs but where wasting is rare. However, in parts of Africa and the Indian subcontinent, the burden is much greater and marked growth retardation prevails and severe wasting is more common (Martorell 1985).

A fundamental principle of pediatrics and of modern public health nutrition is the notion that a child who is growing normally is more likely to be healthy than one who is growing poorly. This is the philosophy behind growth monitoring programs which seek to identify children who are failing to grow adequately in order to intervene with appropriate measures before the situation progresses to wasting and malnutrition (Morley 1976; Rohde et al. 1975).

The rationale for growth monitoring is evidence that children who grow poorly are more likely to be severely ill when infected and more likely to die than children who grow well. Wasting appears to be a stronger predictor of risk than stunting, as one would expect, but indicators of stunting are definitely important, even after controlling for socioeconomic status (Martorell and Ho 1984).

OTHER FUNCTIONAL EFFECTS

A third and related point I would like to make is that the factors which cause growth to be retarded also affect other functional domains as well. One reason growth retardation is predictive of morbidity and mortality is that immunocompetence is impaired, thus rendering the child more vulnerable to infections (Kielmann et al. 1976; McMurray et al. 1981). Physical activity is probably affected even at early stages of energy deficiency but the evidence on this

is lacking. This is unfortunate because activity may be an important factor in child development since it is one determinant of the ability of the child to explore the environment and to learn from it.

There are a number of studies showing strong relationships between stunting and poor psychological test performance (Pollitt and Thomson 1977). The relationship is complex and probably due to third factors, such as those related to poverty, which cause both physical and developmental retardation. The point we should remember is that stunting is a marker for poor psychological performance.

FUNCTIONAL IMPLICATIONS OF STUNTING IN ADULTS

So far I have focused on the functional implications of stunting in children. However, is the child who survives to become a stunted adult healthy? In other words, does stunting in adults have any functional implications? This is the fourth and last point of my presentation.

To answer this question, I would like to focus on two aspects: work capacity and productivity in males, and reproductive performance in females.

In discussing the relationship between body size and work, we should distinguish between capacity and productivity. Work capacity is largely a measure of the biological potential to do work and is determined in the laboratory, whereas productivity is an economic term measured in terms of goods produced per unit time. There is overwhelming evidence showing that stunted men have reduced muscle masses and significantly diminished work capacities (Spurr 1983). However, many jobs in agriculture, manufacturing and industry are not that physically demanding. Also, many factors other than work capacity determine productivity, and among these we can include motivation and training. Hence, one would not necessarily expect small body sizes to be a limiting factor for light to moderate activities. As it turns out, current nutritional status—as measured by weight for height, iron status, and energy intakes—seems to be a better predictor of productivity than height for many types of activities (see Martorell and Arroyave 1988 for a review of the literature). There are, of course, physically demanding tasks such as sugarcane cutting where physical size has been found to be related to productivity. This is to be expected since at a strenuous work load, those with a lower work capacity would be closer to a maximal effort and would function at faster heart rates. Such overtaxed individuals may not be able to maintain the work pace for very long and may produce less (Spurr 1983).

Greater height in women in areas where malnutrition is endemic is associated with an enhanced capacity to conceive, and to deliver a baby more likely to survive and to have better growth and development. The results of a study of maternal stature and infant mortality in several hundred Mayan women illustrate this point (Table 2). Variations in socioeconomic status were minimal because

Table 2 Maternal Stature, Infant Mortality, Parity, and Number of Surviving Children in Mayan Women (*Data from Martorell et al. 1981*)

	Terciles of Height[a]			Analysis of Variance Main Effects	
	Lower (N = 127)	Middle (N = 124)	Upper (N = 129)	F	P
Infant mortality[b]	205	150	101	7.9	<.001
Parity[b]	4.75	4.10	4.22	2.1	.12
Surviving children[b]	2.83	3.02	3.15	1.7	.18

[a]Means and ranges for height (cm) for each of the three groups were as follows: Lower (mean 137.7, range 126.3–140.2), middle (mean 142.0, range 140.3–144.7) and upper (mean 148.2, range 144.8–158.6).
[b]Values standardized for age by analyses of covariance. Adjusted to the mean age of 28.4 years.

all families lived [on] and were employed by owners of coffee plantations, and because all received the same low salaries and small amounts of corn in payment for their labor. Mothers were very short; in fact, the population studied appears to be among the shortest in the world. The mean height was 142.4 cm and the tallest woman was only 158.6 cm or 5 ft 2 in. As shown in Table 2, maternal height was significantly associated with infant mortality which was 205 per 1,000 live births for the shortest group, 150 for the middle group, and 101 for the tallest group. This is not a new finding. Low maternal height is widely recognized as a risk indicator of low birth weight and infant mortality.

Concluding Remarks

It is clear I do not believe small is healthy. This is largely because the process by which children become small is associated with major functional impairment and because its causes are undesirable. I also do not embrace policies which are targeted only at the severely malnourished. Rather, I favor broad public health and nutrition measures which aim to prevent severe malnutrition. Promoting actions which prevent growth failure in young children will reduce the risk of progression to severe malnutrition and death. Throughout my presentation I have emphasized four key points.

First, it is a travesty to call the process of stunting healthy since its causes are deficient diets and infections. To acclaim the end result of the process, small body size, as a desirable attribute of populations is also to affirm that its causes are desirable.

Second, *good growth means good health*. I am not promoting maximal size, but rather insisting that growth retardation is an early warning signal. Linear growth retardation is one of our best indicators that something is going wrong and it should be a call for action.

Third, the stunted child has other unfortunate characteristics such as poor cognitive development. This simply reflects the fact that the harsh conditions which give rise to

markedly reduced stature have other undesirable repercussions as well.

And finally, small body size does have functional implications in adults. Productivity may be limited in small individuals engaged in very strenuous activities, and very short stature in mothers is a powerful predictor of low birth weight and infant mortality.

For all these reasons, small is not healthy. Quite the contrary, poor growth in a child is an indicator of major functional impairment. A society in which a major proportion of its children are stunted is one with serious public health problems.

References

Billewicz, W. Z., and I. A. McGregor 1982 A Birth-to-Maturity Longitudinal Study of Heights and Weights in Two West African (Gambian) Villages, 1951–1975. Annals of Human Biology 9(4): 309–320.

Chen, L. C. 1983 Interactions of Diarrhea and Malnutrition: Mechanisms and Interventions. *In* Diarrhea and Malnutrition: Interactions, Mechanisms, and Interventions. L. C. Chen and N. Scrimshaw, eds. Pp. 3–19. New York: Plenum Press.

Dahlman, N., and K. Petersen 1977 Influences of Environmental Conditions During Infancy on Final Body Stature. Pediatric Research 11:695–700.

FAO/WHO/UNU Joint Expert Consultation 1985 Energy and Protein Requirements. Technical Report Series 724. Geneva, Switzerland: World Health Organization.

Gopalan, C. 1983 Small Is Healthy? For the Poor, Not for the Rich. Nutrition Foundation of India Bulletin, October.

Hauspie, R. C., S. R. Das, M. A. Preece, and J. M. Tanner 1980 A Longitudinal Study of the Growth in Height of Boys and Girls of West Bengal (India) Aged Six Months to 20 Years. Annals of Human Biology 7:429–441.

Kielmann, A. A., I. S. Uberoi, R. K. Chandra, and V. L. Mehra 1976 The Effect of Nutritional Status on Immune Capacity and Immune Responses in Preschool Children in a Rural Community in India. Bulletin of the World Health Organization 54:477–483.

Latham, M. C. 1984 Smallness—a Symptom of Deprivation. Nutrition Foundation of India Bulletin 5(6), July.

Martorell, R. 1985 Child Growth Retardation: A Discussion of Its Causes and Its Relationship to Health. *In* Nutritional Adaptation in Man. Sir Kenneth Blaxter and J. C. Waterlow, eds. Pp. 13–30. London: John Libbey.

Martorell, R., and G. Arroyave 1988 Malnutrition, Work Output and Energy Needs. *In* Capacity for Work in the Tropics. K. J. Collins and D. F. Roberts, eds. Pp. 57–75. Cambridge: Cambridge University Press.

Martorell, R., H. L. Delgado, V. Valverde, and R. E. Klein 1981 Maternal Stature, Fertility, and Infant Mortality. Human Biology 53(3):303–312.

Martorell, R., and J-P. Habicht 1986 Growth in Early Childhood in Developing Countries. *In* Human Growth: A Comprehensive Treatise, 2nd ed. Vol. 3: Methodology: Ecological, Genetic, and Nutritional Effects on Growth. F. Falkner and J. M. Tanner, eds. Pp. 241–262. New York: Plenum Press.

Martorell, R., and T. J. Ho 1984 Malnutrition, Morbidity, and Mortality. *In* Child Survival: Strategies for Research. H. Mosley and L. Chen, eds. Pp. 49–68. Supplement to Volume 10 of the Population and Development Review.

McMurray, D. N., S. A. Loomis, L. J. Casazza, H. Rey, and R. Miranda 1981 Development of Impaired Cell-Mediated Immunity in Mild and Moderate Malnutrition. American Journal of Clinical Nutrition 34:68–77.

Messer, E. 1986 The "Small but Healthy" Hypothesis: Historical, Political, and Ecological Influences on Nutritional Standards. Human Ecology 14(1):57–75.

Morley, D. 1976 Nutritional Surveillance of Young Children in Developing Countries. International Journal of Epidemiology 5(1):51–55.

Pollitt, E., and C. Thomson 1977 Protein-Calorie Malnutrition and Behavior: A Review from Psychology. *In* Nutrition and the Brain, Vol. 2. R. J. Wurtman and J. J. Wurtman, eds. Pp. 261–307. New York: Raven Press.

Rohde, J. E., D. Ismail, and R. Sutrisno 1975 Mothers as Weight Watchers: The Road to Child Health in the Village. Environmental Child Health 21:295–297.

Satyanarayana, K., A. Nadamuni Naidu, M. C. Swaminatham, and B. S. Narasinga Rao 1980 Adolescent Growth Spurt Among Rural Indian Boys in Relation to Their Nutritional Status in Early Childhood. Annals of Human Biology 7:359–366.

———1981 Effect of Nutritional Deprivation in Early Childhood on Later Growth—a Community Study Without Intervention. American Journal of Clinical Nutrition 34(8):1636–1637.

Seckler, D. 1980 Malnutrition: An Intellectual Odyssey. Western Journal of Agricultural Economics 5(2):219–227.

———1982 "Small but Healthy": A Basic Hypothesis in the Theory, Measurement, and Policy of Malnutrition. *In* Newer Concepts in Nutrition and Their Implications for Policy. P. V. Sukhatme, ed. Pp. 127–137. Maharashtra Association for the Cultivation of Science Research Institute. Law College Road, Pune, India.

Spurr, G. B. 1983 Nutritional Status and Physical Work Capacity. Yearbook of Physical Anthropology 26:1–35.

Victora, C. G., J. P. Vaughan, B. R. Kirkwood, J. C. Martines, and L. B. Barcelos 1986 Risk Factors for Malnutrition in Brazilian Children: The Role of Social and Environmental Variables. Bulletin of the World Health Organization 64(2):299–309.

Waterlow, J. C., and I. H. E. Rutishauser 1974 Malnutrition in Man. *In* Early Malnutrition and Mental Development. Symposia of the Swedish Nutrition Foundation XII. J. Cravioto, L. Harnbreaus, and B. Vahlquiest, eds. pp. 13–26. Uppsala, Sweden: Almquist and Wiksell.

CHAPTER 35

Hungry But Not Starving: Functional Consequences of Undernutrition in Adults

Richard L. Bender and Darna L. Dufour

(2012)

It was a small childcare center in a small house in a poor neighborhood of Cali, Colombia. The children were sitting around a table mostly being kids, pushing and shoving and clamoring for attention. All except for one little boy. He was exceptionally quiet and resting on the table. He looked tired and not quite well.

I (D.L.D.) asked, "What's the matter with the little blond boy?"

"He probably came without breakfast," the mother in charge replied. "He'll be Ok when he has his morning snack."

I was stunned. I had read about the low level of physical activity in hungry children, but had not expected to see it so vividly demonstrated. The morning snack came in another half hour or so, and like magic the little boy perked up and started acting like the other little boys.

Many people in the world clearly do not have enough to eat. What does "not enough to eat" actually mean in terms of the quality of life for individuals or populations? What are the functional consequences of undernutrition? This stressor need not reach the level of starvation before adverse effects on health and well-being occur. On the contrary, relatively low levels of undernutrition, which may not even be obvious at first glance to an outside observer, can have a very real impact.

Nutritional anthropologists use a variety of tools to investigate these issues. Traditionally, they use anthropometric measures such as height, weight, skinfold thicknesses, and body circumferences to assess the current nutritional status of the individual. The measured values may be compared to other members of the same population, to a reference population, or to previous measurements taken from the same individual. Anthropometry provides a window into the *history* of an individual's energy balance. In other words, anthropometry represents the physical outcome of the difference (or lack of difference) between energy intake and energy expenditure, on a time scale of months or years.

Additionally, nutritional anthropologists employ *functional indicators* of nutritional status. Functional indicators are meant to assess nutritional status in terms of the individual's performance in a variety of physiological, behavioral, or cognitive "tasks," such as performing physical work or resisting infection (Table 1). The goal is to arrive at a "whole-body" or "whole-individual" view of how people's daily lives are affected by under- and overnutrition. When functional indicators are added to the more traditional measures, we can achieve a fuller picture of the physiological and psychological consequences of chronic or acute under- and overnutrition, and thereby arrive at a more nuanced

Table 1 Functional Indicators of Nutritional Status of the Individual and the Population

Morbidity
Mortality
Growth velocity
Reproduction
Fecundity/fertility
Pregnancy outcome
Lactation performance
Activity
Work capacity
Cognition and behavior
Social performance

Reproduced from Allen, 1984:169

understanding of what it means to have too little or too much to eat.

Here, we focus on two functional consequences of undernutrition in adults. First, we examine how undernutrition affects physical activity levels and, therefore, also the capacity to perform physical work. Second, we examine how undernutrition affects reproductive function.

PHYSICAL ACTIVITY

The human body needs energy for, and expends energy on, several very different things. First, a certain amount of energy is required to maintain organ function and homeostasis. This is known as the basal metabolic rate (BMR). BMR is affected by factors such as sex, age, and body composition—lean tissues require more energy to be maintained than adipose tissues, for example. Second, the body requires energy to digest food. This is known as the thermic effect of food (TEF). Third, the body expends energy in physical activity—moving, working, playing, etc. Additionally, depending on age, sex, and other factors, the body may also expend energy on: growth, fighting diseases, recovering from injury, maintaining reproductive tissues, gestating, and lactating. The sum total of all these types of energy expenditure is known as total daily energy expenditure (TDEE). From the standpoint of functional indicators of nutritional status, the interesting question is whether some components of TDEE are more responsive to undernutrition than others. That is, does undernutrition most likely affect an individual's BMR, TEF, or physical activity?

The available evidence indicates that physical activity is the most variable component of TDEE. Some of the earliest data came out of the Minnesota Experiment, a well-known laboratory study of 36 adult males held in a state of semistarvation for 13 months between 1944 and 1945. The investigators found that this long-term caloric restriction was associated with a decrease in physical activity of all kinds, in addition to many other physiological and psychological effects (Keys et al., 1950). A key conclusion drawn from the study was that

> "the starving man, whether fasting or undergoing semistarvation, is remarkable for his apathy and reluctance to engage in any overt activity [.] The spontaneous reduction in all physical movements and the adoption of energy-sparing postures play a major role in adaptation to a restricted food intake" (Grande, 1964:927–928).

However, the data from the Minnesota Experiment are limited in that no objective measures of physical activity or of TDEE were made (Spurr, 1990). Additionally, the subjects were volunteers in a controlled laboratory setting, rather than a free-living population.

In the early 1970s, Fernando Viteri and colleagues conducted landmark research in Guatemala investigating the physiological effects of long-term undernutrition in a population of agricultural laborers. This research demonstrated that poorly-fed laborers worked more slowly, walked more slowly, rested more frequently and for longer periods, and were less active in non-working hours than their better-fed counterparts (Viteri, 1971; Viteri et al., 1971). Additional research in Guatemala (Torun and Viteri, 1981; Immink et al., 1984) and elsewhere (Rutishauser and Whitehead, 1972; Spurr and Reina, 1989) has also demonstrated the pattern of adults and children responding to undernutrition by decreasing physical activity, or substituting lower-effort activities for higher-effort ones (Gorsky and Calloway, 1983), compared to normally nourished counterparts. Additionally, these effects of undernutrition have been observed in situations where an entire population faces periodic episodes of food shortage. For example, Jenike (1996) observed an increase in resting behavior during seasonal episodes of hunger among Lese subsistence farmers in the Ituri Forest, Zaire.

Also notable is the *rapidity* of this response to undernutrition. For instance, Spurr and Reina (1988) used heart rate as a measure of physical activity to compare energy expenditure between nutritionally normal and marginally malnourished Colombian boys at a summer day-camp. They found that the physical activity level of malnourished boys generally did not keep up with that of their better-nourished counterparts in sports and physical play activities. However, for around two hours immediately following a ~760 kcal midday meal, the malnourished boys were able to increase their level of physical activity to match that of the nutritionally normal boys. This increase in physical activity subsequently dropped again later in the afternoon.

If individuals respond quickly to undernutrition by altering their physical activity patterns, then what is the problem? Is the physical activity shift truly a negative consequence of undernutrition, or is it an effective behavioral response with no long-term repercussions? In fact, there are several reasons why decreased physical activity due to undernutrition should be viewed as a short-term compensatory mechanism or *accommodation* rather than as an *adaptation*. As Scrimshaw and Young (1989:27) point out, physical activity is required not only for work activities but also for "discretionary activities that are essential for household improvement, supplementary economic activities, food procurement, community organization, and the like." Thus, the physiologically driven reduction of physical activity may have adverse social, cultural, and economic consequences.

Ferro-Luzzi (1985) suggested a useful distinction between the direct and indirect consequences of decreased physical activity. Direct consequences include the actual and immediate consequences of inactivity, including refraining from engaging in life-sustaining activity. Indirect consequences include the de-training effects of long-term inactivity, associated with a decline in work capacity and therefore potential productivity.

Work Capacity

Flor sold avocados door to door in the hot midday sun. The idea was to sell them for the noon meal. Not much of a job, but she was poor and there were not many opportunities other than selling food on the street. This was the situation in Cali, Colombia in 1990. One day we went along for the walk—a day that seemed unusually hot and the sun unusually bright. By 1 pm people were eating lunch and no longer buying avocados. We stopped at a small store for a cold drink, some shade, and a bit of rest. Maria and I took stools in the front of the store. I (D.L.D.) was tired. We had been walking for almost two hours. Flor sat on the steps, or rather sprawled on the steps, clearly wanting to lie down but not allowing herself to do so in such a public place. She looked exhausted. I knew from the measurements we had done that she was not well nourished, and her resting posture that day was another indication of her poor nutritional status.

Work capacity is the ability to perform physical work, such as carrying a load or using agricultural tools. In most cases, work capacity is operationally defined as the maximal rate of oxygen uptake, or VO_{2max}. Since active tissues require oxygen in order to function, a higher work rate requires the body to take in a greater amount of oxygen. VO_{2max} is assessed by measuring a subject's oxygen consumption while performing physical exercise at steadily increasing workloads until exhaustion. This type of "fitness" test is considered to be the best measure of an individual's capacity to perform physical work. Ideally, the exercise performed to measure VO_{2max} should be the same or a closely similar type of activity to the actual work commonly performed by the subject, such as traveling long distances by foot, lifting heavy loads, or operating machinery. In practice, however, the test is performed with the subject exercising on a treadmill or a bicycle ergometer.

Since the 1970s, researchers and policy makers have been keenly interested in the impact of poor nutritional status on the capacity to perform work, particularly the physically demanding agricultural or industrial work still done by many in developing countries. From the point of view of national economic development, there is a pragmatic reason for this concern: hungry people cannot work very hard. That is bad news for individuals, since monetary income is often tied directly to work output, and also bad news for the population, since low work output hinders economic growth.

There is ample data to support this concern. Some of the classic studies demonstrating this were conducted in Colombia during the late 1970s and early 1980s. For example, Barac-Nieto et al. (1978) found that VO_{2max} in undernourished Colombian males ranged from 1 to 2 liters of oxygen per minute, whereas normally nourished control subjects averaged 2.75 liters per minute. Spurr (1984), working among male Colombian sugarcane cutters, likewise found that normally nourished subjects had a higher VO_{2max} than undernourished subjects. Additionally, he found that work capacity was positively correlated with productivity, in this case the weight of sugarcane cut per day. In other words, the normally nourished men were not only capable of performing more work, but they actually accomplished more work, and therefore earned more money. Why would a higher maximal work capacity result in greater work output?

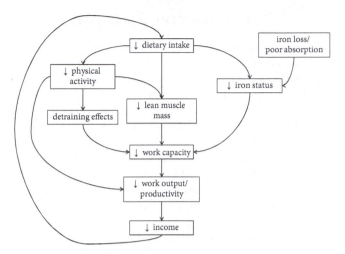

Figure 1 *Positive feedback between insufficient dietary intake and lowered work output/productivity.*

Spurr et al. (1977) found that individuals tended to operate at 35–40% of their VO_{2max} during self-paced work such as sugarcane cutting, regardless of their absolute work capacity. Thus, individuals with a higher maximal work capacity tended to self-pace their work at a higher rate. These findings underline the very real and concrete socioeconomic consequences of undernutrition, especially in situations where income is tied directly to work output.

How does undernutrition impact work capacity? There are several possibilities (Figure 1). First, undernourished individuals are likely to have a lower mass of lean tissue, including muscle (Roubenoff and Kehayias, 1991). Muscle tissue of any kind is metabolically active and the body cannot maintain it without an adequate intake of energy and protein. Low muscle mass limits both the maximal duration and the maximal intensity of work that can be performed.

Second, undernourished individuals often suffer from iron deficiency, most commonly iron deficiency anemia, and work capacity is negatively affected by iron deficiency. Several factors can lead to iron deficiency, including inadequate dietary intake, inadequate absorption of dietary iron, or high loss of iron (e.g., through menstruation, childbirth or serious injury). The ability of red blood cells to transport oxygen to active tissues depends on iron status, among other factors. Iron deficiency anemia lowers oxygen-transport ability, and therefore limits the maximal rate of oxygen intake: VO_{2max}, or maximal work capacity (Haas and Brownlie, 2001). Interestingly, iron deficiency anemia has been shown to negatively affect maximal work capacity not only in physically demanding jobs, but also in less demanding jobs such as factory work (e.g., Li et al, 1994; Untoro et al., 1998). Furthermore, several studies have demonstrated that iron supplementation can increase physical activity, and hence work output, in iron-deficient women (e.g. Edgerton et al, 1979; Li et al, 1994). This is an important finding from a public health standpoint, since iron deficiency is the most common micronutrient deficiency worldwide, affecting about two billion people (Zimmermann and Hurrell, 2007).

REPRODUCTIVE FUNCTION

"Food restriction and energy drain, in the form of exercise, may transiently affect the fertility of malnourished and underweight populations to a far greater extent than has been realized" (Warren, 1983:374).

It has long been known that inadequate food intake is associated with the suppression of reproductive function in humans and other animals. Since the mid-1970s, researchers have noted an increased incidence of amenorrhea, delay of menarche, and other negative reproductive consequences in young women who engage in intensive physical activity, such as ballet dancing (e.g., Warren, 1980) or running (e.g., Dale et al., 1979). Other researchers have associated the suppression of reproductive function in these populations with anthropometric thresholds, such as low percentage of body fat or low weight for height (e.g., Frisch and McArthur, 1974). Yet others have found reproductive suppression in laboratory subjects whose food intake was restricted or decreased (e.g., Williams et al., 1995; Loucks and Thuma, 2003).

Although the physiological mechanism is not well-understood, a common evolutionary explanation is that this suppression of reproductive function is an adaptation. The argument is that since reproductive function is not necessary for individual survival, it is suppressed during periods of energetic stress, allowing the organism to prioritize energy use for more vital functions (Wade and Jones, 2004). Theoretically, this argument is compelling. Methodologically, however, it is challenging to not only assess the adequacy of food energy intake in free-living human populations under natural conditions, but also to relate this to reproductive function.

Reproductive function in humans is usually assessed in females, since male reproductive function (e.g., sperm production) incurs little metabolic cost and seems to be highly insensitive to energetic constraints (Ellison, 2003). On the other hand, female ovarian function appears to be highly sensitive to energetic factors. Additionally, pregnancy is a very energy-expensive state, and lactation is even more energetically expensive. In fact, lactation is the most expensive phase of the reproductive cycle (Dufour and Sauther, 2002). Thus, females are sensitive to changes in energy balance in at least three ways: first, in the energy required to maintain the normal functioning of the reproductive system; second, in the energy required to support a growing fetus during gestation; third, in the energy required to support a growing infant during lactation. Here, we concentrate on the first category, ovarian function, since gestation and lactation appear to be "buffered" against energetic fluctuations to a much greater extent than ovarian function (Ellison, 2003; Figure 2).

Laboratory studies of both recreational and competitive female athletes have demonstrated the suppression of reproductive function in response to energetic stress (reviewed in Dufour, 2009). Williams et al. (1995), for instance, found reproductive suppression in a small sample (n = 4) of runners whose training volume was abruptly increased

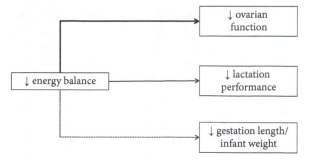

Figure 2 *Effect of negative energy balance on women's reproductive effort. Line weight indicates relative magnitude of effect.*

in conjunction with dietary restriction. In a slightly larger sample (n = 9), Loucks et al. (1998) observed a decline in reproductive function after the subjects underwent a four-day exercise treatment (treadmill walking) without a concurrent increase in the dietary energy intake needed to maintain energy balance. In an additional study, Loucks and Thuma (2003) were able to demonstrate that a dramatic increase in exercise (treadmill walking) did not affect reproductive function as long as subjects consumed a diet designed to maintain energy balance.

Importantly, these studies collectively suggest that the suppression of reproductive function is not caused by the exercise itself, but rather by the concurrent inadequacy of food intake which leads to negative energy balance. In other words, it is the difference between energy intake and energy expenditure—regardless of the absolute value of the energy expenditure—that suppresses reproductive function. These laboratory results are mirrored by the few field studies that have been successful to date.

Assessing reproductive function and changes in energy balance in free-living women going about their normal lives is methodologically very challenging. Despite the difficulty, a number of field studies have attempted it. These field studies used progesterone in the saliva as a biomarker of ovarian function. Progesterone is a steroid (cholesterol-derived) hormone critical to the normal menstrual cycle. Variations in progesterone have been linked to variation in the probability of conception even in the absence of observable changes in menstrual cycling (Ellison, 2003). Thus, progesterone provides a sensitive indicator of female reproductive function.

In the first study, Ellison et al. (1989) found depressed salivary progesterone levels among Lese horticulturalists in Zaire during the season when food availability was low and body weight was declining. The latter observation suggests that the decreased food availability was not compensated by a decrease in energy expenditure (through lowered physical activity, for example), leading to negative energy balance.

In the second study, Panter-Brick and Ellison (1994) found lower than normal salivary progesterone in rural Tamang women in Nepal during the season when physical work in subsistence agriculture was high and body weight seasonally low. Again, the latter suggests that the Tamang were in negative energy balance during this period. These two studies suggest that negative energy balance, whether as the result of decreased energy intake or increased energy expenditure, can suppress women's reproductive function.

In the third study, Jasieńska and Ellison (1998) reported that Polish women farmers showed evidence of lowered salivary progesterone levels in response to a 2-month seasonal increase in farm work. They attributed this suppression of reproductive function to the increase in work-related energy expenditure itself, rather than to negative energy balance because food intake was observed to increase with energy expenditure in this population. However, the possibility that the women were in negative energy balance cannot be excluded with confidence because the methods used in the study may not have been sensitive enough to detect it (Dufour, 2009). In sum, the weight of current evidence suggests that negative energy balance, rather than high levels of physical activity or low food energy intake per se, drives the suppression of ovarian function.

CONCLUSIONS

Starvation is one potential outcome of inadequate food intake, but it is by no means the only one. Undernutrition can in fact have substantial functional consequences for both individuals and populations. A lack of sufficient dietary energy or nutrients leads to lower levels of physical activity, and to a decreased capacity to perform physical work. For many people in the world, physical work output is tied directly to monetary income, and therefore to the ability to obtain food, medical care, and education. This sets the stage for a vicious cycle linking undernutrition to decreased work capacity: hungry people cannot work as hard, so they earn less money, so they have less food, so they become hungrier.

Additionally, undernutrition can negatively affect women's reproductive physiology by suppressing ovarian function or even inducing amenorrhea. This problem is of particular interest in populations that experience seasonal changes in physical work requirements, since the periods of increased physical work (i.e., energy expenditure) are not necessarily associated with increased food availability (i.e., energy intake).

In a way, undernutrition can act as a "hidden stressor" in that its functional consequences for individuals or populations are not always obvious to the casual observer. The consequences are real, though. They affect families and livelihoods, health and well-being. It hurts to be hungry—even when you're not starving.

References

Allen LH. 1984. Functional indicators of nutritional status of the whole individual or the community. Clinical Nutrition 3:169–175.

Barac-Nieto M, Spurr GB, Maksud MG, Lotero H. 1978. Aerobic work capacity in chronically undernourished adult males. Journal of Applied Physiology: Respiratory, Environmental, Exercise Physiology 44:209–215.

Dale E, Gerlach DH, Wilhite AL. 1979. Menstrual dysfunction in distance runners. Obstetrics & Gynecology 54:47–53

Dufour DL. 2009. The energetic cost of physical activity and regulation of reproduction. In Nicholas Mascie-Taylor CG, Rosetta L, eds. Reproduction and Adaptation. Cambridge, UK: Cambridge University Press.

Dufour DL, Sauther ML. 2002. Comparative and evolutionary dimensions of the energetics of human pregnancy and lactation. American Journal of Human Biology 14:584–602.

Edgerton VR, Gardner GW, Ohira Y, Gunawardena KA, Senewiratne B. 1979. Iron deficiency anemia and its effect on workers productivity and activity patterns. British Medical Journal 2(602):1546–1549.

Ellison PT, Peacock NR, Lager C. 1989. Ecology and ovarian function among Lese women of the Ituri forest, Zaire. American Journal of Physical Anthropology 78(4):519–526.

Ellison PT. 2003. Energetics and reproductive effort. American Journal of Human Biology 15:342–351.

Ferro-Luzzi A. 1985. Work capacity and productivity in long-term adaptation to low energy intakes. In Blaxter K, Waterlow JC, eds. Nutritional adaptation in man. London: John Libbey, pp. 61–69.

Frisch RE, McArthur JW. 1974. Menstrual cycles: fatness as a determinant of minimum weight for height necessary for their maintenance or onset. Science 185: 949–951.

Gorsky RD, Calloway DH. 1983. Activity pattern changes with decreases in food energy intake. Human Biology 55:577–586.

Grande F. 1964. Man under caloric deficiency. In Dill DB, Adolph EF, Wilber CG, eds. Handbook of physiology, section 4: adaptation to the environment. Baltimore: Waverly Press, pp. 911–937.

Haas JD., Brownlie T. 2001. Iron deficiency and reduced work capacity: A critical review of the research to determine a causal relationship. Journal of Nutrition 131(2):676S-688S, Sup 2.

Immink MDC, Viteri FE, Flores R, Torun B. 1984. Microeconomic consequences of energy deficiency in rural populations in developing countries. In Pollitt E, Amante P, editors. Current topics in nutrition and disease. New York: Alan R. Liss. p 355–376.

Jasieńska G. and Ellison PT. 1998. Physical work causes suppression of ovarian function in women. Proceedings of the Royal Society of London, Series B, Biological Sciences 265(1408):1847–1851.

Jenike MR. 1996. Activity reduction as an adaptive response to seasonal hunger. American Journal of Human Biology 8:517–534.

Keys A, Brožek J, Henchel A, Mickelsen O, Taylor HL. 1950. The biology of human starvation. Minneapolis: University of Minnesota Press.

Li RW, Chen XC, Yan HC, Deurenberg P, Garby L, Hautvast JGAJ. 1994. Functional consequences of iron supplementation in iron deficient female cotton workers in Beijing, China. American Journal of Clinical Nutrition 59(4):908–913.

Loucks AB, Verdun M and Heath EM. 1998. Low energy availability, not stress of exercise, alters LH pulsatility in exercising women. Journal of Applied Physiology 84: 37–46.

Loucks AB and Thuma JR. (2003). Luteinizing hormone pulsatility is disrupted at a threshold of energy availability in regularly menstruating women. Journal of Clinical Endocrinology and Metabolism 88: 297–311.

Panter-Brick C and Ellison PT. 1994. Seasonality of workloads and ovarian function in Nepali women. Human reproductive ecology-interactions of environment, fertility and behaviour. Book series: Annals of the New York Academy of Sciences 709:234–235.

Roubenoff R, Kehayias JJ. 1991. The meaning and measurement of lean body mass. Nutrition Reviews 49:163–175.

Rutishauser IHE, Whitehead RG. 1972. Energy intake and expenditure in 1–3-year-old Ugandan children living in a rural environment. British Journal of Nutrition 28:145–152.

Scrimshaw NS, Young VR. 1989. Adaptation to low protein and energy intakes. Human Organization 48:20–30.

Spurr GB., Barac-Nieto M, Maksud MG. 1977. Productivity and maximal oxygen consumption in sugar cane cutters. American Journal of Clinical Nutrition 30(3):316–321.

Spurr GB. 1984. Physical activity, nutritional status and work capacity in relation to agricultural productivity. In Pollitt E Amante P, eds. Energy intake and activity New York: Alan R. Liss-United Nations University. pp. 207–261.

Spurr GB, Reina JC. 1988. Influence of dietary intervention on artificially increased activity in marginally undernourished Colombian boys. European Journal of Clinical Nutrition 42:835–846.

Spurr GB, Reina JC. 1989. Energy expenditure/basal metabolic rate ratios in normal and marginally malnourished Colombian children 6–16 years of age. European Journal of Clinical Nutrition 43:515–527.

Spurr GB. 1990. Physical activity and energy expenditure in undernutrition. Progress in Food and Nutrition Science 14:139–192.

Torun B, Viteri FE. 1981. Energy requirements of pre-school children and effects of varying energy intakes on protein metabolism. Food and Nutrition Bulletin 5S1:229–241.

Untoro J, Gross R, Schultink W, Sediaoetama D. 1998. The association between BMI and haemoglobin and work productivity among Indonesian female factory workers. European Journal of Clinical Nutrition 52(2):131–135.

Viteri FE. 1971. Considerations on the effect of nutrition on the body composition and physical working capacity of young Guatemalan adults. In: Scrimshaw NS, Altshull AM, editors. Amino acid fortification of protein foods. Cambridge, MA: MIT Press. p350–375.

Viteri FE, Torun B, Galicia JC, Herrera E. 1971. Determining energy costs of agricultural activities by respirometer and energy balance techniques. American Journal of Clinical Nutrition 24:1418–1430.

Wade GN, Jones JE. 2004. Neuroendocrinology of nutritional infertility. American Journal of Physiology-Regulatory, Integrative and Comparative Physiology 287(6):R1277-R1296.

Warren MP. 1980. The effects of exercise on pubertal progression and reproductive function in girls. Journal of Clinical Endocrinology and Metabolism 51: 1150–1157.

Warren MP. 1983. Effects of undernutrition on reproductive function in the human. Endocrine Reviews 4:363–377.

Williams NI, Young JC, McArthur JW, Bullen BA, Skrinar, GS and Turnbull B. 1995. Strenuous exercise with caloric restriction: effect on luteinizing hormone secretion. Medicine and Science in Sports and Exercise 27: 1390–1398.

Zimmermann MB, Hurrell RF. 2007. Nutritional iron deficiency. The Lancet 370:511–520.

CHAPTER 36

New Variant Famine: AIDS and Food Crisis in Southern Africa

Alex de Waal and Alan Whiteside

(2003)

Despite repeated warnings that AIDS could be a disaster for development, little systematic investigation has been done into the contribution of AIDS to development, and virtually no studies have been undertaken on HIV/AIDS, food security, famine, and nutrition.[1]

Demographic findings show that the secondary effect of a famine or epidemic could be at least as great as the primary effects. For example, a chain reaction of further famines and epidemics or massive out-migration might arise.[2] The food crisis developing in southern Africa could be the first major manifestation of this chain reaction.

Droughts and famines have afflicted large parts of Africa throughout history. In past decades, these food crises have had a characteristic demographic and socioeconomic profile. They have raised crude death rates by two to five fold, with mortality concentrated in very young and elderly people,[3-5] and mortality in males has been higher than in females.[6] However, farmers and pastoralists have developed sophisticated coping strategies[7] that are characterised by considerable resilience—defined as the ability to return to a former livelihood on the basis of diversity of income and food sources—and accumulated skills, including knowledge of wild foods and kinship networks.[8,9] Only when these coping strategies collapse are African societies faced with so-called entitlement failure (inability to command sufficient food to prevent starvation) and outright starvation.[10] Most typically, such extreme crises have arisen in wartime, when armed forces have actively prevented civilian populations from pursuing coping strategies.[11]

The present southern African food crisis confounds many expectations. A cycle of drought is taking place, in which region-wide rainfall failures can be expected about once every decade. The last such drought happened in 1991–92. Despite the fact that the region was economically and politically less well-prepared to withstand a food crisis than nowadays, famine was averted. The main reason for this was the effective coping mechanisms of the affected people.[12] The region is in better shape 10 years on: apartheid has been ended in South Africa, and there is peace in Mozambique and Angola. The exceptions are political and economic crisis in Zimbabwe and mismanaged economic liberalisation in Malawi, in particular the attempt to make the national strategic grain reserve commercially viable by selling off stocks.[13,14]

The present food crisis is more widespread and intractable than its predecessors, and has three distinct features. First, vulnerability is very widely spread, including areas that are not severely affected by drought. The numbers defined as in need by the United Nations are considerably higher than were anticipated after the poor 2001–02 rains. Second, household impoverishment has arisen more rapidly than in earlier droughts. Third, present estimates are that—despite the return of good rains in early 2003—a high level of vulnerability will continue.

The factor that could account for these features is HIV/AIDS. Southern Africa is the location of the world's worst AIDS epidemic, with most countries having a prevalence of HIV in adults in excess of 20%. Zambia, Zimbabwe, and Botswana have recorded very high levels for several years, and AIDS mortality rates are climbing steadily.

THE NEW VARIANT FAMINE HYPOTHESIS

Our hypothesis is that the HIV/AIDS epidemic in southern Africa accounts for why many households are facing food shortage and explains the grim trajectory of limited recovery. Four factors are new: (1) household-level labour shortages are attributable to adult morbidity and mortality, as is the rise in numbers of dependants; (2) loss of assets and skills results from increased adult mortality; (3) the burden of care is large for sick adults and children orphaned by AIDS; and (4) vicious interactions exist between malnutrition and HIV.

AIDS and Decline in Food Production

Table 1 shows the severe food production problem in the region. Reasons for the aggregate decline in food production

Alex de Waal and Alan Whiteside, "New variant famine: AIDS and food crisis in southern Africa." *The Lancet* 362 (2003):1234–1237. Reprinted with permission.

Table 1 Cereal Production in Selected Countries in Southern Africa

Country	Cereal	Year			
		1999	2000	2001	2002
Lesotho	Maize	124 500	97 100	103 000	82 000
Malawi	Maize	2 479 400	2 501 300	1 696 000	1 600 000
Mozambique	Maize	1 246 100	1 019 000	1 143 000	1 240 000
	Sorghum	326 300	252 500	263 000	364 000
Swaziland	Maize	113 000	84 500	73 000	70 000
Zambia	Maize	855 900	881 600	802 000	602 000
Zimbabwe	Maize	1 519 600	2 108 100	1 480 000	509 000
	Sorghum	85 600	103 300	60 700	37 000
	Wheat	320 000	250 000	280 000	213 000

All amounts in metric tonnes. Data from the Food and Agricultural Organization, 1999 and 2000 figures (http://www.fao.org), and SADC Food Security Bulletin and SADC Regional Assessments, 2001 and 2002 figures (http://www.sadcfanr.org.zw).

across southern Africa include drought, floods in some areas, Zimbabwe's land policies, the scarcity of seeds and fertilisers, deterioration in marketing infrastructure, and HIV/AIDS.

Results of household-level studies unequivocally show a decline in agricultural production attributable to the effects of AIDS.[1,15] Households affected by AIDS morbidity and mortality lose income, assets, and skills; those with a chronically-ill member have average reductions in yearly income of 30–35%.[16] The households must change their livelihood strategies, cultivating smaller areas and abandoning more high input high output activities in favour of those that demand less labour.[17,18] One of the few studies of the effect of AIDS on rural cereal production was done in a community in Zimbabwe (before the country's rapid descent into crisis). The results showed that an adult death resulted in a 45% decline in a household's marketed maize, but in cases when the cause of death was identified as AIDS, the fall was 61%.[19] Survey data show a close correlation between household labour availability and access to food.[20] The concurrent and associated tuberculosis epidemic, which also clusters at the household level, further exacerbates the situation.

A sign of impoverishment is that high-value and highly nutritious crops—such as cereals and oilseeds—are replaced by low-value and less nutritious ones, such as cassava. Production of cassava in Malawi, Zambia, and Zimbabwe increased from 880 000 metric tonnes in 1990 to 2 036 000 metric tonnes in 1999, a reversal of previous agricultural development gains (http://www.fao.org).

To explain famine, our concern is less with the overall availability of food and more with the ability of the poorest members of society to grow or buy it. Famines have arisen when no countrywide food availability shortages have been present.[21] Thus, results of micro-level studies of afflicted households struggling to cope indicate the emergence of a new category of poor and vulnerable people, namely those affected by HIV/AIDS. Merely by increasing inequality, AIDS increases vulnerability to famine. Overall food availability figures mask the sharp decline in control over food entitlements among these poorest strata.

THE EFFECT OF AIDS ON LIVELIHOOD COPING STRATEGIES

Changing Dependency Patterns

HIV/AIDS has a great effect on dependency of family members. Projections of the demographic effect of the HIV epidemic in southern Africa do not predict substantial changes in the dependency ratio.[22] This counterintuitive outcome is because the fertility rate is expected to fall, and child mortality rates to rise, because of AIDS. However, this crude dependency ratio stability conceals three important distortions.

First, HIV/AIDS and its effects cluster at the level of households and (to a lesser extent) communities, because of conjugal and mother-to-child transmission. A stable dependency ratio can conceal serious adverse shifts for the affected households, which may lose viability.

Second, the age and sex distribution within the adult population is changed by AIDS; for example, fewer mature adults and more teenagers and people in their early twenties are present in the population. Because women are typically infected with HIV at an age several years younger than men, fewer adult women are present in the population. Those who make the greatest contribution to support of dependants—namely mature adults, especially women—form the smallest proportion of the population, whereas young men and teenagers, who have little role in support of dependants, are more plentiful.

Third, conventional dependency ratio calculations are based on the assumption that all adults are productive. In a generalised AIDS epidemic, a small, but important, number of people are chronically sick, and therefore properly belong in the dependants category.

We therefore introduce two ideas to refine the dependency analysis. First, the dependency separation that relates to the second point above, namely the different roles of age and sex categories in support of dependants. Second, the effective dependency ratio, which captures the effects of inclusion of sick adults in the denominator rather than the numerator of the dependency ratio. When these two adjustments are included, along with the clustering effect, we can identify a new category of AIDS-poor people, defined by an adverse effective dependency ratio and dependency separation. Findings of surveys show these factors are correlated with household food insecurity.[20]

The most graphic manifestation of changing dependency patterns is the rapid growth in number of children orphaned by AIDS. Up to 13% of all children in southern Africa are orphans (defined as having lost their mother or both parents), more than half of whom have been orphaned by AIDS.[23] We have never entered a famine with a comparable level of orphaning, and simply do not know what will be the effect of food shortages, social disruption, and famine-coping strategies on these four million or so unfortunate children (or indeed vice versa).

The scarcity of labour means that affected households face increasing difficulties in pursuing labour-intensive coping strategies, including labouring for money and gathering wild foods.

Loss of Assets and Skills

Many famine-coping strategies need skill, experience, and a positive outlook on the future. An important skill is knowledge of wild foods and how to prepare them, which is handed down from mother to daughter. If young women do not have this key knowledge, they may go hungry because of their ignorance. More widely, planning a year-long strategy for a family to feed itself and protect the basis of its livelihood needs much experience about income-earning opportunities. Without mature adults, these planning skills and networks may be absent. Lastly, the motivation for implementation of a difficult and complex coping strategy is the assumption that things can return to normal. With the reduced adult life expectancy associated with HIV/AIDS and the perception of a downward spiral in standards of living, this motivation may be absent too. Indeed a successful livelihood coping strategy might only postpone the decline by a year or so rather than provide the foundation for a recovery.

The Burden of Care

One of the main factors impoverishing rural Africa is the burden of providing for orphans and sick adults:[1] it is a major expenditure and diversion of labour. Most affected households struggle to cope.[24] Some businesses have responded to the costs of AIDS by reducing sickness and disability benefits and shifting to use of self-employed subcontractors.[25] The unstated assumption is that wider society—mainly women in rural areas—will carry the burden. Furthermore, urban children orphaned by AIDS are usually sent to rural relatives to be cared for. The burden is thus doubled. In the past, rural households could rely on urban relatives for assistance during times of hardship. Nowadays, the flows of assistance have been reversed. The implication is that the preferred and most resilient livelihood coping strategy—of reliance on kinship networks for assistance—is increasingly inoperable.

Malnutrition and HIV

In past famines, adults have reduced their consumption of food and simply gone hungry. People from rural areas time and again showed remarkable physical capacity for work despite very low consumption of food. Relief agencies assumed that famine-affected adults could still look after themselves, and concerned themselves overwhelmingly

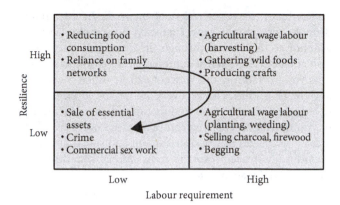

Figure 1 *Course of livelihood coping strategies.*

with young children and their mothers. Findings of the southern African development community survey[20] showed that skipping meals was not only typical in all rural areas but was also more usual in households with a chronically ill adult. For example, 57% of such households had gone entire days without eating in the preceding 2 months.[20]

In so-called new-variant famine, adults cannot be neglected: malnutrition has very different implications. Undernourished individuals are more susceptible to being infected with HIV than are those who are well nourished. Nutritional status is also an important determinant of risks in mother-to-child transmission of HIV.[26]

Adults living with HIV endanger their health by going hungry. Many types of nutritional deficiencies suppress the immune system, and hence make infections more virulent. This is true of HIV, which replicates most rapidly in malnourished individuals, hastening progression from HIV to AIDS.[18,27,28] HIV-positive status inhibits absorption of nutrients, and the body's needs in fighting the infection are considerable. Hence, people living with HIV have higher nutritional needs than normal: protein requirements are usually estimated at 30–50% more, and energy needs about 15% more. Malnutrition thus threatens to accelerate progression from HIV to AIDS for millions of infected individuals.

Conversely, good nutrition delays progression from HIV to AIDS, and is essential for effective antiretroviral treatment—some medication needs to be taken on a full stomach. This fact implies that plans for introduction of antiretroviral treatment on a large scale should be combined with nutritional support programmes.

Overall Implications for Famine-Coping Strategies

The figure shows the course of coping strategies undertaken by a household afflicted by food crisis. HIV/AIDS renders many high resilience strategies impossible (labouring, relying on networks) or dangerous (reducing food consumption), and reduces the effectiveness of them all. In a traditional drought, one might expect affected households to take 2 years or so to descend through the quadrants into destitution and activities such as commercial sex work. In so-called new variant famine, this descent can be much more rapid, and the possibilities for recovery are much reduced. Results of aid-agency surveys are finding rapid rises in the numbers of young women entering commercial sex work in affected areas.[29] Widespread impoverishment and social disruption, including increased resort to transactional sex, threaten to increase HIV transmission.

CONCLUSION

The new-variant famine hypothesis is a plausible idea for analysis of the causes and trajectories of food insecurity in southern African societies. These are societies afflicted by a combination of shocks including a generalised AIDS epidemic, drought, and poverty. The hypothesis cannot be judged proven, but it provides a framework for policy-making, relief provision, monitoring, and research. The hypothesis is lent support by results of the growing number of household-level studies of the effect of AIDS.

The analysis does not neglect the role of factors such as drought and macro-economic disparities and mismanagement. Rather, it points to the way in which HIV/AIDS accentuates existing difficulties, compelling us to confront many simultaneous problems, all of which need resolution. The challenges are daunting. A scaled-up long-term international effort will be needed to deal with the humanitarian needs that will result in southern Africa.

We must face the prospect that this food emergency will become a structural feature of the southern African landscape for many years to come, unless innovative and generous interventions are made now.

Notes

The research for and writing of this paper was in part supported by a knowledge programme of the British Department for International Development, UNICEF, and Justice Africa. The ideas and interpretation are the authors' own.

References

1. Barnett T, Whiteside A. AIDS in the twenty-first century: disease and globalization. Basingstoke: Macmillan Palgrave, 2002.
2. Dyson T. Famine in Berar, 1896–7 and 1899–1900: echoes and chain reactions. In: Dyson T, Gráda CÓ, eds. Famine demography: perspectives from the past and present. Oxford: Oxford University Press, 2002.
3. Watkins SC, Menken, J. Famines in historical perspective. *Popul Dev Rev* 1985; **11**: 647–76.
4. Caldwell JC. Demographic aspects of drought: an examination of the African drought of 1970–74. In: Dalby D, Harrison-Church R, Bezzaz F, eds. Drought in Africa 2. London: International African Institute, 1977.
5. de Waal A. Famine mortality: a case study of Darfur, Sudan, 1984–5. *Popul Stud* 1989; **43**: 5–24.
6. Macintyre K. Famine and the female mortality advantage. In: Dyson T, Gráda CÓ, eds. Famine demography: perspectives from the past and present. Oxford: Oxford University Press, 2002.
7. de Waal A. Famine that kills: Darfur, Sudan, 1984–1985. Oxford: Clarendon Press, 1989.
8. Davies S. Adaptable livelihoods: coping with food insecurity in the Malian Sahel. London: Macmillan Palgrave, 1995.
9. Swift J. New approaches to famine. *IDS Bull* 1993; **24**: 1–5.
10. Sen A. Poverty and famines: an essay on entitlement and deprivation. Oxford: Clarendon Press, 1981.
11. de Waal A. A re-assessment of entitlement theory in the light of the recent famines in Africa. *Dev Change* 1990; **21**: 469–90.
12. Eldridge C. Why was there no famine following the 1992 Southern African drought? The contributions and consequences of household responses. *IDS Bull* 2002; **33**: 79–87.
13. Devereux S. The Malawi famine of 2002. In: Devereux S, ed. The new famines, Sussex. *IDS Bull* 2002; **33**: 88–95.
14. World Development Movement. Structural damage: the causes and consequences of Malawi's food crisis. London: WDM, 2002.
15. Barnett T, Blaikie P. AIDS in Africa: its present and future impact. London: John Wiley, 1992.
16. Webb D, Mutangadura G. The Socio-economic impact of adult morbidity and mortality in households in Kafue District Zambia. *SAfAIDS News* 1999.
17. Baylies C. The impact of AIDS on rural households in Africa: a shock like any other? *Dev Change* 2002; **33**: 611–32.
18. Haddad L, Gillespie S. Effective food and nutrition policy responses to HIV/AIDS: what we know and what we need to know, discussion paper no 112. Washington DC: International Food Policy Research Institute, Food Consumption and Nutrition Division, 2001.
19. Kwaramba P. The Socio-economic impact of HIV/AIDS on communal agricultural production systems in Zimbabwe, working paper 19, economic advisory project. Harare: Friedrich Ebert Stiftung, 1998.
20. Southern Africa development community. Vulnerability assessment community: the impacts of HIV/AIDS on food security in Southern Africa: regional analysis based on data collected from national VAC emergency food security assessments in Malawi, Zambia and Zimbabwe. Harare: Mimeo, 2003.
21. Sen A. Poverty and famines: an essay on entitlement and deprivation. Oxford: Clarendon Press, 1981.
22. Stanecki K, Heaton LM. A descriptive analysis of dependency ratios and other demographic indicators

in population affected by HIV/AIDS. Paper presented to meeting, Empirical Evidence for the Demographic and Socio-Economic Impact of AIDS. Durban, March, 2003.

23. UNICEF, USAID, UNAIDS. Children on the brink 2002: a joint report on orphan estimates and program strategies. Washington: The Synergy Project, 2002.

24. Rugalema G. Coping or struggling? A journey into the impact of HIV/AIDS in Southern Africa. *Rev Afr Polit Econ* 2000; **27**: 537–45.

25. Rosen S, Simon J. Shifting the burden of HIV/AIDS. Boston: Boston University, Center for International Health, 2002.

26. Coutsoudis A, Pillay K, Spooner E, Kuhn L, Coovadia H. Influence of infant feeding patterns on early mother-to-child transmission of HIV-1 in Durban, South Africa: a prospective cohort study. *Lancet* 1999; **354**: 471–76.

27. Semba RD, Tang AM. Micronutrients and the pathogenesis of human immunodeficiency virus infection. *Br J Nutr* 1999; **81**: 181–89.

28. United Nations Administrative Committee on Coordination/Subcommittee on Nutrition of the United Nations. Overview to the feature: nutrition and HIV/AIDS. *SCN News* 1998; **17**: 3–4.

29. Save the Children Fund. The livelihoods of commercial sex workers in Binga. Harare, March 2002.

CHAPTER 37

Child Malnutrition and Responses to Famine in the Nigerien Sahel

Catherine Panter-Brick, Rachel Casiday, Katherine Hampshire, and Kate Kilpatrick

(2010)

Food insecurity, poverty, and risks to health are clearly political and economic issues requiring top-level intervention. An important question is whether intervention efforts launched by humanitarian or governmental structures articulate effectively with the grass-root strategies developed by local communities to face acute, chronic, or acute-upon-chronic food shortages. In addressing food crises and/or chronic poverty, humanitarian agencies, central governments, local communities and individual households may work towards the same critical aims—to protect lives and livelihoods—yet operate within different sets of constraints, worldviews and expectations. For instance, humanitarian agencies have a mandate to step up all efforts in order to manage a transitory "emergency" situation, such as a food crisis on an unprecedented scale, because such crisis demands immediate action to save lives; this level of intervention contrasts with efforts for managing the "silent emergency" of child malnutrition, in communities which suffer chronic, albeit severe, poverty. Local households, however, often cope with severe food shortages as part and parcel of habitual experience; their responses to an acute food crisis are not necessarily *qualitatively* different from the coping responses to everyday poverty, reflecting their dual concern to save both fragile lives and vulnerable livelihoods.

In this chapter we draw upon the example from the Nigerien Sahel at a time of severe food shortage to review macro- and micro-level responses to food insecurity, clarifying the priorities that guide them. We examine how risks to health and survival are operationalized by humanitarian agencies involved in Sub-Saharan famine relief, with reliance on biological (anthropometric and mortality) indicators of child vulnerability to differentiate between different levels of emergency requiring intervention. We also document local responses vis-à-vis emergency nutrition and health programs, how these are embedded in social experience, and what they reveal about indigenous frameworks for understanding vulnerability and resilience in the context of chronic poverty. Issues raised below are integral to research and advocacy within a biocultural framework and within a political economy framework of anthropology.

FOOD INSECURITY AND GRINDING POVERTY IN THE POOREST COUNTRY OF THE WORLD

Niger is a land-locked country in the Sahel region of Central West Africa, ranked as the poorest country in the world on the UN Human Development Index (UNDP 2006). On the new Multidimensional Poverty Index, which assesses poverty using 10 different indicators, Niger has the highest incidence of poverty (93%) of any country in the world, based on 2006 DHS Survey data (Alkire and Santos 2010). Out of a population estimated at 12.4 million in 2005, 63% lived on less than a dollar a day, and 34% lived in extreme poverty (Mousseau and Mittal 2006).

Recent decades have seen very high population growth (3.3 percent annually between 1988 and 2001), and increasing overexploitation of land for agricultural production (May, Harouna, and Guengant 2004, World Bank 2002, World Bank 2010). Population pressure, land degradation, reduced income-generating opportunities, and weak markets all conspire to render the people of Niger vulnerable to food insecurity (Baro and Deubel 2006). Poor harvests result in price explosions of basic grains, making them unaffordable to the poor. Many are forced to borrow and repay at much higher rates after the harvest, creating cycles of indebtedness and food insecurity. Moreover, poor access to health care, high rates of infection and illness, and inappropriate infant feeding practices contribute to worsen the effects of food scarcity on young children (Daulaire 2005, Hampshire, Panter-Brick et al. 2009a).

In 2005, recurrent food insecurity in the Sahel caught international attention, as its impact on human lives and

Updated from work by Casiday, Hampshire, Panter-Brick, and Kilpatrick (2010), published in the edited volume by Moffatt and Prowse with permission from Berghahn Books.

338

livelihoods reached a crisis point—warranting emergency intervention. A severe drought and locust invasion had led to very poor harvests and widespread food shortages in 2004. Although total food production for Niger was only 7.5 percent below the national food requirement, control of the national cereal markets by a few big traders meant that many people were unable to afford the high food prices that year (Mousseau and Mittal 2006). The situation failed to improve in the following year (2005), because communities were left in a precarious position, their livelihoods at risk from having sold their livestock and incurred debts to cope with the food crisis of the preceding year (Daulaire 2005, Kapp 2005).

In some localities, however, the food crisis of 2004–2006 was not necessarily *qualitatively* different from other years. Seasonal hunger and food crises are part and parcel of habitual, "normal" experience. It is even argued that it is the very nature of chronic hunger in this part of the world that resulted in delayed and inadequate responses, on the part of the Nigerien government and of international donors, to the emergency situation of 2004–2005 (Mousseau and Mittal 2006).

Indeed, in 2007 after the food crisis was ostensibly over, Niger's children still suffered a 50% chronic and 10% acute malnutrition rate (Dolan 2007). A new crisis emerged in 2010, following floods in the north in late 2009 and a season of unpredictable rains, then compounded by further flooding in August 2010. In April (2010) the UN called for $190 million to fund an Emergency Humanitarian Action Plan for Niger, of which $22 million was to tackle child malnutrition (UNICEF 2010).

APPRAISAL OF A FOOD CRISIS AND CHILD MALNUTRITION

For Western outsiders, Niger was clearly in an emergency situation during the 2005 Sahelien food crisis. Many Nigerien people endured extreme conditions – during interviews we conducted in 2006, for example, one woman recounted being prostrate on the ground, too weak to get up to meet the Western photographers who were "*clicking and flashing at my face.*" Another woman, whom we asked how villagers had been able to complete the fasting month of Ramadan, replied: "*Ramadan or not, it made no difference—we had nothing to eat.*"

Despite the sudden media attention, some critical reviewers have emphasized that this was "not a transitory emergency but a permanent feature of mounting vulnerability" (Baro and Deubel 2006:529). Indeed Rubin (2006) argued that the country was in fact facing two emergencies, one immediate and the other long-term, and that both demanded intervention.

Humanitarian agencies rely on a standardized set of indicators to classify food crisis situations requiring different levels of humanitarian assistance (SPHERE 2004, Young and Jaspars 2006). Data collection surveys and intervention efforts frequently focus on young children, 6 months

to 5 years of age. Children under 5 have high nutritional requirements per kg body weight and require nutritionally dense foods. These children are also vulnerable to infectious diseases, especially during the process of complementary feeding and when they begin to crawl on dirty surfaces. Nutritional supplementation of babies under 6 months of age presents greater difficulties, given global frameworks of breastfeeding promotion that recommend exclusive breast-feeding for infants under 6 months (WHO 2001).

The most common indicators used to assess the severity of food crises are community prevalence rates of acute malnutrition, together with child mortality rates and other aggravating factors such as infectious disease epidemics (Table 1). *Global acute malnutrition* (GAM) is taken as the percentage of children with weight-for-height z-scores (WHZ) <-2 relative to the reference population; *severe acute malnutrition* (SAM) is taken as WHZ<-3 (Figure 1). Thus indices of acute malnutrition, namely growth *wasting*, rely on measures of child growth expressed as z-scores (standard deviations, SD) from the median of a reference population for children of the same sex and age. Reference populations are typically Western, well-nourished children, although in 2006 the WHO introduced a multicenter reference growth curve based on data from multiethnic (but still well nour-ished) children in Brazil, Ghana, India, Norway, Oman, and the U.S. (WHO 2009). The prevalence and, crucially, the individuals identified as malnourished, will vary depending on which reference is used, so the WHO recommends using less stringent admission criteria for therapeutic feeding interventions in order to encompass children at risk who might not have been identified by earlier criteria (WHO 2009, p. 4). According to the WHO framework, special interventions are required where GAM exceed 15% (indicating a critical situation for community rates of child malnutrition) or 10% (indicating a serious situation), while the presence of aggravating factors serves to trigger interventions from lower thresholds for rates of acute malnutrition (Table 1).

Mid-upper-arm circumference (MUAC) is another helpful indicator of child nutritional status, using a cut-off point of 110 mm for acute childhood malnutrition. Because MUAC changes little between 1 and 5 years of age, and has a stronger association with mortality risk than weight-for-height within this age group (Young and Jaspars 2006), it is often used as a criterion for admission to therapeutic feeding programs. While MUAC is often reported in nutrition surveys alongside WHZ, the two indicators may identify different individual children as acutely malnourished; cau-tion should be employed when comparing prevalence rates of malnutrition based on one indicator against surveys using a different indicator.

In Niger, indicators for child health and mortality are clearly very poor (Table 2), reflecting both a crisis situation and the underlying perennial problem of grinding poverty. Child malnutrition rates regularly fall in the risky to serious categories of the WHO framework (Table 1), representing "a chronic nutritional emergency" (Mousseau and Mittal 2006:3). Nutritional surveys conducted in early 2005 found

Table 1 International Frameworks to Assess the Severity of a Food Crisis

Framework	Médecins Sans Frontières (1995)	World Health Organization (2000)	Action required
Critical/serious situation	>20% GAM among children 6 months to 5 years -OR- 10–19% GAM with aggravating factors	>15% GAM among children 6 months to 5 years -OR- 10–14% GAM with aggravating factors	* General rations * Supplementary feeding for all members of vulnerable groups * Therapeutic feeding for severely malnourished individuals
Risky situation	10–19% GAM -OR- 5–9% GAM plus aggravating factors	10–14% GAM -OR- 5–9% GAM plus aggravating factors	* Supplementary feeding for malnourished individuals in vulnerable groups * Therapeutic feeding for severely malnourished individuals
Acceptable situation	<10% GAM without aggravating factors	<10% GAM without aggravating factors	* Attention to malnourished individuals through regular community services

GAM = global acute malnutrition, weight-for-height z-score <-2.
Aggravating factors = excessive child mortality, epidemic of communicable diseases.
Adapted from Young and Jaspers (2006).

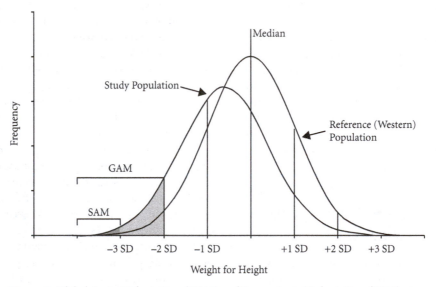

Figure 1 *Global Acute Malnutrition (GAM) and Severe Acute Malnutrition (SAM) at a population level. The shaded portions of the graph represent those children with weight-for-height lower than -2 standard deviations (SD) below the median for the reference population (GAM) and lower than -3 standard deviations below the median (SAM), respectively. Drawn by Rachel Casiday and Matthew Scott.*

GAM rates in excess of 20 percent, far above the threshold defining an emergency situation. In addition to wasting (GAM and SAM) in 2004–2005, there is plentiful evidence of growth *stunting* (global chronic malnutrition, GCM), as indicated by low height-for-age z-scores. Thus indicators of childhood malnutrition clearly reveal an acute-upon-chronic situation.

GOVERNMENT, DONOR AND HUMANITARIAN RESPONSES

Modern analysis of famines has shifted from considering overall food supply to exchange entitlements specific to population groups (Sen 1981). More recently, Devereux (2007) proposed a further conceptual shift to focus on response failure, "or the failure of governments and agencies to intervene to protect household food security following supply and/or demand failures" (Devereux 2009, p. 26). This, he argued, requires a shift in focus from *what* caused the shortage in food, to *who* caused the food shortage to become a famine. "The new famines are *political* because they are almost always *preventable*" (Devereux 2007, p. 11, emphasis in original). Sen (1982) also pointed to the importance of governments in preventing famines, claiming that famines do not occur in countries with a democratic government and free press. However, as Rubin (2009) shows, a

Table 2 Child Health Indicators for Children 6 to 59 Months Old: Malnutrition, Infection, and Mortality Rates

Niger	1996 to 2005[1]	1998[2]	2006[3]	June 2007[6]	June 2008[6]	June 2009[6]
Malnutrition rates (%)						
Wasting: Global Acute Malnutrition (GAM)	13.4–24.0	20.7	10.3	12.3	11.6	12.3
Wasting: Severe Acute Malnutrition (SAM)	1.6–5.4	3.7	1.5	2.5	2.8	2.1
Stunting: Global Chronic Malnutrition (GCM)		38.0	50.0	49.9	47.2	46.3
Infection rates, preceding two weeks (%)						
Fever		48.3	26.8			28.1
Diarrhoea		37.8	20.8			22.2
Acute Respiratory Infections		14.2	13.8			8.4
Mortality rates						
Risk of dying before age 5, per 1,000 (5q0)			257			

Sources: [1] FEWS NET, 2006; [2] DHS 1999; [3] INS and Macro International, 2007; [4] Kokere 2006; [5] Concern Worldwide, 2007; [6] Gouvernement de Niger, WFP, UNICEF, 2009. **Note:** At the time of preparation of this manuscript, no survey data were available to us on the effects of the 2010 food crisis. Global Acute Malnutrition (GAM): weight-for-height z-scores ≤-2; Severe Acute Malnutrition (SAM): weight-for-height z-scores ≤-3; Global Chronic Malnutrition (GCM): height-for-age z-scores ≤-3.

democratically elected government in Niger presided over the escalation of a relatively minor drop in food production into a full-blown famine.

In this light, the 2005 situation in Niger raises a very sensitive question, best phrased by Mousseau and Mittal (2006: 14) in these terms: "Why was the poorest country in the world, with one of the highest levels of malnutrition, so unsuccessful in attracting donors' interest in 2005?" These authors argue that responsibility for this "lies first with the government, which failed to request an adequate level of assistance", but that this crisis had also been "largely ignored by donors" (p.14).

In 1991, a transition government in Niger replaced the 30-year legacy of autocratic regimes, holding free elections and preparing a new constitution, but this government was overthrown by a military coup in 1996. The military dictator was assassinated 3 years later, allowing President Mamadou Tandja to be elected, and "free and fair" presidential and municipal elections held in 2004 (Rubin 2009, p. 289–290). This would appear to challenge Sen's (1982) 'democracy thesis,' although it is not clear that Sen's other condition—a free press—was fully met in this case. Although freedom of speech is enshrined in Niger's constitution, the country has very low literacy, much of the radio media is state-owned, and there was government censorship of journalists dissenting from government policy during the 2005 food crisis (Rubin 2009, p. 290–91). Rubin (2009) argues that the political process failed to work as anticipated by Sen's democracy

thesis for three reasons, namely: government unresponsiveness, failure of the domestic media to play a watchdog role and call for more extensive intervention, and the eventual request for aid coming from the UN rather than the democratically elected government.

In the 2004–2006 crisis, the Nigerien government had first responded with a very limited call for international assistance. Its system of prevention and response to food crises (consisting largely of maintaining a national grain reserve) had been in place since the 1980s; yet in 2004, the government had only 20,000 tons of grain at its disposal, and financial reserves to procure an additional 20,000 tons—against a national deficit of 505,000 tons (Mousseau and Mittal 2006)! In November 2004, the government requested 32.7 million Euros ($42 million U.S.) in additional support, to be used primarily for the procurement of 78,000 tons of food to be sold to those in need at subsidized prices. Not only was this amount woefully inadequate to address the scale of the problem, but less than 10 percent of requested funds had actually been donated by July 2005. Moreover, Médecins Sans Frontières denounced the strategy of offering only subsidized (rather than free) food to the poor, because many could not afford even the subsidized prices and were continuing to starve (Jezequel and Yzebe 2005). Food-for-work and food-for-loan schemes were later implemented, although these also had significant problems: in particular, borrowing food meant incurring debt when grain prices were at their highest and repaying it at 4–5 times the borrowed amount after the harvest, when prices were lowest (Eilerts 2006).

In their detailed case study of the Nigerien food crisis, Mousseau and Mittal stated that donors were finally stirred to action after news of the famine had been broadcast to the world. "In the face of this mounting crisis, international NGOs raced to set up a huge intervention in order to treat 230,000 malnourished children under five—an astonishing number, far higher than any previous relief intervention" (p.13). Yet a comparison of international assistance shows how few funds were devoted to Niger, relative to other emergencies: for example, Niger received 25 times less aid from the U.S. than did Darfur ($6 vs $149 per person affected, respectively), even though the absolute numbers of people affected were much the same (3.2 million in Niger, 3.4 million in Darfur; Mousseau and Mittal, 2006:14).

The reasons for the limited governmental and international donor responses are complex and, to some extent, obscure. Niger's long-term poverty and reliance on foreign aid (with half the national budget dependent on international donors) mean that policy decisions are largely dictated by the development strategies of the World Bank and other funders, requiring recipient countries to implement structural adjustment programs to encourage private-sector economic growth (Drouhin and Defourny 2006, Jezequel and Yzebe 2005, Mousseau and Mittal 2006). Free food distribution, it was argued, would disrupt local and national markets (undercutting farmers' livelihoods) and thus hamper the country's long-term economic development.

The government was fighting significant resourcing issues, limiting its ability to respond to a scaled-up version of donor operations, but was also concerned with preserving a sense of national dignity. In September 2005, Prime Minister Hama Amadou complained: "Our dignity suffered. And we've seen how people exploit images to pledge aid that never arrives to those who really need it" (BBC News Online 2005). The government became extremely sensitive to the charge that it had allowed sections of the population to become critically malnourished. Low expectations may also have played a role in the inadequate response: the limited request for aid perhaps reflected the Nigerien government's (realistic) assessment of what international donors were actually willing to pay for. By contrast, the military coup that overthrew the government in 2010 ushered in a new transparency: one of the first policy decisions was to appeal for $123 million in foreign aid to tackle the still-existing food crisis (Tsai, 2010). Furthermore, the state was visibly working with NGOs, including national NGOs, to address the 2010 crisis (Onimus-Pfortner 2010).

On the part of donors, delay may also have been fuelled by a lack of confidence in the Nigerien government and shortage of existing, on-the-ground relief agencies, which meant that Niger was not sufficiently visible on donor radar screens. More critical voices have argued that the chronic nature of hunger in Niger had made the situation appear inevitable, even "normal" (Drouhin and Defourny 2006, Mousseau and Mittal 2006:4). As Roger Yates, Director for Disaster Risk Management at Plan International, notes of the 2010 food situation, this disaster was multi-causal and slow to evolve, and therefore was less amenable to grabbing media portrayals than other crises of the same year, such as the earthquake in Haiti (Yates 2010).

Several humanitarian agencies implemented programs responding in various ways to the crises. We are most familiar with the work of Concern Worldwide in the 2004–2006 crisis, having had access to a number of their consultancy reports. Concern implemented an emergency nutrition program, adopting a strategy of *community-based therapeutic care* (CTC) broadly in line with the Valid International protocols for CTC (Valid International 2006). There was a hierarchy of response based on the triage of children by age, nutrition, and sickness status. Community workers based in villages were trained in the targeted referral of children. Local centers offered *supplementary feeding programs* (SFP) for the treatment of moderate malnutrition, *outpatient therapeutic programs* (OTP) for the treatment of severe malnutrition, and *onwards referral* to inpatient care for the treatment of severe malnutrition with medical complications in a regional stabilization center (SC).

In villages, children between 6 months and 5 years of age were screened for acute malnutrition using MUAC (middle-upper arm circumference). Children with MUACs of less than 110 mm were admitted directly on to the OTP or to the regional SC. Those with MUACs between 110 mm and 125 mm were referred to feeding centres, where height and weight were measured (Concern Worldwide 2007). Children presenting with moderate or severe malnutrition were admitted onto the SFP or OTP, respectively.

All CTC children were given supplementary rations of Unimix (enriched porridge) and vegetable oil. Severely malnourished children were given, in addition, between two and five daily rations of "Plumpy'nut" sachets (each 500 Kcal), depending on their weight. Plumpy'nut is a specially formulated peanut butter-like product that is nutritionally similar to therapeutic milk formula and can be eaten directly from the package (thus eliminating concerns about mixing the product with contaminated water, and enabling outpatient treatment) (Nutriset 2006). In addition, all CTC children were given a "protection ration" of pre-mixed corn-soya blend, oil and sugar, and their families received a one-off "family ration" of grain, pulses and oil, partly to minimize the sharing of high density food supplements with better-nourished siblings. Basic medical treatment, referral to health centers for vaccination, and limited water and sanitation programs were also provided, as appropriate.

The emergency feeding programs were explicitly short-term relief efforts, targeted at saving the lives of the most vulnerable children as defined by anthropometric measures. Yet many of the agencies involved also ran longer-term development programs. It became increasingly clear that high levels of acute childhood malnutrition were an ongoing problem in Niger: humanitarian agencies begun to shift their focus towards integrating emergency nutrition programs with longer-term state-led health and development initiatives. For example, Concern Worldwide is now working closely with the Ministry of Health at national and regional levels to address some of the constraints that parents face in accessing curative healthcare for their children (Concern Worldwide 2007). While the Government of Niger and humanitarian agencies both stress the importance of the integration of nutritional programming into wider health services, they face considerable operational and resource challenges in achieving sustainable improvements.

In 2010, UNICEF reported the piloting of a very different approach, in which cash was given to every mother of a child under 2 years in the worst affected areas, in addition to a blanket nutritional supplementation for all children under 2 years of age (Curney 2010).

EXPERIENCE ON THE GROUND AND DISJUNCTURE OF WORLD VIEWS

How did intervention programs, deployed in those areas most affected by the food crisis and chronic poverty, articulate with the perspectives of local households? It is important to emphasize that Nigerien families were generally very enthusiastic and supportive of the emergency programs and that they recognized and appreciated the substantial benefits in terms of saving the lives of children who would otherwise have died. Indeed, one longer-term consequence of the programs might have been to heighten parents' sense of agency and control over the fate of their children. In interviews, several parents commented on the fact that children, who had appeared destined to die, had recovered following timely and appropriate treatment.

Nonetheless, there were areas of disjuncture between local perspectives and the practices and experiences of the humanitarian programs. We focus on three aspects of local experience: (a) perspectives about vulnerability and entry into the emergency nutrition programs, (b) household allocation of food rations in relation to management of risk at individual and household levels, and (c) leaving the humanitarian program and concerns about sustainability.

We draw on data collected as part of an anthropological consultancy on behalf of Concern Worldwide in January–February 2006 (some 3 months after the harvest) in two rural districts of Niger: Tahoua and Illela (Hampshire, Panter-Brick et al. 2009a, Hampshire, Panter-Brick et al. 2009b). We used a range of qualitative methods, including participant observation, interviews, and consultation with government health workers and local staff employed by the humanitarian agencies. Sampling was purposive, including households with diverse child nutritional and health status (available from growth/health records), livelihood security, subsistence system, ethnic group, and distance from health services. Semi-structured interviews were conducted with mothers (N=40), other carers (N=6), siblings (N=9), health workers and community leaders (N=38) and focus groups with mothers and grandmothers (N=15 focus groups). We also collected morbidity and feeding histories, with 7-day dietary recall, for children under 5 from their primary carers (N=44), using structured interviews. Analysis of interview material was undertaken in consultation with local field assistants and key informants, enabling juxtaposition of emic and etic perspectives (following Miles and Huberman 1994). This participatory approach to data analysis helps to ensure that data interpretation made sense locally (Young and Jaspars 1995a). In addition, we performed secondary analysis of local survey data, collected by Concern (Kokere 2006).

Vulnerability and Entry into Emergency Nutrition Programs

It was clearly necessary for humanitarian agencies to assess and target the most vulnerable children for assistance. However, some noteworthy obstacles, including a disjuncture with some parental views of vulnerability, prevented some malnourished children from having access to emergency nutrition programs. We give several examples to illustrate these problems.

Local people could not understand why acutely malnourished babies were not accepted at the emergency feeding centers that distributed supplementary food rations. We cannot estimate how many babies might have been affected, given that anthropometric data on infants 0–6 months old are not available, but there was widespread perception of babies denied a right of entry. In the words of one Hausa mother: "*I took him [4 month-old son] to the weighing, but they said he was too young. Look at him—he is so weak and I do not have enough milk to make him strong.*" This mother knew her baby was highly vulnerable, but the baby did not meet the age criteria for entry into the program.

The examples in Box 1 focus on babies less than 6 months old (Case A and Case B). Intervention efforts did not extend to young babies in supplementary feeding or outpatient therapeutic programs, although where appropriate, babies under 6 months could be admitted to the regional stabilization centre. Feeding young babies with supplementary foods presents complex problems, ranging from the suitability of liquid foods for an infant's biological requirement to the enhanced risk of illness with food supplementation, and the possibility of undermining good breastfeeding practice (World Health Organization 2001). The problem is that the prevalence of exclusive breastfeeding in Niger is extremely low. Local surveys for Tahoua and Illéla Districts show that 0% and 11% of mothers, respectively, exclusively breastfed for the first 4 to 6 months of a baby's life (Kokere 2006). The most common reason given for early cessation of breastfeeding is subsequent pregnancy. In addition, some mothers introduce complementary foods at a very young age (a matter of weeks), because they believe that their breastmilk is insufficient or "bad." Mothers make these judgments on the grounds that babies become unhappy or ill. Thus breastmilk is withdrawn or nutritionally poor supplementary foods are given just at a point when children are vulnerable to disease and malnutrition. Babies are also frequently given water-based preparations thought to have medical or health-giving

---

BOX 1 CASE STUDIES OF EARLY/ABRUPT WEANING OF ALREADY VULNERABLE INFANTS

Case A: Early Supplementation due to Perceived Lack of Breastmilk

Zenabu (a Hausa mother) has seven living children and three dead children. Her youngest daughter, Hawa, was 9 months old and malnourished at the time of interview. She began giving each of her children millet water from the age of a few weeks, and here explains why:

Zenabu: *All of my children were ill as young babies. They were born fine, but they all became ill when they drank my milk. I did not have enough milk in my breasts.*

KH: *How did you know you did not have enough milk?*

Zenabu: *I knew because my first two children died when they drank my milk. After they take my milk, they always cry and I know there is not enough for them. Look* [points to Hawa] *– see how small she is because I can't give her enough milk.*

KH: *So, when you found you didn't have enough milk, what did you do?*

Zenabu: *With the first two* [children], *I kept giving them my milk, and they both died. So, since then, I give them millet-water* [the water that millet is cooked in, once it has been drained] *from the time they are one week old.*

Case B: Early Cessation of Breastfeeding due to Perceived "Bad Milk"

Hadiza (a Hausa grandmother) explains why her granddaughter, Jamila, was weaned abruptly at the age of two months:

Hadiza: *Jamila was born weak. Then, when she was two months old, she had difficulties breathing. I thought this had happened because her mother had fallen pregnant again, and so her milk had become bad.*

KH: *Did she say she was pregnant?*

Hadiza: *No, but many women do not want to say if they are pregnant. I thought her milk must be bad and that was why Jamila couldn't breathe properly. So I thought she must stop breastfeeding and I brought her back to live here with me.*

---

properties. In Niger, while health providers say that they regularly counsel mothers to exclusively breastfeed infants younger than 6 months, our data show that only 6% of new mothers reported that they were advised to breastfeed their infant exclusively for the first 6 months of life (Hampshire et al. 2004). More recently, in response to Niger's low rates of exclusive breastfeeding, UNICEF and Niger's Ministry of Public Health have launched a three-year nationwide campaign promoting exclusive breastfeeding through community health promoters, multimedia workshops, radio and television interviews and debates, films, theatre productions, and song (Coen 2010).

A second issue concerns children who were not presented to feeding centers, even though they would be eligible for supplementary feeding, for a variety of reasons related to social status and ethnic identity. Consideration of social status is one reason why relative wealth does not appear to protect children from severe malnutrition (Young and Jaspars 1995b). As illustrated in case study C (Box 2), wealth and status can, under some circumstances, be obstacles to vulnerable children receiving assistance in the form of food supplements. Household expenditures to maintain the position of "big people" with considerable power over village-level decisions may at first seem perverse, but could have far-reaching consequences for their well-being. Case D illustrates how powerful voices within the dominant social group were marginalising other ethnic groups, to harness exclusive access to humanitarian assistance and other development support. Finally, Case E shows how relative wealth does little to protect children against risks of severe malnutrition, given detrimental childcare practices and the lack of suitable complementary foods in the area.

Other practical factors, such as extremely long queues at the gates of feeding and therapeutic centers, prevented some people from accessing the emergency programs. This was particularly true for mothers who had busy work schedules or who were not articulate in Hausa. Mothers and grandmothers told us of having repeatedly tried to get children admitted to the local supplementary feeding center. One mother stated: "*When I take him, there are so many people waiting—I never managed to get to the front of the queue, so I became disheartened.*" One Tuareg woman reported that she had been turned away after staff could not verify the age of her baby, because she could not express his date of birth in Hausa. These difficulties underscore the enormity of the problem faced by the humanitarian agencies in distributing emergency food rations, working with set criteria to manage an enormous number of people queuing for extra food rations.

Humanitarian relief agencies operate under immense fiscal, resource, and staffing constraints and so they must target their efforts to the *most vulnerable*, even if this means that others in need cannot always be helped. It is notoriously difficult in situations of food crisis to ensure that humanitarian aid is effectively delivered to the most in need. Poverty and malnutrition are commonly used as criteria for inclusion in emergency response programs but, particularly in complex emergencies, it has been argued that these do not always capture those most at risk (Jaspars and Shoham 1999). It remains to be seen how the blanket cash and supplementation strategy being piloted to cope with the 2010 food crisis (Curney 2010) will be received. We might expect that some of the dissonances between agency and recipient expectations about entry into the therapeutic programmes would be overcome, while other practical issues associated with accessing the distribution centres are likely to remain. In the blanket intervention piloted, aid is still concentrated on those groups deemed most vulnerable by external parties, this time based on age and geography rather than anthropometry, and careful evaluation will be needed to determine how this policy articulates with recipient needs and expectations.

BOX 2 CONSIDERATIONS OF WEALTH, STATUS AND ETHNIC IDENTITY IN CHILDCARE PRACTICES AND ACCESS TO EMERGENCY FEEDING PROGRAMMES

Case C: Malnourished Child from a High Status Family

Halima (a Tuareg mother) was from a very high status family: she lived in a large courtyard and her husband was one of the big chiefs of the village, and yet her youngest daughter had been severely malnourished. It was clear that the family had been very wealthy, but had recently suffered a change of fortune. However, a strong sense of pride and shame constrained their responses to this newly-found poverty.

Because he had never worked in his fields, Halima's husband continued to hire paid labour to cultivate, even when he could no longer afford to do so. He had to borrow money to pay the labourers, which he repaid by selling a substantial proportion of his grain—at very low post-harvest prices. As a result, the household did not have enough millet to last through the year. When her daughter became very thin and ill, Halima refused to take her along to the weighing. She was too ashamed to admit that her child might be malnourished:

"How could I stand in the queue with all the other women from the village?"

Case D: Ethnic Marginalisation as a Barrier to Accessing Food Programmes

Roukietou (a Mbororo mother) had a 6-month-old son, Boureima, so emaciated he looked on the point of death. The Mbororo are a marginalised group of Fulani; this community lived a few km away from a large Hausa village. When asked if she had taken Boureima to the feeding center, Roukietou replied:

No. When the program people come to [the village], the chief's wife chases us [Mbororo women] away.

Another woman corroborated:

We always miss out on [NGO] programs, because we stay at the edge of the village.

A few minutes after this discussion, the chief's wife and other Hausa women came to chase the Mbororo women away, insisting the interviews should be done with Hausa women instead.

Case E: Severely Malnourished Twins in Wealthy Migrants

One of Bintou's twin children had been admitted for inpatient care at the regional stabilisation centre for treatment of severe malnutrition and medical complications. Bintou was dressed with good clothes and gold jewellery, a sign of substantial wealth. She had lived two years in Abijan, where her husband had a business, but had now returned to live in the village for two years – it was her co-wife's turn to be taken by the head of household to Abidjan.

Bintou explained that because this child was born in the village, she had followed the local custom of giving *boule* (watery porridge) in the first few weeks of life and that did not make the baby strong. For one of her older children, born in Abidjan, she had followed the urban practice of breastfeeding for close to six months. She also remarked that in town, there were plentiful food supplements to give to young children, while in this area, there was nothing but *boule*.

The twin girl was discharged from the stabilisation centre, with rations of plumpy'nut to supplement her and rations of flour and oil for the family. Bintou said she would share the plumpy'nut between the twins – one acutely malnourished and recovering from malaria, the other malnourished but with a weight-for-height just under the threshold of admission qualifying her for individual emergency feeding rations.

Household Allocation of Rations and Management of Risk

The explicit goal of emergency feeding and therapeutic programs is to save the lives of the most vulnerable individuals. By contrast, parents seek to address the vulnerability of *all* of their children and the long-term livelihoods of the whole household (Hampshire, Panter-Brick et al. 2009b).

As we show elsewhere (Hampshire et al. 2009b), it makes sense to spread risks in contexts where children's lives are seen as inherently precarious. There is a sense of powerlessness among parents over the fate of their children, such that even when extra resources are invested (high quality foods, timely medical care, extra supervision time), this will not necessarily guarantee the survival of that child. Furthermore, long-term livelihood insecurity means that families must maintain productive assets (such as livestock), as well as social capital, upon which the future well-being of the whole family depends.

There is a strong local ethos of non-discrimination between children within a household. A widely expressed sentiment was that *"all children are the same."* This ethos is manifested in practices of food sharing and equal distribution of resources within households and applies even when one child is sick or otherwise particularly vulnerable. The lack of positive discrimination to target food and health care

to the most vulnerable children results in a *de facto* discrimination against them (Hampshire, Panter-Brick et al. 2009b). Practices resulting in child neglect, in the Nigerien case, result, perversely, from an ethos of non-discrimination, rather than from willful or benign neglect, as documented elsewhere. Other research has highlighted a failure of health providers in Niger to address the need for sick children to receive special nutritional care, with only 64% of sick children observed in consultations being weighed and only 24% of their caregivers questioned or counselled on feeding (Hampshire et al., 2004) as stipulated in the WHO's Integrated Management of Childhood Illness protocol (WHO 2008).

Sick children are not usually given special foods (high quality or easy to digest). Indeed cultural practices of eating together and sharing food equally between children make it very difficult for parents to single out a child for special treatment. In addition, there is a strong belief that giving a child high quality foods, especially milk, for a temporary period can result in that child falling ill with a serious condition known as anugu (fever and rash) when the extra food is withdrawn. Fear of anugu underlies (or perhaps helps to justify) mothers' reluctance to give high quality foods to sick children.

In relation to the food supplements received from emergency feeding centers, parents' priorities do not, therefore, always coincide with those of the humanitarian agencies:

parents do not always use rations for the purposes intended by donors. Despite the efforts of agencies to persuade parents against this, there were numerous accounts of parents dividing rations equally between all their children, rather than just giving them to the child identified as malnourished, as this focus group exchange between Hausa mothers illustrates:

"No one gives the ration just to the child it is meant for. We have to share between all children."

"And with the neighbours' children too, or we will be criticised for being selfish."

There were also reports of people selling rations, or sharing them with others. One local school-teacher offered us a sachet of Plumpy'nut that she had been given by the parents of one of her pupils. Such behavior may seem perverse, but makes sense from a local perspective of risk-spreading to secure a range of social networks. Plumpy'nut is a highly desirable food. As such, respondents stated that it could be sold to pay for other food for the whole family. Plumpy'nut packets also become currency as a way of acquiring social capital. By giving sachets to influential community figures, parents underscore important social networks that might later prove invaluable in times of crisis.

Leaving the Humanitarian Program: A "Second Weaning"

Finally, what happens to children who leave the feeding or therapeutic programs? Children are discharged when they have re-established sufficient weight and health to leave at-risk categories. However, parents reported that their children become accustomed to the food supplements and, in some cases, even refused to eat normal household foods (a bland, liquid porridge called *boule*) while they are receiving the high density rations. Parents fear that, once the rations are withdrawn, children will be in a worse position than before. One woman compared the discharge from the feeding programme to the customary abrupt cessation of breastfeeding when a mother finds she is pregnant, an abrupt weaning for the second time in the child's life. Another woman expressed similar concerns: *"When Hawa [her baby] is better, they will stop the ration, and I am afraid that she will become ill again. That is what has happened to other babies here."* This fear of potential illness, following sudden withdrawal of a food to which the child has become accustomed, links into beliefs about *anugu*.

Some children are re-admitted to the supplementary feeding programs after discharge, because they cannot thrive at home. Unfortunately, there are few quantitative or qualitative data on re-admissions to emergency programs, an indicator which it has proved difficult to monitor accurately within such large-scale programs. Issues of discharge and re-admission to emergency programs are areas of disjuncture between donor and community perspectives that remain little explored.

CONCLUSION

In tackling the problems of child undernutrition, sickness and mortality in a food crisis situation, relief agencies, governments, and households arguably share an overall goal—protecting children's lives while preserving livelihoods. However, they operate under very different constraints and thus adopt different strategies and priorities toward maximising this goal. First of all, humanitarian interventions in a "crisis situation" are hard-pressed to coordinate with government action: they achieve very substantial results in terms of saving individual lives, but frustrating results in terms of making those individual lives sustainable. Second, governments in very poor countries operate under formidable challenges to achieve equitable and efficient distribution of resources. Last, households operate to spread risks and achieve resilience in the face of chronic poverty. Global and local constraints each make logical sense within their respective parameters; nonetheless, there are important points of disjuncture between them, especially in cases of acute-upon-chronic situations of mounting social and economic vulnerability.

To what extent are these different priorities reconcilable? In Niger, humanitarian agencies, such as Concern Worldwide, are increasingly working with government partners, such as the Ministry of Health, in addressing some of the barriers to treatment-seeking for children's illnesses (particularly malaria, diarrhoea, and acute respiratory infections) that can precipitate malnutrition, as well as working to train health workers in responding to malnutrition. Similarly, given the way that chronic livelihood insecurity underpins parents' risk-averse strategies of investment in vulnerable children, a top priority must be working to develop better linkages between humanitarian emergency programs and longer-term initiatives aimed at sustainable livelihood development (see Hampshire, Panter-Brick et al. 2009a). Building the efficiency and sustainability of health systems is currently a top-ranking global health priority. In particular, the issue of scaling-up nutrition programs to prevent malnutrition is debated at highest levels, e.g. at the World Bank (Blackwell et al. 2010).

Particularly in cases of protracted crisis, it is essential to articulate effectively the position of humanitarian agencies, government structures, and local communities, and variation and contradictions therein. This clarity of purpose, regarding what are their diverse priorities but also their common agenda, is necessary to address the very real constraints of pervasive poverty and to achieve sustainable and mutually-reinforcing improvements in child health and in household livelihoods.

References

Alkire S, Santos ME. 2010. Niger Country Briefing. Oxford Poverty & Human Development Initiative (OPHI)

Multidimensional Poverty Index Country Briefing Series. Available at: www.ophi.org.uk/policy/multidimensional-poverty-index/mpi-country-briefings.

Baro M and Deubel TF. 2006. Persistent hunger: perspectives on vulnerability, famine, and food security in Sub-Saharan Africa. Annual Review of Anthropology 35:521–38.

BBC News Online. 2005. Niger food aid 'no longer needed'. http://news.bbc.co.uk/2/hji/africa/4253060.stm

Blackwell N et al. 2010. Food crisis in Niger: A Chronic emergency. The Lancet 376 (August 7): 416–417.

Casiday RE, Hampshire KR, Panter-Brick C and Kilpatrick K. 2010. Responses to a Food Crisis and Child Malnutrition in the Nigerien Sahel. In Moffat T and Prowse T (Editors), Human Diet and Nutrition in Biocultural Perspective: Past meets Present. Volume 5, Studies of the Biosocial Society. Oxford: Berghahn Books, pp. 152–172.

Coen B. 2010. A campaign to promote exclusive breastfeeding makes strides in rural Niger. UNICEF Newsline (6 August) http://www.unicef.org/infobycountry/niger_55454.html (accessed accessed 30 April 2012).

Concern Worldwide. 2007. Emergency Nutrition Programme: Final Report to DEC ERP Tahoua and Illela Districts 2006–07. Concern Worldwide.

Curney V. 2010. Infusions of cash tackle immediate needs in Niger's drought-affected areas. UNICEF Newsline (6 October) http://www.unicef.org/infobycountry/niger_56364.html (accessed 30 April 2012)

Dolan S. 2007. ECHO and UNICEF promote Plumpy'nut production to improve child nutrition in Niger. UNICEF Newsline (18 May). http://www.unicef.org/nutrition/niger_39675.html (accessed 30 April 2012)

Daulaire N. 2005. Niger: Not just another famine. The Lancet 366:2004.

Devereux S. 2007. Introduction: From "old famines" to "new famines". In: Devereux S, Editor. The new famines. 1–26. Routledge: London.

Devereux S. 2009. Why does famine persist in Africa? Food Security 1:25–38.

DHS. 1999. Enquête Démographique et de Santé 1998. CARE International and Macro International Inc.

Drouhin E and Defourny I. 2006. Niger: taking political responsibility for malnutrition. Humanitarian Exchange 33:20–22.

Eilerts G. 2006. Niger 2005: Not a famine, but something much worse. Humanitarian Exchange 33:17–19.

FEWS NET. 2006. Understanding Nutrition Data and the Causes of Malnutrition in Niger: A Special Report by the Famine Early Warning Systems Network (FEWS NET). FEWS NET.

Gouvernement de Niger, WFP, UNICEF. 2009. Rapport d'enquête nationale: nutrition et survie de l'enfant. Niger, Mai/Juin 2009. http://www.unicef.org/wcaro/wcaro_Enquete_nutrition_Niger_2009_ECHO_UNICEF.pdf. (accessed 30 April 2012).

Hampshire RD, Aguayo VM, Harouna H, Roley JA, Tarini A, Baker SK. 2004. Delivery of nutrition services in health systems in sub-Saharan Africa: opportunities in Burkina Faso, Mozambique and Niger. Public Health Nutr. 2004 7(8):1047–53.

Hampshire K, Casiday R, Kilpatrick K, Panter-Brick C. 2009a. The social context of childcare practices and child malnutrition in Niger's recent food crisis. Disasters 33(1):132–151.

Hampshire K, Panter-Brick C, Kilpatrick K, Casiday R. 2009b. Saving lives, preserving livelihoods: Understanding risk, decision-making and child health in a food crisis. Social Science & Medicine 68(4): 758–765.

Moffatt T and Prowse T, Editors. 2010. Human Diet and Nutrition in Biocultural Perspective: Past meets Present. Volume 5, Studies of the Biosocial Society. Oxford: Berghahn Books.

Howe P and Devereux S. 2004. Famine Intensity and Magnitude Scales: A Proposal for an Instrumental Definition of Famine. Disasters 28(4):353–72.

Institut National de la Statistique (INS) and Macro International. 2007. Résultats Préliminaires de la troisième Enquête Démographique et de Santé et à Indicateurs Multiples du Niger. Calverton, Maryland, USA: INS and Macro International Inc.

Jaspars S and Shoham J. 1999. Targeting the vulnerable: a review of the necessity and feasibility of targeting vulnerable households. Disasters 23:359–372.

Jezequel J-H and Yzebe A. 2005. Niger: The sacrificial victims of development. Messages MSF 137:3–4.

Kapp C. 2005. As Niger's emergency eases, another crisis looms. The Lancet 366:1065–66.

Kokere S. 2006. Anthropometric and Nutritional Survey, Tahoua and Illela Districts, Tahoua Region. Summary Report. 2nd – 12th December 2005. Concern.

May JF et al. 2004. Nourrir, Eduquer et Soigner Tous les Nigeriens, La Demographie en Perspective. Departement du Developpement Humain, Region Afrique, Banque Mondiale.

Miles MB and Huberman AM. 1994. Qualitative Data Analysis: Sage.

Mousseau F and Mittal A. 2006. Sahel: A prisoner of starvation? A case study of the 2005 food crisis in Niger. Oakland: The Oakland Institute.

Nutriset. 2006. "Plumpy'nut." http://www.nutriset.fr/en/product-range/produit-par-produit/plumpynut-ready-to-use-therapeutic-food-rutf.html (accessed 30 April 2012).

Onimus-Pfortner J. 2010. Health centres focus on treatment of undernourished children in Niger. UNICEF Newsline. (18 June 2010) http://www.unicef.org/infobycountry/niger_54022.html (accessed 30 April 2012).

Rubin O. 2009. The Niger famine: A collapse of entitlements and democratic responsiveness. Journal of Asian and African Studies 44(3): 279–298.

Rubin V. 2006. The humanitarian-development debate and chronic vulnerability: lessons from Niger. Humanitarian Exchange 33:22–24.

Sen A. 1981. Poverty and Famines: An essay on entitlement and deprivation. Oxford: Clarendon.

SPHERE. 2004. The Sphere Project: Humanitarian Charter and Minimum Standards in Disaster Response (Revised Edition). Oxford: Oxfam GB.

Tsai TC. 2010. Food crisis no longer taboo in Niger. The Lancet 375(April 3): 1151–1152.

'UNDP. 2006. Human Development Report 2006. United Nations Development Programme. http://hdr.undp.org/en/media/HDR06-complete.pdf (accessed 30 April 2012).

UNICEF. 2010. UNICEF Humanitarian Action Update: Sahel, 3 June 2010. http://www.unicef.org/infobycountry/files/UNICEF_Humanitarian_Action_Update-_Sahel-_3_June_2010(1).pdf (accessed 30 April 2012).

UNICEF Niger. 2006. Bilan Semestriel: Réponse à la Situation Nutritionnelle des Enfants. UNICEF.

Valid International. 2006. Community-Based Therapeutic Care (CTC): A Field Manual. Oxford: Valid International.

World Bank. 2002. Niger Poverty Reduction Strategy Paper and Joint Staff Assessment. World Bank 23483-NIR.

World Bank. 2010. Country summary data: Niger. http://data.worldbank.org/country/niger (accessed 30 April 2012).

World Health Organization. 2001. The Optimal Duration of Exclusive Breastfeeding: Report of an Expert Consultation. WHO WHO/FCH/CAH/01.24.

World Health Organization. 2008. Integrated Management of Childhood Illness chart booklet. http://whqlibdoc.who.int/publications/2008/9789241597289_eng.pdf (accessed 30 April 2012).

World Health Organization and UNICEF. 2009. WHO child growth standards and the identification of severe acute malnutrition in infants and children. Geneva: WHO and UNICEF. http://www.who.int/nutrition/publications/severemalnutrition/9789241598163/en/index.html (accessed 30 April 2012).

Yates, R. 2010. Why not all disasters are equal. The Guardian [online] http://www.guardian.co.uk/commentisfree/2010/sep/06/disasters-donor-fatigue-media-images (accessed 30 April 2012).

Young H and Jaspars S. 1995a. Nutritional assessments, food security and famine. Disasters 19:26–36.

Young H and Jaspars S. 1995b. Malnutrition and poverty in the early stages of famine: North Darfur, 1988–90. Disasters 19:198–215.

Young H and Jaspars S. 2006. Meaning and measurement of acute malnutrition, A Primer for Decision-Makers. Network Paper No 56, Humanitarian Practice Network. Overseas Development Institute.

UNIT IX

DIETARY TRANSITIONS AND GLOBALIZATION

Coca-Cola™ is one of the United States' biggest exports. Like their thirsty cousins in the United States, the average Mexican and Icelander drink almost 8 ounces of Coca-Cola per day. Coca-Cola is not merely a major economic commodity, but a major contributor to diets. As the chapter in this section by Leatherman and Goodman suggests, the drinking of two to three soft drinks in a day by a 10-year-old Mayan boy accounts for about a third of his energy intake.

In the 1980s, a popular movie, *The Gods Must Be Crazy*, centered on an empty bottle of Coca-Cola found by a !Kung San. The soft drink bottle was a well-chosen metaphor for the intrusion of Western culture. It appears that the local and ecologically adapted diets noted in previous chapters, such as the hunting and gathering lifestyle of the Dobe !Kung San, and the entomorphagy of Native Amazonians, are becoming increasingly rare and, at the same time diets all over the world are becoming increasingly similar. Local food production has been on the decline as large scale factory farming has increased. The foods eaten in the new global village are increasingly Western and fast foods. How did this come to be? What are the consequences for culture, environment, and human biology?

Half a millennium ago, each local populace of each region had the serious responsibility for producing food by themselves for the individuals in their region. Food systems developed in response to ecological limits and cultural patterns. For example, in the highlands of Peru, different varieties of potatoes were developed. Some are tastier and others more nutritious and other resist drought. The different varieties meet different needs and desires and at the extreme, they provide a hedge against the worst possible outcomes.

Local independence began to change with long-distance exploration and trade. First, explorers, such as Marco Polo, came back with easily transported spices, teas, and condiments. These exotic items were initially made available to sponsors, and the tastes of the wealthy and the nobility began to change. Full-blown globalization of diets began at about the time of the colonization and conquest of the Americas.

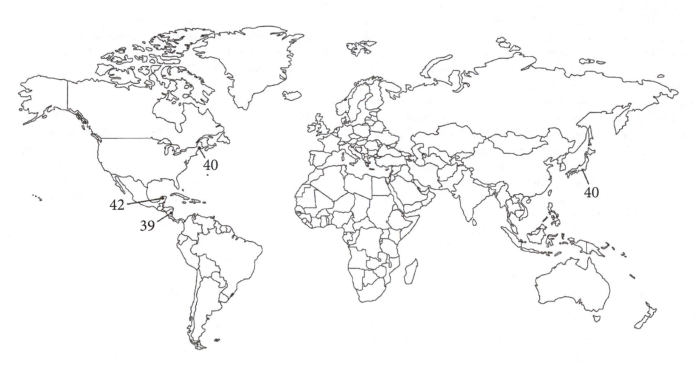

Figure 1 *Map shows the location of the groups referred to in the chapters in this section by chapter number: 39 = Miskito, eastern coast of Nicaragua; 40 = fishermen, coast of Maine, United States and fish marketers, Tokyo, Japan; 42 = Mayan communities, Yucatan, Mexico.*

Increased transcontinental transport provided a means of supplying goods to the middle classes. Staples began to be traded, and seeds of fruits, vegetables, tubers, and grains were transported and replanted in faraway places. Some of these "ecological exchanges" likely failed miserably and became of little historical consequence. Others proved to be great successes, at least initially, as, for example, the migration of the potato from Peru to Ireland.

The chapters in this part focus on various aspects of the key historical trends of dietary delocalization and commoditization. Anthropologists Gretel Pelto and Pertti Pelto (chapter 38) define *delocalization* as "processes in which food varieties, production methods, and consumption patterns are disseminated throughout the world in an ever-increasing and intensifying network of socioeconomic and political interdependency." Commoditization of food systems, a process embedded in dietary delocalization, is defined by Dewey (1989:415) as "the use of agricultural goods for sale rather than home consumption." The chapters that follow illustrate general aspects of these processes with specific examples.

In "Diet and Delocalization: Dietary Changes since 1750," Pelto and Pelto outline the idea of delocalization, how it might vary from place to place, and its potential impact on nutritional status. As stated in their definition of *delocalization*, they view this process as "ever-increasing and intensifying." It is clear that more and more groups are being drawn into national and international markets and systems of trade. Trade agreements such as NAFTA and those of the WTO support this trend.

Delocalization is in reality a number of interrelated processes involving the movement of the diverse things used to produce foods, foods themselves as well as peoples and their ideas. Key processes include new foods being introduced through trade, locally produced foods now purchased in stores, new foods grown locally, and new knowledge and food preferences brought about by migration of individuals and ideologies. Because the mix of sub-processes varies, the consequences of delocalization for diet and nutrition are complex. The end result, however, is typically an increase in energy costs due in part to transportation. Local autonomy is frequently lost because external "market forces" control access and prices. As well, industrial food products have "hidden costs" in their use of fertilizers, in energy for transportation, and loss of freshness and nutrients.

Pelto and Pelto suggest that one means to evaluate delocalization is via its consequence on dietary diversity. *Dietary diversity* is important because more diverse diets are more likely to provide a healthy mix of nutrients. They hypothesize that delocalization has had a positive effect on dietary diversity for wealthy individuals. However, for individuals who cannot afford to purchase exotic foods, delocalization may lead to decreased diversity.

In "When the Turtle Collapses, the World Ends" anthropologist Bernard Nietschmann provides a vivid example of the potentially negative ecological and nutritional consequences of globalization. Nietschmann was working on ethnographic fieldwork with the Miskito Indians of the Atlantic coast of Nicaragua during a time of great change from subsistence agriculture and fishing to exporting turtle to distant world markets. Along with cassava, a high-energy source, green turtle meat had been a dietary staple of the Miskito. Turtle meat was highly esteemed, but there was no need to catch more turtles than could be locally consumed. That changed dramatically in the late 1960s when two export companies began processing turtles for their meat and other products to market in Europe and North America. For the first time, the Miskito Indians had the option of selling turtles—in fact, selling as many as they could catch. Unfortunately, the ecological reality is not "turtles all the way down" (a quote from the opening of Nietschmann's chapter). Turtles are a finite resource. When turtle production declines and/or competition increases, financial yield may decrease and nutrition suffers. What is the lesson to be learned from this chapter? How generalizable is it? What could and should be done to prevent this type of exploitation from occurring in the future?

"How Sushi Went Global" by anthropologist Theodore Bestor provides an excellent example of a global food. Bestor follows bluefin tuna and the individuals involved in economic, culinary, and cultural transactions in turning bluefin into sushi, around the globe. We all know by now that sushi, once a food eaten in Japan but hardly anywhere else, now has a high perch among foods in the global village. But bluefin tuna have been a global commodity for longer than sushi. Bestor takes us to the coast of Maine, where bluefin tuna are caught, driven to New York, and flown to Tokyo. In some cases, the tuna is served the next day as sushi in Japan. More often now, the Tokyo market is just a stop along the way back to North America or some other destination.

As he follows the tuna in its dizzying journey around the globe, Bestor wonders about the meaning of such a global commodity. How has the trade in bluefin tuna influenced how fisherman in Maine think of Japan? And how do all these tuna miles square with the increasing desire to eat locally?

In "Nutrition Transitions," Darna Dufour and Richard Bender ask how we can understand the shifts in diet and physical activity patterns—and the concurrent explosion of obesity rates—that appear to be occurring very rapidly across the globe, first in developed nations and now in poorer nations. The most widely known description of these phenomena is a model called the Nutrition Transition, first proposed by Barry Popkin in the early 1990s (see Popkin 1993). According to this model, the changes in nutrition and health we observe in populations around the world are not haphazard, but follow a distinct sequence of five stages defined by a specific set of dietary practices, physical activity, and health characteristics.

Despite the popularity of the Nutrition Transition, as an explanatory framework among nutritional scientists, epidemiologists and the public health community, Dufour and Bender argue that this model conforms only loosely to anthropological understanding of the nutrition of past human populations: it does not address the great variability we observe both among and even within current populations. This leaves us with some difficult questions. How can we explain broad-scale global shifts in nutrition without losing sight of the richly contextual variability among and within populations? Can we construct a parsimonious general framework that strikes a useful balance between simplicity and complexity?

In an anthropological classic, "Sweetness and Power" (1985), Sidney Mintz demonstrates the key role of one food item—sugar—in the development of England and Europe and the "underdevelopment" of the Caribbean. In Mintz's analysis, the developed taste for sugar among the working class of Europe provided the impetus for an extractive industry that changed the Caribbean forever and helped to fuel the Atlantic slave trade.

Following sugar around the globe, as Mintz does, provides an excellent illustration of the importance of delocalization and commoditization. The production of sugar from sugarcane began in South Asia and was imported to the Caribbean along with enslaved Africans. Sugar production was an industry on new soil (the Caribbean) run by nonlocal, wealthy Europeans and maintained by the labor of enslaved Africans. The dietary consequences are also systemic and delocalized. At the beginning of the seventeenth century, sugar in Britain was a luxury and a medicine. But with mass production and trans-Atlantic trade, by the end of the century it had become a necessity. Everyone wanted sugar, and consumption rates dramatically rose.

Paradoxically, the craving for sugar is expanding still. Sugar has returned to Central American and the Caribbean in a soft drink bottle, as Leatherman and Goodman show in "Coca-colonization of diets in the Yucatan." They studied dietary intakes and nutritional status in three Mayan communities: Coba, an inland community with a tourist based economy due to the presence of the Coba archaeological remains; Yalcoba, a more isolated inland community; and a community that had developed on the coast around a tourist destination. Western foods, of which Coke is both a symbol and a key component, are clearly evident in the diets of individuals in all communities, and not unexpectedly, more so in the diets of those communities with greater contact with the tourist economy of the Yucatan. Is the westernization of diets a good thing? From both an emic and an etic perspective, the answer seems to be yes, no and various degrees in between. More than anything, perhaps, this chapter shows the complexity of nutritional and dietary transitions that are also discussed by Dufour and Bender.

It is easy to envision why subsistence farmers would become increasingly drawn into markets. Selling their crops provides cash that offers the flexibility to buy commodities of choice, as chapter 15 by Elizabeth Finnis nicely demonstrates. In the best of situations, they can increase the intake of nutrient-dense foods. For example, fruits and vegetables that do not grow well in local soils and climates might be purchased. Fish may be brought to inland areas. Additionally, nonfood items can be purchased with money from growing

export foods. More often, delocalization involves the loss of control over pricing, and the amount of funds available for purchasing foods is limited. What is bought may be more a function of the power of advertisement than of family nutritional needs.

Delocalization has prevented starvation and allowed more individuals to be fed. Delocalization has led to wonderfully tasteful mixes of food as sushi joins the ranks of readily available foods and spices and food crops from around the globe merge and blend. If diversity is the spice of life, then delocalization is the spice factory. But globalization and delocalization can go too far and its negative impacts might not be immediately foreseen or equally distributed. Will the pressures to earn wages to pay for other goods pull many peasants worldwide even further away from tending their small gardens and agricultural plots? If local autonomy is lost, then delocalization can have horrific economic, social, and nutritional consequences. Cokes and chips and genetically engineered seeds will replace tortillas and fruits.

In recent years we have seen growing responses to the pace and globalization of food systems toward slow foods and local food movements. Popular writers such as Michael Pollan and Barbara Kingsolver have argued strongly for local foods. In "Looking for Solutions," the final unit of this book, chapters consider initiatives to fight malnutrition, including initiatives to build more sustainable food systems, ones that are affordable, low in food miles, rich in taste, and provides a healthy diet.

SUGGESTIONS FOR THINKING AND DOING NUTRITIONAL ANTHROPOLOGY

1. *The Turtle People* is an older film about the plight of the Miskito Indians as described by Nietschmann (1974). Another view of commoditization is found in the film *Jungle Burger*. View one or both films and consider the consequences of commoditization of systems of exchange.

2. Select a favorite dish that you associate with an ethnic group. Identify each ingredient. Where did each ingredient originate, and how did it become incorporated into this culture?

3. Select a processed food item and trace its origins. Where did the various components originate? Try to identify where they are now grown or produced.

4. Calculate your dietary diversity. As a class, first construct food categories. Your categories should not be too broad (all carbohydrate-based foods) or too narrow (chicken). For three days, place each of your foods into these categories and score the total number of categories you eat from for each day. Compare your diversity to that of fellow students.

5. One of the most serious debates of the coming years will be over the introduction of genetically

engineered foods. Assuming that these foods will be developed, what might be some of the ways to make sure the benefits are shared by those who are most in need?

References

Dewey KG. 1989. Nutrition and the Commoditization of Food Systems in Latin America and the Caribbean. Social Science and Medicine 28: 415–424.

Mintz S. 1985. Sweetness and Power. New York: Viking Press.

Popkin, BM. 1993. Nutritional patterns and transitions. Population and Development Reviews. 19:138–157.

Suggested Further Reading

Daly DC. 1996. The Leaf that Launched a Thousand Ships. Natural History. January: 24–30. Along with other articles in this issue, Daly's is a good starting point on the history of the potato and the "Great Famine" in Ireland.

Kingsolver, B. 2007. Animal, Vegetable, Miracle. Perennial: New York. Essayist and Novelist Barbara Kingsolver writes through a year of her family's attempt to eat locally.

Koeppel, Dan. 2008. Banana. The fate of the fruit that changed the world. Hudson Street Press: New York. A fascinating look at the history of a single crop in crisis.

Kloppenburg J. 1990. First the seed: The political Economy of Plant Biotechnology 1492–2000. New York: Cambridge University Press. Kloppenburg was one of the first and most outspoken critics of the role of multinationals in controlling seed distribution.

Mintz S. 1985. Sweetness and Power. New York: Viking Press. A classic on the role of sugar in world history. Essentially, an expansion of the chapter that is included here.

Plotnicov, L and R. Scaglion. 1999. The globalization of food. Waveland Press: Prospect Heights, Illinois. Readable, short book on globalization of food systems.

Sokolov R. 1991. Why We Eat What We Eat. New York: Simon and Schuster. A lively series of short articles by a food writer on the spread of foods and condiments around the world and the process of increasing hybridity of food traditions.

Viola HJ and Margolis C, editors. 1991. Seeds of Change. Washington, DC: Smithsonian Institution Press. Chapters trace the routes of Old World crops into the Americas and vice versa.

Wilk, Richard, editor. 2006. Fast Food/Slow Food. The cultural economy of the Global Food System. Altimara: New York. Excellent compilations on local and global foods.

CHAPTER 38

Diet and Delocalization: Dietary Changes since 1750

Gretel H. Pelto and Pertti J. Pelto
(1983)

During the past two centuries virtually all of the populations in the world have experienced dramatic changes in their dietary patterns. In the industrialized countries changes in food patterns have been associated with improved levels of nutrition and public health, although some nutrition-related diseases are increasing. Similar processes of change in the less industrialized nations, however, have often had serious negative effects. We examine here some of the primary processes of change in food resources and distribution over the past 250 years, focusing on three main transformations that have had profound effects on global eating patterns. Our primary thesis is:

First, the general direction of transformations in food use throughout the world in the past two or three centuries has involved an increasingly rapid "delocalization" of food production and distribution. By "delocalization" (discussed more fully below) we refer to processes in which food varieties, production methods, and consumption patterns are disseminated throughout the world in an ever-increasing and intensifying network of socioeconomic and political interdependency. From the point of view of individuals and families at any one place on the globe, delocalization means that an increasing portion of the daily diet comes from distant places usually through commercial channels.

Second, in the industrialized nations, delocalization has been associated with an increase in the diversity of available foods and the quantity of food imports, and, therefore, with improved diets. In earlier periods this improvement of diet, especially through diversification, primarily benefited the upper social classes, but during the twentieth century the effects have diffused to a wide spectrum of people in the "developed" world.

Third, in the less industrialized countries of the world, the same processes of delocalization have tended to produce opposite effects on dietary quality, except for the elite. Until recent times many peoples in the Third World have been primarily dependent on locally produced food supplies, which remained largely outside the networks of commerce. As these populations have been drawn more and more into full commercial participation, economic and political forces have encouraged concentration on one or two main cash crops, with an accompanying deterioration of food diversity, as well as a loss of local control over the distribution system. Thus, world-wide food distribution and food-use transformations have occurred at the expense of economically marginal populations.

These general ideas about changes in food availability and dietary patterns have been discussed for a number of years. Here we present them in a manner that is intended to encourage historical research on these associations. To date there has been relatively little careful empirical investigation of the relationships among social change, dietary change, and nutritional status and health. Research questions need to be framed in a manner that permits hypothesis-testing and a refinement of the general model.[1]

THREE MAJOR PROCESSES OF DIETARY CHANGE

The dramatic transformations in dietary patterns that have taken place in the past two and a half centuries are one key aspect of the much larger picture of massive social and economic change that has affected all parts of the world. The specific dimensions have varied widely in relation to particular historical, political, and ecological conditions, but the basic food-use changes of interest to us have largely come about as a result of three fundamental developments:

1. A world-wide dissemination of domesticated plant and animal varieties.
2. The rise of increasingly complex, international food distribution networks, and the growth of food-processing industries.
3. The migration of people from rural to urban centers, and from one continent to another, on a hitherto unprecedented scale, with a resulting exchange of culinary and dietary techniques and preferences.

Gretel H. Pelto and Pertti J. Pelto, "Diet and delocalization: dietary changes since 1750." *Journal of Interdisciplinary History* 14 (1983): 507–528. Reprinted with permission.

Each of these processes has been powerfully influenced by national and international politico-economic forces, cultural and religious movements, and other factors. One fundamental sector of great importance has been the development of new technologies; in particular, transportation and communications technologies have played major roles.

Our rationale for focusing on the three processes listed above rests on a view of the basic elements of delocalization as they affect the behavior of particular local communities. That is, if we picture the dietary possibilities of people in a French rural commune, a small valley in Mexico, or an island in Polynesia, their food selections will change if:

a. New plant and animal varieties are introduced to the community for local production, or locally produced foods are removed from the community for sale elsewhere.
b. New foods are made available through commercial or governmental channels.
c. The people themselves move to a new area, or they receive immigrants from elsewhere, resulting in cultural exchange of culinary/dietary preferences.

Changes may also occur because of purely local developments of new food production or preparation techniques, but such occurrences are generally much less frequent.

Throughout our discussion of dietary change we confront the philosophical question of basic causes. Attempting to isolate clear, necessary and sufficient causes may have some utility in relatively simple systems. However, human behavior is more understandable if we conceptualize a system of complex, interconnected forces (including biological, psychological, economic, political, technological, and other factors), so that a focus on one component as a prime mover rests more on philosophical or stylistic preference rather than on demonstrable, empirical evidence. Understanding the developments in human food use patterns of the past 250 years depends, first of all, on sorting out the primary (descriptive) trends and processes, leaving for the future the search for the more or less clear prime movers.

The Concept of Delocalization

The concept of delocalization, which is central to our analysis of changes in human dietary patterns, is one major aspect of all the historical changes to which people give various labels such as modernization, development, progress, acculturation, and so on. In using the term delocalization we are focusing attention on one fundamental, apparently undirectional tendency in human history, particularly of more recent centuries. Delocalization has many different facets, but there are two that are most important for our discussion here.

First, there is the delocalization that results in the reduction of local autonomy of energy resources, due to dependence on gasoline-driven equipment for transportation, local industry, and other essential processes. In recent times this loss of local energy autonomy has been quite striking in the remoter areas of the globe where motor-driven boats, snowmobiles, and other equipment have been widely adopted.

Second, in more complex urban centers, delocalization is evidenced in the increased sensitivity (of prices, costs, etc.) to political fluctuations in any sector of the world energy and food network, as can be seen, for example, in the world-wide impact of Soviet grain purchasing policies, OPEC price manipulations, coffee and sugar production levels, and the beef consumption demands of the international fast-food industry.

Delocalization and Food Systems

One way to gain an understanding of delocalization in matters of human food use is to consider the opposite—local autonomy. In small-scale hunting and gathering societies, such as those of the Inuit (Eskimo) and the San peoples of the Kalahari, or among our ancestors of preagricultural times, the great bulk of food supplies and other energy resources had to be obtained from the immediate local environment. For that reason hunting-gathering societies have always been rather small—usually no more than 300 to 400 persons in the local group (often much less), with population densities that seldom exceeded ten persons per 100 square miles.

Among a great many small-scale cultivator peoples of central Africa, the Amazon rainforest areas, and the South Pacific, local groups have been largely dependent on their own food and energy resources, although some trading of food and other goods has been common between coastal and inland peoples, and between animal–keeping pastoralists and their more sedentary neighbors; occasionally, trade has been widespread among the various islands of the South Pacific.

Despite the presence of small-scale regional trading, human societies of earlier times were, to a considerable extent, unaffected by the state of food supplies in other areas. If crops failed or herds were decimated by disease in any particular area, famine was the usual result; there was no way to send for disaster relief.

In contrast to small-scale, semi-autonomous communities, peasant populations in Europe, Asia, and Latin America, in past centuries, have been a good deal more dependent on at least some commercial exchanges with other regions and nations. A common feature of peasant societies, however, has been the dependence on a wider marketing system for the purchase of non-food supplies and equipment, in exchange for which local peasant peoples were able to transfer their surplus food production, thus feeding not only themselves but the non-food producing people of the cities. A large proportion of the peasant family's food needs were met from their own farm, even though they were dependent on the commercial system for iron equipment, some clothing, a few luxury items, and (in recent decades) special foods such as sugar, salt, tea or coffee, and spices.

Before the fifteenth century there was a slow and gradual dissemination of certain major crops and food animals into ever-wider parts of the world. For example, the wheat, barley, and dairy food complex spread into all parts of Europe, south into Africa, and eastwards into Asia, from the presumed origins in the Far East. A similar process of diffusion occurred with the rice-growing complex in East and South Asia. These slow processes of diffusion certainly had significant effects on food systems in the world but the impact of changes precipitated by the age of discovery were dramatic and rapid.

WORLD-WIDE DISSEMINATION OF DOMESTICATED PLANTS AND ANIMALS

Beginning with Columbus' voyages to the New World, and other fifteenth-century expeditions into hitherto unknown parts, Europeans acquired knowledge about food crops and production systems that was formerly unavailable to them. At the same time, European settlers, missionaries, and adventurers spread the knowledge (and requisite seeds and other materials) of both Old World and New World animal domesticates to other parts of the world. By the beginning of the seventeenth century the boundaries of the various plant and animal species were transformed, as the major crops and animals were introduced into different ecological zones. By 1700 maize, rice, wheat, barley, oats, and potatoes, as well as cattle and other livestock had spread throughout most of the world, whereas earlier each of these food sources had been grown by only a segment of the world's population.

The consequences of the worldwide dissemination of domesticated plants and animals were dramatic. In Europe the slow but steady adoption of maize, potatoes, and other American cultigens began to have powerful effects by the eighteenth century. The addition of potatoes to the basic subsistence economy has been seen by some researchers as a cause of major changes in demographic patterns. For example, Vanderbroek has claimed that potatoes sustained rapid population expansion in the southern Netherlands in the middle of the eighteenth century. His data indicate that potato cultivation grew rapidly in the 1740s and 1750s, returning a five times greater yield per acre than wheat, which had previously been the main crop. Rapid population increases in that part of the Netherlands contrasts, in his view, with slower population growth in areas where potatoes were not adopted at that time.[2]

In approximately the same period the potato spread to northern Europe, where in Sweden, Finland, and Russia its cultivation was seen as an important hedge against famine. Governmental and private groups propagandized on behalf of potato cultivation, and free seed potatoes were made widely available. In Finland at the end of the eighteenth century the Finnish Economics Society distributed free seed potatoes and gave monetary prizes and medals to potato growers. "A famine and epidemic in 1765 persuaded Catherine the Great of the potential importance of the tuber to Russia, and her government launched a campaign to encourage its cultivation. However, the potato did not become a major crop in central Russia until after the crop failures of 1838 and 1839."[3]

Some writers may have exaggerated the importance of the potato in the economics of Europe, but considerable weight may be given to the remarks of Morineau, who noted that "…the potato, thanks in part to its very real advantages, became the only short-term solution (to increased food needs) everywhere in Western Europe. This it remained, despite some periods of blight, as long as new granaries had not opened in other parts of the world and until, in due course, agricultural science was able to produce much higher grain yields than the traditional agriculture."[4]

Negative consequences of the role of potatoes have been noted, particularly in the great potato famines in Ireland in the nineteenth century.

Ho and other scholars consider American cultigens to have been central to the growth of ecological carrying capacity in China. Ho suggests that by the end of the eighteenth century rice cultivation areas (the wetlands) and the dry region lands of millet and wheat had neared their limits of production, so that any further expansion of Chinese population would have been at the cost of increased nutritional deficiencies and periodic famine. However, the adoption of maize and sweet potatoes significantly increased the food supply.[5]

In presenting these observations concerning the worldwide diffusion of major cultigens, we do not need to subscribe to the theory that new foods caused population expansions in various regions of the world. In fact, it would appear that the causal arrows have often been in the opposite direction, in that population pressures have triggered the intensification of food production techniques. It is plausible that both types of situations have occurred repeatedly in different human populations: at times the fortuitous importation of new food crops or production methods has occurred before population expansion; in other circumstances the reverse has happened.[6]

Europe and Asia were not the only continents that experienced large-scale changes in food production as a result of contacts with new cultigens. Africa was an early recipient of new production ideas, in part because slave traders introduced maize and other crops to West Africa in order to provision their ships. Maize was introduced so early in some parts of Africa that some researchers have argued for its aboriginal development there.[7]

In the Americas the powerful influences of wheat, barley, and other Old World crops have been overshadowed by the effects of the massive infusion of meat animals. Before the coming of the Europeans, the natives of North and South America had only turkeys, dogs, llamas, chickens, and guinea pigs as sources of meat. The meat of pigs, cattle, sheep, and other food animals were quickly included in the diet of both the European settlers and the native inhabitants.

THE RISE OF COMMERCIAL FOOD DISTRIBUTION NETWORKS

A second major process in the delocalization of food occurs with the proliferation of commercial food distribution systems, which now affect virtually all societies. Food patterns in formerly remote communities are powerfully affected by the presence of commercially distributed food.

The growth of commercial food distribution networks has been intricately related to the development of food processing technologies. Food processing involves a wide spectrum of manipulation, from relatively simple preservation, such as canning and freezing, to the preparation of cooked, ready-to-eat meals and a variety of snack foods. The great expansion in commercial food processing has taken place in the twentieth century, although important developments occurred throughout the nineteenth century. French, British, and American inventors all contributed to the development of hermetically sealed canning processes in the 1830s and 1840s, followed by the processing of condensed milk and the mechanization of biscuit making.[8]

Prior to the nineteenth century the scope and scale of commercial operations in foodstuffs were limited. The larger and more important commercial houses dealt mainly in a few specialized items—coffee, sugar, spices, tea, salt, and alcoholic beverages. Some researchers have claimed that liquor and beer were practically the only foodstuffs for which production was responsive to demand before the latter half of the nineteenth century. However exaggerated such a statement, it does serve to highlight the importance of the commercial enterprises, and the more complex food marketing, that came into existence in the middle of the last century.[9]

SUGAR: THE COMMERCIAL FOOD PAR EXCELLENCE

Sugar is one processed food item that has played a major role in dietary transformations since the eighteenth century. The history of sugar documents the growing significance of commercial food marketing over the past 200 years. Like many other food products, cane sugar was known and used for centuries in some parts of the world before it rose to prominence in European trade. Gourmets of ancient India knew sugar, and there was some cultivation of sugar cane in Arab Spain and southern France in the eighth century. However, it was a rare and costly luxury until cane production was initiated in the New World.

The special conditions of the Americas, which combined favorable growing conditions, large acreages, and the importation of relatively low-cost (slave) labor, brought about rapid increases in production. During the eighteenth century it was still a costly commodity, but as production increased there was a fairly steady drop in price, and public demand for sugar rose rapidly. The use of by-products of the sugar cane process in the manufacture of rum contributed to the profitability of the sugar business. By the early years of the nineteenth century the average per capita consumption of sugar in the United States had risen to twelve or thirteen pounds per year. From that point the rise was relatively steady to 1929, when a peak of 109 pounds per capita per year was reached. During the

Great Depression sugar intake decreased but rose again with better economic times. Patterns of consumption in England were similar, with a peak in 1960 of 112 pounds per capita per year.[10]

MIGRATION: RURAL TO URBAN AND CROSS-NATIONAL POPULATION MOVEMENTS

The processes of change discussed thus far all refer to the transfer of ideas and materials—the food products themselves—from one area to another, accompanied by mechanisms of interdependency. The third mechanism is, superficially at least, different because the basic feature is the movement of persons. Migration to urban areas from rural regions, and movements from one nation or continent to another, introduce an additional dimension—food preferences and food knowledge are transferred by the migrants themselves. The migrants may exert their influence simply as individuals (or groups of individuals) with specific food preferences, but they also introduce change by actions, such as the establishment of food stores, restaurants, or other special enterprises.

Ethnic foods were introduced by migrants in earlier centuries and especially in America in the nineteenth century. There is a dual feature to the impact of migrant peoples on dietary practices: on the one hand, emigrés from distant places often preserved their traditional food patterns, so that, for example, Italian immigrants in major United States cities were soon able to maintain their consumption of pasta, sausages, olive oil, and other products in neighborhood cafes and restaurants, as well as in their homes; on the other hand these ethnic foods became available to non-Italians as well, and the growingly sophisticated urban-dwellers could select from a variety of different cuisines.

In most cases the old ethnic diets were not maintained in their traditional forms. Working hours—in factories, shops, and offices—soon made the old schedules (e.g. the large midday meal that is common in many European countries) difficult to continue. Even strongly held religious food patterns (e.g. among orthodox Jews) had to be modified to meet the new conditions.

One of the first ecumenical movements in ethnic food adoption was the spread of French cooking as a high prestige practice among upper-class and middle-class people around the world. Equally significant in influencing multi-cultural sophistication in food has been the spread of Chinese restaurants, which can be found in most major cities of the world today. Many of the international exchanges manifested in ethnic restaurants and grocery stores testify to the final phases of the colonial era, during which increasing numbers of families from "the colonies" established ethnic enclaves and food patterns in Europe: Indonesians in Holland, Indian restaurants and shops in England, and Moroccan and other North African coffee houses in France.

The latest phases of worldwide ecumenical sharing of cuisine (as opposed to dissemination of the raw materials)

has taken the form of an accelerated development of international cooking at home. Also, visible today throughout the world is the rapid spread of multi-national, fast-food chains.

MECHANISMS OF CHANGE AND CONSUMPTION TRENDS

The three main processes outlined above have been vehicles by which longstanding dietary patterns have been more and more radically altered in practically all parts of the world. The results of these changes are reflected in consumption statistics and nutrient profiles, which show, for example, continuing increases in the percentages of sugar consumed as diets become "modernized." In the United States the consumption of flour and cereal products dropped from 680 pounds per capita per year in 1910 to 450 pounds in 1970. During the same period vegetable fat consumption increased from 20 grams per capita per day to nearly 50 grams. Viewed in terms of nutrient consumption (rather than types of foods) in the period from 1910 to 1970 iron has declined from 15.2 mg. per capita per day to 8.0 mg. while riboflavin increased from 1.86 mg. to 2.46 mg.; another eight vitamins showed similar increases during that sixty-year span.[11]

It is difficult to find adequate statistical information on dietary changes in small-scale, non-modern societies because of the paucity of careful, quantitative studies. However, some of the main dimensions of change can be inferred from recent ethnographic studies. For example, in the Alaskan Eskimo community of Napaskiak, Oswalt noted that "everyone regards certain [store foods] as absolute necessities. These include sugar, salt, flour, milk, coffee, tea, tobacco, and cooking fats. Other foods frequently purchased include various canned meats and fish, crackers, candy, carbonated beverages, canned fruits, potatoes, onions, and rice." Similarly, among the Miskito Indians of Nicaragua, store-bought foods already accounted for over 30 percent of the diet in 1969, when Nietschmann made a detailed analysis of their food system. The store purchased foods, including sugar, flour, beans, rice, and coffee, had captured two thirds of the Miskito food economy by 1973, mainly because of the depletion of the green sea turtles, which are now sold to international food companies rather than consumed locally. Since the purchased foods are quite different in nutrient content from the wild foods that they replace and are especially high in carbohydrates, the Miskito, like virtually all small-scale societies, are undergoing rapid dietary change.[12]

The Eskimo and Miskito examples are particularly illustrative because they clearly reflect two different aspects of the worldwide commercial food system: in the Miskito situation commercial food distributors have taken away a primary food resource—the sea turtles—thus forcing the local people to change their food patterns. In the North Alaskan situation the emphasis is on the increased availability of modern foods in the local stores. Even in cases where local traditional food resources are not depleted, the availability of sugar, flour, canned goods, and other store food has a powerful effect on diets.

DELOCALIZATION AND THE FINNISH FOOD SYSTEM

Changes in food use brought about by delocalization are clearly revealed in Finland, which was transformed from an underdeveloped nation into an urban, industrialized society from the 1930s to 1970. Until 1940 the great majority of Finnish families were rural; the major cities, other than Helsinki, were little more than overgrown market centers. In 1950 the infant mortality rate was still 43 per 1,000; before the war it had been considerably higher. In other health and welfare statistics, as well as in its income and occupational profile, Finland contrasted sharply with the more industrialized nations of Europe and America.

The traditional Finnish dietary pattern was heavily dependent on dairy products. Finland still ranks as the leading nation in the world in per capita milk consumption, in addition to which Finns consume large amounts of butter, cheese, buttermilk, and viili, a fermented milk product, which is somewhat akin to yogurt.

Grain products made up another major portion of the diet. Rye, oats, and barley had been the most important cereals in earlier centuries, with increasing amounts of wheat in the nineteenth and twentieth centuries. Potatoes were eaten practically every day in considerable quantity, a pattern that continues today for most of the population. Meat, and to a lesser extent fish, although consumed in modest quantities, have been important sources of protein.[13]

In the pre-World War II Finnish diet a major source of vitamin C was the wild lingonberry (and other berries), gathered in large quantities and stored for use throughout the winter. Also characteristic was a lack of green vegetables and fresh fruit, other than berries. Throughout the 1950s the supplies of imported fresh fruit in Finnish grocery stores was irregular.

During the 1960s the commercial food system changed drastically, as large supermarkets were established by several cooperative associations and by private entrepreneurs. Frozen foods, food freezers in stores and in homes, and many other technological features were introduced. A rapid expansion of the network of paved roads also contributed to these developments. At the same time, Finnish nutritionists and government policy-makers mounted extensive informational campaigns to increase the consumption of vegetables and fruit and decrease the intake of saturated fats and sugar. The nutrition information programs were fueled, in part, by the realization that Finland had, until very recently, the highest rates of cardiovascular disease in the world.[14]

Food consumption trends from 1950 to 1973 show the interesting changes that have occurred during the recent decades of delocalization (see Table 1). These changes reflect delocalization both within the Finnish economy, and in relation to worldwide markets. Much of the increase in fruit and vegetables represents greatly expanded imports from

Table 1 Consumption Trends in Finland, 1950–1973 (annual per capita consumption)

Item	Year					
	1950	1955	1960	1965	1970	1973
Wheat (ks)	81.5	86	75	70	65	60
Meat	60	60	60	60	60	60
Sugar (ks)	28.3	38	40	40	45	45
Rye	48	42	39	32	25	24
Butter/margarine	22	22	22	22	22	22
Fruit/vegetables	33	48	53	52	65	81

SOURCE: *Elinolosuhteet 1950–1975* [Living Conditions 1950–1975], Central Statistical Office of Finland, 86.

Eastern Europe and the Mediterranean countries, made possible by the expansion of the modern European trucking network equipped with refrigeration, air conditioning, and other technological features. Meanwhile producers in Finland have begun to use artificially heated greenhouses (relying on new developments in plastic sheeting) to grow cucumbers and tomatoes, which are now in great demand since the introduction of salads into the Finnish diet.

From 1940 to 1970 Finnish farm families gave up most aspects of their earlier self-sufficiency in basic foods. In short, they changed from being peasants to being commercial farmers. The highly developed system of producers' cooperatives played a major part in these changes, augmented by the growth of private food-producing companies. Meat animals, milk, and cereal grains are now delivered directly to the cooperatives or to private buyers. In turn, the farmers buy back selected meat products at a members' discount. Certain parts of slaughtered animals (including the blood), that were routinely used in the family food economy, are now unavailable or must be purchased in processed form from the cooperatives. Blood pancakes and bloodbread, for example, are now generally made from packaged mixes. Even butter and cheese are usually purchased from the cooperatives to which the farmers sell their raw milk, unlike the pre-war days, when families prepared a large share of their own basic foods, from barn and field to the dinner table.

The changes in utilization of home-produced food in Finnish farming households represents delocalization at the local, or micro-level. Thus delocalization refers not only to the increased availability of foods from distant lands; it also means the giving up of local community control to the regional and national food-processing systems.

Although the impact of delocalization in terms of making new foods available was more dramatic in Finland than in some other Western European countries, the general process has been much the same throughout the industrialized world. The example of Finland is instructive because the major changes have occurred largely in the past fifty years, nearly a century later than in most parts of Western Europe. There have been major differences in some aspects of delocalization, as the pattern of land tenure, differences in

international trading networks, and political processes have all strongly affected the course of developments in food distribution and dietary patterns.

DELOCALIZATION IN THE THIRD WORLD

A major feature of food delocalization in the nineteenth and twentieth centuries has been the transformation of food systems in non-industrialized areas as they have become involved in supplying some of the food needs of Euro-American communities. Sugar plantations were among the first manifestations of a rapidly developing commerce in food products. A large-scale banana trade developed later, mainly in the twentieth century. Shipments of bananas, like many other fruits and vegetables, could not become major world trade commodities until the development of effective storage technologies, in addition to faster shipping times.

In countries such as Jamaica the economic livelihood of many small farmers became tied to the fluctuations in world prices of bananas (or other cash crops), as well as to government policies of encouragement or discouragement of farm production. Jamaica is highly delocalized in terms of food resources, as most of the daily diet depends on imports from North America and other sources. The significance of delocalization for the Jamaican (as an example of the effects of modernization in Third World countries) is illustrated by events in the 1970s. As analyzed in a study by Marchione in the mid-1970s, the cost of food in Jamaica (not adjusted to take account of inflation) soared as a result of the oil crisis and other factors in international markets. In the period from 1973 to 1975 the retail price of wheat flour increased 142 percent, corn meal 100 percent, salt cod 75 percent, rice 65 percent, and sugar 60 percent. Banana prices, however, paid to local, mostly small-scale producers, did not rise.[15]

Marchione studied the impact of a nutrition program in the St. James area of Jamaica during this period and found that world market forces resulted in a return to subsistence crop-growing by many farmers. The expected negative effects of highly inflationary food prices appear to have been offset by increases in home-grown foods. Instead of declining, the nutritional status of small children in the St. James area improved during this period. The research design of the evaluation study made it possible to determine that it was mainly the farmers' food production responses to market conditions, rather than the local nutrition education program, that brought about improved nutritional status in the children.

It is also important, Marchione suggests, to note that during this period the climate of commerce in food was affected by the Jamaican government's policy of striving for greater national self-sufficiency. "Jamaican government policies to ban food exports, levy taxes on foreign-owned bauxite companies, create public service jobs and redistribute or force idle land into production represent concerted efforts to gain local control of energy forms and flows; i.e. power."[16]

Another striking example of the negative consequences of delocalization is the widespread adoption of beef cattle production in many parts of Latin America in response to the growth of hamburger and other fast-food merchandizing in the United States. In Guatemala, beef production nearly doubled from 1960 to 1972, yet domestic per capita consumption of beef fell by approximately 20 percent during the same period. In Costa Rica during the same period total production of beef rose from 53.3 to 108 million pounds, yet the amount available for domestic consumption remained constant (34.8 million pounds), resulting in a reduction of nearly one third in beef consumption while exports climbed from 17.5 to 73.7 millions of pounds.[17]

Analyzing the impact of this large-scale shift to beef production, DeWalt found that large areas of forest in Honduras were being cut down to make room for cattle. From 1952 to 1974 the forested area in southern Honduras was reduced from approximately 74,000 to only 41,000 hectares. During the same period the land area in permanent crops actually declined. DeWalt comments that the "implications of the conversion of southern Honduras into a vast pasture for export-oriented cattle production...are the following: first in the long run fewer individuals will have access to land on which to produce their own subsistence crops. Employment opportunities in the local region will decline because livestock raising is less labor intensive than grain crop production. The permanent and temporary migration that these processes produce can only exacerbate the already explosive social, economic, and political situation that exists in Central America."[18]

These cases are intended to illustrate how world-wide delocalization of food production and distribution has created a complex web of interrelations, changes which place local food-producing populations in serious jeopardy, particularly if they are dependent for their livelihood on one or two principal cash crops. In the developing world, delocalization results in a loss of food resources and flexibility as productive agricultural land is put to use for cash crops in competition with land use for local food production, and national food systems become increasingly dependent on the developed nations for shipments of grain and other basic foods.

DIETARY DIVERSITY, NUTRITIONAL STATUS, AND DELOCALIZATION

Good nutrition depends on adequate consumption of calories, protein, fats, vitamins and minerals. Whereas a sufficient intake of calories (and, to some extent, protein and fat) depends on quantity of food consumed, adequate consumption of other nutrients depends on the utilization of foods that are high in these substances. Because vitamins and minerals are differentially distributed in food, it is generally felt that more varied and diverse diets are more likely to be adequate from a nutritional perspective. A "mixed portfolio" also seems advisable on ecological grounds and may provide some protection from overexposure to mildly toxic components of foods.

When delocalization results in an expanded food supply and greater diversity of available foods, one would hypothesize that there should be an improvement in nutritional status, whereas a reduction in diversity, as well as in the quantity of available foods should be associated with a decline in nutritional status. In the industrialized world, it appears that there have generally been significant improvements in nutrition in the past century. There are several lines of evidence to support this statement. The major vitamin-deficiency diseases have now virtually disappeared in developed countries and, although mineral-deficiency diseases are still prevalent, they tend to be much less severely manifested than in developing countries. Except for anorexia nervosa, obesity rather than emaciation is the primary problem of caloric consumption.

Another indicator of improved nutrition is the secular growth trend that makes modern Europeans and North Americans seem like giants compared to the average size of people in the seventeenth and eighteenth centuries. In 1876 Charles Roberts, a doctor employed in a British factory, noted that "a factory child of the present day at the age of nine years weighs as much as one of ten years did in 1833...each age has gained one year in forty." This comparison was possible because a large-scale program of measurements of children was carried out in 1833 to provide evidence for Parliament to consider the effects of child labor. "At that time, working boys aged ten years averaged 121 cm. in height compared with 140 cm. today; those aged eighteen years averaged 160 cm. compared with 175 cm. today." The recent trends in Japan from 1950 to 1970 show a nearly 3 cm. increase per decade among seven year olds, and a 5 cm. per decade increase in twelve year olds. Other factors, including improved sanitary conditions, have also played a part in these trends, but the role of nutrition seems clear.[19]

Although the secular trends in industrialized countries point to a general improvement in nutrition, it is important to note the complexities that are involved in the interpretation of data on height. The issues are ably discussed by Fogel and his colleagues, who point out the significance of "cycles of height" in the past two centuries in British and American populations. Fogel argues that these fluctuations reflect different levels of nutrition and this supports Tanner's and others' interpretation of the meaning of secular trends in height.[20]

Age at menarche is another measure frequently cited in connection with the overall improved nutrition levels of Europeans, North Americans, and other industrialized populations. Tanner has demonstrated that the average age at menarche for girls in Finland, Norway, and Sweden was between sixteen and seventeen years in the middle of the nineteenth century, from which there has been a progressive decline to the present day. Now, the averages hover around thirteen years.

Increased caloric and protein intakes throughout the nineteenth and twentieth centuries have had major impacts, but the increased diversity of available foods has also played a role. In Britain from 1950 to 1973 total fruit as a component of household consumption increased from 18 ounces to 25 ounces per week per person, while in the same period bread dropped from 56 ounces to 34 ounces. Diversification of protein resources was evident in the rise in poultry consumption.[21]

DELOCALIZATION AND FAMINE

One of the more obvious, yet infrequently noted, results of the delocalization of food products in the industrialized world is the elimination, except during wartime, of disastrous famines. Food catastrophes, such as the Irish potato famine, or the less well-known famine between 1865 and 1867 in northeastern Europe, are no longer a threat in developed nations. Recent Soviet grain purchases and shipments of food to Poland show how modern commercial channels can redistribute food in times of serious regional shortages.

In most of the world the channels of food distribution can be expanded in response to regional shortages, although serious distribution problems still remain. Recent crises in Bangladesh, India, and parts of Africa demonstrate that in extreme situations appropriate foods cannot be transported and distributed effectively enough to the populations in need.[22]

McAlpin notes that population growth rates fluctuated widely in India well into the twentieth century because of the interrelated effects of periodic famine and disease. She points out that the development of an effective railroad network helped reduce the sharp impact of regional food shortages.[23]

Famines still occur in isolated parts of India, as they do in some other parts of Asia, but McAlpin's data indicate that "mortality from famines was not an important force in slowing India's population growth after 1921." Thus, the forces of delocalization—the spread of transportation systems and food distribution networks, plus governmental communications and food relief systems—have effectively eliminated most (but not all) of the impacts of regional crop failures and other disasters that in the past led to severe periodic famine conditions.

DEVELOPING NATIONS: SHORTAGES AND DISTORTIONS

Many of the changes that we have described for the industrialized nations have also affected parts of the Third World. The spread of diverse food resources by means of the New World-Old World exchange of cultigens and livestock has had a powerful impact on most of the world. Thus, potentially, the populations of Latin America, much of Asia, and many parts of Africa could have a greatly expanded diversity of foods. Despite that potential, the lack of economic purchasing power for all but a minority in the most affluent sectors means that the diets of the majority are restricted in quantity and quality.

Inequality of wealth is not the only factor that has contributed to the declines in quality and quantity of food in rural sectors of developing nations. Modern farming practices, including the widespread use of chemicals—pesticides and herbicides—may have unexpected, often unnoticed, side-effects on food use. For example, the widespread use of herbicides in the maize fields of Mexico has resulted in the elimination of a number of "weeds" that had been regular, vitamin-rich additions to the peasant diets.[24]

Global delocalization of food resources involves a number of major cost increases. A large part of the price of food items pays for the processing, packaging, advertising, and shipment of foods, as well as the profits of various entrepreneurs in the food chain. Poor people cannot afford to pay these added costs, and hence they are reduced to a narrower selection of the cheaper foods.

Although there continues to be some argument about "how to define" malnutrition, there is little disagreement that for sheer numbers, there are more millions of malnourished people in the world than ever before. The most telling and shocking statistic is the effect of malnutrition on child mortality. Berg estimates that in 1978 "malnutrition was a factor in the deaths of at least 10 million children."[25]

A discussion of all the complex factors involved in contemporary problems of malnutrition is beyond the scope of this article, but we suggest that the poorer populations in developing countries, especially in rural areas, have experienced declines in total caloric consumption (per capita) and in dietary diversity as traditional subsistence systems have been severely disrupted by the forces of modernization, especially delocalization.

Delocalization captures some of the main dimensions of change in food production and diet over the past 250 years. Historically, the process appears to be unidirectional, as most regions of the world give up local autonomy to increased linkages with global food distribution networks. The example of Jamaica, however, is only one of many national policy attempts to counter delocalization through political encouragement of self-sufficiency. Although the process of delocalization is so complex as to appear to be outside the range of local political decision-making, it may not be an inevitable aspect of development.

In examining the relationship between delocalization and changes in nutrition and health status, we are not claiming that the process has been wholly positive in the industrialized countries and completely negative in the Third World. Increased obesity, problems of food sensitivities, and other, more subtle nutrition-related problems may well be related to delocalization of food patterns in the industrialized countries. At the same time, traditional food systems in developing countries are often far from ideal from a nutritional standpoint, and, in many circumstances, environmental factors severely constrain local food production.

There have been massive changes in local food systems over the past 250 years as the world community has become knit into a tightly inter-connected network of economic, social, and political relations. The effects on nutrition and dietary patterns have been powerful. World-wide food production capabilities have increased greatly. However, serious problems of maldistribution of food resources remain, and some problems are becoming worse, not better. Although a considerable proportion of the global community derives clear benefit from food delocalization, many rural and urban low-income communities are experiencing serious malnutrition.

Further analysis of delocalization of food may help to explicate historical conditions. At the same time, improved understanding of the relationship between delocalization and nutritional status may help to make nutrition planning and policy development more effective in the future.

References

1. Cf. Alan Berg, *The Nutrition Factor* (Washington, D.C., 1973); Frances Moore Lappé and Joseph Collins, *Food First* (Boston, 1977).

2. Christian Vanderbroek. "Aardappelteelt en Aardappelverbruik in de 17e en 18e Eeuw," *Tijdschrift voor Geschiedenis*, LXXXII (1969), 49–68.

3. Alfred W Crosby, Jr., *The Columbian Exchange* (Westport, Conn., 1972). 184.

4. Michel Morineau, "The Potato in the Eighteenth Century," in Robert Forster and Orest Ranum (eds.), *Food and Drink in History* (Baltimore, 1979), 17–36.

5. Ping-ti Ho, *Studies on the Population of China, 1368–1953* (Cambridge, Mass., 1959). Crosby, *Columbian Exchange*, 199–200.

6. Ester Boserup, *The Conditions of Agricultural Growth* (Chicago, 1965). William T. Sanders, "Population, Agricultural History, and Societal Evolution in Mesoamerica," in Brian Spooner (ed.), *Population Growth: Anthropological Implications* (Cambridge, Mass., 1972), 101–153.

7. Carl O. Sauer, *Seeds, Spades, Hearths, and Herbs* (Cambridge, Mass., 1952). Cf. Michael D. Gwynne, "The Origin and Spread of Some Domestic Food Plants of Eastern Africa," in H. Neville Chittick and Robert I. Rotberg (eds.), *East Africa and the Orient: Cultural Synthesis in Pre-Colonial Times* (New York, 1975), 248–271.

8. Waverly Root and Richard de Rochemont, *Eating in America* (New York, 1976), 158; James P. Johnston, *A Hundred Years of Eating: Food, Drink, and Family Diet in Britain Since the Late Nineteenth Century* (Montreal, 1977), 33.

9. Maurice Aymard, "Toward the History of Nutrition," in Forster and Ranum. *Food and Drink*, 1–16.

10. Root and Rochement, *Eating in America*, 418; Richard O. Cummings. *The American and His Food* (Chicago, 1940); Chris Wardle, *Changing Food Habits in the U.K.* (London, 1977).

11. United States Dept. of Agriculture, Report No. 138 (Washington, D.C. (1974); Willis A. Gortner, "Nutrition in the United States-1900 to 1974." *Cancer Research*, XXXV (1975), 3246–3253.

12. Wendell Oswalt, *Napaskiak: An Alaskan Eskimo Community* (Tucson, 1963), 102; Bernard Nietschmann, *Between Land and Water* (New York, 1973).

13. I. Talve, *Suommen Kansanomaisesta Ruokataloudesta* (Turku, 1973).

14. Ancel Keys, *Seven Countries: A Multivariate Analysis of Death and Coronary Heart Disease Rates* (Cambridge, Mass., 1980).

15. Thomas J. Marchione, "Food and Nutrition in Self-Reliant National Development," *Medical Anthropology*, I (1977), 57–79.

16. *Ibid.*, 73.

17. Billie R. DeWalt, "The Cattle are Eating the Forest," unpub. ms. (1981).

18. *Ibid.*, 24–25.

19. J. M. Tanner, *Foetus into Man* (Cambridge, Mass., 1978), 150–151.

20. Robert W. Fogel et al., "Secular Changes in American and British Stature and Nutrition," in this issue.

21. Wardle, *Changing Food Habits*, 72.

22. For a discussion of entitlements, see Louise A. Tilly. "Food Entitlement, Famine, and Conflict."

23. Michelle B. McAlpin, "Famines, Epidemics, and Population Growth: The Case of India," in this issue.

24. Ellen Messer, "The Ecology of Vegetarian Diet in a Modernizing Mexican Community," in Thomas K. Fitzgerald (ed.), *Nutrition and Anthropology in Action* (Amsterdam, 1977), 117–124.

25. Berg, *Malnourished People: A Policy View* (Washington, D.C., 1981), 2.

CHAPTER 39

When the Turtle Collapses, the World Ends

Bernard Nietschmann

(1974)

After delivering a lecture on the solar system, philosopher-psychologist William James was approached by an elderly lady who claimed she had a theory superior to the one described by him.

"We don't live on a ball rotating around the sun," she said. "We live on a crust of earth on the back of a giant turtle."

Not wishing to demolish this absurd argument with the massive scientific evidence at his command, James decided to dissuade his opponent gently.

"If your theory is correct, madam, what does this turtle stand on?"

"You're a very clever man, Mr. James, and that's a good question, but I can answer that. The first turtle stands on the back of a second, far larger, turtle."

"But what does this second turtle stand on?" James asked patiently.

The old lady crowed triumphantly, "It's no use, Mr. James—it's turtles all the way down."

In the half-light of dawn, a sailing canoe approaches a shoal where nets have been set the day before. A Miskito turtle-man stands in the bow and points to a distant splash that breaks the gray sheen of the Caribbean waters. Even from a hundred yards, he can tell that a green turtle has been caught in one of the nets. His two companions quickly bring the craft alongside the turtle, and as they pull it from the sea, its glistening shell reflects the first rays of the rising sun. As two men work to remove the heavy reptile from the net, the third keeps the canoe headed into the swells and beside the anchored net. After its fins have been pierced and lashed with bark fiber cord, the 250-pound turtle is placed on its back in the bottom of the canoe. The turtlemen are happy. Perhaps their luck will be good today and their other nets will also yield many turtles.

These green turtles, caught by Miskito Indian turtle-men off the eastern coast of Nicaragua, are destined for distant markets. Their butchered bodies will pass through many hands, local and foreign, eventually ending up in tins, bottles, and freezers far away. Their meat, leather, shell, oil, and calipee, a gelatinous substance that is the base for turtle soup, will be used to produce goods consumed in more affluent parts of the world.

The coastal Miskito Indians are very dependent on green turtles. Their culture has long been adapted to utilizing the once vast populations that inhabited the largest sea turtle feeding grounds in the Western Hemisphere. As the most important link between livelihood, social interaction, and environment, green turtles were the pivotal resource around which traditional Miskito Indian society revolved. These large reptiles also provided the major source of protein for Miskito subsistence. Now this priceless and limited resource has become a prized commodity that is being exploited almost entirely for economic reasons.

In the past, turtles fulfilled the nutritional needs as well as the social responsibilities of Miskito society. Today, however, the Miskito depend mainly on the sale of turtles to provide them with the money they need to purchase household goods and other necessities. But turtles are a declining resource; overdependence on them is leading the Miskito into an ecological blind alley. The cultural control mechanisms that once adapted the Miskito to their environment and faunal resources are now circumvented or inoperative, and they are caught up in a system of continued intensification of turtle fishing, which threatens to provide neither cash nor subsistence.

I have been studying this situation for several years, unraveling its historical context and piecing together its past and future effect on Miskito society, economy, and diet, and on the turtle population.

The coastal Miskito Indians are among the world's most adept small-craft seamen and turtlemen. Their traditional subsistence system provided dependable yields from the judicious scheduling of resource procurement activities. Agriculture, hunting, fishing, and gathering were organized

Bernard Nietschmann, "When the turtle collapses, the world ends." *Natural History*, June/July 1974:34–42. Reprinted with permission.

in accordance with seasonal fluctuations in weather and resource availability and provided adequate amounts of food and materials—without overexploiting any one species or site. Women cultivated the crops while men hunted and fished. Turtle fishing was the backbone of subsistence, providing meat throughout the year.

Miskito society and economy were interdependent. There was no economic activity without a social context and every social act had a reciprocal economic aspect. To the Miskito, meat, especially turtle meat, was the most esteemed and valuable resource, for it was not only a mainstay of subsistence, it was the item most commonly distributed to relatives and friends. Meat shared in this way satisfied mutual obligations and responsibilities and smoothed out daily and seasonal differences in the acquisition of animal protein. In this way, those too young, old, sick, or otherwise unable to secure meat received their share, and a certain balance in the village was achieved: minimal food requirements were met, meat surplus was disposed of to others, and social responsibilities were satisfied.

Today, the older Miskito recall that when meat was scarce in the village, a few turtlemen would put out to sea in their dugout canoes for a day's harpooning on the turtle feeding grounds. In the afternoon, the men would return, sailing before the northeast trade wind, bringing meat for all. Gathered on the beach, the villagers helped drag the canoes into thatched storage sheds. After the turtles were butchered and the meat distributed, everyone returned home to the cooking fires.

Historical circumstances and a series of boom—bust economic cycles disrupted the Miskito's society and environment. In the seventeenth and eighteenth centuries, intermittent trade with English and French buccaneers—based on the exchange of forest and marine resources for metal tools and utensils, rum, and firearms—prompted the Miskito to extend hunting, fishing, and gathering beyond subsistence needs to exploitative enterprises.

During the nineteenth and early twentieth centuries, foreign-owned companies operating in eastern Nicaragua exported rubber, lumber, and gold, and initiated commercial banana production. As alien economic and ecological influences were intensified, contract wage labor replaced seasonal, short-term economic relationships; company commissaries replaced limited trade goods; and large-scale exploitation of natural resources replaced sporadic, selective extraction. During economic boom periods the relationship between resources, subsistence, and environment was drastically altered for the Miskito. Resources became a commodity with a price tag, market exploitation a livelihood, and foreign wages and goods a necessity.

For more than 200 years, relations between the coastal Miskito and the English were based on sea turtles. It was from the Miskito that the English learned the art of turtling, which they then organized into intensive commercial exploitation of Caribbean turtle grounds and nesting beaches. Sea turtles were among the first resources involved in trade relations and foreign commerce in the Caribbean. Zoologist

Archie Carr, an authority on sea turtles, has remarked that "more than any other dietary factor, the green turtle supported the opening up of the Caribbean." The once abundant turtle populations provided sustenance to ships' crews and to the new settlers and plantation laborers.

The Cayman Islands, settled by the English, became in the seventeenth and eighteenth centuries the center of commercial turtle fishing in the Caribbean. By the early nineteenth century, pressure on the Cayman turtle grounds and nesting beaches to supply meat to Caribbean and European markets became so great that the turtle population was decimated. The Cayman Islanders were forced to shift to other turtle areas off Cuba, the Gulf of Honduras, and the coast of eastern Nicaragua. They made annual expeditions, lasting four to seven weeks, to the Miskito turtle grounds to net green turtles, occasionally purchasing live ones, dried calipee, and the shells of hawksbill turtles (*Eretmochelys imbricata*) from the Miskito Indians. Reported catches of green turtles by the Cayman turtlers generally ranged between 2,000 and 3,000 a year up to the early 1960s, when the Nicaraguan government failed to renew the islanders' fishing privileges.

Intensive resource extraction by foreign companies led to seriously depleted and altered environments. By the 1940s, many of the economic booms had turned to busts. As the resources ran out and operating costs mounted, companies shut down production and moved to other areas in Central America. Thus, the economic mainstays that had helped provide the Miskito with jobs, currency, markets, and foreign goods were gone. The company supply ships and commissaries disappeared, money became scarce, and store-bought items expensive.

In the backwater of the passing golden boom period, the Miskito were left with an ethic of poverty, but they still had the subsistence skills that had maintained their culture for hundreds of years. Their land and water environment was still capable of providing reliable resources for local consumption. As it had been in the past, turtle fishing became a way of life, a provider of life itself. But traditional subsistence culture could no longer integrate Miskito society and

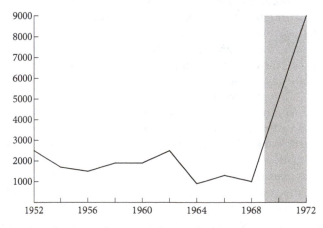

Number of green turtles exported annually from eastern Nicaragua.

environment in a state of equilibrium. Resources were now viewed as having a value and labor a price tag. All that was needed was a market.

Recently, two foreign turtle companies began operations along the east coast of Nicaragua. One was built in Puerto Cabezas in late 1968, and another was completed in Bluefields in 1969. Both companies were capable of processing and shipping large amounts of green turtle meat and by-products to markets in North America and Europe. Turtles were acquired by purchase from the Miskito. Each week company boats visited coastal Miskito communities and offshore island turtle camps to buy green turtles. The "company" was back, money was again available, and the Miskito were expert in securing the desired commodity. Another economic boom period was at hand. But the significant difference between this boom and previous ones was that the Miskito were now selling a subsistence resource.

As a result, the last large surviving green turtle population in the Caribbean was opened to intensive, almost year-round exploitation. Paradoxically, it would be the Miskito Indians, who once caught only what they needed for food, who would conduct the assault on the remaining turtle population.

Another contradictory element in the Miskito—turtle story is that only some 200 miles to the south at Tortuguero, Costa Rica, Archie Carr had devoted fifteen years to the study of sea turtles and to the conservation and protection of the Caribbean's last major sea turtle nesting beach. Carr estimates that more than half the green turtles that nest at Tortuguero are from Nicaraguan waters. The sad and exasperating paradox is that a conservation program insured the survival of an endangered species for commercial exploitation in nearby waters.

Green turtles, *Chelonia mydas*, are large, air-breathing, herbivorous marine reptiles. They congregate in large populations and graze on underwater beds of vegetation in relatively clear, shallow, tropical waters. A mature turtle can weigh 250 pounds or more and when caught, can live indefinitely in a saltwater enclosure or for a couple of weeks if kept in shade on land. Green turtles have at least six behavioral characteristics that are important in their exploitation: they occur in large numbers in localized areas; they are air breathing, so they have to surface; they are mass social nesters; they have an acute location-finding ability; when mature, they migrate seasonally on an overlapping two- or three-year cycle for mating and nesting; and they exhibit predictable local distributional patterns.

The extensive shallow shelf off eastern Nicaragua is dotted with numerous small coral islands, thousands of reefs, and vast underwater pastures of marine vegetation called "turtle banks." During the day, a large group of turtles may be found feeding at one of the many turtle banks, while adjacent marine pastures may have only a few turtles. They graze on the vegetation, rising periodically to the surface for air and to float for awhile before diving again. In the late afternoon, groups of turtles will leave the feeding areas and swim to shoals, some up to four or five miles away, to spend the night. By five the next morning, they gather to depart again for the banks. The turtles' precise, commuterlike behavior between sleeping and feeding areas is well known to the Miskito and helps insure good turtling.

Each coastal turtling village exploits an immense sea area, containing many turtle banks and shoals. For example, the Miskito of Tasbapauni utilize a marine area of approximately 600 square miles, with twenty major turtle banks and almost forty important shoals.

Having rather predictable patterns of movement and habitat preference, green turtles are commonly caught by the Miskito in three ways: on the turtle banks with harpoons; along the shoal-to-feeding area route with harpoons; and on the shoals using nets, which entangle the turtles when they surface for air.

The Miskito's traditional means of taking turtles was by harpoon—an eight- to ten-foot shaft fitted with a detachable short point tied to a strong line. The simple technology pitted two turtlemen in a small, seagoing canoe against the elusive turtles. Successful turtling with harpoons requires an extensive knowledge of turtle behavior and habits and tremendous skill and experience in handling a small canoe in what can be very rough seas. Turtlemen work in partnerships: a "strikerman" in the bow; the "captain" in the stern. Together, they make a single unit engaged in the delicate and almost silent pursuit of a wary prey, their movements coordinated by experience and rewarded by proficiency. Turtlemen have mental maps of all the banks and shoals in their area, each one named and located through a complex system of celestial navigation, distance reckoning, wind and current direction, and the individual surface-swell motion over each site. Traditionally, not all Miskito were sufficiently expert in seamanship and turtle lore to become respected "strikermen," capable of securing turtles even during hazardous sea conditions. Theirs was a very specialized calling. Harpooning restrained possible over-exploitation since turtles were taken one at a time by two men directly involved in the chase, and there were only a limited number of really proficient "strikermen" in each village.

Those who still use harpoons must leave early to take advantage of the land breeze and to have enough time to reach the distant offshore turtle grounds by first light. Turtlemen who are going for the day, or for several days, will meet on the beach by 2:00 A.M. They drag the canoes on bamboo rollers from beachfront sheds to the water's edge. There, in the swash of spent breakers, food, water, paddles, lines, harpoons, and sails are loaded and secured. Using a long pole, the standing bowman propels the canoe through the foaming surf while the captain in the stern keeps the craft running straight with a six-foot mahogany paddle. Once past the inside break, the men count the dark rolling seas building outside until there is a momentary pause in the sets; then with paddles digging deep, they drive the narrow, twenty-foot canoe over the cresting swells, rising precipitously on each wave face and then plunging down the far side as the sea and sky seesaw into view. Once past the breakers, they rig the sail and, running with the land breeze, point the canoe toward a star in the eastern sky.

A course is set by star fix and by backsight on a prominent coconut palm on the mainland horizon. Course alterations are made to correct for the direction and intensity of winds and currents. After two or three hours of sailing the men reach a distant spot located between a turtle sleeping shoal and feeding bank. There they intercept and follow the turtles as they leave for specific banks.

On the banks the turtlemen paddle quietly, listening for the sound of a "blowing" turtle. When a turtle surfaces for air it emits a hissing sound audible for fifty yards or more on a calm day. Since a turtle will stay near the surface for only a minute or two before diving to feed, the men must approach quickly and silently, maneuvering the canoe directly in front of or behind the turtle. These are its blind spots. Once harpooned, a turtle explodes into a frenzy of action, pulling the canoe along at high speeds in its hopeless, underwater dash for escape until it tires and can be pulled alongside the canoe.

But turtle harpooning is a dying art. The dominant method of turtling today is the use of nets. Since their introduction, the widespread use of turtle nets has drastically altered turtling strategy and productivity. Originally brought to the Miskito by the Cayman Islanders, nets are now extensively distributed on credit by the turtle companies. This simple technological change, along with a market demand for turtles, has resulted in intensified pressure on green turtle populations.

Buoyed by wooden floats and anchored to the bottom by a single line, the fifty-foot-long by fourteen-foot-wide nets hang from the surface like underwater flags, shifting direction with the current. Nets are set in place during midday when the turtlemen can see the dark shoal areas. Two Miskito will set five to thirty nets from one canoe, often completely saturating a small shoal. In the late afternoon, green turtles return to their shoals to spend the night. There they will sleep beside or beneath a coral outcrop, periodically surfacing for air where a canopy of nets awaits them.

Catching turtles with nets requires little skill; anyone with a canoe can now be a turtleman. The Miskito set thousands of nets daily, providing continuous coverage in densely populated nocturnal habitats. Younger Miskito can become turtlemen almost overnight simply by following more experienced men to the shoal areas, thus circumventing the need for years of accumulated skill and knowledge that once were the domain of the "strikermen." All one has to do is learn where to set the nets, retire for the night, remove the entangled turtles the next morning, and reset the nets. The outcome is predictable: more turtlemen, using more effective methods, catch more turtles.

With an assured market for turtles, the Miskito devote more time to catching turtles, traveling farther and staying at sea longer. Increased dependence on turtles as a source of income and greater time inputs have meant disruption of subsistence agriculture and hunting and fishing. The Miskito no longer produce foodstuffs for themselves; they buy imported foods with money gained from the sale of turtles. Caught between contradictory priorities—their traditional subsistence system and the market economy—the Miskito are opting for cash.

The Miskito are now enveloped in a positive feedback system where change spawns change. Coastal villages rely on turtles for a livelihood. Decline of subsistence provisioning has led to the need to secure food from local shopkeepers on credit to feed the families in the villages and the men during their turtling expeditions. Initial high catches of turtles encouraged more Miskito to participate, and by 1972 the per person and per day catch began to decline noticeably.

In late 1972, several months after I had returned to Michigan, I received a letter from an old turtleman, who wrote: "Turtle is getting scarce, Mr. Barney. You said it would happen in five or ten years but it is happening now."

Burdened by an overdependence on an endangered species and with accumulating debts for food and nets, the Miskito are finding it increasingly difficult to break even, much less secure a profit. With few other economic alternatives, the inevitable step is to use more nets and stay out at sea longer.

The turtle companies encourage the Miskito to expand turtling activities by providing them with building materials so that they can construct houses on offshore cays, thereby eliminating the need to return to the mainland during rough weather. On their weekly runs up and down the coast, company boats bring food, turtle gear, and cash for turtles to fishing camps from the Miskito Cays to the Set Net Cays. Frequent visits keep the Miskito from becoming discouraged and returning to their villages with the turtles. On Saturdays, villagers look to sea, watching for returning canoes. A few men will bring turtle for their families; the majority will bring only money. Many return with neither.

Most Miskito prefer to be home on Sunday to visit with friends and for religious reasons. (There are Moravian, Anglican, and Catholic mission churches in many of the villages.) But more and more, turtlemen are staying out for two to four weeks. The church may promise salvation, but only the turtle companies can provide money.

Returning to their villages, turtlemen are confronted with a complex dilemma: how to satisfy both social and economic demands with a limited resource. Traditional

Table 1 Distribution of Turtle Meat by Gift and Purchase

Percent of Villagers*	Pounds Received per Person
18	10–14+
28	6–9
32	2–5
22	0–1.9

During the one-month period from April 15 to May 15, 1971, 125 green turtles were caught by the turtlemen of Tasbapauni, Nicaragua. Of these, 91 were sold to turtle companies; the remaining 34 were butchered and the meat sold or given to villagers. In all, 3,900 pounds of turtle meat were distributed, but 54 percent of the villagers received 5 pounds or less, an insufficient amount for adult dietary protein requirements.

*Population of 998 converted to 711 adult male equivalents.

Miskito social rules stipulate that turtle meat should be shared among kin, but the new economic system requires that turtles be sold for personal economic gain. Kin expect gifts of meat, and friends expect to be sold meat. Turtlemen are besieged with requests forcing them to decide between who will or will not receive meat. This is contrary to the traditional Miskito ethic, which is based on generosity and mutual concern for the well-being of others. The older Miskito ask why the turtlemen should have to allocate a food that was once abundant and available to all. Turtlemen sell and give to other turtlemen, thereby insuring reciprocal treatment for themselves, but there simply are not enough turtles to accommodate other economic and social requirements. In order to have enough turtles to sell, fewer are butchered in the villages. This means that less meat is being consumed than before the turtle companies began operations. The Miskito presently sell 70 to 90 percent of the turtles they catch; in the near future they will sell even more and eat less.

Social tension and friction are growing in the villages. Kinship relationships are being strained by what some villagers interpret as preferential and stingy meat distribution. Rather than endure the trauma caused by having to ration a limited item to fellow villagers, many turtlemen prefer to sell all their turtles to the company and return with money, which does not have to be shared. However, if a Miskito sells out to the company, he will probably be unable to acquire meat for himself in the village, regardless of kinship or purchasing power. I overheard an elderly turtleman muttering to himself as he butchered a turtle: "I no going to sell, neither give dem meat. Let dem eat de money."

The situation is bad and getting worse. Individuals too old or sick to provide for themselves often receive little meat or money from relatives. Families without turtlemen are families without money or access to meat. The trend is toward the individualization of nuclear families, operating for their own economic ends. Miskito villages are becoming neighborhoods rather than communities.

The Miskito diet has suffered in quality and quantity. Less protein and fewer diverse vegetables and fruits are consumed. Present dietary staples—rice, white flour, beans, sugar, and coffee—come from the store. In one Miskito village, 65 percent of all food eaten in a year was purchased.

Besides the nutritional significance of what is becoming a largely carbohydrate diet, dependence on purchased foods has also had major economic reverberations. Generated by national and international scarcities, inflationary fallout has hit the Miskito. Most of their purchased foods are imported, much coming from the United States. In the last five years prices for staples have increased 100 to 150 percent. This has had an overwhelming impact on the Miskito, who spend 50 to 75 percent of their income for food. Consequently, their entry into the market by selling a subsistence resource, diverting labor from agriculture, and intensifying exploitation of a vanishing species has resulted in their living off poorer-quality, higher-priced foods.

The Miskito now depend on outside systems to supply them with money and materials that are subject to world market fluctuations. They have lost their autonomy and their adaptive relationship with their environment. Life is no longer socially rewarding nor is their diet satisfying. The coastal Miskito have become a specialized and highly vulnerable sector of the global market economy.

Loss of the turtle market would be a serious economic blow to the Miskito, who have almost no other means of securing cash for what have now become necessities. Nevertheless, continued exploitation will surely reduce the turtle population to a critical level.

National and international legislation is urgently needed. At the very least, commercial turtle fishing must be curtailed for several years until the *Chelonia* population can rebound and exploitation quotas can be set. While turtle fishing for subsistence should be permitted, exportation of sea turtle products used in the gourmet, cosmetic, or jewelry trade should be banned.

Restrictive environmental legislation, however, is not a popular subject in Nicaragua, a country that has recently been torn by earthquakes, volcanic eruption, and hurricanes. A program for sea turtle conservation submitted to the Nicaraguan government for consideration ended up in a pile of rubble during the earthquake that devastated Managua in December, 1972, adding a sad footnote to the Miskito—sea turtle situation. With other problems to face, the government has not yet reviewed what is happening on the distant east coast, separated from the capital by more than 200 miles of rain forest—and years of neglect.

As it is now, the turtles are going down and along with them, the Miskito—seemingly, a small problem in terms of the scale of ongoing ecological and cultural change in the world. But each localized situation involves species and societies with long histories and, perhaps, short futures. They are weathervanes in the conflicting winds of economic and environmental priorities. As Bob Dylan sang: "You don't need a weatherman to tell which way the wind blows."

CHAPTER 40

How Sushi Went Global

Theodore C. Bestor

(2005)

A 40-minute drive from Bath, Maine, down a winding two-lane highway, the last mile on a dirt road, a ramshackle wooden fish pier stands beside an empty parking lot. At 6:00 p.m. nothing much is happening. Three bluefin tuna sit in a huge tub of ice on the loading dock.

Between 6:45 and 7:00, the parking lot fills up with cars and trucks with license plates from New Jersey, New York, Massachusetts, New Hampshire, and Maine. Twenty tuna buyers clamber out, half of them Japanese. The three bluefin, ranging from 270 to 610 pounds, are winched out of the tub, and buyers crowd around them, extracting tiny core samples to examine their color, fingering the flesh to assess the fat content, sizing up the curve of the body.

After about 20 minutes of eyeing the goods, many of the buyers return to their trucks to call Japan by cellphone and get the morning prices from Tokyo's Tsukiji market—the fishing industry's answer to Wall Street—where the daily tuna auctions have just concluded. The buyers look over the tuna one last time and give written bids to the dock manager, who passes the top bid for each fish to the crew that landed it.

The auction bids are secret. Each bid is examined anxiously by a cluster of young men, some with a father or uncle looking on to give advice, others with a young woman and a couple of toddlers trying to see Daddy's fish. Fragments of concerned conversation float above the parking lot: "That's all?" "Couldn't we do better if we shipped it ourselves?" "Yeah, but my pickup needs a new transmission now!" After a few minutes, deals are closed and the fish are quickly loaded onto the backs of trucks in crates of crushed ice, known in the trade as "tuna coffins." As rapidly as they arrived, the flotilla of buyers sails out of the parking lot—three bound for New York's John F. Kennedy Airport, where their tuna will be airfreighted to Tokyo for sale the day after next.

Bluefin tuna may seem at first an unlikely case study in globalization. But as the world rearranges itself—around silicon chips, Starbucks coffee, or sashimi-grade tuna—new channels for global flows of capital and commodities

link far-flung individuals and communities in unexpected new relationships. The tuna trade is a prime example of the globalization of a regional industry, with intense international competition and thorny environmental regulations; centuries-old practices combined with high technology; realignments of labor and capital in response to international regulation; shifting markets; and the diffusion of culinary culture as tastes for sushi, and bluefin tuna, spread worldwide.

GROWING APPETITES

Tuna doesn't require much promotion among Japanese consumers. It is consistently Japan's most popular seafood, and demand is high throughout the year. When the Federation of Japan Tuna Fisheries Cooperative (known as Nikkatsuren) runs ad campaigns for tuna, they tend to be low-key and whimsical, rather like the "Got Milk?" advertising in the United States. Recently, the federation launched "Tuna Day" (Maguro no hi), providing retailers with posters and recipe cards for recipes more complicated than "slice and serve chilled." Tuna Day's mascot is Goro-kun, a colorful cartoon tuna swimming the Australian crawl.

Despite the playful contemporary tone of the mascot, the date selected for Tuna Day carries much heavier freight. October 10, it turns out, commemorates the date that tuna first appeared in Japanese literature, in the eighth-century collection of imperial court poetry known as the Man'yoshu—one of the towering classics of Japanese literature. The neat twist is that October 10 today is a national holiday, Sports Day. Goro-kun, the sporty tuna, scores a promotional hat trick, suggesting intimate connections among national culture, healthy food for active lives, and the family holiday meal.

Outside of Japan, tuna, especially raw tuna, hasn't always had it so good. Sushi isn't an easy concept to sell to the uninitiated. And besides, North Americans tend to think of cultural influence as flowing from West to East: James Dean, baseball, Coca-Cola, McDonald's, and Disneyland have all gone over big in Tokyo. Yet Japanese cultural motifs and material—from Kurosawa's The Seven Samurai to Yoda's Zen and Darth Vader's armor, from Issey Miyake's fashions to Nintendo, PlayStation, and Pokémon—have increasingly

Theodore Bestor, "How sushi went global." In *The Cultural Politics of Food and Eating*. J. I. Watson and M. L. Caldwell, eds. Oxford: Blackwell, 2005, pp. 13–20. Reprinted with permission.

saturated North American and indeed the entire world's consumption and popular culture. Against all odds, so too has sushi.

In 1929, the *Ladies' Home Journal* introduced Japanese cooking to North American women, but discreetly skirted the subject of raw fish: "There have been purposely omitted … any recipes using the delicate and raw tuna fish which is sliced wafer thin and served iced with attractive garnishes. [These] … might not sound so entirely delicious as they are in reality." Little mention of any Japanese food appeared in US media until well after World War II. By the 1960s, articles on sushi began to show up in lifestyle magazines like *Holiday* and *Sunset*. But the recipes they suggested were canapés like cooked shrimp on caraway rye bread, rather than raw fish on rice.

A decade later, however, sushi was growing in popularity throughout North America, turning into a sign of class and educational standing. In 1972, the *New York Times* covered the opening of a sushi bar in the elite sanctum of New York's Harvard Club. *Esquire* explained the fare in an article titled "Wake up Little Sushi!" Restaurant reviewers guided readers to Manhattan's sushi scene, including innovators like Shalom Sushi, a kosher sushi bar in SoHo.

Japan's emergence on the global economic scene in the 1970s as the business destination du jour, coupled with a rejection of hearty, red-meat American fare in favor of healthy cuisine like rice, fish, and vegetables, and the appeal of the high-concept aesthetics of Japanese design all prepared the world for a sushi fad. And so, from an exotic, almost unpalatable ethnic specialty, then to haute cuisine of the most rarefied sort, sushi has become not just cool, but popular. The painted window of a Cambridge, Massachusetts, coffee shop advertises "espresso, cappuccino, carrot juice, lasagna, and sushi." Mashed potatoes with wasabi (horseradish), sushi-ginger relish, and seared sashimi-grade tuna steaks show Japan's growing cultural influence on upscale nouvelle cuisine throughout North America, Europe, and Latin America. Sushi has even become the stuff of fashion, from "sushi" lip gloss, colored the deep red of raw tuna, to "wasabi" nail polish, a soft avocado green.

Angling for New Consumers

Japan remains the world's primary market for fresh tuna for sushi and sashimi; demand in other countries is a product of Japanese influence and the creation of new markets by domestic producers looking to expand their reach. Perhaps not surprisingly, sushi's global popularity as an emblem of a sophisticated, cosmopolitan consumer class more or less coincided with a profound transformation in the international role of the Japanese fishing industry. From the 1970s onward, the expansion of 200-mile fishing limits around the world excluded foreign fleets from the prime fishing grounds of many coastal nations. And international environmental campaigns forced many countries, Japan among them, to scale back their distant water fleets. With their fishing

operations curtailed and their yen for sushi still growing, Japanese had to turn to foreign suppliers.

Jumbo jets brought New England's bluefin tuna into easy reach of Tokyo, just as Japan's consumer economy—a byproduct of the now disparaged "bubble" years—went into hyperdrive. The sushi business boomed. During the 1980s, total Japanese imports of fresh bluefin tuna worldwide increased from 957 metric tons (531 from the United States) in 1984 to 5,235 metric tons (857 from the United States) in 1993. The average wholesale price peaked in 1990 at 4,900 yen (US $34) per kilogram, bones and all, which trimmed out to approximately US $33 wholesale per edible pound.

Not surprisingly, Japanese demand for prime bluefin tuna—which yields a firm red meat, lightly marbled with veins of fat, highly prized (and priced) in Japanese cuisine—created a gold-rush mentality on fishing grounds across the globe wherever bluefin tuna could be found. But in the early 1990s, as the US bluefin industry was taking off, the Japanese economy went into a stall, then a slump, then a dive. US producers suffered as their high-end export market collapsed. Fortunately for them, the North American sushi craze took up the slack. US businesses may have written off Japan, but Americans' taste for sushi stuck. An industry founded exclusively on Japanese demand survived because of Americans' newly trained palates and a booming US economy.

A Transatlantic Tussle

Atlantic bluefin tuna ("ABT" in the trade) are a highly migratory species that ranges from the equator to Newfoundland, from Turkey to the Gulf of Mexico. Bluefin can be huge fish; the record is 1,496 pounds. In more normal ranges, 600-pound tuna, 10 feet in length, are not extraordinary, and 250- to 300-pound bluefin, six feet long, are commercial mainstays.

Before bluefin became a commercial species in New England, before Japanese buyers discovered the stock, before the 747, bluefin were primarily sports fish, caught with fighting tackle by trophy hunters out of harbors like Montauk, Hyannis, and Kennebunkport. Commercial fishers, if they caught bluefin at all, sold them for cat food when they could and trucked them to town dumps when they couldn't. Japanese buyers changed all of that. Since the 1970s, commercial Atlantic bluefin tuna fisheries have been almost exclusively focused on Japanese markets like Tsukiji.

In New England waters, most bluefin are taken one fish at a time, by rod and reel, by hand line, or by harpoon—techniques of a small-scale fisher, not of a factory fleet. On the European side of the Atlantic, the industry operates under entirely different conditions. Rather than rod and reel or harpooning, the typical gear is industrial—the purse seiner (a fishing vessel closing a large net around a school of fish) or the long line (which catches fish on baited hooks strung along lines played out for many miles behind a swift vessel). The techniques may differ from boat to boat and from country to country, but these fishers are all angling for a share of the same Tsukiji yen—and in many cases, some biologists argue, a share of the same tuna stock. Fishing communities often think of themselves as close-knit and proudly parochial; but the sudden globalization of this industry has brought fishers into contact—and often into conflict—with customers, governments, regulators, and environmentalists around the world.

Two miles off the beach in Barbate, Spain, a huge maze of nets snakes several miles out into Spanish waters near the Strait of Gibraltar. A high-speed, Japanese-made workboat heads out to the nets. On board are five Spanish hands, a Japanese supervisor, 2,500 kilograms of frozen herring and mackerel imported from Norway and Holland, and two American researchers. The boat is making one of its twice-daily trips to Spanish nets, which contain captured Mediterranean tuna being raised under Japanese supervision for harvest and export to Tsukiji.

Behind the guard boats that stand watch over the nets 24 hours a day, the headlands of Morocco are a hazy purple in the distance. Just off Barbate's white cliffs to the northwest, the light at the Cape of Trafalgar blinks on and off. For 20 minutes, the men toss herring and mackerel over the gunwales of the workboat while tuna the size (and speed) of Harley-Davidsons dash under the boat, barely visible until, with a flash of silver and blue, they wheel around to snatch a drifting morsel.

The nets, lines, and buoys are part of an *almadraba*, a huge fish trap used in Spain as well as Sicily, Tunisia, and Morocco. The *almadraba* consists of miles of nets anchored to the channel floor suspended from thousands of buoys, all laid out to cut across the migration routes of bluefin tuna leaving the strait. This *almadraba* remains in place for about six weeks in June and July to intercept tuna leaving the Mediterranean after their spawning season is over. Those tuna that lose themselves in the maze end up in a huge pen, roughly the size of a football field. By the end of the tuna run through the strait, about 200 bluefin are in the pen.

Two hundred fish may not sound like a lot, but if the fish survive the next six months, if the fish hit their target weights, if the fish hit the market at the target price, these 200 bluefin may be worth $1.6 million dollars. In November and December, after the bluefin season in New England and Canada is well over, the tuna are harvested and shipped by air to Tokyo in time for the end-of-the-year holiday spike in seafood consumption.

The pens, huge feed lots for tuna, are relatively new, but *almadraba* are not. A couple of miles down the coast from Barbate is the evocatively named settlement of Zahara de los Atunes (Zahara of the Tunas) where Cervantes lived briefly in the late 16th century. The centerpiece of the village is a huge stone compound that housed the men and nets of Zahara's *almadraba* in Cervantes's day, when the port was only a seasonally occupied tuna outpost (occupied by scoundrels, according to Cervantes). Along the Costa de la Luz, the three or four *almadraba* that remain still operate under the control of local fishing bosses who hold the customary fishing rights, the nets, the workers, the boats, and

the locally embedded cultural capital to make the *almadraba* work—albeit for distant markets and in collaboration with small-scale Japanese fishing firms.

Inside the Strait of Gibraltar, off the coast of Cartagena, another series of tuna farms operates under entirely different auspices, utilizing neither local skills nor traditional technology. The Cartagena farms rely on French purse seiners to tow captured tuna to their pens, where joint ventures between Japanese trading firms and large-scale Spanish fishing companies have set up farms using the latest in Japanese fishing technology. The waters and the workers are Spanish, but almost everything else is part of a global flow of techniques and capital: financing from major Japanese trading companies; Japanese vessels to tend the nets; aquacultural techniques developed in Australia; vitamin supplements from European pharmaceutical giants packed into frozen herring from Holland to be heaved over the gunwales for the tuna; plus computer models of feeding schedules, weight gains, and target market prices developed by Japanese technicians and fishery scientists.

These "Spanish" farms compete with operations throughout the Mediterranean that rely on similar high-tech, high-capital approaches to the fish business. In the Adriatic Sea, for example, Croatia is emerging as a formidable tuna producer. In Croatia's case, the technology and the capital were transplanted by émigré Croatians who returned to the country from Australia after Croatia achieved independence from Yugoslavia in 1991. Australia, for its part, has developed a major aquacultural industry for southern bluefin tuna, a species closely related to the Atlantic bluefin of the North Atlantic and Mediterranean and almost equally desired in Japanese markets.

CULTURE SPLASH

Just because sushi is available, in some form or another, in exclusive Fifth Avenue restaurants, in baseball stadiums in Los Angeles, at airport snack carts in Amsterdam, at an apartment in Madrid (delivered by motorcycle), or in Buenos Aires, Tel Aviv, or Moscow, doesn't mean that sushi has lost its status as Japanese cultural property. Globalization doesn't necessarily homogenize cultural differences nor erase the salience of cultural labels. Quite the contrary, it grows the franchise. In the global economy of consumption, the brand equity of sushi as Japanese cultural property adds to the cachet of both the country and the cuisine. A Texan Chinese-American restauranteur told me, for example, that he had converted his chain of restaurants from Chinese to Japanese cuisine because the prestige factor of the latter meant he could charge a premium; his clients couldn't distinguish between Chinese and Japanese employees (and often failed to notice that some of the chefs behind his sushi bars were Latinos).

The brand equity is sustained by complicated flows of labor and ethnic biases. Outside of Japan, having Japanese hands (or a reasonable facsimile) is sufficient warrant for sushi competence. Guidebooks for the current generation of Japanese global *wandervogel* sometimes advise young Japanese looking for a job in a distant city to work as a sushi chef; US consular offices in Japan grant more than 1,000 visas a year to sushi chefs, tuna buyers, and other workers in the global sushi business. A trade school in Tokyo, operating under the name Sushi Daigaku (Sushi University) offers short courses in sushi preparation so "students" can impress prospective employers with an imposing certificate. Even without papers, however, sushi remains firmly linked in the minds of Japanese and foreigners alike with Japanese cultural identity. Throughout the world, sushi restaurants operated by Koreans, Chinese, or Vietnamese maintain Japanese identities. In sushi bars from Boston to Valencia, a customer's simple greeting in Japanese can throw chefs into a panic (or drive them to the far end of the counter).

On the docks, too, Japanese cultural control of sushi remains unquestioned. Japanese buyers and "tuna techs" sent from Tsukiji to work seasonally on the docks of New England laboriously instruct foreign fishers on the proper techniques for catching, handling, and packing tuna for export. A bluefin tuna must approximate the appropriate *kata*, or "ideal form," of color, texture, fat content, body shape, and so forth, all prescribed by Japanese specifications. Processing requires proper attention as well. Special paper is sent from Japan for wrapping the fish before burying them in crushed ice. Despite high shipping costs and the fact that 50 percent of the gross weight of a tuna is unusable, tuna is sent to Japan whole, not sliced into salable portions. Spoilage is one reason for this, but form is another. Everyone in the trade agrees that Japanese workers are much more skilled in cutting and trimming tuna than Americans, and no one would want to risk sending botched cuts to Japan.

Not to impugn the quality of the fish sold in the United States, but on the New England docks, the first determination of tuna buyers is whether they are looking at a "domestic" fish or an "export" fish. On that judgment hangs several dollars a pound for the fisher, and the supply of sashimi-grade tuna for fishmongers, sushi bars, and seafood restaurants up and down the Eastern seaboard. Some of the best tuna from New England may make it to New York or Los Angeles, but by way of Tokyo—validated as top quality (and top price) by the decision to ship it to Japan by air for sale at Tsukiji, where it may be purchased by one of the handful of Tsukiji sushi exporters who supply premier expatriate sushi chefs in the world's leading cities.

PLAYING THE MARKET

The tuna auction at Yankee Co-op in Seabrook, New Hampshire, is about to begin on the second-to-last day of the 1999 season. The weather is stormy, few boats are out. Only three bluefin, none of them terribly good, are up for sale today, and the half-dozen buyers at the auction, three Americans and three Japanese, gloomily discuss the impending end of a lousy season.

In July, the bluefin market collapsed just as the US fishing season was starting. In a stunning miscalculation, Japanese

purse seiners operating out of Kesennuma in northern Japan managed to land their entire year's quota from that fishery in only three days. The oversupply sent tuna prices at Tsukiji through the floor, and they never really recovered.

Today, the news from Spain is not good. The day before, faxes and e-mails from Tokyo brought word that a Spanish fish farm had suffered a disaster. Odd tidal conditions near Cartagena led to a sudden and unexpected depletion of oxygen in the inlet where one of the great tuna nets was anchored. Overnight, 800 fish suffocated. Divers hauled out the tuna. The fish were quickly processed, several months before their expected prime, and shipped off to Tokyo. For the Japanese corporation and its Spanish partners, a harvest potentially worth $6.5 million would yield only a tiny fraction of that. The buyers at the morning's auctions in New Hampshire know they will suffer as well. Whatever fish turn up today and tomorrow, they will arrive at Tsukiji in the wake of an enormous glut of hastily exported Spanish tuna.

Fishing is rooted in local communities and local economies—even for fishers dipping their lines (or nets) in the same body of water, a couple hundred miles can be worlds away. Now, a Massachusetts fisher's livelihood can be transformed in a matter of hours by a spike in market prices halfway around the globe or by a disaster at a fish farm across the Atlantic. Giant fishing conglomerates in one part of the world sell their catch alongside family outfits from another. Environmental organizations on one continent rail against distant industry regulations implemented an ocean away. Such instances of convergence are common in a globalizing world. What is surprising, and perhaps more profound, in the case of today's tuna fishers, is the complex interplay between industry and culture, as an esoteric cuisine from an insular part of the world has become a global fad in the span of a generation, driving, and driven by, a new kind of fishing business.

Many New England fishers, whose traditional livelihood now depends on unfamiliar tastes and distant markets, turn to a kind of armchair anthropology to explain Japan's ability to transform tuna from trash into treasure around the world. For some, the quick answer is simply national symbolism. The deep red of tuna served as sashimi or sushi contrasts with the stark white rice, evoking the red and white of the Japanese national flag. Others know that red and white is an auspicious color combination in Japanese ritual life (lobster tails are popular at Japanese weddings for just this reason). Still others think the cultural prize is a fighting spirit, pure machismo, both their own and the tuna's. Taken by rod and reel, a tuna may battle the fisher for four or five hours. Some tuna literally fight to the death. For some fishers, the meaning of tuna—the equation of tuna with Japanese identity—is simple: Tuna is nothing less than the samurai fish!

Of course, such mystification of a distant market's motivations for desiring a local commodity is not unique. For decades, anthropologists have written of "cargo cults" and "commodity fetishism" from New Guinea to Bolivia.

But the ability of fishers today to visualize Japanese culture and the place of tuna within its demanding culinary tradition is constantly shaped and reshaped by the flow of cultural images that now travel around the globe in all directions simultaneously, bumping into each other in airports, fishing ports, bistros, bodegas, and markets everywhere. In the newly rewired circuitry of global cultural and economic affairs, Japan is the core, and the Atlantic seaboard, the Adriatic, and the Australian coast are all distant peripheries. Topsy-turvy as Gilbert and Sullivan never imagined it.

Japan is plugged into the popular North American imagination as the sometimes inscrutable superpower, precise and delicate in its culinary tastes, feudal in its cultural symbolism, and insatiable in its appetites. Were Japan not a prominent player in so much of the daily life of North Americans, the fishers outside of Bath or in Seabrook would have less to think about in constructing their Japan. As it is, they struggle with unfamiliar exchange rates for cultural capital that compounds in a foreign currency.

And they get ready for next season.

CHAPTER 41

Nutrition Transitions: A View from Anthropology

Darna L. Dufour and Richard L. Bender

(2012)

There is little doubt that human diets and patterns of physical activity have changed over time. There is also a strong sense that these changes have accelerated in the recent past, and are leading to increases in body fatness that negatively impact health. Large-scale dietary changes that affect many different types of populations are collectively referred to as nutrition transitions. The term nutrition here refers to more than diet. It is short for nutritional status, a measure of health that includes shortness/tallness, fatness/thinness, as well as other indicators of under- and overnutrition.

There is an expanding scientific and popular literature focused on current nutrition transitions at global and national levels and in particular the increases in obesity that are occurring in much of the world. While this literature might lead you to conclude that everyone in the world is well-fed and fat, that is not true as there are still millions of people in the world who suffer from hunger and undernutrition. But fatness/obesity has captured the imagination of the public and the concerns of health professionals. The fear is that there is a McDonald's on every corner and that global food chains are delivering the same high fat, high sugar, and highly processed foods to everyone on the planet.

The emphasis on current nutrition transitions implies that these kinds of transitions are novel for humans as a species. They are not. They are just another change in nutrition in our continued evolution as omnivores, animals capable of including a wide variety of foods in their diet. We have probably been through many nutrition transitions, the bigger ones tied to our capacity to control the plants and animals we sought to use as food, and more recently the ability to convert those same plants and animals into a vast array of processed food products.

Nutrition transitions are complex and involve multiple processes and variables. To understand these phenomena, scientists use *models*, or conceptual frameworks to organize empirical data in a parsimonious, theoretically meaningful way. Much of the discussion of nutrition transitions in the historic past, as well as the current context, has been dominated by the "Nutrition Transition," a model proposed by Barry Popkin in the early 1990s. Our goal in this essay is to consider the validity and usefulness of this particular model from an anthropological perspective. We argue that the model ignores the significant variation within and between human populations in the past as well as the present, and in doing so limits our understanding of the very phases and transitions the model proposes to represent. Lastly, we comment on more theoretical issues regarding the Nutrition Transition as a model.

THE NUTRITION TRANSITION—A MODEL

Barry Popkin introduced the Nutrition Transition as "a heuristic framework that accommodates the dynamic nature of diet and the relationship of diet with other aspects of society" (1993:138). The Nutrition Transition model is composed of five distinct stages or patterns: 1) *collecting food,* 2) *famine,* 3) *receding famine,* 4) *degenerative disease,* and 5) *behavioral change*. Each stage is conceived as "a broad pattern of food use and corresponding nutrition-related disease" (Popkin, 1994:285), and is more specifically defined by a) a set of dietary and physical activity characteristics, b) typical short-term, individual-level health outcomes, and c) long-term, population-level health outcomes. Some stages are also described in terms of food economy, or the ways in which a population interacts with its environment to procure or produce food. Due to the current ubiquity and familiarity of this model, we refer to it as the Nutrition Transition, to avoid any confusion with other discussions of dietary or activity transitions in general. The following descriptions of the stages of the Nutrition Transition are drawn principally from Popkin (1994, 2002a), although many other sources are available.

Stage 1, *collecting food,* characterizes both modern and historical hunter-gatherer populations. The diet is high in carbohydrates and fiber and low in fat, particularly saturated fat. Activity levels are very high and little obesity is found.

Stage 2, *famine*, describes a much less varied diet subject to episodic periods of extreme food shortage. During the later phases of this stage, social stratification intensifies and dietary heterogeneity according to social status and gender increases. There was little change in physical activity levels during this period, although the types of activity did change.

Stage 3, *receding famine*, corresponds with an increased consumption of fruits, vegetables, and animal proteins, while starchy staples become less important in the diet. While many early civilizations made substantial progress in alleviating chronic hunger and famines, it is only in the final third of this millennium that these dietary changes became widespread. On the other hand, famines continued well into the 18th century throughout Europe, and remain common in other parts of the world. Activity patterns begin to shift, with inactivity and leisure becoming more common.

Stage 4, *degenerative disease*, is characteristic of most high-income societies, and of increasing proportions of the population in many low- and middle-income societies. The diet is high in total fat, cholesterol, sugar, and other refined carbohydrates, and low in fiber and polyunsaturated fats. This diet, combined with a shift toward sedentary activity patterns, results in an increased prevalence of obesity and contributes to the degenerative diseases that define the final stage of the epidemiological transition.

Stage 5, *behavioral change*, represents an emerging pattern of dietary change driven by the health-conscious desires of individual consumers and government agencies. The diet resembles Stage 1 (*collecting food*) more than Stage 4 (*degenerative disease*), while recreational physical activity increases and sedentary patterns decrease. The focus is on reducing nutrition-related non-communicable diseases and extending "healthy ageing," that is, "postponing infirmity and increasing the disability-free life expectancy" (Popkin, 2002a:94). This stage is unique in that it involves conscious, purposeful changes in nutrition and physical activity.

AN ANTHROPOLOGICAL VIEW OF THE FIRST STAGES

Stage 1, Collecting Food

Populations in Stage 1 of the Nutrition Transition are well-described within the anthropological literature. In fact, they are the hunter-gatherer societies such as the !Kung San of Botswana and Namibia, the Aché of Paraguay, the Inuit and Yupik of northern Canada, Alaska and Greenland, and various Australian aboriginal groups, that have long been classic research targets for anthropologists interested in nutrition, adaptation, and human ecology.

The anthropological interest in hunter-gatherer diets originates from two basic questions. First, how do hunter-gatherers compare to sedentary agricultural populations in terms of nutrition, health, and quality of life? Second, can the dietary ecology of hunter-gatherers help us to understand the costs and benefits of modern, industrialized food systems? Inherent in this question is the idea that modern or

historical hunter-gatherer diets are good analogues for the diets of early humans or human ancestors.

The work of anthropologist Richard B. Lee among !Kung San hunter-gatherers in the mid-1960s and 70s was instrumental in generating widespread interest in these questions. Lee argued that the !Kung San lived a relatively comfortable life in a very harsh, hot, dry environment. They devoted only an average of 12–19 hours per week obtaining food and had considerable leisure time. Though willing to expend considerable time and energy in hunting, their diet consisted mostly of plant foods, with a third of total calories provided by Mongongo nuts (Lee, 1968:40).

Although this optimistic view of the !Kung San lifestyle has been questioned recently (see Chapter 28 by Bogin), researchers have found that many other hunter-gatherer diets followed a similar broad pattern to that described by Lee: a strong reliance on plant foods such as fruits, nuts, or roots, and a secondary—though still important—role for hunted or scavenged animal foods. The animal foods that make it into these diets are typically much leaner than industrially produced meat and possess a higher polyunsaturated-to-saturated fat ratio (Cordain et al., 2005). So, these food intake patterns are accurately described as Stage 1 diets high in carbohydrates, including fiber, and low in fat, particularly saturated fat.

Observations of hunter-gatherer diets have led to a more recent interest in the second question posed above. Are hunter-gatherer diets merely different from modern industrial ones, or are they in fact superior in some quantifiable sense? Eaton and Konner, in a classic 1985 article in *The New England Journal of Medicine*, argued that the most nutritionally sound diet for humans should be the one that they grew up with, in evolutionary terms. The diet of humans during the Paleolithic (from 2.6 million years ago to about 20,000 years before the present) obviously "worked," since we are here to think about it. In contrast, the evolutionarily novel diets introduced more recently by industrialized societies are clearly *not* working, as evidenced by the high rates of obesity and other nutrition-related non-communicable diseases they seem to produce. How can we know what Paleolithic diets looked like? By observing contemporary and historical hunter-gatherers. The dietary ecology of these populations has presumably changed very little over the past several thousand years, and should therefore provide us with a better idea of what early humans were up to, and consequently how we can improve our modern diets.

However, from an anthropological perspective, there is no such thing as "the" hunter-gatherer diet. Instead, the main impression we have of hunter-gatherer diets is one of omnivory, ecological flexibility, and dietary variability. While many hunter-gatherer diets do in fact fit the "classic" model—high in carbohydrates and animal protein, low in animal fats—there are important exceptions to this pattern.

Perhaps the most striking example is the traditional diet of the Inuit and some other high-latitude populations. This diet is composed almost exclusively of meat and fat from marine mammals (e.g., whales, seals), terrestrial mammals (e.g., caribou), or fish, with almost no plant foods. Thus, the diet of these hunter-gatherers is very high in saturated fat, with almost no carbohydrate content—the opposite of that expected for a Stage 1 population. On the other hand, the activity level (or at least, total energy expenditure) is very high, and there is little or no evidence of obesity or other nutrition-related non-communicable diseases.

Overall, then, what does the anthropological data tell us about Stage 1 populations? The description of this stage within the Nutrition Transition model is rather general, and rightly so. Stage 1, or hunter-gatherer, populations are in fact highly variable and demonstrate that humans are able to adapt to a wide range of ecological conditions and maintain good health on nearly any kind of diet imaginable. This means that the connection between diet and health is mediated by myriad other influences such as activity patterns, infectious disease prevalence, environmental conditions, and socioeconomic and political factors.

Stages 2 and 3, Famine and Receding Famine

Populations that clearly fit into Stage 2 or Stage 3 of the Nutrition Transition are more difficult to identify in the anthropological literature. Certainly, there are many populations that fit some or all of the descriptions of these stages, but these populations are highly diverse and scattered across time and geographic space. The main difficulty, as we will show, is that the terms "famine" and "receding famine" do not usefully describe these kinds of populations.

In our interpretation, Stage 2 best describes populations with food economies based on a mixed hunter-gatherer/horticultural strategy, an agricultural economy dependent on the intensive cultivation of one primary plant food such as maize, or perhaps pastoralism. Local food self-sufficiency, or self-reliance, has been a hallmark of these populations. Their temporal and geographic variation is staggering. Well known ethnographic examples include horticulturalists like the Papua New Guinea Tsembaga (Rappaport, 1968) and Wamira (Kahn, 1986), Balinese rice farmers (Lansing, 1991), cash-cropping agriculturalists like the Nigerian Kofyar (Netting et al., 1996) and pastoralists like the East African Turkana (Galvin, 1994). Diets are equally as diverse. They include taro and sweet potato-based diets with minimal animal products (Tsembaga and Wamira), rice-based diets with vegetables and animal products serving as condiments (Balinese), millet, sorghum and yam-based diets (Kofyar), and milk-based diets supplemented by maize meal (Turkana).

Populations in Stage 3, on the other hand, would be those with food economics further along the continuum from local food self-sufficiency to dependence on markets and industrialized food production. We emphasize the notion of continuum here as there are no pure strategies: hunter-gatherers often trade with cultivators, cultivators hunt for meat and gather wild plant foods, and many pastoralists cultivate grains. Furthermore, these characteristics are not set in stone; populations can and do modify their

subsistence strategies in response to changing environmental, economic, or political factors.

How have anthropologists thought about Stage 2 and 3 populations? From a prehistorical perspective, the focus has been on the changes in health and social structure that accompanied the transition from hunter-gatherer to agricultural subsistence strategies in many different part of the world. From a contemporary perspective, the focus has been on the ecologies of pastoralists, horticulturalists, and small-scale agriculturalists, and on their interactions with larger economic communities. We examine these viewpoints in turn.

A Prehistorical View of Stages 2 and 3

The transition from gathering food to producing food through horticulture has long been an important research focus for anthropologists. Although it was characterized by different sets of precedents and consequences in different regions and time periods, some broad patterns have emerged suggesting that a decline in overall health following the initial adoption of intensive agriculture is indeed a general historical trend. For example, Larsen argued that the adoption of agriculture during the Neolithic "led to a reduction in health status and well-being, an increase in physiological stress, a decline in nutrition, and an alteration of activity types and work loads" (Larsen, 1995:204). As evidence for these changes, he cites an increase in the number of dental pathologies including dental caries, enamel defects, and tooth loss, as well as skeletal indices such as reduced stature and cortical bone thickness, and pathologies indicative of iron deficiency like cribra orbitalia/porotic hyperostosis (cranial lesions caused by overproduction of red blood cells in response to anemia). This suite of pathologies is observed in a variety of locations and time periods.

What about the increases in social stratification and dietary heterogeneity according to social status that Popkin includes in Stage 2? The anthropological data does indicate an increase in these phenomena concurrent with the shift toward agriculture. Interestingly, some researchers have suggested that the first domesticated food animals and plants were not dietary staples cultivated for their nutritional qualities, but rather luxury foods to be used during feasts, trading, and other expressions of status and power (Hayden, 2003). The production, distribution, and consumption of food have played a powerful role in the political economy of countless societies around the world, both past and present (Dietler, 1996). Food is simultaneously a great uniter and a great divider. It is a uniter in that any human, regardless of gender, ethnicity, or social status, requires the same basic nutrients as anyone else. It is a divider in that unequal access to food is one of the most fundamental inequalities that humans can impose on one another.

Importantly, however, the adverse health conditions documented by anthropologists in prehistoric agricultural societies are not considered to necessarily be the result of episodic periods of extreme food shortage or famines. On the contrary, these health outcomes can easily emerge from a consistently lower-quality diet, even if it is continually available. Hence, famines do not appear to be a defining nutritional characteristic of these societies. This leads us to a contemporary view of Stage 2 and 3 populations, and to a discussion of the nature of famines.

A Contemporary View of Stages 2 and 3

Stages 2 and 3 of the Nutrition Transition are called *famine* and *receding famine*. So, our conception of these stages depends on our understanding of what exactly is meant by "famine." It is not necessarily obvious what constitutes a famine versus some other phenomenon related to insufficient food. We think of these phenomena as existing along a continuum of severity from hunger, through food insecurity, to severe food shortage, and finally to famine. From our perspective, famines are discrete events that happen to specific populations at specific times. They are characterized by an usually severe food shortage caused by a set of identifiable, quantifiable economic, social, and environmental factors. They have predictable biological and cultural effects, such as starvation, mass emigration, changes in activity patterns, and shifts in the performance of ritual (Dirks, 1980). Famines are not inherent characteristics of certain types of societies—even ones that experience chronic undernutrition or episodic food shortages. On the contrary, famines can and have struck healthy, well organized societies not otherwise characterized by chronic hunger. For example, the devastating Soviet famine of 1932–1933, which killed several million people, is widely acknowledged to be the result of conscious economic and political decisions made by the centralized government of a powerful industrial state (Kuromiya, 2008).

From an anthropological perspective, populations can cope with or adapt to chronic hunger and episodic food shortages, but not famines. Indeed, Colson (1979:18) pointed out long ago that self-reliant societies develop food strategies to maintain dietary adequacy "in good years and in bad." Thus, the terms "famine" and "receding famine" are inappropriate as typological labels, and they do not usefully describe the kinds of populations we would think of as being included in Stages 2 and 3 of the Nutrition Transition.

Inherent in Popkin's definition of Stages 2 and 3 is the notion that a population's susceptibility to famines is directly linked to its subsistence strategy; hence, famines are expected to be common among self-reliant agriculturalists but not among hunter-gatherers. In fact, multiple lines of evidence suggest that the incidence of famine has varied widely within different types of subsistence strategies, and that small-scale agricultural populations are not necessarily more famine-prone than other societies (Benyshek and Watson, 2006; see also Dirks, 1993). To reiterate, famines are things that happen to specific populations at specific times for specific reasons, and are not inherent qualities of certain types of societies like self-reliant agriculturalists.

Before turning to Stage 4 of the Nutrition Transition, we must revisit pastoralism, since this important type of food economy is conspicuously missing from the model. Pastoralists maintain herds of domesticated livestock which provide the majority of dietary intake in the form of milk, blood, or meat. This unique subsistence strategy, which may have originally arisen concurrently with agriculture (Bates and Lees, 1996), does not comfortably fit within the stages of the Nutrition Transition. Pastoralists are certainly not Stage 1 populations since they rely on animal husbandry rather than hunting/gathering and their activity levels are not particularly high (Curran and Galvin, 1999). Pastoralists are also not Stage 2 or 3 populations since they are not characterized by high degrees of social stratification and dietary heterogeneity, although they may experience episodic periods of extreme food shortages (e.g., Fratkin and Roth, 1996; Scoones, 1996). The high proportion of animal source foods in pastoralist diets also does not match the Stage 1 or 2 definitions; it is the closest match to Stage 4. However, unlike Stage 4, obesity is rare. Hence, it is unclear where these anthropologically important and geographically widespread populations should be placed within the Nutrition Transition model.

WHERE ARE WE NOW?

According to the Nutrition Transition model, most of the world's populations are now in Stage 4 (*degenerative disease*), or transitioning into it. This stage has been the focus of most of the research on the Nutrition Transition, and nutrition transitions more generally. We will focus on the past 40–50 years, and on developing countries because that is where changes in diet, physical activity and body composition have been more rapid and profound (Popkin, 2002b), or at least we think they have been more rapid and profound. The term developing countries refers to those countries that have per capita (per person) income levels lower than those of developed countries like the United States, Canada, Japan, Australia, New Zealand and those in the European Union. They are also referred to as low and middle-income countries.

The ongoing Nutrition Transition in developing countries is conceptualized as a process of dietary change leading to diets similar to those currently consumed in the wealthy countries of Europe and North America (Popkin, 2003). These diets, referred to as "western" diets, tend to be high in fat, sugar, animal source foods (ASF) and processed foods, and low in fiber. The transition to "western" diets is conceptualized as occurring in two phases. In the early phase there is typically an increased consumption of vegetable oils and sugar (Drew and Popkin, 1997), and in the later phase an increase in the consumption of ASFs, highly processed foods, and an increase in food consumption away from home (Drewnowski, 2000).

These dietary changes are conceptualized as occurring in parallel with reductions in physical activity, which together lead to outcomes like increases in body weight and the prevalence of obesity. The increases in obesity have been the focus of attention because they are seen as negative outcomes associated with the risk of nutrition-related non-communicable diseases like diabetes and heart disease.

Does the current global nutritional situation reflect the expectations of the Nutrition Transition model? Below we consider some of the available evidence for changes in diet, physical activity and the prevalence of obesity. We focus on data from three nations that are all "developing countries" yet are geographically, culturally, and economically distinct: India, Kenya, and Brazil.

Lines of Evidence—Changes in Diet

Change over time is always difficult to document and analyze because we typically lack data on the earlier time periods we wish to compare to the present. This is also true for nutrition. So what data do we have? For developing countries we have very limited quantitative data on either dietary intake, physical activity or other indicators of nutritional status that go back 50, or even 20 years. The data we do have is typically for small subpopulations that were studied only once at some point of time in the past, and hence do not provide a measure of change over time. Given that limitation, researchers have used the FAO (Food and Agricultural Organization of the United Nations) "food balance sheets" to assess long-term trends at national levels. These food balance sheets provide average food availability per capita in terms of broad categories like cereal grains, starchy roots, ASFs, etc. for all the countries in the world. It is important to note that the data are not actually based on diets, i.e. food consumed, but rather on food available at the national level. These data are not very fine grained, but do provide evidence of global shifts in food availability that fit expectations of Stage 4 of the Nutrition Transition model described above.

We would expect, however, that local economies and histories will influence the timing and dimensions of any transitions in nutrition. In this regard, country-specific examples illustrate the inherent variation and suggest caution in assuming the Nutrition Transition model explains all cases.

Figure 1 shows the major sources of dietary energy for India, Kenya, and Brazil between 1967 and 2007, or roughly the past 40 years. Data for the United States are shown for comparison since U.S. diets are the classic example of the "western" diet toward which developing countries are assumed to be moving. All the data are FAO food availability data. The primary source of calories in the three developing countries has remained cereal grains, but their availability has declined. In contrast most of the available calories in the United States come from ASFs. Beyond the predominance of cereal grains, the plots of the three developing countries look quite different. In India the availability of cereal grains is higher than either Kenya or Brazil (60% or more), and almost half of it is from rice. The availability of other foods is lower and has remained relatively flat. The availability of ASFs and vegetable oils have increased, however, and increased in parallel from about 5% of dietary energy in 1967 to about 8% in 2007. The availability of fruits and vegetables did not change.

Food availability in Kenya and Brazil follows an intermediate pattern. In Kenya, cereal grains, in this case maize, are less important than they are in India. ASFs and vegetable oils have been more important and have been increasing more rapidly. In Brazil the pattern is similar in that ASF and vegetable oil availability has increased dramatically. The decline in the availability of fruits and vegetables has been profound; most of it is due to the decline in pulses and roots.

In summary, the direction of the changes in food availability is toward diets with less cereal grain, fruits and vegetables and more ASFs and vegetable oils. It is clear that these 40-year trends indicate shifts toward "western-style" diets like that of the United States. Also, it is clear that the availability of different types of foods in each country was quite distinct 40 years ago and remained distinct in 2007.

Country-level data are, of course, averages across many groups of people living in different geographical areas, perhaps living very different lifestyles, and likely having different income levels, religious beliefs, etc. You name it. Because any number of these characteristics might be related to

Table 1 Composition of the Diet in Terms of Total Grams (g) and Percent of Food Consumed Per Person Per Day by Income Quartile in Urban India. Percent of Total. Data from Vepa (2004)

Food	Quartile 1		Quartile 2		Quartile 3		Quartile 2	
	g	%	g	%	g	%	g	%
Cereal grains	338	50	354	42	355	32	331	22
ASF	67	10	127	15	223	20	385	25
Vegetables	171	25	211	25	250	22	313	21
Fruit	8	1	13	2	23	25	57	4
Oils	12	2	22	3	26	2	32	2
Sugars	19	3	30	4	37	3	44	3
Beverages & processed foods	61	9	94	11	186	17	351	23
TOTAL	676	100	852	100	1103	100	1517	100

nutrition it is useful to drill down and take a closer look at variations within individual countries. Diet surveys are particularly useful in this regard, and in addition are actually based on what people eat. Unfortunately there are very few of these available. Dietary surveys of urban areas in India are particularly interesting. In these surveys the investigators asked, does diet vary by income level? The data suggest it does (Table 1). These data provide a snapshot taken at a single point in time and show not changes over time, but variability within one subpopulation. The differences in the amount of food consumed are striking: 676 grams per day in the lowest income group and 1517 grams per day in the highest, almost three times as much. The amount

of rice consumed is roughly similar in all income groups, but consumption of everything else increases dramatically from the lowest to the highest income quartile. People in the highest income quartile consume seven times as much fruit and almost six times as much ASF. They also consume almost six times more beverages (including carbonated sugary drinks) and processed foods like bread and biscuits/cookies (Vepa, 2004: 221).

So, even within urban areas in a single developing country people can have very different diets. Diets of the high income groups look like what we would expect based on the Nutrition Transition model, while those of the lower quartile do not (compare data in Table 1 to Figure 1). Hence,

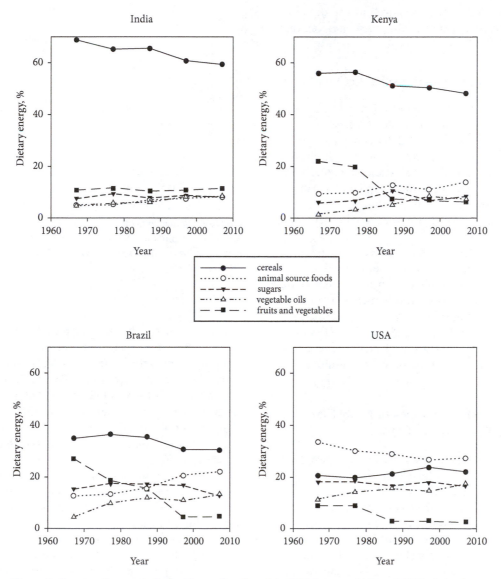

Figure 1 *Sources of energy in India, Kenya, Brazil and the USA between 1967 and 2007. Animal source foods includes all animal products; fruits and vegetables includes pulses and starchy roots. Data shown do not include minor sources of energy in the food supply like oil seeds, stimulants (coffee, tea, chocolate), spices and alcoholic beverages. Data from FAO food balance sheets, accessed December 31, 2010 at http://faostat.fao.org/site/368/DesktopDefault.aspx?PageID=368#ancor*

if the processes of globalization are driving the nutrition transition in India they are impacting income groups in urban areas very differently.

Microlevel case studies, the kind anthropologists do, are another source of data. They do not typically provide dietary intake data, but do provide the ethnographic context of small-scale, highly localized changes in diet and work patterns, and in doing so give us a sense of local nutrition transitions and the processes driving them. For example, one case study from the Kolli Hills region of rural India documents substantial changes in the kinds of cereal grains (rice replacing millets) consumed, as well as the work effort associated with both agricultural production and food processing (Finnis, 2009). Further, the study suggests that these changes in diet and physical activity are the direct results of localized changes in rainfall affecting the crops that can be grown as well as the desire for cash income that can be met by selling cassava rather than millet.

Lines of Evidence—Physical Activity

Unfortunately we do not have good quantitative longitudinal data on changes in physical activity, so researchers make a number of assumptions. The tendency has been to assume, for example, that physical activity has declined as motorized transportation and household appliances like laundry machines have become more available. Further, it is assumed that physical activity has declined as people have migrated from rural to urban settings, which they have been doing in large numbers.

The only actual data we have on changes in physical activity is from a short term interview-based study in China. That study found a reduction in time spent in vigorous physical activity in males in urban sites, 1979–1989. Unexpectedly, time in vigorous physical activity increased in urban females, and both rural males and females in the same time period (Table 2). The unexpected increases were attributed to the economic pressure to hold multiple jobs (Du et al., 2002).

Lines of Evidence for Changes in Body Size and the Prevalence of Obesity

The evidence for increases in body size and the prevalence of obesity is better than it is for either changes in dietary intake or physical activity. Time periods are not the same as they are for the data on food availability, but there is evidence from a number of countries that the prevalence of obesity has increased in the recent past, although it differs greatly from country to country (Figure 2). The term obesity is defined here according to the WHO guidelines as a body mass index (BMI) greater than or equal to 30 kg/m². For the three developing countries we have been considering, India, Kenya, and Brazil, the prevalence of obesity is 0.7%, 6%, and 11%, respectively. For the United States, in contrast, the prevalence is 32% (Table 3). Dramatic

Table 2 Proportion of Total Physical Activity Classified as Vigorous in Adults Ages 20-45 Years in China in 1989 and 1997. Data from the China Health and Nutrition Survey as Reported by Du et al. (2002)

	Males		Females	
Year	Urban	Rural	Urban	Rural
1989	27.1	52.5	24.8	20.8
1997	22.4	59.9	47.4	60.0

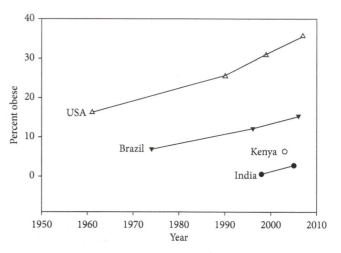

Figure 2 *Change in the prevalence of obesity over time in India, Kenya, Brazil and the USA. Data from WHO: Global Data Base on Body Mass Index. Accessed February 19, 2010 at http://apps.who.int/bmi/index.jsp*

differences. On the flip side, the prevalence of underweight (BMI < 18.5 kg/m²), an indicator of undernutrition, differs just as dramatically. It is 33%, 12%, and 4% for India, Kenya, and Brazil, respectively. For the United States it is 2%. So although there is talk of a global obesity epidemic, implying that all countries of the world are experiencing high rates of obesity, the situation is that not all countries are, and indeed some continue to confront problems of undernutrition.

Again, a closer look at variations within countries provides interesting insights. Figure 3 shows trends in the prevalence of obesity in adults in urban Brazil by income in two different regions. For males, the prevalence increased between 1975 and 1997 in both regions and was highest in the highest income group (quartile 4). The exception was in 1997 in the southeast region, where the prevalence of obesity converged in the three higher income groups. This suggests that in the southeast, the wealthier of the two regions, income was no longer a factor in the prevalence of obesity in 1997, except in the lowest income group.

Table 3 BMI Distributions in Four Countries. Data from WHO: Global Data Base on Body Mass Index. Accessed February 19, 2010 at http://apps.who.int/bmi/index.jsp

Category	BMI	India	Kenya	Brazil	USA
Underweight	< 18.5	33.0	12.3	4.0	2.3
Normal	18.5–24.9	62.6	64.3	55.4	34.3
Overweight	24.9–29.9	3.8	17.2	29.5	30.9
Obese	≥ 30	0.7	6.3	11.1	32.5

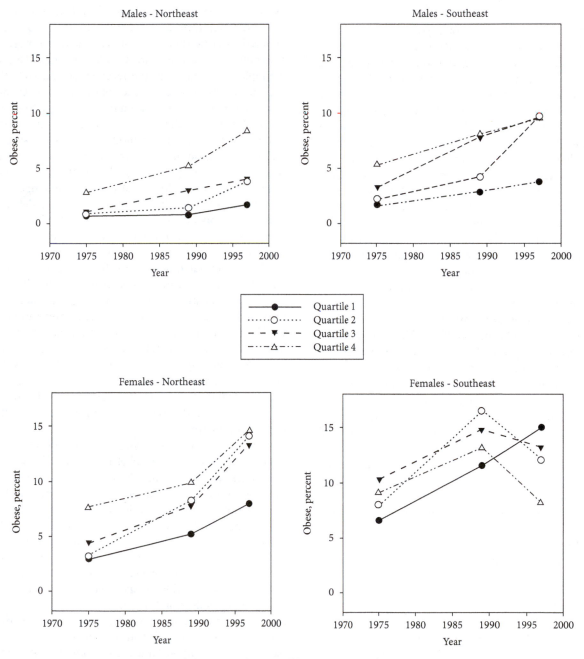

Figure 3 *Trends on the prevalence of obesity in urban Brazil by income quartile (1= lowest income) and region (Northeast and Southeast) for adult males and females. Data from Monteiro et al. (2002).*

For females, the prevalence of obesity also increased between 1975 and 1997, but only in the northeast (less wealthy region), and the lowest income group in the southeast. In the three higher income groups in the southeast, the percentages peaked in 1990 and then declined. This again suggests a weak link between income and the prevalence of obesity, or some kind of nonlinear relationship. That is, does the prevalence of obesity increase with income, and presumably the ability to purchase food, to some point and then actually decline? Does the famous saying, "You can never be too rich or too thin," apply to developing as well as developed countries?

Where Does All This Leave Us?

The available evidence is a bit of a patchwork quilt. We have some data on long term trends in diet, none on long-terms trends in physical activity, and some data on changes in body size. Geographically, the coverage of developing countries is uneven, and there are more data available for the middle income, as opposed to the low-income countries. What we do have available suggests wide variation between and within countries. Some countries, and perhaps groups within countries, fit the expectations of the Nutrition Transition model (Stage 4), others do not. There is very little data for the continent of Africa. Some of the countries in Africa have continued to experience significant problems of undernutrition, and in some cases actual famines (e.g., Niger; see Chapter 37). They are perhaps in earlier phases of the Nutrition Transition, i.e., Stage 3, *receding famine*. So although some say "the world is fat" (Popkin, 2009) it does not seem to be. Perhaps the world only looks fat when viewed from the land of the fat.

The forces driving the current nutrition transitions are not well understood (Popkin, 2006). They are generally assumed to be the forces of globalization, i.e., the increased flow of food, other commodities, information, and financial capital across national borders, and the myriad of processes associated with those flows, like urbanization and increased incomes (Kennedy et al., 2004). However, the linkages between globalization and nutrition have not been well established. The problem lies in understanding how some or all of the phenomena of globalization are actually linked to the local-level outcomes of interest, the nutrition of local populations and subpopulations. To solve it we need richly contextualized, fine-grained case studies that identify the changes in local food environments associated with globalization and the responses, in terms of diet and nutritional status, of different local populations and subpopulations to those changes.

Models and Muddles

Changes in diet and body size over time are well documented in the archaeological and historical records, at least in general terms. The ethnographic record provides evidence of change over time as well. There is little doubt these changes have occurred. What is referred to as the Nutrition Transition proposed by Popkin is a model of these changes. It mirrors the demographic transition (Thompson, 1929) and epidemiological transition (Omran, 1971) models, and shares many of the same advantages and limitations.

All models are simplifications of reality. They are heuristic devices, or tools, and useful to the extent that they generate testable hypotheses (Levins, 1966), or in some way help us understand reality. No single model can explain everything, so any model should be evaluated in terms of what it was meant to do rather than what we wish it would do. As a model, the Nutrition Transition superimposes stages on a continuous process of changes over time and in doing so calls attention to major changes and invites us to make comparisons and test hypotheses regarding the changes. That is useful. The stages are on different time scales; some seem to have lasted many hundreds, maybe thousands of years, and the more recent ones only decades. This characteristic of the model highlights the rapidity of change in the recent past. Indeed, although Popkin's model includes the idea of transitions over the long term, most of the attention is on the recent past 20–50 years.

Unfortunately the model muddles our thinking in a number of ways. First, the model presents the stages as a linear progression moving toward a defined end point. Although Popkin (1994:286) claims the stages are not restricted to specific historical periods, the language used to describe the stages inexorably drives the reader to think in terms of a historical progression, as do the terms "transitions" and "stages." This does not leave room to think about potential deviations and/or reversals in direction such as the declines in nutritional status that have accompanied the HIV/AIDS epidemic in parts of Africa (see de Waal, 2003).

Second, the model predicts the same sequence of stages to occur with the same set of results in any region of the world, and that these changes are independent of particular historical, environmental or ecological contexts. At least with the demographic and epidemiological models there is no indication that this has, or will, happen (Carolina and Gustavo, 2003). Rather we would expect that different populations can take different paths and operate on different, historically contingent, time scales.

Third, there is a troubling "mix and match" flavor to the model. Some stages are labeled in terms of food production, others in terms of health and disease; some stages are described by the level of starches in the diet, others by the level of recreational activity. In addition, the changes characteristic of Stage 4 tend to be described in negative terms whereas those of the other stages are described in neutral terms. This lack of internal consistency to the Nutrition Transition model is unlike that found in the epidemiological and demographic transition models, which engage well-defined and circumscribed independent and dependent variables. For example, the demographic transition model makes specific predictions about a population's growth in size (the dependent variable) based on changes in birth rates and death rates (the independent variables). Each of the stages of the demographic transition is defined in terms of these particular variables, and the theoretical goal of the model is to explain how and why the independent variables change as a population shifts from a pre-industrial to an industrialized economic system.

Fourth, the Nutrition Transition model is limited to a general description of changes over time, and is not a model of the causal mechanisms responsible for those changes. Indeed, the forces responsible for the changes observed are not clearly understood. However, the language and structure of the Nutrition Transition imply that the model is explanatory, rather than descriptive. For instance, it is not useful to simply attribute the increasing incidence of obesity in low- or middle-income countries to the Nutrition Transition as if the model itself were the cause, rather than asking more precisely what social, economic, environmental, and/or dietary factors might have been responsible for the changes observed.

Fifth, the Nutrition Transition model is a generalized model of large-scale changes that obscures variation within subpopulations, and in doing so limits our understanding. It is clear that rural and urban populations within a given country, as well as the rich and the poor, live in separate worlds and hence their experience of nutrition transitions will be different.

CONCLUDING THOUGHTS

The Nutrition Transition model, as developed by Barry Popkin, conforms only loosely to current knowledge of the nutrition of past and present human populations. It is a model, and all models simplify reality, but too loose a coupling between the available evidence and what the model proposes to represent is not useful. We contend that the model represents past populations too simplistically and as too homogeneous. Similarly, the model minimizes the variability inherent in the current situation which blinds us to the reality of a world in which undernutrition and associated morbidity and mortality is all too present. We would argue that understanding variability *within* populations, not just between them, is key to recognizing the factors driving variability and hence the very nutrition transitions we observe. While we acknowledge the need to conceptualize, and model, broad macro-level processes of change, we would also argue the need for models that help us think about how macro-level phenomena translate to the micro-level changes we observe in individual populations. That is, how exactly does globalization lead to changes in diet, physical activity, and the prevalence of obesity in any given population?

Nutrition transitions have happened in the past and they are happening now. That much is clear. What we need to think about now is why these transitions occur, and how they shape the nutritional status of different populations throughout the world.

References

Bates DG, Lees SH. 1996. Pastoralism. In: Bates DG, Lees SH, editors. Case studies in human ecology. New York: Plenum Press. p 153–158.

Benyshek DC, Watson JT. 2006. Exploring the thrifty genotype's food-shortage assumptions: a cross-cultural comparison of ethnographic accounts of food security among foraging and agricultural societies. American Journal of Physical Anthropology 131:120–126.

Carolina MS, Gustavo LF. 2003. Epidemiological transition: model or illusion? A look at the problem of health in Mexico. Social Science and Medicine 57:539–550.

Colson E. 1979. In good years and in bad: food strategies of self-reliant societies. Journal of Anthropological Research 35:18–25.

Cordain L, Eaton SB, Sebastian A, Mann N, Lindeberg S, Watkins BA, O'Keefe JH, Brand-Miller J. 2005. Origins and evolution of the Western diet: health implications for the 21st century. American Journal of Clinical Nutrition 81:341–54.

Curran LS, Galvin KA. 1999. Subsistence, activity patterns and physical work capacity. In: Little MA, Leslie PW, editors. Turkana herders of the dry savanna. New York: Oxford University Press. p 147–163.

De Waal A. 2003. "New variant famine." AIDS and the food crisis in Southern Africa. The Lancet 362:1234–1237.

Dietler M. 1996. Feasts and commensal politics in the political economy: food, power, and status in prehistoric Europe. In: Wiessner P, Schieffenhövel W, editors. Food and the status quest: an interdisciplinary perspective. Providence: Berghahn Books. p 87–125.

Dirks R. 1993. Starvation and famine: cross-cultural codes and some hypothesis tests. Cross-Cultural Research 27:28–69.

Dirks R. 1980. Social responses during severe food shortages and famine. Current Anthropology 21:21–44.

Drewnowski A. 2000. Nutrition transition and global dietary trends. Nutrition. 16: 486–87.

Du S, Lu B, Zhai F, Popkin BM. 2002. The nutrition transition in China. In: Caballero B, Popkin BM, editors. The nutrition transition: diet and disease in the developing world. London: Academic Press. p 205–221.

Eaton SB, Konner M. 1985. Paleolithic nutrition: a consideration of its nature and current implications. The New England Journal of Medicine 312:283–289.

FAO (Food and Agricultural Organization of the United Nations). 2004. Globalization of food systems in developing countries: impact on food security and nutrition. Accessed at ftp://ftp.fao.org/docrep/fao/007/y5736e/y5736e02.pdf

FAO (Food and Agricultural Organization). Food balance sheets, accessed December 31, 2010 at http://faostat.fao.org/site/368/DesktopDefault.aspx?PageID=368#ancor

FAO (Food and Agricultural Organization of the United Nations) and ILSI (International Life Sciences Institute). 1997. Preventing micronutrient malnutrition - a guide to food-based approaches. Accessed at http://www.fao.org/docrep/x0245e/x0245e00.HTM

Finnis E. 2003. "Now I have an easy life": women's accounts of cassava, millets and labor in south India. Culture and Agriculture 31: 88–94.

Fratkin E, Roth EA. 1996. Who survives drought? Measuring winners and losers among the Ariaal Rendille pastoralists of Kenya. In: Bates DG, Lees SH, editors. Case studies in human ecology. New York: Plenum Press. p 159–174.

Galvin KA, Coppoch DL, Leslie PW. 1994. Diet, nutrition and the pastoral strategy. In: Fratkin E, Galvin KA, Roth EA, editors. African pastoral systems. Boulder: Lynne Reinner Publishers Inc. p 113–132.

Hayden B. 2003. Were luxury foods the first domesticates? Ethnoarchaeological perspectives from Southeast Asia. World Archaeology 34:458–469.

Kahn M. 1994. Always hungry, never greedy: food and the expression of gender in a Melanesian society. Prospect Heights, Illinois: Waveland Press. 187 p.

Kennedy G, Nantel G, Shetty P. 2004. Globalization of food systems in developing countries: a synthesis of country case studies. In: Globalization of food systems in developing countries: impact on food security and nutrition. FAO Food and Nutrition Paper 83. Rome: Food and Agricultural Organization of the United Nations. Accessed at ftp://ftp.fao.org/docrep/fao/007/y5736e/y5736e02.pdf

Kuromiya H. 2008. The Soviet famine of 1932–1933 reconsidered. Europe-Asia Studies 60:663–675.

Lansing S. 1991. Priests and programmers: technologies of power in the engineered landscape of Bali. Princeton University Press: Princeton. 183 p.

Larsen CS. 1995. Biological changes in human populations with agriculture. Annual Reviews of Anthropology 24:185–213.

Lee RB. 1968. What hunters do for a living, or, how to make out on scarce resources. In Lee RB, DeVore I, editors. Man the hunter. Chicago: Aldine Publishing Company. p 30–48.

Levins R. 1966. The strategy of model building in population biology. American Scientist 54: 421–431.

Monteiro CA, D'Aquino Benicio MH, da Cruz Gouveia N. 1994. Secular growth trends in Brazil over three decades. Annals of Human Biology 21:381–390.

Monteiro CA, Conde WL, Popkin BM. 2002. Is obesity replacing or adding to undernutrition? Evidence from different social classes in Brazil. Public Health Nutrition 5: 105–112.

Murton B. 2000. Famine. In: Kiple KF, Ornelas KC, editors. The Cambridge world history of food, volume two. Cambridge University Press. p 1411–1427.

Netting RM, Stone MP, Stone GD. 1996. Kofyar cash-cropping: choice and change in indigenous agricultural development. In: Bates DG, Lees SH, editors. Case studies in human ecology. New York: Plenum Press. p 327–348.

Omran AR. 1971. The epidemiologic transition: a theory of the epidemiology of population change. The Milbank Memorial Fund Quarterly 49:509–538.

Popkin BM. 1993. Nutritional patterns and transitions. Population and Development Review 19:138–157.

Popkin BM. 1994. The nutrition transition in low-income countries: an emerging crisis. Nutrition Reviews 52:285–298.

Popkin BM. 2002a. An overview on the nutrition transition and its health implications: the Bellagio meeting. Public Health Nutrition 5:93–103.

Popkin BM. 2002b. The shift in stages of the nutrition transition in the developing world differs from past experiences! Public Health Nutrition 5: 205–214.

Popkin BM. 2003. The nutrition transition in the developing world. Development Policy Reviews 21: 581–597.

Popkin BM. 2006. Global nutrition dynamics: the world is shifting rapidly toward a diet linked with noncommunicable diseases. American Journal of Clinical Nutrition 84:289–98.

Popkin BM. 2009. Global changes in diet and activity patterns as drivers of the nutrition transition. In: Kalhan SC, Prentice AM, Yajnik CS, editors. Emerging societies—coexistence of childhood malnutrition and obesity. Basel: Nestec Ltd., Vevey/S. Karger AG. p 1–14.

Popkin BM. 2009. The world is fat: the fads, trends, policies, and products that are fattening the human race. London: Penguin Books. 233 p.

Popkin BM, Gordon-Larsen P. 2004. The nutrition transition: worldwide obesity dynamics and their determinants. International Journal of Obesity 28:S2-S9.

Ramakrishnan U. 2002 Prevalence of micronutrient malnutrition worldwide. Nutrition Reviews 60:S46-S52.

Rappaport RA. 1968. Pigs for the ancestors: ritual in the ecology of a New Guinea people. New Haven: Yale University Press. 501 p.

Sawaya AL, Martins PA, Martins VJB. 2004. Impact of globalization on the food consumption health and nutrition in urban areas: a case study of Brazil. In: Globalization of food systems in developing countries: impact on food security and nutrition. FAO Food and Nutrition Paper 83. Rome: Food and Agricultural Organization of the United Nations. Accessed at ftp://ftp.fao.org/docrep/fao/007/y5736e/y5736e02.pdf

Scoones I. 1996. Coping with drought: responses of herders and livestock in contrasting savanna environments in southern Zimbabwe. In: Bates DG, Lees SH, editors. Case studies in human ecology. New York: Plenum Press. p 175–194.

Thompson WS. 1929. Population. American Journal of Sociology 34:959–975.

USDA National Database for Windows.

Vepa, S. 2004. Impact of globalization on the food consumption of urban India. In: Globalization of food systems in developing countries: impact on food security and nutrition. FAO Food and Nutrition Paper 83. Rome: Food and Agricultural Organization of the United Nations. Accessed at ftp://ftp.fao.org/docrep/fao/007/y5736e/y5736e02.pdf

WHO Global Data Base on Body Mass Index. Accessed February 19, 2010 at http://apps.who.int/bmi/index.jsp

CHAPTER 42

Coca-Colonization of Diets in the Yucatan

Thomas L. Leatherman and Alan Goodman

(2005)

INTRODUCTION

Throughout Latin America and much of the developing world, nations are turning to tourism as a means for generating foreign capital and economic development. Stonich (1998) notes that international tourism to Central America has grown dramatically since the 1980s, with annual growth rates in arrivals and receipts of 11.5% and 16.8%, respectively, between 1987 and 1991. Mexico is the leader of this trend in Central America, and the primary destination is the Caribbean coast of the state of Quintana Roo in the Yucatan Peninsula. Cancun, the center of this development, grew from a fishing village of about 426 inhabitants in the early 1970s, to the state's most important city with a population of over 400,000 people by the early 1990s (Daltabuit & Leatherman, 1998). In the last three decades, Quintana Roo has experienced a transformation from one of the most economically marginal areas of Mexico into a tourist bonanza, an unqualified economic success for the Mexican government and foreign investors. The tourism industry also brings cash and increased purchasing power to the many Maya who build and maintain the infrastructures and work in tourism's service economy.

Anthropological research on tourism has focused on the economic, social, and cultural impacts on local communities and peoples. Tourism disrupts local subsistence activities as more small producers turn to wage labor, increases economic and social differentiation (and conflicts), and can lead to the "commodification of culture", in which cultural items or rituals become valued primarily in terms of their exchange value (Stronza, 2001). Tourism development can affect environmental degradation, water quality, nutrition, and health (Stonich, 1998). Similarly, tourism research in the Yucatan has concluded that as environmental resources, labor, and food become increasingly commoditized, and symbols of prestige become increasingly western, disruptions to environment, economy, culture, and health are inevitable (Daltabuit & Pi-Sunyer,

1990; Daltabuit & Leatherman, 1998; Pi–Sunyer & Thomas, 1997).

The questions raised in this paper concern how these dynamics of change are linked to the production of health in Mayan families and communities. One set of concerns highlights the economic, socio-cultural, and psychological dimensions of these changes. In their study of tourism in the Yucatan, Pi–Sunyer and Thomas (1997) argued that tourism constitutes a totalizing experience which affects not only families' economic and social activities but also their broader sense of community and cultural identity. A second set of concerns that we address more centrally in our research relates to how tourism-led development has affected Mayan food systems, diets, and nutritional health. One of the major ways that local communities interact with their environment, and reflect and reify culture is through food systems. Hence, changes in food systems and diets are a critical piece of the cultural and social transformations that accompany tourism-led development. In turn, dietary changes directly link development to measurable changes in human nutrition and health. Since the pioneering work by Scrimshaw, Taylor, and Gordon (1968), the negative synergism between nutrition and disease is well known. Macro and micronutrient deficiencies can impact health by affecting growth, physical and cognitive development, working capacity, reproduction, immune systems and disease resistance, and also the absorption and utilization of other nutrients (Allen, 1984, 1993; Martorell, 1980, 1989; Chavez & Martinez, 1982).

Based on our research in the Yucatan since 1989, and work by Daltabuit (1988) and Pi–Sunyer and Thomas (1997), we expected that there might be considerable variation and ambiguity in how tourism-led social, economic, and cultural change affects nutrition, health, and other indicators of well-being. Some individuals spoke of the past 20 years as having been a time of increased income and economic resources, better and more diverse diets, and an improved quality of life. Others noted declines in agricultural productivity and the availability of locally produced foodstuffs, which for them meant a diminished dietary diversity. Studies of child growth, as an indicator of community nutrition and health in the Yucatan Peninsula (Gurri & Balam, 1992; Gurri, Balam & Moran, 2001; Leatherman, Stillman, & Goodman, 2000), have noted an increase in stature and weight over the

Thomas L. Leatherman and Alan Goodman, "Coca-colonization of diets in the Yucatan." *Social Science & Medicine* 61 (2005):833–846. Reprinted with permission.

past few decades indicating improved health and/or nutritional conditions. However, stature is still low, indicating the persistent presence of chronic undernutrition. Gurri and Balam (1992) further note that caloric undernutrition is a lesser problem now than in the past, but that other nutrient deficiencies continue to affect nutritional status in Mayan communities. Also, adult obesity and associated diseases such as hypertension and diabetes are clearly increasing in urban and peri-urban locales in the Yucatan (Dickinson, Castillo, Vales, & Uc, 1993). Dickinson et al. (1993) depict current shifts in Mayan diets in and around Merida (the capital of Yucatan) as indicative of a "double-edged sword of malnutrition," where childhood malnutrition is replaced by adult obesity later in life. Here, we go a step further in suggesting that this doubled-edged problem of micronutrient undernutrition and adult obesity is in part due to coca-colonization.

These ambiguities reflect the manner in which the social, cultural, and health impacts of tourism-led development are distributed unevenly and experienced unequally among Mayan communities, families, and individuals. Much of this variation is influenced by the manner and degree to which communities, households, and individuals articulate with the tourism-based economy and their relative economic success. For example, in households with steady, predictable incomes, an increase in markets can provide access to more foods throughout the year, enhanced dietary diversity, and improved nutritional status. However, past research has more commonly found that a movement away from traditional diets and towards greater market dependency often has the opposite effect: a decline in the dietary diversity and nutritional status of peasant communities (e.g., Pelto & Pelto, 1983; Dewey, 1989). As fewer local foods are produced and reliance on market foods increases, cash poor households are likely to suffer nutritionally.

In this article, we address how tourism-based economic development creates the conditions for new and often unequal social relations, food systems and diets, thereby resulting in differential nutrition and health of Yucatec Mayans. Specifically, we explore the linkages between food commoditization, diet, and nutritional status in Mayan communities and households with qualitatively and quantitatively different involvement in local food production and the tourism economy. High calorie, low-nutrient snack foods are a particularly strong and pernicious example of commercialized processed foods, and we are interested in understanding their increasingly common and widespread consumption and potential impact on child and adult nutritional status.

BACKGROUND

Until relatively recently, the Maya of the Yucatan Peninsula had successfully resisted greater assimilation into the Mexican and Western cultural and economic systems. This is no longer the case. Mayan communities are enmeshed in the broader tourism-based economy as construction workers, tour guides, and artisans, as well as waiters, maids, and gardeners in tourist resorts. The movement of people and goods is facilitated by a recently expanded road network that now connects Quintana Roo with its bordering states. Cancun is linked to Merida by a toll road 'super-highway', and is connected to the world through an international airport that by the mid-1990s was bringing in over 1.5 million foreign tourists each year (Pi–Sunyer & Thomas, 1997). The 126 km of coastline leading south from Cancun to the historic community and ancient Mayan archeological site of Tulum is well on its way to being completely developed. Many of these developments are gated resort communities catering to tourists of specific nationalities, while the beach-front accessible to Mayan residents is quickly diminishing.

While Mayan communities have a long history of articulation with capitalist enterprises in boom and bust economic cycles (e.g., sugar, chicle, and henequen production systems), they have always relied upon and enjoyed the security of slash-and-burn *milpa* agriculture. This locally based production system provided the key staples of corn, beans and squash, complemented with fruits, peppers, herbs, medicinals, chickens, turkeys, and pigs, all grown in home gardens (Kintz, 1980). With the growth of the tourist economy, however, households and communities have become increasingly dependent on the large urban centers for income (Daltabuit & Pi–Sunyer, 1990; Kintz, 1980), and we have observed that reliance on milpa agriculture and home gardens often declines (Daltabuit & Leatherman, 1998). A new generation of Mayans prefer to seek their fortune in "Cancun" (i.e., the tourist economy), rather than in the milpa. Some young men refer to the drudgery of milpa work as "*trabajo rudo*" (coarse, rough work), preferring service jobs or even construction work at tourist centers. Despite a continued practice of patrilocal residence, some young families have ceased to pool resources and labor, or even share food and meal preparation with their parents and in-laws. This reflects a social independence consistent with economic independence for young families; yet for their parents, it reflects an erosion of the very meaning of family and community and, in more practical terms, means an erosion of social and economic security for parental generations, and potentially a scarcity of labor for milpa production and household domestic tasks.

Decreased milpa production and a growth in commoditized food and labor markets have increased Mayan dependence on non-traditional and store-bought foods (Daltabuit, 1988; Daltabuit & Leatherman, 1998). Although shifts from locally produced to market and commercialized foods have been associated with improved levels of nutrition in industrialized nations, such shifts often have a negative impact on nutrition in developing countries (Pelto & Pelto, 1983). In many developing countries, of which Mexico is no exception, rapid economic development leads to large disparities in wealth rather than increased wealth for the population as a whole. Therefore, while growth in markets may increase dietary diversity, much of the population may be unable to afford market prices, and decreased subsistence production coupled with an inability to purchase foods will lead to reduced dietary diversity (Pelto & Pelto, 1983; Dewey, 1989).

The exception to this pattern might be found in households with steady, predictable incomes and hence access to greater dietary diversity. Adequate cash flows provide households with real access to markets, from which they can buy a diversity of better quality foods at less expense and in greater bulk. A steady income can also serve to dampen seasonal variation in the availability of locally produced foods, especially in regions such as the Yucatan with a single main rainy and growing season. Thus, shifts toward commoditized food systems provide a context in which inequalities in access to adequate diets might emerge and increase.

RESEARCH DESIGN AND METHODS

Community Contexts

To examine how the tourism-led economic change has produced different patterns of food systems, diet, and nutritional health in the Yucatan, we have been conducting research in Mayan communities that differ in subsistence base and articulation with the tourist industry. These include two inland communities, Yalcoba and Coba, and two coastal communities, Akumal and Ciudad Chemuyil. We conducted research on health and nutrition in Yalcoba in 1989 and 1991, and a preliminary dietary survey in Coba and Yalcoba in 1994. We then carried out household dietary surveys in the coastal communities in 1996, and in Yalcoba and Coba in 1998, as well as studies of child growth in Yalcoba in 1998. This work has been part of a larger effort of a group of anthropologists studying the social, economic, cultural, and health effects of the rapid growth in the tourist economy in the Yucatan, including students and professors (Brooke Thomas and Oriole Pi–Sunyer of the University of Massachusetts, and Magali Daltabuit of UNAM in Mexico) from the US and Mexico. We draw liberally from their insights, as well as our observations and experiences, in presenting the contexts of research.

One set of communities, Akumal and Ciudad Chemuyil, arose as service villages to popular resorts on the Caribbean coast. Many of the immigrants to these communities came from two inland Mayan communities in the state of Yucatan, Sotuta and Kantunil. Ciudad Chemuyil was designed and built in the 1990s by a consortium of hotels and the Mexican government to house the growing worker population needed for the expanding tourist industry (Pi–Sunyer & Thomas, 1997). It consists of a school, stores, a few restaurants, and about 250 cinderblock homes on small plots of land. Residents have no agricultural land and little land for home gardens, and thus are totally dependent on local markets for access to food.

The community of Akumal first arose as a squatter settlement on land adjacent to the resort of the same name.

Residents were subsequently forced to move to Ciudad Chemuyil, or to another site about 5 km away (also called Akumal), on the other side of the main highway that runs along the coast. The new Akumal community includes stores, a school, and housing plots of different sizes that might allow for a fruit tree or small home gardens.

Kinship relations often connect families from the two communities. Some families have moved back and forth, and intermingle with the local (tourist) economy and food systems in similar ways (e.g., as construction workers, gardeners, waiters, cooks, maids, tourist guides, and small-scale entrepreneurs running businesses oriented toward tourists or fellow residents). Neither has the resources to produce their own food and must rely on local markets. Therefore, despite the distance and the different physical layouts and origin of these two communities, for this paper the households interviewed in each are combined to form a single sample representing a coastal service community.

A third community, Coba, is a farming village of about 900 persons, settled about 50 years ago by immigrants from nearby zones looking for new land (Kintz, 1980). Some residents work in the coastal tourist economy, but far more are involved in the tourist economy through "archeotourism", because Coba is the gateway community to the famous Classic Maya archeological site from which the community takes its name. Taking advantage of the flow of approximately 60,000 tourists per year to the archeological site (Pi–Sunyer & Thomas, 1997), the town of Coba currently hosts a smattering of tourist-oriented businesses including a few restaurants, about a dozen souvenir shops, and two hotels (one budget and the other run by Club Med). By all accounts, tourism in Coba is highly seasonal: some restaurants and stores stay open only during prime tourist season. While there are visible signs of asymmetries in wealth between local entrepreneurs and small-scale producers, real incomes (and improved diet diversity) are reported to vary seasonally based on highs and lows in tourism. Coba has a wealth of land for making milpa, but one informant estimated that only about 50% of *ejiditarios* (individuals with access to communal ejido lands for farming) planted fields in 1998, and that many of those who did hired someone else to plant for them.

Yalcoba, the fourth community, is an old settlement of about 1500 inhabitants, located near the town of Valladolid, toward the center of the Yucatan peninsula. A 16th century church and near-by classic and post-classic Mayan ruins stand as testimony to the long settlement history of the town. In contrast to the other communities, Yalcoba has little direct exposure to tourism, but many of its men and some women work at construction and service jobs in Cancun and other tourism areas. The percent of households involved in the Cancun migration increased steadily between the mid-1980s and mid-1990s from about 45% to over 75% (Daltabuit & Leatherman, 1998). As well, hammock making on consignment has emerged as another source of cash generation. Otherwise, there are few local opportunities for wage work. In contrast to Coba, ejido lands in Yalcoba are limited in size and overworked, making it difficult for young families to engage in home food production. The only way to obtain new lands for the community has been to petition the government for an expanded ejido, but these fields would necessarily be even farther from the community. Already, some younger households with limited access to ejido lands might walk over 12 km to get to fields. Because the community and number of ejiditarios have grown, fields are left fallow for shorter periods between planting, and this leads to decreased productivity. Decreased productivity in farming was a common response by local residents to questions about what they considered major changes in the region over the past three decades.

METHODS

We conducted surveys of 30 coastal households (15 in Akumal and 15 in Cd. Chemuyil), and 30 households each from Coba and Yalcoba. The surveys collected information on household demographic, social, and economic characteristics, food acquisition (e.g., from *milpa* production, home gardens, and purchases in local stores and larger markets), and dietary intake, as well as a variety of perceptions of social change, soft drink consumption, and the quality of local vs. non-local foods. In each community, we also visited most stores and noted the range of foods and products, and the marketing displays of sodas and snack foods. We asked store owners about food purchasing patterns in the community, and supplemented this information with opportunistic observations (30–60 min) of purchasing patterns of visitors to larger stores as part of participant observation. In 1998, we collected anthropometric data on school children in Yalcoba, measuring height, weight, upper-arm circumference, and triceps and sub-scapular skinfolds, according to standard techniques (Frisancho, 1990). Finally, we rely on participant observation and informant interviews, during repeated visits to all communities (but especially Yalcoba) over a 4-year period, to better understand the changing economic strategies, diets, and degree of commercialization of the food system.

The dietary data presented here are derived from a 7-day food frequency and recall from the family: both how often a food item was eaten and the amount consumed over a week. Because recalls of the frequency and quantities of some foods eaten at meals during the week were not precise, some of the data on quantity of consumption was collected in terms of food purchased and prepared for the entire family. For example, the female head of household knew exactly the amount of *masa* (corn meal) used and consumed as tortillas, even if individual members could not recall how many tortillas they ate for a given meal or day.

From earlier pilot surveys, the work of Daltabuit (1988), and information from informants, we developed a food list to prompt for foods eaten regularly, and inquired about other foods consumed in the previous week. Given this background information, and because households consume primarily what is stored from earlier harvests or what

they purchase from local markets, we are confident that all or most foods consumed in the home were recorded. We may have missed some foods consumed out of the household, especially sodas and snack foods consumed by children; thus, these items are likely underestimated in weekly recalls. It is important to note that these dietary data were collected in the summer months (mostly June and July), and, therefore, do not represent the seasonal variation of an annual diet. Also, they are a measure of consumption in the household residence and do not include diets of workers living away from the family during the week.

We analyze and report the data from the household weekly food consumption in three ways. First, we list key food items and their caloric contribution to the diet to illustrate the range of dietary diversity in each community. Dietary diversity is an important measure of dietary quality because more diverse diets tend to be more nutritionally balanced if caloric requirements are met (Allen, Backstrand, & Stanek, 1992). Second, as another measure of diversity and quality of diets, we present the caloric contribution of macronutrients (carbohydrates, fats, proteins) and protein quality in each community. Protein quality (PQ) is an indicator of the availability of protein (and its constituent amino acids) in the diet. A low PQ indicates that one or more amino acids are deficient. Third, we provide an estimate of how rich diets are in micronutrient intakes (i.e., vitamins and minerals) by presenting the amount of select micronutrients standardized to a 2000-kcal daily intake (i.e., amount of micronutrient present in a 2000-kcal diet). Data entry and analyses were done using The Food Processor® Nutrition Analysis Software from ESHA Research, Salem, OR (Version 7.0).

Recent work had suggested that caloric undernutrition among Mayan communities in the Yucatan was much less of a problem than in past decades (Gurri et al., 2000), perhaps a benefit of the market and government-sponsored stores (CONASUP) that now provide basic staples. Hence, attention has turned to micronutrient deficiencies as a critical nutritional problem. These deficiencies have likely always been a problem but received less attention compared to caloric deficiency. Also, the nature of the weekly household food frequency did not consistently yield precise caloric intakes for individual family members, and lent itself better to analyses of nutrient density based on a standardized caloric intake.

In order to evaluate the adequacy of nutrient densities, we compared our results to densities required to meet recommended dietary allowances (RDAs) for a 7–10-year-old child with a caloric requirement of approximately 2000 kcals per day. We chose to estimate adequacy of micronutrient intake in children for three reasons. First, children in the 7–10 age range are less likely to be away from the household for meals during the week. Second, child growth is frequently used to estimate the nutrition and health of entire communities, and thus our estimates of dietary quality and nutritional status are made in roughly similar age groups. Third, by estimating dietary adequacy in children, we are providing a more conservative measure of micronutrient deficiency for the community and household. While children often do not have equal access to all foods served at the family meal, our estimates assume that they do, which may underestimate deficiencies. Two other factors make for conservative estimates of micronutrient deficiency. First, nutrient densities are based on the dietary diversity of a weekly food intake, yet daily diets were substantially less diverse (e.g., meat was often only eaten on weekends). Second, our estimates do not account for reduced bioavailablity (absorption and utilization) of nutrients, a frequent characteristic of less diverse diets.

Child growth and body composition is a commonly used indicator of nutrition and health status for individuals and communities and is presented here as a link between dietary quality and nutritional status. The analysis has two goals. One is to illustrate a potential link between dietary quality, nutrition, and health for at least one community (Yalcoba). The other is to draw suggestive links between tourism-based economic change, diet, and child growth. Because our most complete sample of child growth was obtained in Yalcoba, and data collected previously in Yalcoba is available for comparison (Daltabuit, 1988), we use only the growth data from Yalcoba in the present analysis. Also, we were able to calculate estimates of adult body mass index (BMI) in Yalcoba using stature and weight measurements from clinic records, and this provides data for a broader pattern of growth, body composition, and nutrition for this community.

FOOD COMMODITIZATION

As milpa production has declined and the availability of markets with foods produced outside of the area has increased, Yucatecans are increasingly consuming goods and foods produced out of the area—a process of dietary delocalization. The nature of food commoditization, however, is markedly different for the coastal (Akumal and Ciudad Chemuyil) vs. inland maize-producing communities (Coba and Yalcoba). In the coastal communities, a fully commercial and commoditized system is now in place. Most foods are purchased year round from local stores, weekly markets, and traveling vendors specializing in food stuffs from specific growing regions. For example, fruit is typically purchased from vendors bringing it from Oxkutzcab, a farming and orchard town to the west, while meat is often bought from vendors from Sotuta, a town closer to Merida and the original home of a number of residents. Weekly markets adjacent to the resort community of Akumal and nearby Tulum bring vendors and food from Chiapas and occasionally farther west. Local *tiendas* (small variety stores) sell basic staples, canned goods, sodas, and snack foods. Local restaurants, sandwich shops, and pizzerias offer noon and evening meals for residents and workers. Workers within the resorts purchase soft drinks, candy bars, and chips at tourist prices for morning snacks and noontime meals from tiendas in the resorts.

In the two inland communities, products from the milpa (primarily corn, beans, squash, melons) are harvested and available for consumption seasonally. Most produce is consumed within the household, although the general availability of local products increases during these times. A common complaint in both Coba and Yalcoba is that the productivity of local *ejido* lands had decreased markedly in the past several decades. Very few families grow enough corn to last a year, and more foods of all sorts must be purchased, especially during the summer months leading into the next harvest. We noted no great differences in the degree of food commoditization in Yalcoba and Coba.

By the mid-1980s in Yalcoba, Daltabuit (1988) had already noted a shift from local foods and drinks that had been important in the past (such as honey, tubers, and wild meat) toward commercial foodstuffs (including rice and pasta), of which sodas and snack foods were key elements. This trend was even more pronounced in the 1990s. Even maize and beans, two key staples, are often bought from government-subsidized stores (CONASUP) that import them from Chiapas and beyond. Local tiendas sell small quantities of produce (tomatoes, potatoes, cabbage, carrots, onions, garlic, and peppers) and a few staples (dried beans, rice, and pasta) purchased in larger towns and resold locally. Some households in both communities travel to the nearby city of Valladolid in order to purchase better quality and a wider choice of fruits, vegetables and meat at lower cost. Taxis now regularly make the 24 km trip between Yalcoba and Valladolid, facilitating these trips. Locally grown fruit is available seasonally and other fruits are brought to the villages by vendors in trucks and then distributed on tricycles. Fruits and vegetables do not preserve well in the heat, and the only households able to consume a variety of fruits and vegetables year round are those few with refrigerators (their purchase made possible by the increased cash from wage work). In addition to extending the life of produce and meats, families with refrigerators often stock and sell sodas.

Compared to 10 years ago, a greater variety of foods is available in rural communities, but at a higher cost to households. As one resident of Coba noted "there are more foods available now, but no money to buy them." Thus, many households in the more rural communities of Coba and Yalcoba see the past 20 years as a time of steadily decreasing food availability. Moreover, there is a preference for the taste, quality, and storage capacity of local foods over those bought through CONASUP. A few individuals stated that local foods were fresher and (nutritionally) better than those from other areas. Thus, while a commercialized food system and dietary delocalization is universally accepted, the replacement of local staples and foods by those from another region does not go unnoticed or uncritically accepted.

Coca-Colonization

The most dramatic aspect of the commercialization of food systems in the region is the pervading presence of *Coca-Cola*®, *Pepsi*®, and an assortment of chips, cookies, candies, and other high-sugar, high-fat snack foods, collectively called "*comidas chatarras*" (junk foods). Such foods are frequently labeled as 'empty calories' or 'calorie-dense but nutrient-poor' foods. This does not mean all snack foods have no useful nutrients. For the most part the sodas and candies are 'empty' of nutrients, while chips and cookies provide limited amounts of nutrients. However, the nutrient contributions relative to sugar or fat are small.

While Coca-Cola products have been distributed in Mexico and the Yucatan since the early 20th century, bottled soft drinks became a staple commodity when road networks and electricity—hence refrigeration—were established. This infrastructure development was accelerated in the early 1970s with the development of the coast as a tourist zone. By the 1990s, Mexico had already become one of the world's largest consumers of soft drinks, with an annual per capita consumption of 560 8-oz. servings accounting for over 20% of Pepsi's and 15% of Coke's international sales (Jabbonsky, 1993). In 1999, their annual per capita consumption of 431 servings of Coca-Cola products alone was the highest of any country in the world, and marked a 23% increase over the previous 5 years (Coca–Cola Company, 1999). Mexico, and the Yucatan, is the site of an ongoing "Cola War" between Coke and Pepsi, as executives see it—a fight over the "stomach share" of the Mexican people. Coke's goal and company slogan is "an arm's length from desire"—that is, to make Coke available at every corner in every town or village in every part of Mexico (Pendergrast, 2000). Indeed, this goal seems to be met in Yalcoba, where one can purchase a soft drink, and often a Coke, at over 40 tiendas.

Pepsi has waged their version of the "Cola Wars" using a strategy of "the Power of One". This entails marketing Pepsi soda in conjunction with junk foods. Pepsico's logo is found on the majority of the chips, cookies, candies, and other processed snack foods seen on prominent displays in tiendas. This has been a successful strategy that has helped them capture market shares from Coke. It is likely, then, that Coca-Cola will have no choice but to compete by creating their own linkages between beverages and snacks. If this comes to pass, the fight for "stomach share" will intensify and we can expect to see an even greater penetration of soda and snack foods in the diets of Mexicans and the Yucatec Maya.

Currently in Coba and Yalcoba, both Pepsi and Coke trucks make weekly visits to large and small stores. In order to acquire new clients, company representatives will paint new signs on tiendas, set up display cases, and provide coolers for the sodas. Upon entering almost any tienda, displays of snack food are the first things to catch one's eyes. In addition to sodas and name brand snack foods, jars of cheap candies are found on most counters. Indeed, our observations suggest that most children who enter tiendas leave with some form of candy, chips, or a drink. Moreover, given the few opportunities for small investment in Yalcoba or Coba, many home-based stores have sprung up locally, doing little more than selling sodas. A 5-min walk now puts all but the most isolated households in the community within "an arm's length of desire".

Local distributors of soft drinks in Coba and Yalcoba in 1996 and 1998 reported weekly sales reflecting an average per capita consumption of one soda per day, while in the coastal service villages of Akumal and Chemuyil consumption is at least 50% greater. Also, given that the very young and very old consume fewer soft drinks, these estimates should be higher for children, adolescents, and adults. In 1996, 75 school-aged children in Yalcoba reported average daily intakes of just over one 12 oz. soft drink (mostly Coke or Pepsi), 1.5 packaged snack foods (e.g., chips or cookies), and 1.7 small candies (e.g., suckers). Maximum daily individual consumption rates reported were about four to five sodas, seven snack foods, and six candies. During a morning school break in Yalcoba, it is typical for children to buy a soft drink and a snack. This simple treat accounts for nearly 400 cal, about one-fifth of an elementary school child's daily requirement (Daltabuit, 1988; McGarty, 1995). They are largely consumed away from the household and are consequently underreported in weekly dietary reports.

For our informants, coke is not food (*alimento*): it has no redeeming nutritional qualities, other than being sweet with sugar. Rather it is drunk "*por gusto*"—for pleasure and taste. Indeed, to see a man or woman taking a break from work on a hot afternoon with a cold soda illustrates the role of soft drinks as providing a moment of leisure and pleasure. Yet many feel that one can drink too much, and speak of how consuming too many cokes in one's youth makes one 'accustomed to' wanting a soda. Informants in the two inland communities consider cokes and other sodas too strong and inappropriate for babies and young children; they can cause parasites, gas, and stomach cramps. Nevertheless, it is not uncommon to see a young infant with a coke or another soft drink.

FOOD CONSUMPTION

A community comparison of foods commonly eaten by percent contribution to energy is presented in Table 1. As might be expected, individuals surveyed from the coastal resort service communities of Akumal and Chemuyil have a greater dietary diversity; eight types of foods contribute at least 5% of total caloric intake, compared to four to five foods in the two inland communities. Compared to inland communities, weekly food frequencies in the two coastal communities include half the tortillas, three times the sodas and snack foods, three times dairy, twice the fruits, and from one and a half to four times the meat contribution to calories. For each of these food items, and for sugar, the differences among the communities is significant (Anova, $p < .02$), and the difference is primarily based on values in the coastal vs. inland communities. The two inland communities differ significantly only in meat and sugar consumption (*t*-test, $p < .01$).

Maize tortillas are the major contributor to caloric intake in all communities, but especially in Coba and Yalcoba (Table 1). Oil and lard are next, followed by soft drinks and

Table 1 Commonly Consumed Foods and Macronutrients

	COASTAL (N = 26)	COBA (N = 30)	YALCOBA (N = 24)
Food items			
Tortillas	23.0	44.0	46.0
Oil/lard	12.0	10.5	9.5
Sodas/snacks	12.0	4.5	4.0
Sugar	4.0	6.0	4.0
Beans	5.0	6.0	6.0
Meat	8.0	2.0	5.0
Rice/pasta	4.5	5.5	3.0
Bread/crackers	5.0	4.0	3.0
Fruits	6.0	3.0	3.0
Eggs	3.0	2.5	2.0
Dairy	3.5	1.0	1.0
Macronutrients			
Carbohydrate	62.5	69.3	68.6
Fat	29.2	23.3	23.2
Protein	11.6	10.6	11.0
Protein quality	79.0	67.0	73.0

The top part of this table lists the percent contribution of commonly consumed food to total caloric intake (median value) and the bottom part provides the percent estimated total contributions of macronutrients to energy and protein quality scores.

snack foods. Together, sugar and these snack foods account, on an average, for 16% of calories in the coastal communities, compared to 10.5% in Coba and 8% in Yalcoba. Beans and rice/pastas are fairly evenly represented in the three communities. Meat and eggs (combined) comprised 11% in coastal diets, 7% of Yalcoba, and only 4.5% in Coba. The greater meat consumption in Yalcoba was due to more local production of pigs and beef, and the closer proximity of Yalcoba to markets in Valladolid. The main source of dairy in both inland communities is powdered milk, often consumed as a chocolate drink for breakfast. Fruit consumption during the survey was comprised almost entirely of locally produced fruits, specifically mangoes in Yalcoba and guayas in Coba.

The percent of calories coming from the basic macronutrients (carbohydrate, protein, and fat) is subtly different in the three locales (Anova, $p < .01$). The relative contributions of protein and fat are higher on the coast, and more of the protein comes from meat and other animal products. Hence, PQ scores of coastal diets are higher than in Yalcoba and Coba (Anova, $p < .01$). Yalcoba and Coba do not significantly differ in macronutrient contribution to caloric intake, but Yalcoba does have significantly greater PQ scores ($p < .03$, t-test).

The smaller consumption of tortillas in the coastal communities is both a material and symbolic reflection of dietary change. Part of the difference is based on incomes and the role of tortillas as an inexpensive staple that can be used to feed and fill the stomachs of large families with limited resources. In coastal communities, we failed to find a relationship between tortilla consumption and household economic status, or between consumption of tortillas and other foods. In the two inland communities, however, higher tortilla consumption is a sign of relative decreased consumption of most other staples (oil, rice/pasta, dairy in Coba, and rice/pasta, meat sugar, beans, and fruit in Yalcoba; $p < .05$), and is indirectly a sign of relative poverty. Yet, tortillas are also culturally and symbolically important. While watching government trucks unload corn and other foodstuffs following a major hurricane and drought in 1991, a friend in Yalcoba muttered, "How many of us will starve this year?" We commented on the quantity of corn being unloaded, and she replied that this corn was not suitable for making good tortillas. For her, and others, without tortillas there is no real meal, amounting to symbolic and psychological (if not nutritional) starvation.

Not only are fewer tortillas eaten in coastal communities but increasingly those consumed are processed soft white flour tortillas, as opposed to corn tortillas typical of most rural areas and both Yalcoba and Coba. This shift, accompanied by greater consumption of bread, crackers, and other replacement starches, reflects the marked shifts in preferences and dietary styles, as well as coastal community lifestyles. If we consider the cultural position of locally made tortillas in inland farming communities, the same sort of communities from which coastal residents emigrated, then these shifts in consumption patterns on the coast can provide a metaphor for broader cultural transformations and lifestyles that have occurred in a relatively short time.

MICRONUTRIENT PROFILES

Micronutrient adequacies are based on a 7-day food record and estimates of nutrient adequacy for a 7–10-year-old child consuming 2000 kcals daily (Table 2). The more diverse diets of the service communities on the coast provide greater density and adequacy for most nutrients compared to the inland communities (Anova, p <.01 for vitamins A, B2, B12, and E). The only exception is zinc, which is also low in Coba and Yalcoba. Our analyses detected other potential deficiencies in Coba and Yalcoba: vitamin B2 or riboflavin, B12 (cobalamin) and vitamin E in Yalcoba; and vitamins A, B2, and B12 in Coba. In both the inland communities, tortilla consumption, as an indirect reflection of poverty, is negatively correlated with a number of micronutrients such as vitamins A, B12, C, E, and specifically with PQ scores in Coba, and vitamins B12 and E in Yalcoba (p <.05). In addition, the high phytate content of corn greatly decreases the bioavailability of zinc and iron (Allen et al., 1992).

The greater vitamin A (retinol) intake in Yalcoba compared to Coba (p <.03, t-test) is almost entirely due to the widespread availability of mangos from local *solares* (home gardens) and the relative paucity of mangos and other locally available fruits in Coba. Both the inland communities ingest adequate levels of vitamin C due in part to regular consumption of 'chaya', a leafy plant grown in home gardens, that is high in protein and several micronutrients, including vitamin C. The contribution of mangos and *chaya* to local diets illustrates the critical importance of home gardens to diets, and specifically to micronutrient profiles.

The importance of incomes for shaping diets and nutrient profiles is illustrated by comparing households from Yalcoba with steady employment in the tourist economy (and relatively higher incomes) and others relying on local subsistence production and irregular wage work to meet basic needs (Table 3). Households with steady incomes eat 20% fewer tortillas, over twice the amount of meat/eggs, fruit, and other sources of complex carbohydrates (rice, pasta, breads, crackers). The percent contribution of protein to calories (11.8%) and the median PQ score (80.5) is slightly higher in these higher-income families than the average for the coastal communities (Tables 1 and 3). Due to small sample sizes, significant differences are found only for tortilla, bread, and fruit consumption, and for PQ (p <.01, t-test). Households with steady incomes also have relatively higher levels of vitamins A, B2, and B12 but are not immune to the generally low levels of vitamin E and zinc (all nutrient comparisons not statistically significant). These comparisons also suggest that families in Yalcoba relying on irregular wage work and milpa production may be experiencing deficiencies in vitamin A, as well as deficiencies in the B vitamins, vitamin E, and zinc.

Households with steady employment can purchase a variety of foods year round, while others households are more dependent on the local harvest and temporary wage jobs. And given a string of poor harvests and natural disasters, most families depended on wage jobs to acquire the foods they ate. Yet employment in the tourist industry is often unpredictable, both in availability of work and adequacy of wages. Temporary work in Cancun without benefits or health care is usually available, but the kind of steady employment with a living wage associated with improved dietary diversity and micronutrient profiles is more rare, and is dependent on skills, interpersonal relationships, and luck. Besides regular access to cash, another key difference we saw in economically successful households was owning a refrigerator, which enabled these families to consume meats,

Table 2 Percent RDA's for Micronutrient Intake Based on US Child, 7–10 Years (Median Value)

Micronutrients	% RDA		
	Coastal %	Coba %	Yalcoba %
Vitamin A	> 100	53.1	85.1
Riboflavin	> 100	74.9	74.5
Vitamin B12	> 100	63.8	76.7
Vitamin C	> 100	> 100	> 100
Vitamin E	> 100	87.7	59.9
Iron	> 100	> 100	> 100
Zinc	69.6	72.1	79.5

Data are based on weekly food frequencies questionnaires.

Table 3 Diet Composition and Nutrition in Yalcoba Households of Different Economic Positions (% RDA's for US Child 7–10 Years: Median Values)

Dietary component	Steady income "Cancun" (N = 10)	Milpa production and irregular wages (N = 14)
Foods (% kcals)		
Tortillas	31.5	51.5
Oil/lard	10.0	9.0
Sugar/sodas/snacks	9.0	8.0
Meat & Eggs	7.0	3.0
Beans	6.0	5.0
Rice/pasta	5.0	3.0
Bread	5.0	1.0
Fruits	6.5	2.5
Dairy	1.5	0.0
Macronutrient (% kcals)		
Carbohydrate	65.3	70.0
Fat	25.9	22.6
Protein	11.8	10.7
Protein quality	80.5	69.5
%RDA of micronutrients		
Vitamin A	91.8	71.1
Riboflavin	78.1	73.9
Vitamin B12	82.6	69.7
Vitamin E	59.9	60.1
Zinc	81.6	77.9

fruits, and vegetables more regularly and to buy in greater quantities at more economical markets in larger towns.

In contrast to Yalcoba, we found no clear differences in diet and nutrient profiles between households of different economic status in Coba. We believe one reason for this was that the timing of the dietary surveys coincided with a summer planting–growing season, and a slow-down in tourism. As one relatively wealthy individual observed, "restaurant and other tourist-based business owners are on equal footing with poorer households during the off seasons. They might eat meat every day during peaks in the tourist season, but are lucky to eat it once a week in the off-season." One teacher related how school children are awake, attentive, and energetic during the peaks in the tourist season. During the summer months, many come to school with no morning meal, and are sleepy, inattentive, and lethargic.

We also found no association between occupation and food consumption in the coastal communities. It appeared that all households had sufficient incomes to purchase adequate diets, and while differences might exist in the number of meals eaten away from home or in the number of more

expensive foodstuffs consumed, basic staples and micronutrient profiles were roughly similar.

In summary, inland diets look somewhat like historical Mayan diets, but with clear differences too. A broader array of fruits, dairy, meat, alternative complex carbohydrates, and sodas and snack foods are now available. Also, some foods and dishes historically important in local diets (e.g., honey, wild meat, *atole*, etc.) are now rarely consumed in the communities studied. Coastal diets exhibit an even broader array of foods available and regularly consumed, none of which are produced locally; all are commercialized, and many are processed.

It appears that caloric intakes are generally adequate, a great improvement over recent decades (Daltabuit, 1988; Daltabuit & Leatherman, 1998; Gurri et al., 2001). Protein intake appears to be adequate in quantity, but less so in quality. In the case of Coba, for example, where only 10.6% of calories come from protein and with a PQ score of only .67, one might suspect some functional consequences. Thus limits in protein, PQ and micronutrients such as zinc might be responsible for the continued presence of stunting, even though caloric intake may be generally adequate and average heights have increased over previous decades (see below, and Gurri et al., 2001).

While caloric intakes appear to be generally adequate, the dietary profile suggests potential micronutrient deficiencies in vitamins A, B2, B12, E, and zinc for the two inland communities. In Yalcoba households with a source of steady income, only vitamin E and zinc appear to be low, while in poorer families without steady incomes, levels of each of these micronutrients evaluated are near or below 75% of the RDA, suggesting micronutrient deficiencies.

The requirements and bioavailablity of micronutrients also vary with other dietary components that might exacerbate existing deficiencies. Plant-based diets high in fiber and phytates are associated with low bioavailablity of a number of micronutrients such as zinc, iron, calcium, and vitamin B12 (Allen et al., 1992; Calloway, Murphy, Beaton, & Lein, 1993). Also, as dietary phosphorous and protein increases, zinc requirements increase (Sandstead, 1982). All communities met their RDAs for protein, and far exceeded RDAs for phosphorous (between 200% and 240%) and fiber (140–175%). Hence it is likely that requirements for zinc are elevated and bioavailablity is limited by the dietary structures in all communities, but especially in the two inland communities of Coba and Yalcoba. The potential micronutrient deficiencies described here gain importance in high maize diets and when considering the shifts in dietary diversity toward the consumption of more soft drinks. When the remaining "non-maize" calories in a "high maize" diet come from sugar, soft drinks, and snack foods, it is likely that marginal nutrition will become worse.

NUTRITIONAL STATUS

In order to evaluate the nutritional status of individuals from these communities, anthropometric data on school children were collected and compared to earlier studies from the region. Children were classified for stature and body composition based on the US National Center for Health Statistics (NCHS) reference data, and the classification systems of Waterlow

(1984) for stature, and Frisancho (1990) for weight-for-height. Individuals are classified as stunted if they fall at or below two standard deviations from the NCHS reference data for stature within 1-year age groups [calculated as Z-scores: (individual value–mean of NCHS reference standard)/standard deviation of reference standard]. This is roughly equivalent to falling at or below the third percentile of the US population. Frisancho (1990) classifies children within age groups as below average if they are at or below the 15th percentile, and above average if they are above the 85th percentile based on US reference data from the NCHS, and we use his standards to evaluate weight-for-height in the children.

A comparison of Yucatec Mayan children's heights in 1938, 1987, and 1998 revealed significant increases in child growth, especially in the last decade (Leatherman et al., 2000). Yet the increase in height of approximately 2.6 cm between surveys conducted in 1987 and 1998 in Yalcoba is only about half the rate of increase observed for Mayan children migrating to the US (Bogin & Loucky, 1997). The children remain short for their ages compared to US and Mexican standards. Over 65% percent of Yalcoba children were stunted in 1998, and 20% were very stunted (Table 4A). In contrast, only about 7.5% were underweight, but 13.4% were classified as overweight based on their weight-for-height (Table 4B).

Thus, while overall child growth has improved in the past decade, levels of stunting indicate that the prevalence of chronic, mild-to-moderate malnutrition remains high; this can be interpreted as an indicator of chronically marginal health and low protein and/or micronutrient status. It appears likely that either poor PQ and/or low zinc bioavailablity could be partly responsible for the stunting that persists in association with increased weight gain in the Yalcoba children. The fact that almost twice as many children were above average in weight-for-height, as below, suggests that caloric intakes are in excess for some children. However, none of these children were obese, and excessive weight gain in children does not appear to be a problem at this time.

While there is still concern for childhood undernutrition, adult overnutrition, obesity, and diabetes are of major

Table 4 Anthropometric Assessment of Nutritional Status in Yalcoba Children (1998)

Z-score	N	Percent (%)
A. *Height-for-Age in Children 6–18 years (N=456)*		
Normal (> −2.0)	157	34.4
Stunted (≤ −2.0 to−2.99)	208	45.6
Very stunted (≤ −3.0)	91	20.0
B. *Weight-for-height in children 6–11 years (N=224)*		
Above Average > 85th percentile	30	13.4
Normal 15.1–85th percentile	192	79.0
Below average ≤ 15th percentile	17	7.5

concern in urban settings in the Yucatan (Arroyo, Pardio, Fernandez, Vargas–Ancona, Canul, & Loria, 1999; Dickinson et al., 1993). Dickinson et al. (1993) conducted studies in the vicinity of Merida and report that 86% of urban women are overweight and about 50% are obese. Using slightly more conservative standards, Arroyo et al. (1999) found that 45% of urban Yucatec men and 73% of women are overweight and at or near obesity (BMI>27.8 and >27.3), and that 2% of men and 12% of women are severely obese (BMI>35+). Moreover, diabetes, a common correlate of obesity, is the fourth leading cause of death in the Yucatan (Arroyo et al., 1999).

As early as 1986, Daltabuit (1988) found a dietary pattern in Yalcoba where younger females had very low intakes of calories and protein, while older women were above standard. We collected heights and weights from clinic records (most from the 1990s), obtaining a sample of 83 adult males and 214 females, and from these assessed the prevalence of overweight and obese adults. About 40% of the men were overweight and 10% were obese (BMI > 25 and BMI > 30, respectively); whereas 64% of the women were overweight and 20% were found to be obese. These levels fall short of those from urban centers in the Yucatan, but begin to approach Mexico City estimates (Arroyo et al., 1999) (Table 5).

The overall pattern of child and adult growth and nutritional status suggests a trend towards what Dickinson et al. (1993, p.315) have described as a double-edged sword of malnutrition: undernourished and stunted children grow up to be obese adults. A fast growing body of literature now links early under-nutrition to chronic disease in adulthood (Henry & Ulijaszek, 1996). One obvious concern is whether and when growing tendencies toward overweight and obese adults in these communities become associated with the diabetes and hypertension that already plague urban Yucatec Maya. We have no direct evidence to suggest that the rates of diabetes are increasing in Yalcoba. However, diabetes has become a point of local discussions of health. On our last field visit in 1998, two older men told us within the first hour of entering the community that their wives had died in the preceding months, and both identified diabetes as a contributing factor.

DISCUSSION

The massive penetration of tourism in Quintana Roo and the rest of the Yucatan has irrevocably transformed Mayan environment, economy, society, and culture. We have presented a small slice of what these transformations might bring in terms of diet and nutrition, two important, but little studied, factors in assessing consequences of change. We are *not* arguing that tourism-led development is necessarily a harbinger of either poverty or prosperity, or of improved or worsening health and nutrition. It can be both, largely depending on how individuals, households, communities, and regions interface with and respond to the sort of economic, cultural, and ecological changes brought about by international tourism. Several studies have argued that those individuals and households who have successfully integrated into the tourist-based market economy are among the best off in rural villages (Kintz & Ritchie, 1999; Dufresne & Locher, 1995). Growth in food markets and increased access to a diversity of products may benefit families with steady incomes and a real living wage. We are impressed that child growth has increased in the past decade. Yet others suffer without access to a steady wage and market foods, and with less local produce available. Moreover, increased consumption of commercial foods also means that a greater proportion of caloric intake is met through sodas and snack foods. This change may prove to be particularly detrimental. Ultimately, the broader pattern of childhood undernutrition and adult overnutrition foreshadows chronic diseases that concern us.

Local residents have little sense of the microchanges in diets that might have occurred over the past 20 years. Nor do they express concerns over dietary change explicitly in terms of health. This is not surprising because for the Maya, and many other cultures, health is but one dimension of an overdetermined web of relationships and realities that are not easily separated out, but rather are interwoven into a broader sense of lived experiences. If we are to adequately problematize the meaning of health and the conditions that produce health differences in such contexts of rapid change, it is important that we broaden our conceptions of health and well-being, as well as the multiple dimensions of change. There are other, and perhaps greater, costs of change in Maya communities, including declining production systems, loss of indigenous knowledge, and an altered sense of identity, community, and family relations. Milpa production has declined, and diets are shifting away from a base in local produce to commercialized foodstuffs. A younger generation of Cancun migrants sees the work of the milpa as crude, "*trabajo rudo*", and shares little sense

Table 5 Body Mass Index (BMI) and Overweight and Obese Adults in Yalcoba

Weight level (BMI)	Percent of males (N = 83)	Percent of females (N = 214)
Underweight (BMI < 20)	8	3
Normal (BMI ≥ 20 and < 25)	52	33
Overweight (BMI ≥ 25)	40	64
Obese (BMI > 30)	10	20

with their parents of its importance to the fabric of social and community life. Home gardens are less expansive, less diverse, and less relied upon as a cornerstone for diet. Since foods from these gardens have historically been a major source for vitamins and minerals, and can make up for seasonal shortfalls in the intermittent tourist economy, the dietary and nutritional consequence of this decline warrants further research. Villagers also tie a sense of dietary quality and health to consumption of locally grown corn, beans, vegetables, and fruits. They note the lesser quality and taste of foods they now consume from outside their community, much as they note the decline in milpa as a way of life and the necessity of Cancun to their families' livelihoods.

The state has strongly promoted regional integration, transportation and market infrastructure, as well as a shared greater national identity via education, social relief programs, and the media. Yet there is a question of priorities for promoting social and biological well-being in these villages. Social welfare programs such as the *Solidaridad* program of President Carlos Salinas invested very little in food-based poverty programs (1%) and health services (7%) (Laurell & Wences, 1994). The rural communities in which we worked had limited access to clean running water and no sewage or sanitation infrastructure, but they did have cable TV service bringing US baseball, *telenovelas* (soap operas) depicting the urban elite of Mexico City, and a barrage of advertisements for food, toys, clothing, and other commodities, and for sun-and-sand tourism. Of course, advertisements for *Coca-Cola* and *Pepsi* appeared with increased frequency amid their cola war, and presented compelling images and reasons to consume their products. These are images difficult to combat. One teacher in Coba told us how nutrition education efforts in the classroom could not compete with Coke and Pepsi commercials. Her students responded to lectures on nutritional education and the ills of junk food with observations that the people on TV drinking coke are rich and successful, and coke cannot be all bad.

In summary, there are indications that while tourism-led economic change has raised economic and some health indicators, it also carries environmental, social, and health costs for many Mayan households. Local populations recognize the potential damage that tourism brings to all aspects of their lives, but also recognize that it brings the much-needed jobs that provide an income to meet the basic needs of their families. As many say, "We would starve without Cancun."

Perhaps the biggest problem is that the Maya have been granted little input in the planning and development process. They are primarily seen as sources of cheap labor and ethnic backdrop at tourist sites. They are absent from regulatory bodies and middle management strata. It is not too extreme to say that this economic development is transforming the Maya into a peripheral element in their own homeland, a situation that has powerful political and social implications, and complex consequences on health.

Note

The authors appreciate the considerable help they received from numerous students and colleagues during the course of the project, including Jamie Jones, Carol Hudak, Ashley Lebner, Jose Martinez, Erica Seeber, Tobias Stillman, R. Brooke Thomas (University of Massachusetts), Magali Daltabuit (CRIM and UNAM), and Federico Dickinson (CINVESTAV, Merida). The Centro de Investigaciones Ecologica in Akumal facilitated the research in the coastal communities. We also thank two anonymous reviewers for their insightful comments which have added clarity to this article. Finally we offer our deepest gratitude to the people of Yalcoba, Coba, Cd. Chemuyil, and Akumal for their help and friendship over the years. The research was funded by a University of South Carolina Research and Productive Scholarship Award and a Grant from the Wenner-Gren Foundation for Anthropological Research.

References

Allen, L. (1984). Functional indicators of nutritional status of the whole individual or the community. *Clinical Nutrition, 3*(5), 169–174.

Allen, L. (1993). The nutrition CRSP: what is marginal malnutrition, and does it affect human function. *Nutrition Reviews, 51*(9), 255–267.

Allen, L., Backstrand, J. R., & Stanek, E. J. (1992). The interactive effects of dietary quality on the growth of young Mexican children. *American Journal of Clinical Nutrition, 56*, 353–364.

Arroyo, P., Pardio, J., Fernandez, V., Vargas-Ancona, L., Canul, G., & Loria, A. (1999). Obesity and cultural environment in the yucatan region. *Nutrition Reviews, 57*(5), S78–S82.

Bogin, B., & Loucky, J. (1997). Plasticity, political economy, and physical growth status of Guatemala Maya children living in the United States. *American Journal of Physical Anthropology, 102*, 17–32.

Calloway, D., Murphy, S. P., Beaton, G. H., & Lein, D. (1993). Estimated vitamin intakes of toddlers: predicted prevalence of inadequacy in village populations in Egypt, Kenya, and Mexico. *American Journal of Clinical Nutrition, 58*, 376–384.

Chavez, A., & Martinez, C. (1982). *Growing up in a developing community*. Mexico: Instituto Nacional de la Nutricion.

Coca-Cola Company. (1999). *Annual Report of the Coca-Cola Company for 1999*.

Daltabuit, M. (1988). *Mayan women, work, nutrition and child care*. Ph.D. dissertation, University of Massachusetts, Amherst, MA.

Daltabuit, M. & Leatherman, T. (1998). The biocultural impact of tourism on Mayan communities. In A. Goodman, T. Leatherman (Eds.), *Building a new biocultural synthesis: political-economic perspectives on human biology*. pp. 317–338. Ann Arbor: University of Michigan Press.

Daltabuit, M., & Pi-Sunyer, O. (1990). Tourism development in Quintana Roo, Mexico. *Cultural Survival Quarterly, 14*(1), 9–13.

Dewey, K. (1989). Nutrition and the commoditization of food systems in Latin America. *Social Science & Medicine, 28*, 415–424.

Dickinson, F., Castillo, M. T., Vales, L., & Uc, L. (1993). Obesity and women's health in two socioeconomic areas of Yucatan, Mexico. *Colloquia Antropologia, 2*, 309–317.

Dufresne, L., & Locher, U. (1995). The Mayas and Cancun: migration under conditions of peripheral urbanization. *Labour, Capital and Society, 28*(2), 176–202.

Frisancho, A. R. (1990). *Anthropometric standards for the assessment of growth and nutritional status.* Ann Arbor: University of Michigan Press.

Gurri, F. D., & Balam, G. (1992). Regional integration and changes in nutritional status in the central region of Yucatan, Mexico: a study of dental enamel hypoplasia and anthropometry. *Journal of Human Ecology, 3*(2), 417–432.

Gurri, F. D., Balam, G., & Moran, E. (2001). Well-being changes in response to 30 years of regional integration in Maya populations from Yucatan, Mexico. *American Journal of Human Biology, 13*, 590–602.

Henry, C. K. J., & Ulijaszek, S. (Eds.). (1996). *Long-term consequences of early environment: growth, development and the lifespan developmental perspective.* New York: Cambridge University Press.

Jabbonsky, L. (1993). The Mexican resurrection. *Beverage World, 112*(1547), 38–40.

Kintz, E. (1980). *Life under the tropical canopy.* Fort Worth, TX: Holt, Reinhart, & Winston.

Kintz, E. & Ritchie, A. (1999). The transformation of paradise: deep, social, and political ecology among the Yucatec Maya of Coba, Quintana Roo, Mexico. A dialogical approach. *Meetings of the American Anthropological Association.* Chicago, IL.

Laurell, A. C., & Wences, M. I. (1994). Do poverty programs alleviate poverty? The case of the Mexican National Solidarity Program. *International Journal of Health Services, 24*(3), 381–401.

Leatherman, T.L., Stillman, J.T., Goodman, A.H. (2000). The effects of tourism-led development on the nutritional status of Yucatec Mayan children. Paper presented at the Annual Meeting of the American Association of Physical Anthropologists, April, 2000. San Antonio, TX; *American Journal of Physical Anthropology* Supplement, *30*, 207.

Martorell, R. (1980). Interrelationship between diet, infectious disease and nutritional status. In Greene, L., & Johnston, F. (Eds.), *Social and biological predictors of nutritional status, physical growth, and neurological development* (pp. 81–106). New York: Academic Press.

Martorell, R. (1989). Body size, adaptation and function. *Human Organization, 48*(1), 15–20.

McGarty, C.A. (1995). *Dietary delocalization in a Yucatecan resort community in Quintana Roo, Mexico: junk food in paradise.* Honor's thesis, School of Nursing, University of Massachusetts, Amherst.

Pelto, G. H., & Pelto, P. J. (1983). Diet and delocalization: dietary changes since 1750. *Journal of Interdisciplinary History, 14*, 507–528.

Pendergrast, M. (2000). *For god, country and coca-cola: the unauthorized history of the great American soft drink and the company that makes it.* New York: Charles Scribner's Sons.

Pi-Sunyer, O., Thomas, R.B. (1997). Tourism, environmentalism and cultural survival in Quintana Roo, Mexico. In B. Johnston (Ed.), *Life and death matters, human rights and the environment at the end of the millennium* (pp. 187–212). Walnut Creek, CA: Altamira Press.

Sandstead, H. (1982). Availability of zinc and its requirement in human subjects. In Prasad, A. S. (Ed.), *Clinical, biochemical and nutritional aspects of trace elements* (pp. 83–101). New York: Alan R. Liss, Inc.

Scrimshaw, N., Taylor, C.E., Gordon, J.E. (1968). *Interactions of nutrition and infections.* Geneva: WHO Series No. 57.

Stonich, S. (1998). Political ecology of tourism. *Annals of Tourism Research, 25*(1), 25–54.

Stronza, A. (2001). Anthropology of tourism: forging new ground for ecotourism and other alternatives. *Annual Review of Anthropology, 30*, 261–283.

Waterlow, J. C. (1984). Current issues in nutritional assessment by anthropometry. In Brozek, J., & Scherch, R. (Eds.), *Malnutrition and behavior: critical assessment of key issues.* Lausanne: Nestle Foundation.

UNIT X

CULTURAL ECOLOGY OF INFANT AND YOUNG CHILD FEEDING

Together with the rest of the mammalian world, human females have the capacity to produce milk, a complete food, to meet the needs of their newborn offspring. As would be expected for a substance that is so central to survival, the composition of mammalian milks is finely adapted to the specific nutrient requirements of offspring. Human milk is no exception. In addition to containing the appropriate balance of essential nutrients, human milk also contains antibodies and other substances that help to protect infants from potentially life-threatening infection. Although the milk of other animals is not ideal for human infants, it is possible for babies to consume and derive nutrients from it. This feature of human adaptability has led to the use of other animal milks to supplement or replace breastmilk. Bottle-feeding is not a new invention, and the use of feeding bottles and animal milks was known in classic Greek and Roman times. However, it did not become a common practice across the populations of the world until this century, in particular after the Second World War.

The significance of the massive culture change in infant feeding practices with the growth of bottle-feeding began to be carefully studied in the 1960s and 1970s. The more that biological, medical, and social scientists discovered about breastfeeding, the more serious were the concerns about the consequences of the major behavioral change from breastfeeding to bottle-feeding. In much of the world bottle-feeding cannot be safely practiced, and children who are bottle-fed are at massively increased risk of morbidity and mortality. Conversely, the more breastmilk an infant receives, the better the health outcome.

Breastfeeding is not only beneficial for infants; it is also good for mothers. In the immediate post-delivery period, the action of infant suckling helps the uterus to contract, which stems postpartum bleeding. Most important from the perspective of women's health is the contraceptive effect of exclusive or intensive breastfeeding. Although the protection is not absolute, on average, women who breastfeed intensively and who are not taking other contraceptive measures are protected from a new pregnancy for nearly a year. This biological protection is particularly important in our species, in which the danger of too short a spacing between births is high because there are no cycles of sexual receptivity and because the adult male-female couple is the fundamental unit of social organization.

The paper "Evolution of Infant and Young Child Feeding: Implications for Contemporary Public Health," by Daniel Sellen in this section is a classic example of applying a biocultural approach to understand a fundamental human behavior. It shows the kinds of insights that can be gained by examining human behaviors as an interactive process involving both biological and sociocultural dimensions. This paper is also a seminal piece with respect to placing human lactation within the larger perspective of comparative analysis with other mammalian species. Here we learn about the similarities and differences between human breastfeeding and lactation patterns in other animals, and the factors that help to explain them. Sellen introduces the concept of "life history" to help reveal the predictable changes that occur over time, as infants (and mothers) move through the stages from birth to physiological independence. Finally, Sellen takes on the important issue of the positive and negative consequences of the inevitable shift from exclusive breastfeeding to the introduction of other foods into infant diets, a process that is now referred to as "complementary feeding."

The paper "Premastication: The Second Arm of Infant and Young Child Feeding for Health and Survival?" by Gretel Pelto, Yuanyuan Zhang, and Jean-Pierre Habicht continues the biocultural approach utilized by Sellen. Here we encounter the benefits of a cultural adaptation that begins out of a specific biological challenge—namely the problem of neotany. Neotany refers to the delayed maturation in human infants compared to other animal species. Of particular concern in relation to infant feeding is the fact that human infants do not have the capacity to chew the foods that comprise contemporary adult diets at the time they begin to need nutrients from non-breastmilk sources, and certainly did not have capacity to chew the wild foods that comprised the diets of our hunting-gathering ancestors. This paper is another example of a classic type of biocultural analysis. The authors lay out an argument to support their hypothesis that premastication represents an adaptation that evolved to cope with a fundamental survival challenge.

Pelto and colleagues go beyond the nutritional implications of giving children pre-chewed foods that are high in essential nutrients to discuss the implications of exposing children to saliva. In contrast to the usual biomedical orientation of regarding saliva primarily as a carrier of disease, they show that saliva contains all of the positive, non-nutritional elements (e.g., enzymes, antibodies) that breastmilk contains, and thus consuming pre-chewed foods extends infants' acquisition of these elements through the complementary feeding period when a diminution in breastmilk intake would otherwise reduce them. Moreover, the authors turn the interpretation of the disease issue on its head. Rather than viewing disease exposure as entirely a bad thing they suggest that this early, controlled exposure plays an important role in the development of a healthy immune system. Premastication may, in fact, have been an aspect of child survival. Not all disease exposure is a good, of course. The slight potential for the HIV virus to be transmitted through premastication if both the adult caregiver and the infant have open, bleeding sores in their mouths suggests that this practice should be discouraged for HIV positive caregivers, just as it is better to discourage breastfeeding, but only when safe alternative breastmilk substitutes are consistently available.

Another aspect of the paper by Pelto and colleagues that is worth noting is the use of two different types of research methods—the Cross Cultural Method and generational interviewing. The specific features of these two techniques are described in some detail in the paper. These methods are used to examine the ways in which premastication has survived or failed to survive across and within societies and subgroups around the world.

The degree to which mothers complement breastmilk with other foods as the child makes the transition to the family diet is influenced by many factors. In industrialized societies, as well as in many developing countries, the recommendations of health care providers are an important influence on caregivers' decisions to begin adding other foods to infants' diets. Beliefs about how to introduce infants to "food" can be found in virtually every society. In some societies, the introduction of the first food is recognized with a formal ritual, much like naming ceremonies, infant circumcision, baptism, or the first birthday are ritual occasions in the life of children. Apart from ritual or beliefs related to people's ideas about child health, the introduction of complementary foods is often influenced by women's work roles. For example, a number of years ago, Nerlove (1974) examined information about the age of introduction of complementary foods available for a sample of 83 traditional cultures, ranging from hunting-gathering groups to peasant agriculturalists. She found that in societies where there was a high level of women's participation in food production, complementary foods were often introduced before one month of age. A corollary of this finding is that the frequency of breastfeeding is also affected by women's work roles, and in some traditional societies women leave their infants in the care of others while they engage in agricultural work.

The research for the paper by Gretel Pelto, Emily Levitt, and Lucy Thairu, "Feeding Babies: Practices, Constraints and Interventions," was originally undertaken in preparation for an international conference on complementary feeding, convened by WHO and UNICEF. Within the context of the conference, the paper had several purposes. One purpose was to review what was known about patterns of complementary feeding around the world as a systematic review had not previously been done. A second purpose related to determinants of complementary feeding behaviors. Prior to the first decade of the 21st century the focus of nutrition research and program activities in complementary feeding was almost exclusively on the biological aspects of complementary feeding; at the time of the conference there was a growing recognition of the importance of behavioral aspects, not only in relation to nutritional outcomes, but also for the design of intervention programs. Therefore, a second purpose of the paper was to identify and describe some of the determinants of variations in practices from one social setting to another. A third purpose was to examine the nature of feeding behaviors in relation to the concept of "responsivity." What kinds of caregiver feeding behaviors promote positive nutritional and psychological outcomes? The paper examines this question from the perspective of "best practice recommendations."

The version of the paper presented here has been adapted from the original version, which was much longer because it contained descriptions of 18 country case studies in the form of an extended appendix. The current version contains all the sections of the original paper, but in a condensed form. The paper is an example of an anthropological approach, including the application of anthropological research methods, to a fundamental nutrition issue. It is also an example of one of the ways in which anthropological research (in this case producing a synthesis paper) can enter the arena of policy and action in the "real world."

In summary, in this section you will find an overview of the biocultural challenges and responses that humans have made in the area of feeding infants and young children. Ensuring that their offspring are well-nourished is a fundamental challenge for all species, and we humans are no exception. In this section you will encounter the fundamental principles of human lactation as well as for feeding infants when breastmilk alone becomes inadequate. The intricate relationships of biology and behavior are described. The section also provides insights into the diversity of ways in which families around the globe, historically and in the contemporary world, manage the complex process of nutritional care for their youngest members. As editors of the volume, we hope this section will elicit and build your respect for the extraordinary job the people everywhere accomplish to nourish their infants and young children and bring them safely through this nutritionally challenging part of their lifespan.

SUGGESTIONS FOR THINKING AND DOING NUTRITIONAL ANTHROPOLOGY

1. From art history books, museum catalogs, and books on archaeological sites, put together a collection of pictures that illustrate cultural values about breastfeeding.

2. Using magazine and newspaper stories and advertising, identify the types of messages concerning infant feeding that Americans receive through these mass media sources. What kinds of practices are being promoted? What practices are being discouraged?

3. Replicate the study that was carried out in China (c.f. Pelto, Zhang, and Habicht). Create a short questionnaire and then interview your mother, father, or whoever was responsible for feeding you when you were about a year old. Find out what kinds of food you were given, where they came from (store, home-made, fast food restaurant). Compare your results with other classmates. What are the similarities and differences?

Reference

Nerlove S. 1974. Women's workload and infant feeding practices: A relationship with demographic implications. Ethnology 13:207–2 14.

Suggested Further Reading

Dettwyler KA. 1994. *Dancing skeletons: Life and death in West Africa.* Prospect Heights, Ill.: Waveland Press. A personal account of Dettwyler's research in Mali on infant nutrition.

Stuart-Macadam P & Dettwyler K (Eds.). 1995. *Breastfeeding: Biocultural perspectives.* Chicago: Aldine. A wide-ranging set of articles on the evolution of infant feeding and current health, nutrition, and social issues.

Van Estrick P. 1989. *Beyond the breast and bottle controversy.* New Brunswick, N.J.: Rutgers University Press. An anthropological perspective on issues underlying the promotion of bottle-feeding in the developing world.

http://www.iycn.org/ A website sponsored by USAID that provides extensive information about infant and young child feeding across the world.

http://www.pronutrition.org/ A website for organizations that are interested in and involved with nutrition and agricultural projects that often have a strong infant and young child feeding component.

CHAPTER 43

Evolution of Infant and Young Child Feeding: Implications for Contemporary Public Health

Daniel W. Sellen

(2007)

Two observations about the patterns of infant and young child feeding (IYCF) in contemporary human societies are puzzling for nutritionists and anthropologists, respectively. First, the proportion of newborns that breastfeed exclusively for six months, receive timely and appropriate complementary foods, and continue to breastfeed into their third year is small, even though overwhelming evidence suggests such a pattern is optimal for most healthy, term infants (including low-birth-weight infants born at >37 weeks gestation). Second, humans tend to wean their babies significantly earlier than most other apes do, even though children depend on others for subsistence much longer than do the offspring of any other mammal (172). This article reviews zoological, anthropological, and nutritional data that suggest these two apparently paradoxical observations are evolutionarily linked. It summarizes recent conclusions about the unique characteristics of human life history and discusses how they may be related to unique characteristics of human lactation biology. It briefly reviews data on variation in lactation patterns among nonhuman patterns and data on variation in IYCF among preindustrial human societies and ancient populations. The aim is to provide an evolutionary perspective on why optimal IYCF is so rare and difficult to promote in modern human societies that are far removed from the original conditions shaping human adaptation.

COEVOLUTION OF LIFE HISTORY AND LACTATION BIOLOGY

It is possible to distinguish the evolutionarily derived features of human life history (44) and lactation biology from those that are shared with other mammals by using the comparative methods of zoology and drawing on physiological and epidemiological data that signal an evolved, optimal pattern of human IYCF.

VARIATION AMONG MAMMALS

Mammals vary in age at weaning, as well as in many other characteristics that together describe their life history (109), such as age at first reproduction, gestation length, interbirth intervals, and age at death. Much of this variation is linked to more or less species-typical patterns of growth and development, and is associated with variation in body size, demography, sociality, and ecology (36, 39, 153, 171, 187). Evolutionary theory suggests life history variation is an adaptive response to natural selection within physiological, ecological, and social constraints (37, 38, 44, 74, 186, 216).

Lactation probably evolved between 210 and 190 million years ago (mya) (20, 41, 91, 127, 145, 147) and prior to the origin of another defining characteristic of mammals, specialized hair and fur (143). Lactation probably evolved initially as an adaptation to transfer immune factors to offspring (99) and later as an adaptation to make efficient use of maternal body fat and other stored nutrients in feeding offspring and spacing births (45, 178, 179).

Significant diversity exists in the species-specific characteristics of lactation biology and their relation to life history (29, 91, 98, 152). Milk immune components (82), milk energy density (169), milk yield (168, 185), relative milk energy yield (152), and milk composition (79) vary among species with disease risk, body size, litter size and mass, maternal diet, maternal use of body stores, suckling patterns, and care behavior. This diversity reflects phylogenetic differences in the selective response to shifts in disease ecology, foraging opportunities, and constraints on growth and development. Table 1 summarizes some key trends linking variation in lactation biology and life history across mammals.

Nevertheless, all surviving mammals retain lactation as a key adaptation that contributes to the organization of life history characteristics (88). Four basic functions of lactation present as plesiomorphies are summarized in Table 2. Also highly conserved are similar mechanisms of lactogenesis (67, 89), mammary development (32), immunological activity (82), milk transport proteins (158), and metabolic adaptation during lactation (228).

Daniel W. Sellen, "Evolution of infant and young child feeding: implications for contemporary public health." *Annual Review of Nutrition* 27 (2007):123–148. Reprinted with permission.

Table 1 Key Trends Linking Variation in Lactation Biology and Life History Across Mammals

1. Marsupials commonly overlap lactation with gestation of younger offspring, whereas most placental species do not.

2. The period between first solid food consumption and weaning is long in species with single, precocial young, and provisioning may occur, whereas first solid food is usually eaten near weaning in polytokous species with altricial young (98).

3. Milk energy concentration decreases with maternal and neonatal size.

4. Milk fat and protein concentration are positively correlated, and both are negatively correlated with sugar, which is associated with suckling frequency.

5. Milk energy output at peak lactation scales with basal metabolic rate according to Kleiber's Law.

Table 2 Basic Functions of Lactation Present in All Extant Mammal Species

1. Transfer protective functions of fully developed immune system across generations.

2. Optimize litter size to allow titration of maternal investment across sib sets.

3. Facilitate efficient reproduction in unpredictable environments lacking special foods for young.

4. Increase behavioral flexibility and opportunities for learning.

SIMILARITIES AMONG NONHUMAN PRIMATES

More is known about the range of life history variation observed among nonhuman primates and hominids (40, 80, 92, 93, 140, 141, 176, 211–214, 227) than about variation in primate lactation biology (204, 242).

Life History

Recent work suggests the common ancestor of primates weighed between 1 and 15 g and therefore had high metabolic, reproductive, and predation rates, and that body size remained below 50 g during the early Eocene primate radiations (78). Extant primates, however, range in size by an order of magnitude (92). Compared with other mammals, they are characterized by a slow life history and low postnatal growth rates (40, 92, 93). The few available data on variation in primate lactation biology suggest all species share common adaptations to meet infant nutritional needs conditioned by this characteristically slow life history.

Milk Composition

Most previous reviews conclude that the gross composition of milk does not vary widely across nonhuman primate species with differences in body size, reproductive rates, patterns of maternal care, or other life history characteristics (32, 57, 69, 117, 173, 180). A single recent study reports variation in milk protein within a species in relation to parasitic infection (108). Primates are unusual among mammals because the milk they produce is lower in volume, more dilute, lower in energy, fat, and protein, and higher in lactose than would be predicted by body size (152), and because length of lactation is relatively long and always exceeds that of gestation (91).

It has long been hypothesized that these shared characteristics of primate milk coevolved with low reproductive rates and slow life histories relative to body size (15, 138, 167). Thus, a lower protein concentration of primate milks coevolved with slower growth rates (168, 169); lower fat concentration coevolved with the behavioral ecology of continuous infant carrying (which facilitates frequent suckling and is unusual in any other order of mammals) (15, 152, 170, 220); and a relatively high lactose content coevolved with the lower fat storage in adult females and low fat content of milk, and may also be linked to faster rates of postnatal brain growth. There is, however, no evidence that levels of long-chain polyunsaturated fatty acids (LCPUFAs) increase among primates with rates of postnatal brain growth (192).

Juvenile Feeding Ecology

One correlate of a relatively slow life history is the relatively slow development and early maturation of the gastrointestinal tract in primates (195). This means that there is little clustering of gut maturational changes around the species-typical age at birth and age at weaning. Primates are therefore able to begin consuming milk even if born preterm and are generally viable from about 70% of the length of gestation without intensive neonatal care.

Nevertheless, from a nutritional perspective, nonhuman primate postnatal life can be divided into three phases (exclusive suckling, transitional feeding, and weanling) separated by two key life history markers (first consumption of solid food and weaning) that can be used to define two life history variables (age at first solid food and age at weaning) that increase with body size. Thus, nonhuman primates conform to a generalized mammalian pattern linking life history to feeding ecology (Figure 1). Juvenile daily intake of energy and specific nutrients increases from birth and is entirely due to greater milk intake during exclusive suckling.

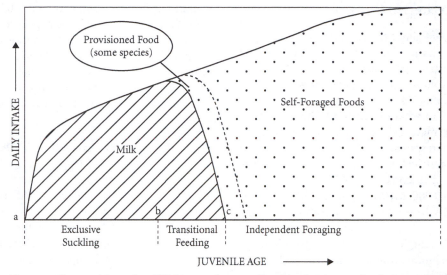

Figure 1 *Key nutrition-related life history phases and markers for a generalized mammal.*

After weaning, further increase in total intake occurs by means of independent foraging or maternal provisioning.

Transitional Feeding

Variation in transitional feeding has yet to be fully described and explained and may be substantial both within and between species (136–138). There are few data with which to assess the length of transitional feeding in primates or the relative nutritional contribution of milk versus foraged foods (205). It has been hypothesized that relative length of transitional feeding is inversely related to adult diet quality (205), but available data are insufficient properly to test this. In the absence of good observational data it has been generally assumed that nonhuman primate infants wean relatively abruptly and begin to forage on foods similar to those selected by the mother, processing them largely for themselves. However, the transition to weaning is a gradual process in at least one ape, the orangutan (226), and possibly chimpanzees (165). Similarly, although it is commonly assumed that parental provisioning of juveniles is rare or absent in most species (75, 114, 122), there is limited evidence that it occurs in apes (166).

Weaning

Last suckling is very difficult to observe directly in the wild, but captive data indicate that nonhuman primate weaning age is scaled to other life history traits, such as gestation length (92), birth weight (133, p. 245; 139), and adult weight (40), and developmental events such as age at molar eruption (193, 211, 212). However, such traits do not reliably predict age at weaning for all primate species, suggesting that age at weaning is labile. Studies of nonhuman primate behavioral ecology suggest that weaning age is plastic in most species and sensitive to ecological factors that constrain maternal ability to meet the increasing energy needs of growing offspring and the ability of infants to survive without mother's milk (4, 5, 136, 137, 139).

Infant Requirements

Few data are available on age-specific changes in energy requirements of nonhuman primates, of the total energy costs of growth and maintenance during infancy, or of the proportion met by milk consumed. Observation of ad libitum intakes among several captive large bodied cercopithecine species yields estimates of average infant energy requirements in the range 0.837–1.255 MJ/kg/d (160, 163). Such intakes are likely to differ from either average requirements or usual intakes in the wild, however. A study of free-living yearling baboons (*Papio cynocephalus*) estimated minimum total energy requirements for growth and maintenance at 0.871 MJ/d, or 0.383 MJ/kg/d (8).

It is difficult to identify studies that estimate the concentration of key nutrients such as vitamin A, vitamin D, iodine, calcium, and essential LCPUFAs in the milk of nonhuman primates (180). At present few conclusions can be drawn for any species about how milk nutrient content varies with maternal diet or about the extent to which exclusive suckling and milk consumption during transitional feeding satisfy age-specific nutrient requirements. Although evolved associations between feeding ecology and milk composition might be predicted across species, the data are too scant to test nutritional ecological hypotheses. For example, it is not known whether primate species that are nocturnal or obligatory carnivores (such as tarsiers) secrete milk richer in vitamin D levels in their milk as they are (no sun exposure) and are similar to felids. The milk of diurnal monkeys and apes is not reported as a rich source of vitamin D, and it is currently assumed that this is because endogenous synthesis satisfies the requirement.

Maternal Costs

Relatively little is known about the reproductive ecology of wild nonhuman primate mothers. Evidence that they can accommodate the costs of protecting their infants against fluctuations in milk volume and composition when conditions are adverse is scant (57).

It is also unclear to what extent nonhuman primates share a capacity for maternal accommodation of lactation performance in response to moderate decreases in maternal energy or nutrient intakes. Free-living yearling baboons are estimated to consume 2.251 MJ/d, of which approximately 40% (0.900 MJ/d) comes from milk, suggesting their mothers bear the cost of minimal energy requirement (8).

Available data indicate that lactation places a significant metabolic demand on mothers and that limited mechanisms exist to accommodate this (6, 7, 57, 86, 135). Field observations of several species indicate that lactating females increase their intake of high-energy foods (27), overall food energy (196, 215), and time allocated to foraging (4, 58), particularly when forage quality is poor (59). Indirect evidence from captive studies suggests that in some species, energetic costs of lactation are accommodated by energy-sparing adaptations, physiological adaptations (17, 191), reductions in physical activity (17, 87), and shared care of infants (219, 242). No studies have shown conclusively that lactating nonhuman primate mothers are able to reduce the daily costs of milk production using fat stored during pregnancy.

Maternal Reproductive Ecology

Among wild great apes, female reproductive biology seems designed to avoid conception under food stress rather than to protect mothers from nutritional deficiency during lactation. Lactation, nutritional intake, energy expenditure, and net energy balance appear to be key influences on fecundity (16, 164). Field observations indicate conception is more likely to occur during periods of positive maternal energy balance because food availability is so unpredictable that conception cannot be timed so that birth will occur during periods of highest food availability (122).

DERIVED CHARACTERISTICS OF HUMANS

Table 3 summarizes some key differences in life history parameters among the great ape species, using values obtained for wild apes and hunter-gatherers with natural fertility. Table 4 summarizes the shared and derived characteristics of human lactation biology.

Life History

There has been considerable debate about whether and why human life history differs from the typical primate pattern (25, 28, 77, 97, 105, 107, 119, 148, 229, 230, 239). A consensus has recently emerged that, in comparison to other primates, humans have evolved four distinctive life history traits: slow maturation, long lifespans with slow aging, postmenopausal longevity, and weaning before independent feeding (95).

Although not the largest living ape, humans have the slowest life history. This is evidenced by a markedly later age at maturity (marked by age at first birth), a longer period of nutritionally "independent" growth between weaning and maturity, longer maximum lifespan, and longer potential adult lifespan. Not all aspects of human life history are slowed, however. Duration of gestation is similar for all living ape species despite appreciable variation in size at maturity.

Table 3 Phylogenetic Relationships of Great Ape Species and Average Values for Selected Life History Parameters

	Estimated time of divergence from hominid lineage, mya	Adult female weight (range), kg	Gestation length, years	Birth interval, years	Age at weaning, years	Age at first birth, years	Maximum independent lifespan, years	Period of growth, years	Potential adult lifespan, years	Neonate weight/ maternal weight, %	Weaning weight/ maternal weight, %
Human, *Homo sapiens*	–	47.0 (38–56)	0.7	3.7	2.8	19.5	85.0	16.7	65.5	5.9	0.21
Chimpanzee, *Pan trogolodytes*	5–7	35.0 (25–45)	0.6	5.5	4.5	13.3	53.4	8.8	40.1	5.4	0.27
Bonobo, *Pan paniscus*	5–7	33.0 (27–39)	0.7	6.3	–	14.2	50.0	–	35.8	4.2	–
Gorilla, *Gorilla gorilla*	6–8	84.5 (71–98)	0.7	4.4	2.8	10.0	54.0	7.2	44.0	2.3	0.21
Orangutan, *Pongo pygmaeus* and *Pongo abelii*	12–15	36.0	0.7	8.1	7.0	15.6	58.7	8.6	43.1	4.3	0.28

Adapted from Sources Cited in Reference 193.

Healthy human neonates are relatively large for gestational age and relative to maternal body size, indicating faster fetal growth rates. Estimates of human weaning age and relative weaning weight are at the short end of the range for great apes.

Most striking, human birth interval is exceptionally short, both in absolute time and relative to body size. Average birth intervals rarely exceed four years in human populations without effective technological means of controlling fertility (232). In marked contrast, half of all randomly selected closed birth intervals exceed four, five, and eight years in wild gorillas, chimpanzees, and orangutans, respectively (75). Since fertility ends at similar ages in human and chimpanzee females, the "species-typical" rate of human reproduction is higher (25).

Milk Composition

A recent review (205) suggested that humans have retained a number of features of lactation biology that are plesiomorphic with mammals and synapomorphic with nonhuman primates. These shared characteristics include the four basic functions of lactation, similar spectra for the immune components of milk (82), and similar features of gross milk composition (22, 115, 117, 161, 167, 173). These design similarities are likely linked to recurring patterns of pathogen exposure, dietary ecology, and constraints on growth and development that shaped the adaptive radiation of primates. They must have been present in our last common ancestor with apes (which lived approximately 6–7 mya) and in all subsequent hominid species including those ancestral to humans (i.e., various members of the genera *Ardipithecus, Australopithecus,* and *Homo*).

Thus, all evidence suggests that the basic composition of human milk, its basic functions in the infant, and its mechanism of secretion and delivery remained unchanged during seven million years of human evolution. This is striking given that during this period there occurred a shift to bipedal locomotion, radical dental and cranial adaptations to a more omnivorous diet, a large increase in brain size, a doubling of adult body size, an even larger increase in the length of the juvenile period and of total lifespan, a shortening of birth intervals, and an increase in female postreproductive lifespan.

Juvenile Feeding Ecology

Current international recommendations (49–51, 55, 234, 237) based on clinical and epidemiological data (31, 49, 52, 125) provide a compelling model for the evolved pattern of human IYCF practices because they are predictive of optimal growth and development of healthy newborn humans

Table 4 Summary of Shared and Derived Characteristics of Human Lactation Biology

	Plesiomorphic shared with other mammals	Symplesiomorphic shared with other primates	Apomorphic unique to humans
Postnatal immune defense	X		
Optimal postnatal nutrition	X		
Fertility regulation	X		
Developmental window for learning	X		
A period of exclusive lactation yields optimal benefits to mothers and offspring	X		
Low protein and fat and high lactose milk content		X	
Frequent suckling, high cost of infant carrying		X	
Slow infant growth		X	
A period of transitional feeding yields optimal benefits to mothers and offspring		?	
Age at weaning highly labile relative to other life history traits		?	
Complementary feeding			X
Increased plasticity in length of lactation relative to body size			X
Reduced infant energy needs			?
Significant buffering of lactation by fat storage in pregnancy			?

in favorable environments (76, 202, 204). By this reasoning, the evolved template for human IYCF includes (*a*) initiation of breastfeeding within an hour of birth; (*b*) a period of exclusive breastfeeding followed by introduction of nutrient-rich and pathogen-poor complementary foods at about six months of infant age; (*c*) introduction of high-quality family foods, usually prepared from a variety of raw sources using some form of processing, heat treatment, and mixing; (*d*) continued breastfeeding at least until the third year; and (*e*) a package of "responsive caregiving" throughout the period of nutritional dependency but particularly during the transition to complementary feeding. This evolved human pattern is based on what is optimal for the child in terms of clinical outcomes and is schematized in Figure 2. Comparison of Figures 1 and 2 suggests that important apomorphic features of human lactation biology include (*a*) complementary feeding and (*b*) early and flexible weaning (i.e., increased plasticity in the length of lactation).

Complementary Feeding

The most remarkable change is the human use of complementary foods, which is unique among mammals (122) and results in a pattern of transitional feeding that appears to be fundamentally different from that of other primates.

Overwhelming clinical and epidemiological evidence demonstrates that infants have not evolved to make efficient use of other foods before six months (53, 54, 126) and may suffer deficits and increased morbidity if not exclusively breastfed (42, 125). A wealth of data on the trajectory of infant development of feeding competency and changes in the nutritional needs of growing infants in relation to maternal milk supply supports the hypothesis that humans evolved to begin consuming complementary foods at approximately six months of age (205).

After approximately six months of age, complementary and family foods (235) increasingly contribute to the diet (131), as chewing (210, 211, 217), tasting (14, 47, 142), and digestive (134, 194) competencies develop. Frequency of suckling and volume of milk consumed do not necessarily diminish after six months in healthy babies, and the complementary feeding phase continues at least until the third year of life, during which breast milk remains an important, relatively sterile source of nutrients and immune protection.

Ethnographic evidence from preindustrial societies indicates that the duration of exclusive breastfeeding is extremely variable (201). Some indicators suggest that the age-related pattern for introduction of complementary foods in preindustrial societies concords loosely with the current clinical recommendations for normal, healthy children (203). The modal age of introduction of liquid and solid foods in a sample of published ethnographic reports was six months, suggesting a sizeable proportion of infants in these populations may have been exclusively breastfed for six months.

Early and Flexible Weaning

Humans are the only primates that wean juveniles before they can forage independently (94). The targeting and sharing of high-yield, nutrient-dense foods that entail high acquisition and processing costs is a specialization of human foragers (18), as is the use of heat treatments and combination of raw foods in "cuisine" (43, 240). We are also unusual in the extent to which we recruit and distribute help among conspecifics, including young child feeding and care (23, 221). Thus, weaning marks a shift to allo-caregiver support, not feeding independence.

Given the potential flexibility and observed variation in weaning age, it is difficult to conclude that humans have

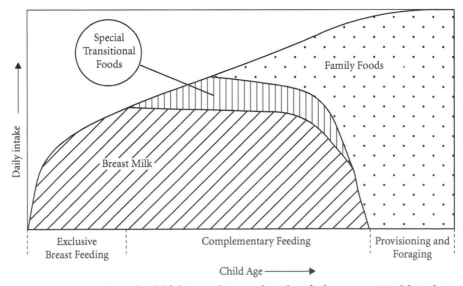

Figure 2 *Key nutrition-related life history phases and markers for humans, optimal for infants and young children.*

evolved a species-specific, global optimum weaning age. The clinical model suggests that there is no upper age limit at which breastfeeding ceases to be of some benefit to children (66, 151). Current international recommendations are based on evidence that infants benefit from breastfeeding into the third year (238). Continued breastfeeding must have remained a strongly selected component of ancestral maternal strategies because of its powerful anti-infective properties (100, 128, 157) and nutritional or physiological benefits to infants (19, 46) and mothers (10, 129, 223, 224).

The degree of flexibility in age at weaning is unusual among primates and probably a distinctive, derived characteristic. The diversity in human breastfeeding and complementary feeding patterns has long been a focus of lactation researchers (91). The duration of human lactation, if initiated at all, ranges from a few hours to more than five years in recent and contemporary societies (48, 121, 201, 202, 218). This spans most of the range observed for all other species of mammal (90). Ethnographic evidence from recent and contemporary foraging populations indicates that human weaning age is extremely variable within and between groups and that the process of weaning could be gradual (73, 123) or (less commonly) abrupt (71, 72). Humans also wean over a wide range of infant sizes; even among hunter-gatherers human infants are weaned after relatively smaller postnatal weight gain (11).

Nevertheless, some indicators suggest that the age-related pattern for termination of breastfeeding concords with the current clinical recommendations for normal, healthy children. It is estimated that breastfeeding beyond two years was the norm in between 75% (162) and 83% (12) of small-scale societies and that the modal age at weaning was approximately 30 months (201, 203). This suggests a sizeable proportion of infants in these populations may have been partially breastfed for more than two years, a pattern known to be optimal for growth and development. Rigorously collected data from hunter-gatherer populations suggest mean weaning age of 2.8 years (9). Even if we accept that the latest reliable estimate of modal age of weaning reported [four years among the !Kung (124)] is an indication of a species-typical value, it is well below the five to seven years predicted for primates with our life history parameters (48).

Archaeologists and skeletal biologists have made recent progress in developing approaches to estimating the timing of the trophic shifts associated with complementary feeding and weaning. Their studies use isotopic ratios in bony remains from juvenile and adult skeletons (21, 60, 197–200) and estimate childhood diet from tooth enamel recovered from adult remains (102, 120, 159). Results of such studies show that children in past populations often shifted to solid foods before two years of age while continuing to breastfeed.

Infant Energy Requirements

Cumulative energy requirements for male babies average 374.2 MJ between birth and 6 months and 959.4 MJ between birth and 12 months (data recalculated from data in Reference 34). Depending on age and sex, estimated mean total energy requirements for growth and maintenance in the first year range between 0.351 and 0.372 MJ/kg/d (1.347 and 3.519 MJ/d). These estimates are regarded as universally valid because healthy infants from different geographic areas show relative uniformity of growth, behavior, and physical activity (33, 76). They fall below the estimates for free-living yearling baboons (8) and well below those for captive large-bodied cercopithecines (160, 163). Thus, although comparative data are scant, human infants appear to have low energy requirements in comparison with other primates. This is likely due to comparatively slower growth.

Maternal Energy Cost

Human peak milk volume corresponds to a mean infant energy intake of 2.87 MJ/d (183), which is well in excess of healthy infant requirements in the first six months. The crude energetic costs of human lactation estimated from measurements of daily milk intake among predominantly breastfed infants observed for two years postpartum is ~1686 MJ, more than half of which is borne in the first year of infant life (recalculated from data in Reference 183). This corresponds to a mean daily additional cost of approximately 2.3 MJ/d [actually 2.7 MJ/d in the first six months (183)]. Thus, the daily cost of lactation is potentially high (~25%–30%) in a mother compared with average total energy expenditure for a moderately active nonpregnant, nonlactating woman of average size (calculated from equations in Reference 70). However, two mechanisms allow mothers to accommodate the cost of lactation, both of which appear to be derived for humans relative to our nonhuman primate ancestors.

First, depletion of the maternal fat laid down before and during pregnancy has the potential to subsidize lactation by ~118.6 MJ (0.325 MJ/d) in the first year. Fat storage demands the largest proportion (~71%) of additional energy needed to sustain a healthy pregnancy in nonchronically energy-deficient women (62, 132, 183). Nevertheless, reductions in basal metabolic rates and physical activity (61, 183) ensure that for many women average daily costs of pregnancy (~0.7 MJ/d) are low (~8%) in relation to the usual dietary energy intakes and requirements of healthy nonpregnant, nonlactating women (~8.78 MJ/d). In favorable conditions, the average woman begins lactation with approximately 125 MJ of additional fat accumulated during pregnancy.

Second, feeding of nursing infants using safe and nutritionally adequate complementary foods can result in maternal energy savings of almost 1.8 MJ/d in the first year.

Together, healthy fat depletion and complementary feeding reduce the actual cost of lactation estimated to satisfy infant and young child needs for two years by 1023.6 MJ, or almost 61%. On a daily basis this reduces the net additional costs from ~2.3 MJ/d to ~0.9 MJ/d. For many women, this represents between 10% and 20% of usual total energy expenditure. Healthy people unconstrained in their access to food or choice of activities can comfortably increase energy intake, decrease physical activity, or both to accommodate increases in daily energy requirement of up to 30%. Despite these adaptations, however, the average daily energetic cost of human lactation is potentially higher than that of pregnancy (~2.3 MJ/d versus ~0.7 MJ/d).

One corollary is that human lactation performance is well buffered from fluctuations in maternal condition and nutrient supply (3, 112, 113, 181, 189). Aerobic exercise and gradual weight loss have no adverse impact on milk volume or composition, infant milk intake, infant growth, or other metabolic parameters (56, 144, 154, 155). A single intervention study has suggested that milk production can be improved by maternal food supplementation during exclusive lactation (83). However, most studies suggest lactation is rarely compromised even when mothers are multiparous, marginally undernourished, engaged in high levels of physical activity, and lose weight and fat with age and by season (1, 30, 146, 182, 184, 231).

Maternal Reproductive Ecology

Lactation, nutritional intake, energy expenditure, and net energy balance are the key influences on fecundity among humans (64, 65, 233). Reproductive endocrinology responds adaptively to maternal nutrient flux and behavioral ecology to schedule reproductive effort across the life span. Flexibility in weaning age reflects an evolved maternal capacity to vary reproduction in relation to ecology (23, 35, 63), the availability of alternate caregivers (110, 123, 150), and other environmental and social factors affecting the costs and benefits of weaning to mothers and infants (156). It has been hypothesized that the maternal cost of reproduction has likely been reduced in humans by the increased availability of help from older offspring [linked to the evolution of long childhood (24, 26)] and grandparents and other elders [linked to the evolution of greater longevity and vigorous postreproductive lifespan in females (96, 174)]. Observation in contemporary human societies shows lactation behavior is sensitive to maternal workload and the availability of cooperative childcare and feeding (13, 203). Weaning age is later among foragers than among subsistence herders and farmers (207), among whom women often do more of the kind of work that separates them from their infants for extended periods.

DEMOGRAPHIC IMPLICATIONS

The early age at weaning suggests that ancestral humans evolved an unusual capacity to reduce the length of exclusive and transitional feeding without increasing mortality. In humans, an inverse relationship between birth interval and child survival is mediated by breastfeeding (149, 209, 236). Birth intervals below two years are risky for older sibs. Nevertheless, as a species we are particularly good at keeping young alive in a peculiarly wide range of habitats. Infant and weanling survival is much greater among human foragers [60%–70% (103, 130)] than among apes [25%–50% (106, 107, 121)], and greater still in nonindustrial herding

and farming economies (103, 104, 118, 164, 206). These simple demographic differences, which are based in part on differences in juvenile feeding ecology, have had enormous impact. The human population now exceeds six billion, whereas total populations of great ape species are estimated in the low thousands (122).

Shortened birth interval is currently regarded by anthropologists as one of the most evolutionarily significant human deviations from the expected pattern of great ape life history (75, 121, 122, 193, 204). Among our female ancestors, shortening of the periods of exclusive lactation or transitional feeding, or both, likely reduced birth intervals (by accelerating the return of ovarian cycling) and may have improved subsequent birth outcomes (by reducing maternal depletion). Shortened birth spacing would have increased maternal fitness only if it did not increase offspring mortality. Reduced juvenile mortality could be achieved only if many of the nutritional components of breast milk were provided by other kinds of foods or if infant development were accelerated so that the period of nutritional dependency was shortened (68, 85, 175).

IMPLICATIONS FOR CONTEMPORARY PUBLIC HEALTH

Despite burgeoning biomedical (81) and anthropological (225) research on human lactation in recent decades, few scholars have asked broader evolutionary questions about which characteristics of human lactation biology reflect evolutionarily conserved design features and which aspects, if any, reflect a distinctively human phenotype (204, 241). An evolutionary perspective provides insight into why contemporary patterns of IYCF often deviate from the optimal pattern indicated by clinical and epidemiological evidence. Human mothers are physiologically and behaviorally adapted to exercise more choice in the patterns and duration of full and partial breastfeeding than do other primates.

The evolution of the use of complementary foods to facilitate physiologically appropriate early weaning relative to other species has created potential for physiologically inappropriate early weaning and introduction of foods that are not complementary for breastfed infants. One recent and powerful manifestation of this potential is the development and widespread use of commercial infant formulas that meet some of the nutritional needs but none of the immunological needs of infants.

Contemporary human caregivers tend to titrate breastfeeding, complementary feeding, and child care in response to shifts in ecology, subsistence, and social environment. Across cultures, underlying attitudes and values about child feeding are often broadly concordant with optimal practice, but focus more explicitly on tradeoffs between infant/child and maternal/caregiver needs. More often missing are the material conditions conducive for optimal breastfeeding and complementary feeding. Mismatch between optimal and actual infant feeding practices in contemporary populations is widespread and

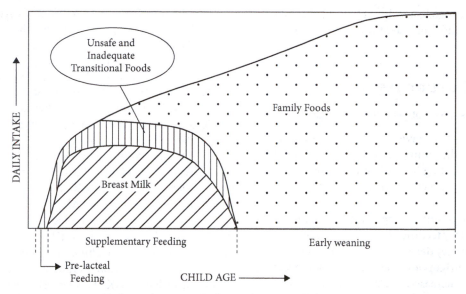

Figure 3 *Commonly observed pattern of infant and young child feeding, not optimal for child outcomes.*

presents a major public health challenge (111, 188, 208, 222). Common practices such as discarding of colostrum (84, 190), use of prelacteal feeds (2, 177), reduced breast milk intake due to early introduction of formula and other substances, and early weaning (101) are associated with infant illness and death (116). These suboptimal practices are schematized in Figure 3.

CONCLUSION

Unlike other species, the life histories of mammals have coevolved with the special adaptive advantages and physiological demands of lactation biology. This review has suggested that human patterns of lactation and complementary feeding are intimately linked with the evolution of a distinctive set of human life history variables. Complementary feeding and fat storage in pregnancy probably evolved in the past 5–7 million years as unique and important human adaptations that together reduce the energetic and opportunity costs of lactation for mothers and the potential fitness costs of relatively early transitional feeding and weaning for infants and young children. The human lactation span is comparatively short. The lower bound for safe complementary feeding has been set at around six months for normal-term and preterm babies by constraints on the evolution of physiological factors such as the growth and maturation of infant systems affecting immune, feeding, and digestive competency. The upper bound for safe weaning has been set above two years of infant age by similar constraints, but the evolution of complementary feeding, together with many other distinctively human evolutionary changes, has introduced enormous behavioral flexibility in maternal response to social and ecological constraints.

This evolutionary perspective provides insight into why, in today's world, young child feeding practices are

clinically suboptimal for most children and their mothers, and why many people in both rich and poor societies fail to adopt recommended feeding practices. Understanding the ultimate evolutionary causes of human variability in young child feeding can provide insights on the proximate causes of patterns of breastfeeding and complementary feeding that subsequently lead to poor health outcomes for mothers and babies. Such insight may help in the design of interventions to promote improved infant feeding practices.

SUMMARY POINTS

1. Human use of highly processed, nutrient-rich, complementary foods is hypothesized as unique among primates.
2. Complementary feeding is an evolutionarily derived (i.e. apomorphic) species characteristic that coevolved with changes in life history and physiology that reduce the maternal costs of lactation and with distinctive patterns of human foraging, parenting, social behavior, growth, and development.
3. The evolution of complementary feeding occurred because it made exclusive lactation relatively shorter and reduced birth intervals without increasing maternal or infant mortality.
4. Behavioral and physiological shifts during the evolution of complementary feeding enabled human infants to survive without breast milk at a relatively younger age and at a smaller size than infant apes.
5. Contemporary public health challenges arising from this evolutionary history include a strong behavioral tendency among humans to reduce

the length of exclusive breastfeeding beyond the lower bounds consistent with optimal infant outcomes.

FUTURE ISSUES

The following issues have not yet been resolved:

1. The extent of behavioral and physiological variation in the timing and dietary impact of transitional feeding in nonhuman primates and its socioecological correlates (such as quality of adult diet).

2. The absolute timing of steps in the evolution of complementary feeding and the relation of these steps to other key derived human characteristics (such as the origins and maintenance of bipedal locomotion, increased brain size, reduced sexual dimorphism, tool use, food sharing, cooking, and allo-parenting).

3. How humans evolved to overcome the physiological and psychosocial challenges to successful establishment of exclusive breastfeeding that are observed in contemporary populations.

4. How humans evolved to meet the complex challenge of introducing appropriate complementary foods in a timely manner while satisfying other demands on caregivers.

5. How human lactation biology evolved to protect low-birth-weight and premature infants, and to reduce the risks of maternal-to-child transmission of pathogens.

Note

Support for the author's work was furnished by the Canada Research Chairs Program (CRC), the Canadian Institutes of Health Research (CIHR), and the Canadian Foundation for Innovation (CFI).

References

1. Adair LS, Pollitt E, Mueller WH. 1983. Maternal anthropometric changes during pregnancy and lactation in a rural Taiwanese population. *Hum. Biol.* 55:771–87

2. Akuse RM, Obinya EA. 2002. Why healthcare workers give prelacteal feeds. *Eur. J. Clin. Nutr.* 56:729–34

3. Allen LH. 1994. Maternal micronutrient malnutrition: effects on breast milk and infant nutrition, and priorities for intervention. *SCN News* 11:21–24

4. Altmann J. 1980. *Baboon Mothers and Infants.* Cambridge, MA: Harvard Univ. Press

5. Altmann J, Alberts SC. 2003. Variability in reproductive success viewed from a life history perspective in baboons. *Am. J. Hum. Biol.* 14:401–9

6. Altmann J, Altmann SA, Hausfater G. 1978. Primate infant's effects on mother's future reproduction. *Science* 201:1028–30

7. Altmann J, Samuels A. 1992. Costs of maternal care: infant carrying in baboons. *Behav. Ecol. Sociobiol.* 29:391–98

8. Altmann SA. 1998. *Foraging for Survival: Yearling Baboons in Africa.* Chicago: Chicago Univ. Press. 609 pp.

9. Alvarez HP. 2000. Grandmother hypothesis and primate life histories. *Am. J. Phys. Anthropol.* 113:435–50

10. Am. Dietet. Assoc. 2005. *Position of the American Dietetic Association: Promoting and Supporting Breastfeeding.* Chicago/Washington, DC: Am. Dietet. Assoc.

11. Ball HL, Hill CM. 1996. Reevaluating "twin infanticide." *Curr. Anthropol.* 37:856–63

12. Barry H III, Paxson LM. 1971. Infancy and early childhood: cross-cultural codes 2. *Ethnology* 10:466–508

13. Baumslag N, Michels DL. 1995. *Milk, Money, and Madness: The Culture and Politics of Breastfeeding.* Westport, London: Bergin & Garvey. 256 pp.

14. Beauchamp GK, Cowart BL. 1987. Development of sweet taste. In *Sweetness*, ed. J Dobbing, pp. 127–38. Berlin: Springer-Verlag

15. Ben Shaul DM. 1962. The composition of the milk of wild animals. *Int. Zool. Yearbook* 4:333–42

16. Bentley GR. 1999. Aping our ancestors: comparative aspects of reproductive ecology. *Evol. Anthropol.* 7:175–85

17. Bercovitch FB. 1987. Female weight and reproductive condition in a population of olive baboons (*Papio anubis*). *Am. J. Primat.* 12:189–95

18. Bird DW. 2001. Human foraging strategies: human diet and food practices. In *Encyclopedia of Evolution*, ed. M Pagel. New York: Oxford Univ. Press

19. Black RF, Bhatia J. 1998. The biochemistry of human milk. In *The Science of Breastfeeding*, ed. RF Black, L Jarman, JB Simpson, pp. 103–52. Boston, MA: Jones & Bartlett

20. Blackburn DG. 1993. Lactation: historical patterns and potential for manipulation. *J. Dairy Sci.* 46:3195–212

21. Blakely RJ. 1989. Bone strontium in pregnant and lactating females form archaeological samples. *Am. J. Phys. Anthropol.* 80:173–85

22. Blaxter KL. 1961. Lactation and growth of the young. In *Milk: The Mammary Gland and Its Secretion*, ed. SK Kon, AT Cowie, pp. 305–61. London: Academic

23. Blurton Jones N. 2002. The lives of hunter-gatherer children: effects of parental behavior and parental reproductive strategy. In *Juvenile Primates: Life History, Development, and Behavior*, ed. ME Pereira, LA Fairbanks, pp. 309–26. New York: Oxford Univ. Press. 2nd ed.

24. Blurton Jones N. 2005. Introduction: Why does childhood exist? See Ref. 104a, pp. 105–8

25. Blurton Jones N, Hawkes K, O'Connell JF. 1999. Some current ideas about the evolution of the human life history. In *Comparative Primate Socioecology*, ed. PC Lee, pp. 140–66. London: Cambridge Univ. Press

26. Bock J, Sellen DW. 2002. Childhood and the evolution of the human life course: an introduction. *Hum. Nat.: An Interdiscip. J.* 13:153–59

27. Boinski S. 1988. Sex differences in the foraging beahvior of squirrel monkeys in a seasonal habitat. *Behav. Ecol. Sociobiol.* 32:177–86

28. Bribiescas RG. 2001. Reproductive ecology and life history of the human male. *Yearbook Phys. Anthropol.* 44:148–76

29. Bronson FH. 1989. *Mammalian Reproductive Biology.* Chicago: Chicago Univ. Press

30. Brown KH, Akhtar NA, Robertson AD, Ahmed MG. 1986. Lactational capacity of marginally nourished mothers: relationships between maternal nutritional status and quantity and proximate composition of milk. *Pediatrics* 78:909–19

31. Brown KH, Dewey KG, Allen L. 1998. *Complementary Feeding of Young Children in Developing Countries: A Review of Current Scientific Knowledge.* Geneva: World Health Org. 178 pp.

32. Buss DH. 1971. Mammary glands and lactation. In *Comparative Reproduction of Nonhuman Primates*, ed. ESE Hafez, pp. 315–33. Springfield, IL: Thomas

33. Butte NF. 1996. Energy requirements of infants. *Eur. J. Clin. Nutr.* 50:S24–36

34. Butte NF, Henry CJK, Torun B. 1996. Report of the working group on energy requirements of infants, children and adolescents. *Eur. J. Clin. Nutr.* 50:S188–89

35. Caro TM, Sellen DW. 1990. On the reproductive advantages of fat in women. *Ethol. Sociobiol.* 11:51–66

36. Charnov EL. 1991. Evolution of life history variation among female mammals. *Proc. Natl. Acad. Sci. USA* 88:1134–37

37. Charnov EL. 1993. *Life History Invariants: Some Explorations of Symmetry in Evolutionary Ecology.* London: Oxford Univ. Press

38. Charnov EL. 1997. Trade-off-invariant rules for evolutionarily stable life histories. *Nature* 387:393–94

39. Charnov EL. 2001. Evolution of mammal life histories. *Evol. Ecol. Res.* 3:521–35

40. Charnov EL, Berrigan D. 1993. Why do female primates have such long lifespans and so few babies? Or life in the slow lane. *Evol. Anthropol.* 1:191–94

41. Cifelli RL, Rowe TB, Luckett WP, Banta J, Reyes R, Howes RI. 1996. Fossil evidence for the origin of the marsupial pattern of tooth replacement. *Nature* 379:715–18

42. Cohen R, Brown KH, Canahuati J, Rivera LL, Dewey KG. 1994. Effects of age of introduction of complementary foods on infant breast milk intake, total energy intake, and growth: a randomised intervention study in Honduras. *Lancet* 344:288–93

43. Conklin-Brittain N, Wrangham R, Smith CC. 2002. A two-stage model of increased dietary quality in early hominid evolution: the role of fiber. In *Human Diet: Perspectives on Its Origin and Evolution*, ed. PS Ungar, MF Teaford, pp. 61–67. Westport, CT: Greenwood

44. Daan S, Tinbergen JM. 1997. Adaptation of life histories. In *Behavioral Ecology: An Evolutionary Approach*, ed. JR Krebs, NB Davies, pp. 311–33. Oxford: Blackwell Sci.

45. Dall SRX, Boyd IL. 2004. Evolution of mammals: Lactation helps mothers to cope with unreliable food supplies. *Proc. R. Soc. Lond. B Biol. Sci.* 271:2049–57

46. Dept. Health Human Serv. Off. Women's Health. 2003. Benefits of breastfeeding. *Nutr. Clin. Care* 6:125–31

47. Desor JA, Bauchamp GK. 1987. Longitudinal changes in sweet preference in humans. *Physiol. Behav.* 39:639–41

48. Dettwyler KA. 2004. When to wean: biological versus cultural perspectives. *Clin. Obstetr. Gynecol.* 47: 712–23

49. Dewey K. 2003. *Guiding Principles for Complementary Feeding of the Breastfed Child.* Geneva: World Health Org.

50. Dewey K. 2005. *Guiding Principles for Feeding Nonbreastfed Children 6–24 Months of Age.* Geneva: World Health Org.

51. Dewey KG. 2002. *Guiding Principles for Complementary Feeding of the Breast Fed Child.* Geneva: Pan Am. Health Org./World Health Org. 37 pp.

52. Dewey KG, Brown KH. 2003. Update on technical issues concerning complementary feeding of young children in developing countries and implications for intervention programs. *Food Nutr. Bull.* 24:5–28

53. Dewey KG, Cohen RJ, Brown KH, Rivera LL. 1999. Age of introduction of complementary foods and growth of term, low-birth-weight, breast-fed infants: a randomized intervention study in Honduras. *Am. J. Clin. Nutr.* 69:679–86

54. Dewey KG, Cohen RJ, Brown KH, Rivera LL. 2001. Effects of exclusive breastfeeding for four versus six months on maternal nutritional status and infant motor development: results of two randomized trials in Honduras. *J. Nutr.* 131:262–67

55. Dewey KG, Cohen RJ, Rollins NC. 2004. Feeding of nonbreastfed children from 6 to 24 months of age in developing countries. *Food Nutr. Bull.* 25:377–402

56. Dewey KG, Lovelady CA, Nommsen LA, McCrory MA, Lonnerdal B. 1994. A randomized study of the effects of aerobic exercise by lactating women on breast-milk volume and composition. *New Engl. J. Med.* 330: 449–53

57. Dufour DL, Sauther ML. 2002. Comparative and evolutionary dimensions of the energetics of human pregnancy and lactation. *Am. J. Hum. Biol.* 14:584–602

58. Dunbar RIM, Dunbar P. 1988. Maternal time budgets of gelada baboons. *Anim. Behav.* 36:970–80

59. Dunbar RIM, Hannah-Stewart L, Dunbar P. 2002. Forage quality and the costs of lactation for female gelada baboons. *Anim. Behav.* 64:801–5

60. Dupras TL, Schwarcz HP, Fairgrieve SI. 2001. Infant feeding and weaning practices in Roman Egypt. *Am. J. Phys. Anthropol.* 115:204–12

61. Durnin JV, McKillop FM, Grant S, Fitzgerald G. 1985. Is nutritional status endangered by virtually no extra intake during pregnancy? *Lancet* 2:823–25

62. Durnin JV. 1987. Energy requirements of pregnancy: an integration of the longitudinal data from the five-country study. *Lancet* 2:1131

63. Ellison PT. 1994. Advances in human reproductive ecology. *Annu. Rev. Anthropol.* 23:255–75

64. Ellison PT. 2001. *On Fertile Ground: A Natural History of Human Reproduction.* Cambridge, MA: Harvard Univ. Press

65. Ellison PT. 2003. Energetics and reproductive effort. *Am. J. Hum. Biol.* 15:342–51

66. Fewtrell MS. 2003. The long-term benefits of having been breast-fed. *Curr. Paediatr.* 14:97–103

67. Fleet IR, Goode JA, Hamon MH, Laurie MS, Linzell JL, Peaker M. 1975. Secretory activity of goat mammary glands during pregnancy and the onset of lactation. *J. Physiol.* 251:763–73

68. Foley R. 1995. Evolution and adaptive significance of hominid behavior. In *Motherhood in Human and Nonhuman Primates*, ed. CR Pryce, RD Martin, SD, pp. 27–36. Basel, Switz.: Karger

69. Fomon SJ. 1986. Breast-feeding and evolution. *J. Am. Dietary Assoc.* 86:317–18

70. Food Nutr. Board. 1989. Energy. In *Recommended Dietary Allowances*, ed. National Research Council, pp. 24–38. Washington, DC: Natl. Acad. Press

71. Ford CS. 1945. *A Comparative Study of Human Reproduction.* New Haven, CT: Yale Univ. Press

72. Fouts HN, Hewlett BS, Lamb ME. 2005. Parent-offspring weaning conflicts among the Bofi farmers and foragers of central Africa. *Curr. Anthropol.* 46:29–50

73. Fouts HN, Lamb ME. 2005. Weanling emotional patterns among the Bofi foragers of Central Africa: the role of maternal availability. See Ref. 104a, pp. 309–21

74. Futuyma DJ. 1998. The evolution of life histories. In *Evolutionary Biology*, pp. 561–78. Sunderland, MA: Sinauer

75. Galdikas BMF, Wood JW. 1990. Birth spacing patterns in humans and apes. *Am. J. Phys. Anthropol.* 83:185–91

76. Garza C. 2006. New growth standards for the 21st century: a prescriptive approach. *Nutr. Rev.* 64:S72–91

77. Geary DC. 2002. Sexual selection and human life history. *Adv. Child Dev. Behav.* 30:41–101

78. Gebo DL. 2004. A shrew-sized origin for primates. *Phys. Anthropol.* 47:40–62

79. Gittleman JL, Thompson SD. 1988. Energy allocation in mammalian reproduction. *Am. Zool.* 28:863–75

80. Godfrey KM, Samonds KE, Jungers WL, Sutherland MR. 2001. Teeth, brains, and primate life histories. *Am. J. Phys. Anthropol.* 114:192–214

81. Goldman AS. 2001. Breastfeeding lessons from the past century. *Pediatr. Clin. North Am.* 48:xxiii–xxv

82. Goldman AS, Chheda S, Garofalo R. 1998. Evolution of immunologic functions of the mammary gland and the postnatal development of immunity. *Pediatr. Res.* 43:155–62

83. Gonzalez-Cossio T, Habicht JP, Rasmussen KM, Delgado HL. 1998. Impact of food supplementation during lactation on infant breast-milk intake and on the proportion of infants exclusively breast-fed. *J. Nutr.* 128:1692–702

84. Gunnlaugsson G, Einarsdottir J. 1993. Colostrum and ideas about bad milk—a case-study from Guinea-Bissau. *Soc. Sci. Med.* 36:283–88

85. Hammel EA. 1996. Demographic constraints on population growth of early humans. *Hum. Nat.* 7:217–55

86. Harcourt AH. 1987. Dominance and fertility among female primates. *J. Zool. Lond.* 213:471–87

87. Harrison MJS. 1983. Age and sex differences in the diet and feeding strategies of the green monkey, *Cercopithecus sabaeus. Anim. Behav.* 31:969–77

88. Hartmann P, Morgan S, Arthur P. 1986. Milk letdown and the concentration of fat in breast milk. In *Human Lactation 2: Maternal and Environmental Factors*, ed. M Hamosh, AS Goldman, pp. 275–81. New York: Plenum

89. Hartmann PE. 1973. Changes in the composition and yield of the mammary secretion of cows during the initiation of lactation. *Endocrinology* 59:231–47

90. Hartmann PE, Arthur PG. 1986. Assessment of lactation performance in women. In *Human Lactation 2: Maternal and Environmental Factors*, ed. M Hamosh, AS Goldman, pp. 215–30. New York: Plenum

91. Hartmann PE, Rattigan S, Prosser CG, Saint L, Arthur PG. 1984. Human lactation: back to nature. In *Physiological Strategies in Lacation*, ed. M Peaker, RG Vernon, CH Knight, pp. 337–68. London: Academic

92. Harvey PH, Clutton-Brock TH. 1985. Life history variation in primates. *Evolution* 39:559–81

93. Harvey PH, Martin RD, Clutton-Brock TH. 1987. Life histories in comparative perspective. In *Primate Societies*, ed. BB Smuts, DL Cheney, RM Seyfarth, RW Wrangham, TT Struhsaker, pp. 181–96. Chicago: Univ. Chicago Press

94. Hawkes K. 2006. Life history and the evolution of the human lineage: some ideas and findings. See Ref. 97, pp. 45–94

95. Hawkes K. 2006. Slow life histories and human evolution. See Ref. 97, pp. 95–126

96. Hawkes K, O'Connell JF, Blurton Jones NG, Alvarez H, Charnov EL. 1998. Grand-mothering, menopause, and the evolution of human life histories. *Proc. Natl. Acad. Sci. USA* 95:1336–39

97. Hawkes K, Paine RL, eds. 2006. *The Evolution of Human Life History.* Santa Fe, NM: School Am. Res. Press

98. Hayssen V. 1993. Empirical and theoretical constraints on the evolution of lactation. *J. Dairy Sci.* 76:3213–33

99. Hayssen VD, Blackburn DG. 1985. Alpha-lactalbumin and the evolution of lactation. *Evolution* 39:1147–49

100. Heinig MJ. 2001. Host defense benefits of breastfeeding for the infant: effect of breast-feeding duration and exclusivity. *Pediatr. Clin. North Am.* 48:105–23

101. Heinig MJ, Nommsen LA, Peerson JM, Lonnerdal B, Dewey KG. 1993. Intake and growth of breast-fed

and formula-fed infants in relation to the timing of introduction of complementary foods: the DARLING study. *Acta Paediatr.* 82:999–1006

102. Herring DA, Saunders SR, Katzenberg MA. 1998. Investigating the weaning process in past populations. *Am. J. Phys. Anthropol.* 105:425–39

103. Hewlett BS. 1991. Demography and childcare in pre-industrial societies. *J. Anthropol. Res.* 47:1–37

104a. Hewlett BS, Lamb ME. 2005. *Hunter-Gatherer Childhoods: Evolutionary, Developmental, and Cultural Perspectives.* Piscataway, NJ: Aldine Trans.

104. Hewlett BS. 2005. Introduction: Who cares for hunter-gatherer children? See Ref. 104a, pp. 175–76

105. Hill K. 1993. Life history theory and evolutionary anthropology. *Evol. Anthropol.* 2:78–88

106. Hill K, Hurtado AM. 1995. *Ache Life History: The Ecology and Demography of a Foraging People.* New York: Aldine de Gruyter

107. Hill K, Kaplan H. 1999. Life history traits in humans: theory and empirical studies. *Annu. Rev. Anthropol.* 28:397–430

108. Hinde K. 2006. Milk composition varies in relation to the presence and abundance of *Balantidium coli* in the mother in captive rhesus macaques (*Macaca mulatta*). *Am. J. Primatol.* 69:1–10

109. Horn HS. 1978. Optimal tactics of reproduction and life history. In *Behavioral Ecology: An Evolutionary Approach*, ed. JR Krebs, NB Davies, pp. 272–94. Oxford: Blackwell Sci.

110. Hrdy S. 1999. *Mother Nature: A History of Mothers, Infants and Natural Selection.* New York: Pantheon. 944 pp.

111. Huffman SL, Martin LH. 1994. First feedings: optimal feeding of infants and toddlers. *Nutr. Res.* 14:127–59

112. Inst. Med. (U.S.) Subcomm. Nutr. During Lactation. 1991. Milk composition. In *Nutrition During Lactation*, pp. 113–52. Washington, DC: Natl. Acad. Sci.

113. Inst. Med. (U.S.) Subcomm. Nutr. During Lactation. 1991. Milk volume. In *Nutrition During Lactation*, pp. 80–112. Washington, DC: Natl. Acad. Sci.

114. Janson CH, Van Schaik CP. 2002. Ecological risk aversion in juvenile primates: Slow and steady wins the race. In *Juvenile Primates: Life History, Development and Behavior*, ed. ME Pereira, LA Fairbanks, pp. 56–76. New York: Oxford Univ. Press. 2nd ed.

115. Jenness R. 1974. Biosynthesis and composition of milk. *J. Invest. Dermatol.* 63:109–18

116. Jones G, Steketee RW, Black RE, Bhutta ZA, Morris SS, Bellagio Child Suriv. Study Group. 2003. How many child deaths can we prevent this year? *Lancet* 362:65–71

117. Kanazawa AT, Miyazawa T, Hirono H, Hayashi M, Fujimoto K. 1991. Possible essentiality of docosahexaenoic acid in Japanese monkey neonates: occurrence in colostrum and low biosynthetic capacity in neonate brains. *Lipids* 26:53–57

118. Kaplan H, Hill K, Hurtado AM, Lancaster J. 2001. The embodied capital theory of human evolution. In *Reproductive Ecology and Human Evolution*, ed. PT Ellison, pp. 293–317. New York: Aldine de Gruyter

119. Kaplan H, Hill K, Lancaster J, Hurtado AM. 2000. A theory of human life history evolution: diet, intelligence, and longevity. *Evol. Anthropol.* 9:156–84

120. Katzenberg MA, Herring DA, Saunders SR. 1996. Weaning and infant mortality: evaluating the skeletal evidence. *Yearbook Phys. Anthropol.* 39:177–99

121. Kennedy GE. 2005. From the ape's dilemma to the weanling's dilemma: early weaning and its evolutionary context. *J. Hum. Evol.* 48:123–45

122. Knott CD. 2001. Female reproductive ecology of the apes: implications for human evolution. In *Reproductive Ecology and Human Evolution*, ed. PT Ellison, pp. 429–63. New York: Aldine de Gruyter

123. Konner M. 2005. Hunter-gatherer infancy and childhood: The !Kung and others. See Ref. 104a, pp. 19–64

124. Konner MJ. 1977. Infancy among the Kalahari Desert San. In *Culture and Infancy*, ed. PH Leiderman, SR Tulkin, A Rosenfeld, pp. 69–109. New York: Academic

125. Kramer M, Kakuma R. 2002. The optimal duration of exclusive breastfeeding: a systematic review. *Cochrane Database System. Rev.* 1. http://www.update-software.com/Abstracts/ab003517.htm

126. Kramer MS, Guo T, Platt RW, Sevkovskaya Z, Dzikovich I, et al. 2003. Infant growth and health outcomes associated with 3 compared with 6 mo of exclusive breastfeeding. *Am. J. Clin. Nutr.* 78:291–95

127. Kumar S, Hedges B. 1998. A molecular timescale for vertebrate evolution. *Nature* 392:917–20

128. Labbok M, Clark D, Goldman A. 2005. Breastfeeding: maintaining an irreplaceable immunological resource. *Breastfeeding Rev.* 13:15–22

129. Labbok MH. 2001. Effects of breastfeeding on the mother. *Pediatr. Clin. North Am.* 48:143–58

130. Lamb ME, Hewlett BS. 2005. Reflections on hunter-gatherer childhoods. See Ref. 104a, pp. 407–15

131. Lartey A, Manu A, Brown KH, Peerson JM, Dewey KG. 1999. A randomized, community-based trial of the effects of improved, centrally processed complementary foods on growth and micronutrient status of Ghanaian infants from 6 to 12 mo of age. *Am. J. Clin. Nutr.* 70:391–404

132. Lawrence M, Lawrence F, Coward WA, Cole TJ, Whitehead RG. 1987. Energy requirements of pregnancy in the Gambia. *Lancet* 2:1072

133. Lawrence RA. 1989. *Breastfeeding: A Guide for the Medical Profession.* St. Louis, MO: Mosby

134. Lee MF, Krasinski SD. 1998. Human adult-onset lactase decline: an update. *Nutr. News* 56:1–8

135. Lee PC. 1987. Nutrition, fertility and maternal investment in primates. *J. Zool. Lond.* 213:409–22

136. Lee PC. 1996. The meanings of weaning: growth, lactation, and life history. *Evol. Anthropol.* 5:87–96

137. Lee PC. 1999. Comparative ecology of postnatal growth and weaning among haplorhine primates. In *Comparative Primate Socioecology*, ed. PC Lee, pp. 111–39. London: Cambridge Univ. Press

138. Lee PC, Bowman JE. 1995. Influence of ecology and energetics on primate mothers and infants. In *Motherhood in Human and Nonhuman Primates*, ed. CR Pryce, RD Martin, D Skuse, pp. 47–58. Basel, Switz.: Karger

139. Lee PC, Majluf P, Gordon IJ. 1991. Growth, weaning and maternal investment from a comparative perspective. *J. Zool.* 225:99–114

140. Leigh SR, Blomquist G. 2007. Life history. In *Primates in Perspective*, ed. CJ Campbell, A Fuentes, KC MacKinnon, M Panger, SK Beader, pp. 396–407. Oxford, UK: Oxford Univ. Press

141. Leigh SR, Shea BT. 1996. Ontogeny of body size variation in African apes. *Am. J. Phys. Anthropol.* 99:43–65

142. Liem DG, Mennella JA. 2003. Heightened sour preferences during childhood. *Chem. Senses* 28:173–80

143. Long A. 1972. Two hypotheses on the origin of lactation. *Am. Natural.* 106:141–44

144. Lovelady CA, Lonnerdal B, Dewey KG. 1990. Lactation performance of exercising women. *Am. J. Clin. Nutr.* 52:103–9

145. Luckett WP. 1993. An ontogenetic assessment of dental homologies in therian mammals. In *Mammal Phylogeny, Vol. 1: Mesozoic Differentiation, Multituberculates, Monotremes, Early Therians, and Marsupials*, ed. FS Szalay, MJ Novacek, MC McKenna, pp. 182–204. New York: Springer

146. Lunn PG. 1985. Maternal nutrition and lactational infertility: the baby in the driving seat. In *Maternal Nutrition and Lactational Infertility*, ed. J Dobbing, pp. 41–64. Vevey/New York: Nestlé Nutr./Raven

147. Luo ZX, Crompton AW, Sun AL. 2002. A new mammal form from the early Jurassic and evolution of mammalian characteristics. *Science* 292:1535–40

148. Mace R. 2000. Review: evolutionary ecology of human life history. *Anim. Behav.* 59:1–10

149. Manda SOM. 1999. Birth intervals, breastfeeding and determinants of childhood mortality in Malawi. *Soc. Sci. Med.* 48:301–12

150. Marlowe FW. 2005. Who tends Hadza children? See Ref. 104a, pp. 177–90

151. Marquis GS, Habicht J. 2000. Breastfeeding and stunting among toddlers in Peru. In *Short and Long Term Effects of Breast Feeding on Child Health*, ed. B Koletzko, KF Michaelsen, O Hernell, pp. 163–72. New York: Kluwer Acad./Plenum

152. Martin RD. 1984. Scaling effects and adaptive strategies in mammalian lactation. *Symposia Zool. Soc. Lond.* 51:87–117

153. Martin RD, MacLarnon AM. 1985. Gestation period, neonatal size and maternal investment in placental mammals. *Nature* 313:220–23

154. McCrory MA. 2000. Aerobic exercise during lactation: safe, healthful, and compatible. *J. Hum. Lactat.* 16:95–98

155. McCrory MA. 2001. Does dieting during lactation put infant growth at risk? *Nutr. Rev.* 59:18–27

156. McDade TW, Worthman CM. 1998. The weanling's dilemma reconsidered: a biocultural analysis of breastfeeding ecology. *J. Dev. Behav. Pediatr.* 19:286–99

157. McGuire E. 2005. *An Exploration of How Mother's Milk Protects the Infant*. East Malvern, Victoria, Australia: Austral. Breastfeed. Assoc. Lactat. Resource Cent.

158. Messer M, Weiss AS, Shaw DC, Westerman M. 1998. Evolution of the monotremes: phylogenetic relationship to marsupials and eutherians, and estimation of divergence dates based on α-lactalbumin amino acid sequences. *J. Mammalian Evol.* 5:95–105

159. Moggi-Cecchi J, Pacciani E, Pinto-Cisneros J. 1994. Enamel hypoplasia and age at weaning in nineteenth century Florence, Italy. *Am. J. Phys. Anthropol.* 93:299–306

160. Natl. Acad. Sci. 1989. *Nutrition and Diarrheal Diseases Control in Developing Countries*. Washington, DC: Natl. Acad. Press. 14 pp.

161. Natl. Res. Counc. Natl. Acad. Sci. 2003. *Nutrient Requirements of Nonhuman Primates, Table 9-4*. Washington, DC: Natl. Acad. Press. 286 pp.

162. Nelson EAS, Yu LM, Williams S, Int. Child Care Pract. Study Group. 2005. International Child Care Practices study: breastfeeding and pacifier use. *J. Hum. Lactat.* 21:289–95

163. Nicolosi RJ, Hunt RD. 1979. Dietary allowances for nutrients in nonhuman primates. In *Primates in Nutritional Research*, ed. KC Hayes, pp. 11–37. New York: Academic

164. Nishida T, Corp N, Hamai M, Hasegawa T, Hiraiwa-Hasegawa M, et al. 2003. Demography, female life history, and reproductive profiles among the chimpanzees of Mahale. *Am. J. Primatol.* 59:99–121

165. Nishida T, Ohigashi H, Koshimizu K. 2000. Tastes of chimpanzee plant foods. *Curr. Anthropol.* 41:431–38

166. Nishida T, Turner LA. 1996. Food transfer between mother and infant chimpanzees of the Mahale Mountains National Park, Tanzania. *Int. J. Primatol.* 17(6):947–68

167. Oftedal OT. 1984a. Body size and reproductive strategy as correlates of milk energy output in lactating mammals. *Acta Zool. Fennica* 171:183–86

168. Oftedal OT. 1984b. Milk composition, milk yield and energy output at peak lactation: a comparative review. *Symposia Zool. Soc. Lond.* 51:33–85

169. Oftedal OT. 1986. Milk intake in relation to body size. In *The Breastfed Infant: A Model for Performance*, ed. LJ Filer Jr, SJ Fomon, pp. 44–47. Columbus: Ross Lab.

170. Oftedal OT, Iverson SJ. 1987. Hydrogen isotope methodology for measurement of milk intake and

energetics of growth in suckling young. In *Marine Mammal Energetics*, ed. AC Huntley, DP Costa, GAJ Worthy, MA Castellini, pp. 67–96. Lawrence, KS: Allen

171. Pagel MD, Harvey PH. 1993. Evolution of the juvenile period in mammals. In *Juvenile Primates: Life History, Development, and Behavior*, ed. ME Pereira, LA Fairbanks, pp. 528–37. New York: Oxford Univ. Press

172. Paine RR, Hawkes K. 2006. Introduction. See Ref. 97, pp. 3–16

173. Patino EM, Borda JT. 1997. The composition of primate's milks and its importance in selecting formulas for hand rearing. *Lab. Primate Newsl.* 36:8–9

174. Peccei J. 2001. A critique of the Grandmother Hypothesis: old and new? *Am. J. Hum. Biol.* 13:434–52

175. Pennington RL. 1996. Causes of early human population growth. *Am. J. Phys. Anthropol.* 99:259–74

176. Pereira ME, Fairbanks LA, eds. 2002. *Juvenile Primates: Life History, Development, and Behavior*. Chicago: Univ. Chicago Press

177. P'erez-Escamilla R, Segura-Mill'an S, Canahuati J, Allen H. 1996. Prelacteal feedings are negatively associated with breast-feeding outcomes in Honduras. *J. Nutr.* 126:2765–73

178. Pond CM. 1984. Physiological and ecological importance of energy storage in the evolution of lactation: evidence for a common pattern of anatomical organization of adipose tissue in mammals. *Symposia Zool. Soc. Lond.* 51:1–31

179. Pond CM. 1997. The biological origins of adipose tissue in humans. In *The Evolving Female*, ed. ME Morbeck, A Galloway, AL Zihlman, pp. 47–162. Princeton, NJ: Princeton Univ. Press

180. Power ML, Oftedal OT, Tardif SD. 2002. Does the milk of callitrichid monkeys differ from that of larger anthropoids? *Am. J. Primatol.* 56:117–27

181. Prentice A. 1986. The effect of maternal parity on lactational performance in a rural African community. In *Human Lactation 2: Maternal and Environmental Factors*, ed. M Hamosh, AS Goldman, pp. 165–73. New York: Plenum

182. Prentice A, Paul A, Prentice A, Black A, Cole T, Whitehead R. 1986. Cross-cultural differences in lactational performance. In *Human Lactation 2: Maternal and Environmental Factors*, ed. M Hamosh, AS Goldman, pp. 13–43. New York: Plenum

183. Prentice A, Spaaij C, Goldberg G, Poppitt S, van Raaij J, et al. 1996. Energy requirements of pregnant and lactating women. *Eur. J. Clin. Nutr.* 50:S82–111

184. Prentice A, Whitehead R, Roberts S, Paul A. 1981. Long-term energy balance in child-bearing Gambian women. *Am. J. Clin. Nutr.* 34:2790–99

185. Prentice AM, Prentice A. 1988. Energy costs of lactation. *Annu. Rev. Nutr.* 8:63–79

186. Promislow D. 2003. Mate choice, sexual conflct, and evolution of senescence. *Behav. Genet.* 33:191–201

187. Promislow DE, Harvey PH. 1990. Living fast and dying young: a comparative analysis of life-history variation among mammals. *J. Zool. Lond.* 220: 417–37

188. Quandt S. 1985. Biological and behavioral predictors of exclusive breastfeeding duration. *Med. Anthropol.* 9(2):139–51

189. Rasmussen KM. 1992. The influence of maternal nutrition on lactation. *Annu. Rev. Nutr.* 12:103–17

190. Rizvi N. 1993. Issues surrounding the promotion of colostrum feeding in rural Bangladesh. *Ecol. Food Nutr.* 30:27–38

191. Roberts SB, Cole TJ, Coward WA. 1985. Lactational performance in relation to energy intake in the baboon. *Am. J. Clin. Nutr.* 41:1270–76

192. Robson SL. 2004. Breast milk, diet, and large human brains. *Curr. Anthropol.* 45:419–24

193. Robson SL, van Schaik CP, Hawkes K. 2006. The derived features of human life history. See Ref. 97, pp. 17–44

194. Sahi T, Isokoski M, Jussila J, Launiala K. 1972. Lactose malabsorption in Finnish children of school age. *Acta Paediatr. Scand.* 61:11–16

195. Sangild PT. 2006. Gut responses to enteral nutrition in preterm infants and animals. *Exp. Biol. Med.* 231:1–16

196. Sauther ML. 1994. Changes in the use of wild plant foods in free-ranging ring-tailed lemurs during pregnancy and lactation: some implications for human foraging strategies. In *Eating on the Wild Side: The Pharmacologic, Ecologic and Social Implications of Using Noncultigens*, ed. NL Etkin, pp. 240–46. Tucson: Univ. Arizona Press

197. Schurr MR. 1997. Stable nitrogen isotopes as evidence for the age of weaning at the Angel site: a comparison of isotopic and demographic measures of weaning age. *J. Archaeol. Sci.* 24:919–27

198. Schurr MR. 1998. Using stable nitrogen-isotopes to study weaning behavior in past populations. *World Archaeol.* 30:327–42

199. Schurr MR, Powell ML. 2005. The role of changing childhood diets in the prehistoric evolution of food production: an isotopic assessment. *Am. J. Phys. Anthropol.* 126:278–94

200. Schwarcz HP, Wright LE. 1998. Stable carbon and oxygen isotopes in human tooth enamel: identifying breastfeeding and weaning in prehistory. *Am. J. Phys. Anthropol.* 106:1–18

201. Sellen DW. 2001a. Comparison of infant feeding patterns reported for nonindustrial populations with current recommendations. *J. Nutr.* 131:2707–15

202. Sellen DW. 2001b. Of what use is an evolutionary anthropology of weaning? *Hum. Nat. Interdiscip. J.* 12:1–7

203. Sellen DW. 2001c. Weaning, complementary feeding, and maternal decision making in a rural east African pastoral population. *J. Hum. Lactat.* 17:233–44

204. Sellen DW. 2006b. Lactation, complementary feeding and human life history. See Ref. 97, pp. 155–97

205. Sellen DW. 2007. Evolution of human lactation and complementary feeding: implications for understanding contemporary cross-cultural variation. *Adv. Exper. Med. Biol.* In press

206. Sellen DW, Mace R. 1999. A phylogenetic analysis of the relationship between subadult mortality and mode of subsistence. *J. Biosoc. Sci.* 31:1–16

207. Sellen DW, Smay DB. 2001. Relationship between subsistence and age at weaning in "preindustrial societies." *Hum. Nat. Interdiscip. J.* 12:47–87

208. Sellen DW. Sub-optimal breast feeding practices: ethnographic approaches to building "baby friendly" communities. *Adv. Exper. Med. Biol.* 503:223–32

209. Shahidullah M. 1994. Breast-feeding and child survival in Matlab, Bangladesh. *J. Biosoc. Sci.* 26:143–54

210. Sheppard JJ, Mysak ED. 1984. Ontogeny of infantile oral reflexes and emerging chewing. *Child Dev.* 55:831–43

211. Smith BH. 1991. Dental development and the evolution of life history in Hominidae. *Am. J. Phys. Anthropol.* 86:157–74

212. Smith BH. 1992. Life history and the evolution of human maturation. *Evol. Anthropol.* 1:134–42

213. Smith BH, Crummett TL, Brandt KL. 1994. Ages of eruption of primate teeth: a compendium for aging individuals and comparing life histories. *Yearbook Phys. Anthropol.* 37:177–231

214. Smith RJ, Jungers WL. 1997. Body mass in comparative primatology. *J. Hum. Evol.* 32:523–59

215. Stacey PB. 1986. Group size and foraging efficiency in yellow baboons. *Behav. Ecol. Sociobiol.* 18:175–87

216. Stearns SC. 1992. *The Evolution of Life Histories.* Oxford: Oxford Univ. Press

217. Stevenson RD, Allaire JH. 1991. The development of normal feeding and swallowing. *Pediatr. Clin. North Am.* 38:1439–53

218. Sugarman M, Kendall-Tackett K. 1995. Weaning ages in a sample of American women who practice extended breastfeeding. *Clin. Pediatr.* 34:642–47

219. Tardif SD, Harrison ML, Simek MA. 1993. Communal infant care in marmosets and tamarins: relation to energetics, ecology, and social organization. In *Marmosets and Tamarins: Systematics, Behavior, and Ecology,* ed. AB Rylands, pp. 220–34. New York: Oxford Univ. Press

220. Tilden CD, Oftedal OT. 1997. Milk composition reflects pattern of maternal care in prosimian primates. *Am. J. Primatol.* 41:195–211

221. Trevathan WR, McKenna JJ. 1994. Evolutionary environments of human birth and infancy: insights to apply to contemporary life. *Child. Environ.* 11:88–104

222. Underwood BA, Hofvander Y. 1982. Appropriate timing for complementary feeding of the breast-fed infant. *Acta Paediatr. Scand.* S294:5–32

223. U.S. Breastfeeding Comm. 2002a. *Benefits of Breastfeeding.* Raleigh, NC: U.S. Breastfeeding Comm.

224. U.S. Breastfeeding Comm. 2002b. *Economic Benefits of Breastfeeding.* Raleigh, NC: U.S. Breastfeeding Comm.

225. van Esterik P. 2002. Contemporary trends in infant feeding research. *Annu. Rev. Anthropol.* 31:257–78

226. van Noordwijk MA, van Schaik CP. 2005. Development of ecological competence in Sumatran orangutans. *Am. J. Phys. Anthropol.* 127:79–94

227. van Schaik CP, Barrickman N, Bastian ML, Krakauer EB, van Noordwijk MA. 2006. Primate life histories and the role of brains. See Ref. 97, pp. 127–54

228. Vernon RG, Flint DJ. 1984. Adipose tissue: metabolic adaptation during lactation. *Symposia Zool. Soc. Lond.* 51:119–45

229. Walker R, Gurven M, Migliano A, Chagnon N, Djurovic G, et al. 2006. Growth rates, developmental markers, and life histories in 20 small-scale societies. *Am. J. Hum. Biol.* 18:295–311

230. Walker R, Hill K, Burger O, Hurtado AM. 2006. Life in the slow lane revisited: ontogenetic separation between chimpanzees and humans. *Am. J. Phys. Anthropol.* 129:577–83

231. Winkvist A, Jalil F, Habicht JP, Rasmussen KM. 1994. Maternal energy depletion is buffered among malnourished women in Punjab, Pakistan. *J. Nutr.* 124:2376–85

232. Wood JW. 1990. Fertility in anthropological populations. *Annu. Rev. Anthropol.* 19:211–42

233. Wood JW. 1994. *Dynamics of Human Reproduction: Biology, Biometry, Demography.* New York: Aldine de Gruyter

234. World Health Org. 1979. *Joint WHO/UNICEF Meeting on Infant and Young Child Feeding: Statement and Recommendations.* Geneva: World Health Org.

235. World Health Org. 2000a. *Complementary Feeding: Family Foods for Breast Fed Children.* Geneva: World Health Org.

236. World Health Org. 2000b. Effects of breastfeeding on infant and child mortality due to infectious diseases in less developed countries: a pooled analysis. *Lancet* 355:451–55

237. World Health Org. 2001. Global strategy for infant and young child feeding: the optimal duration of exclusive breastfeeding. *Rep. A54/INF.DOC./4.* Geneva: World Health Org.

238. World Health Org., U.N. Children's Fund. 2003. *Global Strategy for Infant and Young Child Feeding.* Geneva: World Health Org.

239. Worthman CM, Kuzara J. 2005. Life history and the early origins of health differentials. *Am. J. Hum. Biol.* 17:95–112

240. Wrangham R, Jones JH, Laden G, Pilbeam D, Conklin-Brittain N. 1999. The raw and the stolen: cooking and the ecology of human origins. *Curr. Anthropol.* 40:567–94

241. Wray J. 1991. Breast-feeding: an international and historical review. In *Infant and Child Nutrition Worldwide: Issues and Perspectives,* ed. F Falkner, pp. 62–117. Boca Raton, FL: CRC Press

242. Wright P. 1990. Patterns of paternal care in primates. *Int. J. Primat.* 11:89–102

CHAPTER 44

Premastication: The Second Arm of Infant and Young Child Feeding for Health and Survival?

Gretel H. Pelto, Yuanyuan Zhang, and Jean-Pierre Habicht

(2010)

As with all mammals, lactation provided a secure base for infant survival during the course of homo sapiens evolution; however, it did not solve the problem of what to do when breastmilk alone becomes inadequate to meet the growing infant's nutritional needs. This paper presents the argument for the second arm of the solution to how humans, as a biological and culture-producing species, met the extraordinary challenge produced by selection pressures for neoteny beginning with our early homo sapiens ancestors. "Neoteny" refers to the reduction in the rate of somatic development, relative to other species, which has permitted the evolution of critical human capacities, especially related to brain size and upright posture (McNamara 2002). Humans develop more slowly, in utero and post-natally, and achieve the characteristics necessary to survive independently later than other mammalian species. This is particularly evident with respect to the dentition that is required to bite off and chew the foods of an omnivorous diet. As part of general neoteny, tooth eruption in humans is significantly delayed compared to other mammals, including other primates (Smith 1989).

Our closest primate relatives, who were not challenged to find an adaptation to the nutritional threat to infants created by late eruption of teeth, solve the problem of ensuring infant nutrition with two adaptations: (1) prolonged lactation and (2) early tooth eruption, which together provide offspring with the capacity to start consuming the adult diet while they are still consuming maternal milk (Sellen 2007). In humans, breastfeeding is not as prolonged as our life history parameters would predict (Sellen 2007) and becomes inadequate as the exclusive source of nutrition to the infant at about 6 months of age (WHO recommendation). Our teeth develop late, especially our molars, which only erupt at about 18–24 months and which are essential for consuming an adult diet. Thus, our evolving ancestors must have found another solution to making up for the shortfall in breastmilk.

The hypothesis of this paper is that a behavioral solution, premastication (pre-chewing), of adult diets by infants' caregivers provided the solution, a second arm following the first arm of breastfeeding. The idea of feeding infants premasticated foods seems as inappropriate today as breastfeeding seemed to many people only 40 years ago, yet without it, it is unlikely that our hunting-gathering ancestors would have survived to establish the agricultural revolution that permitted the development of other modes of infant feeding. In fact, however, from the perspective of ensuring infant nutrition, plant domestication did not provide an adequate solution to the challenge of providing infants with nutritionally adequate diets before they were able to meet their nutritional requirements from the family diet. The paps and gruels of earlier farming cultures, like the unfortified complementary foods in use today, did not contain sufficient micronutrients to meet infants' biological requirements.

Even today and even in wealthy, industrialized countries, the micronutrient content of usual complementary foods is problematic. For example, with respect to iron the PAHO/WHO document on Guiding Principles for Complementary Feeding of the Breastfed Child (2003), notes that the "average intakes of breastfed infants in industrialized countries would fall short of the recommended intake of iron if iron-fortified products were not available" (p. 25). Moreover, as they are readily subject to inappropriate dilution, the paps and gruels made from the staples created by plant domestication set the stage for energy and protein undernutrition in infancy and early childhood. It is generally recognized that reliance on them as the primary or exclusive complement to breastmilk not only leads to kwashiorkor, but is implicated as a major cause of growth faltering and significant undernutrition in poor populations today. Moreover, malnutrition subsequent to the loss of hunting-gathering was exacerbated and rendered more fatal (Pelletier et al. 1993) by increased exposure to infectious disease (Cohen 1989) due to higher population densities that fostered not only the transmission of diseases, but also the development of new diseases.

Gretel H. Pelto, Yuanyuan Zhang, and Jean-Pierre Habicht, "Premastication: the second arm of infant and young child feeding for health and survival?" *Maternal & Child Nutrition*, 2010, 6:4–18. Reprinted with permission.

The rationale for the premastication hypothesis involves the following:

1. The need for energy, protein, and micronutrients from non-breastmilk dietary sources occurs before dental development is sufficiently adequate to permit infants to consume family foods.
2. During our long evolution as a hunting-gathering species foods were not easily processed into a form that children without a full set of teeth could consume.
3. Populations in which adults pre-chewed (premasticated) foods and fed them to infants had a strong survival advantage to such an extent that this behavioral trait was sustained through selection.
4. In agriculture-based populations the continuation of premastication prevented malnutrition by providing protein and nutrient-dense foods to supplement carbohydrate-based paps and gruels. It also supported other aspects of infant health through maternal-infant saliva transfer.
5. The disappearance of premastication as a usual practice is recent and has occurred in populations that either have access to modern food processing techniques or in which traditional practices have been lost as a consequence of culture change and economic impoverishment. The abandonment of premastication is reinforced by modern, biomedical concepts of hygiene, which have labeled the practice as "unhygienic" and "dangerous."

As there are no longer any groups of people who are living exclusively as hunter-gatherers, it is not possible to determine whether premastication prevented malnutrition in such societies. However, it is possible to use ethnographic data to provide some insights into where and how it has been practiced historically. Sections I and II present the results of two empirical studies we conducted to examine the hypothesis that premastication was wide spread. The first study is a cross-cultural examination, using the Human Relations Area Files (HRAF) to obtain ethnographic data on the occurrence of premastication in human societies. The second study is a qualitative survey of the infant feeding practices experienced two decades ago by students in an elite Chinese University, which was undertaken to assess the potential for serious under-reporting of the practice in the HRAF files, and to describe specific features of it. Section III is a discussion of the potential risks and benefits of infant exposure to maternal saliva.

THE CROSS-CULTURAL STUDY

The cross-cultural method, in which societies are treated as units of analysis, was initially developed by anthropologists in the first half of the 20th century. It has been used by social scientists to study the distribution of social and cultural traits and to test hypotheses descriptively through the examination of associations among traits. The method uses information from a large body of descriptive ethnographic research monographs, which are products of the primary research mode of cultural anthropologists from the inception of the discipline. Anthropologists set out to develop ethnographies that contained rich description of the culture, behaviors and lifeways of a geographically delimited social group. Typically the description is produced as the result of long-term field research in a specific location in which the anthropologist obtains data through a combination of interviews and observations. Often data collection is based on the method of "participant-observation," in which the ethnographer engages directly in daily or ritual behaviors in order to learn, first-hand, the complexities of cultural performance. Data are recorded in written form, on tape, on film, and in videos. From these sources the ethnography is written, typically organized in chapters that cover different aspects of social and cultural life.

Several databases have been constructed to facilitate cross-cultural research, of which the best known and most comprehensive is the Human Relations Area Files (HRAF). This ambitious endeavor "...currently contains over 800,000 pages of indexed information on over 370 different cultural, ethnic, religious, and national groups around the world.... [It] ... contains mostly primary source materials—mainly published books and articles, but it also includes some unpublished manuscripts and dissertations. The files contain studies on cultures or societies in all of the regions in the world" (Ember & Ember http://www.yale.edu/hraf/basiccc.htm). Every page in each document is indexed and assigned subject category codes according to a classification scheme contained in the Outline of Cultural Materials (OCM) (Murdock et al. 1987). One can search documents by subject codes, as well as by key words and phrases.

A few investigators have used the cross-cultural method to address nutritional questions. For example, Sarah Nerlove (1974) studied the relationship between women's workload and infant feeding practices, and found that infants tend to begin receiving supplementary foods earlier in cultures in which women are more active in agricultural subsistence activities. Dan Sellen (Sellen and Smay 2001; Sellen 2001) applied the cross-cultural method to examine the ages when "exclusive" breastfeeding ceased in order to compare cultural patterns to current feeding recommendations.

Methods

For this study we used e-HRAF. This is an electronic version of the files that contains all of the documents (monographs, journal articles) for a subset of 155 cultures that were selected by the HRAF organization as a geographically representative sample, containing materials that conform to a pre-specified standard of methodological soundness. We began by identifying texts that included OCM numbers 853 ("infant feeding") and 862 ("weaning"). We also searched

Table 1 Occurrence of Premastication in e-HRAF Reports

Geographic area	No. of cultures with information on code "853" (infant feeding)	No. of cultures reporting premastication
Africa	24	4
North and Middle America	37	9
South America	17	8
Asia	21	10
Europe and Middle East	11	2
Oceania	9	5
Total	119	38

using different combinations of words related to premastication, such as "chew," "chewing" and "pre-chewing." All texts that contained one or more of the relevant codes were read and coded for presence of premastication. In ethnographies in which a mention or description of premastication occurred, additional variables were coded to capture information on what foods were premasticated, when the practice was initiated and terminated, who chewed the foods, and the ethnographer's stated purpose for the practice. All relevant pages were also photocopied in order to ensure that original text was available for subsequent review.

Results

From the total of 155 cultures in the HRAF online database, the OCM codes for infant feeding and/or weaning occurred in 119 (77%). The information ranged from a couple of lines to extensive discussion. Of the 119 cultures in which there was text to review, premastication was reported in 38; that is, nearly one-third of the cultures in which the ethnographer included some mention or discussion about feeding of infants includes a reference to premastication. Table 1 shows the geographic distribution by region of the world.

According to the ethnographers who reported the practice the primary reason for engaging in premastication was to provide children with food, but occasionally other motivations (cultural and spiritual beliefs, and disease prevention and healing) were mentioned. In 31 out of 38 cultures, premastication is reported to be practiced solely for the purpose of providing foods to babies. In 4 cultures, infants and young children were given specific premasticated foods to facilitate a beneficial outcome that originated in religious and cultural beliefs. In 2 cultures, premasticated herbs were used medicinally to cure disease, and in 1 to prevent disease. In one other culture, the purposes were both to provide food and to induce a beneficial outcome related to a cultural belief.

Information about the ages at which the practice of premastication were initiated and terminated is sparse. For age at initiation, there are data for only 13 of the 38 cultures.

Table 2 Age of Introducing Premasticated Foods in e-HRAF Reports

Age in months	No. of cultures
1–2	2
3–4	3
5–6	3
7–8	–
9–10	1
11–12	3
>12	1

These results, shown in Table 2, illustrate wide variability, with a median age of 6 months. It was impossible to estimate precisely the age at which premastication ended, but the descriptions suggest that it continued into the second year of life. When it had a spiritual dimension it may continue into adulthood, as in the following quotation from a Blackfoot: "...This would be some special old lady—one with a lot of power to doctor or put up Sun Dances. She would chew my meat and then give it to me to swallow. This was a blessing for me, just like getting part of her life. Whenever we had any spare change we were taught to give it to old people like that" (Hungry Wolf, 1980).

In 30 of the 38 cultures we could ascertain the type of individual who pre-chewed the infant's food. In the majority of cases it was only the mother (25 out of 30). In 5 cultures, other individuals—fathers, grandparents, siblings or a spiritually important person—also were reported to premasticate food for the child.

A wide variety of foods were reported to be premasticated. The level of detail varies considerably in the reports, but typically is quite general, with foods being reported in broad categories, such as "meat," "fish," "roots," etc. Table 3 summarizes the diverse list by plant and animal food

Table 3 Premasticated Foods Reported in e-HRAF Reports

Plant foods	Animal Foods
Nuts	Game
Legumes	Domesticated meat
Maize	Fish
Rice	
Tubers	
Fruit	
Roots	

groups. Below are two examples to illustrate how data on foods are reported in ethnographies:

The Kung San of the Kalahari (Africa):

"The !Kung have no milk from cows or goats and no cereals to feed an infant, and they…[feed]…by chewing their tough meat, harsh roots, and nuts and feed the infant premasticated food from their own mouths"

—MARSHALL 1976

The Garo (Asia)

"…with a banana leaf beside her containing food which she chews mouthful by mouthful, before spitting it into her hand and placing it in the baby's mouth. Gradually she tries feeding the baby meat, dried fish, and all the other Garo foods"

—BURLING 1963

Discussion

The data in the ethnographies provide evidence that premastication has been practiced on all continents and in every type of subsistence system, from hunter-gatherers, through horticultural societies to complex societies based on intensive agricultural. Although it is difficult to determine with precision, it appears that the types of foods that are pre-chewed for infants by their caregivers reflect the household diets consumed by other family members. They include animal-source foods, fruits, vegetables and nuts, as well as the staples of agricultural societies.

Can we conclude that, leaving aside the 25% of societies for which we have no information, one-third of the societies in this representative sample of human groups practiced premastication? On one hand, this is an impressive finding. It provides evidence that it was commonly practiced in different types of societies and environments. Its occurrence in widely different cultural traditions and environments indicates that it was not a unique invention of a particular cultural group, which then spread to neighboring societies. One-third is also significant in that it indicates that a substantial portion of humanity experienced this practice over the course of human history.

On the other hand, one-third is far from universal. Is this proportion actually correct? The cross-cultural method has several problems that affect the ability of researchers to investigate hypotheses (Bernard 2006). A major weakness in using the HRAF files to address a nutritional question is the problem of missing information. Ethnographers focus on describing social and cultural features in human societies, and nutrition has not been highly salient for most of them. It is surprising, therefore, to find that the majority of ethnographies actually have an entry for the OCM code for infant feeding. However, on closer inspection one finds that the level of detail is so poor that it is difficult to come to any conclusions about nutritionally relevant questions (Pelto et al. 2003). Ethnographers are not trained in nutrition, and what they observe and report reflects the common wisdom and perceptions about what was important to note about food and nutrition issues that were extant at the time of their work.

Given the lack of attention to the details of infant feeding practice in most ethnographies, it is probable that premastication is under-reported in the ethnographic literature. To test this hypothesis, we turned to a specific culture area for more in-depth investigation of the magnitude of a potential reporting problem. We began by conducting a study of all the ethnographies of Han societies in Mainland China in the full HRAF files, as contrasted with the reduced numbers in the electronic version. There are a total of 8 Han societies in the files, representing groups in North China, Northwest China, Central China, East China, Southwest China, South China, and Inner Mongolia. Seven of these 8 contain information under the OCM subject code 853 ("infant feeding"). Not a single description of premastication is found in the texts on any of these 8 societies.

If we conclude that premastication is not under-reported in the ethnographic reports, we would also have to conclude that the practice is a very recent cultural introduction in Mainland China because we know from personal observation that it is currently practiced there. In fact, one of us (Zhang) has not only seen it, but personally experienced it, having received premasticated foods from her medically trained, cardiologist mother and her grandmother.

A QUALITATIVE SURVEY OF INFANT FEEDING AMONG STUDENTS IN AN ELITE CHINESE UNIVERSITY

To provide some indication of the degree of underreporting in the HRAF files, we undertook a study to examine premastication in Han cultures in China. A review of the non-ethnographic nutrition literature on infant feeding in China provided no insights about feeding behaviors. Studies reported information about nutrient intake but not about how the foods containing the nutrients were fed. Since a large field study was not feasible, we decided to conduct a qualitative survey to determine whether our (Zhang's) experience was aberrant or whether premastication was widespread in the student population. We reasoned that if it was widespread, such a finding would indicate that premastication is underreported in the ethnographic literature.

Methods

Students were recruited from the biological sciences, agronomy and biotechnology in a large, elite university in Beijing. The student interviewers were initially recruited from friends who were part of Zhang's personal network and then by snowball sampling. The students came from all parts of China. Clearly a volunteer sample of university students is not a random sample, but if premastication was reported at all in this group, it is probably practiced by other social groups in China as well, especially as most of the students came from well-educated families whose feeding practices 20 years ago would represent acceptable "modern" practices including premastication.

We asked the students to interview their parents and/or grandparents, with the focus on how they (the interviewers) were fed as infants. We gave them an interview schedule to follow in conducting the interview. The interview schedule was pilot tested with Chinese students studying at Cornell and, by telephone, with their mothers in China. Decisions about face and content validity were based on feedback from the pilot process.

The interviews were conducted by telephone (in most cases) because students came from all over the country and usually return home only for holidays. If a student returned home during the period of data collection, the interview was conducted face-to-face. As premastication is generally discouraged by physicians and nurses, we felt it was necessary to embed questions about this practice within a larger set of questions about infant feeding. The study design and the interview protocol were approved by the Cornell University Human Subjects Committee. Procedures to ensure anonymity were carefully followed, and in accord with the assurance of privacy, we do not disclose the name of the university from which the student investigators and their respondent caregivers were recruited.

Results

One hundred twenty copies of the interview schedule were distributed, and 104 were returned and used for this analysis. The interviewers ranged in age from 20 to 24 years of age, of which 54 were female and 50 were male. The university recruits students from all over the country, and the 104 child/parent pairs of respondents represented 27 out of 34 provinces, autonomous regions, and municipalities. The sample did not include respondents from Nignxia Hui, Xinjiang Uigur, Qinghai, or Tibet.

The parent respondents were 90 female and 14 males, of which 89 were mothers of the interviewers, 14 were fathers and 1 was a grandmother. The median age of the parent respondents was 48 years old. As expected the education levels of respondents were high, far beyond the average of their age group in China. Only 4 out of 104 caregiver respondents had not received any formal education. Nearly 32% had received a college level education or above; another 38% had received a high-school-level education. At the time of the child's birth, 23 mothers had no outside job, while 79 were employed full time outside the home; 52 out of 77 (68%) of the working mothers had a maternal leave equal to or less than 3 months, 17 mothers (24%) had a maternal leave of 4–6 months, and only 7 (9%) mothers had a maternal leave of 6–12 months.

Virtually all of the students were breastfed: 102 of the 104. The 2 mothers who did not breastfeed said that this was due to lack of breastmilk. Seventy two percent of the mothers started breastfeeding within the first day of their children's birth. The median duration of breastfeeding was 12 months, with a minimum of one month and a maximum of 48 months.

Premastication was a common practice. Only 37% of respondents (39 of 104) reported that they never gave premasticated food to the infant. Of the 65 families who reported practicing premastication 22% said they used this practice "often" or "very often."

The start of premastication ranged from 1 month to 24 months with a median of 8 months (Table 4). The range in reported cessation was from 5 months to 48 months with a median of 24 months. Parents with less education were more likely to give premasticated foods (P<.001). There was no difference in reporting the practice in nuclear compared to extended families, but infants had a higher likelihood of receiving premasticated food if someone other than the parents was involved in their feeding (p<.002).

The most frequently premasticated food was meat, followed by rice, other grains, other "tough foods" and nuts. Table 5 lists all the items reported by parent respondents as foods they premasticated before giving it to their infants.

Discussion

The findings provide confirmation that premastication was undoubtedly seriously under-reported in the ethnographies on Chinese societies in the HRAF files. None of

Table 4 Age of Introduction of Complementary Foods by Premastication Status in Chinese Student Study

Age of introduction of complementary food in months	Premastication Reported		
	Yes	No	Total
1–2	6	2	8
3–4	19	11	30
5–6	11	12	23
7–8	9	3	12
9–10	2	1	3
11–12	5	4	9
>12	6	4	10
Missing information	7	2	9
Total respondents	65	39	104

Table 5 Premasticated Foods Reported by Parents of Students in an Elite University in China

Animal Foods	Fresh Fruits and Vegetables
Meat	Apple
Dried meat	Orange
Fish	Tomato
Dried fish	Tangerine
Eggs	
Staples	**Nuts**
Rice	Walnuts
Millet	Peanuts
Porridge	
Noodles	**Other**
Potato	Dumplings
Corn bread	Cookies
Steamed buns	

the ethnographies mentioned this practice, but we found that it was practiced by a majority of families in a sample that would be least likely to give premasticated food to their babies. It is unlikely that the discrepancy for China is unique to that country, particularly in view of the fact that nearly all of the China cultures (7 of 8) reported data under the "infant feeding" OCM numbers and none identified premastication.

In addition to providing support for the hypothesis that premastication is significantly under-reported in ethnographic accounts, the study in China also provided some information about the nature of premastication within the context of infant feeding practices in generally well-educated Chinese families two decades ago. These include:

1. Premastication happened in all parts of China, in large cities and provincial areas.
2. It was practiced in both nuclear and extended families, so it was not limited to older generation grandparents.
3. Parents with more education were less likely to premasticate foods for their babies, as would be expected since they are less likely to have been exposed to the counsel of pediatricians.

SALIVA: NON-NUTRITIONAL BENEFITS AND RISKS OF PREMASTICATION

An evaluation of the role of premastication as a behavioral adaptation to ensure infant nutrition must also examine the practice in relation to other aspects of health. There are no systematic reviews relating the biological aspects of saliva to the benefits and risks of premastication. However, the results of our initial exploration were surprising to us, as they will probably be for many readers. They raise interesting issues that need further attention. In this section we sketch out some of the issues that warrant further examination.

In their thorough review of the literature, Humphrey and Williamson (2001) enumerate the composition and describe the functions of saliva, primarily in relation to oral health. Saliva contains electrolytes, immunoglobulins, proteins, enzymes, mucins, and nitrogenous products that are important in the promotion of oral health, mastication, swallowing and pre-gastric digestion. Apart from its well-recognized functions in oral health, of particular interest with respect to premastication are its potential digestive health promoting properties, which need to be weighed against its potential to transmit diseases.

With respect to digestion, Humphrey and Williamson note the role of saliva in early stages of digestion, particularly of starches (Mandel 1987) and fats (Valdez and Fox 1991). The ability to digest complex carbohydrates develops slowly in infants. At birth there is a physiologic deficiency of pancreatic amylase. It is not until 9 months of age that adult values are reached (Lebenthal and Lee 1980; Zhang et al. 1996). Premastication, therefore, may facilitate absorption of foods that are given to the young infant in this manner.

Saliva also contains multiple growth factors that can enhance the body's repair mechanisms after tissue injury and may also have protective functions (Kongara and Soffer 1999). Table 6 presents a list of the many health-promoting substances that are found in both breastmilk and saliva. There are some substances in breastmilk that have not been reported for saliva, including bifidus factor, α1-antichymotrypsin, α1-antitrypsin, calcitonin, parathyroid hormone, erythropoietin, IgF binder, and thyroxine binder. Similarly, some substances found in saliva have not been reported as present in breastmilk, including gonadotropins, basic fibroblast growth factor (bFGF), peroxidase, proteases and peptidases, salivary acid phosphatase A, salivary acid phosphatase B, N acgtylmuramyl-alanine, amidase, NAD(P)H dehydrogenase-quinone, and Glucose-6-phosphate isomerase. However, the striking feature of Table 6 is how many substances the two body fluids – breastmilk and saliva – have in common. In short, the substances in maternal saliva, like the substances in breastmilk, have many potential beneficial roles for infant health.

However there is also the potential for harm from ingestion of saliva. A number of pathogens that have been isolated from maternal saliva are thought to be transmitted to their children. These include *H. pylori* (Bassily et al. 1999), Hepatitis B (Armstrong 2001), Human herpes virus 6 (HHV-6) (Yamanishi 2000), and human herpes virus 8 (HHV-8) (Brayfield 2003).

Saliva has also been linked to the contamination of premasticated foods. Imong and colleagues (1995) examined the bacterial contamination of infant weaning foods in a study in Thailand and found that in households who reported practicing premastication the weaning food samples were significantly higher in bacterial content than households who did not premasticate foods. The authors speculate that the diseases that could be introduced through premastication could include, among others, leprosy and tubercle mycobacterium, hemolytic streptococci, and respiratory tract viruses. However, a finding of increased

Table 6 Health-Promoting Factors in Breastmilk and Saliva[1]

Antimicrobial factors	Cytokines and anti-inflammatory factors
secretory IgA, IgM, IgG (Norhagen et al 1989) lactoferrin (Tenovuo, 1989), lysozyme (Tenovuo, 1989), complement components (Andoh, 1997), leucocytes (Wright, 1959), lipids and fatty acids (Tenovuo, 1989), antiviral mucins, GAGs (Shugars, 1999), oligosaccharides (Rosenblum, 1988), thiocyanate (breastmilk: Kirk, 2006; saliva: (Schultz, 1996)	tumour necrosis factor (Pezelj-Ribaric, 2004), interleukins (Dugue, 1996), interferon-γ (Sfriso, 2003), prostaglandins (Kasinathan, 1995), platelet-activating factor: acetyl hydrolase (Ribaldi, 1998)

Hormones	Growth Factors
insulin (Marchetti, 1986), prolactin (Vining, 1986) thyroid hormones (Vining, 1986) corticosteroids: ACTH (Lowe, 1983) oxytocin (Carter, 2007)	epidermal (EGF) (Kagami, 2000), nerve (NGF) (Kagami, 2000), insulin-like (IGF) (Kagami, 2000), transforming (TGF) (Kagami, 2000), taurine (Soderling, 2002), polyamines (Venza, 2001)

Digestive enzymes	Transporters
amylase (Tenovuo, 1989) esterase (Tenovuo, 1989) lipases (Tenovuo, 1989)[2]	lactoferrin (Fe) (Komine et al. 2007) folate binder (Verma, 1992) cobalamin binder (Hippe, 1972) corticosteroid binder (Groschl, 2004)

[1] Breastmilk factors, except for thiocyanate, are from a major review by Prentice (1996). All other references in parentheses are references for presence of these factors in saliva.

[2] Lipase may have a different form of aggregation in breastmilk and saliva (Larson et al, 1996) but whether this results in different functions has not been established.

bacterial count without further specification of which bacteria were involved does not tell us whether there is a greater risk of infection. Moreover, the authors present no rationale for their list of specific diseases or any evidence that these were present in their samples.

The presence of pathogens in saliva does not necessarily mean that they are infectious, especially because saliva contains IgG, IgM, and especially secretory IgA, which contain antibodies to viruses and bacterial antigens, and inhibit bacterial attachment to host tissues, thus controlling bacterial, fungal, and viral colonization. A case in point is human immunodeficiency virus (HIV), which can be isolated in saliva. A substantial body of research has shown that there are mechanisms which reduce the infectivity of HIV in saliva (Baron et al. 1999) thus making the risk of transmission low (Campo et al. 2006), lower than in breast milk. A recent meta-analysis of oro-genital transmission confirms that genital exposure to saliva of HIV positive partners is associated with low risk (Baggaley et al. 2008). The potential importance of premastication as a risk factor for HIV in infants and young children appears to be likely to be negligible.

There is better evidence to suggest that saliva transfer between mothers and their children is a cause of child infections with *H. pylori* (Taylor and Blasser 1991). The evidence for maternal transmission of *Streptococcus mutans* and *Streptococcus sobrinus*, the primary microorganisms associated with dental caries, is well established and it seems likely that transmission occurs through saliva (Berkowitz 1981).

As part of an assessment of the risks and benefits of premastication from the perspective of disease transmission it is useful to compare saliva to breastmilk. To date many more pathogens have been identified in breastmilk than in saliva, but this reflects the greater attention that has been given to breastmilk as a potential source of disease transmission to infants. The fact that pathogens can be identified in both breastmilk and saliva raises two important points: (1) Virtually all biological adaptations have downsides, and to put these into perspective requires a risk/benefit analysis; (2) Research on breastfeeding demonstrated that the risks of disease transmission were so small relative to the advantages that nobody would recommend curtailing breastfeeding except in very unusual and specific situations (e.g., HIV in wealthy populations). Similar results may pertain for premastication in view of the fact that, in addition to saliva's role in providing nutrients, premastication may play other positive roles in infant health. The extent to which maternal to infant transfer of saliva conveys specific antibody protection and promotes immunological health needs to be studied.

The potential for disease transmission leads to another question: Is transmission of disease agents from mother to child through saliva (or breastmilk) unequivocally bad? This question deserves careful consideration. When diseases are widespread and kill early, they prevent reproduction; therefore mechanisms that promote acquired immunity in childhood that either prevent or attenuate severity of disease in reproductively active adults would be advantageous. This has indeed occurred for many widespread pathogens, including rubeola (measles), varicela-zoster (chicken pox), paramyxovirus (mumps) and poliovirus (poliomyelitis), in which the diseases are significantly more serious when they occur in adulthood. The potential role of late exposure to Epstein-Barr (HHV-4) in the genesis of several cancers is currently attracting research attention (Stoppler 2008) and, with the development of further knowledge, may join the list of pathogens for which early exposure reduces adult health risks.

Apart from infectious disease, there is increasing evidence that early exposure to modern sanitary environments markedly increases the risk of atopic diseases, including asthma (Eder et al. 2006). In other words early exposure to a rich microbial environment is important in priming the immune system. In a similar vein, early exposure to potential food allergens in premasticated foods, particularly when the infant is still breastfeeding, may also have a role in reducing allergic responses to foods.

In summary, the argument for potential benefits from saliva exposure through premastication is strong. If the positive characteristics of saliva are sustained through infancy, then, apart from its nutritional aspects, it may be an important mechanism for supporting child, and even adult, health. At present, there is simply insufficient information to permit an estimate of the trade-offs between the potentially positive and negative features.

CONCLUSIONS

In a seminal paper on the evolution of infant and young child feeding, Sellen (2007) lays out two related paradoxes in the relationship of lactation and the role of foods in complementing and/or replacing breastmilk in human societies. These are: (1) although humans have the longest period of dependence on others for subsistence compared to other mammals, they generally do not maximize the period of exclusive breastfeeding, and (2) they wean their infants sooner than do other apes. He also highlights "The most remarkable change [in the evolution of human infant feeding compared to other animals] is the human use of complementary foods, which is unique among mammals, and results in a pattern of transitional feeding that appears to be fundamentally different from that of other primates" (p. 130).

To find an explanation for the apparent paradoxes in human management of infant feeding Sellen examines the energetic costs of lactation in relation to other critical features of reproductive success using a comparative life history analysis of humans and other apes. He points out that "Lactation, nutritional intake, energy expenditure, and net energy balance are the key influences on fecundity among humans" (p. 133). Focusing on the physiologic costs of lactation in relation to other aspects of reproduction, and the potential to share child complementary feeding with other caregivers, Sellen concludes that "Flexibility in weaning age reflects an evolved maternal capacity to vary reproduction in relation to ecology, the availability of alternate caregivers and other environmental and social factors affecting the costs and benefits of weaning to mothers and infants" (p. 135). In other words, the paradoxes are, ultimately, explained by the energetic costs of reproduction in relation to the alternative behavioral solutions that humans were able to evolve.

Sellen ends the article with a set of issues about our understanding of the evolution of infant and child feeding that have not yet been resolved. Among these he identifies: "How humans evolved to meet the complex challenge of introducing appropriate complementary foods in a timely manner while satisfying other demands on caregivers" (p. 136). We believe that the key to this understanding lies in premastication.

If premastication poses significant dangers from the perspective of disease transmission, then it is unlikely that it would have been sustained through the course of cultural evolution. Although there are examples of negative practices that become deeply embedded in cultural repertoires, these are not usually widely dispersed across all regions of the world. In addition to the empirical evidence, cultural-ecological theory would also predict that the behavior could not have been sustained.

If premastication was an integral part of the evolutionary process associated with selection for neoteny, one would expect to find bio-behavioral traits in adults and infants that reinforced it. We believe there are such traits, which are still observable today. When infants of complementary feeding age are face-to-face with adults, they often reach for the adult's mouth, in preference to other parts of the face, pulling on his/her lips and sticking their fingers into the adult's mouth. The typical response of the adult is to suck playfully on the tiny fingers, often pretending to chew them lightly. The response, in turn, provokes laughter and smiles from both infant and adult. Another common adult behavior that might be related to reinforcement of premastication is the tendency for adults to nuzzle their head and mouth into or close to the lower part of a baby's face or neck.

It is also the case, as was apparent in the comments from Hungry Wolf quoted above, that premastication can be viewed as a form of expressing affection. In informal interviews with mothers of young children, we have encountered women who describe or justify premastication as a way of showing affection and reinforcing the special bond they have with their infants. As one young mother recently put it "I know I probably shouldn't because of germs and all, but it's a way of sharing my love with my baby."

If both nutrition and immunological health are involved in the evolutionary benefits of premastication, then it is probable that it also has implications with respect to the synergistic relationship of nutrition and disease on child mortality (Pelletier et al. 1993). A behavior that simultaneously supports better nutrition and better immunological status would be expected to reduce the risk of mortality during the period when infants and young children are at high risk of dying. Until recently diarrhea was been the primary killer of children throughout the developing world, and it still remains a major cause of mortality (Boschi-Pinto et al. 2007). The incidence of diarrhea in young children peaks during the period of complementary feeding when infants are exposed to contaminated foods. Thus, the sharp rise in diarrhea that occurs when complementary foods are added can be seen as due to a trade-off between meeting nutritional needs and increasing the risk of life-threatening illness through ingestion of contaminated foods. This trade-off is called the "the weanling's dilemma" (Gordon et al. 1963, Rowland 1986). If it is correct that premastication neutralizes contamination it may be that the "weanling dilemma" is a consequence of lack of premastication. Worldwide, half of deaths from infectious diseases today, including diarrhea (Caulfield et al. 2004), occur because children are malnourished. This is compounded by the fact that diarrhea exacerbates malnutrition (Lutter et al. 1989). Thus there is promise that premastication could reduce, or even eliminate, the "weanling dilemma" by both improving nutrition and reducing infection.

In summary, did premastication protect children from the devastating consequences of diarrhea associated with the introduction of complementary foods by improving their nutritional status? Did the additional immunological substances transferred through saliva improve their ability to prevent and fight infections? Are the present high rates of diarrheal disease-related mortality the results of widespread loss of premastication as a basic childcare practice?

Issues for Further Investigation

Current understanding of the biology and biochemistry involved in premastication promises a potential for improving infant feeding in poor populations. However to assess this potential requires a concerted research effort. At the level of understanding evolutionary processes, the loss of adaptive behaviors that conferred survival advantage for our ancestors and shaped our evolution as a biological and social species continues to be a subject of considerable scholarly concern. Modern humans' departure from the dietary patterns of our predecessors has been linked to the development of diet-related chronic disease and obesity (cf. Cohen 1989; Eaton et al. 1989). Continued research in this area will contribute to understanding the place of premastication.

Of critical importance to assessing the public health implications is an examination of the *nutritional* benefits of premastication founded on empirical clinical and epidemiological research. In view of the ubiquitous prevalence of iron deficiency in infancy (Beard and Stoltzfuss 2001), and the fact that humans have evolved with greater iron requirements than can be met from breastmilk alone (PAHO/WHO 2003), as well as the fact that infants experience declining iron stores before they are physically capable of consuming heme iron from external sources, an area of special interest is the role of premastication in preventing iron deficiency in infants and young children. Iron is just one of several nutrients whose adequacy in infancy may have relied on premastication. In practice, it is likely that the potential nutritional benefits are going to be related to the diet of the adult who is feeding the child, and this raises the issues of the best foods for premastication feeding and their accessibility.

The subject of early immunological health and its relationship to health outcomes of older children and reproductively active adults is becoming increasingly better understood (Barrett at al. 1998; von Hertzen 2000). What is required is evidence for the role of premastication specifically for present and future health.

Another research issue of central importance is a systematic examination of the health and other benefits and risks to infants of receiving premasticated foods from their mothers. An early probe of the issue would be to undertake, for premastication, the kind of survey and analysis that demonstrated that breast-feeding saved lives (Habicht et al. 1986), and had high enough plausibility that intervention trials were warranted.

When one considers the reasons for contemporary departures from evolution-shaped practices, it is readily apparent that they are extremely complex and restoring or sustaining them in the contemporary world presents major, some would argue, insurmountable, challenges. However, at least with respect to infant feeding, the resurgence of breast-feeding in populations where there were severe declines in the prevalence of this essential health practice provides clear evidence that human societies are capable of re-institutionalizing adaptive practices.

The aversion with which many people today regard the very thought of premastication is similar to the negative views of breastfeeding that characterized many people's view of breastfeeding until recently. Fortunately, as research has demonstrated the benefits of breastfeeding, and as these benefits have become widely understood and accepted, negative attitudes about breastfeeding have largely disappeared. Whether or not premastication should be considered as part of a larger strategy to improve infant feeding and health, the second arm requires, as a first step, a research investment similar to the investments in breastfeeding, which have so richly paid off in supporting improvements in infant survival and health.

References

Andoh A., Fujiyama Y., Kimura T., Uchihara H., Sakumoto H., Okabe H., Bamba T. (1997) Molecular characterization of complement components (C3, C4, and factor B) in human saliva, *Journal of Clinical Immunology*, 17 (5): 404–407.

Armstrong G.L., Mast E. *et al.* (2001) Childhood hepatitis B virus infection in the United States before hepatitis B immunization. *Journal of Pediatrics* 108, 1124–1128.

Bagaglio S., Sitia G., Prati D., Cella D. (2002) Mother-to-child transmission of TT virus: sequence analysis of non-coding region of TT virus in infected mother-infant pairs. *Archives of Virology* 147:803–812.

Baggaley R.F, White R.G., Boily M-C. (2008) Systematic review of orogenital HIV-1 transmission probabilities. *International Journal of Epidemiology*, 37: 1255–1265.

Baron S., Poast J., Cloyd, M.W. (1999) Why is HIV rarely transmitted by oral secretions? Saliva can disrupt orally shed, infected leukocytes. *Archives of Internal Medicine* 159: 303–310.

Barrett R., Kuzawa C., McDade T., Armelagos G.J. (1998) Emerging and re-emerging infectious diseases: the third epidmiologic transition. *Annual Review of Anthropology* 27, 247–271.

Bassily S., Frenck W.R., Moharebe E.W. et al. (1999) Seroprevalence of Helicobacter Pylori Among Egyptian Newborns and Their Mothers: a Preliminary Report. *The American Journal of Tropical Medicine and Hygiene* 61 (1) 37–40.

Beard J. & Stoltzfus R. (2001) Iron-deficiency anemia: reexamining the nature and magnitude of the public health problem. Proceedings of the Belmont Conference. Published as a Supplement to the *Journal of Nutrition* 131 No. 2S-II.

Berkowitz R.J., Turner J., & Green P. (1981), Maternal salivary levels of streptococcus mutans and primary oral infection of infants. *Archives of Oral Biology* 26(2):147–149.

Bernard H.R. (2006). *Research Methods in Anthropology. Qualitative and Quantitative Approaches.* Alta Mira Press: New York.

Boschi-Pinto C., Velebit L., Shibuya K. (2007) Estimating child mortality due to diarrhoea in developing countries. *WHO Bulletin,* 86 (9):50–54.

Brayfield B.P., Phiri S., Chipepo K. *et al.* (2003) Postnatal human herpesvirus 8 and human immunodeficiency virus type 1 infection in mothers and infants from Zambia. *Journal of Infectious Disease* 187:559–568.

Burling R. (1963) *Rengsanggri: Family and Kinship in a Garo Village.* University of Pennsylvania Press: Philadelphia.

Campo J., Perea M.A., del Romero J., Cano J., Hernando V., Bascones A. (2006) Oral transmission of HIV, reality or fiction? An update. *Oral Disease.*12, 219–228.

Carter C.S., Purnajafi-Nazarloo H., Kramer K.M., Ziegler T.E., White-Traut R., Bello D Schwertz D. (2007) *Annals of the New York Academy of Sciences,* vol.1098:312–322.

Cohen M.N. (1989) *Health and the Rise of Civilization.* Yale University Press: New Haven.

Caulfield LE, de Onis M, Blössner M, Black RE. (2004) Undernutrition as an underlying cause of child deaths associated with diarrhea, pneumonia, malaria, and measles. *AmJ Clin Nutr* 80: 193–98.

Dugue B., Ilardo C. Aimone-Gastin I., Gueant J.L., Mouze-Amady M., Cnockaert J. C., Mur J-M., Grasbeck R. (1996) Cytokines in saliva. Basal concentrations and the effect of high ambient heat (sauna), *Stress Medicine,*12 (3):193–197.

Eaton S.B., Shostak M, Konner M. (1989) *The Paleolithic Prescription: A Program for Diet and Exercise and a Design for Living.* Harper Collins: New York.

Eder W., Ege MJ, von Mutius E. (2006) The asthma epidemic. *New England Journal of Medicine* 355: 2226–2235.

Ember C.R. & Ember, M. User's Guide: HRAF Collection of Ethnography. http://www.yale.edu/hraf/basiccc.htm Retrieved on 2007–3–15.

Gordon JE, Chitkara ID, Wyon JE. (1963) Weanling diarrhea. *Am J Med Sci.* 246:245–51.

Gröschl M., Köhlera H., Topfa H-G., Rupprecht T., Rauha M. (2008) Evaluation of saliva collection devices for the analysis of steroids, peptides and therapeutic drugs. *Journal of Pharmaceutical and Biomedical Analysis* 47 (3): 478–486.

Habicht, J-P., DaVanzo, J. and Butz, W. P.: (1986) Does breastfeeding really save lives, or are apparent benefits due to biases? *American Journal of Epidemiology,* 123 (2): 279–290.

Hippe E. (1972), Studies on the Cobalamin-Binding Protein of Human Saliva: *Scandinavian Journal of Clinical and Laboratory Investigation,* 29 (1):59–68.

Hungry Wolf (1980) *The Ways of My Grandmothers.* William Morrow: New York.

Imong S.M., Jackson D.A., Rungruengthanakit K., Wongsawasdii L., Amatayakul K., Drewett R.F., Baum J.D. (1995) Maternal behaviour and socio-economic influences on the bacterial content of infant weaning foods in rural northern Thailand, *Journal of Tropical Pediatrics.* 41(4): 234–40.

Humphrey S.P., Williamson R. T. (2001) A review of saliva: normal composition, flow, and function. *Journal of Prosthetic Dentistry* 85:162–169.

Kagami H., Hiramatsu Y., Hishida S.,Okazaki Y., Horie K., Oda Y., Ueda M. (2000) Salivary growth factors in health and disease, *Adv Dent Res* 14:99–102.

Kasinathan C., Sundaram R., William S. (1995) Effects of prostaglandins on tyrosylprotein sulfotransferase activity in rat submandibular salivary glands, *General Pharmacology,* 26 (3): 577–580.

Kirk A.B., Dyke J.V., Martin C.F., Dasgupta1 P.K. (2007). Temporal patterns in perchlorate, thiocyanate, and iodide excretion in human milk, *Environ Health Perspect.* 115(2): 182–186.

Komine K., Kuroishi T, Ozawa A., Komine Y., Minami T., Shimauchi H., Sugawara S. (2007) Cleaved inflammatory lactoferrin peptides in parotid saliva of periodontitis patients, *Molecular Immunology,* 44 (7): 1498–1508.

Kongara K.R., Soffer E.E. (1999) Saliva and esophageal protection. *American Journal of Gastroenterology* 94, (6): 1446–1452.

Larsen C.S. (2002) Post-Pleistocene Human Evolution: Bioarcheology of the agricultural transition. In: *Human Diet: Its Origin and Evolution.* P. S. Unger and M. F. Teaford, eds. pp.19–36. Greenwood Press: Westport, CT.

Larsson B., Olivecrona G., Ericson T. (1996) Lipid in human saliva. *Archives of Oral Biology,* 41(1):105–110.

Lebenthal E, Lee PC. Development of functional responses in human exocrine pancreas. Pediatrics 1980; 66: 556–60.

Lowe JR., Dixon JS. (1983). Salivary kinetics of prednisolone in man. *J Pharm Pharmacol* 35:390–391.

Lutter, C. K., Mora, J. O., Habicht, J-P., Rasmussen, K. M., Robson, D. S., Sellers, S. G., Super, C. M. and Herrera, M. G.: (1989) Nutritional supplementation: Effects on child stunting because of diarrhea. *American Journal of Clinical Nutrition*, 50: 1–8.

Mandel I.D. (1987) The function of saliva. *Journal of Dental Research* 66:623–627.

Marchetti P., Benzi L., Masoni A., Cecchetti P., Giannarelli R., Di Cianni G., et al. (1986). Salivary insulin concentrations in type 2 (non-insulin-dependent) diabetic patients and obese non-diabetic subjects: relationship to changes in plasma insulin levels after an oral glucose load. *Diabetologia* 29:695–698.

Marshall L. (1976), *The !Kung of Nyae Nyae*. Harvard University Press: Cambridge, MA.

McNamara, K. J. (2002) Sequential hypermorphosis: stretching ontogeny to the limit. In: N. Minugh-Purvis and K. McNamara, eds. Human Evolution Through Development Change. Baltimore: JHU Press pp. 102–121.

Murdock G.P. *et al.* (2004) *Outline of Culture Materials*, fifth edition. Human Relations Area Files Press: New Haven.

Nerlove S.B. (1974) Women's workload and infant feeding practices: a relationship with demographic implications. *Ethnology* 13: 207–214.

Norhagen G.E. Engström P.E. Hammarström L., Söder P.O., Smith C.I.E. (1989) Immunoglobulin levels in saliva in individuals with selective IgA deficiency: Compensatory IgM secretion and its correlation with HLA and susceptibility to infections. *Journal of Clinical Immunology*, 9(4) 279–286.

Pan American Health Organization and World Health Organization. Guiding Principles for Complementary Feeding of the Breastfed Child. (2003). Washington and Geneva.

Pelletier D.L., Frongillo, E.A., Habicht, J-P. (1993) Epidemiologic evidence for a potentiating effect of malnutrition on child mortality. *American Journal of Public Health*, 83(8): 1130–1133

Pelto G.H., Levitt E., Thairu L. (2003) Improving feeding practices: current patterns, common constraints and the design of interventions. *Food and Nutrition Bulletin* 24(1): 45–82.

Pezelj-Ribaric S., Brekalo Prso I., Abram M., Glazar I., Brumini G., Simunovic-Soskic M., (2004) Salivary levels of tumor necrosis factor-alpha in oral lichen planus. *Mediators Inflamm.* 13(2): 131–133.

Prentice A. (1996) Constituents of human milk, *Food and Nutrition Bulletin*, 17 (4): 305–312.

Ribaldi E., Guerra M., Mezzasoma A., Staffolani N., Goracci G., Gresele P. (1998) PAF levels in saliva are regulated by inflammatory cells, *Journal of Periodontal Research* 33(4): 237–241.

Rowland MG. (1986) The weanling's dilemma: Are we making progress? *Acta Paediatr Scan.* 323(suppl):33–42.

Rosenblum J.L., Irwin C.L., Alper D.H. (1988) Starch and glucose oligosaccharides protect salivary-type amylase activity at acid pH, *Am J Physiol Gastrointest Liver Physiol* 254: G775–780.

Schultz C., Ahmed K., Dawes C., Mantsch H. (1996), Thiocyanate levels in human saliva: Quantitation by Fourier transform infrared spectroscopy. *Analytical Biochemistry* 240: 7–12.

Sellen D.W. (2007) Evolution of infant and young child feeding: implications for contemporary public health. *Annual Review of Nutrition*, Volume 27. pp 123–148.

Sellen D.W. & Smay D.B. (2001) Relationship between subsistence and age at weaning in "pre-industrial societies." *Human Nature* 12:47–87.

Sellen D.W. (2001) Comparison of infant feeding patterns reported for non-industrial populations with current recommendations. *Journal of Nutrition.* 131:2707–2715.

Sfriso P., Ostuni P., Botsios C., Andretta M., Olivviero F., Punzi L., Todesco S. (2003) Serum and salivary neopterin and interferon-γ in primary Sjögren's syndrome: Correlation with clinical, laboratory and histopathologic features, *Scandinavian Journal of Rheumatology*, 32 (2): 74–78.

Shugars D.C. (1999), Endogenous Mucosal Antiviral Factors of the Oral Cavity. *Journal of Infectious Diseases* 179:S431–S435.

Sinha S.K., Martine B, Gold B.D., Nyren Q., Granstrom M. (2001) Helicobacter pylori infection in Swedish school children lack of evidence of child-to-child transmission outside the family. *Gastroenterology.* 121:310–316.

Smith B.H. (1989) Dental development as a measure of life history in primates. *Evolution*, 43 (3):683–688.

Soderling E., Parto K., Simell O., (2002) Saliva flow rate and composition in lysinuric protein intolerance, *Braz J Oral Sci.* 1(1): 40–44.

Stoppler M.C. (2008) The broad spectrum of EBV disease. Medicinenet.com

Taylor D.N., & Blaser M.J. (1991) The epidemiology of helicobacter pylori infection. *Epidemiologic Review* 13, 42–59.

Tenovuo J.O. (1989) *Human Human Saliva: Clinical Chemistry and Microbiology*. Volume 1, New York: CRC Press.

Valdez I.H., Fox P.C. (1991) Interactions of the salivary and gastrointestinal systems: I. The role of saliva in digestion. *Digestive Diseases and Sciences* 9 (3): 125–32.

Venza M., Visalli M., Cicciu D., Teti D. (2001) Determination of polyamines in human saliva by high-performance liquid chromatography with fluorescence detection, *Journal of chromatography. B, Biomedical sciences and applications* 757 (1): 111–117.

Verma R.S., Antony A.C. (1992) Immunoreactive folate-binding proteins from human saliva. Isolation and comparison of two distinct species. *Biochem J.* 286 (3): 707–715.

Vining RF., McGinley RA. (1986). Hormones in saliva. *Crit Rev Clin Lab Sci* 23:95–146.

Von Hertzen L.C. (2000) Puzzling associations between childhood infections and the latter occurrence of asthma and atopy. *Annuals of Medicine*, 32 (6), 397–400.

Wright D.E. (1959) A note on leucocytes in saliva. *J. Microsc Soc.* 77:139–41.

Yamanishi K. (2000) Human Herpesvirus 6: An evolving story. *Herpes* 7 (3), 70–75.

Zhang B, Khin-Maung-U, Lu R, Hill ID, Lebenthal E. (1996) Age-related changes in exocrine pancreatic function in infants and children. *International Pediatrics* 11:23–6.

CHAPTER 45

Feeding Babies: Practices, Constraints, and Interventions

Gretel H. Pelto, Emily Levitt, and Lucy Thairu

(2003)

The nutritional care of the young is a major challenge for many animal species, and humans are no exception. From the time the umbilical cord is cut to the point at which the child can obtain all of its nutritional requirements from an adequate share of the household diet is a difficult period for caregivers, regardless of their level of household food security. The activities that occur during this period consist of multiple behavioral and physiological events. The totality of these events constitutes the weaning process, in which the young child moves from total nutritional dependence on his or her mother to relative independence.

Among mammals, the solution to the challenge of feeding new offspring is maternal milk, which is augmented at some stage of their development with other foods. In contemporary nutritional parlance, these other foods are referred to as "complementary foods," which carries the implication that their function is to augment the nutrients received from maternal milk. When the offspring are no longer receiving any maternal milk, it is common practice to refer them as weaned.

The mechanisms for delivering complementary foods to dependent offspring and the forms in which such foods are provided vary from one species to another and depend on a number of factors, including the degree of physiological maturity and the methods of protecting the young from predators. Throughout the course of our sociocultural evolution from a hunting-gathering lifestyle to industrial societies, premastication of vegetable and animal foods has been a primary technique for humans. This technique has continued into modern times. In addition to techniques that permit parents to feed family foods to infants and young children, another strategy to provide complementary foods is the creation of special transitional foods.

This paper examines the behavioral aspects of complementary feeding. The aim is to assist the process of planning interventions to improve feeding practices during the period before children can meet their nutritional requirements

from the household diet. In breastfed infants, this will typically be the period from the age of 6 months to about 24 to 30 months.

BACKGROUND

Growth Faltering as a Marker of Inadequate Nutrition

The presentation of a child's growth as a smooth line that rises steeply in early childhood, then more slowly until adolescence when there is another sharp rise, after which it flattens as adult height is reached, is, to some extent, a convention of the time units of data presentation. The more frequently measurements are made, the easier it is to see the unevenness in growth in a healthy, well-growing child. But in healthy children whose growth is not constrained by an inadequate nutrient intake or illness, the periods of no apparent growth are very short. As a result, the calculated growth rate for a population of well-growing children shows that a steady increment in size is the normal condition when growth is not constrained by exogenous factors. It is the nature of young children to grow and develop rapidly and steadily. When they are not, something is wrong.

A large body of anthropometric data shows the existence of significant constraints to normal growth that have affected millions of children, almost entirely in developing countries. Anthropometric data also provide evidence of when children in different populations are most likely to be affected by these constraints. Regardless of how protracted or short the period of risk is, in virtually all populations in which growth is constrained, the period of greatest vulnerability is the second semester of life (6 to 12 months of age) and into the second year (until 18 months of age and often longer). It begins when maternal milk is no longer adequate to supply all of the child's needs and continues until he or she is able to meet nutritional requirements through consumption of the usual family diet and requires no special assistance with eating.

The anthropometric evidence of growth faltering has fueled an international research effort that has been aimed mainly at understanding its biological determinants. Epidemiological and social research has also been directed

Gretel H. Pelto, Emily Levitt, and Lucy Thairu. "Feeding babies: practices, constraints and interventions." Adapted from: Improving Feeding Practices: Current Patterns, Common Constraints, and the Design of Interventions. *Food and Nutrition Bulletin*, 2003, 24: 45–82. Reprinted with permission.

to this problem, although less extensively. At the same time, evaluations of programs to prevent or ameliorate faltering have contributed further knowledge about this pervasive public health problem.

Changing Perspectives on the Determinants of Growth Faltering

Nutrition intervention programs reflect public health professionals' and policy-makers' views about the determinants of growth faltering and are aimed at correcting them. Previously programs focused exclusively on improving the quality of food and diet, improving the household food supply, engaging in educational activities to provide information on appropriate foods, and education on hygienic food preparation. Today, additional concerns are leading to new program directions. For example, the recognition of the importance of intra-household food distribution means that supplementary feeding programs provide food to other household members and administrators appear to be less concerned about "leakage." Other important new directions are the result of an expanding concern with the behavioral aspects of infant and young child feeding.

THE ROLE OF THE CAREGIVER'S BEHAVIOR AS A PRIMARY DETERMINANT OF NUTRITION

Historical Developments

Historically, there has been a longstanding, but poorly coordinated, interest in how the behavior of the caregiver affects nutrition. Before 1990, when the concept of "care" was given formal recognition in the UNICEF conceptual framework (see below), there were pioneering efforts to provide empirical data linking the caregiver's behavior to nutritional outcomes. For example, in the early 1970s Muñoz de Chavez et al, attempted to identify specific behaviors that protected children from malnutrition in a Mexican community in which malnutrition was endemic (Muñoz de Chavez et al. 1974). The work of Zeitlin et al. under the rubric of "positive deviance" similarly sought to isolate specific behaviors that supported child growth in conditions where poor growth was normative (Zeitlin et al. 1989; Zeitlin et al. 1990). Engle et al. (1987) reported on "caretaker competence," and Pelto et al. (1989) suggested that the significant associations between indicators of "maternal management" and growth, which they found in their work in central Mexico, reflected the operation of differential caregiving behaviors. A study in southern Brazil demonstrated that unobtrusive indicators of maternal behavior, which also reflect caregiving, were risk factors for persistent infant diarrhea and malnutrition. Such was the expanding level of interest that, by the late 1980s, Pelto (1989:729) claimed that "the concept of 'maternal caregiving' has received increasing attention as a primary intervening or proximal factor in nutrition". She went on to suggest

that "among the components of care-giving for which direct links to nutrition can be traced are food selection and preparation practices, which affect food safety and nutrient density, feeding practices, management of illness, and an array of psychosocial actions that influence endocrine responses and other physiological functions in the child" (Pelto 1989:729).

In 1990, UNICEF published a document, "Strategy for improved nutrition of children and women in developing countries," in which they introduced the "UNICEF conceptual framework for determinants of nutritional status." This framework has had a major impact on current thinking about childhood malnutrition. In the original model, which has since been modified and elaborated, inadequate dietary intake and disease are the most proximate (immediate) causes of malnutrition. The underlying causes, which give rise to the immediate causes, are grouped into three main categories: insufficient household food security, inadequate maternal and child care, and insufficient health services and unhealthy environments. These, in turn, are the product of the basic causes that rest in economic structures and political and ideological superstructures, which affect resources and controls. In the model, education is placed in a mediating position between the basic and the underlying causes.

The framework has helped to clarify thinking about the relationships of macro-level to micro-level factors in affecting nutritional status. By laying out the levels of determinants from basic, through underlying, to immediate causes, the model helps both investigators and program personnel to situate their particular activities within the larger framework of causation.

The focus on "care" as it relates to childhood malnutrition and the intellectual development of this concept can be traced through a series of papers and meetings. At the International Conference on Nutrition in 1992 the first steps toward defining care were made (FAO/WHO 1992; Engle 1992). This was followed, in 1995, by a conference held at Cornell University for the purpose of reviewing available knowledge related to child care, growth, and development. The concept was further advanced and developed by research activities undertaken by the International Food Policy Research Institute (Engle et al. 1996; Arimond and Ruel 2001).

Other strands of research have made important contributions to the emerging emphasis on the behavioral components of infant feeding. Beginning with her research in India on household responses to diarrhea, Bentley and colleagues (1988; 1991a,b; 1999) undertook a series of investigations into the relationships of complementary feeding behaviors and feeding styles to cultural beliefs and household conditions.

In their studies of American mothers, Birch and Fischer (1995) distinguished three feeding styles, to which they gave the labels "controlling," "laissez-faire," and "responsive." A controlling feeding style is characterized by behaviors that are intended to control when and how much the child eats. Birch and Fisher found that some children who experience this style of feeding are unable to self-regulate their energy intake. They suggested that the intermediate position between highly controlling and non-interactive is appropriately characterized as responsive. A laissez-faire feeding style refers to the type of non-interactive behavior that has been described for a number of cultural settings (Dettwyler 1989; Gittelsohn et al. 1998).

Another strand of research that directs attention to the significance of complementary feeding behaviors consists of investigations of the relationships of maternal education, socioeconomic status, and nutrition of young children in developing countries. The relationships of maternal education to child health and nutrition outcomes have been extensively documented over a considerable period of time (Cleland and Van Ginneken, 1988). However, survey data analyses generally have not provided a means of understanding the underlying dynamics of these associations. In the last decade, a series of epidemiological and observational studies aimed at identifying the mechanisms by which the caregiver's education is translated into better growth and health outcomes points to the fundamental role played by maternal caregiving behaviors, particularly in connection with complementary feeding (e.g., Ruel et al. 1992; Reed et al. 1996).

The Expanding Dimensions of Complementary Feeding

The introduction of "care" (or caregiving) into our understanding of complementary feeding requires a broadening of activities in research and programmatic action. Several additional dimensions need to be added to augment the focus on *what* is fed. These additional dimensions can be described as *how* food is fed, *when* food is fed, *where* food is fed, and *who* is giving the food. The dimension labeled *how* involves several aspects, including feeding style, the utensils that are used to offer the food, and food preparation and preservation activities. *When* refers primarily to the scheduling of feeding and requires attention to frequency and degree of flexibility. *Where* is concerned with the feeding environment and includes issues of distraction, safety, comfort, and potential for interaction. *Who* directs attention to the relationship of the child with the individual who is feeding him or her, whether it is the mother or an adult to whom the infant has a primary attachment, or another familiar adult, an older child, a day-care worker, or a hired caregiver.

"Complementary feeding practices" can be defined as consisting of two main components: the biological component, which is concerned with what is being fed, and the behavioral component, which is concerned with issues of how, who, when, and where.

Feeding Behaviors that Reflect Principles of Care

The original UNICEF (1990) conceptual model defined care as "the provision in the household and the community of time, attention, and support to meet the physical, mental, and social needs of the growing child and other household members." In the theme paper prepared for the International Conference on Nutrition (ICN), Engle (1992) amplified the basic definition with a categorization of types of care behaviors. She identified six categories of care: care for pregnant and lactating women, breastfeeding and the feeding of very young children, psychosocial stimulation of children and support for their development, food-preparation and food-storage behavior, hygiene behavior, and care for children during illness, including care-seeking behavior.

At the heart of this conception is the idea of "psychosocial care." In their 1996 paper on "Care and nutrition: concepts and measurement," Engle et al. (1996: 34) provide a definition of psychosocial care as "the provision of affection and warmth, responsiveness to the child, and the encouragement of autonomy and exploration." A primary feature of this definition is that it calls attention to the fact that there are two parties involved in psychosocial care—the adult caregiver and the young child. The actions are not one-way arrows from the adult to the child; to the contrary, the child's needs for autonomy and freedom to explore are also highlighted. It is in the interaction in the adult-child dyad that psychosocial care is grounded.

The fundamental principles of psychosocial care include accurately perceiving and interpreting the child's signals, responding adequately and promptly, and using "scaffolding" in interactions. Scaffolding here refers to a mode of interaction in which the adult's behavior is adjusted over time to the emerging skills of the young so that the child is adequately challenged but not overwhelmed and is able to use his or her behavioral and expressive skills.

When principles of psychosocial care are integrated with other aspects of caregiving, a different paradigm emerges. We have proposed the concept of "responsive parenting" as a way of capturing or expressing the dyadic nature of effective caregiving (Pelto 2000). This phrase is intended to call attention to the interactive nature of caring for infants and young children, in which the caregiver and the child are engaged in mutually reinforcing positive (and occasionally negative) actions.

When the foregoing principles are applied to the domain of complementary feeding and integrated with emerging knowledge about the conditions that promote adequate intake of complementary foods, we can begin to construct a set of "best-practice feeding behaviors." These behaviors should be based on the hallmark principles of attending to and responding to the child's signals. They can also take advantage of the essential and repeated act of feeding to promote the evolution of the child's development through "scaffolded interactions." These behaviors sustain and reinforce the strong affective ties that develop between mother and infant during breastfeeding and provide a means for extending these ties to other primary adults in the infant's world. The set below is offered as a first approximation. It is intended as a catalyst for future work.

Some best-practice feeding behaviors:

- Feeding with a balance between giving assistance and encouraging self-feeding, as appropriate to the child's level of development.
- Feeding with positive verbal encouragement, without verbal or physical coercion.
- Feeding with age-appropriate as well as culturally appropriate eating utensils.
- Feeding in response to early hunger cues.
- Feeding in a protected and comfortable environment
- Feeding by an individual with whom the child has a positive emotional relationship and who is aware of and sensitive to the child's individual characteristics, including his or her changing physical and emotional states.

This set of best-practice behaviors needs to be joined with another set of behaviors that specify best-practice guidelines from the perspective of food safety and hygiene. The augmented behavioral guidelines can then be melded with recommendations on what to feed (designated from a biological perspective) to create a set of generic guidelines for complementary feeding practices to promote child growth and well-being. We emphasize that global guidelines are, by definition, generic. To be useful for programmatic action or for research, they must always be translated to a specific context.

CROSS-CULTURAL PATTERNS IN FEEDING AND YOUNG CHILD FEEDING PRACTICES

Case Studies of Complementary Feeding

The purpose of this section is to review current feeding practices around the world in order to provide a basis for comparing the current situation with "best practices" and identify the most significant deviations.

Methods

To obtain an illustrative group of case studies, we began by screening the Human Nutrition database for records published within the last 20 years that contained information on "weaning" and "culture." The following search terms were used; weaning, weaning foods, community, cultural practice, culturally appropriate, culturally sensitive, wean, food, complementary foods, complementary feeding, infant diet. These results were augmented by a search in the BIOSIS Previews database using the following search terms: medical anthropology, infant feeding, infant diet, behavior. The anthropological literature was explored using the Eureka database of the Tozzer Library of Harvard University. In addition we reviewed medical anthropology journals (e.g., Medical Anthropology and Medical Anthropology

Quarterly) for articles related to child nutrition. Finally, other studies were located in bibliographies of articles and monographs identified with the previous methods. Our first criterion for selection of cases was the availability of at least some data on nutrition-related care practices. That is, we examined the studies for evidence of information on the caregiver (who), the feeding style (how), the feeding environment (where), and the frequency and scheduling of feeding (when). Since it is not our intention in this paper to review the biological aspects of food practices, the inclusion of detailed data on what is being fed and the schedule of introduction of complementary foods was not a criterion for case selection. With respect to why (the determinants of feeding practices), we examined studies for information on the following, potentially modifiable, determinants of care practices: maternal time allocation and competing demands on women's time; beliefs, knowledge, and perceptions; the health of the caregiver and other family members; and social pressures, social support, and normative expectations. (The rationale for this selection of determinants is provided below.)

In addition to the adequacy or richness of information, our final selection of cases was based on geographic distribution. The 18 ethnographic studies are distributed by region as follows: Africa (4 cases); Latin America (4 cases); Asia (4 cases); Oceania (3 cases); North America (3 cases). The sample of 18 case studies is not a representative sample in the technical sense, as they were not randomly selected from the larger database of ethnographic studies. Rather, they are random in the colloquial sense of common English usage, reflecting the coincidence of where investigators with an interest in complementary feeding behaviors happened to conduct their research. We relied almost entirely on articles from peer-reviewed journals, which reflect another selection process, including the motivation of the investigators to publish their observations in a readily accessible source. No doubt there is a considerable body of useful data on the behavioral aspects of complementary feeding in postgraduate theses and in unpublished reports.

Results Related to Behavioral Components of Complementary Feeding Practices

Virtually all of the reports have significant information gaps in relation to the framework. Nonetheless they are informative about current practices and permit some examination of commonalities and divergences in complementary feeding behaviors. Tables 1, 2, and 3 provide summaries of the key parameters across the 18 studies.

Modifiable Determinants of Complementary Feeding Practices

We selected four categories of determinants: maternal time allocation and competing demands on women's time; beliefs, knowledge, and perceptions; health of the caregiver and other

Table 1 How Complementary Food Is Fed[a]

Manner of feeding	Case study[b]																	
	1	2	3	4	5	6	7	8	9	10	11	12	13	14	15	16	17	18
Vehicle																		
Caregiver's hand	x				x				x	x	x							
Caregiver's mouth											x			x				
Bottle						x		x		x		x		x		x		
Cup, bowl, or spoon		x	x	x		x	x			x		x	x	x		x	x	x
Child's hand										x								
No information															x			
Method																		
Spoon held by caregiver				x								x				x		
Food placed in child's hand					x									x				
Caregiver premasticates											x			x	x	x		
Caregiver force-feeds if child is resistant	x																	
Child expected to self-feed			x				x										x	
No information		x				x		x	x				x					
Feeding style																		
Inadequate information to specify		x		x		x		x	x			x	x	x	x	x		x
Possibly interactive, but cannot judge whether the caregiver is responsive					x					x	x							
Controlling	x																	
Laissez-faire			x				x										x	

[a] Except for the rows with no information, x indicates that the practice was explicitly reported by the investigator.

[b] 1 Nigeria (Oni et al., 1991); 2 Tanzania (Mabilia, 1996); 3 Mali (Dettwyler, 1987a,b); 4 Zimbabwe (Cosminsky et al., 1993); 5 Brazil (Wright and Dutra de Oliveira, 1988); 6 Guatemala (Izurieta and Larson-Brown, 1995); 7 Peru (Bentley et al., 1995; Creed Kanishiro et al., 1991); 8 Dominican Republic (McClennan, 1994); 9 Bhutan (Bohler and Staffan, 1995); 10 Bangladesh (Guldan et al., 1993); 11 Nepal (Levine, 1988); 12 Philippines (Acuin, 1992); 13, Papua New Guinea (Conton, 1985); 14 Solomon Islands (Alan, 1985); 15 Trobriand Islands (Montague, 1984); 16 Maryland, USA (Bentley et al., 1999); 17 Kentucky, USA (McLorg and Bryant, 1989); 18 Pennsylvania, USA (Adair, 1983).

Table 2 Who Feeds Complementary Foods

Caregiver	1	2	3	4	5	6	7	8	9	10	11	12	13	14	15	16	17	18
Mother is with the child during the day																		
Mother	x			x	x	x		x	x				x					x
Mother + grandmother														x			x	
Mother + adult female relative										x				x	x		x	
Mother + older sibling							x			x				x			x	
Mother + father														x	x	x		
Child feeds self			x															
Mother is away during the day; child has another caregiver																		
Grandmother		x										x				x		
Other adult female relative											x	x			x			
Sibling		x									x							
Unrelated caregiver	x																	x

[a] 1 Nigeria (Oni et al., 1991); 2 Tanzania (Mabilia, 1996); 3 Mali (Dettwyler, 1987a,b); 4 Zimbabwe (Cosminsky et al., 1993); 5 Brazil (Wright and Dutra de Oliveira, 1988); 6 Guatemala (Izurieta and Larson-Brown, 1995); 7 Peru (Bentley et al., 1995; Creed Kanishiro et al., 1991); 8 Dominican Republic (McClennan, 1994); 9 Bhutan (Bohler and Staffan, 1995); 10 Bangladesh (Guldan et al., 1993); 11 Nepal (Levine, 1988); 12 Philippines (Acuin, 1992); 13, Papua New Guinea (Conton, 1985); 14 Solomon Islands (Alan, 1985); 15 Trobriand Islands (Montague, 1984); 16 Maryland, USA (Bentley et al., 1999); 17 Kentucky, USA (McLorg and Bryant, 1989); 18 Pennsylvania, USA (Adair, 1983).

Table 3 Frequency of Feeding Complementary Food[a]

Frequency	1	2	3	4	5	6	7	8	9	10	11	12	13	14	15	16	17	18
1/day									x									
2/day		x				x	x											
3/day											x	x			x			
≥4/day			x		x	x				x						x		
Explicit mention of snacks			x					x								x		
No information, or difficult to determine from the report	x			x				x					x	x			x	x

There was not enough information on scheduling of feeding to permit tabulation from the case studies.

[b] 1 Nigeria (Oni et al., 1991); 2 Tanzania (Mabilia, 1996); 3 Mali (Dettwyler, 1987a,b); 4 Zimbabwe (Cosminsky et al., 1993); 5 Brazil (Wright and Dutra de Oliveira, 1988); 6 Guatemala (Izurieta and Larson-Brown, 1995); 7 Peru (Bentley et al., 1995; Creed Kanishiro et al., 1991); 8 Dominican Republic (McClennan, 1994); 9 Bhutan (Bohler and Staffan, 1995); 10 Bangladesh (Guldan et al., 1993); 11 Nepal (Levine, 1988); 12 Philippines (Acuin, 1992); 13, Papua New Guinea (Conton, 1985); 14 Solomon Islands (Alan, 1985); 15 Trobriand Islands (Montague, 1984); 16 Maryland, USA (Bentley et al., 1999); 17 Kentucky, USA (McLorg and Bryant, 1989); 18 Pennsylvania, USA (Adair, 1983).

family members; and social pressures and social support, particularly in the caregiver's immediate social network. The selection of these categories was based on an initial thematic analysis of the descriptive ethnographic reports, as well as a broad, if diffuse, body of social science theory, and, most importantly, the fact that these determinants are potentially amenable to change through various types of intervention activities. Thus, they provide an important link between the insights that can be gained from ethnographic description and the development of programs. However, in focusing on these categories it is not our intention to suggest that they constitute the definitive set of proximal, modifiable determinants. We believe that they are likely to be important, to varying degrees, in many different cultural settings. Other determinants may also be significant, and the identification of specific constraints must be sought in each local context. Moreover, the focus on these specific areas of caregiver and household-level factors does not imply that interventions should be directed solely to caregivers and households. To the contrary, both the design and implementation of interventions demand attention to the social context, particularly the community context, where both the resources and constraints to behavior change are likely to be found.

Maternal Time Allocation and Competing Demands on Women's Time

To understand a mother's ability to satisfy the needs of her child, one must know about the range of her competing responsibilities and their compatibility with child-care practices. Although women's activities vary greatly across geographic and cultural regions, and in relation to economic conditions, the model of the mother-as-domestic-homemaker is becoming increasingly rare, even in societies where this was formerly a common situation. In most societies today, a significant proportion of women with small children must engage in some form of income-producing activities, which are typically structured in a manner that creates powerful constraints on caring. Even in more traditional, subsistence-oriented communities, food-production responsibilities and other domestic, non-child-care activities place heavy time-allocation demands on women.

Beliefs, Knowledge, and Perceptions

When public health and nutrition professionals from Euro-American societies and cultures first encountered the diversity of cultural beliefs and perceptions about food, health, and well-being, there was a tendency to invest them with strong deterministic power in the explanation of why people ate as they did. The concept that "ignorance" or bizarre cultural beliefs explained why people in other societies "ate poorly" or had "bad dietary habits" was an explanation that permitted Euro-Americans to ignore the role of poverty and resource constraints as causes of malnutrition. It put a premium on inventions designed to teach people better nutritional habits.

On the other hand, clinical and research professionals with greater sensitivity to the conditions of daily life in poor communities countered with economic, materialist explanations, and questioned whether beliefs had any causal role, at least in undernutrition. To the extent that the materialist position entertained any acknowledgment of cultural factors, there was a tendency to stress the wisdom of traditional cultural knowledge, with little room for any role for educational interventions.

A more balanced view is that cultural beliefs, knowledge, and perceptions influence food behaviors to varying degrees, except under the most severely constrained economic conditions. Many aspects of culturally shared understandings and interpretations are positive with respect to current scientific knowledge, some aspects are best regarded as neutral, and some are counterproductive from the perspective of contemporary biomedical theory.

Health of the Caregiver and Other Family Members

Ethnographic reports contain many examples of cultural perceptions about the effects of the mother's state, including illness, on the quality of breastmilk. If a mother is angry, tired, or ill, her milk can become spoiled or tainted, and illness in the breastfeeding infant is often attributed to such conditions in the mother. Much less is known about how the mother's health is perceived to affect complementary feeding. Is it that investigators have failed to ask, or are such ideas absent in most cultural systems? From observational and epidemiological data there is evidence that the caregiver's health (physical and mental) has important effects on the outcome for the child. Currently, there is much concern about this determinant with respect to HIV/AIDS. A few of the case studies contain relevant material on the influences of the caregiver's health and the health of other family members on behaviors related to complementary feeding.

Social Networks, Social Pressure, and Normative Expectations

The importance of social support and social expectations for infant feeding decisions and behaviors became very clear with the advent of systematic research on breastfeeding versus bottle-feeding (Pelto 1981; Allen and Pelto 1985; Van Esterik 1989). Examination of the effects of the immediate social group on complementary feeding behavior is less fully reported and less well understood. As with breastfeeding, it is likely that the social group surrounding the caregiver-child dyad can exert both positive and negative pressures on complementary feeding behaviors. These, in turn, reflect more widely shared, normative expectations. On the other hand, the significance of medical and health personnel in influencing caregivers' practices represents the introduction of new ideas and new sources of social pressure.

GENERALIZATIONS CONCERNING THE CASE STUDIES

The ethnographies contain few surprises, but they illustrate and reinforce a number of issues that have previously been identified. They are particularly useful because of the nature of the research process that underlies many of the studies—namely, the use of in-depth interviews rather than preset questions. In some cases the investigator used directed questions, such as "Is there anyone you consulted concerning advice on how to feed your child?" Such open-ended questions are clearly valuable, and they are essential for deriving quantitative estimates of beliefs, attitudes, and behaviors. But there is also a role for less directed methods. Many of the data reported in the articles were obtained by the investigators through thematic analysis of field notes from interviews and observations. Thus they present more "emic" views (the perspective of individuals who are "insiders" to their culture) than is typical of most of the data in epidemiologically oriented nutrition research. That is, they reflect the beliefs, values, and experiences of the local community and the people who are being interviewed to a greater degree than is usual in the case of preformed questionnaires, even when the latter are open-ended. Among the themes and generalizations that can be derived from the case studies, we would like to draw attention to the following.

Feeding Infants Is a Family Affair

The significance of the effects of male partners, friends, and women of older generations on breastfeeding has been well documented in research in the last two or three decades. To date, the importance of the family in complementary feeding has been less clearly revealed. However, in almost all of the case studies, we found that complementary feeding of the infant or young child is very much a family affair. As can be seen in Table 2, mothers generally have the primary responsibility for preparing and feeding complementary foods, but other people are also involved, and often (although not always) these other people are family members. Some family member involvement is in the form of affecting what the mother can do, including constraints on her decisions as well as her behaviors. One could label this as "advice with a bite" because it reveals the authority of other family members to determine the feeding practices in which mothers are engaged.

Another form of family involvement is in the preparation of complementary foods. Perhaps the most common form of family participation in complementary feeding is the family's role in the actual feeding of infants and young children. We have no quantitative data across the globe on what proportion of infants receive what proportion of their complementary food from someone who is not their mother, but it is probably safe to say that it is not negligible. The significance of these alternative caregivers for child growth outcomes is unknown, and it is unlikely that it can be derived from existing sources of data. The ethnographic reports suggest that there are potentials for both positive and negative consequences. For example, emotionally engaged grandmothers in families where mothers are experiencing situations and pressures that affect their ability to carry out effective complementary feeding may provide the type of care that the young child needs. On the other hand, there may also be negative consequences. For example, the public health community has voiced concern that artificial nipples on feeding bottles interfere with breastfeeding by affecting the babies' preferences. What are the effects of unpleasant, controlling, or nonresponsive feeding of complementary food by alternative caregivers with more attenuated relationships to the child than that of the mother? In theory, these experiences may be very disruptive of the development of good feeding behaviors on the part of the child.

Balancing the Demands Engendered by Complementary Feeding Against All the Other Demands and Needs of an Adult Woman's Life Is a Fundamental Issue for Mothers

One of the most consistent themes in the case studies was the problem of time and the relationship of complementary feeding activities to other, competing demands. The problem of not having enough time for all of the work and other activities in which people engage is a litany of professional life in industrialized countries. But it is equally salient for mothers in situations as diverse as the Nepalese highlands, Bamako, or peri-urban Manila. Women select complementary foods that can be prepared quickly, not only to save fuel, but also to save time. They change traditional food-preparation techniques in favor of those that are less time-consuming. They feed quickly or non-interactively in order to save time and to use the time taken by the child for eating to accomplish other tasks. They feed less often in order to save time for other tasks. They prepare complementary foods early in the day to avoid disrupting other work by having to prepare complementary foods just before feeding them. The time factor thus affects the selection of foods, their preparation, and feeding style.

The issue is not simply time, but time in relation to other activities, other responsibilities, and other demands. Thus, the themes that emerge are related to larger issues of household economic organization and domestic social management tasks, resources, and the expectations of self and others, and the degree of flexibility to make adjustments during the period in which their infants and young children require complementary feeding.

Mothers and Other Adults Have Conceptual Frameworks in Terms of Which They Make Decisions About Complementary Feeding (What to Feed, How to Prepare It, and How to Feed It)

The case studies provide rich descriptive evidence of the "theories-in-use" that guide people's behaviors with respect to what, when, where, and how to feed their children. These can be characterized as "conceptual frameworks" that structure the multiple decisions that people have to make in relation to feeding and caring for their children. Some elements of this framework are directly economic. They concern decisions about how to use household resources and involve giving foods that are affordable, avoiding foods that are regarded as too expensive, and generally structuring the infant's diet in relation to the larger economic issues in the family.

Apart from economic considerations and other issues of time and resource allocation, caregivers' conceptual frameworks are reflected in the data in their concerns about what is good for children. The following examples paraphrase some of the ideas that we found in the ethnographic reports: "It is good to give foods that are light foods because heavy foods can make a child sick, irritable, and not active;" "It is good to give infants bits of adult food so that he or she will learn to like them;" "It isn't good to give too many different kinds of foods because the child will then expect them later and as we can't afford them, he or she will be unhappy and difficult;" "Children need to feed themselves from the very beginning, so they learn to be independent and are able to take care of themselves;" "The child knows whether he or she is hungry, so it is not good to try and make him or her eat more."

Independently of any assessments one might make about the "correctness" of these views from a biomedical viewpoint, a primary generalization that can be drawn from the case studies is that complementary feeding is structured by local theories of child well-being and the role of feeding in achieving that.

In Most Communities, Common Patterns of Complementary Feeding Behaviors Do Not Conform to Best-Practice Feeding Behaviors (as Derived from Principles of Psychosocial Care)

The data in the case studies are very thin from the perspective of revealing the nature and extent of best-practice feeding behaviors. Consequently, it is difficult to examine these themes in the ethnographic reports. Part of the problem is that ethnographers of feeding practices have had no reason to report on these, because there is no larger theoretical structure in nutrition that would direct their attention to them. A further problem is that the reports tend to focus on common, normative patterns, with much less attention to intercultural or intragroup diversity. Undoubtedly, in every community there are families whose feeding practices reflect principles of psychosocial care, but it appears that, in general, the common practices in many communities are less than optimal.

"Feeding with a Balance between Giving Assistance and Encouraging Self-feeding, as Appropriate to the Child's Level of Development." In a few of the case studies, it appears that assistance in feeding is inadequate because caregivers are actively encouraging early independence or assume that the infant can manage without help. This may be the situation with bottle-propping, as well as with a laissez-faire mode of feeding with spoon, bowl, or the child's hand. At the other extreme is a case of forced feeding, in which there is no assistance but rather insistence. It is difficult to judge the extent to which a balance occurs in other environments.

"Feeding with Positive Verbal Encouragement, Without Verbal or Physical Coercion." Apart from the potential for physical coercion in the case of forced hand-feeding, it is difficult in the case studies to gauge the extent of encouragement that children are given. Where parents adhere to the belief that children "know" whether or not they are hungry, it is probable that there is no verbal encouragement to eat. On the other hand, some of the parental concerns and behavioral changes that accompany feeding children who are ill may include greater verbal encouragement.

"Feeding with Age-Appropriate as well as Culturally Appropriate Eating Utensils." There is so little information concerning this feature that it is very difficult to assess the frequency of this best-practice behavior.

"Feeding in Response to Early Hunger Cues." Although many of the studies provided at least passing reference to the number of times per day that children receive food, there is almost no information on how feeding is scheduled. It appears that in many situations the feeding of complementary food occurs in connection with family meals, which presumably are scheduled not in relation to young children's hunger but to adult work schedules. There are clear exceptions to this, as for example in the study in Baltimore, where it is likely that children's hunger cues are the basis for offering foods.

"Feeding in a Protected and Comfortable Environment." Protecting infants and young children from environmental hazards emerges clearly as a priority in virtually all of the case studies, and in difficult environments it may actually function to reduce child mobility and opportunities for exploration. However, none of the studies documents a concern for providing a feeding environment that is free of distractions, which may be of significance to intake during the period of complementary feeding. Again, this is an area for which there is so little information that informed generalizations cannot be made.

"Feeding by an Individual with Whom the Child Has a Positive Emotional Relationship and Who Is Aware of and Sensitive to the Child's Individual Characteristics, Including His or Her Changing Physical and Emotional States." There are virtually no data on this aspect of best-practice behavior in the case study materials. As noted above, the situation of multiple caregivers can be either positive or negative, and the descriptions do not readily permit generalizations about

this. However, it seems likely that when young children are left with older siblings who are themselves still children, sensitivity to the young child's needs and skill in meeting them may not always be present.

Implications of the Case Studies for Interventions

Best-Practice Feeding Behaviors in the Case Studies

Analyses in which the dietary intakes of infants and young children are compared with nutritional recommendations have consistently identified significant problems (Brown et al., 1998). The contribution of poor feeding practices to the ubiquitous growth faltering that characterizes most poor populations is generally assumed to be a primary source of the problem. In the language of the framework we proposed earlier, we would say that the problem of inadequate quality and quantity in complementary feeding is fundamentally a problem of "what." When the focus is mainly on "what," planning of interventions is directed to improving access to food and educational activities that emphasize better food selection and preparation. Although we did not undertake a systematic description of the "what" component of feeding practices in the case studies, there is ample evidence to argue for the value of interventions that improve access and increase families' understanding of children's nutritional needs and how to meet them. As we suggested above, the arguments for attention to best-practice feeding behaviors should not be viewed as a substitute for "what" but as a call for attention to other factors that can have significant effects on child nutrition, growth, and development. These are in addition to the potential benefits of improving food selection and preparation. What is not clear from the present state of scientific knowledge is whether the benefits will be additive or synergistic.

Even in earlier periods when ethnographers adhered to a philosophy of holistic description, investigators were concerned about selection bias and looked to theory for guidance on what to record in their field notes and report in their monographs. As nutrition theory emphasizes dietary intake, one would expect to find more details about foods in nutritionally oriented ethnographic studies. With respect to infant and young child feeding, one would therefore expect to see more descriptions of what is fed than other aspects of feeding-related behaviors. This expectation is fulfilled in the case studies, although the level of quantification is usually frustratingly low. On the other hand, some components of complementary feeding, particularly the feeding environment and the feeding schedule, have only recently been recognized as important, so one would not expect to find rich detail in descriptive studies. Thus, our capacity to evaluate these features in the case studies is seriously constrained by lack of data.

To the extent that global judgments can be made for the case materials, there is evidence that care-related practices need to be improved in many cultural settings. The descriptions of common and normative behaviors with respect to care-related components are often suboptimal when viewed through the lens of current theory.

In general the "how" aspects of feeding styles tend toward the laissez-faire end of the spectrum, whereas the more dramatic opposite pole (controlled feeding or forced feeding) is rare. Both ends of the continuum—laissez-faire and controlled feeding—reflect a theme that is common throughout the case studies: the view that feeding children during the period from 6 to 24 months is time-consuming and interferes with what are implicitly viewed as more pressing and more important demands. Patient, engaged interactive feeding is not culturally normative in most places.

Scheduling of breastfeeding during infancy is often described in ethnographic reports and is usually reported as frequent and on-demand. After solid foods are added, the continuation of on-demand breastfeeding appears to be typical in situations where the mother and child remain together during the day. At the same time, the common situation with respect to scheduling is to feed solids two or three times a day. However, the relationship of breastfeeding (or feeding of breastmilk-substitutes by bottle) to feeding of solids is generally not well reported, particularly in situations in which the child is not with his or her mother for long periods during the day. Although the evidence is not as clear as one would wish, it is probably the case that in most settings the "when" of complementary feeding does not meet the recommendations promoted through the Integrated Management of Childhood Illness (WHO/FCH/CAH, 2000): at 6 to 12 months, three times a day for breastfed children, and five times a day for children who are not breastfed; at 12 to 24 months, five times a day.

Detailed information on the feeding environment is almost nonexistent in the case reports. This omission is to be expected since there has been very little systematic investigation of the effects of the feeding environment on child consumption. On the other hand, investigators generally tend to report the practice of leaving children routinely at home while the mother goes out to attend to other activities. This information is usually provided in the context of descriptions of who is taking care of the child. Two types of arrangements are common when the mother is not the sole caregiver: care is provided by adult women relatives (grandmothers, sisters, or sisters-in-law) or by older siblings (sometimes by another child who may be only a few years older). It is less common to find that fathers or unrelated adults are caring for young children, either in the child's home or in a day-care home or day-care center. However, the importance of day care as the place where children are fed and otherwise cared for is expanding throughout the world, particularly in urban areas. The quality of feeding care behaviors by alternative caregivers is very difficult to assess in case studies, but it is probably safe to conclude that these vary across a spectrum from excellent to very poor, and in many situations it is likely that this compromises dietary intake in early childhood.

Some of the reports about the "where" and "who" of young child care also document the ambivalence with which women leave the care (including nutritional care) of their young children to others. In every society, families worry about the safety, health, and well-being of their young children. For a preverbal infant, families are usually quick to respond to crying and often interpret it as a sign of hunger, unless there are clear signs that point to another source of distress. On the other hand, competing demands on an adult's time, particularly mothers, requires compromises. These compromises are reflected in statements of ambivalence and concern, some of which are evident in the case studies we reviewed.

Implications of the Findings for Interventions

In the preceding paragraphs we suggested that, in many settings, there are features of common caregiving practices that do not support the optimal growth and development of children. The implications of this analysis are the following:

- There is a need for interventions to improve nutrition-related caregiving practices during the period of complementary feeding.
- Nutrition-related caregiving behaviors are always embedded in a much larger complex of family and caregiver activities and a broad sociocultural context.
- Therefore, interventions undertaken for the purpose of changing specific behaviors must be designed in relation to their sociocultural context and in relation to situation-specific determinants.

Many years ago, Gordon et al. (1963) called attention to the problem of "weanling diarrhea," thereby setting off a series of investigations and discussions concerning the tradeoff between the consumption of complementary foods and the increased risk of diarrhea, which is often referred to as "the weaning dilemma" (Hibbert and Golden, 1981; Rowland, 1986; Martines et al., 1994). The weaning dilemma extends beyond the arena of nutrients and disease. It includes a series of dilemmas for caregivers as well as babies. One of the most difficult is balancing the demands on mothers to feed effectively in relation to other demands, particularly time demands. These time and resource dilemmas have been present in every social system, but they are exacerbated in contemporary societies, whether because of wage-labor and other income-earning conflicts or because of conflicts in food-production. Feeding styles have evolved that stress speed over psychosocial interaction.

Another recent factor that may have influenced the development of non-interactive feeding styles is the loss of premastication as a primary technique for transforming adult foods into a form that can be consumed by the young child. Although older ethnographies are not as detailed as one would wish, it appears that premastication occurs as a bite-by-bite technique, which requires the caregiver to follow the child's pace.

Regardless of the initial determinants, the effect of changing norms and expectations about feeding style is that even in household situations where the tradeoffs are less clear, there may be tendencies to adopt style that are suboptimal. One of the major challenges for the development of locally appropriate intervention will be to find ways to balance demands on the caregiver's time with the promotion of a responsive feeding style.

Another major challenge that needs to be addressed in the development of behavior change interventions is what methods to use to promote learning new food-related, childcare behaviors. According to Raphael (1976) Margaret Mead and colleagues were among the first to point out that breastfeeding is not a natural behavior that women automatically know how to do well. They pointed out that it is a complex behavior that requires learning and modeling. They identified the significance of the role of the *doula* (the traditional breastfeeding counselor) and pointed out that in many communities this vital role had disappeared. Thus, they attributed some of the decline in breastfeeding to the loss of the doula and advocated social interventions to replace this role. In the past two to three decades, the promotion of breastfeeding has focused heavily on teaching, modeling, and the provision of supportive structures. The success of this strategy is becoming widely understood.

The feeding of complementary foods is also a complex behavior, even more complex than breastfeeding, not least because it also depends on the availability of food. ("Availability" is used here in multiple senses, including the knowledge and skills to prepare and feed foods so that they are truly available to the young child, and availability in the larger sense of having resources to access them.) Like breastfeeding, complementary feeding needs to be learned through behavioral modeling, as well as through the acquisition of knowledge. Like breastfeeding, it also requires social support. In short, we need doulas for complementary feeding. Developing systems to provide them will be one of the significant challenges for complementary feeding interventions.

Adequate complementary feeding is obviously contingent on the availability of appropriate foods. An essential component of any intervention program is to ensure that behavioral-change interventions are undertaken in a context in which access to appropriate foods is assured.

As with all activities that are undertaken with the goal of improving well-being, the planning of interventions to improve feeding practices needs to follow basic principles of community action. These principles include:

- Obtaining knowledge about current behaviors.
- Obtaining an understanding about the key context conditions and determinants of current behaviors.
- Working with communities to design interventions that are responsive to the context and to local values.
- Building on principles and strategies of individual, familial, and community behavior change.

Finally, we need to remember that feeding infants and young children is a complex challenge for all species, including our own, and now, when rapid social and cultural change has become the human condition, we no longer have the advantage of long-term cultural evolution to guide our management of the process. In the past few decades we have developed a number of strategies to support the first part of the process—breastfeeding—although there are still many challenges, particularly in relation to exclusive breastfeeding. While continuing to work on these, it is essential to develop more creative and effective support for the continuation of the process so that the young child is protected through the entire journey from the cutting of the umbilical cord to the point at which he or she can be adequately nourished from the family pot.

References

Acuin CCS. 1992. Emic and etic perspectives on maternal care-giving and their relationship to infant nutrition. Master's thesis, Department of Anthropology, University of Connecticut, Storrs, Conn, USA.

Adair L. 1983. Feeding babies: mother's decisions in an urban U.S. setting. Med Anthropol 4:1–19.

Alan KG. 1985. Women's work and infant feeding: traditional and transitional practices on Malaita, Solomon Island. Ecol Food Nutr 16:55–73.

Allen L, Pelto GH. 1985. Research on determinants of breastfeeding duration: suggestions of biocultural studies. Med Anthropol 9:97–105.

Arimond M, Ruel M. 2001. Assessing care: progress towards the measurement of selected childcare and feeding practices, and implications for programs. FCND Discussion Paper No. 119. Washington, DC: Food Consumption and Nutrition Division, International Food Policy Research Institute.

Bentley ME, Pelto GH, Straus WL, et al. 1988. Rapid ethnographic assessment: applications in a diarrhea management program. Soc Sci Med 27: 106–16.

Bentley ME, Dickin KL, Mebrahtu S, et al. 1991. Development of a nutritionally adequate and culturally appropriate weaning food in Kwara State, Nigeria: an interdisciplinary approach. Soc Sci Med 33:1103–11.

Bentley ME, Stallings, RY, Fukumoto M, Elder JA. 1991. Maternal feeding behavior and child acceptance of food during diarrhea, convalescence, and health in the Central Sierra of Peru. Am J Public Health 81:43–7.

Bentley ME, Elder J, Fukumoto M, Stallings RH, Jacoby E, Brown K. 1995. Acute childhood diarrhea and maternal time allocation in the Northern Central Sierra of Peru. Health Pol Plan 10:60–70.

Bentley ME. 1999. Caretaker style of infant feeding as a determinant of dietary intake: the need for promotion of "interactive" feeding. FASEBJ 13:A211.

Bentley M, Gavin L, Black MM, Teti l. 1999. Infant feeding practices of low-income, African American, adolescent mothers: an ecological, multigenerational perspective. Soc Sci Med 49:1085–1100.

Birch LL, Fisher JA. 1995. Appetite and eating behavior in children. Pediatr Clin North Am 42:931–53.

Bohler E, Staffan B. 1995. Premature weaning in East Bhutan: only if mother is pregnant again. J Biosoc Sci 27: 253–65.

Brown KB, Dewey K, Allen LH. 1998. Complementary feeding of young children in developing countries: a review of current scientific knowledge. Geneva: World Health Organization.

Cleland JG, Van Ginneken JK. 1988. Maternal education and child survival in developing countries: the search for pathways of influence. Soc Sci Med 27:1367–8.

Conton I. 1985. Social, economic and ecological parameters of infant feeding in Usino, Papua New Guinea case. Ecol Food Nutr 16:39–54.

Cosminsky S, Mhykiyi M, EwbankD. 1993. Child feeding practices in a rural area of Zimbabwe. Soc Sci Med 36:937–47.

Creed Kanishiro H, Fukumoto M, Bentley ME, Jacoby E, Verzosa C, Brown KH. 1991. Use of recipe trials and anthropological techniques for the development of a home-prepared weaning food in the Central Highlands of Peru. J Nutr Educ 23:30–5.

Dettwyler KA. 1987a. Infant feeding in Mali, West Africa: variations in belief and practice. Soc Sci Med 23: 651–64.

Dettwyler KA. 1987b. Breastfeeding and weaning in Mali: cultural context and hard data. Soc Sci Med 24:633–44.

Dettwyler KA. 1989. Styles of infant feeding: parental/caretaker control of food consumption in young children. Am Anthropol 91 :696–703.

Engle P. 1987. Caretaker competence. Abstracts of the 86th Annual Meeting of the American Anthropological Association. Washington, DC: American Anthropological Association.

Engle PL. 1992. Childcare and nutrition. Theme Paper for the International Conference on Nutrition. New York: UNICEF.

Engle PL, Menon P, Haddad L. 1996. Care and nutrition: concepts and measurement. Food Consumption and Nutrition Division Discussion Paper No. 18. Washington, DC: International Food Policy Research Institute.

Food and Agriculture Organization of the United Nations and World Health Organization. 1992. Major issues for nutrition strategies. International Conference on Nutrition. Rome and Geneva: FAO and WHO.

Gittelsohn J, Shankar AY, West KP, et al. 1998. Child feeding and care behaviors are associated with xerophthalmia in rural Nepalese households. Soc Sci Med 36:925–35.

Gordon JE, Chitkara ID, Wyon JE. 1963. Weanling diarrhea. Am J Med Sci 246:245–51.

Guldan GS, Zeitlin MF, Beiser AS, Super CM, Gershoff SN, Datta S. 1993. Maternal education and child feeding practices in rural Bangladesh. Soc Sci Med 36:925–35.

Hibbert JM, Golden MH. 1981. What is the weanling's dilemma? J Trop Pediatr 27:255–8.

Izurieta LM, Larson-Brown LB. 1995. Child feeding practices in Guatemala. Ecol Food Nutr 33:249–62.

Levine NE. 1988. Women's work and infant feeding: a case from rural Nepal. Ethnology 27:231–51.

Mabilia M. 1996. Beliefs and practices in infant feeding among the Wagogo of Chigongwe (Dodoma rural district), Tanzania: weaning. Ecol Food Nutr 35:209–17.

Martines JC. 1988. The interrelationships between feeding mode, malnutrition and diarrhoeal morbidity in early infancy among the urban poor in southern Brazil. London: Human Nutrition Department, London School of Hygiene and Tropical Medicine, University of London.

Martines JC, Habicht JP, Ashworth A, Kirkwood BR. 1994. Weaning in southern Brazil: Is there a "weanling's dilemma"? J Nutr 124:1189–98.

McClennan JD. 1994. Infant feeding practices in a poor district of Santo Domingo. Ecol Food Nutr 32:167–79.

McLorg PA, Bryant CA. 1989. Influence of social network members and health care professionals on infant feeding practices of economically disadvantaged mothers. Med Anthropol 10:265–78.

Montague SF. 1984. Infant feeding and health care in Kaduwaga village, the Trobriand Islands. Ecol Food Nutr 14:249–58.

Muñoz de Chavez M, Arroyo P, Perez Gil S, Hernandez M, Quiroz S, Rodriquez M, de Hermelo M, Chavez A. 1974. The epidemiology of good nutrition in a population with a high prevalence of malnutrition. Ecol Food Nutr 3:223–30.

Oni GA, Brown KH, Bentley ME, Dickin KL, et al. 1991. Infant feeding practices and prevalence of hand feeding of infants and young children in Kwara State, Nigeria. Ecol Food Nutr 25:209–19.

Pelto GH. 1981. Perspectives on infant feeding: decision making and ecology. Food Nutr Bull 3:16–29.

Pelto GH. 1989. Maternal care-giving and nutrition. In: Young et al, editors. Proceedings of the 14th International Congress of Nutrition. Seoul, Korea: Fourteenth International Congress of Nutrition Organizing Committee. p 729–33.

Pelto GH. 2000. Improving complementary feeding practices and responsive parenting as a primary component of interventions to prevent malnutrition in infancy and early childhood. Pediatrics 106:1300–1.

Raphael D. 1976. The tender gift. New York: Schocken Books.

Reed BA, Habicht J-P, Niameogo C. 1996. The effects of maternal education on child nutritional status depend on socio-environmental conditions. Int J Epidemiol 25:585–92.

Rowland MG. 1986.The weanling's dilemma: Are we making progress? Acta Paediatr s323:33–42.

Ruel MT, Habicht J-P, Pinstrup-Andersen P, Grohn Y. 1992. The mediating effect of maternal nutrition knowledge on the association between maternal schooling and child nutritional status in Lesotho. Am J Epidemiol 35:904–14.

UNU (United Nations University). 1995. Special issue on care and nutrition of the young child. Food Nutr Bull 16(4):281–412.

UNICEF. 1990. Strategy for improved nutrition of children and women in developing countries. New York: UNICEF.

Van Esterik P. 1989. Beyond the breast-bottle controversy. New Brunswick, NJ, USA: Rutgers University Press.

WHO (World Health Organization). 2000. IMCI Handbook. WHO/ FCH/CAH/00.12. Geneva: WHO.

Wright MM, Dutra de Oliveira JE. 1988. Infant feeding in a low-income Brazilian community. Ecol Food Nutr 23:1–12.

Zeitlin M, Hollser R, Jolmson Fe. 1989. Active maternal feeding and nutritional status of 8–20-month-old Mexican children. Kansas City, Mo, USA: Society for Research in Child Development.

Zeitlin ME. 1996. Child care and nutrition: the findings from positive deviance research. Nutrition Monograph Series No. 27. Ithaca, NY: Cornell International Nutrition Program.

Zeitlin MF, Ghassemi H, Mansour M. 1990. Positive-deviance in child nutrition. Tokyo: United Nations University.

UNIT XI

OVERNUTRITION AND HUNGER IN LANDS OF PLENTY

The nutrition of individuals in the United States and other "lands of plenty" is seemingly paradoxical. There is both overnutrition and hunger, sometimes in the very same individual and group. Overnutrition is manifested as obesity and its prevalence is increasing in the United States as well as around the world. In 2007–2008 over 30% of the U.S. adult population was defined as obese (Flegal et al. 2010). The simple equation for the etiology of obesity is that more energy (calories) is consumed than is expended. But why does this seem to happen so easily? How do we explain obesity at a deeper and more meaningful level? Why is it so easy to gain weight, and so hard to reverse the gain? How could it be that overweight and obesity are signs of health and beauty among some groups, whereas just the opposite is true among many ethnicities and classes in the United States?

Even as the rising tide of obesity dominates the news, some families have difficulty providing a nutritious diet for themselves and their children. Deficient quality, rather than deficient quantity, is usually the problem. For many families in poverty, the diet is dominated by lower cost, often processed, foods that are high in fat and low in nutrient density (the ratio of micronutrients to calories). These are diets that can result in deficiencies in micronutrients (vitamins and minerals), and if available in sufficient quantity, simultaneously promote obesity.

Hunger is a term with multiple meanings. It refers to the physiological craving for food, the discomfort that accompanies inadequate food intake, as well as the perception that food intake is inadequate. Hunger is quickly alleviated by inexpensive, high sugar snacks, such as a soft drink, but returns rapidly. Hunger co-exists with poverty. It occurs in households and individuals that are "food insecure," that is, those unable to provide enough food for their family members or themselves due to a lack of resources. In 2009, about 15% of U.S. households were classified as food insecure, and about 6% of those had "very low food security" in which food intake was reduced or disrupted due to a lack of resources (Nord et al. 2010).

While perhaps not as obvious and severe as the problems faced by individuals living in extreme poverty in some developing countries, the nutritional problems in lands of plenty like the United States demand a better understanding. The chapters in this section explore the dimension of the complex problems of obesity and hunger.

In "Big Fat Myths," Alexandra Brewis takes a broad anthropological view of the so called obesity "problem." She argues that to understand it requires an approach that integrates social and biological dimensions of body fatness over time and across populations. To demonstrate the value of this approach she dissects five conventional ideas about obesity, ideas she considers myths. They are beliefs that obesity is genetic, losing weight is easy, excess body fat is deadly, fat people are perceived to be less worthy, and lastly, that thin-is-beautiful.

Leslie Sue Lieberman's paper, "Evolutionary and Anthropological Perspectives on Optimal Foraging in Obesogenic Environments," is also an anthropological look at obesity, in which she approaches the question of the high rates of obesity in modern populations from an evolutionary perspective. She considers ecological foraging theory, a set of cost/benefit models that link food-related behaviors to characteristics of the environment. Her basic thesis is that humans continue to use cues from their evolutionary past in accessing and consuming food. The problem is that these cues lead to overconsumption in modern environments where the costs of accessing food are minimal because food is ubiquitous and bountiful, processing costs are minimal because foods are sold ready-to-eat, and foods of high energy density (high caloric content per unit weight) are highly visible in the environment and available 24-hours a day throughout the year. These kinds of modern food environments are referred to as obesogenic, i.e., tending to cause obesity. They are qualitatively different than the food environments of most of the peoples described in this volume: the !Kung San of southern Africa, the rice farmers in Laos, Tukanoan Indians in the Amazon, Maasai Pastoralists in East Africa, and the Malaiyalis of rural India among others.

Humans are not the only primates susceptible to weight gain in environments with easy access to lots of energy dense foods. In the chapter "Junk Food Monkeys," Robert Sapolsky demonstrates that nonhuman primates, in this case wild baboons, respond the same way as human do to obesogenic environments.

"The Pima Paradox" by Malcolm Gladwell is a case study on obesity in one human group - the Pima of Arizona and northern Mexico. Gladwell travels around the Gila River reservation of the Pima, into the world of diet books and weight-loss drugs, and finally over the Mexican border to the world of the Mexican Pima. Along the way, he evaluates the conflicting set of explanations for why certain people gain weight so readily and what can be done about it. It is no wonder that most of us are confused about weight. The main lesson he shares is from the Mexican Pima, the southern cousins of the Gila River Pima. The Mexican Pima appear to be genetically indistinguishable from their U.S. cousins. But unlike the Gila River Pima, who live on a reservation and have very low activity levels, the Mexican Pima still subsist by maintaining small farms. They are active and thin. What is the lesson to be learned from the Pima? What does this say for the health care system's approach to obesity?

The first two chapters in this section are focused on children. The paper by Deborah Crooks, "Trading Nutrition for Education: Nutritional Studies and the Sale of Snack Foods in an Eastern Kentucky School," is a case study of the food environment and specifically the sale of snack foods in an elementary school. It is a curious case of school officials concerned about the quality of the school lunches, but willing to sell snack foods (mostly candy, chips and soft drinks), even though they recognize them as unhealthy. Why do they do it? They do it because it is the only source of funding for educational programs they believe the children deserve. This bakesale approach to funding education has come under increasing scrutiny as childhood obesity has continued to rise.

The first chapter in the section, "Children's Experiences of Food Insecurity Can Assist in Understanding Its Effect on Their Well-Being," causes us to pause and remember that obesity is not the only nutritional problem in the United States. Hunger and undernutrition are also problems. In this chapter, Carol Connell and co-authors discuss the perceptions of children living in food insecure families, families that have limited or inadequate access to the quality and quantity of food needed to maintain health. The children they studied were from families categorized as food insecure. They had experienced the family running out of food at the end of the month, and described how eating patterns changed at home and at school, as well as the shame they experienced.

Does it seem incongruous that overweight and hungry people in the United States depend on the same food production system to move food from farmers' fields to dinner plates? Is it just purchasing power that differentiates them? Hunger has been with us for a very long time, maybe forever, but obesity on the scale we are experiencing it now is a new phenomenon. What has changed? How could it be that some states in the United States have much higher rates of obesity than others? Michigan, for example, has a prevalence rate of 31% as compared to Colorado that has a rate of 21%. See Centers for Disease Control (CDC) for more information on obesity rates by state (http://www.cdc.gov/obesity/data/trends.html).

SUGGESTIONS FOR THINKING AND DOING NUTRITIONAL ANTHROPOLOGY

1. Compare the energy density (kilocalories per unit weight) of 10 foods you commonly consume. Use information on food packages or the USDA website (http://www.nal.usda.gov/fnic/foodcomp/search/) to calculate energy density as kcal/oz. For example, *Smartfood* cheddar cheese popcorn has 240 kcal per 1.5 oz bag, which is 160 kcal/oz (i.e., 240/1.5). How variable are the energy densities of the foods you eat? Could the energy densities of processed foods be contributing to the obesity epidemic?
2. What is your BMI? See Appendix 2 for help in calculating BMI.
3. Travel around a neighborhood. What is easier to purchase: beer, soft drinks or a fresh orange?

References

Flegal KM, Carroll MD, Ogden CL, Curtin LR. 2010. Prevalence and Trends in Obesity Among US Adults, 1999–2008. Journal of the American Medical Association 303(3):235–24.

Nord, Mark, Alisha Coleman-Jensen, Margaret Andrews, and Steven Carlson. *Household Food Security in the United States, 2009.* ERR-108, U.S. Dept. of Agriculture, Econ. Res. Serv. November 2010. http://www.ers.usda.gov/Publications/ERR108/ERR108.pdf (accessed June 20, 2011).

Suggested Further Reading

Brewis A. 2011. Obesity: Cultural and Biocultural Perspectives. New Brunswick: Rutgers University Press. Book length treatment of beliefs surrounding obesity in different societies.

De Garine I and Pollock NJ (Eds.). (1995). Social Aspects of Obesity. New York: Gordon and Breach. A good source of readings on the social milieu of obesity worldwide.

Maurer D and Sobal J, Eds. 1995. Eating Agendas: Food and Nutrition as Social Problems. New York: Aldine de Gruyter. A wide-ranging set of chapters on social aspects of food, especially pertaining to obesity, hunger, and body image.

CHAPTER 46

Children's Experiences of Food Insecurity Can Assist in Understanding Its Effect on Their Well-Being

Carol L. Connell, Kristi L. Lofton, Kathy Yadrick,

and Timothy A. Rehner

(2005)

During the late 1980s and early 1990s, research focused on understanding the experience of food insecurity and hunger from the perspective of adults, particularly families with children living at home (1,2). This research resulted in a conceptualization of food insecurity and hunger that was grounded in the experience of adults and included 4 broad components at 2 levels of food insecurity, the individual level and the household level. The first component was a quantity aspect, including food depletion at the household level and insufficient food intake at the individual level. The second component was a quality component composed of unsuitable food at the household level and an inadequate diet at the individual level. The third, a psychological component, included anxiety about the household food supply and individual feelings of deprivation or lack of choice. The fourth, a social component, included acquiring food through socially unacceptable means at the household level and disrupted eating patterns at the individual level (1,3). This conceptualization was then used in the development of the current measure of household food security (4).

A number of studies have attempted to assess the effect of household food insecurity on the nutritional, physical, and mental well-being of children using household level measures of food insecurity. In short, these studies reported associations between household food insecurity and adverse emotional, behavioral, academic, and cognitive measures as well as poorer mental and physical quality of life measures among children (5-17). Studies of the associations between food insecurity and child well-being to date have used household levels of food insecurity as reported by adult respondents. Little if any research has been conducted to assess children's own perceptions of or experience with

food insecurity. An understanding of the experience of food insecurity by children is essential for better measurement and assessment of the effect of food insecurity on children's health and quality of life. Therefore, the purpose of this research was to explore children's perceptions of household food insecurity and use their descriptions of food insecurity to define components of the experience of food insecurity for children.

SUBJECTS AND METHODS

This study was the first phase of a 3-phase research project designed to develop a food security survey module that could be administered directly to children. The research was approved by the Institutional Review Board at the University of Southern Mississippi. The second and third phases of the study consisted of cognitive testing of the questions developed from the results of the study reported here and then piloting the questions and conducting scaling analyses to assess the internal validity and reliability of the child food security survey module (18). The research design for this phase was a qualitative approach that explored children's perceptions of household food insecurity and the language they used to describe experiences associated with it. The study population consisted of a purposeful sample of children aged 11–16 y who were likely to have experienced food insecurity. Children were recruited from 2 after school programs targeting low-income children in a mid-size central city (urban) and from a rural middle school within a Metropolitan Statistical Area with a high rate of eligibility for free and reduced-price school meals (rural). Parental consent and child assent were obtained before the interviews. Individual semistructured interviews were conducted by the first 2 authors who were trained by an expert in child qualitative marketing research to conduct interviews with children. The training included didactic and experiential instructional methods under the guidance of the expert.

Carol L. Connell, Kristi L. Lofton, Kathy Yadrick, and Timothy A. Rehner, "Children's experiences of food insecurity can assist in understanding its effect on their well-being." *The Journal of Nutrition* 135(2005):1683–1690. Reprinted with permission.

Questions used in the semistructured interviews were developed with assistance from food security experts and an expert in qualitative marketing research with children. The questions were designed to assess children's perception of food insecurity by asking what happened when food supplies in the house began to get low and what they thought led to that situation, as well as about anxiety over the family's food supply. Questions and interview methods were pretested with the guidance of a child marketing research expert, with 10 children aged 10–12 y old who resided in a local apartment complex housing primarily graduate and/ or married university students. The pretest resulted in a few minor changes to the qualitative questions, inclusion of more probes, addition of a nonthreatening opening question to introduce the topic of food and meals, 2 transition questions leading into the primary questions related to food insecurity, and a closing question designed to diffuse tension that might have been created from the discussion about running out of food (Table 1). The questions were used as a guide for the conversation about food insecurity with children. Probes were used if children were hesitant in answering a question or to clarify what children were expressing in the conversation about food insecurity. The food insecurity questions (Q4–Q6) are the focus of this article.

Individual children were interviewed either at the after school centers or the middle school in an empty room to allow for privacy. Interviews were tape-recorded; to ensure trustworthiness of the data, both researchers conducting the interviews debriefed one another immediately after the interviews to compare themes that seemed to be emerging from the interviews (19). Tape-recorded interviews were then transcribed. The constant comparative method was used to identify common themes that emerged from the children's discussions on food insecurity during the debriefing sessions and from the transcripts of the interviews (20). In short, statements that appeared to be describing similar behaviors and responses were grouped together into behaviors/responses of children and behaviors/responses of adults as perceived and described by children. These groups were then categorized by the researchers into 3 broad themes: eating behaviors, emotional responses, and social behaviors. Behavior and response frequencies were noted for the number of interviews in which they appeared, the frequency within the urban or rural context in which they appeared, and the number of times across all interviews that they appeared. In the final step, statements about children's reactions and adults' reactions were classified according to the components of food insecurity described in the earlier literature using systematic comparison (21). This was done in anticipation of developing food insecurity questions for children in the second phase of this research.

RESULTS

Description of Study Participants

The qualitative interviews were concluded after interviewing 32 children because similar answers were being obtained

---

Table 1 Semistructured Interview Questions Used in Qualitative Interviews with 11–16 Y Old Children

1. Icebreaker question: If you were going to cook a meal tonight for supper, what would you make?

   (Probe: What types of foods would you have?)

2. Transition question: Tell me about the last time you were hungry.

   (Probe: What was going on then? Why did it happen?)

3. Transition question: When you worry about being hungry, what sorts of things do you worry about?

   (Probe: What is happening that you know you need to worry?)

4. Food insecurity question: Have you ever known kids from a family that almost ran out of food before the end of the month?

   (Probes: What made that happen? What did the grown-ups say that let the kids know there wasn't enough money to get more food? What did the grown-ups do that let the kids know there wasn't enough money to get more food?)

   (May probe for: changes in type of foods eaten, meals got smaller, frequency of meals changed.)

5. Food insecurity question: Have you ever known kids from a family that worried that their food would run out and they wouldn't have enough money to get more?

   (Probe: How did the kids in the family know they were worried?

   What did grown-ups say that let the kids know they were worried?

   What did the grown-ups do that let the kids know they were worried?)

   (May probe for: Did the kind of meals the family ate change when they were worried? How did they change? Did the amount of food the family ate change when they were worried about having enough? How did it change?)

6. Food insecurity question (clarification): If child answers yes to question 4, but no to question 5, ask: You said earlier that you knew families that sometimes didn't have enough money to eat right. Could you help me understand a little better? Did they not worry about running out of food before it happened?

7. Diffusion question: Tell me about your favorite holiday or birthday meal.

from children who had knowledge of food insecurity. Our sample of children was somewhat smaller than the average sample size reported in a review of qualitative research sample extensiveness by Sobal (22). However, purposeful sampling of children likely to have experience with food insecurity allowed us to reach data repetitiveness, informational redundancy, and thus theoretical saturation with 32 individual interviews (21,23,24). Even though 4 children were not willing/able to answer questions related to household food insecurity, there were consistent answers across the remaining children who had knowledge of food insecurity. The study sample was equally divided between boys and girls (Table 2). Similarly, Black children and White children, and rural and nonrural children were fairly equally distributed. The majority of the Black children lived in the mid-size inner city (urban), whereas all of the White children lived in the rural community. The children ranged in age from 11 to 16 y old; the majority (65%) were 13–14 y old.

Children's Behavioral Descriptions of Food Insecurity

Because it became clear in the early interviews that we could not ask children whether they had direct experience with food insecurity, we asked them if they knew of a child whose family who had run out of food before there was money to buy more. Eighteen of the children stated they had known kids from other families who nearly ran out of food before the end of the month. Despite our purposeful sample and the fact that we asked about "other kids," there were still a small number of children who said they did not know other kids who had this problem. However, when probed further, 10 of these children described situations that indicated they were well aware of

Table 2 Demographics of Children Participating in Semistructured Interviews

Characteristic	n (%)
Gender	
Male	16 (50)
Female	16 (50)
Race	
Black	17 (53)
White	15 (47)
Age, y	
11–12	8 (25)
13–14	21 (65)
15–16	3 (9)
Setting	
Rural (within MSA[1])	17 (53)
Mid-size inner city	15 (47)

[1] Metropolitan Statistical Area.

"others" who had problems running out of food. From this, we concluded that 28 children had some experience, either directly or indirectly, with food insecurity (data not shown). Children across all ages that we interviewed were able to describe situations in which families had "almost run out of food before the end of the month." Most used behaviors to describe how they came to know these families were running out of food. Children who appeared to be the most comfortable expressing their thoughts freely described situations of food insecurity. They talked about how families got in a food shortage situation and described what other kids said/did to let them know they were running out of food. They also reported what grown-ups said/did when food supplies were getting low

Causes of food insecurity. Resource constraints were mentioned as the cause of food insecurity in 17 of the interviews (data not shown). These are illustrated in the following quotes:

> "His daddy died and his mama didn't have a job."
>   "Say that we don't have enough food stamps. If we are working on food stamps, you got that card and it runs out of money. That is bad."
>   "…it was the bills. They had so many bills that they had to pay and had to cut back on some stuff."

In 7 interviews, other reasons given were the parent(s)/caregiver smoking, drinking alcohol, or buying drugs or clothes rather than buying food.

Children's behaviors and responses associated with food insecurity. Children indicated they did not routinely talk to each other about running out of food. They used behaviors to describe how they could tell when another child or family was running out of food (Table 3). We categorized the statements related to children's behaviors and responses associated with family food insecurity into the 3 broad themes noted in the Methods. Within the theme of children's eating behaviors, eating less was mentioned in 14 interviews, eating food that was less desirable because there was no other choice in 13 interviews, and eating larger amounts or faster than normal in 7 interviews. Eating all of the school lunch or eating the school lunch very fast were behaviors 2 children told us indicated others were running out of food at home. Over twice as many children in the rural setting mentioned eating less compared with the urban group. Children mentioned being ashamed or fearful of being labeled as "poor" 14 times in 7 interviews, primarily during the urban interviews. We categorized this under the theme of emotional responses to the family running out of food. Within the theme of social behaviors, children eating with other family, friends, or neighbors or borrowing food or money to buy food was mentioned in 12 interviews. A similar behavior, "sharing" food, was mentioned in 5 interviews. Eating with others, borrowing, or sharing was mentioned in >4 times the number of urban interviews compared with rural interviews. Statements indicative of these behaviors/responses were:

Table 3 Children's Descriptions of Food Insecurity in Terms of the Number of Times in Which the Behavior or Response Appeared

	Interviews in which the variable appeared			Total times variable appeared (all interviews)
	All	Urban	Rural	
			n	
Children				
Eating behaviors				
Eat less[1]	14	4	10	19
Eat less desirable foods[2]	9	5	4	12
Eat larger amounts/faster[3]	7	4	3	7
Emotional responses				
Worry	3	3	0	4
Ashamed/afraid of being labeled "poor"	7	6	1	14
Social behavior				
Eat with others; borrow food, money	12	10	2	29
Share food	5	4	1	5
Other				
Stealing, losing weight, sad or anxious appearance	7	3	4	9
Adults				
Eating habits				
Eat less so children have enough	3	3	0	5
Buy/prepare less desirable foods	2	2	0	3
Emotional responses				
Try to hide situation from children	10	4	6	11
Tell children only when necessary	8	5	3	12
Tell child to "wait" or go play	3	3	0	7
Worry	4	2	2	4
Family stress	7	6	1	7
Social behaviors				
Encourage child to eat with others, borrow food or money	4	4	0	5
Limit child's activities	6	2	4	7

[1] Eating less in either quantity of food or frequency of meals.
[2] Less desirable foods were foods that the children would eat only if there was no other choice.
[3] Eating larger amounts of food or faster than normal was mentioned as occurring at times when food was available.

Eating less: "*They will just start cutting back on what they're eating.*"

Eating less desirable foods: "*...change to lower class meals like eatin' a whole lot of canned food instead of fixin' up some proper meals.*"

Eating with others/sharing: "*...they ask if they can spend the night over to our house and I tell them yes...*"

Shame/fear: "*They be like ashamed or whatever.*"

Children's descriptions of adults' behaviors and responses associated with food insecurity. Children also mentioned adult's behaviors related to food insecurity; we categorized behaviors of adults as described by children into the same 3 broad themes of "eating behaviors," "emotional responses," and "social behaviors" (Table 3). Statements about eating behaviors related to parents' eating less food themselves to save food for the children. Comments about adults were most often in the category of emotional responses or social behaviors. Within the theme of emotional responses, the most frequently mentioned were trying to hide the situation from children (10 interviews), telling the child about the lack of money or food only when necessary (8 interviews), and indications of family stress related to running out of food (7 interviews). We classified trying to hide the situation or telling the child only when necessary in the emotional responses category because statements made about these responses indicated that parents/caregivers were experiencing stress related to trying to protect children from experiencing hunger. Social behaviors included encouraging the child to eat with others or to borrow food or money, and limiting the child's activities. Parents encouraging children to eat with someone else or borrow money/food was mentioned only in the urban interviews. Examples of statements associated with these behaviors were:

> Hide situation: *"Sometimes they just lie to protect them (the younger kids) so they don't scare the children."*

> Family stress: *"They (children) start looking sad and everything and their (parents') attitudes get worse 'cause the kids get real hungry and the parents start to get madder and madder 'cause the kids' beggin'."*

> Limiting activities: *"My mom just tells me straight out that we don't have the money to do [this] and we don't have the money to do that."*

Components of the Food Insecurity Experience of Children

Because the statements about adult behaviors were part of the child's perception of family food insecurity, child and adult themes that were similar were collapsed. These groups were then categorized into 4 components of food insecurity previously described by Radimer et al. (1) that the researchers judged also captured components of the food insecurity experience of children (Table 4).

Quantity Components

Eating less (quantity and frequency). This component of the food insecurity experience of children included eating less, being told to "wait" to eat, losing weight due to eating less, and adults eating less so children could have food. Eating less food than desired or less frequently than usual was mentioned 24 times. Statements representing this component of the food insecurity experience of children were:

Table 4 Components of Children's Food Insecurity Experiences[1]

Component	Times themes mentioned
	n
Quantity	
Eating less (children and adults)	24
Eating more/fast when food available	7
Quality	
Use of few kinds of low-cost foods[2]	15
Psychological	
Worry/Anxiety/Sadness (children and adults)[3]	14
Feelings of "no choice" (eating less desirable foods)[2]	15
Shame/fear of being labeled "poor"[3]	14
Attempts to shield children[3]	20
Inability to shield children[3]	19
Social	
Use of social networks for food acquisition (sharing/borrowing/eating with others)	39
Social exclusion (limited participation in other activities)	7
Family stress[3]	7
Other (stealing, losing weight, parent working extra job)	7

[1] Numbers in themes may not match those from same themes in Table 3 due to overlap and collapsing of themes into the components that make up the experience of children's food insecurity as interpreted by the authors.
[2] These two themes overlapped. During the course of the interviews, children talked about eating a few foods that were not what they really wanted because there was no choice.
[3] These themes overlapped. Discussions around worry, shame, attempts to shield children, and inability to shield children often suggested stress within the family although it may not have been expressed as such by the children.

"They sort of ration the food…say that if you have a large meal and food begins to run out, you go to a medium meal, then a small meal and they get smaller."

"They [parents]…organize all their food or eat one time and find ways to supplement food and stuff…the parents might eat once a day and the kids eat regular like they do everyday."

Eating more or fast when food is available. Although only 7 interviews contained this theme, it was interesting that individual children in different settings talked about it. It was mentioned in both urban and rural interviews. Children mentioned eating all of the school lunch or "eating real fast" as indications that another child was running out of food at home.

"Yeah, 'cause when they get food they try to eat it all up so that it will take a long time before they get hungry again."

"…they eat all of their food [at school] and people make fun of them, that they eat all their food."

"…eat a lot at school and then when you come home you won't be hungry for another hour or 4 hours."

Quality Component

Use of a few kinds of low-cost ("cheap") foods. It appeared that this component of the food insecurity experience overlapped considerably with the psychological aspect of the experience in that children talked about eating foods they did not necessarily like, but that were the only foods in the house. Children generally named canned foods when talking about eating only a few kinds of low-cost foods. This theme appeared 15 times in the course of 11 interviews and included children eating less desirable foods or only a few items and parents preparing less desirable or only a few foods. Statements associated with this theme were:

"They eat bologna or vegetables in the can…"

"Little small foods or like just 3 things to eat and drink…toast, sausage, and peas."

Psychological Components

Worry/anxiety/sadness about the family food supply. Two themes we placed in the psychological component of children's food insecurity overlapped with social components of the experience as well. These overlapping components included worry/anxiety, shame/fear, attempts to shield children, and family stress. Statements that appeared to overlap were counted in each of the themes. Statements made by children in 14 interviews indicated worry, anxiety, or sadness about the family food situation either on the part of the parent or child. For parents, expressing worry was exemplified by this quote:

"…she would tell them she has to pray about it and pray that everything would get better because they are not giving her enough food stamps to supply her and her kids."

The term "look sad" was used to describe children who were running out of food. Children who talked about other children running out of food told us they knew this by the way the child looked. Two very shocking examples of children describing other children's anxiety and sadness (or their "look") were:

"They make those sad faces."
"They will look crazy and try to borrow food."

Feeling there is "no choice." This theme overlapped with the quality component theme of use of a few kinds of low-cost foods. Children who talked about eating less desirable foods usually discussed it in the context of eating a few foods that they would not have chosen had there been another choice. The concept of lack of choice was reflected in statements such as:

"…She just cook…something we don't like and says this is all we have."

"…the parents would say that they were running out of food and that they had to cut back on the meals…and that they should be grateful for the meals they had to eat; it was better than having nothing."

Shame/fear of being labeled as "poor." This theme focused on shame about the family's situation and fear of being labeled as "poor." The children indicated that they did not routinely talk to each other about running out of food. One or two said they might tell their best friend that they were low on food at home, but most of them "just knew" when "other kids" were food insecure or hungry by their behaviors or "looks" as noted above. Several children said it would be embarrassing to tell others that food was running out in the household and that other kids would make fun of children who had this problem.

"…some of them be like ashamed or whatever."

"…well, where we stay, they will [tease them]…push them in the head and talk about them. They will bring up something like that that they had to come to their house and eat their food."

"they don't want their friends to think bad of them or think that they are a poor family…yeah, a whole lot of people would take that as an advantage over you…if he tells the truth [about not having food] in a class of boys, they will take that to their advantage."

Attempts to shield children. We labeled statements related to "sharing" food as attempts to shield children from hunger in addition to being part of the informal network for food acquisition. In addition, we included adults trying to hide the situation from children and encouraging children to eat with others or borrow money in this theme. Several children indicated that adults and even older siblings would try to hide food insecurity from younger children.

"...I go in my house and I do everything that I can for my little brother, my little sister, and my friends so I just bring them something to eat."

Inability to shield children. Statements made by children indicated that parents tell them about the food situation at home only when the situation has reached a critical point and there is not enough food for them. We chose to separate this theme from attempts to shield children and labeled it "inability to shield children." It included parents telling the child to "wait until I get paid" or telling him/her to "go play" when the child asked for something to eat.

Social Components

Use of informal social networks for food acquisition. Sharing, borrowing food or money to buy food, and eating with other families were mentioned most frequently by children in the 2 after school programs. Parents encouraging these behaviors were mentioned directly in 4 urban interviews but not rural ones. We labeled these behaviors "use of informal social networks for food acquisition." Only 1 child in the rural interviews mentioned being "loaned" some money that he then used for food. Statements related to this were:

"They send you to borrow some flour. Our neighbor do that all the time. She borrow flour and eggs all the time so that she can finish cooking. We borrow flour all the time. We always run out."

"...she gets food stamps but they like run out like in the middle of the month so my mama gives her some chicken or something."

"...they go ask my mama because they know that she gonna feed them and they can just stay and get fed."

Limited participation in social activities. Parents limiting children's social activities due to limited resources was categorized as a social component of the experience of food insecurity because children in the interviews indicated this was a way they knew families were running out of money.

DISCUSSION

The child development literature indicates that children are emotionally and psychologically affected by their parent/caregiver experiences. In fact, Bandura (25–27) argues that children capable of cognition watch others and selectively imitate adult behaviors. He defined this as modeling and observational learning (28,29). Therefore, we utilized previous literature from qualitative studies of adult experiences with food insecurity to inform our exploration of children's experience with food insecurity. We used semi-structured individual interviews that were guided, rather than prescribed, by a series of questions related to families

running out of food or worrying that food would run out to allow children the opportunity to more freely discuss what they had experienced relative to these 2 questions. The primary purpose of this phase of the research study was to use children's descriptions of their experience with food insecurity to define components of that experience for children with the eventual goal of developing a valid instrument for the direct measurement of child food insecurity.

Children's responses spanned the severity range of food insecurity from the psychological aspect of worry to the quantitative aspect of eating less (1). The most frequent responses were related to using informal social networks for food acquisition, having no choice in the foods eaten, and eating less. Only 2 children indicated they or "other kids" had gone hungry and no child talked about going a whole day without eating. This supports earlier work indicating that most children are spared from hunger by adults except at the most severe level of household food insecurity (1,2,14). It also may reflect the important role of the school breakfast and lunch programs in providing nourishment for children because a few children talked about eating all of the school lunch to keep from being hungry later. One child said other food insecure kids would eat the school lunch to keep from being hungry even if it was something they did not want.

We expected the interviews to be somewhat sensitive. We discovered in the pretest that children would not answer questions that were directed toward them personally; we had to ask about "kids from a family..." Somewhat surprising was the magnitude of the psychological responses, emotional strain, and social ramifications created for the children "running out of food." A growing body of literature suggests an association between household food insecurity and children's adverse outcomes related to emotional and mental health (8,12,13,17) as well as cognitive, academic, and psychosocial development (10). The remainder of the discussion will focus on the emotional responses and social ramifications that may add to the current knowledge related to food insecurity and child well-being. Additionally, there were some obvious differences in the responses of urban vs. rural children that will be discussed.

Bandura's work in social learning and, later, social cognitive theory, suggests that children not only are affected by their parents' stressors, but in fact mirror and replicate their parents' responses to the same stressors (25,28,29). Thus, children capable of cognition can understand issues such as inadequate food supplies within their households even if the gravity of the situation was not directly explained to them. Responses from children in this study indicated they were well aware of parental attempts to manage the food supply as well as the parental anxiety created by diminishing food supplies and constrained financial resources to acquire more food. Adult behaviors such as "praying about it," getting madder "cause the kids' beggin," and "they stop talking (at meals)" related to food insecurity as reported by the children in this study mirror the Hamelin et al. (30) report of sociofamilial perturbations in reaction to food insecurity as reported by adults. In the present study, even attempts to hide the food situation from children were noticed as indicated by statements such as "they [parents] lie to protect the children" and "they [try to hide it] because they don't want their kids to think they cannot trust their parents."

The anxiety and frustration of the parents/caregivers were mirrored in the children as indicated by statements about other children such as "they make those sad faces" and "they look crazy and will try to borrow food." This also suggests that children in this situation have learned to recognize behaviors exhibited by other children related to food insecurity and use these behaviors to make judgments about the child. This observation can then lead to fear on the part of the food-insecure child of being labeled as "poor" by other children. This was a theme that was vocalized among the urban children with statements about being teased for having to eat with another family in the neighborhood or being made fun of for eating all the school lunch. Further it suggests that behaviors indicate to other children that there is something "different" about the food-insecure child that prevents him/her from participating fully in social activities. This exclusion, termed "alienation" by Hamelin et al. (30) was also reported among food-insecure adults and again fits within Bandura's framework of modeling and observational learning on the part of children (28,29). One rural child noted that kids would not want their friends to think "bad" of them or think they were a "poor" family, implying that a person who is poor is somehow "bad" and that poverty was a situation of that person's making. An indication that the stigma associated with poverty was a constant, albeit perhaps subconscious, concern to these children was embodied in statements made by one child related to the best way to administer a similar survey to other children.

> Child: *"Like you wouldn't go in their house or nothin' you would just ask them if you run out of food we can help you?"*
>
> Interviewer: *"No, we wouldn't go in their house…"*
>
> Child: *"We can ask their parents if they want to come to a place with their children where you be healthier and never be poor again."*

Adults and elders reported feelings of shame and embarrassment related to their inability to adequately provide the necessary food for their families or themselves (30,31). Similarly, shame and embarrassment about the family's food situation were expressed verbally and nonverbally by the children in this study. However, their shame and embarrassment appeared to be relative to others "discovering" that their family was poor rather than their own inability to provide food for themselves. Statements such as "they be like ashamed or whatever" and "some [kids] won't tell anybody [they are hungry]" are indicative of the shame, embarrassment, and need for secrecy that food-insecure children feel. Six urban children verbally expressed these feelings but only 1 rural child mentioned this. Rural interviews became more tense once Q4 was asked compared with urban interviews.

Rural children took on a more defensive posture and were more guarded in responding to questions about families running out of food than urban children, nonverbal indications that these children also felt shame about their family's food situation and its social implications if discovered by their peers.

Research with low-income food-insecure adults revealed several strategies used to manage the household food supply and feed families such as sending children to eat with relatives or friends, borrowing food or money, or buying food on credit (1,30). Our findings add to this by revealing that children adopt similar strategies, often at the behest of parents, to cope with food insecurity themselves. In some cases, the coping strategies assisted in acquisition of food and at the same time alleviated the fear of being labeled as poor. Urban children most frequently mentioned strategies such as eating with other relatives or friends and borrowing food or money. Statements such as "They (parents) send you to borrow some flour" and "…our neighbor do that all the time. She borrow flour and eggs all the time so she can finish cookin' " reveal that mothers have developed a "code" of how to ask for food (borrowing to finish cooking) that can both garner needed supplies and spare the child the embarrassment of admitting the family ran out of food. It also means that adults avoid being labeled as "poor parents" or being accused of child neglect if they ask for food or money themselves. This was exemplified in one child's story of a neighbor who lost 2 of her "babies" to the "welfare people" because she "ran out of food." Therefore, sending children to borrow flour and eggs "to finish cooking" may deflect accusations of child neglect.

Social learning theory suggests that modeling and observational learning influence children's behavior. One way children are influenced is when they are placed in parental roles in which they supervise their younger siblings and are likely to engage in the same type of "protective" behaviors that they have seen their parents/caregivers model for them relative to the family's food situation (25–29). Some of the statements made by children indicate they adopt similar strategies of coping behaviors to those of their parents. Statements such as "I go in my house…and I just bring them some food" and "I gave him 3 pieces of chicken and he fried it…" embody the construct of borrowing from neighbors. However, these actions were independent of encouragement from parents and we labeled them "sharing" food among children. Additionally, both of the above statements were in reference to what 2 children were doing for younger children, indicating that as children age, they begin to model their parents' attempts to shield younger children from hunger.

There were 2 apparent differences between the urban and the rural interviews. More rural children reported the behavior of eating less and more urban children reported using informal social networks for food acquisition. Several possible explanations for these differences exist. Relative to "eating less," rural children may be modeling the rural pride in self-sufficiency they see in their parents, which may include resistance to asking for assistance from others outside the family and reluctance to use government food assistance programs other than the school lunch program. Therefore, they are more likely to "go without" or eat less rather than admit that they need assistance. Others have reported food insecure rural elders to exhibit this characteristic and to be more resistant to asking for assistance from outsiders and less likely to participate in food assistance programs because of an unfavorable view of food assistance as "welfare" (31–33). Only 2 rural children made statements indicating their parents used food stamps; 3 rural children made statements indicating they thought parents should "get a second job" or the "wife might have to go to work" to provide more income to get enough food for the family. This is perhaps further evidence for the self-sufficiency modeling of children in the rural setting.

Relative to using informal social networks, urban children in this study lived primarily in subsidized housing apartments and therefore were likely in closer proximity to friends and neighbors than rural children. This would make it easier to ask others outside the family to "borrow flour." Similarly, extended families lived in the same apartment complex, which made it easier to "go to your uncle's or grandma's to eat." Urban children were also together for longer periods of time after school during participation in the after school programs as well as playing together in the neighborhood on weekends. Therefore, they were likely better able to observe each other and offer to "share" food with their friends. However, the sense of shame and embarrassment about the family food situation and the implications it had relative to poverty were still apparent among urban children as they verbalized in their descriptions of "running out of food." Without further research, we cannot say whether these differences were truly urban vs. rural or whether they were ethnically or culturally based because we did not interview any urban White children and only 2 rural Black children.

The detailed probes for Q4 and Q5, listed in Table 1 as "may probe for...," had the potential to lead children to answer in a particular way. Therefore we avoided using these probes except when children hesitated or had difficulty verbalizing their thoughts or to clarify an answer. We used these probes in only 10 of the interviews, indicating that for the most part, children were telling us their own direct or indirect experience with food insecurity. Similarly, the transition questions related to the last time the child was hungry had the potential to impress upon the child that the interviews were only about being physically hungry rather than about food insecurity, which may or may not include hunger as an outcome. However, the change in the children's demeanor and the atmosphere of the interviews from relaxed to tense and strained when we introduced the first food insecurity question indicated that the children understood the intent of the interviews.

Our research was limited in its purpose, which was to understand children's perceptions of food insecurity and the language they use to describe it, allowing us to develop a direct measure of child food insecurity. This goal was accomplished (18). However, this central purpose limited our inquiry into the emotional responses and social ramifications of child food insecurity, and therefore our ability to more fully illuminate emotional and social facets of a child's experience of food insecurity. Nonetheless, we found that children's experiences of food insecurity bear a strong resemblance to those of adults, and that children do in fact experience physical, psychological, and social dimensions of food insecurity that could in turn contribute to adverse outcomes in children in each of these dimensions. Our work thus provides a foundation for the further exploration of the relation between food insecurity and children's emotional and mental well-being.

Note

Mark Nord, Economic Research Service/United States Department of Agriculture and Kathy Radimer, National Center for Health Statistics, are acknowledged for their guidance and early contributions to the development of the questions used in the semistructured interviews. Kathy Doyle, Doyle Research Associates, is acknowledged for her expertise in qualitative marketing research with children, for assistance in development of the questions and interview guide used in the semistructured interviews, and for her valuable training of the first 2 authors in interviewing children.

References

1. Radimer, K. L., Olson, C. M., Greene, J. C., Campbell, C. C. & Habicht, J. P. (1992) Understanding hunger and developing indicators to assess it in women and children. J. Nutr. Educ. 24: 36S–45S.
2. Wehler, C. A., Scott, R. I. & Anderson, J. J. (1995) Community Childhood Hunger Identification Project. Food Research and Action Center, Washington, DC.
3. Radimer, K. L., Olson, C. M. & Campbell, C. C. (1990) Development of indicators to assess hunger. J. Nutr. 120: 1544–1548.
4. Bickel, G., Andrews, M. & Klein, B. (1997) Measuring food security in the United States: a supplement to the CPS. In: Nutrition and Food Security in the Food Stamp Program (Hall, D. & Stavrianos, M., eds.), pp. 91–111. United States Department of Agriculture, Food and Consumer Service, Washington, DC.
5. Casey, P., Goolsby, S., Berkowitz, C., Frank, D., Cook, J., Cutts, D., Black, M. M., Zaldivar, N., Levenson, S., et al. (2004) Maternal depression, changing public assistance, food security and child health status. Pediatrics 113: 298–304.
6. Oh, S. Y. & Hong, M. J. (2003) Food insecurity is associated with dietary intake and body size of Korean children from low-income families in urban areas. Eur. J. Clin. Nutr. 57: 1598–1604.
7. Matheson, D. M., Varady, J., Varady, A. & Killen, J. D. (2002) Household food security and nutritional status

of Hispanic children in fifth grade. Am. J. Clin. Nutr. 76: 210–217.

8. Alaimo, K., Olson, C. M. & Frongillo, E. A. (2002) Family food insufficiency, but not low family income, is positively associated with dysthymia and suicide symptoms in adolescents. J. Nutr. 132: 719–725.

9. Casey, P. H., Szeto, K., Lensing, S., Bogle, M. & Weber, J. (2001) Children in food-insufficient, low-income families. Prevalence, health, and nutrition status. Arch. Pediatr. Adolesc. Med. 155: 508–514.

10. Alaimo, K., Olson, C. M., Frongillo, E. A., Jr. & Briefel, R. R. (2001) Food insufficiency, family income and health in US preschool and school-aged children. Am. J. Public Health 91: 781–786.

11. Cutts, D. B., Pheley, A. M. & Geppert, J. S. (1998) Hunger in Midwestern inner-city young children. Arch. Pediatr. Adolesc. Med. 152: 489–493.

12. Kleinman, R. E., Murphy, J. M., Little, M., Pagano, M., Wehler, C., Regal, K. & Jellinek, M. S. (1998) Hunger in children in the United States: potential behavioral and emotional correlates. Pediatrics 101: e3.

13. Murphy, J. M., Wehler, C. A., Pagano, M. E., Little, M., Kleinman, R. E. & Jellinek, M. S. (1998) Relationship between hunger and psychosocial functioning in low-income American children. J. Am. Acad. Child Adolesc. Psychiatry 37: 163–170.

14. Rose, D. & Oliveira, V. (1997) Nutrient intakes of individuals from food-insufficient households in the United States. Am. J. Public Health 87: 1956–1961.

15. Bhattacharya, J., Currie, J. & Haider, S. (2004) Poverty, food insecurity, and nutritional outcomes in children and adults. J. Health Econ. 23: 839–862.

16. Knol, L. L., Haughton, B. & Fitzhugh, E. C. (2004) Food insufficiency is not related to the overall variety of foods consumed by young children in low-income families. J. Am. Diet. Assoc. 104: 640–644.

17. Casey, P. H., Szeto, K. L., Robbins, J. M., Stuff, J. E., Connell, C., Gossett, J. M. & Simpson, P. M. (2005) Child health-related quality of life and household food security. Arch. Pediatr. Adolesc. Med. 159: 51–56.

18. Connell, C. L., Nord, M., Lofton, K. L. & Yadrick, K. (2004) Food security of older children can be assessed using a standardized instrument. J. Nutr. 134: 2566–2572.

19. Krefting, L. (1991) Rigor in qualitative research: the assessment of trustworthiness. Am. J. Occup. Ther. 45: 214–222.

20. Glaser, B. G. & Strauss, A. L. (1967) The Discovery of Grounded Theory: Strategies for Qualitative Research. Aldine de Gruyter, New York, NY.

21. Strauss, A. & Corbin, J. (1998) Basics of Qualitative Research: Techniques, and Procedures for Developing Grounded Theory, 2nd ed., Sage Publications, Thousand Oaks, CA.

22. Sobal, J. (2002) Sample extensiveness in qualitative nutrition education research. J. Nutr. Educ. Behav. 33: 184–192.

23. Curtis, S., Gesler, W., Smith, G. & Washburn, S. (2000) Approaches to sampling and case selection in qualitative research: examples in the geography of health. Soc. Sci. Med. 50: 1001–1014.

24. Kuzel, A. J. (1992) Sampling in qualitative inquiry. In: Doing Qualitative Research (Crabtree, B. F. & Miller, W. L., eds.), pp. 31–44. Sage, Newbury Park, CA.

25. Bandura, A. (1986) Social Learning Theory. Prentice-Hall, Englewood Cliffs, NJ.

26. Bandura, A. (1989) Social cognitive theory. Ann. Child. Dev. 6: 1–60.

27. Bandura, A. (1992) Perceived self-efficacy in cognitive development and functioning. Educ. Psychol. 28: 117–148.

28. Bandura, A. (1967) Behavioral psychotherapy. Sci. Am. 216: 78–86.

29. Bandura, A. (1977) Social Learning Theory. Prentice-Hall, Englewood Cliffs, NJ.

30. Hamelin, A. M., Beaudry, M. & Habicht, J. P. (2002) Characterization of household food insecurity in Quebec: food and feelings. Soc. Sci. Med. 54: 119–132.

31. Wolfe, W. S., Frongillo, E. A. & Valois, P. (2003) Understanding the experience of food insecurity by elders suggest ways to improve its measurement. J. Nutr. 133: 762–769.

32. Wolfe, W. S., Olson, C. M., Kendall, A. & Frongillo, E. A., Jr. (1996) Understanding food insecurity in the elderly: a conceptual framework. J. Nutr. Educ. 28: 92–100.

33. Quandt, S. A., Arcury, T. A., McDonald, J., Bell, R. A. & Vitolins, M. Z. (2001) Meaning and management of food security among rural elders. J. Appl. Gerontol. 20: 356–376.

CHAPTER 47

Trading Nutrition for Education: Nutritional Status and the Sale of Snack Foods in an Eastern Kentucky School

Deborah L. Crooks

(2007)

In the United States, there is increasing public health concern over what is being called an "epidemic of overweight" among children (Strauss and Pollack 2001). Over the last 20 years, children have become fatter and are exhibiting what were formerly thought of as adult diseases associated with overweight (e.g., type 2 diabetes, dislipidemia, and elevated blood pressure) (Deckelbaum and Williams 2001; Dietz and Gortmaker 2001). In addition, evidence continues to mount for an association between childhood and adolescent overweight and adult overweight (Deckelbaum and Williams 2001). Overweight in adults is associated with a variety of chronic diseases, including cardiovascular disease, hypertension, diabetes, and certain cancers (Pi-Sunyer 1993).

Although there is some indication of a genetic component to overweight, as Dietz and Gortmaker (2001) point out, there has not been a major change in the gene pool in the last 20 years, thus the factors influencing the rapid increase in overweight must be environmental. The uneven distribution of overweight across the social and geographical landscapes in the United States suggests that the nutrition environment is complex and multifactorial. Based on an analysis of national survey data, Richard Strauss and Harold A. Pollack (2001:2846) report a higher prevalence of overweight among African American and Hispanic children, among boys, and among children living in southern states; and they report an association between income and overweight that varies by ethnicity. With respect to dietary patterns that shape nutritional status, K. D. Reynolds et al. (1999) report ethnic, gender, and regional variation in consumption of fruits and vegetables; Susan J. Crockett and Laura S. Sims (1995) note that economic status, ethnicity, and region are all predictors of nutritional risk among children.

Cara B. Ebbeling et al. (2002) identify a number of interacting environmental influences on diet, activity, and family practices in the United States that promote overweight and poor nutritional status among children and that make long-term improvement in nutritional status difficult to attain. Important among these influences are aggressive marketing of low-quality foods to children, reduced opportunities for physical activity resulting from a cultural "premium on convenience," environmental structures that mitigate against children's play, and long work hours for parents. In addition, they comment that underfunding of schools may lead to reductions in or elimination of physical education classes, the contracting out of food services to companies that often sell low quality fast foods, and/or the placement of vending machines in schools for the sale of soft drinks, and, as others point out (Wechsler et al. 2001), low quality, high calorie snack foods.

Recently, the school nutrition environment has received a great deal of attention, not only from the health community, but from the general population as well, and the sale of soft drinks and other snack foods in schools has come under political fire in many states and individual school districts. Interest in the school nutrition environment has accelerated along with the rise of child overweight, and it is increasingly recognized that schools are important shapers of children's nutritional status in two ways. First, children spend a great deal of time in school, where they may consume up to one-third of their daily food intake (Wechsler et al. 2001; Wildey et al. 2000). Second, schools are a primary source of learning about nutrition and appropriate diet through classroom teaching and they provide a venue for modeling and practicing those lessons during the school day (Dietz and Gortmaker 2001; Wechsler et al. 2001).

This article presents the findings of school-based nutritional anthropological research in a community in eastern Kentucky. Understanding the production of nutritional status in Kentucky is particularly important because Kentuckians exhibit some of the highest rates in the country

Deborah L. Crooks, "Trading nutrition for education: nutritional status and the sale of snack foods in an eastern Kentucky school." *Medical Anthropology Quarterly* 17(2007):182–199. Reprinted with permission.

of mortality from chronic diseases in which diet is implicated (i.e., heart disease, stroke, diabetes, all cancers, lung cancer, and colorectal cancer), and Kentucky is in the mid-range of states for deaths among women due to breast cancer (Centers for Disease Control, September 25, 2002: www.cdc.gov/nccdphp/burdenbook2002). In addition, Kentucky adults have the highest, or among the highest, rates of reported behavioral risk factors for chronic diseases, including overweight, inactivity, and low consumption of fruits and vegetables (Centers for Disease Control, September 25, 2002, www.apps.need. cdc.gov/BurdenBook/DeathCause.asp?state=ky).

The original aims of the research project were to: (1) document the growth and nutritional status of elementary school children in the community; (2) document the dietary intake and activity patterns contributing to nutritional status; and (3) gain an understanding of environmental factors that shape dietary intake. Early on in the fieldwork, my ethnographic gaze became focused on the school nutrition environment and the use of snack foods in the school, including the sale of snack foods to children. Although this practice is becoming common in U.S. schools, the reasons behind it are not always clear. In this school, the sale of snack foods is linked to poverty in the community and the constraints it places on educational success. To provide a higher-quality education to help poor children lift themselves out of poverty as adults, the principal supplements the school's budget with revenues from the sale of snack foods, bringing the production of a good education into opposition with the production of good nutritional status for all children in the school.

THE RESEARCH APPROACH

In this research, I used a combination of theory and method from cultural and biological anthropology. Research in nutritional anthropology has long been guided by a biocultural approach, one that recognizes that cultural ideologies and social and ecological circumstances come together to shape food-related behaviors and consequent nutritional status (Pelto et al. 2000; Quandt and Ritenbaugh 1986). In an early publication establishing the field of nutritional anthropology, Randy F. Kandel et al. (1980:3–4) pointed out that nutritional anthropology is organized around a combination of four lines of inquiry: dietary survey studies, food habits and foodways, the cognitive aspects (or meaning) of food, and ecological theory. Additional lines of inquiry also come from biological anthropology, because food and foodways interact with human biology and affect anthropometric measures of growth and nutritional status.

Biocultural approaches to understanding health and nutrition are varied (Crooks 1996, 1997; Dressler 1995), but in most cases, biocultural research combines ethnography with quantitative measures of human biological outcome to better determine how human/environment interactions shape health and nutritional status. This necessitates

a broadening of perspective on the human environment compared to more traditional, ecological approaches to better account for the influence of social and cultural factors. Thus, to adopt a phrase from R. Levins and R. Lewontin (1985), many biocultural researchers view "human biology as socialized biology," a perspective that guides this research.

THE RESEARCH SETTING: BRIDGES COUNTY, KENTUCKY, AND BRIDGES ELEMENTARY SCHOOL

This research took place in a community in eastern Kentucky, in the region known as Central Appalachia. The Appalachian Regional Commission designates Bridges County[1] as "severely distressed,"[2] but it was not always so. The area now known as Bridges County had an early history of economic viability resulting from its location along prominent Native American paths connecting major villages in the north and south. European farmers moved into the area in the 1700s, followed by mining concerns and producers of iron and manufactured iron products in the 1800s. By the time of its establishment as a county in the mid-1840s, Bridges had a vital economy based on resource extraction, milling, forging, and agriculture (Coleman 1978; Collins 1874; Lee 1981; Verhoeff 1911). However, since the 1800s, the economy of Central Appalachia, including Bridges County, has waxed and waned and economic development has always been uneven in the region.

Policies to create business-friendly environments have brought industry to parts of Appalachia, but wages were often low and work conditions hazardous (Fisher 1993; Gaventa et al. 1993b). Economic restructuring in the 1980s continued to create jobs in Appalachia that were low-wage and without benefits (Couto 1994; Fisher 1993; Gaventa et al. 1993a, 1993b), and Bridges County was no exception to this. At the time of the research, the unemployment rate in Bridges County was above the national average at 10 percent compared to 5.8 percent, and for many who were employed, wages were low and/or jobs were seasonal. As a result, the poverty rate in Bridges County at the time of the research exceeded the national rate at 25 percent versus 15 percent, with a child poverty rate of 35 percent versus 22.7 percent (Good Samaritan Foundation, Inc. 1997; U.S. Census Bureau 1995).

Bridges County has three elementary schools, and the vast majority of research activities took place in the school that serves the poorest section of the county. Bridges Elementary School is a modern, one-story, brick school building, with grades K–5, serving approximately two hundred and fifty children at the time of the research. The staff and teachers at Bridges Elementary School seem dedicated to providing a high-quality education, seeing education as the key to overcoming poverty. During my time at Bridges, parent volunteers assisted in this endeavor, contributing much to the learning environment. They assisted teachers in the classroom and on field trips; they created art and craft displays for the school corridors; and they helped with various school events and celebrations. Thus, the school was the site of numerous in-class and other activities designed to provide a welcoming environment and the best education possible for Bridges children.

The School Nutrition Environment

Like other schools in the United States (Baxter 1998), food and nutrition are important aspects of the school environment at Bridges Elementary School, and the school administration places great emphasis on the quality of food in the cafeteria. Many teachers and school administrators told me that "good food" is especially important at Bridges because 76 percent of the children qualify for free or reduced-price lunch (i.e., they come from poor households). As a result, the teachers and administrators are concerned that many Bridges children do not have access to high-quality food on a constant basis at home. In addition to the provision of food through school breakfasts and lunch, nutrition and health are also important components of the school's curriculum at Bridges Elementary School. As in most U.S. schools, Bridges children are taught about food, nutrition, appropriate food choices, and the relationship between nutrition and health. Because questions about nutrition and health are included on statewide standardized exams in Kentucky, the results of which can translate to monetary and/or other benefits to educators and schools, lessons on food and nutrition gain additional importance.

Food also serves purposes at the school apart from its nutritional aspects. As in most societies, food is an important element of celebrations and other social events in the United States. During the research, children at Bridges Elementary celebrated holidays with classroom parties at which snack foods played a prominent role; cookies and soft drinks were provided at after-school or evening parent-teacher activities at which children were present; and food was central to a number of fund-raising activities, including the annual "Chili Supper" and the sale of candy-grams on Valentine's Day. But the largest income-generating activity involving food at Bridges Elementary School was the sale of snack foods from the "snack room" in the afternoons.

The snack room is located at the end of a corridor in a small room that has been converted to a "store." Shelves in the room are filled with a variety of snacks, mostly candy and chips, but crackers and granola bars are often available. In addition, a soft drink machine is located just outside the snack room door. Most children purchase snacks, but for those without money, teachers provide a snack (usually a small candy), or children share. As a result, most children at Bridges Elementary School have access to afternoon snacks, either directly or indirectly, because of the presence of the snack room.

METHODS

The majority of data collection took place during the 1994–95 school year (August–May) and the beginning of the 1995–96 school year (September–October). The University of Kentucky Institutional Review Board and the Bridges Elementary School Family Resource Center (FRC)[3] Advisory Council approved data-collection procedures; the council also approved the dissemination of the results of the research. The research was conducted through the FRC, and data were gathered with the help of the director.

Because research in school settings takes time away from classroom activities, we took care to administer our research protocols with as little disruption to classroom learning activities as possible. To ensure confidentiality, pseudonyms are used for the research site and surrounding towns; children were assigned identification numbers and all children's data are stored according to those numbers; no names are used in the presentation of any data associated with this project; and, finally, identifiers such as job titles are used only where necessary. No one was paid for participating in the research.

A letter sent home via all children in grades 1–5 requested children's participation in the research. Written consent of parents was required, along with verbal assent of the children. From the approximately two hundred and thirty letters sent, we received 102 positive responses. Eleven children moved out of the area during the school year, and another three were eliminated because of unreliable data. A subsample of 54 children, those in grades 3–5, provided the anthropometric and dietary data in this report; children in grades 1–2 were eliminated from this portion of the research because the collection of dietary data from younger children is problematic (see below). I cannot establish if the final sample is representative of all children in grades 3–5 in all aspects; however, the sample is representative in terms of socioeconomic status (78 percent qualified for the federal lunch program versus 76 percent for the entire school).

Teachers and staff provided written consent following a presentation in which I explained the research and provided time for questions and answers. All present were invited to participate and all agreed to do so. In addition, as I participated in the daily activities of the school, I was always careful to state my position as a researcher to parents, volunteers, staff, and children.

Data collected were both quantitative and qualitative. Quantitative data are anthropometric and dietary measures (see Crooks [1999, 2000] for full explanations of data-collection procedures). Children's height was measured without shoes via a portable stadiometer. Weight was measured following removal of shoes and extra clothing (sweaters, coats, etc.) via a digital scale that was calibrated daily. Remaining clothing was noted and approximate weights were later subtracted from the measured weight. Growth and nutritional status were assessed by comparing sample data to the National Center for Health Statistics references for stature and weight (Anthro Software, Centers for Disease Control, Atlanta, Georgia) and the National Health and Nutrition Examination Survey (NHANES) I and II references for body mass index (Frisancho 1990).

Food-consumption data were collected from children in grades 3–5 via four 24-hour dietary recalls, spaced over a year to account for day of the week and seasonal variation. Dietary data-collection techniques are difficult to accomplish with children and can yield inaccurate data (Baranowski et al. 1986; Frank et al. 1977). To increase accuracy, children were verbally "walked" through their day; prompts (analogous to interview probes) assisted them in recalling foods eaten in various daily contexts—at home, school, and elsewhere (Frank 1994). Food models and a large variety of sample plates, cups, etc. assisted in estimating portion sizes. Recalls were not validated by other methods. Food consumption data were entered into a computerized program (Nutritionist V, First DataBank, Inc., San Bruno, California) for analysis, and then all numerical data were entered into SPSS Version 8.0 for Windows (SPSS, Inc., Chicago, Illinois).

Qualitative data were gathered through participant observation in the school and through semistructured and unstructured interviews, as indicated below. Over the course of the research, I spent many days observing and participating in the activities of the FRC, in classrooms I went to, and in schoolwide assemblies and other events at which school children, staff, and parents were present in various combinations and to varying degrees. Some events were school-only events at which children, teachers, and staff, but no parents, were in attendance; others were daytime events at which a few parents (for the most part, those who were volunteers) were present. Still others were evening events, which brought parents and their children into the school for a variety of activities. Other times, I participated in conversations that took place among teachers, staff, parents, and administrators, for example, over lunch, or helping out in the school's kitchen, or when taking the children on field trips.

I conducted semistructured interviews with the head of Social Services in Bridges County and the administrator and nurse at the County Health Department in which I asked them to talk about the health, nutrition, and education of Bridges County children. These interviews took place in their respective offices. I also participated in unstructured

interviews with other community members, including one minister, the president of the local Jay Cees, two staff members of the local Agricultural Extension office, and a representative from the area Girl Scouts. These discussions took place in various locales. Finally, given that FRCs in Kentucky are charged with assisting families in overcoming barriers to education, I participated in semistructured and unstructured interviews with the director of the FRC, the main FRC staff member, and the school counselor on what they perceived these barriers to be. These conversations took place in the school, sometimes in a private room or office, but at other times in the FRC, the cafeteria, or as we moved through the corridors engaging in the daily activities of the school.

ANALYSIS AND RESULTS

Previously Published Results of Anthropometric and Dietary Analyses

Two goals of the greater research project were to (1) assess the growth and nutritional status, and (2) assess the diets of children at Bridges Elementary School. Analyses of the anthropometric and dietary data for the 54 children in grades 3–5 have been reported in detail elsewhere (Crooks 2000). However, because those analyses are highly relevant to this article, I reiterate some of the findings here. Bridges sample children tend to be slightly taller and heavier than the reference group, with higher BMIs (Table 1). BMI percentiles are often used to assess overweight, and although there is some variation in the literature, most researchers now use the 85th percentile to indicate "at risk for overweight," with the 95th percentile to indicate "overweight" (see fuller discussion in Crooks 2000).

Using these categories, 14.8 percent of sample children are at risk for overweight, with an additional 18.5 percent overweight (Table 2). Focusing only on the 95th percentile category, the rate of overweight children at Bridges Elementary School is well above that for the NHANES III nationally representative samples reported in *Morbidity and Mortality Weekly* (MMWR 1997) at 14 percent and in Richard P. Troiano et al. (1995) at 10.9 percent.

Comparing the Bridges data to the NHANES data by gender and ethnicity, far more Bridges boys are overweight

Table 1 Mean Height-for-Age (HAZ), Weight-for-Age (WAZ), and Body Mass Index (BMIZ) Z-Scores for Sample Children (Standard Deviations in Parentheses)

	Full sample (*n* = 54)	Boys only (*n* = 54)	Girls only (*n* = 54)
HAZ	0.43** (0.95)	0.21 (0.92)	0.62** (0.95)
WAZ	0.70*** (1.30)	0.90** (1.41)	0.53* (1.19)
BMIZ	0.57** (1.31)	0.90** (1.42)	0.29 (1.14)

*Differs significantly from 0 at $p \leq .05$
**Differs significantly from 0 at $p \leq .01$
***Differs significantly from 0 at $p \leq .001$

at 28 percent compared to 13.2 percent for the NHANES III boys (category "White, non-Hispanic," MMWR 1997) and 10.4 percent (category "Non-Hispanic White," Troiano et al. 1995). The girls' data are closer to those reported by MMWR and Troiano et al. at 10.3 percent for Bridges girls compared to 11.9 percent (MMWR) and 9.8 percent (Troiano et al. 1995). The elevated rate of overweight among Bridges children compared to NHANES children is consistent with Strauss and Pollack's (2001) report that overweight is increasing faster among boys than girls (actual prevalence rates were not provided), and among children from the south compared to the west (17.1 percent in southern states compared to 10.8 percent in the west, prevalence data for other regions were not included in the report).

The earlier analysis of the 24-hour dietary recalls (Crooks 2000) indicated that Bridges children are not meeting the recommended daily servings from the five food groups according to the food guide pyramid. Table 3 shows low consumption in every food category, with the exception of the milk, yogurt, and cheese group, which shows adequate consumption, and the fats, oils, and sweets group, which shows extremely high consumption. Although there is individual variation among Bridges children, on average, sample children appear to be consuming high-fat and sugary foods at the expense of other, more healthful foods such as fruits and vegetables.

Research indicates U.S. children commonly have low-quality diets, with particularly low consumption of fruits and vegetables and high consumption of sugar and fat (Brady et al. 2000; Kennedy 1998; Munoz et al. 1997). Using national data from the U.S. Department of Agriculture, Munoz et al. (1997) report consumption of 2.4 servings of vegetables and 1.3 servings of fruit by 6–11-year old boys, compared to 1.80 servings of vegetables and 0.96 servings of fruits for Bridges boys; and they report consumption of 2.4 servings of vegetables and 1.4 servings of fruit for 6–11-year old girls, compared to 1.79 and 0.91 for Bridges girls. Brady et al. (2000) report 2.5 servings of vegetables and 0.90 servings of fruits for 7–14-year-old boys from Birmingham, Alabama, with 2.3 and 0.80 for girls. Both of these studies report high consumption of sugar and fat by sample children; however, the type of analysis used is not comparable with that of this study, therefore, comparisons cannot be made.

Another goal of nutritional analysis is to assess the consumption of certain nutrients compared to the dietary guidelines. Percent of calories from fat, saturated fat, and carbohydrates, and the amount of fiber consumed are important for long-term health (Kimm et al. 1990). The

Table 2 Distribution of Sample Children Who Are at Risk for Overweight (≥ 85th percentile BMI) and Overweight (≥ 95th Percentile BMI), NHANES I and II References. [Crooks 2000]

	Full sample (*n* = 54)		Boys only (*n* = 25)		Girls only (*n* = 29)	
	n	*percent*	*n*	*percent*	*n*	*percent*
At risk:	8	14.8	5	20.0	3	10.3
Overweight:	10	18.5	7	28.0	3	10.3

Table 3 Mean Daily Consumption of Food Groups Servings by Bridges Elementary School Children Based on an Average of Four (4) 24-Hour Diet Recalls, Compared with Recommendations in the Food Guide Pyramid; Standard Deviations in Parentheses. [Crooks 2000]

Food groups in Food Guide Pyramid	Recommended # of servings	Sample mean (sd)	Boys only	Girls only
Bread, cereal, rice, and pasta	6–11	5.49 (1.73)*	6.10 (1.77)**	4.97 (1.55)**
Vegetables	3–5	1.80 (0.94)**	1.80 (0.87)**	1.79 (1.01)**
Fruits	2–3	0.93 (0.98)**	0.96 (1.13)**	0.91 (0.85)**
Milk, yogurt, and cheese	2–3	2.57 (1.44)	2.62 (1.20)**	2.53 (1.64)
Meat, poultry, fish, dry beans, eggs, and nuts	2–3	1.80 (0.63)*	1.92 (0.60)	1.69 (0.64)*
Fats, oils, and sweets	sparingly	23.53 (10.55)	24.84 (9.97)	22.41 (11.08)

*Differs significantly from recommendation at $p \leq .05$
**Differs significantly from recommendation at $p \leq .001$

earlier analysis of the dietary recalls indicates that sample children's average consumption of calories from fat (over the four days) is significantly greater than the recommendation (36.3 percent compared to the recommended 30 percent, $p \leq .001$), with consumption of saturated fat also above the recommendation (13.12 percent compared to 10 percent, $p < .001$). The percent of calories consumed from carbohydrates is below the recommendation (51.83 percent compared to 55–60 percent, $p < .001$), as is the average daily consumption of fiber (12.43 grams, compared to 25 grams, $p < .001$; 10–13 g/1,000 kcal, based on a 2000 kcal diet). These figures are similar to other U.S. children reported in Kimm et al. (1990) at 35–36 percent calories from fat, 13 percent from saturated fat, and 49–51 percent from carbohydrates (based on NHANES II–data; fiber was not reported).

The Contribution of Snacks to Diet and Nutritional Status

Although the earlier report revealed few significant associations between overweight and food consumption, perhaps because of small sample size and high variability, as well as the difficulties of ascertaining usual food consumption for individuals, it did find that overweight children consume a greater mean number of daily servings from the fats, oils, and sweets food group (28.29 versus 22.17, $p < .10$) compared to nonoverweight children. Snacks are an important source of fat and sugar in the U.S. diet (Jahns et al. 2001; Zizza et al. 2001). Table 4 provides information on consumption of snacks by Bridges children.[4]

Sample children report an average of 1.70 snacks per day, contributing an average of 763.94 calories to the daily diet or 36.71 percent of daily calories. Snacks contribute 27.22 grams of fat to the daily diet, and account for 31.92 percent of daily fat consumption. Boys consume more calories and fat from snacks than do girls, but the differences are not significant. Although more snacking occurs at home than school, children report a daily average of 0.46 school snacks, contributing 134.70 calories to the daily diet. School snacks contribute 4.41 grams of fat to the daily diet, which is 5.56 percent of the total daily fat consumption. Girls consume slightly more school snacks than do boys, as well as more calories and fat from school snacks.

The distinction between total snacks consumed in a day and snacks consumed at school is important. School is a primary source of information about good nutrition, thus offering snack foods in school provides a contradictory message, one that can affect snack consumption outside of school and has the potential to undermine both short- and long-term nutrition goals (Cline and White 2000; Wechsler et al. 2001). In addition, at Bridges, sample boys "at risk" for overweight report a higher average daily consumption of school snacks compared to other boys, 0.48 versus 0.35 snacks (Table 5), with higher consumption of calories (146.33 versus 83.54 kcal) and carbohydrates (27.00 versus 14.31 g.) from school snacks. These relationships do not hold for girls, perhaps because of the small number of girls who are overweight, making statistical comparison of nonoverweight to overweight girls difficult.

These results indicate that school snacks are an important source of calories for sample children, and, among

Table 4 Mean Daily Consumption of Snack Foods by Bridges Sample Children Based on the Average of Four 24-Hour Dietary Recalls; Standard Deviations in Parentheses

Total snacks:	Sample mean	Boys only	Girls only
Snacks consumed:	1.70 (0.47)	1.68 (0.49)	1.72 (0.46)
Calories from snacks:	763.94 (342.60)	797.35 (289.19)	735.14 (385.53)
Percent of total calories from snacks:	36.71 (13.60)	37.51 (13.97)	36.02 (13.48)
Fat (g) from snacks:	27.22 (17.47)	27.68 (13.22)	26.83 (20.67)
Percent of total fat from snacks	31.92 (18.46)	33.52 (17.05)	30.54 (19.79)
School snacks:	**Sample mean**	**Boys only**	**Girls only**
Snacks consumed:	0.46 (0.19)	0.41 (0.19)*	0.50 (0.18)*
Calories from snacks:	134.70 (89.15)	113.68 (91.0)	152.83 (84.9)
Percent of total calories from snacks:	6.79 (4.44)	5.27 (3.88)**	8.10 (4.54)**
Fat (g) from snacks:	4.41 (4.58)	3.16 (3.20)**	5.48 (5.32)**
Percent of total fat from snacks	5.56 (5.59)	4.05 (4.20)*	6.86 (6.33)*

*Indicates significant difference between boys and girls at $p \leq .10$
**Indicates significant difference between boys and girls at $p \leq .05$
***Indicates significant difference between boys and girls at $p \leq .01$

Table 5 Mean Snack Consumption (Average of Four 24-Hour Recalls) by Overweight Status (NOW = not Overweight, BMI < 85th Percentile NHANES References, OW = Overweight, BMI ≥ 85th Percentile) Among Sample Boys and Girls, Evaluated via Student T-tests (Standard Deviations in Parentheses)

| | Boys | | Girls | |
	NOW	OW	NOW	OW
Total snacks	1.67(0.46)	1.69(0.53)	1.175(0.48)	1.63(0.41)
School snacks	0.35(0.19)*	0.48(0.17)	0.51(0.18)	0.46(0.19)
Snack calories (kcal)	850.15(297.59)	740.17(281.06)	756.83(351.94)	652.00(526.23)
School snack calories (kcal)	83.54(66.61)*	146.33(104.83)	146.61(81.54)	176.67(101.37)
Snack carbs (g)	130.46(41.64)	120.92(48.10)	114.35(49.45)	102.50(40.00)
School snack carbs (g)	14.31(11.51)**	27.00(18.96)	25.43(13.21)	26.33(15.62)
Snack fat (g)	31.08(13.92)	24.00(11.90)	27.78(16.24)	23.17(34.83)
School snack fat (g)	2.62(2.66)	3.75(3.72)	4.91(3.91)	7.67(9.18)

*Indicates significant difference between NOW and OW at p ≤ .10
**Indicates significant difference between NOW and OW at p ≤ .05

boys, they contribute to the risk for overweight. In addition, the large number of servings from the fats, oils, and sweets food group, and the low number of servings from the fruits and vegetable food groups, suggests that snacks are substituting for more healthful foods in the daily diet, possibly leading to underconsumption of many nutrients associated with good nutrition and health. Given the recognized association between diet and chronic disease, and the high levels of adult chronic disease in Kentucky, it makes sense to ask why snack foods are being sold at Bridges Elementary School.

The Sale of Snacks at School

The sale of snack foods in U.S. schools is becoming increasingly common (Wechsler 2001), but the practice is controversial. At Bridges Elementary School, teachers and parents express a variety of concerns over the sale of snack foods to children. One afternoon, when her students left the classroom to purchase their snacks, a teacher criticized the principal for selling snack foods because she felt that the excess sugar provided by these foods contributed to the unruliness of children.[5] At a Parent–Teacher Forum, a parent expressed a similar concern, "What about more nutritious snacks? This stuff hypes them up for the ride home." Another parent was concerned that snacks were not available to all children because of the cost. She stated, "About the snack issue—these are not free, therefore, they're not for all." The principal responded that most children have money for snacks, noting that when they do not, teachers provide snacks. As she continued to be questioned, the principal registered the parents' concern, and although she agreed that the nutritional quality of snacks was important for children, for her, the more important issue was the quantity of funds generated from snack food sales. As she explained:

These things [snack foods] pay the telephone bill. Also supplies for the office and teacher's equipment, like slide projectors. Also, trips for kids who can't afford them. Parents don't understand all the expenses at the school—snacks bring in $7,000–$8,000 per year. Teachers only have to ask for something and they get it.

In support of the principal's position, a parent stated, "It's worth selling snacks—it gives money for the paper [the construction paper used in the many wall displays created by parent volunteers], and other things." The principal added, "and props for plays, too; and for the school calendars we send home." But the discussion ended with a comment on the nutritional quality of the snacks. Although the commenting parent agreed that the funds generated by the sale of snack foods were important, she added, "Still. I would prefer nutritious snacks—juice boxes, fruit, and milk from the cafeteria." In a separate conversation with the principal, I asked about the sale of snack foods versus some other kind of food or commodity. She responded that she had tried other things, but candy, chips, and pop were the best income generators.[6]

The principal and the teachers at Bridges Elementary School seemed very aware of the relationship between food, nutrition, and health—nutrition is taught in the classrooms; school administrators and teachers talk about it over lunch and in the school's kitchen while preparing food for special events. Teachers and school administrators are parents, too, and they often discuss how to get children to eat better and how one finds the time to cook good meals. Physical education programs focus on fitness and wellness; the physical education teacher often creates individual programs for children who need to lose weight and/or exercise more. It is clear from these and other examples that the educators at Bridges Elementary School consider good nutrition and nutritional status to be important elements of the school environment.

But even more important, and the primary objective at Bridges, is the provision of a quality education for *all* children. As the director of the FRC told me, this requires additional funding for programs to fill in the "gaps between what is provided in the community and parental, teacher and kid needs." In her opinion, as well as that of the principal and many teachers, these gaps result from a low funding base due to high poverty in the community and the increased educational needs of those Bridges children who grow up in poverty. Comparing the situation of Bridges Elementary School to two other schools in the same county, one teacher told me,

> All schools are not treated equally, because there is difference in the local contribution of money to the schools. Bridges, for instance, has lots of poverty—little money for the school. Rockridge probably has more [money], and Hill Valley certainly does. Therefore, Bridges is particularly strapped for cash for programs.[7]

At Bridges Elementary School, the programs funded through the sale of snacks are perceived to be fundamental to the education of Bridges children, especially those who come from poor families. When speaking of the importance of field trips, one school administrator told me,

> They don't get out to see things outside of Bridges County walls. The low income kids are everywhere…lots have never been past Hill Valley—to plays, museums, shopping malls. There is a different culture from here to Hill Valley.…Hill Valley is more included with common things—Cub Scouts, Girl Scouts, library, and courthouse.…How can we relate to something in a book if we haven't seen it?

This inability to relate to "common" things for many Bridges children is perceived as a barrier to school success by this administrator, who believes it contributes to the high drop-out rate in Bridges County, continuing the "cycle of poverty" for some families. Therefore, programs that can help break the cycle are considered of primary importance at the school, and funds for those programs must be found, despite the costs.

CONCLUSION: TRADING NUTRITION FOR EDUCATION

Rebecca A. Huss-Ashmore and R. Brooke Thomas (1997) argue that gaining an understanding of how humans perceive their environments is important in biocultural research because perceptions structure responses that may have biological impact. At Bridges Elementary School, the realities of historically constituted poverty shape the school leaders' perceptions of the environment in which many children grow and develop, and it structures their responses to the challenge of providing a good education where needs may be greater and resources fewer than in more affluent communities. One response is to sell snack foods to fund activities and programs to enrich the life experiences of poorer children, enabling them to compete on a par with richer children once they move on to middle school.

But the sale of snack foods is not without biological cost for children across the socioeconomic range at Bridges. On the whole, Bridges children exhibit higher rates of overweight than the general population, with boys at particular risk; and Bridges children consume low-quality diets, irrespective of gender. At Bridges, overweight boys consume more snack foods than nonoverweight boys, increasing their risk for elevated blood pressure, dyslipidemia, insulin resistance, and type II diabetes (Deckelbaum and Williams 2001; Dietz and Gortmaker 2001). And although the same relationship does not hold for girls, snacks are probably displacing higher-quality foods in the diets of both genders, increasing nutritional risk from micro-nutrient deficiencies, many of which are implicated in cardiovascular disease, osteopenia, and bone fractures, and colon, breast, and other cancers (Fletcher and Fairfield 2002; Key et al. 2002). Finally, although children consume more snacks at home than school, school is, nevertheless, a powerful influence on children's behavior in all life settings (Dietz and Gortmaker 2001). Because nutritional conditions and food-related behaviors track from childhood to adulthood (Devine et al. 1998; Dietz 1998), establishing healthy food behaviors early on may lead to reductions in the excessive rates of chronic disease seen among Bridges County adults.

Because of the "epidemic of overweight" among U.S. children and the seeming intractability of adult chronic illnesses related to overweight and poor nutritional status, the nutrition environment in which children live and grow is coming under increased scrutiny. In the past, undernutrition was the nutritional problem of concern for U.S. children, and the National School Lunch Act was created in 1946 to help protect children against undernutrition. However, because of the rising prevalence of overweight, the act was amended in 1994, requiring school meals to adhere to the Dietary Guidelines for Americans (DGA), to reduce the fat, sodium, and sugar content, and meet the RDAs for a variety of nutrients (Wechsler et al. 2001).

Many (not all) schools have accomplished this change, but school meals are only one aspect of the school nutrition environment that contributes to children's nutritional status. Recently, the American Dietetic Association took the position that "school and community have a shared responsibility to provide all students with access to high-quality foods and nutrition services as an integral part of the total education program" (reported in Cline and White 2000). This level of "nutrition integrity" in the schools necessitates that *all* foods be consistent with the DGAs, not just school meals, and that schools provide positive nutrition experiences as a part of everyday school experiences (Cline and White 2000).

But all over the country, school districts and school administrators are making the decision to sell foods in their schools that are of limited nutritional value and that compete with higher-quality foods (Wechsler et al. 2001). Although there is ample documentation of the sale of snack foods in U.S. schools, there is near silence in the literature as to why. Agnes Molnar (2000:403) points out that snack food sales are the "inevitable response to decades of inadequate funding for schools," but like others (Miller 1994; Wildey et al. 2000), she suggests the funds generated are usually applied to "noneducation" or "extra-curricular" activities, such as music, art, and sports. The case of Bridges Elementary School indicates that these revenues may be put to more fundamental uses, especially in schools situated in high-poverty areas. A recent report of Kentucky's Coalition on Type 2 Diabetes and Overweight in Children (now the Lt. Governor's Task Force on Childhood Nutrition and Fitness) (Tietyen n.d.; Tietyen et al. 2002) shows that vending machines in Kentucky's schools generate an average of $6,016 per school surveyed, and school stores generate $7,788. Revenues are used for sports equipment, music programs, guest speakers, field trips, and student awards and incentives, but also for books, instructional materials, computers, paper supplies, and even the school lunch or cafeteria fund.

Therefore, if we consider the school nutrition environment as one element of a greater environment, we can begin to understand the decision by some administrators to sell snack foods. As Rebecca A. Huss-Ashmore and R. Brooke Thomas (1997) point out, environmental negotiations to produce well-being often involve competing goals and motivations that are not biological, but that may have biological costs. Like all schools, Bridges Elementary is charged with providing the best possible education for children so they can grow up to be productive members of the community. But the funds with which to carry out this charge are inadequate. To augment those funds, the principal sells a commodity that generates high revenue (i.e., snack foods), because the cost of a less-than-adequate education appears greater than the cost of poor nutritional status. In other words, the decision to sell snack foods is a decision about education, not biology; and in Kentucky, "Education Pays";[8]—it is seen as the key to overcoming poverty for poor families and communities in the commonwealth. In this context, trading nutrition for education can make sense; at least, it may appear to be the better of a bad choice.

Notes

Acknowledgments. The research for this article was funded by a National Institutes of Health Fellowship, grant number 5 F32 HD097620; the writing was facilitated by a University of Kentucky Summer Research Fellowship in 2001 and sabbatical leave during the Fall semester, 2002. I extend my appreciation to the *MAQ* reviewers for their many insightful comments on the manuscript, and especially to Mac Marshall for exemplary editorial guidance. I thank the principal, the teachers, and the staff of Bridges Elementary School for their help and their patience while I conducted the research. I particularly thank the children who participated in the research and their parents for allowing them to do so. My special thanks goes to the director of the Family Resource Center, without whom this research would not have been possible.

1. Bridges County is a pseudonym; I take the name from my grandfather who was also from the Appalachian Mountains.

2. "Distressed" is an official designation of the Appalachian Regional Commission. It is based on three criteria: poverty, market income, and unemployment.

3. According to the director of the Family Resource Center at Bridges, FRCs are funded by the Commonwealth of Kentucky to act as liaison between community services and poorer families. The intent is to help children overcome barriers to school success.

4. Although snacks and snacking are variably defined in the literature, I define snacks here as between-meal eating events, irrespective of foods consumed; however, most foods were those typically identified as snack foods—cookies, candy, pop, chips, etc. One reviewer raised a concern that by utilizing "snacking" in this way, I was presuming that three meals a day was the best nutrition strategy for children, for example, as opposed to "grazing." That is not my intent. For the most part, these children are following the breakfast/lunch/supper meal pattern that is fairly common in the United States, in addition to which they are consuming what would commonly be termed "snack-foods." Whether or not this is a pattern of grazing versus meals-plus-snacks would make an interesting discussion, but it is outside the scope of the article and requires additional research to sort out.

5. The notion that sugar contributes to hyperactivity in children is a common misconception.

6. Snacks (i.e., chips, candy, and soda pop) are desired commodities on the part of children and their parents. This may be due, in part, to the intensive advertising campaigns that directly target children. At the time of the research, the snack food market in the United States was worth $15 billion dollars per year; the children's food market was worth $9 billion, and marketers were targeting beverages and candy as two growth areas within that market (Littman 1998).

7. Hill Valley and Rockridge are pseudonyms for other towns and their elementary schools in Bridges County.

8. "Education Pays" is a promotional campaign in Kentucky aimed at decreasing dropout rates and encouraging continuing education. This slogan can be seen on billboards and in other public relations venues throughout the commonwealth.

References

Baranowski, Tom, Rosalind Dworkin, Janice C. Henske, Donna R. Clearman, J. Kay Dunn, Philip R. Nader, and Paul C. Hooks. 1986. The Accuracy of Children's Self-Reports of Diet: Family Health Project. Journal of the U.S. Dietetic Association 86:1381–1385.

Baxter, Suzanne Domel. 1998. Are Elementary Schools Teaching Children to Prefer Candy but Not Vegetables? Journal of School Health 68:111–114.

Brady, L. M., C. H. Lindquist, S. L. Herd, and M. I. Goran. 2000. Comparison of Children's Dietary Intake

Patterns with U.S. Dietary Guidelines. British Journal of Nutrition 84:361–367.

Cline, Tami, and Gene White. 2000. Position of the American Dietetic Association: Local Support for Nutrition Integrity in Schools. Journal of the American Dietetic Association 100:108–111.

Coleman, "Squire" J. Winston, Jr. 1978. 200 Years in Kentucky. Frankfort, KY: America's Historic Records, Inc.

Collins, Richard H. 1874. History of Kentucky. Vol. 2. Covington, KY: Collins and Company.

Couto, Richard A. 1994. An American Challenge: A Report on Economic Trends and Social Issues in Appalachia. Commission on Religion in Appalachia. Dubuque, IA: Kendall/Hunt Publishing Company.

Crockett, Susan J., and Laura S. Sims. 1995. Environmental Influences on Children's Eating. Journal of Nutrition Education 27:235–249.

Crooks, Deborah L. 1996. Biocultural Anthropology. In The Encyclopedia of Cultural Anthropology. David Levinson and Melvin Ember, eds. Pp. 130–133. New York: Holt Publishing.

———. 1997. Biocultural Factors in School Achievement for Mopan Children in Belize. American Anthropologist 99:586–601.

———. 1999. Child Growth and Nutritional Status in a High-Poverty Community in Eastern Kentucky. American Journal of Physical Anthropology 109:129–142.

———. 2000. Food Consumption, Activity and Overweight among Elementary School Children in an Appalachian Kentucky Community. American Journal of Physical Anthropology 112:159–170. New York: Holt Publishing.

Deckelbaum, R. J., and C. L. Williams. 2001. Childhood Obesity: The Health Issue. Obesity Research 9:239S–243S.

Devine, Carol M., Margaret Connors, Carole A. Bisogni, and Jeffery Sobal. 1998. Life-Course Influences on Fruit and Vegetable Trajectories; Qualitative Analysis of Food Choices. Journal of Nutrition Education 30:361–370.

Dietz, William H. 1998. Health Consequences of Obesity in Youth: Childhood Predictors of Adult Disease. Pediatrics 101:518–525.

Dietz, William H., and S. L. Gortmaker. 2001. Preventing Obesity in Children and Adolescents. Annual Review of Public Health 22:337–353.

Dressler, William W. 1995. Modeling Biocultural Interactions: Examples from Studies of Stress and Cardiovascular Disease. Yearbook of Physical Anthropology 38:27–56.

Ebbeling, Cara B., Dorota B. Pawlak, and David S. Ludwig. 2002. Childhood Obesity: Public-Health Crisis, Common Sense Cure. Lancet 360:473–482.

Fisher, Steve. 1993. National Economic Renewal Programs and Their Implications for Appalachia and the South. In Communities in Economic Crisis, Appalachia and the South. John Gaventa, Barbara Ellen Smith, and Alex Willingham, eds. Pp. 263–277. Philadelphia: Temple University Press.

Fletcher, R. H., and K. M. Fairfield. 2002. Vitamins for Chronic Disease Prevention in Adults: Clinical Applications. JAMA 287:3127–3129.

Frank, Gail C. 1994. Environmental Influences on Methods Used to Collect Dietary Data from Children. U.S. Journal of Clinical Nutrition 59:207S–211S.

Frank, Gail C., Gerald S. Berenson, Prentiss E. Schilling, and Margaret C. Moore. 1977. Adjusting the 24-Hr. Recall for Epidemiologic Studies of School Children. Journal of the American Dietetic Association 71:26–31.

Frisancho, A. Roberto. 1990. Anthropometric Standards for the Assessment of Growth and Nutritional Status. Ann Arbor: University of Michigan Press.

Gaventa, John, Barbara Ellen Smith, and Alex Willingham. 1993a. Introduction. In Communities in Economic Crisis, Appalachia and the South. John Gaventa, Barbara Ellen Smith, and Alex Willingham, eds. pp. 3–14. Philadelphia: Temple University Press.

———. 1993b. Toward a New Debate: Development, Democracy, and Dignity. In Communities in Economic Crisis, Appalachia and the South. John Gaventa, Barbara Ellen Smith, and Alex Willingham, eds. pp. 279–291. Philadelphia: Temple University Press,

Good Samaritan Foundation, Inc. 1997. County Profiles in Health for the Commonwealth of Kentucky, vols. 1–3. Lexington, KY: Good Samaritan Foundation, Inc.

Huss-Ashmore, Rebecca A., and R. Brooke Thomas. 1997. The Future of Human Adaptability Research. In Human Adaptability: Past, Present and Future. Stanley J. Ulijaszek and Rebecca A. Huss-Ashmore, eds. Pp. 295–319. Oxford: Oxford University Press.

Jahns, L., A. M. Siega-Riz, and B. M. Popkin. 20010. The Increasing Prevalence of Snacking among U.S. Children from 1977 to 1996. Journal of Pediatrics 138:493–498.

Kandel, Randy F., Gretel H. Pelto, and Norge W. Jerome. 1980. Introduction. In Nutritional Anthropology: Contemporary Approaches to Diet and Culture. Norge W. Jerome, Randy F. Kandel, and Gretel H. Pelto, eds. pp. 1–12. Pleasantville, NY: Redgrave Publishing.

Kennedy, Christine M. 1998. Childhood Nutrition. Annual Review of Nursing Research 16:3–38.

Key, Timothy J., Naomi E. Allen, Elizabeth A. Spencer, and Ruth C. Travis. 2002. The Effect of Diet on Risk of Cancer. The Lancet 360:861–868.

Kimm, S. Y., P. J. Gergen, M. Malloy, C. Dresser, and M. Carroll. 1990. Dietary Patterns of U.S. Children: Implications for Disease Prevention. Preventive Medicine 19:432–442.

Lee, Lloyd G. 1981. A Brief History of Kentucky and Its Counties. Berea, KY: Kentucky Kentucke Imprints.

Levins, R., and R. Lewontin. 1985. The Dialectical Biologist. Cambridge, MA: Cambridge University Press.

Littman, Margaret. 1998. Youth Will Be Served (Niche Marketing for Children of All Ages). Prepared Foods 167:21–24.

Miller, Hilary S. 1994. School Soft Drink Sales Debate Resurfaces. Beverage Industry 85:18.

MMWR. 1997. Update: Prevalence of Overweight among Children, Adolescents, and Adults—United States, 1988–1994. Morbidity and Mortality Weekly 46:199–202.

Molnar, Agnes. 2000. Soft Drinks in Schools. Public Health Reports 115:403.

Munoz, Kathryn A., Susan M. Krebs-Smith, Rachel Ballard-Barbash, and Linda E. Cleveland. 1997. Food Intakes of U.S. Children and Adolescents Compared with Recommendations. Pediatrics 100:323–329.

Pelto, Gretel H., Alan H. Goodman, and Darna L. Dufour. 2000. The Biocultural Perspective in Nutritional Anthropology. *In* Nutritional Anthropology: Biocultural Perspectives on Food and Nutrition. Alan H. Goodman, Darna L. Dufour, and Gretel H. Pelto, ed. Pp. 1–9. Mountain View, CA: Mayfield Publishing.

Pi-Sunyer, F. Xavier. 1993. Medical Hazards of Obesity. Annals of Internal Medicine 119:655–660.

Quandt, Sara A., and Cheryl Ritenbaugh. 1986. Introduction. *In* Training Manual in Nutritional Anthropology. Sara A. Quandt and Cheryl Ritenbaugh, eds. pp. 1–2. Washington, DC: American Anthropological Association.

Reynolds, K. D., T. Baranowski, D. B. Bishop, R. P. Farris, D. Binkley, T. A. Nicklas, and P. J. Elmer. 1999. Patterns in Child and Adolescent Consumption of Fruit and Vegetables: Effects of Gender and Ethnicity across Four Sites. Journal of the American College of Nutrition 18:248–254.

Strauss, Richards, and Harold A. Pollack. 2001. Epidemic Increase in Childhood Overweight, 1986–1998. The Journal of the American Medical Association 286:2845–2849.

Tietyen, Janet. N.d. Kentucky School Nutrition Environment Survey. Unpublished manuscript.

Tietyen, Janet L., Maria G. Boosalis, Jody L. Clasey, Kim Ringley, and Stephen L. Henry. 2002. Kentucky Children at Risk: The War on Weight. Position Paper for the Coalition on Type 2 Diabetes and Overweight in Children. January 2002.

Troiano, Richard P., Katherine M. Flegal, Robert J. Kuczmarski, Stephen M. Campbell, and Clifford L. Johnson. 1995. Overweight Prevalence and Trends for Children and Adolescents: The National Health and Nutrition Examination Surveys, 1963 to 1991. Archives of Pediatric and Adolescent Medicine 149:1085–1091.

U.S. Bureau of the Census. 1995. Current Population Reports. Washington, DC: U.S. Government Printing Office.

Verhoeff, Mary. 1911. The Kentucky Mountains: Transportation and Commerce 1750–1911, a Study in the Economic History of a Coal Field, vol. 1. Filson Club Publication 26. Louisville, KY: John P. Morton and Company.

Wechsler, Howell, Nancy D. Brener, Sarah Kuester, and Clare Miller. 2001. Food Service and Foods and Beverages Available at School: Results from the School Health Policies and Programs Study 2000. Journal of School Health 71: 313–324.

Wildey, Marianne B., Sacha Z. Pampalone, Robin L. Pelletier, Michelle M. Zive, John P. Elder, and James F. Sallis. 2000. Fat and Sugar Levels Are High in Snacks Purchased from Student Stores in Middle Schools. Journal of the U.S. Dietetic Association 100:319–322.

Zizza, C., A. M. Siega-Riz, and B. M. Popkin. 2001. Significant Increase in Young Adults' Snacking between 1977–1978 and 1994–1996 Represents a Cause for Concern! Preventive Medicine 32:303–310.

CHAPTER 48

Big Fat Myths

Alexandra A. Brewis
(2012)

Obesity is here, moved in, and sitting on our couches eating pizza. According to the World Health Organization, there are well over 1 billion overweight adults globally, and at least 300 million of us are obese. There are a good number of countries, mostly in the Pacific and Middle East, where more than 60 percent of the adult population is overweight or obese. In the United States, rates are around 66 percent and have doubled in just one generation. Many of the middle income developing countries, such as China and India, have not had any discernible obesity until the last couple of years, but estimates suggest they and much of the rest of the world will match current U.S. figures by 2020. It is reported that the costs of health care, absenteeism, and lost productivity associated with obesity are already in the billions or even trillions of dollars annually, and according to Philip James, chair of the International Obesity Task Force, this trend threatens to "overwhelm every medical system in the world." Panic around the topic of obesity has in a very short time become part of the fabric of modern life (Campos 2004).

Given this level of concern about obesity, and especially the amount of money being spent globally to address it, we need sophisticated understandings of obesity as part of the human experience that allow us to best prioritize our concerns and create the most effective strategies. Here I discuss five different ideas about obesity that are currently influential in medical and public thinking that are challenged as "myths" by applying an anthropological perspective. An anthropological approach integrates knowledge about both social and biological dimensions of the human condition in the contexts of the widest sweep of human history and diversity, and this can help clarify when and exactly how we should be concerned about this "problem" of obesity.

Obesity is a term bantered about in many domains of contemporary life, so it important to start with some consistent notion of what we mean. In the most general sense, obesity refers to an excess of adipose (fat) tissue on the body, and often understood to be a level of fat that impedes health and functioning. In terms of using a standard cut-off for defining people as obese or not, the most commonly applied classification in medicine and public health is based on body mass index or BMI of 30 or higher.

Overweight or at-risk-for-obesity is generally represented by a BMI of 25–29.9, and "normal" or "ideal" weight as a BMI of 18.5–24.9. BMI is not a direct measure of body fat, but rather roughly estimates it by comparing someone's ratio of body weight to their height using the formula BMI = weight in kilos/height in meters^2.

MYTH 1: IT'S ALL IN OUR GENES

There is a burgeoning and highly publicized scientific literature cataloging genetic variants that explain person-to-person differences in propensity to obesity. Single genes that determine obesity seem to occur only very rarely; an example is Prader-Willi syndrome, a condition in which affected children are driven to excessive eating and have low metabolic needs. Association studies, which examine genetic differences between obese and non-obese people, have identified several dozen inherited variants that appear to explain some intra-individual differences in risk. These multiple genes are tied to such factors as appetite, metabolic rate, how the body responds to exercise, and fat storage, rather than obesity per se (Bouchard 2007). Family, twin and adoption studies show that obesity certainly has a strong heritability, even once you control for shared environments (Musani et al. 2008).

Studies looking for genetic bases of across-population variation in obesity risk, such as the high historical rates of obesity seen in some Native American and Pacific Island groups, have, by comparison with the person-to-person studies, had little or no success. For example, the Arizona Pima have had very high rates of obesity and diabetes in the last two generations, and a long-favored explanation was that such groups have a distinctive "thrifty genotype" coding for different metabolic profile that places them at particular risk for obesity and diabetes when food and exercise environments change (e.g., Knowler et al. 2005). However, after decades of study there has emerged no good evidence the Pima are genetically different in any way that would count (e.g., Norman et al. 1998). Further, rates of diabetes and obesity are one-tenth as common for men and less than one-third as common for women among the closely genetically related Mexican Pima (Shulz et al. 2006). Many of the factors that appear to explain their risk are those also identified for other groups—low birth weight, less breast-feeding of infants, relative physical inactivity in leisure and work time, lower fiber and higher fat diets, and ready access to mechanization and mass-produced food (e.g., Smith-Morris 2006).

Perhaps the most telling findings suggesting a lack of explanatory power provided by the genetic bases to widespread obesity are those related to its socioeconomic patterning. Socioeconomics (SES) are one of the most noticeable predictors of obesity risk within and across countries, and increasingly obesity is a condition of poverty. The survey of the studies examining the relationship between obesity and wealth conducted by Sobal and Stunkard (1989) showed that in the developing countries higher SES predicted more overweight and obesity. By contrast in developed countries the pattern was SES-neutral or negative, meaning higher SES women tended to be slimmer. More recent reviews suggest the SES gap is closing (Wang and Beydoun 2007), higher SES people in developed countries are nonetheless becoming fatter, but that the rise in availability of cheap, processed, high calorie foods globally (Popkin 2009) is creating a burgeoning in obesity in the lower income sectors of developing and developed countries alike (McClaren 2007).

Where you live is also a critical determinant of obesity risk, and provides a non-genetic explanation for why minorities might be at more risk, such as African Americans in the United States who have higher rates of obesity compared to other ethnic groups. Notably, people who are lower income tend to be clustered into specific neighborhoods, so that spatial and economic factors tend to run together. That is, poorer people, many of them minorities, tend to live in the most obesogenic (high calorie, sedentary, fat-promoting) environments. When we examine the pattern of distribution of obesity in modern American cityscapes for example, higher BMIs can be found in poverty-affected (usually inner city) "food deserts," where residents (many of whom lack transportation options) are provided with fewer options for purchasing health food at a reasonable cost such as fresh produce and fast food, high fat options are simultaneously cheaper and more easily accessed (e.g., Larsen and Gilliland 2008). The quality of built environments also appears to pattern our risk across neighborhoods. A number of studies have shown that minority neighborhoods in the United States have higher BMI and limited or no access to safe and pleasant local parks or pleasant walkable streets that would otherwise encourage people to exercise (e.g., Lindsay et al. 2001, Cutts et al. 2010). These factors of course can affect everyone living in an area: Manhattan is a relatively low BMI city given its demographics, because the way in which the city is laid out discourages car ownership and encourages walking (Rundle et al. 2007).

Another quite different example of how social factors shape obesity is related to who you make and stay friends with. Christakis and Fowler (2007) used data from a heart study in Massachusetts collected over many years to show that if your closer (especially same-sex) friends gain weight as they age, you will also, and over time this creates a clustering of overweight and obese people together (as well as slimmer people in other clusters). Christakis and Fowler could not explain the exact mechanism driving this, but it could be that we are influenced over time by other's attitudes toward exercise, eating, or body image.

This does not mean genes have no role in our understanding of obesity, but rather they do not do a good job explaining the macro-level patterns of who becomes obese (such as across a social network, a city, or across populations). Genetic factors around our capacities for weight gain and loss probably emerged a very long time ago, and the place of genetics in the explanation of contemporary obesity makes more sense when viewed in evolutionary perspective. This brings us to myth #2.

MYTH 2: LOSING WEIGHT IS EASY

At any time, apparently two thirds of Americans are dieting in some fashion to lose or control weight. Yet, most of those trying to lose weight either fail to do so, or lose it and gain it back, often plus some. Weight loss is a multi-billion dollar industry based on the key idea anyone can be slim if they want to simply by applying a little self-discipline (and the right product). Essentially, obesity is a disease or condition understood by many to be entirely under personal control. The perspective provided by looking at the idea of weight loss in relation to the long term, evolutionary history of our species suggests, in stark contrast, that losing weight should not be especially easy because the capacity to gain and maintain fat on our bodies is a particular and important human adaptation and fundamental part of our biology (Wells 2006). Thus efforts at weight loss are often fighting against our bodies' most basic tendencies.

To understand why humans might be evolved to conserve fat, we need to begin with the environmental conditions to which human bodies originally adapted: hunter-gathering lifestyles on an increasingly seasonal African savannah. Humans lived on wild game, plant foods such as fruit, nuts, and leaves, drank only water, and walked or ran everywhere they needed to go. Under these conditions, weight gain is not easy, and the capacity to retain fat can help even out energy needs when food sources become limited or energy demands go up (such as during illness or pregnancy and lactation). After the emergence of sedentary agriculture some 10,000 years ago, the ability to put on weight and keep it on may have been even more important, because reliance on a more limited number of food sources such as specific crops can mean even more vulnerability to seasonal or periodic famine. This historical view provides a large-scale perspective on why people in the new millennium are so commonly overweight—because we have a fat metabolism designed to react to plenty by storing for shortages to come, but now we never have the shortages. Modern environments filled with plenty of cheap, high-fat and high-sugar calories are toxic for our fat-seeking hunter-gatherer biologies.

Epigenetic effects, meaning the interaction between our evolved genotype and environmental triggers or shapers during development, appear to have some profound effects on our energy metabolism and also our ability to lose weight under specific ecological conditions. The "thrifty phenotype" draws on the idea that the fetus should be programmed to do best or adapt to possibly variable hunter gatherer conditions. Fetuses that were short on nutrition in-utero appear to develop a physiological profile (such as in fat or sugar metabolism) that prepares them to process and store energy reserves efficiently when they are adults. A mismatch between that fetal programming and the food environments of adults is what explains why some people seem more at risk of being obese and less able to lose weight than others—their bodies have developmental adaptations designed to help them deal with expected food shortages (Gluckman and Hanson 2005). And of course this is tied in complex ways to the issues raised by myth #1: many of the socioeconomic changes happening in developing nations mean that babies born to mothers suffering from undernutrition are now growing up in highly obesogenic environments, so we are seeing the emergence of many more people with both growth stunting (compensatory shorter adult heights linked to undernutrition) combined with obesity (Jehn and Brewis 2009).

MYTH 3: FAT IS DEADLY

There is a key idea that dominates most medical and public health discourse about obesity: it is inherently dangerous. There is a long list of awful diseases any doctor can rattle off that obesity is thought to trigger: including type-II (adult-onset) diabetes, heart disease, hypertension, various cancers, liver disease, and osteoarthritis. And it is credited with hastening millions of deaths a year. Yet, the evidence of the relationship between obesity and elevated mortality and morbidity risk is surprisingly contradictory and confusing. While there is no doubt that those classified as obese have higher rates of all these (and many other diseases), there are also many obese people who have very good health. For example, in one study that pooled the results of 250,000 people from other studies (termed a meta-analysis), people in the obese category were no more likely to die than those in the "normal" weight category, and actually had better survival odds than those classified as underweight (Romero-Corral et al. 2006). Other studies focused on the metabolic profiles have shown that many of those classified as obese by their BMI have healthy profiles, while many in the health ("normal") weight category have the profile that one might otherwise expect from someone very obese, such as high blood pressure, triglycerides, and blood sugar (Wildman et al. 2008, Romero-Corral et al. 2008).

There are probably a variety of reasons for these types of contradictory findings. An important one is that BMI is a very imprecise measure of actual level of body fat. For example, you can have people with high BMI because they are muscular rather than fat, such as professional athletes and George Clooney. Second, it is not just overall level of fat that seems to make a difference to obesity's role as a predictor of ill-health, but where on your body the fat is located. More fat around the mid-section ("apple shaped") appears to predict a worse metabolic profile compared to that around the buttocks and hips ("pear shaped"). There are also the issues of confounding factors such as cigarette smoking and other lifestyle factors (Lindsted et al. 1991). This suggests the important question of whether talking about health-risks in relation to BMI-based categories of obesity is even warranted.

The unwillingness to uncouple obesity from its health effects, and the idea that obesity should be understood as a disease and treated through primarily medical approaches (such as the mushrooming bariatric surgeries and lipo-suction) is actually a very recent and quite cultural phenomenon. Until the last century, being large and fat was not seen as a particular health problem, and many doctors recommended their patients fatten up for health's sake. Rather, it was skinny bodies that were diagnosed with nervous exhaustion, with a standard prescription of more food and less activity to treat it (Pool 2000). The distinction between being large and being unhealthy has however become severely blurred in both medical and popular contemporary understandings and hence responses to obesity. In part, this is promulgated by the powerful social messages of moral failing that have become attached to obesity in contemporary society, which leads us to myth #4.

MYTH 4: FAT IS BAD

There is no scientific evidence to suggest that obese people are more lazy or stupid than everyone else. Yet in many places the meanings of "fat" have become entwined with these and other personal failings, including lack of self-control, dirtiness, lack of sexuality, and unattractiveness. By contrast, being slim is linked conceptually to all that is good—beauty, discipline, intelligence, and strength of character. For example, using implicit association tests in which people are asked to link words together at high speed, Schwartz et al. (2006) showed how a sample of U.S. respondents consistently associated fat with lazy. In the same study, they also show how people would make some serious trade-offs to avoid being known as obese by others: some 15% of adults would rather give up 10 years or more of life to avoid being obese, and 25% said they would rather be infertile. Some even said they would prefer to be blind or lose a limb. Obese women frame much of their entire sense of self around their large bodies and judge their worth in line with this type of thinking (Bordo 1993:203). There is probably little way to avoid or resist this in societies like the mainstream United States where our bodies have become a primary anchor for our social identities (Becker 1995).

In this manner, self and others' negative reactions to obesity as a sign of deep personal failing underpins its status as arguably the last socially acceptable form of targeted discrimination (Puhl and Brownell 2001). The pattern of this humiliation and denegation is so widespread and so tolerated that some have termed it "civilized oppression" (Rogge et al. 2004). Obese people in Western countries consistently have less educational opportunity, less options for employment, are paid less, and more likely to be fired or passed over for promotion (Puhl and Huer 2009). Perhaps most concerning is that the medical profession appears to hold some truly profound negative attitudes toward the obese, and obese people get significantly lower quality care (Puhl and Huer 2001). Following myth #2, many doctors and nurses describe their obese patients as non-compliant, meaning they understand the failure of patients to lose weight as a sign of their lack of effort or concern to do so. Many medical staff say they would rather not treat obese people at all. Hardly surprisingly, obese people express reluctance to even seek health care (Puhl and Brownell 2001). Essentially, the "fat is bad" belief runs together with the "fat is unhealthy" one in shaping medical responses to obesity (Nordholm 1980).

One of the interesting insights offered by studies of the social problems people with obesity face is that much of the suffering around obesity can be understood as emotional rather than physical. Many obese people have higher rates of depression and anxiety (Simon et al 2006). Some cope to the social rejection through isolating themselves from others, and others cope by limiting their close relationships to other "sympathetic stigma sufferers," i.e., people the same size who are coping with the same judgments (Brochu and Morrison 2007, Carr and Friedman 2006).

Myth 5: Fat-Loving Societies

Historically, there is good documentation that many societies, perhaps most, valued plump bodies, and the slim-idealism so common in the West is something of an historic and cross-cultural aberration. In an oft-cited review of the cross-cultural record, based on the ethnographically diverse Human Relations Area Files generated by anthropologists prior to the 1980s, Brown and Konner (1987) estimated that 81% of the included human societies preferred plump or fat bodies to thin ones. The cultural and social contexts surrounding fat-preferring societies have been detailed in a number of ethnographies by cultural anthropologists since. One of the most detailed and clear examples is Rebecca Popenoe's (2004) study of women's extreme fatness among Azawagh Arabs in West Africa. Girls are force-fed large bowls of millet porridge and milk, and show their commitment and discipline through eating, with the ultimate goal of building beautiful rolls of fat around their bodies that enhance their attractiveness and marriageability. Eileen Anderson-Fye's (2004) study of women living in a tourist town on a cay in Belize discusses how women value their curves, with the ideal shaped like a glass Coca-Cola bottle. Elisa Sobo's (1994) ethnographic study of Jamaican communities explains how being thin is understood to represent social and physical decay or sickness, a miserly

or mean person, and someone who is unloved by others. Big Jamaican bodies by contrast denote happiness, youth, power, vitality, and exude sexuality. These types of ethnographic examples alongside the Brown and Konner review suggest the "fat is bad" belief is limited in its global impact, and that there are plenty of societies in which fat bodies are seen as an index of a morally good, marriageable, and attractive person.

However, this probably does not well represent the current ethnographic spectrum, and it seems that the situation is changing rapidly throughout the world. In mid 2009, our research team conducted a survey of cultural ideas about obesity in ten different settings: East Africa (Tanzania), Latin America (Paraguay, Mexico, Argentina), Europe (United Kingdom, Iceland), Oceania (New Zealand), and the US and territories (Arizona, Puerto Rico, American Samoa). Several of these settings (such as American Samoa and Puerto Rico) are contexts in which large bodies were traditionally valued for their positive social messages. We found that people in all these different places expressed a shared cultural model of obesity that highlighted the ideas of fat-as-bad and fat-as-unhealthy. Perhaps most pointedly, when we looked solely at the negative moral attributions people placed on obesity (such as "people are obese because they are lazy"), the highest frequency of these stigmatizing beliefs was in the middle income developing nation of Paraguay. The second highest—and most surprising—was American Samoa, since Pacific Island societies in particular have long been touted for their fat-positive beliefs. Thus, there may be a few isolated social settings where fat remains positively viewed, but the fat-as-unhealthy and fat-as-bad messages appear to be globalizing very fast. The range of cultural variation in how people respond to big bodies appears to be narrowing, and human suffering (created by the widespread nature of myth #4) is probably growing along with this.

Conclusion

So what does our different anthropological take on these five conventional ideas about obesity suggest for prevention, intervention and policy? First, we very much need to move beyond a "blame the victim" mentality around obesity. We need health practitioners to understand their reactions to obese patients are often more cultural than medical in origin, and everyone to understand that obese people grow fat for very many reasons, and many of those reasons are completely beyond their control. This suggests we should focus on systemic, rather than behavior-focused obesity interventions. Much of the current focus on weight loss and weight control is about pushing individuals to eat less and exercise more, and cursing their failures a lack of commitment to the task at hand. We need more effort to make our everyday environments healthier by having them promote healthy eating choices and exercise, and in ways that make these advantages fairly distributed to everyone, not just the well-to-do. An evolutionary perspective, which understands us as "stone agers in the fast lane" (Eaton et al. 1988), provides a good basic set of clues about the sorts of foods and exercise environments that likely trigger the most healthful metabolic profiles as our children grow. The thrifty phenotype addition to this thinking suggests we should especially focus on diet and exercise environments during pregnancy. Finally, we need to carefully assess when and if there is a need to panic about obesity, or if the hype is just taking over.

References

Anderson-Fye, EP. 2004. A Coca-Cola shape: Cultural change, body image, and eating disorders in San Andrés, Belize. Culture, Medicine, and Psychiatry 28:561–595.

Becker AE. 1995. Body, Self and Society: The View from Fiji. Philadelphia: University of Pennsylvania Press.

Bordo S. 1993. Unbearable Weight: Feminism, Western Culture and the Body. Berkeley, CA: University of California Press.

Bouchard C. 2007. The biological predisposition to obesity: beyond the thrifty genotype scenario. International Journal of Obesity 31:1337–1339.

Campos P. 2004. The Obesity Myth: Why America's Obsession with Weight Is Hazardous to Your Health. New York: Penguin.

Carr D, Friedman MA. 2005. Is obesity stigmatizing? Body weight, perceived discrimination, and psychological well-being in the United States. Journal of Health and Social Behavior 46:244–259.

Christakis NA, Fowler JH. 2007. The spread of obesity in a large social network over 32 years. New England Journal of Medicine 357(4): 370–379.

Cutts B, Darby K, Boone C, Brewis A. 2009. City structure, obesity, and environmental justice: An integrated analysis of physical and social barriers to walkable streets and park access. Social Science and Medicine 69(9):1314–1322.

Eaton SB, Konner M, Shostak M. 1988. Stone agers in the fast lane: chronic degenerative diseases in evolutionary perspective. Am J Men 84:739–49.

Gluckman P, Hanson M. 2005. The Fetal Matrix: Evolution, Development and Disease. Cambridge: Cambridge University Press.

Jehn M, Brewis A. 2009. Paradoxical malnutrition in mother-child pairs: Untangling the phenomenon of over- and under-nutrition in underdeveloped economies. Economics and Human Biology 7:28–35.

Knowler W, Pettitt D, Bennett P, Williams R. 2005. Diabetes mellitus in the Pima Indians: Genetic and evolutionary considerations. American Journal of Physical Anthropology 62:107–14.

Larsen K, Gilliland J. 2008. Mapping the evolution of 'food deserts' in a Canadian city: supermarket accessibility in London, Ontario, 1961–2005. International Journal of Health Geographics 7:16.

Lindsey G, Maraj M, Kuan S, 2001. Access, equity, and urban greenways: an exploratory investigation. The Professional Geographer 53:332–346.

Lindsted K, Tonstad S, and Kuzma J. 1991. Self-report of physical activity and patterns of mortality in Seventh-Day Adventist men. Journal of Clinical Epidemiology 44(4–5):355–364.

McLaren L. 2007. Socioeconomic status and obesity. Epidemiological Reviews 29:29–48.

Musani SK, Erickson S, and Allison DB. 2008. Obesity—still highly heritable after all these years. American Journal of Clinical Nutrition 87:275–276.

Nordholm LA. 1980. Beautiful patients are good patients: evidence for the physical attractiveness sterotype in first impressions of patients. Soc Sci Med 14:81–3.

Norman R, Tataranni P, Pratley R, Thompson D, inter alia. 1998. Autosomal genomic scan for loci linked to obesity and energy metabolism in Pima Indians. American Journal of Human Genetics 62(3):659–668.

Popkin B. 2009. The World Is Fat: The Fads, Trends, Policies, and Products That Are Fattening the Human Race. New York: Avery.

Pool R. 2000. Fat: Fighting the Obesity Epidemic. New York: Oxford University Press.

Popenoe R. 2004. Feeding Desire: Fatness, Beauty, and Sexuality among a Saharan People. London, New York: Routledge.

Puhl R., Brownell K. 2001. Bias, discrimination, and obesity. Obesity Research 9:788–805.

Puhl R, Heuer C. 2009. The stigma of obesity: A review and update. Obesity Research 17(5):941–964.

Rogge M, Greenwald M, Golden A. 2004 Obesity, stigma, and civilized oppression. Adv Nurs Sci 27:301–15.

Romero-Corral A., Montori V, Somers V, Korinek J, Thomas R, Allison T, Mookadam F, López-Jiménez F. 2006. Association of bodyweight with total mortality and with cardiovascular events in coronary artery disease: a systematic review of cohort studies. Lancet 368:666–678.

Romero-Corral, A., Somers V, Sierra-Johnson J, Thomas R, Collazo-Clavell M, Korinek J, Allison T, Batsis J, Sert-Kuniyoshi F, López-Jiménez F. 2008. Accuracy of body mass index in diagnosing obesity in the adult general population. International Journal of Obesity 32:959–966.

Rundle A, Diez Roux AV, Freeman LM, Miller D, Neckerman KM, Weiss CC. 2007. The urban built environment and obesity in New York City: a multilevel analysis. Am J Health Promot. 21:326–334.

Schwartz, M, Vartanian L, Nosek B, Brownell K. 2006. The influence of one's own body weight on implicit and explicit anti-fat bias. Obesity 14:440–447.

Shulz L. Bennett P, Ravussin E, Kidd J, Kidd K, Esparza J, and Valencia V. 2006. Effects of traditional and western environments on prevalence of type 2 diabetes in Pima Indians in Mexico and the U.S. Diabetes Care 29(8):1866–1871.

Simon, G., Von Korff M, Saunders K, Miglioretti D, Crane P, van Belle G, Kessler R. 2006. Association between obesity and psychiatric disorders in the U.S. adult population. Archives of General Psychiatry 63:824–830.

Sobal J., and Stunkard A. 1989. Socioeconomic status and obesity: A review of the literature. Psychological Bulletin 105:260–275.

Sobo E. 1994. The sweetness of fat: Health, procreation, and sociability in rural Jamaica. In Many Mirrors: Body Image and Social Meaning, ed. N. Sault, 132–154. New Brunswick, N.J.: Rutgers University Press.

Wang Y, Beydoun M. 2007. The obesity epidemic in the United States – gender, age, socioeconomic, racial/ethnic, and geographic characteristics: A systematic review and meta-regression analysis. Epidemiology Review 29:6–28.

Wells, JCK. 2006. The evolution of human fatness and susceptibility to obesity: An ethological approach. Biological Reviews 81:183–205.

Wildman R, Muntner P, Reynolds K, McGinn A, Rajpathak S, Wylie-Rosett J, Sowers MR. 2008. The obese without cardiometabolic risk factor clustering and the normal weight with cardiometabolic risk factor clustering: Prevalence and correlates of 2 phenotypes among the U.S. population (NHANES 1999–2004). Archives of Internal Medicine 168:1617–1624.

CHAPTER 49

The Pima Paradox

Malcolm Gladwell

(1998)

1

Sacaton lies in the center of Arizona, just off interstate 10, on the Gila River reservation of the Pima Indian tribe. It is a small town, dusty and unremarkable, which looks as if it had been blown there by a gust of desert wind. Shacks and plywood bungalows are scattered along a dirt-and-asphalt grid. Dogs crisscross the streets. Back yards are filled with rusted trucks and junk. The desert in these parts is scruffy and barren, drained of water by the rapid growth of Phoenix, just half an hour's drive to the north. The nearby Gila River is dry, and the fields of wheat and cushaw squash and tepary beans which the Pima used to cultivate are long gone. The only prepossessing building in Sacaton is a gleaming low-slung modern structure on the outskirts of town—the Hu Hu Kam Memorial Hospital. There is nothing bigger or more impressive for miles, and that is appropriate, since medicine is what has brought Sacaton any wisp of renown it has.

Thirty-five years ago, a team of National Institutes of Health researchers arrived in Sacaton to study rheumatoid arthritis. They wanted to see whether the Pima had higher or lower rates of the disease than the Blackfoot of Montana. A third of the way through their survey, however, they realized that they had stumbled on something altogether strange—a population in the grip of a plague. Two years later, the N.I.H. returned to the Gila River Indian Reservation in force. An exhaustive epidemiological expedition was launched, in which thousands of Pima were examined every two years by government scientists, their weight and height and blood pressure checked, their blood sugar monitored, and their eyes and kidneys scrutinized.

In Phoenix, a modern medical center devoted to Native Americans was built; on its top floor, the N.I.H. installed a state-of-the-art research lab, including the first metabolic chamber in North America—a sealed room in which to measure the precise energy intake and expenditure of Pima research subjects. Genetic samples were taken; family histories were mapped; patterns of illness and death were traced from relative to relative and generation to generation. Today, the original study group has grown from four thousand people to seven thousand five hundred, and so many new studies have been added to the old that the total number of research papers arising from the Gila River reservation takes up almost forty feet of shelf space in the N.I.H. library in Phoenix.

The Pima are famous now—famous for being fatter than any other group in the world, with the exception only of the Nauru islanders of the West Pacific. Among those over thirty-five on the reservation, the rate of diabetes, the disease most closely associated with obesity, is fifty per cent, eight times the national average and a figure unmatched in medical history. It is not unheard of in Sacaton for adults to weigh five hundred pounds, for teen-agers to be suffering from diabetes, or for relatively young men and women to be already disabled by the disease—to be blind, to have lost a limb, to be confined to a wheelchair, or to be dependent on kidney dialysis.

When I visited the town, on a monotonously bright desert day not long ago, I watched a group of children on a playing field behind the middle school moving at what seemed to be half speed, their generous shirts and baggy jeans barely concealing their bulk. At the hospital, one of the tribe's public-health workers told me that when she began an education program on nutrition several years ago she wanted to start with second graders, to catch the children before it was too late. "We were under the delusion that kids didn't gain weight until the second grade," she said, shaking her head. "But then we realized we'd have to go younger. Those kids couldn't run around the block."

From the beginning, the N.I.H. researchers have hoped that if they can understand why the Pima are so obese they can better understand obesity in the rest of us; the assumption is that obesity in the Pima is different only in degree, not in kind. One hypothesis for the Pima's plight, favored by Eric Ravussin, of the N.I.H.'s Phoenix team, is that after generations of living in the desert the only Pima who survived famine and drought were those highly adept at storing fat in times of plenty. Under normal circumstances, this disposition was kept in check by the Pima's traditional diet: cholla-cactus buds, honey mesquite, povertyweed, and prickly pears from the desert floor; mule deer, white-winged dove, and black-tailed jackrabbit; squawfish from the Gila River; and wheat, squash, and beans grown in irrigated desert fields. By the end of the Second World War, however,

Malcolm Gladwell, "The Pima paradox." *The New Yorker*, 2 February 1998:44–57. Reprinted with permission.

the Pima had almost entirely left the land, and they began to eat like other Americans. Their traditional diet had been fifteen to twenty per cent fat. Their new diet was closer to forty per cent fat. Famine, which had long been a recurrent condition, gave way to permanent plenty, and so the Pima's "thrifty" genes, once an advantage, were now a liability. N.I.H. researchers are trying to find these genes, on the theory that they may be the same genes that contribute to obesity in the rest of us. Their studies at Sacaton have also uncovered valuable clues to how diabetes works, how obesity in pregnant women affects their children, and how human metabolism is altered by weight gain. All told, the collaboration between the N.I.H. and the Pima is one of the most fruitful relationships in modern medical science–with one fateful exception. After thirty-five years, no one has had any success helping the Pima lose weight. For all the prodding and poking, the hundreds of research papers describing their bodily processes, and the determined efforts of health workers, year after year the tribe grows fatter.

"I used to be a nurse, I used to work in the clinic, I used to be all gung ho about going out and teaching people about diabetics and obesity," Teresa Wall, who heads the tribe's public-health department, told me. "I thought that was all people needed—information. But they weren't interested. They had other issues." Wall is a Pima, short and stocky, who has long, straight black hair, worn halfway down her back. She spoke softly. "There's something missing. It's one thing to say to people, 'This is what you should do.' It's another to actually get them to take it in."

The Pima have built a new wellness center in downtown Sacaton, with a weight room and a gymnasium. They now have an education program on nutrition aimed at preschoolers and first graders, and at all tribal functions signs identify healthful food choices—a tray of vegetables or of fruit, say. They are doing, in other words, what public-health professionals are supposed to be doing. But results are hard to see.

"We've had kids who were diabetic, whose mothers had diabetes and were on dialysis and had died of kidney failure," one of the tribe's nutritionists told me. "You'd think that that would make a difference—that it would motivate them to keep their diet under control. It doesn't." She got up from her desk, walked to a bookshelf, and pulled out two bottles of Coca-Cola. One was an old glass bottle. The other was a modern plastic bottle, which towered over it. "The original Coke bottle, in the nineteen-thirties, was six and a half ounces." She held up the plastic bottle. "Now they are marketing one litre as a single serving. That's five times the original serving size. The McDonald's regular hamburger is two hundred and sixty calories, but now you've got the double cheeseburger, which is four hundred and forty-five calories. Portion sizes are getting way out of whack. Eating is not about hunger anymore. The fact that people are hungry is way down on the list of why they eat." I told her that I had come to Sacaton, the front lines of the weight battle, in order to find out what really works in fighting obesity. She looked at me and shrugged. "We're the last people who could tell you that," she said.

In the early nineteen-sixties, at about the time the N.I.H. team stumbled on the Pima, seventeen per cent of middle-aged Americans met the clinical definition of obesity. Today, that figure is 32.3 per cent. Between the early nineteen-seventies and the early nineteen-nineties, the percentage of preschool girls who were overweight went from 5.8 per cent to ten per cent. The number of Americans who fall into what epidemiologists call Class Three Obesity—that is, people too grossly overweight, say, to fit into an airline seat—has risen three hundred and fifty per cent in the past thirty years. "We've looked at trends by educational level, race, and ethnic group, we've compared smokers and non-smokers, and it's very hard to say that there is any group that is not experiencing this kind of weight gain," Katherine Flegal, a senior research epidemiologist at the National Center for Health Statistics, says. "It's all over the world. In China, the prevalence of obesity is vanishingly low, yet they are showing an increase. In Western Samoa, it is very high, and they are showing an increase." In the same period, science has unlocked many of obesity's secrets, the American public has been given a thorough education in the principles of good nutrition, health clubs have sprung up from one end of the country to another, dieting has become a religion, and health food a marketing phenomenon. None of it has mattered. It is the Pima paradox: in the fight against obesity all the things that worked in curbing behaviors like drunk driving and smoking and in encouraging things like safe sex and the use of seat belts—education, awareness, motivation—don't seem to work. For one reason or another, we cannot stop eating. "Since many people cannot lose much weight no matter how hard they try, and promptly regain whatever they do lose," the editors of The New England Journal of Medicine wearily concluded last month, "the vast amount of money spent on diet clubs, special foods and over-the-counter remedies, estimated to be on the order of $30 billion to $50 billion yearly, is wasted." Who could argue? If the Pima—who are surrounded by the immediate and tangible consequences of obesity, who have every conceivable motivation—can't stop themselves from eating their way to illness, what hope is there for the rest of us?

In the scientific literature, there is something called Gourmand Syndrome—a neurological condition caused by anterior brain lesions and characterized by an unusual passion for eating. The syndrome was described in a recent issue of the journal Neurology, and the irrational, seemingly uncontrollable obsession with food evinced by its victims seems a perfect metaphor for the irrational, apparently uncontrollable obsession with food which seems to have overtaken American society as a whole. Here is a diary entry from a Gourmand Syndrome patient, a fifty-five-year-old stroke victim who had previously displayed no more than a perfunctory interest in food.

After I could stand on my feet again, I dreamt to go downtown and sit down in this well-known restaurant. There I would get a beer, sausage, and potatoes. Slowly my diet improved again and thus did quality of life. The day after discharge, my first trip brought me to this restaurant, and here I order potato salad, sausage, and a beer. I feel wonderful. My spouse anxiously registers everything I eat and nibble. It irritates me. A few steps down the street, we enter a coffee-house. My hand is reaching for a pastry, my wife's hand reaches between. Through the window I see my bank. If I choose, I could buy all the pastry I wanted, including the whole store. The creamy pastry slips from the foil like a mermaid. I take a bite.

2

Is there an easy way out of this problem? Every year, millions of Americans buy books outlining new approaches to nutrition and diet, nearly all of which are based on the idea that overcoming our obsession with food is really just a matter of technique: that the right foods eaten in the right combination can succeed where more traditional approaches to nutrition have failed. A cynic would say, of course, that the seemingly endless supply of these books proves their lack of efficacy, since if one of these diets actually worked there would be no need for another. But that's not quite fair. After all, the medical establishment, too, has been giving Americans nutritional advice without visible effect. We have been told that we must not take in more calories than we burn, that we cannot lose weight if we don't exercise consistently, that an excess of eggs, red meat, cheese, and fried food clogs arteries, that fresh vegetables and fruits help to ward off cancer, that fibre is good and sugar is bad and whole-wheat bread is better than white bread. That few of us are able to actually follow this advice is either our fault or the fault of the advice. Medical orthodoxy, naturally, tends toward the former position. Diet books tend toward the latter. Given how often the medical orthodoxy has been wrong in the past, that position is not, on its face, irrational. It's worth finding out whether it is true.

Arguably the most popular diet of the moment, for example, is one invented by the biotechnology entrepreneur Barry Sears. Sears's first book, "The Zone," written with Bill Lawren, sold a million and a half copies and has been translated into fourteen languages. His second book, "Mastering the Zone," was on the best-seller lists for eleven weeks. Madonna is rumored to be on the Zone diet, and so are Howard Stern and President Clinton, and if you walk into almost any major bookstore in the country right now Sears's two best-sellers—plus a new book, "Zone Perfect Meals in Minutes"—will quite likely be featured on a display table near the front. They are ambitious books, filled with technical discussions of food chemistry, metabolism, evolutionary theory, and obscure scientific studies, all apparently serving as proof of the idea that through careful management of "the most powerful and ubiquitous drug we have: food" we can enter a kind of high-efficiency, optimal metabolic state—the Zone.

The key to entering the Zone, according to Sears, is limiting your carbohydrates. When you eat carbohydrates, he writes, you stimulate the production of insulin, and insulin is a hormone that evolved to put aside excess carbohydrate

calories in the form of fat in case of future famine. So the insulin that's stimulated by excess carbohydrates aggressively promotes the accumulation of body fat. In other words, when we eat too much carbohydrate, we're essentially sending a hormonal message, via insulin, to the body (actually to the adipose cells). The message: "Store fat."

His solution is a diet in which carbohydrates make up no more than forty per cent of all calories consumed (as opposed to the fifty per cent or more consumed by most Americans), with fat and protein coming to thirty per cent each. Maintaining that precise four-to-three ratio between carbohydrates and protein is, in Sears's opinion, critical for keeping insulin in check. "The Zone" includes all kinds of complicated instructions to help readers figure out how to do things like calculate their precise protein requirements in restaurants. ("Start with the protein, using the palm of your hand as a guide. The amount of protein that can fit into your palm is usually four protein blocks. That's about one chicken breast or 4 ounces sliced turkey.")

It should be said that the kind of diet Sears suggests is perfectly nutritious. Following the Zone diet, you'll eat lots of fibre, fresh fruit, fresh vegetables, and fish, and very little red meat. Good nutrition, though, isn't really the point. Sears's argument is that being in the Zone can induce permanent weight loss—that by controlling carbohydrates and the production of insulin you can break your obsession with food and fundamentally alter the way your body works. "Weight loss...can be an ongoing and usually frustrating struggle for most people," he writes. "In the Zone it is painless, almost automatic."

Does the Zone exist? Yes and no. Certainly, if people start eating a more healthful diet they'll feel better about themselves. But the idea that there is something magical about keeping insulin within a specific range is a little strange. Insulin is simply a hormone that regulates the storage of energy. Precisely how much insulin you need to store carbohydrates is dependent on all kinds of things, including how fit you are and whether, like many diabetics, you have a genetic predisposition toward insulin resistance. Generally speaking, the heavier and more out of shape you are, the more insulin your body needs to do its job. The Pima have a problem with obesity and that makes their problem with diabetes worse—not the other way around. High levels of insulin are the result of obesity. They aren't the cause of obesity. When I read the insulin section of "The Zone" to Gerald Reaven, an emeritus professor of medicine at Stanford University, who is acknowledged to be the country's leading insulin expert, I could hear him grinding his teeth. "I had the experience of being on a panel discussion with Sears, and I couldn't believe the stuff that comes out of this guy's mouth," he said. "I think he's full of it."

What Sears would have us believe is that when it comes to weight loss your body treats some kinds of calories differently from others—that the combination of the food we eat is more critical than the amount. To this end, he cites what he calls an "amazing" and "landmark" study published in 1956 in the British medical journal Lancet. (It should be a tipoff that the best corroborating research he can come up with here is more than forty years old.) In the study, a couple of researchers compared the effects of two different thousand-calorie diets—the first high in fat and protein and low in carbohydrates, and the second low in fat and protein and high in carbohydrates—on two groups of obese men. After eight to ten days, the men on the low-carbohydrate diet had lost more weight than the men on the high-carbohydrate diet. Sears concludes from the study that if you want to lose weight you should eat protein and shun carbohydrates. Actually, it shows nothing of the sort. Carbohydrates promote water retention; protein acts like a diuretic. Over a week or so, someone on a high-protein diet will always look better than someone on a high-carbohydrate diet, simply because of dehydration. When a similar study was conducted several years later, researchers found that after about three weeks—when the effects of dehydration had evened out—the weight loss on the two diets was virtually identical. The key isn't how you eat, in other words; it's how much you eat. Calories, not carbohydrates, are still what matters. The dirty little secret of the Zone system is that, despite Sears's expostulations about insulin, all he has done is come up with another low-calorie diet. He doesn't do the math for his readers, but some nutritionists have calculated that if you follow Sears's prescriptions religiously you'll take in at most seventeen hundred calories a day, and at seventeen hundred calories a day virtually anyone can lose weight. The problem with low-calorie diets, of course, is that no one can stay on them for very long. Just ask Sears. "Diets based on choice restriction and calorie limits usually fail," he writes in the second chapter of "The Zone," just as he is about to present his own choice-restricted and calorie-limited diet. "People on restrictive diets get tired of feeling hungry and deprived. They go off their diets, put the weight back on (primarily, as increased body fat) and then feel bad about themselves for not having enough will power, discipline, or motivation."

These are not, however, the kinds of contradiction that seem to bother Sears. His first book's dust jacket claims that in the Zone you can "reset your genetic code" and "burn more fat watching TV than by exercising." By the time he's finished, Sears has held up his diet as the answer to virtually every medical ill facing Western society, from heart disease to cancer and on to alcoholism and PMS. He writes, "Dr. Paul Kahl, the same physician with whom I did the AIDS pilot study"—yes, Sears's diet is just the thing for AIDS, too—"told me the story of one of his patients, a fifty-year-old woman with MS."

Paul put her on a Zone-favorable diet, and after a few months on the program she came in for a checkup. Paul asked the basic question: "How are you feeling?" Her answer was "Great!" Noticing that she was still using a cane for stability, Paul asked her, "If you're feeling so great, why are you still using the cane?" Her only response was that since developing MS she always had. Paul took the cane away and told her to walk to the end of the hallway and back. After a few tentative steps, she made the round trip quickly. When Paul

asked her if she wanted her cane back, she just smiled and told him to keep it for someone who really needed it.

Put down your carbohydrates and walk!

It is hard, while reading this kind of thing, to escape the conclusion that what is said in a diet book somehow matters less than how it's said. Sears, after all, isn't the only diet specialist who seems to be making things up. They all seem to be making things up. But if you read a large number of popular diet books in succession, what is striking is that they all seem to be making things up in precisely the same way. It is as if the diet-book genre had an unspoken set of narrative rules and conventions, and all that matters is how skillfully those rules and conventions are adhered to. Sears, for example, begins fearful and despondent, his father dead of a heart attack at fifty-three, a "sword of Damocles" over his head. Judy Moscovitz, author of "The Rice Diet Report" (three months on the Times bestseller list), tells us, "I was always the fattest kid in the class, and I knew all the pain that only a fat kid can know....I was always the last one reluctantly chosen for the teams." Martin Katahn, in his best-seller "The Rotation Diet," writes, "I was one of those fat kids who had no memory of ever being thin. Instead, I have memories such as not being able to run fast enough to keep up with my playmates, being chosen last for all games that required physical movement."

Out of that darkness comes light: the Eureka Moment, when the author explains how he stumbled on the radical truth that inpired his diet. Sears found himself in the library of the Boston University School of Medicine, reading everything he could on the subject: "I had no preconceptions, no base of knowledge to work from, so I read everything. I eventually came across an obscure report..." Rachael Heller, who was a co-author of the best-selling "The Carbohydrate Addict's Diet" (and, incidentally, so fat growing up that she was "always the last one picked for the team"), was at home in bed when her doctor called, postponing her appointment and thereby setting in motion an extraordinary chain of events that involved veal parmigiana, a Greek salad, and two French crullers: "I will always be grateful for that particular arrangement of circumstances....Sometimes we are fortunate enough to recognize and take advantage of them, sometimes not. This time I did. I believe it saved my life." Harvey Diamond, the co-author of the three-million-copy-selling "Fit for Life," was at a music festival two thousand miles from home, when he happened to overhear two people in front of him discussing the theories of a friend in Santa Barbara: "'Excuse me,' I interrupted, 'who is this fellow you are discussing?' In less than twenty-four hours I was on my way to Santa Barbara. Little did I know that I was on the brink of one of the most remarkable discoveries of my life."

The Eureka Moment is followed, typically within a few pages, by the Patent Claim—the point at which the author shows why his Eureka Moment, which explains how weight can be lost without sacrifice, is different from the Eureka Moment of all those other diet books explaining how weight can be lost without sacrifice. This is harder than it appears. Dieters are actually attracted to the idea of discipline, because they attribute their condition to a failure of discipline. It's just that they know themselves well enough to realize that if a diet requires discipline they won't be able to follow it. At the same time, of course, even as the dieter realizes that what he is looking for—discipline without the discipline—has never been possible, he still clings to the hope that someday it might be. The Patent Claim must negotiate both paradoxes. Here is Sears, in his deft six-paragraph Patent Claim: "These are not unique claims. The proponents of every new diet that comes along say essentially the same thing. But if you're reading this book, you probably know that these diets don't really work. "Why don't they work? Because they "violate the basic biochemical laws required to enter the Zone." Other diets don't have discipline. The Zone does. Yet, he adds, "The beauty of the dietary system presented in this book is that . . . it doesn't call for a great deal of the kind of unrealistic self-sacrifice that causes many people to fall off the diet wagon. . . . In fact, I can even show you how to stay within these dietary guidelines while eating at fast-food restaurants." It is the very discipline of the Zone system that allows its adherent to lose weight without discipline.

Or consider this from Adele Puhn's recent runaway bestseller, "The 5-Day Miracle Diet." America's No. 1 diet myth, she writes, is that "you have to deprive yourself to lose weight":

> Even though countless diet programs have said you can have your cake and eat it, too, in your heart of hearts, you have that "nibbling" doubt: For a diet to really work, you have to sacrifice. I know. I bought into this myth for a long time myself. And the fact is that on every other diet, deprivation is involved. Motivation can only take you so far. Eventually you're going to grab for that extra piece of cake, that box of cookies, that cheeseburger and fries. But not the 5-Day Miracle Diet.

Let us pause and savor the five-hundred-and-forty-degree rhetorical triple gainer taken in those few sentences:

(1) the idea that diet involves sacrifice is a myth;
(2) all diets, to be sure, say that on their diets dieting without sacrifice is not a myth;
(3) but you believe that dieting without sacrifice is a myth;
(4) and I, too, believed that dieting without sacrifice is a myth;
(5) because in fact on all diets dieting without sacrifice is a myth;
(6) except on my diet, where dieting without sacrifice is not a myth.

The expository sequence that these books follow—last one picked, moment of enlightenment, assertion of the one true way—finally amounts to nothing less than a conversion narrative. In conception and execution, diet books are self-consciously theological. (Whom did Harvey Diamond meet after his impulsive, desperate mission to Santa Barbara? A man he will only identify, pseudonymously and mysteriously, as Mr. Jensen, an ethereal figure with "clear eyes, radiant skin, serene demeanor and well-proportioned body.") It is the appropriation of this religious narrative that permits the suspension of disbelief.

There is a more general explanation for all this in the psychological literature—a phenomenon that might be called the Photocopier Effect, after the experiments of the Harvard social scientist Ellen Langer. Langer examined the apparently common-sense idea that if you are trying to persuade someone to do something for you, you are always better off if you provide a reason. She went up to a group of people waiting in line to use a library copying machine and said, "Excuse me, I have five pages. May I use the Xerox machine?" Sixty per cent said yes. Then she repeated the experiment on another group, except that she changed her request to "Excuse me, I have five pages. May I use the Xerox machine, because I'm in a rush?" Ninety-four per cent said yes. This much sounds like common sense: if you say, "because I'm in a rush"—if you explain your need—people are willing to step aside. But here's where the study gets interesting. Langer then did the experiment a third time, in this case replacing the specific reason with a statement of the obvious: "Excuse me, I have five pages. May I use the Xerox machine, because I have to make some copies?" The percentage who let her do so this time was almost exactly the same as the one in the previous round—ninety-three per cent. The key to getting people to say yes, in other words, wasn't the explanation "because I'm in a rush" but merely the use of the word "because." What mattered wasn't the substance of the explanation but merely the rhetorical form—the conjunctional footprint—of an explanation.

Isn't this how diet books work? Consider the following paragraph, taken at random from "The Zone":

> In paracrine hormonal responses, the hormone travels only a very short distance from a secreting cell to a target cell. Because of the short distance between the secreting cell and the target cell, paracrine responses don't need the long-distance capabilities of the bloodstream. Instead, they use the body's version of a regional system: the paracrine system. Finally, there are the autocrine hormone systems, analogous to the cord that links the handset of the phone to the phone itself. Here the secreting cells release a hormone that comes immediately back to affect the secreting cell itself.

Don't worry if you can't follow what Sears is talking about here—following isn't really the point. It is enough that he is using the word "because."

3

If there is any book that defines the diet genre, however, it is "Dr. Atkins' New Diet Revolution." Here is the conversion narrative at its finest. Dr. Atkins, a humble corporate physician, is fat. ("I had three chins.") He begins searching for answers. ("One evening I read about the work that Dr. Garfield Duncan had done in nutrition at the University of Pennsylvania. Fasting patients, he reported, lose all sense of hunger after forty-eight hours without food. That stunned me.... That defied logic.") He tests his unorthodox views on himself. As if by magic, he loses weight. He tests his unorthodox views on a group of executives at A.T. & T. As if by magic, they lose weight. Incredibly, he has come up with a diet that "produces steady weight loss" while setting "no limit on the amount of food you can eat." In 1972, inspired by his vision, he puts pen to paper. The result is "Dr. Atkins' Diet Revolution," one of the fifty best-selling books of all time. In the early nineties, he publishes "Dr. Atkins' New Diet Revolution," which sells more than three million copies and is on the Times best-seller list for almost all of 1997. More than two decades of scientific research into health and nutrition have elapsed in the interim, but Atkins' message has remained the same. Carbohydrates are bad. Everything else is good. Eat the hamburger, hold the bun. Eat the steak, hold the French fries. Here is the list of ingredients for one of his breakfast "weight loss" recommendations: scrambled eggs for six. Keep in mind that Atkins is probably the most influential diet doctor in the world.

> 12 link sausages (be sure they contain no sugar)
> 1 3-ounce package cream cheese
> 1 tablespoon butter
> 3/4 cup cream
> ¼ cup water
> 1 teaspoon seasoned salt
> 2 teaspoons parsley
> 8 eggs, beaten

Atkins' Patent Claim centers on the magical weight-loss properties of something called "ketosis." When you eat carbohydrates, your body converts them into glycogen and stores them for ready use. If you are deprived of carbohydrates, however, your body has to turn to its own stores of fat and muscle for energy. Among the intermediate metabolic products of this fat breakdown are ketones, and when you produce lots of ketones, you're in ketosis. Since an accumulation of these chemicals swiftly becomes toxic, your body works very hard to get rid of them, either through the kidneys, as urine, or through the lungs, by exhaling, so people in ketosis commonly spend a lot of time in the bathroom and have breath that smells like rotten apples. Ketosis can also raise the risk of bone fracture and cardiac arrhythmia and can result in light-headedness, nausea, and the loss of nutrients like potassium and sodium. There is no doubt that you can lose weight while you're in ketosis. Between all that protein and those trips to the bathroom, you'll quickly become dehydrated and drop several pounds just through water loss. The nausea will probably curb your appetite. And if you do what Atkins says, and suddenly cut out virtually all carbohydrates, it will take a little while for your body to compensate for all those lost calories by demanding extra protein and fat. The weight loss isn't permanent, though. After a few weeks your body adjusts, and the weight—and your appetite—comes back.

For Atkins, however, ketosis is as "delightful as sex and sunshine," which is why he wants dieters to cut out carbohydrates almost entirely. (To avoid bad breath he recommends carrying chlorophyll tablets and purse-size aerosol breath fresheners at all times; to avoid other complications, he recommends regular blood tests.) Somehow, he has convinced himself that his kind of ketosis is different from the bad kind of ketosis, and that his ketosis can actually lead to permanent weight loss. Why he thinks this, however, is a little unclear. In "Dr. Atkins' Diet Revolution" he thought that the key was in the many trips to the bathroom: "Hundreds of calories are sneaked out of your body every day in the form of ketones and a host of other incompletely broken down molecules of fat. You are disposing of these calories not by work or violent exercise—but just by breathing and allowing your kidneys to function. All this is achieved merely by cutting out your carbohydrates." Unfortunately, the year after that original edition of Atkins' book came out, the American Medical Association published a devastating critique of this theory, pointing out, among other things, that ketone losses in the urine and the breath rarely exceed a hundred calories a day—a quantity, the A.M.A. pointed out, "that could not possibly account for the dramatic results claimed for such diets." In "Dr. Atkins' New Diet Revolution," not surprisingly, he's become rather vague on the subject, mysteriously invoking something he calls Fat Mobilizing Substance. Last year, when I interviewed him, he offered a new hypothesis: that ketosis takes more energy than conventional food metabolism does, and that it is "a much less efficient pathway to burn up your calories via stored fat than it is via glucose." But he didn't want to be pinned down. "Nobody has really been able to work out that mechanism as well as I would have liked, "he conceded.

Atkins is a big, white-haired man in his late sixties, well over six feet, with a barrel chest and a gruff, hard-edged voice. On the day we met, he was wearing a high-lapelled, four-button black suit. Given a holster and a six-shooter, he could have passed for the sheriff in a spaghetti western. He is an intimidating figure, his manner brusque and impatient. He gives the impression that he doesn't like having to explain his theories, that he finds the details tedious and unnecessary. Given the Photocopier Effect, of course, he is quite right. The appearance of an explanation is more important than the explanation itself. But Atkins seems to take this principle farther than anyone else.

For example, in an attempt to convince his readers that eating pork chops, steaks, duck, and rack of lamb in abundance is good for them, Atkins points out that primitive Eskimo cultures had virtually no heart disease, despite a high-fat diet of fish and seal meat. But one obvious explanation for the Eskimo paradox is that cold-water fish and seal meat are rich in n-3 fatty acids—the "good" kind of fat. Red meat, on the other hand, is rich in saturated fat—the "bad" kind of fat. That dietary fats come in different forms, some of which are particularly bad for you and some of which are not, is the kind of basic fact that seventh graders are taught in Introduction to Nutrition. Atkins has a whole chapter on dietary fat in "New Diet Revolution" and doesn't make the distinction once. All diet-book authors profit from the Photocopier Effect. Atkins lives it.

I watched Atkins recently as he conducted his daily one-hour radio show on New York's WEVD. We were in a Manhattan town house in the East Fifties, where he has his headquarters, in a sleek, modernist office filled with leather furniture and soapstone sculpture. He sat behind his desk— John Wayne in headphones—as his producer perched in front of him. It was a bravura performance. He spoke quickly and easily, glancing at his notes only briefly, and then deftly gave counsel to listeners around the region.

The first call came from George, on his car phone. George told Atkins his ratio of triglycerides to cholesterol. It wasn't good. George was a very unhealthy man. "You're in big trouble," Atkins said. "You have to change your diet. What do you generally eat? What's your breakfast?"

"I've stopped taking junk foods," George says. "I don't eat eggs. I don't eat bacon."

"Then that's—See there." Atkins' voice rose in exasperation. "What do you have for breakfast?"

"I have skim milk, cereal, with banana."

"That's three carbs!" Atkins couldn't believe that in this day and age people were still consuming fruit and skim milk. "That's how you are getting into trouble!...What you need to do, George, seriously, is get ahold of 'New Diet Revolution' and just read what it says."

Atkins took another call. This time, it was from Robert, forty-one years old, three hundred pounds, and possessed of a formidable Brooklyn accent. He was desperate to lose weight—up on a ledge and wanting Atkins to talk him down. "I really don't know anything about dieting," he said. "I'm getting a little discouraged."

"It's really very easy," Atkins told him, switching artfully to the Socratic method. "Do you like meat?"

"Yes."

"Could you eat a steak?" "Yes."

"All by itself, without any French fries?"

"Yes."

"And let's say we threw in a salad, but you couldn't have any bread or anything else."

"Yeah, I could do that."

"Well, if you could go through life like that....Do you like eggs in the morning? Or a cheese omelette?"

"Yes," Robert said, his voice almost giddy with relief. He called expecting a life sentence of rice cakes. Now he was being sent forth to eat cheeseburgers. "Yes, I do!"

"If you just eat that way," Atkins told him, "you'll have eighty pounds off in six months."

When I first arrived at Atkins' headquarters, two members of his staff took me on a quick tour of the facility, a vast medical center, where Atkins administers concoctions of his own creation to people suffering from a variety of disorders. Starting from the fifth floor, we went down to the third, and then from the third to the second, taking the elevator each time. It's a small point, but it did strike me as odd that I should be in the headquarters of the world's most popular weight-loss expert and be taking the elevator one floor at a time. After watching Atkins' show, I was escorted out by his public-relations assistant. We were on the second floor. He pressed the elevator button, down. "Why don't we take the stairs?" I asked. It was just a suggestion. He looked at me and then at the series of closed doors along the corridor. Tentatively, he opened the second. "I think this is it," he said, and we headed down, first one flight and then another. At the base of the steps was a door. The P.R. man, a slender fellow in a beautiful Italian suit, peered through it: for the moment, he was utterly lost. We were in the basement. It seemed as if nobody had gone down those stairs in a long time.

4

Why are the Pima so fat? The answer that diet books would give is that the Pima don't eat as well as they used to. But that's what is ultimately wrong with diet books. They talk as if food were the only cause of obesity and its only solution, and we know, from just looking at the Pima, that things are not that simple. The diet of the Pima is bad, but no worse than anyone else's diet.

Exercise is also clearly part of the explanation for why obesity has become epidemic in recent years. Half as many Americans walk to work today as did twenty years ago. Over the same period, the number of calories burned by the average American every day has dropped by about two hundred and fifty. But this doesn't explain why obesity has hit the Pima so hard, either, since they don't seem to be any less active than the rest of us.

The answer, of course, is that there is something beyond diet and exercise that influences obesity—that can make the consequences of a bad diet or of a lack of exercise much worse than they otherwise would be—and this is genetic inheritance. Claude Bouchard, a professor of social and preventive medicine at Laval University, in Quebec City, and one of the world's leading obesity specialists, estimates that we human beings probably carry several dozen genes that are directly related to our weight. "Some affect appetite, some affect satiety. Some affect metabolic rate, some affect the partitioning of excess energy in fat or lean tissue," he told me. "There are also reasons to believe that there are genes affecting physical-activity level." Bouchard did a study not long ago in which he took a group of men of similar height, weight, and life style and overfed them by a thousand calories a day, six days a week, for a hundred days. The average weight gain in the group was eighteen pounds. But the range was from nine to twenty-six pounds. Clearly, the men who gained just nine pounds were the ones whose genes had given them the fastest possible metabolism—the ones who burn the most calories in daily living and are the least efficient at storing fat. These are people who have the easiest time staying thin. The men at the other end of the scale are closer to the Pima in physiology. Their obesity genes thriftily stored away as much of the thousand extra calories a day as possible.

One of the key roles for genes appears to be in determining what obesity researchers refer to as setpoints. In the classic experiment in the field, researchers took a group of rats and made a series of lesions in the base of each rat's brain. As a result, the rats began overeating and ended up much more obese than normal rats. The first conclusion is plain: there is a kind of thermostat in the brain that governs appetite and weight, and if you change the setting on that thermostat appetite and weight will change accordingly. With that finding in mind, the researchers took a second step. They took those same brain-damaged rats and put them on a diet, severely limiting the amount of food they could eat. What happened? The rats didn't lose weight. In fact, after some initial fluctuations, they ended up at exactly the same weight as before. Only, this time, being unable to attain their new thermostat setting by eating, they reached it by becoming less active—by burning less energy.

Two years ago, a group at Rockefeller University in New York published a landmark study essentially duplicating in human beings what had been done years ago in rats. They found that if you lose weight your body responds by starting to conserve energy: your metabolism slows down; your muscles seem to work more efficiently, burning fewer calories to do the same work. "Let's say you have two people, side by side, and these people have exactly the same body composition," Jules Hirsch, a member of the Rockefeller team, says. "They both weigh a hundred and thirty pounds. But there is one difference—the first person maintains his weight effortlessly, while the second person, who used to weigh two hundred pounds, is trying to maintain a lower weight. The second will need fifteen per cent fewer calories per day to do his work. He needs less oxygen and will burn less energy." The body of the second person is backpedalling furiously in response to all that lost weight. It is doing everything it can to gain it back. In response to weight gain, by contrast, the Rockefeller team found that the body speeds up metabolism and burns more calories during exercise. It tries to lose that extra weight. Human beings, like rats, seem to have a predetermined setpoint, a weight that their body will go to great lengths to maintain.

One key player in this regulatory system may be a chemical called leptin—or, as it is sometimes known, Ob protein—whose discovery four years ago, by Jeff Friedman, of the Howard Hughes Medical Institute at Rockefeller University, prompted a flurry of headlines. In lab animals, leptin tells the brain to cut back on appetite, to speed up metabolism, and to burn stored fat. The theory is that the same mechanism may work in human beings. If you start to overeat, your fat cells will produce more leptin, so your body will do everything it can to get back to the setpoint. That's why after gaining a few pounds over the holiday season most of us soon return to our normal weight. But if you eat too little or exercise too much, the theory goes, the opposite happens: leptin levels fall. "This is probably the reason that virtually every weight-loss program known to man fails," José F. Caro, vice-president of endocrine research and clinical investigation at Eli Lilly & Company, told me. "You go to Weight Watchers. You start losing weight. You feel good. But then your fat cells stop producing leptin. Remember, leptin is the hormone that decreases appetite and increases energy expenditure, so just as you are trying to lose weight you lose the hormone that helps you lose weight."

Obviously, our body's fat thermostat doesn't keep us at one weight all our adult lives. "There isn't a single setpoint for a human being or an animal," Thomas Wadden, the director of the Weight and Eating Disorders Clinic at the University of Pennsylvania, told me. "The body will regulate a stable weight but at very different levels, depending on food intake—quality of the diet, high fat versus low fat, high sweet versus low sweet—and depending on the amount of physical activity." It also seems to be a great deal easier to move the setpoint up than to move it down—which, if you think about the Pima, makes perfect sense. In their long history in the desert, those Pima who survived were the ones who were very good at gaining weight during times of plenty—very good, in other words, at overriding the leptin system at the high end. But there would have been no advantage for the ones who were good at losing weight in hard times. The same is probably true for the rest of us, albeit in a less dramatic form. In our evolutionary history, there was advantage in being able to store away whatever calorific windfalls came our way. To understand this interplay between genes and environment, imagine two women, both five feet five. The first might have a setpoint range of a hundred and ten to a hundred and fifty pounds; the second a range of a hundred and twenty-five to a hundred and eighty. The difference in the ranges of the two women is determined by their genes. Where they are in that range is determined by their life styles.

Not long after leptin was discovered, researchers began testing obese people for the hormone, to see whether a fat person was fat because his body didn't produce enough leptin. They found the opposite: fat people had lots of leptin. Some of the researchers thought this meant that the leptin theory was wrong—that leptin didn't do what it was supposed to do. But some other scientists now think that as people get fatter and fatter, their bodies simply get less and less sensitive to leptin. The body still pumps out messages to the brain calling for the metabolism to speed up and the appetite to shrink, but the brain just doesn't respond to those messages with as much sensitivity as it did. This is probably why it is so much easier to gain weight than it is to lose it. The fatter you get, the less effective your own natural weight-control system becomes.

This doesn't mean that diets can't work. In those instances in which dieters have the discipline and the will power to restrict their calories permanently, to get regular and vigorous exercise, and to fight the attempt by their own bodies to maintain their current weight, pounds can be lost. (There is also some evidence that if you can keep weight off for an extensive period—three years, say—a lower setpoint can be established.)

Most people, though, don't have that kind of discipline, and even if they do have it the amount of weight that most dieters can expect to lose on a permanent basis may be limited by their setpoint range. The N.I.H. has a national six-year diabetes-prevention study going on right now, in which it is using a program of intensive, one-on-one counselling, dietary modification, and two and a half hours of exercise weekly to see if it can get overweight volunteers to lose seven per cent of their body weight. If that sounds like a modest goal, it should. "A lot of studies look at ten-percent weight loss," said Mary Hoskin, who is coordinating the section of the N.I.H. study involving the Pima. "But if you look at long-term weight loss nobody can maintain ten per cent. That's why we did seven."

On the other hand, now that we're coming to understand the biology of weight gain, it is possible to conceive of diet drugs that would actually work. If your body sabotages your diet by lowering leptin levels as you lose weight, why not give extra leptin to people on diets? That's what a number of drug companies, including Amgen and Eli Lilly, are working on now. They are trying to develop a leptin or leptin-analogue pill that dieters could take to fool their bodies into thinking they're getting fatter when they're actually getting thinner. "It is very easy to lose weight," José Caro told me. "The difficult thing is to maintain your weight loss. The thinking is that people fail because their leptin goes down. Here is where replacement therapy with leptin or an Ob-protein analogue might prevent the relapse. It is a subtle and important concept. What it tells you is that leptin is not going to be a magic bullet that allows you to eat whatever you want. You have to initiate the weight loss. Then leptin comes in."

Another idea, which the Hoffmann-La Roche company is exploring, is to focus on the problems obese people have with leptin. Just as Type II diabetics can become resistant to insulin, many overweight people may become resistant to leptin. So why not try to resensitize them? The idea is to find the leptin receptor in the brain and tinker with it to make it work as well in a fat person as it does in a thin person. (Drug companies have actually been pursuing the same strategy with the insulin receptors of diabetics.) Arthur Campfield, who heads the leptin project for Roche, likens the process by which leptin passes the signal about fat to the brain to a firemen's bucket brigade, where water is passed from hand to hand. "If you have all tall people, you can pass the bucket and it's very efficient, "he said. "But if two of the people in the chain are small children, then you're going to spill a lot of water and slow everything down. We want to take a tablet or a capsule that goes into your brain and puts a muscular person in the chain and overcomes that weakness. The elegant solution is to find the place in the chain where we are losing water."

The steps that take place in the brain when it receives the leptin message are known as the Ob pathway, and any number of these steps may lend themselves to pharmaceutical intervention. Using the Ob pathway to fight obesity represents a quantum leap beyond the kinds of diet drugs that have been available so far. Fen-phen, the popular medication removed from the market last year because of serious side effects, was, by comparison, a relatively crude product, which worked indirectly to suppress appetite. Hoffmann-La

Roche is working now on a drug called Xenical, a compound that blocks the absorption of dietary fat by the intestine. You can eat fat; you just don't keep as much of it in your system. The drug is safe and has shown real, if modest, success in helping chronically obese patients lose weight. It will probably be the next big diet drug. But no one is pretending that it has anywhere near the potential of, say, a drug that would resensitize your leptin receptors.

Campfield talks about the next wave of drug therapy as the third leg of a three-legged stool—as the additional element that could finally make diet and exercise an easy and reliable way to lose weight. Wadden speaks of the new drugs as restoring sanity: "What I think will happen is that people on these medications will report that they are less responsive to their environment. They'll say that they are not as turned on by Wendy's or McDonald's. Food in America has become a recreational activity. It is divorced from nutritional need and hunger. We eat to kill time, to stimulate ourselves, to alter our mood. What these drugs may mean is that we're going to become less susceptible to these messages." In the past thirty years, the natural relationship between our bodies and our environment—a relation that was developed over thousands of years—has fallen out ofbalance. For people who cannot restore that natural balance themselves—who lack the discipline, the wherewithal, or, like the Pima, the genes—drugs could be a way of restoring it for them.

5

Seven years ago, Peter Bennett, the epidemiologist who first stumbled on the Gila River Pima twenty-eight years earlier, led an N.I.H. expedition to Mexico's Sierra Madre Mountains. Their destination was a a tiny Indian community on the border of Sonora and Chihuahua, seven thousand feet above the desert. "I had known about their existence for at least fifteen years before that," Bennett says. "The problem was that I could never find anyone who knew much about them. In 1991, it just happened that we linked up with an investigator down in Mexico." The journey was a difficult one, but the Mexican government had just built a road linking Sonora and Chihuahua, so the team didn't have to make the final fifty- or sixty-mile trek on horseback. "They were clearly a group who have got along together for a very long time," Bennett recalls. "My reaction as a stranger going in was: Gee, I think these people are really very friendly, very cooperative. They seem to be interested in what we want to do, and they are willing to stick their arms out and let us take blood samples." He laughed. "Which is always a good sign."

The little town in the Sierra Madre is home to the Mexican Pima, the southern remnants of a tribe that once stretched from present-day Arizona down to central Mexico. Like the Pima of the Gila River reservation, they are farmers, living in small clusters of wood-and-adobe rancherías among the pine trees, cultivating beans, corn, and potatoes in the valleys. On that first trip, the N.I.H. team examined no more than a few dozen Pima. Since then, the team has been back five or six times, staying for as many as ten days at a time. Two hundred and fifty of the mountain Pima have now been studied. They have been measured and weighed, their blood sugar has been checked, and their kidneys and eyes have been examined for signs of damage. Genetic samples have been taken and their metabolism has been monitored. The Mexican Pima, it turns out, eat a diet consisting almost entirely of beans, potatoes, and corn tortillas, with chicken perhaps once a month. They take in twenty-two hundred calories a day, which is slightly more than the Pima of Arizona do. But on the average each of them puts in twenty-three hours a week of moderate to hard physical labor, whereas the average Arizona Pima puts in two hours. The Mexican Pima's rates of diabetes are normal. They are slightly shorter than their American counterparts. In weight, there is no comparison: "I would say they are thin," Bennett says. "Thin. Certainly by American standards."

There are, of course, a hundred reasons not to draw any great lessons from this. Subsistence farming is no way to make a living in America today, nor are twenty-three hours of hard physical labor feasible in a society where most people sit at a desk from nine to five. And even if the Arizona Pima wanted to return to the land, they couldn't. It has been more than a hundred years since the Gila River, which used to provide the tribe with fresh fish and with water for growing beans and squash, was diverted upstream for commercial farming. Yet there is value in the example of the Mexican Pima. People who work with the Pima of Arizona say that the biggest problem they have in trying to fight diabetes and obesity is fatalism—a sense among the tribe that nothing can be done, that the way things are is the way things have to be. It is possible to see in the attitudes of Americans toward weight loss the same creeping resignation. As the world grows fatter, and as one best-selling diet scheme after another inevitably fails, the idea that being slender is an attainable—or even an advisable—condition is slowly receding. Last month, when The New England Journal of Medicine published a study suggesting that the mortality costs of obesity had been overstated, the news was greeted with resounding relief, as if we were all somehow off the hook, as if the issue with obesity were only mortality and not the thousand ways in which being fat undermines our quality of life: the heightened risk of heart disease, hypertension, diabetes, cancer, arthritis, gallbladder disease, trauma, gout, blindness, birth defects, and other aches, pains, and physical indignities too numerous to mention. What we are in danger of losing in the epidemic of obesity is not merely our health but our memory of health. Those Indian towns high in the Sierra Madre should remind the people of Sacaton—and all the rest of us as well—that it is still possible, even for a Pima, to be fit.

CHAPTER 50

Junk Food Monkeys

Robert M. Sapolsky

(1989)

Few of us think much about Jean-Jacques Rousseau these days. We remember his noble savage, his idealized view of mankind in its primordial splendor, when life was gentle, innocent, and natural. Not that most of us reject Rousseau's thinking; it's just that amid the bustle and ambition of the Me Generation and Reagan's eighties, it no longer seems fashionable to ponder the possibly superior moral state of primordial humans.

Their possibly superior physical state, however, is an issue of more than passing concern, and here a Rousseauean view of sorts continues to hold sway—a view, that is, with an eighties spin. As a society that spends billions of dollars on medical care, health clubs, and looking good, what we want to know is: How was the physical health of primordial humans? What was their secret workout regimen for achieving their beautiful precivilized bodies? What were cholesterol levels like in the Garden of Eden?

Many think that in certain respects early humans fared better than we do. When you subtract the accidents, infections, and infantile diseases that beset them, our forebears might not have had it so bad. In a 1985 article in the *New England Journal of Medicine*, physician-anthropologists S. Boyd Eaton and Melvin Konner did an ingenious job of reconstructing the likely diet of our Paleolithic ancestors, and they concluded that there was much to be said for the high-fiber, low-salt, low-fat diet their evidence suggested.

Anthropologists studying the hunter-gatherers in the Kalahari Desert, a group that's believed to retain the way of life of earlier humans, have come to similar conclusions. Among the !Kung, for example, some maladies that we view as a normal part of human aging are proving not to be obligatory after all: hearing acuity is not lost, blood pressure and cholesterol levels do not rise, degenerative heart disease doesn't seem to develop. As we sit here amid our ulcers and hypertension and hardening arteries, it is getting harder for us to avoid the uncomfortable suspicion that we have fallen from a state of metabolic grace.

For the past decade I have been observing a group of some of our closest relatives as they fell from their own primordial metabolic grace into something resembling our nutritional decadence. My subjects are olive baboons living

in the Masai Mara National Reserve in the Serengeti Plain of Kenya.

Chiefly I'm interested in the relationships between their social behavior and dominance rank, the amount of social stress the baboons experience, and how their bodies react to it. Certainly I didn't set out to investigate the relevance of eighteenth-century French philosophy to twentieth-century American life by looking at a timeless primate society in the African plains. But to study the questions I am interested in, I have to combine extensive behavioral observations with some basic lab work: drawing the animals' blood, measuring hormones, monitoring blood pressure, and conducting other clinical tests to find out how their bodies are functioning. And in this context Rousseau reared his worrisome head.

Masai Mara is a wonderful place to be a researcher. It's a fairly idyllic place to be a baboon: a vast untouched landscape of savannas and woodlands and one of the last great refuges for wild animals left on Earth. Herds of wildebeest roam on the open plains, lions lounge beneath the flat-topped acacia trees, giraffes and zebras drink side by side at the watering places. Inevitably Masai Mara has also become an attractive place to tourists, resulting in all the usual problems that occur when large fluxes of people descend on previously virgin wilderness.

One of the biggest problems here, as in our own national parks, is what to do with the garbage. The solution so far has been to dump much of it into large pits, 5 feet deep by 30 feet wide, hidden among trees in out-of-the-way areas. Brimming with food and refuse rotting in 100-degree heat, infested with flies and circled by vultures and hyenas, the pits look like a scene from a Hieronymus Bosch painting. One of the baboon troops I study had such a garden of earthly delights dumped right in the middle of its territory.

For the baboons this was a major change in fortune, the primatological equivalent, perhaps, of winning the lottery. A major concern in any wild animal's life is getting sufficient food, and an average baboon in the Serengeti spends 30 to 40 percent of each day foraging—climbing trees to reach fruits and leaves, digging laboriously in the ground to unearth tubers, walking five or ten miles to reach sources of food. Their diet is Spartan: figs and olives, grass and sedge parts, corms, tubers, and seedpods. It's unusual for them to hunt

Robert M. Sapolsky, "Junk food monkeys." *Discover*, September 1989:48–51. Reprinted with permission.

or scavenge, and meat accounts for less than one percent of the food they consume. So the typical baboon diet teems with fiber and is very low in fat, sugar, and cholesterol.

For the nouveau riche Garbage Dump troop, life changed dramatically. When I started observing them, in 1978, they had recently discovered the dump's existence and were making an occasional food run. By 1980 the entire group—some 80 animals, ranging from 25-year-old adults to newborn infants—had moved into new sleeping quarters in the trees surrounding the dump. Instead of stirring at dawn, these animals would typically stay in the trees, snoozing and grooming, and only rouse themselves in time to meet the 9 A.M. garbage tractor. The day's feeding would be finished after half an hour of communal frenzy over the pickings. But it was the pickings themselves that made the biggest difference in the baboons' lives.

Once, in the name of science, I donned lab gloves, held my breath, and astonished the tractor driver by methodically sifting through his moldering garbage. The refuse was certainly a far cry from tubers and leaves: fried drumsticks or a slab of beef left over by a tourist with eyes bigger than his stomach; fruit salad gone a bit bad, perhaps left too long on the sun-drenched buffet table; fragments of pies and cakes, and alarming yellow dollops of custard pudding, nibbled at by a disciplined dieter—processed sugars, fat, starch, and cholesterol, our modern Four Horsemen of the Apocalypse.

And what were the physiological consequences for these baboons in Utopia? First the good news: Young baboons grew faster, reaching developmental landmarks such as puberty at earlier ages. These beneficial changes were exactly what one would expect of humans switching from a lean subsistence diet to a more affluent Westernized fare. In the countries of the West the age of first menstruation has declined from an estimated 15 years during the 1800s to our current average of about 12 and a half.

The trend in baboons has been particularly well documented by Jeanne Altmann of the University of Chicago, a biologist studying both foraging and garbage-eating troops in another park in Kenya. Among her animals, eating garbage has led to the onset of puberty at age three and a half instead of age five. Females now typically give birth for the first time at age five, a year and a half earlier than before. Moreover, because the infants develop faster, they are weaned earlier; consequently, females start menstruating again that much sooner, and once they resume, they conceive more quickly. Indeed, Altmann's garbage eaters have had something of a baby boom compared with their foraging cousins.

Another advantage of garbage eating became clear during the tragic East African drought of 1984. During that period wild game found life extremely difficult. The luckier animals merely spent more time and covered more distance in search of food. The less lucky starved and succumbed to diseases previously held in check. However, tourists did not starve, and neither did baboons living off their detritus.

So, at first glance, from the evolutionary standpoint of reproductive fitness, some daily custard pudding appears to do wonders, increasing reproductive rates and buffering the troop from famine. But now here's the bad news: some of the same lousy changes seen in humans eating Westernized fare also occurred in baboons.

Your average wild baboon eating a natural diet has cholesterol levels that would shame the most ectomorphic triathlete. University of Texas pathologist Glen Mott and I have studied a number of troops and found cholesterol levels averaging 66 milligrams in 100 cubic centimeters of blood among adult males. Not only that, but more than half the total cholesterol was in the form of high-density lipoproteins, the "good" type. In humans, cholesterol levels less than 150 with a third of the total in the high-density form are grounds for bragging at the health club.

But when we studied the Garbage Dump baboons, a different picture emerged. Cholesterol levels were nearly a third higher, and most of the increase was attributable to a rise in damaging low-density lipoproteins, the type that builds up plaque on artery walls.

Joseph Kemnitz, a primatologist at the Wisconsin Regional Primate Research Center, analyzed blood samples from these animals and found that levels of insulin were more than twice as high in the Garbage Dumpers as in those eating a natural diet. This hormone is secreted by the pancreas in response to eating, especially eating rich, sugary food, and its function is to tell cells to store glucose for future use as energy.

If insulin levels rise too high, however, cells become inured to its message; instead of being stored, glucose is left circulating in the bloodstream. It's this state of affairs that can eventually lead to adult-onset diabetes, a distinctly Western malady. Since the Garbage Dumpers came from gene stocks similar to those of the natural foragers, genetic differences couldn't account for their much higher insulin levels. The most likely suspect was their junk-food diet and their relative inactivity.

Are the Garbage Dumpers now at risk for diabetes and heart disease, candidates for celebrity diets and coronary bypasses? It is hard to tell; no one has ever reported adult-onset diabetes in wild baboons, but, then, no one has ever looked. Surprisingly, people have looked at the cardiovascular systems of wild baboons and found fatty deposits in their blood vessels and heart. Garbage Dumpers presumably run a higher risk of depositing fat in their arteries, but whether it will affect their health and life spans remains to be seen.

One major impact on the health of Garbage Dumpers became clear in a grim way, however. If you are going to spend your time around human garbage, you are going to have to deal with whatever that garbage has become infected with. And if these infectious agents are new to you, your immunological defenses are not likely to be very good.

A few years ago my Garbage Dump animals began to become dramatically ill. They wasted away, coughing up blood, losing the use of their limbs. Three veterinarians from the Institute of Primate Research in Nairobi—Ross Tarara, Mbaruk Suleman, and James Else—investigated the outbreak and traced it to bovine tuberculosis, probably from eating contaminated meat. It was the first time the disease had been reported in wild primates, and by the time it abated it had killed half the Garbage Dump troop. For them, there had been no free lunch after all.

Has the Westernization of these animals' diets thus been good or bad? This is much the same as questioning the benefits of our own Westernization. Toxic wastes and automatic weapons strike me as bad developments; on the other hand, vaccines, thermal underwear, and 70-year life expectancies seem like marvelous improvements upon the Middle Ages. All things considered, we seem to have benefited, at least from a health perspective.

For the baboons, too, the answer must be carefully considered. Growing fat is unwise if you plan to sit in an arboreal armchair but very wise if you're about to face a dry season. Similarly, a nice piece of meat is a fine thing during a famine, but not such a hot idea if it's contaminated.

It is platitudinous to say that this is a complicated issue, but it is clear that life for the foraging baboon is not one of pure Rousseauean ease, nor life for the garbage eaters one of unambiguous decline. My bias is that the latter's health has, on the whole, suffered from their garbage trove. But what has struck me in these studies is that there are also benefits and the judgment is somewhat difficult to make. It seems that for the baboon, just as for us, there are few unambiguous rules for figuring out what to do with the choices life throws in our lap.

CHAPTER 51

Evolutionary and Anthropological Perspectives on Optimal Foraging in Obesogenic Environments

Leslie Sue Lieberman

(2006)

Ninety-eight percent of hominid existence has been shaped by hunting and foraging with selection for cognitive and behavioral repertories, nutritional requirements and physiological patterns adapted to harsh environments with fluctuations in food availability, food shortages and periodic high energy expenditures (Chakravarthy & Booth, 2004; Eaton, Shostak & Konner, 1988; Kuzawa, 1998; Loos & Rankinen, 2005; Mann, 2004). In this environment, an advantage accrued to hominids who had biological and behavioral mechanisms that insured (over)consumption of available food to meet immediate physiological needs as well as efficient storage of energy and macro- and micronutrients (Chakravarthy & Booth, 2004; Kuzawa, 1998).

These once adaptive cognitive, behavioral and physiological genotypes and phenotypes persist today in evolutionary-novel environments characterized by an abundance of supersized energy-dense foods with low energy-cost availability (Boon, Stroebe, Schut & Jansen, 1998; Booth, Pinkston & Poston, 2005; Brownell & Horgan, 2003; Nestle, 2003; Speakman, 2004). Modern environments, especially urban settings, afford lifestyles conducive to a surfeit of calories and consequent obesity (Popkin, 2001; Popkin & Gardon-Larson, 2004; Winterhalder & Smith, 1981).

This epidemic of overweight and obesity has now reached more than 1.1 billion persons worldwide with some adult populations reaching a prevalence of nearly 80% (International Obesity Task Force, 2004; Kuczmarski, Flegal, Campbell & Johnson, 1994; Lobstein, Baur, Uauy, & IASO International Obesity Task Force, 2004). In 2000, the World Health Organization (2000, 2003) estimated that worldwide there were 22 million overweight children and adolescents. A number of studies indicate that 15–30% of children in developed countries are overweight with percentages in developing countries rapidly rising (de Onis & Blossner, 2000; International Obesity Task-force, 2004; Lobstein et al., 2004). This paper addresses this pandemic by using models from evolutionary behavioral ecology to

elucidate obesogenic features and human behaviors in contemporary environments.

FORAGING THEORY APPLIED TO THE OBESOGENIC ENVIRONMENT

Foraging theory is a component of behavioral ecology that utilizes cost/benefit models to predict food-related behaviors, prey (including plants)–predator interactions and characteristics of the environment. Most cost/benefit models use energy as the currency. Because food is essential to meet nutrient and energy requirements for survival, growth and reproduction, foraging theory provides explanatory models linking the environment through adaptive food-related behaviors that, theoretically, maximize inclusive fitness or reproductive success (MacArthur & Pianka, 1966; Mann, 2004). Illius, Tolkamp, and Yearsley (2002) question whether or not humans have become too 'successful' and now face new selective pressures that compromise fitness. They speculate that in modern environments, obesity and its sequelae, such as type 2 diabetes, are new intrinsic costs or trade-offs that reduce physiological and reproductive fitness. Overly nourished populations have decoupled predicted demographic and epidemiological trends by decreasing their production of offspring and living longer but metabolically challenged lives (Eaton & Eaton, 1999; Popkin, 1994, 2001; Popkin & Gordon-Larson, 2004).

These are interesting speculations but difficult to assess since many factors can influence fitness and there are many critiques of overly enthusiastic adaptation scenarios (Senervo, 1997). Instead, this paper examines proximate food-related behaviors and characteristics of the obesogenic environment that promote the operation of our cognitive and behavioral legacies. The thesis is that humans "continue to use cues from their food and foraging that were part of a previously successful foraging strategy which, in modern conditions, is counterproductive" (Illius et al., 2002, p. 470).

For example, prehistoric and historic external constraints such as the availability of food resources, the travel time between patches of food and the energy costs of hunting, gathering and processing food have all drastically

Leslie Sue Lieberman, "Evolutionary and anthropological perspectives on optimal foraging in obesogenic environments." *Appetite* 47 (2006): 3–9. Reprinted with permission.

diminished in most modern environments. In addition, food processing has significantly reduced or altered intrinsic constraints such as gastric capacity, gut transit times, the need for endogenous production of specific digestive enzymes, and the presence of parasites and toxins. Dietary modernization universally involves increased energy intake with processed energy-dense, fat-rich and fiber-poor foods, and both increased quantity and ingestion frequency. (Chakravarthy & Booth, 2004; Lieberman, 2003; Popkin, 2001).

Globalized 'Fast food meals' are often a combination of low bulk, fiber-poor starches, fatty or oily foods and highly sugared drinks. Relative to Paleolithic diets, these foods produce metabolic impacts that are obesity-enhancing such as high insulin and glucose levels, alterations in lipid profiles, and the blunted satiating effect of some frequently consumed ingredients, such as high-fructose corn syrup (Melanson, 2004). Metabolic efficiency in past environments was advantageous but in modern environments, it has created a perverse normalcy of excessive weight gain.

OPTIMAL FORAGING: ENERGY COSTS AND PROFITABILITY

A central theorem of foraging theory is that animals operate to increase energy intake and reduce energy costs (MacArthur & Pianka, 1966). Profitability defined as energy gain per unit time or effort has markedly increased in modern environments. Foraging in obesogenic landscapes requires little energy expenditure to acquire big energy payoffs (Popkin & Gordon-Larsen, 2004; Winter-halder & Smith, 1981). A number of factors account for this.

First, search time is significantly reduced because of the ubiquitous presence of colorful food advertising, signs and signals (e.g., McDonalds's golden arches). Second, travel and search time are further reduced because there is a high density of food patches or outlets where food is available 24 hours a day in restaurants, gas stations, vending machines, kiosks, supermarkets, fast food outlets, schools and homes, etcetera. For example, McDonalds alone has more than 31,000 stores worldwide, Subway 22,000, Pizza Hut 20,000 and Kentucky Fried Chicken 12,000 (in approximate numbers) (Spurlock, 2005; various Internet data sources). Global Information System technology would be helpful in plotting patch density, travel routes and time versus energy intakes. Third, availability is assured and reliable. Fast food establishments and chain restaurants have the same menus so patches rarely move and they are rarely seasonal. Fourth, travel time to patches is short because of the use of cars or public transportation. Fifth, these modes of transport use little human energy. While an hour of cooking and doing domestic chores is scored as 2.1–2.3 PAR (= physical activity ratio, representing multiples of the basal metabolic rate (BMR), so cooking and domestic chores require about two times the energy expenditure as the BMR), walking without a load is 3.2 PAR, an hour of eating is only about 1.5 PAR and driving a car 2.0 PAR (Cordain, Gotshall, Eaton, & Eaton,

1998; Jenike, 2001). Overall, physical activity levels (PAL = total daily energy expenditure/BMR) for hunting and foraging groups averages 1.15–2.15 PALs compared to sedentary office workers averaging 1.16–1.18 9 PALs (Jenike, 2001). Sixth, the time spent in the patches to obtain food is short (e.g., drive-in service, fast food restaurants, home delivered meals, supermarkets). Foods are readily available, prepackaged and arrayed in the patch in ways that facilitate easy and quick 'capture'. The trade journal *Progressive Grocer* presents supermarket layouts that are designed to increase customer exposure, access and purchases. Seventh, food processing or preparation time and energy costs are low because foods are purchased already highly processed and ready-to-eat. Americans increasingly value convenience, low time and energy investments in food preparation (Rozin, 2005). In a recent survey, 34% of Americans indicated that they preferred to 'dine out' or have a meal catered in their home for Thanksgiving and Christmas, dinners that traditionally have involved extensive preparation time (Hales, 2005). Daily, 40% of US adults eat in restaurants. Sales exceeded $440 billion or $920/person for food consumed with little time or energy spent on food acquisition, preparation, service or cleaning up after the meal (Hales, 2005). Eighth, processed foods are calorie-dense, low in fiber and other bulking components, and thereby allow large intakes. Fast foods appeal to hominid preferences for sweet tastes and fatty creamy or crunchy textures (Rozin, 2005). Fast foods are inexpensive relative to their caloric density. For example, a hamburger (120 g), small French fries (105 g) and soft drink (355 ml) costs about $2.00US or 300 kcals/$1.00. Drewnowski and Spector (2004) demonstrated that energy-dense fast foods provide more calories per dollar than more expensive watery fruits and vegetables. This positive cost/benefit ratio can be invoked to explain the 'paradox' of high rates of obesity in low-income populations in the US. Furthermore, lower income neighborhoods have a higher per capita concentration of fast food restaurants (i.e., higher patch density), lower concentration of supermarkets, and fewer opportunities for safe exercising than do higher income neighborhoods (Booth et al., 2005).

OPTIMAL FORAGING: MARGINAL VALUE THEOREM

The Marginal Value Theorem describes decisions about when, where and how long to stop for a feeding bout among widely scattered food patches (Sinervo, 1997). Under most circumstances, as animals and humans feed, the energy gain declines as the food becomes scarcer in the patch. However, in obesogenic environments there is an endless supply of food, there is no decreasing rate of return for time invested. There are often few time constraints as food is available 24 hours a day with little seasonal variation. As noted above, often very little time is spent in or near the patch, for example, drive-in or pick-up service is designed to acquire more food and faster. Meals are also delivered to people's homes. The tendency to maximize the net rate of energy gain (i.e., calories per unit time) is accomplished in part by supersizing, ready-to-eat, energy-dense, low fiber, easily digested foods.

A corollary involves the quality of the foods in the patch. Animals seek out patches of high quality and will move among patches until their sampling effort finds the highest rate of gain. The same reasoning may apply to humans. So, there is an advantage for restaurants to offer both larger portion sizes and more variety. Fast food restaurants and other restaurant chains replicate themselves, reducing travel time among them and enticing customers who know that they will be a entering a high-quality patch with the anticipated 'prey'. Capture efficiency is almost always high and risks (e.g., a car accident, food poising) are low. Exploiting these food patches does not deplete them. They are endlessly renewable; thereby, negating a need to consider moving one's residence to reduce travel time to a dependable patch.

CONVENIENCE AND THE BUILT ENVIRONMENT

The built environment, daily habits and cultural values can make small but consistent differences in energy intake and expenditure that lead to big differences in obesity prevalence. For example, Frenchmen are physically active based on necessities of the built environment (e.g., few elevators), convenient walking distances (e.g., small markets in mixed residential and commercial neighborhoods) and traditions of walking and biking (Rozin, 2005). These aspects of lifestyle account, in part, for the three-fold difference (11% versus 30%) in French versus American obesity prevalence (Rozin, 2005).

Industrialized nations are marvels of ergonomic efficiency with remote controls and cordless or cellular phones. The number of hours of sedentary activities such as watching television and DVD's or playing videogames is positively correlated with weight gains for both children (Rachagan, 2004) and adults (Stroebele & de Castro, 2004). The Kaiser Family Foundation (1999, 2003) documented that children aged 2–18 years spent an average of 5 h and 29 min/day using media of which 2 h and 46 min were spent watching television and over two-thirds of children under 2 years of age spent a little over 2 h a day watching television. In a study of six Asian countries, 30% for Malaysian but only 2% for Pakistani children watched 8 h or more of television during school vacation days (Rachagan, 2004).

GLOBALIZED FOOD TRENDS AND DIETARY BREADTH

As big-brained omnivores, we enjoy and seek dietary variety to balance nutrient requirements. Plant and animal evidence from Paleolithic sites to the present documents dietary breadth and geographic and seasonal dietary variation (Eaton et al., 1988; Unger & Teaford, 2002). Extensive studies of three species of apes show that they consume an average of 94 plant species while a classic hunting and foraging population, the !Kung of the Kalahari desert, consume 110 species of plants (Lee & Devore, 1968; Rodman, 2002).

Dietary diversity is an important factor increasing consumption (Rolls et al., 1981; Wansink, 2004b). Satiation, the feeling that you have eaten enough, is achieved more quickly when food choices are limited because dietary monotony produces sensory-specific satiety (Melanson, 2004; Wansink, 2004a, b). For example, people eat more at buffets than in other food service settings or when food is served 'family style' in bowls on the table providing numerous food cues. In a series of experiments with jelly beans, people given a bowl of jelly beans with six different colors ate about 60% more than those given a bowl with jelly beans of only four colors even though both bowls had the same number of jelly beans and all the colors tasted the same (Wansink, 2004b).

Fast food giants such as McDonalds have responded to the popularity of low-carbohydrate diets by adding salads and other healthful options to their menus; thus, increasing choices and profits (Brownell & Horgan, 2003; Nestle, 2003; Schlosser, 2001). One strategy is to produce a cuisine with novel fusions of food items and spice appealing to local tastes. Pizza Hut produces a *kung pao* chicken pizza in Taiwan and a *kimchi* pizza in Korea and KFC serves soup and dumplings in China (Rachagan, 2004). Even specialty foods (i.e., high protein bars, low calorie drinks) are produced in multiple flavors and sizes. In 2004, 948 new reduced-sugar products were introduced into the US food market (Spurlock, 2005, p. 258). More products mean increased consumption and higher profits (Schlosser, 2001; Wansink, 2004a).

This diversity in the food supply may, in part, be subjected to what some evolutionary biologists and psychologists postulate is a search image composed of a small number of salient cues used to identify foods (Sinervo, 1997). Advertising defines and manipulates these cues to increase variety and increased consumption (Wansink 2004a, b). Interestingly, the food industry has evolved foods with elaborate cryptic adaptations such as tofu turkeys, sugar-free products that taste sweet or fat-free foods with the correct mouthfeel (Fellows, 2000). Rozin (2005) asserts that in ancestral environments, appearance equaled reality but that modern populations, particularly those in (sub)urban environments, have lost their intimacy with food.

GLOBALIZED FOOD TRENDS: LARGE PORTION SIZES

Larger portion sizes of foods characterize obesogenic environments. Supersizing, which began in the 1990s, costs the industry pennies because most of the cost is in advertising, packaging and labor (Brownell & Horgan, 2003; Nestle, 2003; Spurlock, 2005). Therefore, larger portions are actually more profitable for the fast food companies; consumers expect them and get more food for their money (Spurlock, 2005).

Portion size is a potent environmental determinant of how much a person eats (Diliberti, Bordi, Conklin, Roe & Rolls, 2004; Rolls, 2003; Wansink, 2004a, b; Young & Nestle, 2002). People given large buckets of movie theater popcorn ate 50% more than those given smaller buckets. When both groups were asked to estimate the amount or the calories they had eaten, there was no significant difference in their reported intakes (Wansink, 2004a, b). In an M&M candy experiment, people given 1 lb bags of M&M's ate 120 M&M's compared to people given a ½ lb bag, who ate 63 M&M's while watching a videotape. A number of researchers suggest that the size of the package or portion gives people a perceptual consumption cue as to what is 'normal' or acceptable (Grier & Rozin, 2005; Wansink, 2004b) regardless of the amount they actually consume. Unit size perceptions are deceptive. For example, a single-packaged large muffin would appear to be single serving although the label informs the consumer that the 660 kcal muffin is really three servings (Nestle, 2003). Furthermore, normative or standard sizes have increased. For example, the retail 'standards' for fruit drinks, carbonated beverages and ice teas have increased from 240 ml to nearly 1000 ml over the last decade.

A large body of research on portion size shows that individuals miscalculate portion sizes for all types of food items (Godwin, Chambers, & Cleveland, 2004). Even with the aid of measuring devices and training, people continue to miscalculate portion sizes (Furbisher & Maxwell, 2003). Cross-cultural and ethnic differences on culturally salient 'common' measures have not been well researched. From an evolutionary perspective, there may have been little selection pressure favoring accurate and precise judgments about portion sizes because the natural environment already constrained the size and amount of available food (Jenike, 2001; Ungar & Teaford, 2002).

GLOBALIZED FOOD TRENDS: UBIQUITOUS VISUAL FOOD CUES

Modern environments are filled with an array of visual stimuli of actual food items, their representations in the media, and universally recognized iconic images and logos (e.g., McDonald's golden arches). These images transcend cultural and linguistic boundaries. The visual appeal is purposeful and effective because vision is the primary primate mode of perception (Jones, Martin & Pilbeam, 1992). As the architecture of the primate face evolved, rotation of the eye orbits to the front of the face necessitated to reduction of the snout and the olfactory sense. Hence, vision is the primary sense used to negotiate the current obesogenic environment. Vision of palatable stimuli can initiate the cephalic phase of digestion by increasing gastric motility and the secretion of saliva, gastric acid, gastrointestinal hormones and pancreatic enzymes (Katschinski, 2000). These stimuli signal learned messages about the nutritional and physiological effects of particular foods. For primates, initial food cues are often visual with color as a primary salient property (Dominy & Lucas, 2004; Post, 1962).

Primate brains have neurological features that result in excellent depth perception as well as input to higher cortical areas involved in attention to visual stimuli and perception of movement, position, color and visual learning (Jones et al., 1992). Vision and visual memory are used to locate and exploit food patches. Natural selection favored depth perception, color vision, grasping hands and coordinated eye–hand movements for tree-dwelling, insect, flower, fruit and seed-eating primates (Cartmill, 1974).

Color vision aids fruit-eating primates in determining the ripeness of fruit; and thereby, signals changes in taste (sweeter with more sugars); nutrient quantity and bioavailability; presence of phytochemicals; texture (density and softness); and aroma (Dominy & Lucas, 2004; Vorobyev, 2004). Color provides clues to the physiological consequences of ingestion, such as the production and/or release of insulin or increase in body temperature. Dichromatic monkeys and colorblind humans have difficulty in visually distinguishing between immature and ripe fruit (Vorobyev, 2004). Leaf maturity is also signaled by color change from reddish to green and used by leaf-eating primate species to select edible, young leaves often containing more protein and micronutrients, lower levels of toxins and less fiber than older leaves (Dominy & Lucas, 2001, 2004). Clearly, all these variables have implications for survival and reproductive fitness for all primates. Post (1962) has postulated that color vision conferred a selective advantage to human hunters and foragers because they could see prey more readily. The average frequency of colorblindness for males in 12 groups of contemporary hunters and foragers (e.g., Eskimo, Australian Aborigines, Native Americans) is less than 2% but ranges from 5–10% among agricultural–industrial groups.

Humans use color changes to signal when food is cooked (e.g., lobsters turn red, beef turns brown). Applying heat and observing color changes can indicate when pathogenic bacteria, other micro organisms and parasites have been killed. Food that is spoiling will change color (e.g., browning of lettuce leaves). Certain colors are cues for particular nutrients (e.g., orange and yellow are associated with carotene or pro-vitamin A). Food technology is used to enhance and retain natural color in fruits, vegetables, fish and meat (Fellows, 2000). Supermarkets display fruits and vegetables in colorful arrangements. Restaurant food displays, plastic food models and menus with color pictures are common throughout the world. Restaurant drive-ins place colorful food pictures on marquees near ordering stations. Full color food ads in magazines and newspapers, billboards, hand flyers and cookbooks are common. Colorful television and computer Internet ads for foods are abundant. Billions of dollars are spent on food advertising in visual media. For example, in 2004, $13 billion of an approximately $144 billion fast food advertising budget was spent on food advertising for children (Spurlock, 2005). US children watch an average of 20–40,000 TV commercials per year and 11–19 commercials per hour on food on Saturday mornings (Story & French, 2004). Children in the Philippines and Malaysia watch 20 min of advertising per hour and 40–75%

of these are for food and beverages high in sugar, fat and/or salt (Rachagan, 2004). Multinational food companies have begun to exploit other visual technologies for advertising: cell phones, iPods, Mp3 players and DVD's are used to build brand loyalty among children (Hawkes, 2004; Lang & Heasman, 2004; Schlosser, 2001; Spurlock, 2005).

Americans select fresh products based on color, size, shape and blemish-free appearance. This visual inspection occurs at a distance, well before aroma and after-purchase taste are used to assess palatability of the choices. US strawberries are a prime example of market demands for visually appealing but taste-compromised produce. Supermarkets reduce aromas by prepackaging foods, placing fresh food in refrigerated displays or freezing them.

The paradox of relying on visual cues is that they are very good for induction of eating but distractibility is a prime factor in overconsumption of food. Supersized, high-energy-dense foods and a high threshold to satiation further promote overconsumption. Once food is purchased, it is often packaged in ways or eaten under circumstances (e.g., in cars, watching television) that do not allow the consumer to monitor consumption rate or amount. People will continue to eat until the food is consumed or external signals terminate ingestion (Wansink, 2004b). The lack of sensitivity to internal cues of satiation may have been advantageous in feast and famine dietary environments (Melanson, 2004).

CONCLUSION

In summary, in obesogenic environments, the foraging costs are low (minimized) and the benefits in caloric intake are high (maximized) relative to prehistoric and historic feeding patterns. The demographic shift to urban and suburban environments affords both adults and children access to energy-saving conveniences, inexpensive processed foods and sedentary leisure activities. Optimal foraging models in these environments with abundant visual food cues predict behaviors in high density and easily accessible food patches. Evolution has honed human proclivities for voluminous eating and physiological capacities for energy storage that, coupled with modern lifestyles of energy-saving conveniences and rapid globalization of fast foods, promotes weight gain and obesity. Children are particularly vulnerable and are a primary marketing target. This confluence of modern lifestyles provides the opportunity, purveyors of fast foods provide the means and evolution has provided the physiological motive for the obesity pandemic. It is unclear what forces could compel an alteration in this trajectory.

References

Boon, B., Stroebe, W., Schut, H., & Jansen, A. (1998). Food for thought: Cognitive regulation of food intake. *British Journal of Health Psychology, 3*, 27–40.

Booth, K. M., Pinkston, M. M., & Poston, W. S. C. (2005). Obesity and the built environment. *Journal of the American Dietetic Association, 105*, 110–117.

Brownell, K. D., & Horgan, K. B. (2003). *Food fight: The inside story of the food industry, America's obesity crisis and what we can do about it.* New York: McGraw Hill.

Cartmill, M. (1974). Arboreal adaptations and the origins of the Order Primates. In H. R. Tuttle (Ed.), *The functional and evolutionary biology of primates* (pp. 97–122). Chicago: Aldine Atherton.

Chakravarthy, M. V., & Booth, F. A. (2004). Eating, exercise, and "thrifty" genotypes: Connection the dots toward an evolutionary understanding of modern chronic diseases. *Journal of Applied Physiology, 96*, 3–10.

Cordain, L., Gotshall, R. W., Easton, S. B., & Eaton, S. B., III (1998). Physical activity, energy expenditure and fitness: an evolutionary perspective. *International Journal of Sports Medicine, 19*, 328–335.

de Onis, M., & Blossner, M. (2000). Prevalence and trends of overweight among preschool children in developing countries. *American Journal of Clinical Nutrition, 72*, 1032–1039.

Diliberti, N., Bordi, P. L., Conklin, M. T., Roe, L. S., & Rolls, B. J. (2004). Increased portion size leads to increased energy intake in a restaurant meal. *Obesity Research, 12*, 562–568.

Dominy, N. J., & Lucas, P. W. (2004). Significance of color, calories, and climate to the visual ecology of catarrhines. *American Journal of Primatology, 62*, 189–207.

Drewnowski, A., & Spector, S. E. (2004). Poverty and obesity: The role of energy density and energy costs. *American Journal of Clinical Nutrition, 79*, 6–16.

Eaton, S. B., & Eaton, S. B., III (1999). The evolutionary context of chronic degenerative diseases. In S. Stearns (Ed.), *Evolution in health and disease* (pp. 251–259). Oxford: Oxford University Press.

Eaton, S. B., Shostak, M., & Konner, M. (1988). *The Paleolithic prescription: A program of diet and exercise and a design for living.* Philadelphia, PA: Harper & Row.

Fellows, P. (2000). *Food processing technology—Principles and practice* (2nd ed.). New York: CRC Press.

Furbisher, C., & Maxwell, S. M. (2003). The estimation of food portion sizes; a comparison between using descriptions of portion sizes and a photographic food atlas by children and adults. *Journal of Human Nutrition and Dietetics, 16*, 181–188.

Godwin, S. L., Chambers, E., IV, & Cleveland, L. (2004). Accuracy of reporting dietary intake using various portion-size aids in-person and via telephone. *Journal of the American Dietetic Association, 104*, 585–594.

Grier, A.B., & Rozin, P. (2005). Unit bias: a new heuristic that helps explain the effect of portion size on food intake. *Psychological Science*, in press.

Hales, D. (2005). What America really eats. *Parade Magazine*, November, 13, pp. 4–5.

Hawkes, C. (2004). *Marketing food to children: The global regulatory environment.* Geneva, Switzerland: WHO.

Illius, A. W., Tilkamp, B. J., & Yearsley, J. (2002). The evolution of the control of food intakes. *Proceedings of the Nutrition Society, 61*, 465–472.

International Obesity Task Force. (2004). http://www.iotf. org, Retrieved January 2004.

Jenike, M. R. (2001). Nutritional ecology: Diet, physical activity and body size. In C. Panter-Brick, R. Layton, & P. Rowley-Conwy (Eds.), *Hunter-gatherers: An interdisciplinary perspective* (pp. 205–238). Cambridge, UK: Cambridge University Press.

Jones, S., Martin, R., & Pilbeam, D. (1992). *The Cambridge encyclopedia of human evolution.* Cambridge University Press.

Kaiser Family Foundation. (1999). *Kids & media @ The New Millenium.* Menlo Park, CA: Henry J. Kaiser Family Foundation.

Kaiser Family Foundation. (2003). *Zero to six: Electronic media in the lives of infants, toddlers and preschoolers.* Menlo Park, CA: Henry J. Kaiser Family Foundation.

Katschinski, M. (2000). Nutritional implications of cephalic phase gastrointestinal responses. *Appetite, 34,* 189–196.

Kuczmarski, R. J., Flegal, K. M., Campbell, S. M., & Johnson, C. L. (1994). Increasing prevalence of overweight among US adults. The National Health and Nutrition Examination Surveys, 1960 to 1991. *Journal of the American Medical Association, 272,* 205–211.

Kuzawa, C. W. (1998). Adipose tissue in human infancy and childhood: An evolutionary perspective. *Yearbook of Physical Anthropology, 41,* 177–209.

Lang, T., & Heasman, M. (2004). *Food wars—The global battle for mouths, minds, and markets.* London UK & Sterling, VA: Earthscan.

Lee, R. B., & Devore, I. (1968). *Man the hunter.* Chicago: Aldine Press.

Lieberman, L. S. (2003). Dietary, evolutionary and modernizing influences on the prevalence of type 2 diabetes. *Annual Review of Nutrition, 23,* 345–377.

Lobstein, T., Baur, L., Uauy, R. & IASO International Obesity Task Force. (2004). Obesity in children and young people: a crisis in public health. *Obesity Reviews, 5,* 4–104.

Loos, R. J. F., & Rankinen, T. (2005). Gene–diet interactions on body weight changes. *Journal of the American Dietetic Association, 105,* 29–34.

MacArthur, R. H., & Pianka, E. (1966). An optimal use of a patchy environment. *American Naturalist, 100,* 603–609.

Mann, N. J. (2004). Paleolithic nutrition: What can we learn from the past? *Asia Pacific Journal of Clinical Nutrition, 13,* S17.

Melanson, K. J. (2004). Food intake regulation in body weight management: A primer. *Nutrition Today, 39,* 203–213.

Nestle, M. (2003). *Food politics: How the food industry influences nutrition and health.* Berkeley/Los Angeles, CA: University of California Press.

Popkin, B. M. (1994). The nutrition transition in developing countries: An emerging crisis. *Nutrition Reviews, 52,* 285–298.

Popkin, B. M., & Gordon-Larson, P. (2004). The nutrition transition: Worldwide obesity dynamics and their determinants. *International Journal of Obesity and Related Metabolic Disorders, 28,* S2–S9.

Popkin, P. M. (2001). The nutrition transition and obesity in the developing world. *Journal of Nutrition, 131,* 871–873.

Post, R. H. (1962). Population differences in red and green color vision deficiency: A review and a query on selection relaxation. *Eugenic Quarterly, 9,* 31–146.

Rachagan, S. S. (2004). *The junk food generation: A multicountry survey of the influence of television advertisements on children.* London: Consumers International Asian Pacific Office.

Rodman, P. S. (2002). Plants of the apes: Is there a hominoid model for the origins of the hominid diet? In P. S. Unger, & M. F. Teaford (Eds.), *Human diet: its origins and evolution* (pp. 77–109). South Hadley, MA: Bergin & Garvey.

Rolls, B. J. (2003). The supersizing of America. *Portion size and the obesity epidemic. Nutrition Today,, 38,* 42–53.

Rolls, B. J., Rowe, E. A., Rolls, E. T., Kingston, B., et al. (1981). Variety in a meal enhances food intake in men. *Physiological Behavior, 26,* 215–221.

Rozin, P. (2005). The meaning of food in our lives: A cross-cultural perspective on eating and well-being. *Journal of Nutrition Education and Behavior, 37,* S107–S112.

Schlosser, E. (2001). *Fast food nation.* Boston: Houghton Mifflin.

Sinervo, B. (1997). *Optimal foraging theory.* http://bio. research.ucsc.edu/barrylab/classes/animale_behavior/ FORAGING.HTM; Accessed January 2006.

Speakman, J. R. (2004). Obesity: The integrated roles of environment and genetics. *Journal of Nutrition, 134,* S2090–S2105.

Spurlock, M. (2005). *Don't eat this book: Fast food and the supersizing of America.* New York: Putnam.

Story, M., & French, S. A. (2004). Food advertising and marketing directed at children and adolescents in the US. *International Journal Behavior, Nutrition and Physical Activity, 1,* 1–21.

Stroebele, N., & de Castro, J. M. (2004). Television viewing is associated with an increase in meal frequency in humans. *Appetite, 42,* 111–113.

Ungar, P. S., & Teaford, M. F. (2002). Perspectives on the evolution of human diet. In P. Unger, & M. Teaford (Eds.), *Human diet: Its origin and evolution* (pp. 1–6). South Hadley, MA: Bergin & Garvey.

Vorobyev, M. (2004). Ecology and evolution of primate colour vision. *Clinical and Experimental Optometry, 87,* 230–238.

Wansink, B. (2004a). *Marketing nutrition.* Champaign, IL: University of Illinois Press.

Wansink, B. (2004b). Environmental factors that increase the food intake and consumption volume of unknowing consumers. *Annual Review of Nutrition, 24,* 455–479.

Winterhalder, B., & Smith, E. A. (1981). *Hunter-Gather foraging strategies. Ethnographic and archaeological analyses.* Chicago: University of Chicago Press.

World Health Organization. (2000). *The Asia-Pacific perspective: Redefining obesity and its treatment.* Geneva, Switzerland: WHO.

World Health Organization. (2003). *Obesity and Environmental Fact Sheet* 02. http://www.who.int/hpr/NPH/doc/gs_obesity.pdf.

Young, L. R., & Nestle, M. (2002). The contribution of expanding portion sizes to the US obesity problem. *American Journal of Public Health, 92,* 246–249.

UNIT XII

LOOKING FOR SOLUTIONS

Today's world is one of extremes and contradictions as far as food and nutrition go. There is more food in some places than people need, and some wear the excess calories around their middles. The United States comes to mind. In other places there is less food than people need, and some live with the gnawing discomfort that is hunger. Niger comes to mind. There are consequences at both ends of the spectrum. The health consequences of obesity are well recognized and publicized, at least in developed countries. See the unit of this volume, "Overnutrition and Hunger in Lands of Plenty." The health consequences of undernutrition are also well known. They may be less visible on the global stage but they are just as real. See the unit in this volume, "Undernutrition and Its Discontents."

Food production systems are of course linked to diet and hence to nutritional consequences. There are industrialized food production systems in the United States and other developed countries that can produce vast quantities of food, but are energetically inefficient and probably unsustainable. And there are food production systems where people produce most of their own food with their own human labor, but may still not get enough to eat. See the unit of this volume, "Variation in Contemporary Food Systems: Pluses and Minuses."

Not everyone is a farmer; most buy their food from the multitude of trade networks that move food from the farm to the table. These trade networks can be local, but are increasingly national and global in reach. Global networks move luxury foods like coffee and tea, as well as staple foods, like grains, from producing to consuming countries. For example, the people of Egypt have a diet heavily reliant on wheat bread, but Egypt is dependent on global trade for 40% of its wheat. This dependency can lead to a crisis in food availability if the global price of wheat rises unexpectedly as it did in 2008. See chapter 17 by David Himmelgreen, "Anthropological Perspectives on the Global Food Crisis."

The four chapters in this section provide examples of potential solutions to contemporary diet and nutrition problems. We start with farming, the very basis of food production systems where solar energy is converted to green plants, and with Africa where food production is not adequate to meet local demand.

"I enjoy farming very much. It is a very noble profession," said Winifred Omoding, a smallholder (small-scale)

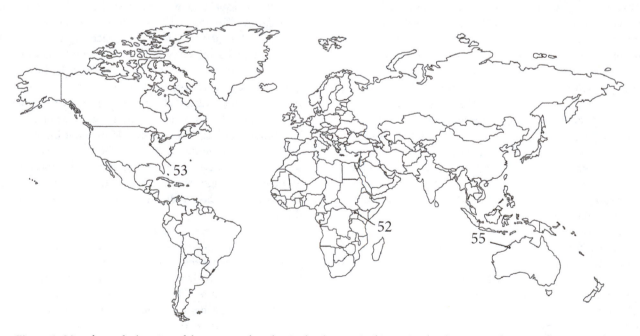

Figure 1 *Map shows the location of the groups referred to in the chapters in this section by chapter number: 52 = farmer, northern Uganda; 53 = farmers, Illinois, United States; 55 = Australian Aborigines, Derby, Australia.*

farmer in Uganda. Her story of achieving success in farming is told by science writer Gaia Vince in the chapter "From One Farmer Hope—and Reason to Worry." Omoding turned to farming after years of civil war had left her few other choices. She suffered repeated crop failures, and could not grow enough food to feed her own family—a situation not unusual in a country where 21% of the population is undernourished (FAO, 2010). Finally, with help from a government agricultural research institute in the form of seeds developed to thrive in the dry climate of northern Uganda, plus a microloan, her farm began to prosper. The story is a good illustration of the realities facing farmers in countries like Uganda, where science and technology alone are not the solution to problems of food security. It takes more. It takes political stability, good governance, economic support and most of all, the hard work of farmers like Winifred Omoding.

In agricultural areas of countries like Uganda there is a direct link between food production and diet, and farmers are members of the local community. The situation in the United States is different. Most of the farms are large, highly mechanized, technologically sophisticated operations that produce enormous quantities of food and sell it to consumers who may live thousands of miles away and not know or care where their food comes from, or who has produced it. But some people have become part of a social movement to change that. They are the farmers interested in producing food for their local community. They are the consumers who care where their food comes from and how it is cultivated. One of the ways they are changing the food production system in the United States is described in the chapter "Direct from Farm to Table: Community Supported Agriculture in Western Illinois," by Heather McIlvaine-Newsad and co-authors. Community supported agriculture (CSA) is a kind of small-scale agriculture organized by farmers who sell "shares" of their harvest to local consumers and in doing so ask consumers to assume some of the risks and rewards of the agricultural season. In exchange, CSA farmers dedicate themselves to bringing their share-holders, and others in the community, organically grown fruits, vegetables, meats and other products. The focus is on food, local food, but along with it comes a connection between farmers and consumers, and a stronger sense of community. A good example of the economic and cultural benefits of a return to local food production is provided by the story of Hardwick, Vermont. See recommended reading, "The Town that Food Saved...."

Whether or not CSA-type small-scale farming could produce enough food to feed the current U.S. population is an unanswered question. Consider, for example, the fact that over 40% of the calories in the U.S. diet are from cereal grains (primarily wheat and corn) and sugar, foods that do not fit the CSA model very well. Another question is cost. Industrialized farms which can produce food at a lower cost are an advantage for people on restricted budgets.

The cost advantage does not of course factor in the true costs of industrialized farming in terms of environmental degradation, and the unsustainable use of fossil fuels and water. Maybe the sustainability of the industrialized farms is really the problem that needs to be resolved?

The chapter by Eric Stokstad, a science writer, takes us to the important question of global food security. He asks, "Could Less Meat Mean More Food?" This is the idea that if the rich ate less meat there would be more grain available to feed the poor and global food security would increase. The idea is based on the fact that animals consume a significant portion of the grain harvests in countries like the United States, grain that could feed people instead. However, Stokstad argues, as intuitively appealing as the idea might be, it is more complicated. One of the complications is the fact that maize is the grain fed to animals, and not everyone in the world eats maize. Some people eat rice. Some people eat wheat. There could also be unintended consequences: eating less meat could result in eating more wheat which could drive up the price of wheat on global markets and increase food insecurity in countries dependent on wheat imports. One of those countries would be Egypt. Stokstad does not really address the high energy cost of meat production in the United States, a point made by Michael Pollan in his paper in this volume, "Power Steer." Imagine if you can a dinner table conversation between Stokstad and Pollan at a steak house.

The last paper in this section addresses one health consequence of too much food, or perhaps too much of the wrong kind of food: type II diabetes. The paper by Kerin O'Dea, "Marked Improvement in Carbohydrate and Lipid Metabolism in Diabetic Australian Aborigines After Temporary Reversion to Traditional Lifestyle," describes a very direct and dramatic approach to reducing the symptoms associated with type II diabetes in Australian Aborigines. The approach: return to a traditional hunter-gather lifestyle (diet and level of physical activity). That lifestyle included a mixed animal and vegetable diet that was high in variety and dependent on season. It had no refined grains or sugars, except for honey. It was also a diet that required significant travel (walking) from place to place in order to find the foods that were naturally available in the local environment. Aborigines, the original inhabitants of Australia, were hunter-gatherers when Europeans arrived some 225 years ago and some maintained that lifestyle until 30 or 40 years ago. Now they live in rural "communities" or urban areas and suffer high rates of obesity and type II diabetes.

In the experiment described by O'Dea a small group of Aborigines reverted to their former hunter-gather lifestyle for seven weeks. After seven weeks the Aborigines showed a loss of body weight and improvements in markers of diabetes like blood sugar and insulin levels. The authors do not describe what happened after the study ended so we are left to wonder if the subjects were able to incorporate any aspects of the more healthful diet and level of physical activity into their everyday lives.

The O'Dea et al. experiment was a dramatic one done with a small number of subjects. The results, however, agree with larger scale clinical trials demonstrating that weight loss, a low fat diet and exercise can reverse the metabolic abnormalities associated with type II diabetes. One of those clinical trials used a hunter-gatherer, or "Paleolithic" type diet based on lean meat, fish, fruits, vegetables and nuts (Jonsson, et al. 2009). The possible benefits of a Paleolithic type diet bring us around full circle to the idea of a biological baseline and the kinds of diets humans probably evolved with. See the unit in this volume, "The Biological Baseline."

In summary, the chapters in this section are examples of potential solutions to some of the problems of food and nutrition described in this book. The problems they address all share a mind-boggling degree of complexity, but they are also very different from each other in many ways. One of Uganda's problems is food insecurity; the solution discussed was how to ramp up local food production by small-scale farmers. One of the problems in the United States is the concentration of food production in a few, large-scale industrialized farms and hence the need to transport food long distances. It is one way to feed a large population but results in a disconnect between people and their food. The solution presented here is to revitalize local small-scale food production in ways that reconnect people with the source of their food and rekindles interest in healthier diets. Another problem in the United States is better understanding the impacts of our diets, and especially meat consumption, on global food security. Lastly, a problem for all populations confronting increased rates of obesity and related chronic disease, is identifying and encouraging healthier lifestyles.

SUGGESTIONS FOR THINKING AND DOING NUTRITIONAL ANTHROPOLOGY

1. Talk to a farmer about the food crops they grow, why they grow what they grow, and how much work it involves. If you cannot find a farmer, an interesting situation in itself, talk to a backyard gardener.
2. Try a recipe from Uganda based on the kinds of crops Winifred Omoding was growing in her fields.
3. Record how much beef you eat over a 7-day period, and use that record to estimate how much you probably eat in a year. Calculate how much

grain it would take to produce that much beef. If you are a vegetarian, record a friend's meat intake and use that figure. Use the corn to beef conversion factors available the Colorado State University website: http://www.extension.org/pages/35850/on-average-how-many-pounds-of-corn-make-one-pound-of-beef-assuming-an-all-grain-diet-from-backgrounding. Explain how you arrived at your estimate. Do you agree with the conclusion arrived at by Eric Stokstad in "Could Less Meat Mean More Food?"

References

FAO (Food and Agriculture Organization of the United Nations). 2010 State of Food Insecurity in the World. Addressing food insecurity in protracted crises. Rome: Food and Agriculture Organization of The United Nations.http://www.fao.org/docrep/013/i1683e/i1683e.pdf (accessed June 21, 2011).

Jonsson T, Granfeldt Y, Ahren B, Branell UC, Palsson G, Hansson A, Soderstrom M, Lindeberg S. 2009. Beneficial effects of a Paleolithic diet on cardiovascular risk factors in type 2 diabetes: a randomized cross-over pilot study. Cardiovascular Diabetology 8 # 35:1–14. doi:10.1186/1475–2840–8–35.

Suggested Further Reading

FAO (Food and Agriculture Organization of the United Nations). 2010. 925 million in chronic hunger worldwide. http://www.fao.org/news/story/en/item/45210/icode/ (accessed June 15, 2011).

Herrero M, Thornton PK, Notenbaert AM, Wood S, Msangi S, Freeman HA, Bossio D, Dixon J, Peters M, van de Steeg J, Lynam J, Pathasarathy Rao P. Macmillan S, Gerard B, McDermott J, Seré C, Rosegrant M. 2010. Smart investments in sustainable food production: Revisiting mixed crop-livestock systems. Science 327:822–825.

Hewitt, Ben. 2010. The Town that Food Saved: How One Community Found Vitality in Local Food. New York: Rodale, Inc.

Pollan M. 2008. Farmer in chief. New York Times. http://www.nytimes.com/2008/10/12/magazine/12policy-t.html (accessed June1, 2009).

Schnell SM. 2007. Food with a farmer's face: community-supported agriculture in the United States. The Geographical Review 97: 550–564.

CHAPTER 52

From One Farmer, Hope—and Reason for Worry

Gaia Vince

(2010)

Olagara, Uganda—In this harsh, dry landscape, Winifred Omoding's fields are a welcome burst of color. Her neighbors' plots are pitifully brown, with shriveled maize and sorghum clinging to half-height stalks. Omoding's, however, are an embarrassment of green. Her sunflower, sesame, and cassava thrive amid the cacti and dust that surround this village of 500 people.

Just a few years ago, Omoding's prospects looked bleak. Civil war had left her life in disarray, her crops were failing, and she was struggling to feed her family. Now, the 41-year-old farmer not only produces enough food for her husband and nine children but also makes a healthy profit selling the excess.

"I enjoy farming very much," Omoding says as she weeds sunflowers that tower over her head. "It's a very noble profession: the backbone of our country."

It's just the kind of success story that food-security experts say needs to be replicated if fast-growing populations in Uganda and other developing nations are to avoid widespread hunger. Already, analysts estimate that nearly 2 million of Uganda's 31 million people experience food insecurity due to supply problems or rising prices. Nearly 80% of the people in Omoding's region, for instance, depend on food aid to survive. Such problems could worsen as Uganda's population, which has been increasing at more than 3% per year, surges to an estimated 100 million by 2050. To keep pace, Uganda's farmers will need to at least triple current harvests.

Omoding's story offers some cause for optimism that they can meet that challenge. And it highlights the important role that scientists can play in boosting yields by helping farmers get the most from fundamental resources, such as water, soil, and seeds. But her experience also underscores the complex social, economic, and psychological challenges raised by food insecurity; science alone didn't enable Omoding to transform her fields from brown to green—nor will it do so for her neighbors.

FARMING FROM NEED

Like many developing-world farmers, Omoding fell into farming out of desperation. Her parents were schoolteachers and she had hoped to follow them into the classroom. But that dream ended with the political violence that enveloped her homeland for nearly 20 years starting in the 1980s. "Whenever we heard shootings, we would run into the bush and hide," she recalls. "The rebels killed my older sister and my dad. They burnt our house, took our seven cows and goats and sheep, destroyed our crops."

After Omoding married, she and her husband, Ephrem, inherited about 3 hectares of land. That is a large farm by Ugandan standards, but the couple struggled through the 1990s. Traditional farming practices, which rarely allow fields to lie fallow, had reduced the fertility of their soil. Poor-quality seeds bought at local markets often failed to thrive. A parasitic weed called striga sapped their sorghum crop, reducing yields. With no animals to help plow the hard ground, the couple "appealed to some of the men in the village, who tied their hands to the harness of the plow," recalls Omoding. "It was a terrible time. Many people went hungry and many children died."

The couple's fortunes changed with the return of political stability in the early 2000s. The men gave up soldiering and could help in the fields. And in 2003, aid groups helped Omoding and other Olagara women form an agricultural "microloan" cooperative. In exchange for making small deposits into the co-op, the women could get small loans. Omoding used her first one to hire oxen to plow and weed her fields.

Such help didn't end the crop failures, however, so in 2006 Omoding traveled to the nearby town of Soroti to seek help from scientists at the government's new National Semi-Arid Resources Research Institute (NaSARRI), created as part of a 2005 overhaul of Uganda's agricultural research system. "She was in a terrible way with her harvest having just failed again," recalls NaSARRI's Florence Olmaikorit-Oumo, an outreach worker who helps connect farmers to institute scientists.

The timing was right. The scientists were developing new crop varieties customized to prosper in places like Olagara, which typically gets less than 800 millimeters of rain annually (and much less recently). They were also looking for local farmers to help fieldtest and multiply the seeds. Omoding was a prime candidate, says Olmaikorit-Oumo: "You could see that she really wanted to learn."

Gaia Vince, "From one farmer, hope—and reason for worry." Science 327(2010):798–799. Reprinted with permission.

Institute staff began giving Omoding advice on which crops to grow. Maize was out (too thirsty); sorghum, cassava, and millet were in. They also showed her new ways to restore soil fertility, such as by plowing postharvest leftovers back into the soil. And Omoding got access to the institute's latest seeds, which she bought using a microloan.

She saw immediate results. The first harvest was so successful that she had a surplus—and a few kilos of desirable new seed—to sell through a marketing network created by NaSARRI. Since then, farm profits have allowed her family to add land, send their children to boarding schools, and start building a brick house. "Before, I farmed to feed my children," Omoding says. "Now, I think of it as a way to make our lives better and to become more rich."

Success has also given her the security to experiment with new crops. One is a drought-tolerant sunflower that yields a high-quality oil and a "cake" that farmers can feed to livestock. She's also planting a new drought-tolerant sesame. "It is ready to harvest in just 4 months rather than 6 months like the local variety," she says as she wades through a ripe bumper crop.

DUPLICATION CHALLENGE

To ensure food security in Uganda, however, many more farmers will soon need to duplicate Omoding's success. And that could be a problem if the many struggling farms around Olagara are any guide. Even as the Omodings and others have changed their practices and prospered, many neighboring farmers have not—and understanding why will be key to ensuring food security.

Omoding herself believes one important difference is her willingness to take risks and embrace new ideas. "Whatever the scientists tell me, I try it and see if it works," she says. "I am not happy with just planting the same seeds every year and hoping, like others in the village."

To overcome that mindset, NaSARRI officials have launched efforts to have innovative farmers teach their neighbors—a model that has worked well elsewhere. But progress has been slow, they say, perhaps in part because so many people here are still recovering from decades of traumatic violence and crop failures that sapped hope for the future. It can seem pointless to put in the hard work necessary to rebuild soil fertility or dig a well, for instance, if you fear being uprooted from your home or losing your crop to weather or pests you can't control.

Omoding, however, is looking ahead with confidence. "I always ask how I can do better," she says. "I want my crops to be bigger." She wants to plant an orange grove, for instance, to supply a planned juice factory. To get the needed water, she's already gotten a loan for a treadle pump and is saving up to build a shallow hand-dug well. Eventually, she'd also like to start buying the fertilizers, pesticides, and tractors that farmers in industrialized nations take for granted.

Those dreams, however, rest on a shaky foundation. Part of Omoding's income, for instance, still comes from aid groups that buy part of her sunflower harvest in order to help jump-start the industry. That income could disappear if the donors withdraw. Reliable water supplies also remain a major challenge, which could get worse with climate change. And experts say Uganda's government will need to spend much more to develop the infrastructure—from better roads and irrigation systems to reliable banks and markets—needed to give rural farmers incentives to increase yields and connect them to important urban markets.

Still, those trying to ensure food security in Uganda and elsewhere take some hope from Winifred Omoding. If one woman from a small village can create food from the dust, they say, perhaps the challenge of feeding 9 billion of the planet's future inhabitants becomes a little less daunting.

CHAPTER 53

Direct from Farm to Table: Community Supported Agriculture in Western Illinois

Heather McIlvaine-Newsad, Christopher D. Merrett, and Patrick

McLaughlin

(2004)

INTRODUCTION: NOW THAT TASTES LIKE A TOMATO[1]

There are not many people in the U.S. who farm anymore. Less than 25% of the population live in rural areas and fewer than 3% farm for a living (USDA 2002). Some people consider the shift in our once agrarian lifestyle to be an economic and social victory, while others view this as an indicator of cultural and fiscal deterioration (Hanson 2000). Many of those individuals who fall into the latter category are members of the CSA or community supported agriculture movement. At the core of the CSA philosophy is the production of organic fruits, vegetables, meats, poultry, and other products, which are purchased by local consumers. With the average tomato in the U.S. traveling over 1,300 miles from farm to plate (Lacy 2000; Pirog and Benjamin 2003), CSA not only seeks to redefine agriculture, as we know it, but also attempts to establish personal relationships between farmers, consumers, and specific places, thus fostering a sense of community that is lacking in our modern world.

There are currently over 1,000 registered CSA farms[2] producing food throughout the U.S. and Canada (Van En 2002). In terms of their geographic distribution, CSA farms are found in almost every state. However, they tend to be clustered in three regions: (1) the Northeast near large metropolitan centers such as New York, Boston, and Philadelphia, (2) the upper Midwest and along the upper half of the Mississippi Valley, and (3) the West Coast states of California, Oregon and Washington. According to the USDA (2003) there are 16 registered CSA farms in Illinois. All but four are located near metropolitan centers. This is a trend replicated throughout the United States. According to the first nationwide census of CSA farms carried out in 1999 (Lass et al. 2003), 80% of all CSAs are located near large

metropolitan centers. CSA producers in rural areas, like those highlighted in this paper, are in the minority and face some unique challenges maintaining their livelihoods.

A recent survey of 366 CSAs conducted by the authors of this paper[3] asked what portion of their produce was grown organically. One-hundred percent of the 248 CSAs who responded to the question reported growing organic goods (IIRA 2003). Once thought to be a fringe movement, the general public is embracing organic food. Organic food sales have increased 20–25% since 1996, with sales reaching $7.8 billion in 2001 (Barkley 2002). On October 21, 2002 the USDA announced a new label that will help consumers identify organic foods in supermarkets (Becker 2002). While the USDA typically does not certify the food produced by CSA farms, these farms are the foundation of the organic food movement in North America. In this paper we examine the cultural role of two CSA farms in McDonough County, Illinois. By exploring the hurdles and catalysts encountered by these two particular farms in starting and maintaining the CSA endeavor, we raise some questions about the role of community building as well as the long-term sustainability of the CSA movement in rural areas like western Illinois.

GOING ORGANIC: CSA FARMS AND FREE TRADE

The Roots of CSA

While CSA is a relatively new form of agricultural production in the U.S., the first recorded CSA farms, known as *teikei* started in Japan in 1965 (Broydo 2001; Goland 2002; McLaughlin and Merrett 2002; Van En 2002; Wells, Gradwell, and Yoder 1999). The word *teikei* in its most literal translation means "partnership" or "cooperation." The degree to which subscribers partner or cooperate with growers is one of the concerns of many in the CSA movement who regret that the community in CSA is often less than tangible. On a philosophical level, *teikei* means "food with the farmer's face on it" (Henderson and Van En 1999:xiv). Japanese women

Heather McIlvaine-Newsad, Christopher D. Merrett, and Patrick McLaughlin, "Direct from farm to table: community supported agriculture in western Illinois." *Culture & Agriculture* 26(2004):149–163. Figure has been omitted. Reprinted with permission.

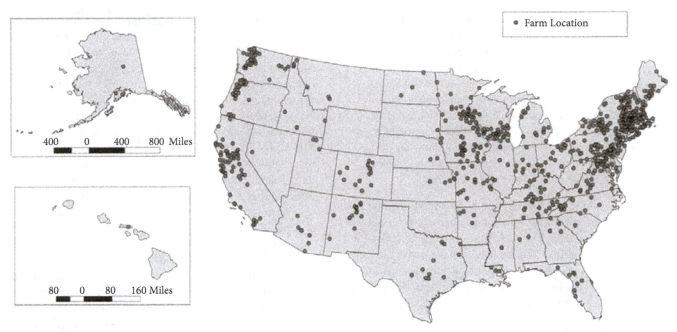

Figure 1 *Location of CSA Farms in the United States, 2002.*

who were concerned with the increased use of pesticides, environmental degradation, and the decrease of rural populations forged a cooperative agreement with local farmers to provide nutritious organic foods for their households.

In 1984 the movement was introduced to the U.S. via a Swiss farmer, Jan Vander Tuin. Vander Tuin along with John Root, Jr., Charlotte Zanecchia, and Robyn Van En formed the first core group of CSA farmers on Indian Line Farm in Egremont, Massachusetts with a small apple orchard. Over the next several years they gradually introduced the "share the harvest" concept to the local community. In 1986, Hugh Ratchliffe joined the group and the first shares of vegetables were offered to the community (Van En 2002).

A Reaction to Globalization?

Agriculture in the U.S. has changed drastically over the past fifty years. As the notion of "development" spread after World War II, the concept and practice of agriculture changed worldwide (Esteva 1992). In the 1940s and 1950s, factories that had been designed to produce gunpowder for the war effort began manufacturing inexpensive nitrogen fertilizers for agriculture. Scientists who had previously worked on inventing technologies for chemical warfare now focused their research on generating agricultural pesticides. These changes allowed farmers to take much of the risk out of farming, and farms began to function like factories rather than dynamic ecological systems that they are (Ikerd 2002). Philip McMichael (2000:21) writes that,

> As such, development became associated with industrial rationality. It viewed nature as an unproblematic human laboratory and rendered rural society as a residual

domain: supplying labor for urban industrial ventures as agro-industrialization expelled rural populations from their local agricultural communities. In this movement, food was removed from its direct link to local ecology and culture, and became an input in urban diets and industrial processing plants.

In the U.S., farmers were encouraged to specialize, not diversify. Those farmers who could not afford to expand their operations, in terms of both land base and/or technological inputs, were forced out of agriculture. The number of farmers decreased, yet the size of farms increased. McMichael (2000:23) claims,

> In the US, two percent of the farms grow fifty percent of agricultural produce, the average family farm earns only fourteen percent of its income from the farm, and ninety-five percent of American food is a corporate product. The food industry is the largest American industrial sector, but it doesn't produce food security, as thirty million Americans are hungry. Huge conglomerates virtually monopolize sales—ConAgra, for example, accounts for twenty-five percent of sales in foodstuffs, feed, and fertilizers, fifty-three percent of sales of refrigerated foods, and twenty-two percent of grocery products.

Until approximately a decade ago, American farmers were the most competitive farmers in the world. Recently, however, the U.S. share of global agricultural exports has plummeted, farm profits have fallen, and confidence in the American farmer's ability to compete has been questioned (Ikerd 2002a). In addition to the success of farmers from countries like Brazil and Argentina, other factors impeding American farmers ability to maintain their primary position in the world market include:

rising costs of land and labor [which] are destroying the traditional competitive advantage of American farmers in world markets. Growing demand for land in rural areas for residential purposes, as America's affluent urbanites acquire more living space, will make even good farmland too costly to farm. Employment opportunities arising from the 'new economy' will make the economic sacrifice of an occupation in farming too high. Cornfields can't compete with condominiums for land and the Missouri Valley can't compete with the Silicone Valley for labor. [Blank 1999 in Ikerd 2002a]

While Blank and Ikerd paint a pessimistic future for American agriculture, one factor neither considers is the role of the increasingly aware and concerned consumer. Consumers in Europe and elsewhere have proven to represent powerful economic and political forces, which have influenced current international agricultural trade patterns. As McMichael (2000:21) notes,

The series of IMF food riots over the last two decades attest to the power of food to generate a substantial critique of the myth of free trade markets. And just as the fiction of money is sustained by the credibility, or sheer power, of the US dollar (as a global force), the fiction of what the corporate world chooses to call 'genetically improved' foods is only sustainable through the complexity of governments, scientists, and agro-chemical corporations in concealing ingredients from consumers and biological hazards from citizens.

The authors of this paper suggest that not all consumers have allowed themselves to become passive clients of faceless corporations. Rather, there is a certain group of consumers that wants to be involved, at differing levels, in the important decisions about the crop and livestock genetics and with whom and where food is produced and marketed. We see the emergence of the CSA movement in North America as one response to the perceived threats of globalization.

Reclaiming the Soul of Farming and Community

The CSA movement in North America appears to be growing in light of, or perhaps in response to globalization, as growing consumer concerns (especially in Europe and developing nations) over GMOs (genetically modified organisms), and the loss of biological and cultural diversity becomes ever more prevalent. In addition to the production of organic food, CSA purports to "provide(s) a social and economic alternative to the conventional, large-scale corporately managed food system" (DeLind and Ferguson 1999:191). Vandana Shiva and others have written extensively about the "corporate hijacking of food and agriculture" in developing countries and the social and environmental consequences that have resulted (Shiva 2000, 1997a, 1997b; Plant 1997; Plant 1990). This "stolen harvest," to use Shiva's terminology, is not restricted to developing nations. In North America

the mosaic of farmland ownership has changed dramatically over the last one hundred years. Geisler and Daneker (2000) report that in the United States from 1940 to 1992, the number of farms decreased by 75% and the ownership of farms declined by 50%. Yet, during the same time period the average size of farms increased three fold (McLaughlin 2002; Geisler and Daneker 2000). This farm consolidation has caused economic and demographic decline in the rural Midwest. CSAs, by promoting small-scale agriculture, may help stabilize communities by providing another profit center for small farms, while creating new social connections between the farm and non-farm community.

McDonough County Illinois, the home of the two case study CSA farms in this paper, follows this national trend. According to information compiled by the IIRA (Illinois Institute for Rural Affairs[4]) in 1987 there were 1,018 farms located in the county. In 1997 the number had dropped to 824 (IIRA 2001). In this same time period the average size of farms in McDonough County increased from 342 to 413 acres (IIRA 2001). In addition to the change in ownership and size of farms in U.S. and McDonough County in particular, the types of crops produced have also changed. Vandana Shiva (2000:7) notes that this homogenization of crop production is a global trend.

Small farms and small farmers are pushed to extinction, as monocultures replace biodiverse crops, as farming is transformed from the production of nourishing and diverse foods into the creation of markets for genetically engineered seeds, herbicides, and pesticides.[] ... farmers are transformed from producers into consumers of corporate-patented agricultural products, as markets are destroyed locally and nationally but expanded globally. ...

Many "conventional" farmers like the father and brother of one of the authors, who farm in southern Ohio, lament the loss of ecological diversity on the farm, and acknowledge that their choices for crop production are limited. While SKM Farms is among the relatively few family farms to survive the national farm crisis of the 1980s, the notion of what farming is and its subsequent practice has changed. Over the course of thirty years, SKM Farms has gone from being a diverse livestock and grain farm, to specializing in the production of corn and soybeans. In order to survive economically as a conventional farmer in the U.S., farmers need to continue to increase the acreage under production and plant what the market dictates. This is what farms like SKM Farms have done in order to remain competitive. Today that market is controlled by ten corporations who command 32% of the commercial seed market, valued at $23 billion, and 100% of the market for genetically engineered, or transgenic, seeds (Shiva 2000:7; Lappé and Bailey 1998). As noted by McLaughlin and Merrett (2002) and Halweil (2000), the number of Midwestern counties in the U.S. with more than 55% of their acreage in soybean or corn production has tripled since 1972. This, as is the case with SKM Farms, results in a loss of crop diversity. As conventional farmers concentrate on fewer crops, their productivity increases. As farmers produce more commodities, the prices for commodities drop, prompting farmers to seek new strategies to survive. Farmers are on the "technological treadmill," where they have to adopt new technologies and increase farm size to remain viable because increased productivity drives down commodity prices and profit margins (Cochrane 1979:389). CSAs may offer a way for some farmers to get off of the treadmill and embrace a form of agriculture that is more compatible with rural communities and the environment.

In addition, the plight of the family farm has not been aided by American farm policy, which has been historically biased toward larger farms (McLaughlin and Merrett 2002). U.S. agricultural policy is designed not to promote the sustainability and development of rural areas, but rather to supply the urban population with an adequate, safe, and most importantly, an affordable supply of food. Government programs are designed to offer tax breaks and incentives on the volume, not the diversity, of food produced. CSA farms, which run counter to the current agricultural trend in the U.S., represent an alternative to the contemporary agricultural landscape. CSA consumers dictate that these farmers produce a wide variety of crops. The seasonal heterogeneity of CSA produce is one of the elements that captivates and retains local subscribers. The socio-economic status of the subscribers also influences the pricing of farm shares. It is not unheard of for subscription prices in metropolitan areas to run $500 per season, compared to the same size shares in rural areas costing closer to $325. Unlike and yet similar to conventional agriculture, the market, albeit a local rather than global market, influences the financial viability of CSA producers.

With the ubiquity of the 24-hour, warehouse-style grocery stores that carry food ranging from avocados from California, mangos from the Dominican Republic, to *molé* from Mexico, CSA farms provide local consumers with locally grown, season-specific food. The growers agree to do their best to provide the consumers with a sufficient quantity and quality of food to meet the needs and expectations of the consumers at a reasonable price (Lamb 1996). Inherent to this agreement is the understanding that both farmers and consumers share the risks and rewards of farming (DeLind and Ferguson 1999).

Cultivating Community

Community and community building are essential elements of the CSA philosophy. "Yet looking back, it is apparent that 'community' has often been viewed naively, or in practice dealt with, as a harmonious and internally equitable collective" (Guijt and Shah 1998:1). This mythical notion of community cohesion and shared ideology continues to permeate the CSA movement. Still minimal consideration has been given to the differing needs, goals, and aspirations for those operating and participating in CSAs. In her most recent work on CSAs, DeLind (2003:194) writes that while CSAs

have been successful at "serving as a market instrument for small diversified farmers and conscientious consumers," its third goal of building "community may exist more as a metaphor than a fact." The authors postulate that the question DeLind and others may really be asking is what is community and how is it understood by growers and subscribers?

At the heart of the CSA movement is the notion that growers are raising food, not commodities (DeLind 2003: 194). According to scholars like Polanyi (1977) and Zsolnai (2002) this understanding of farming clearly places CSAs within the category of substantive economics rather than formal economics. Share prices are not driven by the global economy, but rather by what the local community needs and can afford. In addition, those who purchase farm shares know who grows their food, and perhaps have some kind of relationship with them. Yet, we know that there are different types of interactions between growers and consumers. There are CSA farms which produce upwards of 500 shares for subscribers in distant urban centers, versus smaller CSAs with fewer than twenty shareholders. Therefore, the degree to which subscribers participate in on-farm activities and know their farmers varies based on the type of CSA arrangement.

Many of the distinctions between CSA farms and subscriber relationships are related to the resources (land, labor, and capital) of the farmers as well as the desires and expectations of the consumers. As such, the practical arrangements vary from farm to farm. However, there are four basic CSA arrangements (Broydo 2001):

(1) Subscription or Farmer-driven CSAs: Farmers organize the CSA and make most of the management and production decisions. The shareholder or subscriber is generally not involved in the day-to-day production activities. This type of CSA is the most prevalent type found today throughout North America.

(2) Shareholder or Consumer-driven CSAs: Consumers organize the CSA and hire a farmer to grow what they want. The shareholders, while not involved day-to-day production activities, do decide what will be grown. This type of CSA is most commonly found in the Northeastern part of the U.S.

(3) Farmer Cooperatives: This is a variation of the farmer-driven cooperative that pools the resources of two or more farmers. This agreement allows local producers to offer a wider variety of food to local consumers, thus extending the subscription period or growing season. Such arrangements often include vegetable farmers and dairy or meat producers working together.

(4) Farmer-consumer cooperatives: Under this arrangement farmers and consumers co-own land and resources and work together on almost all aspects of food production.

All CSA farms, regardless of their production structure share three underlying goals. These aspects include (1) providing consumers with healthy locally grown food, (2) reconnecting the consumer with the producer, and (3) fostering a sense of local environmental and human stewardship. These goals meet the stated goals of sustainable agriculture that seeks to promote "environmental health, economic profitability, and social and economic equity" (University of California 1997). The end goal of sustainable agriculture includes both the development of environmentally sound agricultural practices and the movement away from the negative social and environmental results of our current industrialized food production systems (Hinrich 2000; McLaughlin 2002).

Many of us, the authors' of this paper included, share the notion that being part of a CSA means that as subscribers we participate *to some extent* in the cultivation of our food. In the act of assisting to grow our food, we are also building community. Yet, we know that the majority of CSA subscribers do not regularly participate in on-farm activities. DeLind (1999) writes extensively on how her experiences as a new CSA organizer and member left her wiser to the complexities of community building. Most CSAs, rural and urban alike, deliver the farm shares to their subscribers, either in their homes or at specific drop off points. One question to ponder is, are there characteristics of subscribers who participate in on-farm activities which distinguish them from those who do not?

From on-farm participant observation in two rural Illinois CSAs, the authors have observed that the household composition of subscribers is a major variable influencing the degree to which shareholders participate in community building activities. The subscribers of *Ana's Garden CSA* can be divided into two basic groups: (1) households with children who have lived in the area for a number of years, and (2) single individuals or childless households new to the area who are seeking not only fresh produce, but also a sense of community.

The first group of subscribers generally tends to have their baskets delivered to them. When asked why they selected this delivery option, convenience was the most common answer. Most of the households in this group have young children who are involved in a multitude of activities. Adding a 40 mile roundtrip drive each week to pick up fresh produce would tax their already busy lives. These subscribers did participate in the mid and end of the year on-farm activities, and often brought their children along. One might speculate that one motivating factor for this group of subscribers was not to build a new community, but to support and broaden the community to which they already belonged.

Michael Nash and partner Solvig Hanson (2004), CSA growers in rural Iowa, bring some insight from the producer perspective to this question. When asked how actively involved the subscribers to *Sunflower Fields* are in day-to-day activities of the farm they commented:

> There are lots of illusions about people in rural areas wanting to participate in on-farm activities. But we haven't found it to be true, because unlike folks from the urban areas, being on a farm isn't a novelty. Work days aren't real popular because people can go and work on their own farms.

Regarding the notion of community building as an integral part of rural CSAs, Nash and Hanson (2004) responded that in their experience:

> The need for community and its definition is different. Their community is defined by a geographic location and centers around high school sports, the school, and the churches. With rural communities, there isn't that sense of searching that you might find in the urban areas. They don't want to hear that we are going to do a little community building. They want us to contribute to the community in ways that benefits the community they have already been working a lifetime to build. And as farmers, they want us to be economically successful.

The owners and subscribers of *Good Eats Gardens* follow the basic pattern outlined by Nash and Hanson. Located at the opposite end of McDonough County, *Good Eats Gardens* delivers all of their subscriber baskets. When asked why community building is not a larger component of their CSA operation they offered the following:

> Our subscribers are generally older retired farmers. They have been gardening their entire lives, but can no longer do so. They don't get out often, but they certainly look forward to our weekly deliveries. Being part of our CSA offers them an opportunity to continue to support agriculture in the area, even if they aren't involved in the day to day production and stay involved in the community without leaving their homes.

As Nash and Hanson (2004) commented, rural CSAs are often not about the food: "Our boxes are almost secondary to most of these folks. They care about bending our ear, they aren't just customers. They are also our friends." Misunderstanding or not recognizing the diversity of needs and desires of individuals who participate in a CSA community can often lead to the negative feelings about the community building aspect of the movement. This is especially true in the changing face of rural America. The use of the term community is in essence a conceptual problem, which has been discussed at length among scholars who work in the realm of participatory development. "Well over a century ago, the idea of a culturally and politically homogeneous participatory local social system gained acceptance" (Guijt and Shah 1998:7). Yet, we know that communities are neither homogeneous in their composition, or concerns, nor are they harmonious in their relationships (Guijt and Shah 1998:8). Why do we assume that a community of CSA subscribers will be any different? Regardless of this knowledge, we seem perplexed to find that the community building aspect of CSAs often leaves something to be desired.

METHODOLOGY

The data for the ethnographic portion of this paper was collected between August 2000 and October 2002 in McDonough County Illinois. The study began initially with Ana's Garden and in the spring of 2002 expanded to include Good Eats Gardens.[5] These two CSA farms were selected because they are within close geographic vicinity of Western Illinois University and the Illinois Institute of Rural Affairs where the authors' work or were enrolled in graduate studies.

The McDonough County data was obtained using a variety of ethnographic methods. These included participant observation—working on the Ana's Garden farm, attending CSA sponsored events, and being present at farmers' markets and other distribution sites; multiple in-depth face-to-face ethnographic interviews; and numerous telephone conversations with the owners of both farms.

National level data was collected through a survey of CSAs in the United States. The survey was conducted between November 2002 and January 2003. The list of respondents came from a directory of CSAs on the Van En (2002) website, as well as from Internet searches, archival data, and field research. The survey protocol included an initial survey mailing, a reminder postcard, and a second survey mailing. Of 755 valid addressees, we received 366 responses for a 48.5% response rate (IIRA 2003).

THE FINDINGS: THE FARMERS AND THE FARMS

Good Eats Gardens: A Family Venture

The Delaney family, who own and operate Good Eats Gardens, like many people in this part of Illinois, have lived in the area for generations and come from an agricultural background. In November 2002 they ended their sixth year of CSA operations, about average for CSAs in the survey (Table 1). It was not the best of years, according to Marianne, the matriarch of the family, who laughed that they "fought mother nature all the way."

The Delaney's farm covers 40.8 acres and they own all but 6.2 acres of the land currently in production. In 2002, 10.8 acres were dedicated to the CSA gardens (4.6 acres in strawberries) and an additional 30 acres produced organic corn, hay, and pasture for the 200 head of sheep that Marianne also raises. The amount of land the Delaneys devote to the CSA is close to the national average (Table 1). The Delaneys practice a diversified farm management strategy and the 20-plus CSA subscribers reap the benefits of their endeavors. Last season they produced over 30 varieties of vegetables— "everything from A to Z"—and also supplied their members with fresh eggs for several weeks of the 21-week season. The Delaneys utilize the composted sheep manure, which they compost for four years, as fertilizer for the gardens and in the spring and summer the chickens roam the gardens as a form of natural pest management. While Marianne is also interested in offering their subscribers organic lamb, they are currently unable to do so because of the presence of scrapie among goats and sheep in the Midwest.[6]

Good Eats Gardens allows the Delaneys to continue to farm their family's land. Six years ago, Gordon Delaney approached his wife and two children about the future of the farm. According to Marianne, though Gordon had been farming for over twenty years growing and selling vegetables at local farmers' markets, the future for continuing to farm as they had been was not promising. As a family, including their two then teenage children, they decided that it was important to try and hold onto their rural lifestyle. While they could not afford to expand the land under cultivation, they could afford to intensify and diversify what they produced.

The Delaneys experience as CSA producers runs counter to the majority of CSA farmers who responded to the authors' survey (IIRA 2003), as well as findings presented by Lass (2003) on the 1999 CSA survey. According to the IIRA survey, of the 325 farmers who responded to the question, "Were you raised on a farm?," 77% were not. Of those who were raised on a farm, only 29.3% were still living on a farm. This is a surprising result given assumptions that CSAs might represent an attempt to sustain small family farms.

Table 1 Average Characteristics of CSA Operators

Characteristics	National Mean	CSA Survey (Median)	Delaney CSA	Hendrix CSA
Current Age	44.6	(45.0)	48	32
Starting Year	1996.6	(1997)	1997	2003
Acres Devoted to CSA	11.4	(4.0)	10.8	1
Number of Subscribers	103.7	(50.0)	22	20
Subscription Cost ($)	360.74	(375.00)	350.00	300.00
Number of Crops	46.3	(39.5)	30	32
CSA Share (%) of Total Household Income	37.6	(25.0)	5.0 (Estimated)	25.0

Source: Based on calculations from IIRA (2003).

In a majority of cases, the CSAs are operated by relatively young, first generation farmers who rely on a second income to make ends meet (IIRA 2003). The average CSA operator in this survey was 44.6-years old (Table 1). In contrast, the average traditional farmer is 54.3-years old (U.S. Census of Agriculture 1997).

In other ways, the Delaney CSA mirrors results in the IIRA (2003) survey because success over the last six years is influenced in part by their vested interest in seeing their CSA succeed as both a business and lifestyle. When we asked Marianne what motivated them to make a change in production techniques, she replied that they had read several articles about the benefits of bioregionalism and the success of CSA farms in the Northeast, and thus decided to venture into new territory. This resulted in some major changes in the roles and responsibilities of all of the family members. For Marianne, "buying into the business," meant that she would give up her job and the steady income it offered as a nurse in a nearby community.

While maintaining that she never once regretted the decision to stop working off farm, she did say that as a family and a business there were tense times in which the "cash flow wasn't flowing in the right direction." In addition, Marianne makes it clear that they never would have been able to undertake this venture if they had not had the support of their extended family to help care for the children while they were younger. The social network of friends and family who were willing and able to care for their children during the startup years of the operation proved to be a valuable contribution to the success of their business. For the Delaney offspring, the business venture meant giving up some extra-curricular activities and spending long hours working alongside their parents in the gardens. While many teenagers do not relish spending time with their parents, the Delaney offspring seem to truly enjoy their parents' company and count them as friends. For Gordon, the changes resulted in being able to spend more time with his children, pass on the values that his parents had instilled in him, and continue to do a job he loved.

Economics versus Lifestyle. Good Eats Gardens' prices are reasonable, if not under priced. Subscribers pay $350 for a 21-week season and senior citizens subscribe for $275.00—prices which are below the national average (Table 1). This slightly lower-than-average cost could be attributed to the fact that the Delaney CSA offers fewer than average crop varieties. The produce is delivered to the subscriber's door weekly, and the typical share provides enough fresh produce for a family of four. The senior citizen share is somewhat reduced in volume, but not diversity.

In addition to the CSA subscriber income, the Delaneys sell their produce at various farmers markets in the region. Five days a week you can find a Good Eats Garden booth either in Macomb and Galesburg, Illinois or in Burlington, Iowa. In addition, the Delaneys maintain a small roadside shop located next to the gardens. Therefore, while all of the Delaney income is generated from agricultural production, the CSA portion represents only a small percentage of the entire income. This trend is similar to the one noted in the nationwide survey, where respondents reported that an average of 37% of their annual household income was generated through CSA production (IIRA 2003). The remainder of the income was generated by non-CSA farming activity.

The Good Eats Gardens also contradicts the study conducted by Cone and Myers (2000), because the income generated from the Delaney diversified marketing strategy is sufficient to maintain the household, and allows all of the household members, with the exception of the son who is employed as a teacher and has formed his own household, to work fulltime on the farm. The Delaneys hope to be able to maintain this trend. Despite that fact that all four household members work fulltime on the farm during the summer season, they still need to hire extra labor. For the past several seasons two teenage neighbors have worked fulltime in the gardens and another local teenager has worked part time. The youngest Delaney, the daughter, is currently enrolled in a nearby college as an ag-business major. Though she intends to complete her degree, she is committed to making her living as farmer. For Theresa, as with other household members, farming is not about the money, but the lifestyle.

> Where else can I work with my best friend, my mom, all day long? We have such fun at work. I mean, it's not really work is it, when you are throwing strawberry kisses (rotten strawberries) at each other and laughing until your sides hurt and you have tears streaming down your face? Besides, we don't want for anything. We don't have money to throw away, but we do laugh a lot.

As with many CSA farmers, the contributions to and the benefits from belonging to a closely-knit community are also important. Small farms have been shown to bolster not only biodiversity of plants and animals and promote the sustainable use of farmland, but to also foster cultural diversity and provide a platform for the maintenance and building of cultural traditions (Lobao 1995).

The Delaney's motivations for operating a CSA mirror those driving other CSA operators. In the CSA survey, respondents were asked to rate the importance of several factors prompting them to operate a CSA on a scale of 1 to 5, where 1 = unimportant and 5 = very important. Results show that while profit is an important consideration (3.39 out of 5.00), other factors relating to growing wholesome food (4.79), sustainable agriculture (4.65), environmental stewardship (4.53), lifestyle (4.37) and community (4.24) were significantly more important issues motivating people to operate a CSA (Table 2).[7]

Small farms promote self-empowerment and community responsibility, and they provide families a place to pass on the values of hard work and responsibility for the land (NCSF 1998). These values were evident while talking to the Delaneys. The Delaney daughter's comment makes this clear.

> Making deliveries is probably one of the highlights of my week. I have the chance to talk to people I might not ever talk to otherwise. I have learned a lot from the people I

deliver to. Some of our older subscribers talk about ways to can and preserve the produce that never would have occurred to me. In fact, they are the ones who never waste a thing.

Unlike the studies conducted by Kane and Lohr (1998), Cone and Myhre (2000) and Goland (2002), the Delaneys do not have difficulties retaining or satisfying their subscribers. For the past six years the subscriber base has been steady between 18 and 25 subscribers, and generally consist of return subscribers who like the idea of fresh, healthy produce but either do not have the time to or can no longer garden. Perhaps it is because the subscribers are themselves rural residents that they are not confused by the wide variety of food they find in their shares. The Delaneys reported the only confusion or dissatisfaction among shareholders centered on kohlrabi and their unfamiliarity with it. Goland (2002) reported in her study of CSA farms in Ohio that the "exoticness" or unfamiliarity with food is a major stumbling block for shareholder retention; however this does not appear to be the case with the Delaneys. They routinely have to turn away interested shareholders because they feel that they would not be able to provide for more than the current number. As Gordon stated, "The varieties that are grown in the gardens are selected first for flavor and second for yield." Thus, it appears that the Delaneys, now entering the seventh year as a CSA farm, have been able to strike a balance which is benefiting farm, family, community, and the environment.

Ana's Garden: Let's Give This a Try

On the other side of the county, Ana's Garden is preparing for their second season as a CSA farm. Unlike the Delaneys,

Table 2 Factors Motivating CSA Operators

Motivating Factors[a]	Average Rating[b]	N
Providing wholesome food in the community	4.79	328
Promoting sustainable agriculture	4.65	331
Land stewardship/ Environmental concerns	4.53	330
Life style	4.37	325
Community development/ Quality of life	4.26	324
The CSA helps generate a sense of community	4.24	335
Profit	3.39	330
Keeping farmland within the family	3.10	301

[a] Respondents were asked to rate each factor using a Likert scale of 1 to 5, where 1 = not important and 5 = very important.
[b] A chi-square test was conducted to determine if responses were non-random. All averages reported are significantly non-random at $p < .001$.
Source: Based on calculations from IIRA (2003).

Michael and Ana Hendrix are not originally from the area, although both of Michael's parents grew up here and his grandparents still live nearby. Thus, they are representative of the majority (77.8%) of CSA farmers we surveyed (IIRA 2003). The Hendrixs came to Macomb as graduate students on Return Peace Corps fellowships at Western Illinois University. Intrigued by the opportunity to settle near Michael's family and raise their own family of five in a safe, rural environment, they have lived in the area since 1998. Ana had grown up in an urban center in southern California and knew that she did want a different kind of childhood for her children than she had had. When Michael inherited 40 acres of land from his grandfather, a retired farmer, they built their house and decided to build their CSA gardens.

Currently, Ana's Garden has approximately three-quarters to one acre under intensive production. At first glance, this may seem small. But the national median CSA size is only four acres, and the national average is 11.4 acres (Figure 1). As a graduate of the Land Institute in Kansas, Michael believes in utilizing as much vertical space as possible to grow a wide variety of crops in a compact area. For the last several years the garden beds have been prepared, nourished with compost and cover crops, and most recently fitted with water lines for efficient irrigation. For several years the Hendrixs sold their organic produce at the local farmer's market in Macomb, but were not satisfied with the experience. This year, after negotiating a three-quarter-time schedule with the principle and superintendent at the high school where he is employed as an ESL (English as a Second Language) teacher, Michael and Ana decided to act upon their dream.

Building on the experience of their last three growing seasons, Ana's Garden plans to offer subscribers 32 varieties of fresh produce over an 18-week season. Like the Delaneys, the Hendrixs practice a diversified farm management strategy, which includes chickens. Unlike Good Eats Gardens, however, Ana's Garden does not produce all of the compost materials it uses on the gardens. Rather, horse manure, hay, and other compost ingredients are acquired from Michael's grandfather's farm or other neighboring farms. As with the Good Eats Gardens, the Ana's Garden venture will mean a change in roles and responsibilities for Michael and Ana. The Hendrix children, ages 5, 3, and 8 months are yet not able to work in the gardens, although it is expected that in the years to come, they will become contributing members. Ana, with a half-time job in Macomb, says:

> The garden is Michael's domain. I help out with the selection of what to plant and what not to plant, but I don't actually do the gardening. I am responsible for the people part of the operation. I developed the brochure, calculated the prices, and have set up our website. I am also going to put together the shareholder baskets, but the actual gardening is up to him. It is what he enjoys doing.

This situation reflects a typical gender division of labor for a male-operated CSA. The IIRA (2003) survey asked respondents to identify whether they or a spouse/partner were responsible for specific tasks related to CSA operations. For each task, a simple ratio was calculated to determine the extent to which the operator did the task or delegated the responsibilities. The higher the ratio, the less likely the task was shared with a spouse. Survey results suggest that if responsibilities are shared in a male-operated CSA, the male tends to focus on field tasks such as seed selection and planting. The spouse or partner, on the other hand, tends to focus on the business-related tasks such as book keeping, marketing, public relations and education (Table 3).[8]

Their previous experience with the local farmer's market has taught them that while Michael may want to do the gardening by himself, an extra set of hands is useful. Because Ana's time is occupied with the business and educational aspects of the CSA, a part-time job in town and helping to take care of the children, Michael has enrolled the help of a friend to work in the gardens in exchange for a share of the produce for his contributions. While this individual does not have the same level of expertise in organic farming as Michael, he brings other much needed skills to the operation.

The two CSAs described here offer a hint that gender roles on CSAs are more flexible than in conventional agriculture. For example, the case of Good Eat's Gardens shows that women are involved in the day to day operation of the garden, including planting and harvesting. In order to explore the gender division of labor and ownership more closely, the survey asked CSA operators to identify their sex. Results show that CSAs are very different from conventional farms. According to the 1997 Census of Agriculture, about 8.6% of conventional farms are operated by women (U.S. Census 2000). The survey results show that of 339 valid responses, 163 (48.1%) were operated by men, while 176 (51.9%) were operated by women. The fact that more

than half of the respondents in the CSA survey were women suggests that the CSA approach may offer a less patriarchal strategy for women to be involved in agriculture.

In order to further explore gender dynamics on CSA farms, we compared male and female operated CSAs to see how they differed on their gender divisions of labor (Table 3). Again, we are interested in the ratios of operator to spouse for eight assigned tasks, where the higher the ratio, the less likely a task is shared with the spouse. A comparison of ratios shows that men are less likely to share the tasks of crop planning, seed selection, planting and weeding with their spouses or partners than women do on their CSAs. In contrast, women are less likely to share marketing, book keeping, harvesting, and public relations tasks than men do on their CSAs. The highest ratio occurs on female operated CSAs for the book keeping task. When the overall sharing of tasks is examined, results show that slightly less sharing of tasks occurs on female-operated CSAs (2.30 for women versus 2.22 for men). This finding, coupled with the fact that over half of the CSAs in this survey were operated by women, supports the notion that CSAs represent a strategy for women to farm in a less patriarchal setting where they can have more control over the operations and finances of the farm.

Economics versus Lifestyle

Beginning a new business venture is a scary prospect, and one that has not gone unnoted by the Hendrixs. Thus, the prices for the 35 shares in their CSA garden are calculated to replace the salary lost when Michael negotiated his three-quarter-time schedule. The prices also reflect Ana's dedication to making the educational component of their CSA a prominent feature. There are three delivery options and the prices reflect the philosophical aspect of "putting a farmer's face on the food." Subscribers who wish to pick up their

Table 3 Gender Division of Labor on Male and Female Operated CSA Farms

	Frequency Distribution of Tasks on Male-Operated CSA Farms			Frequency Distribution of Tasks Task on Female-Operated CSA Farms		
	CSA Operator	Spouse or Partner	Operator to Spouse Ratio	CSA Operator	Spouse or Partner	Operator to Spouse Ratio
Crop planning	143	39	3.67	135	64	2.11
Seed Selection	143	46	3.10	138	59	2.34
Planting	143	55	2.60	143	79	1.81
Weeding	134	63	2.10	140	77	1.81
Marketing	143	70	2.04	143	51	2.80
Book Keeping	96	53	1.81	132	32	4.13
Harvesting	133	76	1.75	145	80	1.81
Public Relations	127	76	1.67	151	47	3.21
Totals	1,062	478	2.22	1,127	489	2.30

Data are ranked by column 4, the ratio of operator to spouse for male operated CSA farms.
Source: Based on calculations from IIRA (2003).

share of produce at the gardens will pay $300 for the season. For those who decide on the individual home delivery option will pay $400. However, if five or more subscribers select a single location for delivery, the subscription price is reduced to $350 for the season.

Many CSA farms encourage their subscribers to participate in farm activities. Ana's Garden plans to have several "extra" events to encourage shareholders to connect with the people and the land that produces their food. In fact, some of the subscribers to Ana's Gardens are former subscribers to Good Eats who decided to make the change because they wanted to have more interaction with their CSA. Two retired widowers who formerly belonged to the Good Eats CSA have decided to subscribe to Ana's Gardens this year, saying that they "were looking forward to meeting people they wouldn't normally meet," thereby increasing their community involvement. Some of the social events include hosting potluck gatherings where subscribers can meet each other and learn how to make salsa, string hot peppers for drying, or make homemade tomato juice. Ana also plans to produce a weekly newsletter, which will be included in the shareholders basket containing recipes, tips for storage, and what to expect in next week's share. Other plans include the possibility of hosting weekly dinners for ten couples prepared by a friend of the Hendrixs. The menu would be based on the produce available in the garden that week. This event would provide an additional source of income, as well as offering subscribers and non-subscribers the opportunity to eat locally produced food and socialize, thus fostering a sense of community. These plans may seem ambitious for a second year CSA farm, and both Michael and Ana are cautious about promising too much. Ana comments:

> We worry a lot about keeping our subscribers happy. We want them to be satisfied with their shares, but we also really want to work on the community building aspect that is central to the CSA movement.

Unlike the Delaneys, Ana's Garden has no plans to sell additional produce at local farmers' markets. Though they would eventually like to have the CSA as their only source of income, the Hendrixs, like the majority of CSA farmers we surveyed, continue to rely on off-farm sources of income in addition to that earned from the CSA. In the IIRA (2003) survey, 242 of 366 responded to the question asking what percentage of CSA profits contributed to total household income. On average, a CSA operation contributes about 37.6% of household income—the median contribution was 25%. The Hendrixs realize that they will either have to increase their subscriber base or continue to rely, at least in some part, on off-farm employment in order to meet the economic needs of their young family. Conversations about who would work off-farm lead to an interesting observation on Michael's behalf.

> I don't want to get too big. Of course we will have to expand and hope to have the subscribers to support us. But, some of these CSAs with 200 or more members

aren't really CSAs anymore are they? How can you know that many subscribers? Can the subscribers tell you what their farmer looks like?

While it is unlikely that the community of Macomb and the surrounding area would ever be able to provide a CSA farm with 200 or more subscribers, there is no doubt that Ana's Garden will be able to fill the 35 shares they are offering for the 2004 season. Two weeks after the initial brochure was distributed, Ana reported that more than half of the shares had been reserved. When I asked if she worried about competing with the Delaneys for customers she commented:

> I don't think that we will attract the same people. From what I understand, we are targeting a different group of people. Most of our contacts are at WIU or from the Unitarian Church. So, I don't think that we are even talking to the same people.

CONCLUDING THOUGHTS: THE DILEMMA OF FARMING

The CSA movement affords small farmers (especially female farmers) and consumers the opportunity to address many of the dilemmas of our modern world. As our technologically advanced and highly specialized society forces the compartmentalization of lives and demands that individuals narrowly focus the scope of their work, the CSA farmers in Macomb, Illinois and in the national survey demonstrated a wide variety of skills that were shared by men and women alike. As in the Cone and Myhre study (2000) the Delaneys and Hendrixs grew a wide variety of crops timed to provide subscribers with ample produce over an 18–22 week period; they explored ways to foster environmental stewardship and build a sense of community and place; while balancing the everyday economic needs of their households, emphasizing a more flexible gender division of labor than might be found in conventional agriculture.

One thing both CSA farms were emphatic about was the role of family and community and its influence on their choice of lifestyle. Anthony Giddens (1991:18 in Cone and Myhre 2000:1395) defines modernity as the "'lifting out' of social relations from local contexts and their re-articulation across large social tracts of time and space." For both CSA farms, connection to a particular place that had been in their families for generations was an important catalyst for undertaking and sustaining the CSA venture. They were also dedicated to making the personal connection between farmer and consumer. Knowing that their efforts were positively affecting peoples' lives was important. Knowing that their produce would travel directly from farm to table was deeply gratifying. Yet the manner in which the producers and subscribers interact in both CSAs varies tremendously, based on their understanding of community. While McDonough County is small in area and population, the diversity is great. Different people want different things from their 'community' and approach community building or broadening their community through various levels of participation.

In its brief history in the U.S., the CSA movement has been successful, yet there are many challenges facing CSA farms and agriculture in general. CSA is not the answer for all that ails the agrarian landscape. There are many holes in the model as a social movement, one of which is its failure to recognize the diversity of the communities it serves. As Victor Davis Hanson writes about the general state of agriculture and the family farm in this country (2000:23–24):

> Farmers are in a dilemma. We proclaim that we don't like modernism, yet we rely on it, indeed often enjoy, the technology of the age. We are going broke, but the nation at large is affluent. We say that we are crucial to the country, but America has found a way to feed itself quite comfortable without the presence of the family farmer; indeed, the rise of cheap food and corporate farms are perhaps explicable in part because of America's very wealth and serenity…We are uneasy with cities and with corporate America, not out of ideological prejudice, but simply because we feel their life is not ours. We, who embody the values that made our culture majestic and whose failure is symptomatic of what has made the country materially rich, appear at odds with everyone and have no idea where to go or what to do. So mostly, we farmers dream of the past, lie about the future, or rail about the present.

Family farms and CSA farms in particular will continue to face the many challenges resulting from our complex society. With hard work, a strong sense of dedication and a commitment to putting the community back in agriculture, CSA farms may provide a select number of farmers and consumers with an alternative to the current state of agriculture.

Notes

1. We would like to express gratitude to the Illinois Council for Food and Agricultural Research and the Illinois Value-Added Rural Development Center which provided, respectively, financial and logistical support for this research.
2. The authors acknowledge that the number of "registered" CSAs does not reflect the true number of CSAs currently operating in North America.
3. At the time that the IIRA administered the CSA survey, no data from prior nationwide surveys of CSA farms were available. Only after the data from the IIRA survey were analyzed was subsequent data from prior surveys available.
4. Located at Western Illinois University, the Illinois Institute for Rural Affairs is a multi-disciplinary staffed research center designed to improve the quality of life in rural areas by developing public-private partnerships with local agencies on community development projects in rural areas. The Institute works on projects including rural economic and community development (including value-added agriculture), rural health care, rural education, rural public transportation, public management policies, housing, and technology.
5. The names of the CSA farms and farm owners have been altered to protect their privacy.
6. Scrapie is a degenerative and eventually fatal disease affecting the central nervous system of sheep and goats. It is associated with the presence of an abnormal protein called *prion*, which is also related to bovine spongiform encephalopathy (BSE) or so-called mad cow disease in cattle and Cruetzfeldt-Jakob disease in humans. Although scrapie has never been linked with humans, recent publicity, coupled with limited scientific knowledge about these diseases, has heightened public concerns.
7. A paired samples t-test was used to determine if the average rating for the profit motive was significantly different from the average ratings for the other motivations in Table 2. In all instances, the profit rating was found to be significantly different from the other motivations at $p < .01$.
8. There is an important gender division of labor to consider within the CSA movement as a whole. While women only operate 8.6% of the typical family farms in the United States, women play a much more significant role within the CSA movement (USDA 2003, 517). For example, of the 366 responses in the IIRA (2003) survey, 339 responded to the gender identification question. Of those who responded, 176 or 51.9% were women.

References

Barkley, A. 2002. Organic Food Growth: Producer Profits and Corporate Farming. Risk and Profit Conference, Manhattan, Kansas.

Becker, E. 2002. Organic Gets an Additive: A USDA Seal. New York Times October 21.

Blank, J. 1999. The End of Agriculture in the American Portfolio. Westport, CT: Quorum Books.

Broydo, L. 2001. Buying the Farm: Consumers Give "Share cropping" a Whole New Meaning. Mother Jones (March/April).

Cochrane, Willard. 1979. Development of American Agriculture: An Historical Analysis. Minneapolis: University of Minnesota Press.

DeLind, L. 1999. Close Encounters with a CSA: The Reflections of a Bruised and Somewhat Wiser Anthropologist. Agriculture and Human Values 16(1):3–9.

———. 2003. Considerably More than Vegetables, A Lot Less than Community: The Dilemma of Community Supported Agriculture. *In* Fighting for the Farm: Rural America Transformed, Jane Adams, ed. Pp. 192–206. Philadelphia: University of Pennsylvania Press.

DeLind, L., and A. Ferguson. 1999. Is This a Women's Movement: The Relationship of Gender to Community-Supported Agriculture in Michigan. Human Organization 58(2):190–200.

Esteva, G. 1992. Development. *In* The Development Dictionary: A Guide to Knowledge as Power. Wolfgang Sachs, ed. Pp. 6–25. Atlantic Highlands, NJ: Zed Books.

Geisler, C., and G. Daneker, eds. 2000. Property and Values: Alternatives to Public and Private Ownership. Washington, DC: Island Press.

Giddens, A. 1991. Modernity and Self-Identity: Self and Society in the Late Modern Age. Stanford, CA: Stanford University Press.

Goland, C. 2002. Community Supported Agriculture, Food Consumption, and Member Commitment. Culture and Agriculture 24 (1):14–25.

Guijt, I., and M.K. Shah. 1998. The Myth of Community: Gender Issues in Participatory Development, London: Intermediate Technology Publications.

Halweil, B. 2000. Where Have All the Farmers Gone? World Watch 13:12–28.

Henderson, E., and R. Van En. 1999. Sharing the Harvest. White River Junction, VT: Chelsea Green Publishing Company.

Hinrichs, C. 2000. Embeddedness and Local Food Systems: Notes on Two Types of Direct Agricultural Market. Journal of Rural Studies 16:295–303.

IIRA. 2001. Strategic Agricultural Visioning and Economic Development: McDonough County. Macomb: Illinois Institute of Rural Affairs.

———. 2003. Survey of Community Supported Agriculture (CSA) Programs. Macomb: Illinois Institute for Rural Affairs.

Ikerd, J. 2002. Painting a New Picture: The New American Farm. <http://www.ssu.missouri.edu/faculty/jikerd/papers>.

———. 2002a. The Real Costs of Globalization to Farmers, Consumers, and Our Food System. <http://www.ssu.missouri.edu/faculty/jikerd/papers>.

Kane, D., and L. Lohr, eds. 1999. The Dangers of Space Turnips and Blind Dates: Bridging the Gap Between CSA Shareholders' Expectations and Reality. Stillwater, NY: CSA Farm Network.

Lacy, W. 2000. Empowering Communities Through Public Work, Science, and Local Food Systems: Revisiting Democracy and Globalization. Rural Sociology 65:3–26.

Lamb, G. 1996. Community Supported Agriculture: Can it become the basis for a new associative economy? CSA Farm Network:12–19.

Lappé, M., and B. Bailey. 1998. Against the Grain: Biotechnology and the Corporate Takeover of Your Food. Monroe, ME: Common Courage Press.

Lass, D. et al. 2003. CSA Across the Nation: Findings from the 1999 CSA Survey. <http://www.wisc.edu/cias/pubs/csaacross. pdf>.

Lobao, L. 1995. Organizational, Community, and Political Involvement as Responses to Rural Restructuring. In Beyond the Amber Waves of Grain: An Examination of Social and Economic Restructuring in the Heartland. P. Lasley, F. Leistritz, L. Lobao, and K. Meyer, eds. Pp. 183–206. Boulder, CO: Westview Press.

McLaughlin, P. 2002. How Does Location Impact the Viability of Community Supported Agriculture (CSA) Farms in the United States? Proposal for MA Degree. Department of Geography, Western Illinois University.

McLaughlin, P., and C. Merrett. 2002. Community Supported Agriculture: Connecting Farmers and Communities for Rural Development. Macomb: Illinois Institute for Rural Affairs.

McMichael, P. 2000. The Power of Food. Agriculture and Human Values 17:21–33.

Nash, M., and S. Hanson. 2004. Interviewed by Heather McIlvaine-Newsad. Western Illinois University, 2 March 2004.

NCSF. 1998. A Time to Act: A Report of the USDA National Commission on Small Farms. Washington, DC: U.S. Department of Agriculture.

Pirog, Richard and Andrew Benjamin. 2003. Checking the Food Odometer: Comparing Food Miles for Local versus Conventional Produce Sales to Iowa Institutions. Ames: Leopold Center, Iowa State University.

Plant, J. 1990. Searching for Common Ground: Ecofeminism and Bioregionalism. In Reweaving the World: The Emergence of Ecofeminism. I. Diamond and G. Orenstein, eds. Pp. 155–161. San Francisco: Sierra Club Books.

———. 1997. Learning to Live with Differences: The Challenge of Ecofeminist Community. In Ecofeminism: Women, Culture, Nature. K. Warren, ed. Pp. 120–139. Bloomington: Indiana University Press.

Shiva, V. 1997a. Biopiracy: The Plunder of Nature and Knowledge. Boston, MA: South End Press.

———. 1997b. Western Science and its Destruction of Local Knowledge. In The Post-Development Reader. M. Rahnema and V. B. Rahnema, eds. Pp. 161–167. London: Zed Books, Ltd.

———. 2000. Stolen Harvest: The Hijacking of the Global Food Supply. Cambridge, MA: South End Press.

Stoll, S. 2002. Postmodern Farming, Quietly Flourishing. Chronicle of Higher Education June 21:B7–B9.

University of California. 1997. What is Sustainable Agriculture? Sustainable Research and Education Office.

U.S. Census of Agriculture. 1997. Historical Highlights: 1997 and Earlier Census Years. Washington, DC: USDA.

U.S. Census Bureau. 2000. Statistical Abstract of the United States, 2000. Washington, DC: Department of Commerce.

———. 2003. Statistical Abstract of the United States, 2002. Washington, DC: Department of Commerce.

USDA. 2002. What is Rural? Defining Rural: Available Resources. Washington, DC: National Agricultural Library.

———. 2003. CSA Farms in Illinois. Washington, DC: USDA.

Van En, R. 2002. Robyn Van En Center for Community Supported Agriculture. <http://www.csacenter.org/>

Wells, B., S. Gradwell, and R. Yoder. 1999. Growing Food, Growing Community: Community Supported Agriculture in Rural Iowa. Community Development Journal 34(1):38–46.

CHAPTER 54

Could Less Meat Mean More Food?

Erik Stokstad

(2010)

Here's a simple idea you may have heard for improving food security: Eat less meat.

The logic—articulated by groups that include the Vegetarian Society of the United Kingdom and the United Nations Environment Programme—goes like this. From chicken cordon bleu to bacon double cheeseburgers, people in the developed world eat a huge amount of animal protein. And consumption of meat, eggs, and milk is already growing globally as people in poorer nations get richer and shift their diets. That's a problem because animals are eating a growing share of the world's grain harvests—and already directly or indirectly utilize up to 80% of the world's agricultural land. Yet they supply just 15% of all calories. So, the argument goes, if we just ate less meat, we could free up a lot of plants to feed billions of hungry people and gain a lot of good farmland.

Some food-security researchers, however, are skeptical. Although cutting back on meat has many potential benefits, they say the complexities of global markets and human food traditions could also produce some counterintuitive—and possibly counterproductive—results. "It's not this panacea that people have put forward," says Mark Rosegrant of the International Food Policy Research Institute (IFRPI) in Washington, D.C. One provocative forecast: If people in industrialized nations gave up half their meat, more Asian children could become malnourished.

PROTEIN-RICH

Scholars on all sides of the meaty issue agree on one thing: Just as the rich use more energy than the poor, they also eat more meat. The United States, for instance, has just 4.5% of the world's population but accounts for about 15% of global meat consumption. Americans consume about 330 grams of meat a day on average—the equivalent of three quarter-pound hamburgers. In contrast, the U.S. Department of Agriculture recommends that most people consume just 142 to 184 grams of meat and beans daily. In the developing world, daily meat consumption averages just 80 grams.

Those numbers suggest that people living in the United States and other wealthy nations could increase world grain supplies simply by forgoing that extra burger or chop. But it's not that simple. Figuring out the full impact of meat consumption on global food security requires sophisticated computer models that can track how buying decisions ripple out across farming systems, global supply chains, and food markets.

One of those models is called IMPACT, and in 1998 IFPRI's Rosegrant and colleagues used it to study what might happen in 2020 if rich nations cut their per capita demand for meat to half of what it was in 1993. First, the simulation found that as demand for meat fell, prices declined and meat became more affordable worldwide. As a result, in the developing world, per capita meat consumption actually *increased* by 13% as poorer consumers could buy more. That's good news for what could be called "meat equity," because increasing animal-protein consumption among the very poor can provide substantial nutritional benefits, particularly for children.

Surprisingly, however, when the rich halved their meat habit, the poor didn't necessarily get that much more grain—their largest source of calories. According to the model, per capita cereal consumption in developing nations rose by just 1.5%. That's enough grain to ease hunger for 3.6 million malnourished children—but nowhere near the kinds of gains many expect from curbing meat consumption.

One big reason is the mismatch between human and animal diets. In rich countries, farmers usually feed their livestock corn or soybeans. When the farmers produce less meat, demand for corn and soy drops and the grains become more affordable. That's good for people in the parts of Africa and Latin America where corn is a dietary staple. But people in many developing countries, particularly in Asia, don't eat much corn; they eat rice and wheat. So falling corn and soy prices don't directly help them. (It's true that as demand for corn drops, some farmers might start growing wheat instead. In general, however, climate, soil, or water availability often limit a farmer's ability to switch crops easily. Iowa soybean growers, for instance, can't start growing rice, which requires heavy irrigation.)

Eating less meat could even backfire and make food insecurity worse, suggested the simulation, which was published in the *Proceedings of the Nutrition Society*. For

Erik Stokstad, "Could less meat mean more food?" *Science* 327(2010):810–811. Reprinted with permission.

instance, when consumers in developed countries replaced meat with pasta and bread, world wheat prices rose. That actually increased malnutrition slightly in developing countries such as India that rely on wheat. "It's a big deal when wheat prices go up," Rosegrant says.

When all the pluses and minuses are added up, Rosegrant is confident that cutting meat consumption could ultimately help improve global food security. But "it's a small contribution, like changing to fluorescent light bulbs" to fight global warming, he says.

CHANGING APPETITES

Given the world's voracious and growing appetite for animal products, however, how could people be persuaded to eat less? One approach, scholars say, is to raise the price to reduce demand. If meat prices reflected the true ecological and climate costs of raising farm animals, for instance, many people would buy less, suggests Lester Brown of the Earth Policy Institute in Washington, D.C. He'd like to see taxes that are tied to meat's carbon footprint. Beef might get higher taxes than chicken or catfish, he says, predicting that such levies "would free up grain for those further down the food chain."

A similar approach calls for removing subsidies—both obvious and hidden—for meat producers. Beef exporter Brazil, for instance, indirectly subsidizes meat consumption by not charging consumers for the tropical forests destroyed by ranching, argues Sjur Kasa, a sociologist at the University

of Oslo. Ending subsidies would be "the most powerful tool for curbing meat consumption," Kasa says, but it would be "a very difficult battle." So far, however, the battle hasn't been joined. "There are really no big victories when it comes to making people eat less meat for sustainability reasons," he says.

Campaigns directed at consumers, emphasizing the health benefits of reducing calories and animal fats, could prove a winner, says Danielle Nierenberg of the Worldwatch Institute in Washington, D.C. She notes that concerns about health care costs and a greater focus on preventing disease have helped spur a number of innovative efforts. In 2003, for instance, the Johns Hopkins Bloomberg School of Public Health started "Meatless Mondays," an initiative to reduce U.S. meat consumption by 15%. The organizers were inspired in part by government campaigns during World War I and II to ration meat for troops. In May 2009, the city council of Ghent, Belgium, proclaimed that its citizens should avoid eating meat on Thursdays. And last fall, Baltimore became the first city to serve only vegetarian meals 1 day a week in public schools.

So far, it's hard to know if these small-scale efforts have had any significant impact. And Rosegrant has an overarching concern: "What worries me is that people will think that's all we need to do." To truly ensure global food security, he says we'll also need much greater investment in agricultural research to boost yields and more economic development that increases incomes in poorer nations. "We have to go beyond personal responsibility," he says, "to policy action."

CHAPTER 55

Marked Improvement in Carbohydrate and Lipid Metabolism in Diabetic Australian Aborigines After Temporary Reversion to Traditional Lifestyle

Kerin O'Dea

(1984)

The high prevalence of diabetes in urbanized Australian Aboriginal communities[1-3] represents a serious and growing public health problem that has not responded to conventional therapies for a variety of cultural, historic, and economic reasons. In a previous study, we demonstrated that healthy, lean, young Aborigines from a community in which diabetes is highly prevalent among the people over 40 yr of age exhibited mild impairment of glucose tolerance, hyperinsulinemia, and elevated very-low-density lipoprotein (VLDL) lipids.[4] It is possible that these metabolic characteristics in some way facilitated survival in the traditional hunter-gatherer lifestyle (the "thriftygene"[5]), but render these people highly susceptible to non-insulin-dependent (type II) diabetes mellitus when they change to a westernized lifestyle.[6] In both short-term (2 wk) and longer-term (3 mo) studies, we have shown that temporary reversion to traditional diet and lifestyle in nondiabetic Aborigines was associated with improvement in glucose tolerance, reduction of hyperinsulinemia, and reduction in total plasma triglyceride concentrations.[7,8] The change from an urban to a traditional lifestyle involves several factors that directly affect insulin sensitivity: increased physical activity, reduced energy intake and weight loss, and changes in the overall dietary composition. All of these factors improve insulin sensitivity and should, therefore, be of benefit to the insulin-resistant diabetic. In this way it is possible to link urbanization directly to the increasing prevalence of type II diabetes among Aborigines. The rationale of the present study was that temporarily reversing the urbanization process should improve all aspects of diabetic carbohydrate and lipid metabolism that are linked with insulin resistance.

A group of established diabetic subjects from the Mowanjum Community, Derby, in the northern Kimberley region of Western Australia agreed to be tested before and after living for 7 wk as hunter-gatherers in their traditional country in an isolated location in that region of Australia.

MATERIALS AND METHODS

Subjects

Ten diabetic (5 women, 5 men) and four nondiabetic (2 women, 2 men), full-blood Aborigines from the Mowanjum Community (Derby, Western Australia) participated in this study. The mean age of the diabetic subjects was 53.9 ± 1.8 yr and of the nondiabetic subjects, 52.3 ± 4.3 yr. All subjects were weight stable before the study. The initial mean body weight of the diabetic subjects was 81.9 ± 3.4 kg, equivalent to a body mass index (BMI) of 27.2 ± 1.1 kg/m². The nondiabetic subjects had an initial mean body weight of 76.7 ± 3.4 kg, equivalent to a mean BMI of 25.3 ± 0.7 kg/m². Of the 10 diabetic subjects, only one was being treated with oral hypoglycemics (tolbutamide) before the study and none was on insulin. This subject's medication was withdrawn beginning on the morning of the baseline metabolic test. The same subject was also on antihypertensive medication (atenolol, amiloride, and hydrochlorothiazide) that was withdrawn under close supervision. This subject and another were also on thyroxine, which was continued. One previously undiagnosed case of severe hypertension was revealed during routine blood pressure measurements as part of the baseline studies in one of the nondiabetic subjects. She was treated with metoprolol for the duration of the 7-wk study. Five of the diabetic subjects (2 women, 3 men) were moderate-to-heavy drinkers in the urban setting, while the others were nondrinkers. Three of the four nondiabetic subjects were heavy drinkers in the urban setting.

Field Study

The field study was carried out at Pantijan, the Mowanjum Community's cattle station and traditional country of many of the Aborigines now resident at Mowanjum. It is an extremely isolated location north of Derby, 1.5 days'

Kerin O'Dea, "Marked improvement in carbohydrate and lipid metabolism in diabetic Australian Aborigines after temporary reversion to traditional lifestyle." *Diabetes* 33(1984):596–603. Reprinted with permission.

travel by four-wheel drive vehicle or 1 h by light plane. The Aborigines had no access to store foods or beverages from the time they left Derby until when they returned 7 wk later. This investigator was present throughout the study to ensure strict compliance with the experimental diet. The only food eaten after leaving Derby was that hunted or collected by the participants. They traveled from Derby to Pantijan by vehicle. The 7-wk period was spent as follows: en route to Pantijan, 1.5 wk; at the coastal location, 2 wk; and inland, 3.5 wk.

Experimental Diet

During the 10-day trip from Derby to the coastal location, the diet was mixed and included locally killed beef, since supplies of bush food were inadequate: meat (beef, kangaroo), fresh-water fish and turtle, vegetables, and honey. It was estimated that beef comprised 75% of the energy intake during this 10-day period and the overall dietary composition was estimated to be: protein 50%, fat 40%, and carbohydrate 10%. No further beef was consumed once the group arrived at the coastal location.

During the 2-wk period spent on the coast, the diet was derived predominantly from seafood with supplements of birds and kangaroo. The lack of vegetable food in this area eventually precipitated the move inland to the now-abandoned site of the old homestead. The estimated dietary composition while on the coast was: protein 80%, fat 20%, and carbohydrate <5%.

At the inland location, which was on a river, the diet was much more varied: kangaroo, fresh-water fish and shellfish, turtle, crocodile, birds, yams, figs, and bush honey. A detailed analysis of the food intake was conducted over a 2-wk period during this phase of the study (Table 1). All food was weighed before it was eaten and samples were collected and stored in liquid nitrogen before being flown back to Melbourne for analysis. Energy intake over this period averaged 1200 kcal/person/day. In terms of total dietary energy consumed over the 2-wk period, kangaroo accounted for 36%, fresh-water bream 19%, and yams 28%. The remaining 17% was made up from wild honey, figs, birds, turtle, crocodile, and yabbies. The dietary composition in terms of total energy was 54% protein, 13% fat, and 33% carbohydrate. Animal foods accounted for 64% of total energy with vegetable foods making up the remaining 36%.

Urban Diet

The main dietary components were flour, sugar, rice, carbonated drinks, alcoholic beverages (beer and port), powdered milk, cheap fatty meat, potatoes, onions, and variable contributions of other fresh fruit and vegetables. At the time of the study the composition of the diet was estimated to be: carbohydrate 50%, fat 40%, and protein 10%. There was considerable variation within the group depending on the contribution of alcohol to the diet. The nondrinkers were more concerned about their diet in the urban environment and tended to eat more fresh fruit and vegetables and wholemeal bread.

Table 1 Design of the Study and Composition of the Diet During the 7-Wk Lifestyle Change Period

Phase of study	Traveling		Coast		Inland	
Main foods (as % total calories)	Beef	75%	Fish	80%	Kangaroo	36%
					Fresh-water fish (bream)	19%
					Yams	28%
	Kangaroo		Birds		Honey, figs	
	Turtle		Kangaroo	20%	birds, crocodiles	17%
	Bream	25%	Crocodile		turtle, yabbies	
	Yams					
	Honey					
Composition of diet	Estimate only		Estimate only		Measured over a 2-wk period	
Carbohydrate	10%		< 5%		33%	
Protein	50%		80%		54%	
Fat	40%		20%		13%	
Energy (cal/person/day)	1100–1300		1100–1300		1200	

Week	0	1	2	3	4	5	6	7
	↑							↑
	Baseline metabolic studies						Follow-up metabolic studies	

Metabolic Tests

Immediately before the 7-wk experimental period, baseline metabolic studies were performed in the Derby Regional Hospital after a 12-h overnight fast. No alcohol had been consumed by the subjects for at least 24 h before the test. Two of the diabetic subjects (7 and 9) and 3 of the nondiabetic subjects (11, 13, and 14) had been drinking 2 days before the baseline OGTT, while 3 diabetic subjects (1, 4, and 10) had abstained for 2 days or more. The remaining subjects (2, 3, 5, 6, 8, and 12) were nondrinkers (Table 2). An indwelling i.v. cannula was inserted into a vein in the forearm and kept patent with heparinized saline. A 20-ml fasting blood sample was taken before the 75-g glucose load (Glucola) was consumed. Ten-milliliter blood samples were taken 0.5, 1, 2, and 3 h postprandially. At the conclusion of the 7-wk experimental period, the subjects were flown back to Derby at dawn and the metabolic studies repeated.

Measurements During the Field Study

Fasting blood glucose was measured weekly in the diabetic subjects using a battery-operated Ames Glucometer and Dextrostix. Blood pressure and body weights were monitored weekly in all subjects. Physical activity was assessed daily over a 2-wk period on a scale of 1 to 5: 1 being equivalent to sleeping for most of the day and 5 being equivalent to hunting or digging for yams at least 6 h.

Analytic Methods

Glucose concentrations were measured in fluoride oxalate plasma by the glucose-oxidase method. Immunoreactive insulin concentrations in heparinized plasma were measured using dextran-coated charcoal for precipitation of free hormone after reaction of insulin with commercially available antiserum (Burroughs-Wellcome). Human insulin (Novo) was used as the standard. The range of the assay was 5–200 mU/L insulin and the interassay coefficient of variation was 5% at 50 mU/L. Fasting triglyceride concentrations were determined enzymatically after enzymatic hydrolysis using a Technicon autoanalyzer. The normal range for triglyceride concentrations in fasting plasma was 0.5–2 mmol/L. Total cholesterol concentration in fasting plasma was measured colorimetrically after reaction with acetic anhydride and concentrated sulphuric acid using a commercially available kit (Boehringer). The normal range for cholesterol concentration in fasting plasma from Caucasoids is 3.5–6.5 mmol/L.

Cholesterol and triglyceride concentrations were also measured by automated enzymic techniques in very-low-density lipoproteins (VLDL) and in high-density lipoproteins (HDL). VLDL were separated by 16-h ultracentrifugation of plasma at 40,000 rev/min in a Beckman L-50 centrifuge. HDL were separated from other plasma lipoproteins that had been precipitated by heparin manganese

Table 2 The Changes in Body Weight and Fasting Plasma Triglyceride and Cholesterol Concentrations in 10 Diabetic and 4 Nondiabetic Aborigines After 7 wk of Traditional Lifestyle

Subject		1	2	3	4	5	6	7	8	9	10	Mean	±	SEM	11	12	13	14	Mean	±	SEM
													Diabetic subjects					Nondiabetic subjects			
Sex		F	F	F	F	F	M	M	M	M	M				F	F	M	M			
Age	(yr)	57	51	48	62	50	48	50	62	52	59	53.9	±	1.8	49	47	48	65	52.3	±	4.3
Height	(cm)	176	173	172	161	162	174	169	187	177	185	174	±	3	168	171	186	172	174	±	4
Weight	(kg) pre	88.5	81.7	69.0	73.2	86.1	95.7	64.5	96.7	82.7	80.6	81.9	±	3.4	76.6	73.6	86.1	70.4	76.7	±	3.4
	post	78.2	72.6	63.9	65.4	77.3	83.7	59.9	86.7	74.1	77.5	73.8	±	2.8	72.2	64.5	79.2	67.8	70.9	±	3.2
Body Mass Index	(kg/m²) pre	28.7	27.2	23.4	28.4	32.8	31.6	22.6	27.6	26.4	23.7	27.2	±	1.1	27.1	25.2	24.9	23.8	25.3	±	0.7
	post	25.4	24.2	21.7	25.0	29.4	27.6	21.0	24.7	23.7	22.8	24.5	±	0.8	25.6	22.1	22.9	22.9	23.4	±	0.8
Plasma triglyceride	(mmol/L) pre	3.95	3.50	4.41	5.54	2.64	6.67	2.21	2.60	5.20	3.50	4.02	±	0.46	1.69	–	1.76	1.27	1.57	±	0.15
	post	0.90	1.10	1.31	1.62	1.51	1.08	1.40	0.76	1.02	0.75	1.15	±	0.10	1.08	1.04	0.59	0.59	0.83	±	0.13
Plasma cholesterol	(mmol/L) pre	5.08	3.78	5.70	6.06	5.81	4.66	7.41	4.77	6.42	5.31	5.65	±	0.23	4.35	–	3.99	3.99	4.11	±	0.12
	post	5.23	4.56	4.23	7.61	5.39	4.95	5.70	4.43	4.56	4.58	4.98	±	0.34	4.64	3.76	3.21	4.77	4.10	±	0.37
Physical activity level*		3.2	2.5	2.9	3.2	3.3	2.1	1.3	2.3	2.5	1.0				2.1	2.9	2.8	3.4	2.8	±	0.27
Alcohol consumption† (prestudy)		+	–	–	++	–	–	++	–	++	+				++	–	++	++			

*Assessed on a scale of 1–5 (inactivity to hard work)
† –, nondrinker; +, moderate alcohol intake; and ++, heavy alcohol intake.

chloride.[9] Lipids in low density lipoproteins (LDL) were calculated from the differences between whole plasma and VLDL plus HDL.

Diagnostic Criteria for Diabetes

The criteria chosen for definition of diabetes were those of the National Diabetes Data Group[10] for venous plasma glucose. Diabetes: fasting > 7.8 mmol/L and 2-h oral glucose tolerance test > 11.1 mmol/L; impaired glucose tolerance: fasting < 7.8 mmol/L and 2-h oral glucose tolerance test between 7.8 and 11.1 mmol/L; and normal glucose tolerance: 2-h oral glucose tolerance test < 7.8 mmol/L.

Statistical Methods

Statistical analysis of the results was carried out using Student's *t* test for unpaired data. The areas under the curves for insulin and glucose were calculated using the trapezoidal rule. Incremental areas under the curve were calculated by subtracting the total area from the baseline area.

RESULTS

The overall design of the study and composition of the diet over the 7-wk lifestyle change period is presented in Table 1. Animal foods comprised 90% of the energy intake during the first phase (traveling), essentially all of the energy intake on the coast, and 64% during the final (inland) phase of the study. When the Aborigines were eating wild animal foods exclusively (coast and inland, 5.5 wk) the diet was low in fat due to the low fat content of wild animals and fish.[11,12] This would have been an important factor in their weight loss. During the one period when their energy intake was accurately measured (2 wk in the third phase of the study), it was found to average 1200 kcal/person/day. Since weight loss was constant over the 3 phases of the study (Figure 1), it was assumed that the energy intake was also fairly constant (1100–1300 kcal/person/day) over the 7-wk period.

The mean change in body weight of the 10 diabetic subjects is shown in Figure 1. Initial and final body weights for all subjects are reported in Table 2. All subjects lost weight steadily over the 7-wk period: the mean total weight loss was 8.0 ± 0.9 kg (range 3.1–12.0 kg). The three leanest diabetic subjects (baseline BMI < 24 kg/m²) lost the least weight (3.1–5.1 kg), while the remaining seven diabetic subjects (baseline BMI > 26 kg/m²) lost between 7.8 and 12.0 kg. Weight loss was highly correlated with baseline BMI (r = 0.819, P < 0.01). Despite this impressive weight loss, most of the diabetic subjects were still overweight at the end of the study (BMI > 24 kg/m²). Physical activity over the two periods of assessment (weeks 5 and 6) did not correlate with total weight loss.

Fasting plasma glucose concentrations in the 10 diabetic subjects fell from 11.6 ± 1.2 mmol/L before the study

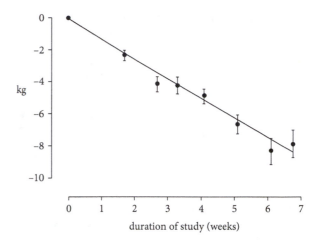

Figure 1 *Fall in body weights of the 10 diabetic Aborigines over the 7-wk period of traditional lifestyle (mean ± SEM).*

to 6.6 ± 0.5 mmol/L after it (P < 0.001, Table 3). Overall, glucose tolerance showed a striking improvement (P < 0.001, Figure 2). In addition to the lower glucose concentration in the basal state, there was also an improvement in glucose removal after glucose ingestion, as shown by the significant reduction in the postprandial rise in glucose concentration in the glucose tolerance test (P < 0.005, Figure 3). This is highlighted by the total and incremental areas under the curve (AUC) for glucose, which were reduced by 37% (P < 0.001) and 22% (P < 0.005), respectively (Table 3). However, in the final analysis, the marked reduction in basal glucose concentration contributed more to the improvement in glucose tolerance than did the improved glucose removal postprandially. Glucose tolerance also improved in the non-diabetic subjects (P < 0.05, analysis of variance, Table 3). However, there was no change in the fasting glucose concentration in the nondiabetic subjects.

Fasting plasma insulin also fell significantly in the diabetic subjects (23 ± 3 mU/L before, 12 ± 1 mU/L after the study, P < 0.005, Table 3). Although there was no significant difference in the peak postprandial insulin concentrations before and after the study (Figure 2), the actual insulin response (increase above fasting values) was significantly improved (Figure 3). This is brought out more clearly by comparing the total AUC for insulin, which was not changed by 7 wk of traditional lifestyle, with the incremental AUC for insulin, which was increased by 72% (P < 0.05, Table 3). The insulin response to a given blood glucose concentration was markedly improved in the diabetic subjects. There was no significant change in either the fasting insulin concentration or the insulin response to glucose in the nondiabetic subjects (Table 3).

The diabetic subjects were extremely hypertriglyceridemic before the study (Table 2), with the bulk of their excess triglycerides being carried in the very-low-density

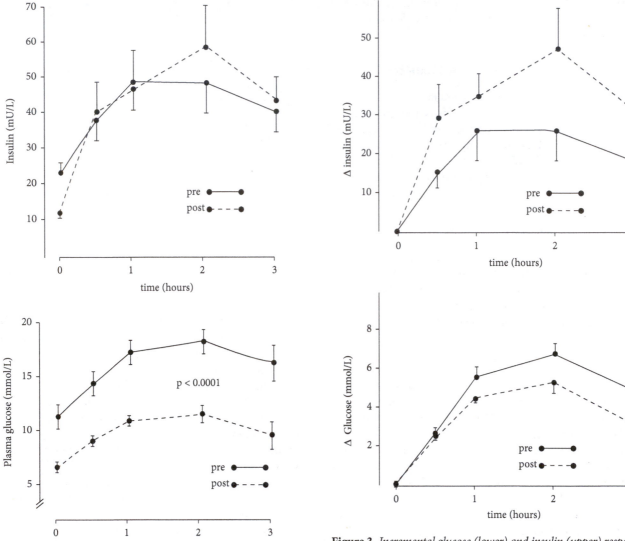

Figure 2 *Change in plasma glucose (lower) and insulin (upper) concentrations in 10 diabetic Aborigines after 75 g oral glucose before and after 7 wk of traditional lifestyle (mean ± SEM).*

Figure 3 *Incremental glucose (lower) and insulin (upper) responses to 75 g oral glucose in 10 diabetic Aborigines before and after 7 wk of traditional lifestyle (mean ± SEM).*

lipoprotein (VLDL) fraction (Table 4). There were striking falls in total plasma triglycerides by the end of the study (P < 0.001, Table 2), the most marked being in the VLDL fraction, which fell to one-tenth its baseline concentration (P < 0.001, Table 4). Similar, although less marked, changes were observed in the nondiabetic subjects.

Total plasma cholesterol concentrations, which were not high initially, did not fall significantly (Table 4). However, there was a change in the distribution of cholesterol between the different lipoprotein fractions that may have occurred, at least partly, to compensate for the greatly reduced contribution of VLDL to the total lipids at the end of the experimental period. Both VLDL and HDL cholesterol fell significantly, while LDL cholesterol tended to rise (Table 4). HDL cholesterol was highest initially in the heavy drinkers but fell in all subjects (including the nondrinkers) at the end of the study.

DISCUSSION

The major finding in this study was the marked improvement in glucose tolerance in 10 diabetic Aborigines after a 7-wk reversion to traditional hunter-gatherer lifestyle. There were two components to this improvement: a striking fall in the basal (fasting) glucose concentration and a less marked, but nevertheless significant, improvement in glucose removal after oral glucose. Associated with the improvement in basal glucose metabolism was a significant fall in the fasting insulin concentration in the diabetic subjects. Although peak postprandial insulin concentrations were no different before and after the temporary lifestyle change, the fall in fasting insulin concentrations indicated that the actual insulin response to oral glucose had increased in these diabetic subjects. This increased response occurred despite the markedly reduced glycemic stimulus.

Table 3 The Changes in Plasma Glucose and Insulin Concentrations in 10 Diabetic and 4 Nondiabetic Aborigines After 75 g Oral Glucose Before and After 7 Wk of Traditional Lifestyle

Subject		1	2	3	4	5	6	7	8	9	10	Mean	±	SEM	11	12	13	14	Mean	±	SEM
		Diabetic subjects													Nondiabetic subjects						
Plasma glucose (mmol/L)																					
Baseline	0 h	14.4	17.5	15.7	7.1	7.7	13.3	9.8	9.0	13.8	7.8	11.6	±	1.2	5.2	5.3	5.2	4.6	5.1	±	0.2
	½ h	16.5	19.7	18.0	9.2	11.3	15.5	12.9	11.6	17.9	11.1	14.4	±	1.1	8.1	8.8	6.8	7.7	7.9	±	0.4
	1 h	19.1	21.7	21.1	12.7	13.8	18.9	17.1	13.7	21.5	13.9	17.4	±	1.1	10.6	8.5	6.5	9.0	8.7	±	0.9
	2 h	21.1	23.9	21.9	12.6	13.6	20.4	21.9	16.9	19.8	13.3	18.5	±	1.3	9.2	4.7	6.9	8.3	7.3	±	1.0
	3 h	19.7	23.6	21.6	9.2	10.9	19.3	22.1	16.0	16.1	8.7	16.7	±	1.7	5.8	4.1	5.1	3.3	4.6	±	0.6
7 wk	0 h	5.6	9.0	8.3	5.6	6.3	5.7	8.3	5.7	5.5	5.5	6.6	±	0.5	5.6	4.8	5.5	4.9	5.2	±	0.2
	½ h	8.5	11.9	10.1	7.0	8.9	8.1	10.1	8.4	9.2	8.9	9.2	±	0.5	7.3	7.2	6.6	6.5	6.9	±	0.2
	1 h	9.8	12.5	13.1	10.4	10.4	10.0	13.1	11.0	10.6	9.2	11.1	±	0.5	7.8	7.2	7.3	5.1	6.9	±	0.6
	2 h	12.5	12.1	15.3	8.2	11.4	9.8	15.3	11.4	11.5	9.6	11.9	±	0.9	5.0	6.4	5.2	4.4	5.3	±	0.4
	3 h	10.7	11.6	16.3	4.9	9.0	5.3	16.3	7.3	9.0	7.1	10.0	±	1.4	5.3	5.0	6.2	2.0	4.6	±	0.9
Area under glucose curve (mmol/L/h)																					
Total	baseline	57.1	66.2	61.5	33.1	37.0	55.3	54.7	43.2	56.4	35.6	50.0	±	3.8	25.4	18.9	19.0	21.7	21.3	±	1.5
	7 wk	30.9	35.5	40.4	23.4	29.7	25.4	45.0	28.9	29.9	25.9	31.5	±	2.2	18.9	19.1	18.5	13.7	17.6	±	1.3
Incremental	baseline	13.9	12.2	14.4	11.8	13.9	15.4	25.3	16.2	15.0	12.2	15.0	±	1.2	9.8	3.0	3.4	7.9	6.0	±	1.7
	7 wk	14.1	8.5	15.4	6.6	10.8	8.3	18.9	11.8	13.4	9.4	11.7	±	1.2	1.8	4.7	3.7	1.0	2.8	±	0.9
Plasma insulin (mU/L)																					
Baseline	0 h	29	20	18	21	18	30	5	18	42	31	23	±	3	22	26	9	5	16	±	5
	½ h	27	26	18	49	40	49	11	42	46	70	38	±	6	51	165	107	53	94	±	27
	1 h	32	30	18	101	48	50	11	60	53	86	49	±	9	96	270	66	83	129	±	48
	2 h	35	27	13	109	48	37	19	50	80	69	49	±	9	143	81	72	69	91	±	18
	3 h	42	24	25	91	36	46	18	37	47	44	41	±	6	80	30	31	9	38	±	15
7 wk	0 h	7	16	8	13	15	10	9	11	16	12	12	±	1	20	38	8	3	17	±	8
	½ h	19	48	13	22	51	33	25	33	49	111	40	±	9	126	74	59	58	79	±	16
	1 h	29	38	19	47	42	49	30	67	57	85	47	±	6	166	58	77	63	91	±	25
	2 h	29	33	16	95	75	73	50	44	46	129	59	±	11	175	75	32	58	85	±	31
	3 h	26	25	19	46	67	23	52	28	54	99	44	±	8	135	52	40	8	59	±	27
Area under insulin curve (mU/L/h)																					
Total	baseline	101	80	53	260	127	130	43	139	177	198	131	±	21	286	388	193	164	256	±	51
	7 wk	75	102	48	168	173	141	113	128	144	301	139	±	22	436	191	141	139	227	±	71
Incremental	baseline	14	20	−2	197	73	40	28	85	51	105	61	±	18	220	310	166	149	211	±	36
	7 wk	54	54	24	129	128	110	86	95	964	265	104	±	21	375	77	117	130	174	±	68

Table 4 Changes in the Triglyceride and Cholesterol Concentrations in Total Plasma and Lipoprotein Fractions in 10 Diabetic Subjects After the 7-wk Lifestyle Change

		Pre	Post
Total	cholesterol	5.65 ± 0.23	4.98 ± 0.34
	triglyceride	4.02 ± 0.46	1.15 ± 0.03†
VLDL	cholesterol	1.01 ± 0.15	0.18 ± 0.03†
	triglyceride	2.31 ± 0.31	0.20 ± 0.03†
LDL	cholesterol	3.34 ± 0.27	4.10 ± 0.32
	triglyceride	0.95 ± 0.23	0.64 ± 0.07
HDL	cholesterol	1.29 ± 0.16	0.69 ± 0.06*
	triglyceride	0.76 ± 0.08	0.29 ± 0.03†

*$P < 0.005$; †$P < 0.001$.

The data in the present study indicate that there have been improvements in two of the major metabolic defects in type II diabetes (insulin secretion and insulin action) as a result of the lifestyle change. The improvement in insulin response to oral glucose was not as striking as the reduction in basal insulin concentrations. Nevertheless, it is consistent with numerous other reports that reducing hyperglycemia in type II diabetic subjects restores, at least in part, the pancreatic β-cell secretory function.[13-16] Despite the improved insulin response to glucose, which was evident in the diabetic subjects at the end of the study, this response remained clearly defective relative to that of the nondiabetic subjects.

The lifestyle changes operating in the present study encompassed three main factors that are known to improve insulin sensitivity: weight loss, low-fat diet, and increased physical activity.[17-20] Theoretically at least, they could all have contributed to the improved metabolic control evident in these diabetic subjects at the end of the study. The marked weight loss that occurred in all subjects was probably a major factor in the improvement. However, it should be emphasized that the type II diabetic subjects in the present study were neither grossly overweight initially (BMI 27.2) nor slim by the end of the study (BMI 24.5). In this respect, the present study differs from other reports of reversal of type II diabetes, in which the subjects have tended to be considerably more obese initially.[14-16] The results of this study support the concept of a multifactorial basis for the improvements in carbohydrate and lipid metabolism. Under the conditions of this study it is difficult to separate out effects of dietary composition, low energy intake, and weight loss. Reduced stress in the traditional lifestyle may also have contributed to the improvements; however, it was not possible to accurately assess this variable in the present study.

The role of increased physical activity in mediating these benefits is difficult to assess. Physical fitness per se was not assessed in this study. However, the mean daily activity estimated on a scale of 1 to 5 over a 2-wk period indicated that the level of physical activity during the study period was not particularly high, despite being greater than in the urban setting. There was no correlation between level of physical activity and improvement in any of the metabolic parameters. This may, of course, have been due to lack of appropriate data on true level of physical activity or improved physical fitness.

The striking fall in VLDL triglyceride concentrations that was also observed in the diabetic subjects at the end of this study is consistent with improved insulin sensitivity in these people.[21] Elevation of VLDL triglyceride concentrations to the levels evident in this group before the study are generally considered to arise from a combination of increased hepatic production and reduced peripheral clearance.[22 23] A recent study on VLDL triglyceride metabolism in diabetic Pima Indians revealed normal VLDL production rates but defective clearance.[24] In this latter group of diabetic subjects, the triglyceride concentrations were not elevated to anywhere near the same extent as the baseline values of the diabetic Aborigines in the present study, although the two groups did exhibit very similar degrees of fasting hyperglycemia. Although alcohol intake may have contributed to the high prestudy triglyceride concentrations, the lower concentrations in the heavy drinking, nondiabetic subjects and the high concentrations in several of the nondrinking, diabetic subjects indicate that diabetes was the major contributing factor to the hypertriglyceridemia. The complete normalization of both total plasma and VLDL triglyceride levels by the end of the study was consistent with lower basal insulin levels, since hyperinsulinemia has been shown to stimulate triglyceride production in man.[25] However, an alternative explanation would be that the glucose intolerance and insulin resistance were secondary to the hypertriglyceridemia, and that the very-low-fat diet, together with the weight loss achieved, were responsible for the dramatic reductions in VLDL levels that, in turn, mediated the improvement in glucose tolerance.[26]

Although HDL cholesterol levels were highest initially in the heavy drinkers, they had fallen in all subjects, including the nondrinkers, by the end of the study. Low HDL cholesterol levels, associated with low total cholesterol levels, have been reported in numerous nonurbanized populations including Australian Aborigines.[4,27,28] The general fall in HDL cholesterol (even in the nondrinkers) may have been partly in response to the greatly reduced VLDL concentrations in all subjects at the end of the study. Similarly, the rise in LDL cholesterol (although not statistically significant) may have occurred to compensate for the greatly reduced VLDL. Thus, although total cholesterol did not fall significantly (despite a trend in that direction) there was a change in the distribution of cholesterol between the different lipoprotein fractions.

The three most striking metabolic changes that occurred in this study, namely the reductions in fasting glucose, insulin, and triglyceride concentrations to normal or near-normal levels, were almost certainly interrelated. Hyperinsulinemia and insulin resistance are associated, ipso facto, with a reduced ability of a given concentration of insulin to stimulate glucose uptake or inhibit lipolysis.[28] However, hepatic triglyceride synthesis does not appear to be subject to insulin resistance.[25,30] As a consequence, the co-existent elevations in insulin, glucose, and free fatty acids in insulin-resistant states provide the setting for increased hepatic triglyceride synthesis and increased VLDL triglyceride secretion. Ameliorating the insulin resistance (by any combination of weight loss, low-fat diet, and increased physical activity) should reverse these processes by improving glucose uptake, inhibiting lipolysis, and lowering basal insulin concentrations, thereby removing the conditions previously promoting excessive VLDL triglyceride production and secretion.

However, the interpretation of the results of the present study is complicated by the observation that despite the marked improvement in basal glucose homeostasis, postprandial glucose clearance was only moderately improved. This is perhaps even more unexpected in view of the improvement in postprandial insulin secretory response. It is interesting to note that this pattern of response has been reported in other studies of the dietary treatment of diabetes. The improvement in glucose tolerance in diabetic subjects after a high-carbohydrate, high-fiber diet was largely accounted for by falls in basal glucose concentrations and not by improved postprandial glucose clearance per se.[31,33]

In summary, all of the metabolic abnormalities of type II diabetes were either greatly improved (glucose tolerance, insulin response to glucose) or completely normalized (plasma lipids) in a group of diabetic Aborigines by a relatively short (7 wk) reversion to traditional hunter-gatherer lifestyle. The public health implications of these results are far-reaching: diabetes is potentially preventable in these people. It should be emphasized that although it is not necessary to revert totally to traditional lifestyle in order to prevent or attempt to reverse diabetes, certain characteristics of that lifestyle must be incorporated into any future public health programs: high physical activity, low-fat diets, and control of body weight.

Notes

This work was supported by grants from the Australian Institute of Aboriginal Studies and the National Health and Medical Research Council of Australia.

Of fundamental importance to the success of this study were the people from Mowanjum Aboriginal Community who participated directly and those who provided help and support in other ways. Their good-humored cooperation and help is gratefully acknowledged. My gratitude also to Dr. R. M. Spargo and staff at Kimberley Health who were instrumental in keeping the study going, to Frank Haverkort and staff in the Pathology Laboratories at Derby Regional Hospital, to Ames Pharmaceuticals for their help in transporting supplies to and from the field, to Janice Turton for her excellent laboratory work and Margaret O'Connor for her help and advice with the lipid analyses, and to Dr. R. G. Larkins for his helpful discussions during the preparation of this manuscript.

References

1. Wise, P. H., Edwards, F. M., Thomas, D. W., Elliot. R. B., Hatcher, L., and Craig, R.: Diabetes and associated variables in the South Australian Aboriginal. Aust. NZ J. Med. 1976; 6.191–96.

2. Bastian, P.: Coronary heart disease in tribal Aborigines—the West Kimberley Survey. Aust. NZ J. Med. 1979. 9:284–92.

3. Duffy, P., Morris, H., and Neilson, G.: Diabetes mellitus in the Torres Strait region. Med. J. Aust. 1981; 1:8–11.

4. O'Dea, K., Spargo, R. M., and Nestel, P. J.: Impact of westernization on carbohydrate and lipid metabolism in Australian Aborigines. Diabetologia 1982; 22:148–53.

5. Neel, J. V.: Diabetes mellitus: a "thrifty" genotype rendered detrimental by progress? Am. J. Hum. Genet. 1963; 14:353–62.

6. Reaven, G. M., Bernstein, R., Davis, B., and Olefsky, J. M.: Nonketotic diabetes mellitus: insulin deficiency or insulin resistance? Am. J. Med. 1976; 60:80–88.

7. O'Dea, K., Spargo, R. M., and Akerman, K.: The effect of transition from traditional to urban lifestyle on the insulin secretory response in Australian Aborigines. Diabetes Care 1980; 3:31–37.

8. O'Dea, K., and Spargo, R M.: Metabolic adaptation to a low carbohydrate-high protein ("traditional") diet in Australian Aborigines. Diabetologia 1982; 23:494–98.

9. Albers. J. J., Warnick, G. H., and Cheung, M. C.: High density lipoprotein quantitation. Lipids 1978: 13:926–32.

10. National Diabetes Data Group: Classification and diagnosis of diabetes mellitus and other categories of glucose intolerance. Diabetes 1979; 18:1039–57.

11. Sinclair, A. J., Slattery, W. J., and O'Dea, K.: The analysis of polyunsaturated fatty acids in meat by capillary gas-liquid chromatography. J. Sci. Food Agric. 1982; 33:771–76.

12. O'Dea, K., and Sinclair, A. J.: Increased proportion of arachidonic acid in plasma lipids after two weeks on a diet of tropical seafood. Am. J. Clin. Nutr. 1982; 36:868–72.

13. DeFronzo, R. A., Ferrannini, E., and Koivisto, V.: New concepts on the pathogenesis and treatment of non-insulin-dependent diabetes mellitus. In The Role of Insulin Resistance in the Pathogenesis and Treatment of Non-insulin-dependent Diabetes Mellitus. Reaven, G. M., Ed. Am. J. Med. 1983; 72 (Suppl.):52–81.

14. Savage, P. J., Bennion, L. J., Flock, E. V., Nagulesparan, M., Mott, D., Roth, J., Unger, R., and Bennett, P. H.: Diet-induced improvement of abnormalities in insulin and glucagon secretion and in insulin receptor binding in diabetes mellitus. J. Clin. Endocrinol. Metab. 1979; 48:999–1007.

15. Doar, J. W. H., Thompson, M. E., Wilde, C. E., and Sewell, P. F. J.: Influence of treatment with diet alone on oral glucose tolerance and plasma sugar and insulin levels in patients with maturity onset diabetes. Lancet 1975; 1:1263–66.

16. Stanik, S., and Marcus, R.: Insulin secretion improves following dietary control of plasma glucose in severely hyperglycemic obese patients. Metabolism 1980; 29: 346–50.

17. Ruderman, N. B., Ganda, O. P., and Johansen, K.: The effect of physical training on glucose tolerance and plasma lipids in maturity-onset diabetes. Diabetes 1979; 28 (Suppl. 1):89–92.

18. Lohmann. D., Liebold, F., Heilmann, W., Senger, H., and Pohl, A.: Diminished insulin response in highly trained athletes. Metabolism 1978; 27:521–24.

19. Himsworth, H. P.: The dietetic factor determining the glucose tolerance and sensitivity to insulin in healthy men. Clin Sci. 1935; 2:67–94.

20. Olefsky, J., Reaven, G. M., and Farquhar, J. W.: Effects of weight reduction in obesity. Studies of lipid and carbohydrate metabolism in normal and hyperlipoproteinemic subjects. J. Clin. Invest. 1974; 53:64–76.

21. Reaven, G. M., and Greenfield, M. S.: Diabetic hypertriglyceridemia. Evidence for three clinical syndromes. Diabetes 1981; 30 (Suppl. 2):66–75.

22. Brunzell, J. D., Porte, D., and Bierman, E. L.: Abnormal lipoprotein lipase-mediated plasma triglyceride removal in untreated diabetes mellitus associated with hypertriglyceridemia. Metabolism 1979; 28:901–907.

23. Greenfield, M., Kolterman, O., Olefsky, J., and Reaven, G. M., Mechanism of hypertriglyceridemia in diabetic subjects with fasting hyperglycemia. Diabetologia 1980; 18:441–46.

24. Howard, B. V., Reitman, J. S., Vasquez, B., and Zeeh, L. A.: Very-low-density lipoprotein triglyceride metabolism in non-insulin-dependent diabetes mellitus. Diabetes 1983; 32:271–76.

25. Tobey, T. A., Greenfield, M., Kraemer, F., and Reaven, G. M.: Relationship between insulin resistance, insulin secretion, very low density lipoprotein kinetics and plasma triglyceride levels in normotriglyceridemic man. Metabolism 1981; 30:165–71.

26. Randle, P. J., Hales, C. N., Garland, P. B., and Newsholme, E. A.: The glucose fatty-acid cycle. Its role in insulin sensitivity and the metabolic disturbances of diabetes mellitus. Lancet 1963; 1:785–89.

27. Nestel, P. J., and Zimmet, P.: HDL levels in populations with low coronary heart disease prevalence. Atherosclerosis 1981; 40:257–62.

28. Connor, W. E., Cerqueira, M. T., Connor, R. W., Wallace, R. B., Malinow, M. R., and Casdorph, H. R.: The plasma lipid lipoproteins and diet of the Tarahumara Indians of Mexico. Am. J. Clin. Nutr. 1978; 31: 1131–42.

29. Crettaz, M., and Jeanrenaud, B.: Postreceptor alteration in the state of insulin resistance. Metabolism 1980; 29:467–73.

30. Terrattaz, J., and Jeanrenaud, B.: In vivo hepatic and peripheral insulin resistance in genetically obese (fa/fa) rats. Endocrinology 1983; 112:1346–51.

31. Simpson, R. W., Mann, J. I., Eaton, J., Moore, R. A., Carter, R., and Hockaday. T. D. R.: Improved glucose control in maturity-onset diabetes treated with high-carbohydrate-modified fat diet. Br. Med. J. 1979; 1:1753–56.

32. Simpson, H. C. R., Simpson, R. W., Lousley, S., Carter, R. D., Geekie, M., Hockaday, T. D. R., and Mann, J. I.: A high carbohydrate leguminous fibre diet improves all aspects of diabetic control. Lancet 1981; 1:1–5.

33. Davis. B. M., Bernstein, R., Kolterman, O., Olefsky, J. M., and Reaven. G. M.: Defect in glucose removal in non-ketotic diabetic patients with fasting hyperglycemia. Diabetes 1978; 28:32–34.

APPENDIX A

Dietary Guidelines

Food and nutrition are hot topics these days, and the sheer amount of information available can be confusing. A good starting point for understanding the scientific basics of nutrition is the Centers for Disease Control (CDC) website: http://www.cdc.gov/nutrition/everyone/index.html.

More detailed recommendations for food and nutrient intakes for those living in the United States are available in two forms. One is based on types and relative amounts of food that are understood to be consistent with good health. These food-based dietary guidelines are the Dietary Guidelines for Americans 2010 published by the U.S. Department of Agriculture's Department of Health and Human Services. They are updated periodically. The current version can be found on the web by searching for Dietary Guidelines for Americans 2010, or going to http://www.nutrition.gov/.

The other form of dietary recommendation is based on nutrient requirements. Nutrients are the substances that provide energy, structural materials and other substances needed to maintain health. They include macro nutrients (protein, fats, carbohydrates), vitamins, minerals and water. The nutrient-based guidelines are the Dietary Reference Intakes (DRI) published by the Food and Nutrition Board of the Institute of Medicine (IOM), which is part of the National Academy of Sciences. These are recommendations for healthy people, and based on a review of the scientific literature, updated periodically. The set of recommendations includes:

- Estimated Average Requirements (EAR). This is the level of dietary intake expected to satisfy the needs of 50% of the people in each age and gender group. It is an estimated average requirement, i.e., what the average person of a given age and gender might need. Any individual might need more or less.
- Recommended Dietary Allowances (RDA). This is the daily dietary intake level of a nutrient considered sufficient to meet the requirements of nearly all (97–98%) healthy individuals in each age and gender group. It is based on the EAR, plus about 20% more. Adequate Intake (AI) is the level of intake that is assumed to be all right when there is no established RDA to cover everyone in the

demographic group. Manganese is an example of a nutrient with an AI.
- Tolerable upper intake levels (UL). This is the highest level of consumption that has been shown to be safe.

The most recent DRI tables are available on the web. Search for Dietary Reference Intake tables or go to http://fnic.nal.usda.gov. Look for links to DRI tables and Dietary Reference Intakes: Recommended Intakes for Individuals.

The estimated energy requirements (EER) are defined by age and gender as well as level of physical activity. They are available at http://www.health.gov/dietaryguidelines/dga2005/report/html/table_d3_1.htm.

Outside of the US, other countries also have both nutrient-based and food-based dietary guidelines; most have only the latter. The FAO (Food and Agricultural Organization of the United Nations) encourages countries around the globe to establish food-based dietary guidelines, and publishes them on the web. Examples are available at the FAO website: http://www.fao.org/ag/humannutrition/nutritioneducation/fbdg/en/.

Some of the guidelines for other countries look similar to those for North America, others do not. For example, the guidelines for Namibia are:

- Eat a variety of foods.
- Eat vegetables and fruit every day.
- Eat more fish.
- Eat beans or meat regularly.
- Use whole-grain products.
- Use only iodized salt, but use less salt.
- Eat at least three meals a day.
- Avoid drinking alcohol.
- Consume clean and safe water and food.
- Achieve and maintain a healthy body weight.

These guidelines give you the sense that the nutritional situation in Namibia is different than it is in North America. The guideline to eat at least three meals a day makes sense in a country with widespread undernutrition among children less than 5 years of age as well as significant undernutrition among women. The guideline to use iodized salt also makes sense since a high proportion of the population suffers from iodine deficiency and goiter. Check out the Nutrition Profile for Nambia on the FAO website.

APPENDIX B

Assessing Nutritional Status

Nutritional status refers to the biological state of the organism with regard to nutrition in the broadest sense. The various measures that collectively comprise the construct of "nutritional status" are the result of complex processes that reflect dietary intake, energy expenditure, the processes of absorption and utilization of nutrients, in interaction with genetic and non-genetic characteristics and conditions, including diseases. The commonly used measures of nutritional status include: (1) anthropometric measures of body size and composition, like weight and height; (2) biochemical measures, such as serum (blood) vitamin C; (3) clinical indicators like hair pigmentation, bone density, or edema.

For adults the most common anthropometric measures are: weight, height and BMI (body mass index), a ratio of weight to height squared. For children, growth is a key consideration and hence anthropometric measures must be normalized for age. The common measures are: length or height-for-age (length in infants and children less than 2 years); weight-for-age; weight-for-length, BMI and upper arm circumference.

Interpreting anthropometric data requires the use of "standards" or "reference data." Standards are values that apply to all populations. Reference data, on the other hand, are data on specific populations that can serve purposes of comparison.

For adults the assessment of BMI is based on standards set by the World Health Organization (WHO): underweight is less than 18.5 kg/m^2; normal weight is 18.5 to 25.0 kg/m^2; overweight is 25.0 to 29.9 kg/m^2 is obese greater than 30.0 kg/m^2. Centers for Disease Control (CDC) provides a handy calculator for BMI at http://www.cdc.gov/healthyweight/assessing/bmi/.

For children, assessment of nutritional status relies on growth charts. The current recommendation is to use the WHO charts which are growth standards describing the growth of healthy children in optimal conditions in many countries across the world. The WHO also provides a *Training Course on Child Growth Assessment* on the application of the WHO Child Growth Standards. The course materials are available at http://www.who.int/childgrowth/training/en/.

GLOSSARY

Acculturated: Adopting the cultural or social traits of another group, especially a dominant one

Adipose: Body fat tissue

Adiposity: The state of being fat; obesity

Aflatoxin: A potent toxin produced by a mold (*Aspergillus flavus*) that may grow on grains and peanuts

Albumins: A class of water-soluble proteins found in many foods as well as in human blood (serum albumin)

Allometry: Also referred to as scaling. The relationship between the sizes of various anatomical structures relative to body size during development

Ameloblast: Enamel-forming cells in teeth

Antiatherosclerotic: Preventing the formation of plaque deposits on the lining of artery walls. *See* Atherosclerosis

Anisotropic: Refers to the directional properties of a material

Anthropogenic: Caused or produced by humans

Anthropometry: Refers to the measurement of metric traits in living humans or skeletons. Common measures include height, weight, circumference and skinfold thickness in living people

Apanados: Breaded fried foods typical of Ecuador

Araceae: Family of plants with large leaves, includes *Philodendrum* (a common house plant), taro (an important food crop in tropical Asia and the main ingredient in the Hawaiian dish *poi*), and mafafa (a food crop in tropical South America)

Atherosclerosis: A common disorder which occurs when fat, cholesterol or other substances build up in the walls of arteries, forming hard structures called plaques which block blood flow through the blood vessels

Atole: A hot beverage made with masa, water, sugar and sometimes chocolate. Traditionally consumed in Mexico and Central America

Basal Metabolic Rate (BMR): The rate of energy required to maintain normal organ function in a fasting state, and at rest. Usually expressed as kcal/kg/hour.

Bioavailability: The extent to which a nutrient is absorbed by the body

Biogeography: The study of the geographic distribution of an organism and the environmental factors which have influenced the distribution

Bioprospecting: The search for native plant or animal species that can be exploited commercially

Brassica: Genus of plants, one species of which (*Brassica oleracea*) includes cabbage, kale, Brussels sprouts, cauliflower, broccoli, and kohlrabi

Cannaceae: Family of plants with edible roots

Cassava: *Manihot esculenta Crantz.* A starchy root commonly eaten in the tropics. Source of tapioca. Also known as manioc

Catechists: Individuals who teach the basic principles of a religion in a question-and-answer form

Ceviche: A typical South American dish consisting of small pieces of raw fish or shellfish marinated in lime juice and often flavored with onions and peppers

Chirimoya: A tropical fruit also known as anon; species *Anona cherimolia*

Churrascos: Spanish for "grilled beef steaks"

Cissus: Family of plants with edible roots

Commoditization: The process in which the commercial value of a resource (food, environmental, cultural) takes precedence over its traditional use or value

Complementary foods: Foods which are acquired and processed by a caregiver and fed to infants and toddlers in addition to breastfeeding

Concomitant: Occurring with something else; accompanying

Corm: Underground stem of a plant

Cribra orbitalia: Porosity in the bone within the eye orbits which can result from anemia, parasitic infection or genetic disease

Cyanogenic: Cyanide-producing

Cyanogenic glucoside: Cyanide-containing compounds found in plants, especially cassava

Cysteine: One of the two amino acids with sulfur groups

Degenerative pathologies: Diseases like arthritis that are age-related and worsen over time

Detritus: Disintegrated material; debris

Diacritica: Things distinguishing one group from another

Diet Quality: Refers to the energy and nutrient density of a diet based on the relative proportion of plant parts and animal derived foods

Disulfide linkage: A chemical bond formed by two sulfur atoms

Docosahexaenoic (DHA): A fatty acid required for normal brain growth in mammals

Dyad: A pair; a couple

Ectomorphic: Referring to a person with a thin, linear body build (contrasts with mesomorphic—referring to a muscular, stocky body build; and endomorphic—referring to a heavy body build)

Edaphic: Pertaining to the chemical and physical characteristics of the soil

Ejiditarios: Individuals who have access to communal farming lands

Ejido: Refers to communal farming land in Mexico

Emic: Refers to a participant's (insider) point of view.

Encephalization: Increases in brain size relative to body size

Endogamous: Marriage that occurs within a particular social, ethnic, or religious group

Endogenous: Resulting from internal conditions; occurring or produced within

Epigenetic: Changes in gene function that occur in without a change in the DNA sequence.

Etic: Refers to an outsider's point of view.

Etiologic: Refers to the cause or origin of a disease

Fallback foods: Refers to foods which are consumed when softer preferred foods are not available

Faunivore: Refers to animal eaters, including insectivores

Finados: A celebration for the dead observed by traditional people throughout the Andes of South America

Food security: "Exists when all people, at all times, have physical, social and economic access to sufficient, safe and nutritious food that meets their dietary needs and food preferences for an active and healthy lifestyle. Household food security is the application of this concept to the family level, with individuals within households as the focus of concern" (from FAO 2010)

Forbs: Herbaceous (not woody-stemmed) plants, except for grasses

Ganbaru: Japanese term meaning "persevere" or "hang in there"

Genus: The main subdivision of a family in biological classification; includes one or more species; the genus name is capitalized and precedes the species name, which is not capitalized (example: *Homo sapiens*)

Geophagy: Practice of eating earth, particularly clay

Geral: A South American language

Globulins: A class of proteins soluble in salty solutions and found in both plant and animal tissues

Glutelin: A single protein found in grain seeds

Gluten: The component of wheat and other grains that give dough a sticky texture; composed mainly of the proteins gliadin and glutenin

Gluten enteropathy: A condition resulting in malabsorption of food from the gastrointestinal tract; usually controlled by eliminating gluten from the diet; same as celiac disease in adults

Gourmand syndrome: A neurological condition characterized by an unusual passion for eating

Grenadilla: Spanish for "pomegranate"

Hegemonic: Dominating

Hemoglobinopathies: Disorders such as sickle-cell anemia caused by abnormal forms of hemoglobin, the iron-containing protein in red blood cells

Heuristic: A device encouraging a person to discover and learn on his or her own

Homeorrhetic: Pertains to the growth pattern seen in malnourished children, in which children have a normal weight for height but are unusually short in stature

Homeostatic system: A system, such as a physiological system, that is capable of maintaining internal stability or equilibrium

Hominin: (also hominid) Taxonomic classification which includes living humans and all fossil human ancestors

Humoral: Pertaining to body fluids or substances in them

Hydrolysis: A chemical reaction in which a compound is split into other compounds or elements by reacting with water

Hyperinsulemia: A condition in which a person has excess insulin in the blood. Often associated with type II diabetes

Hypoplasia: An abnormal deficiency of cells or structural elements (example: dental hypoplasia is a deficiency in enamel)

Immunocompetence: Having the ability to develop an immunological response

Interfluvial: Between rivers

Isocaloric: Similar food energy intake

Isoleucine: One of the essential amino acids

Isotope: A chemical element which has the same atomic number (same number of protons) as another element, but has a different atomic mass (different number of neutrons)

Jeepney: Public transportation in the Philippines known for their elaborate decoration and crowded seating. The first Jeepney's were developed from US military surplus Jeeps after WWII

Kii: Class of high-cyanide-containing varieties of cassava used by Tukanoan Indians in the Amazon. These varieties are also referred to as "bitter"

Kilocalorie (kcal): A unit by which the energy of food is measured. One kilocalorie is the amount of heat needed to raise the temperature of 1 kg of water 1°C

Kwashiorkor: A form of severe undernutrition in infancy or early childhood that results from inadequate protein intake

Lactase: Enzyme responsible for the hydrolysis (breakdown) of lactose (milk sugar) in digestion

Lacustrian: Pertains to lakes, and/or lake resources

Laser ablation: A technique which removes a very small sample of enamel from a fossil tooth in order to measure stable isotope values of the tooth.

Leptin: A protein that acts as a hormone and is involved in the regulation of appetite and energy expenditure

Leucine: One of the essential amino acids

Limiting nutrient: An essential nutrient in shortest supply in the diet, relative to the amounts needed by the body

Linamarase: Enzyme in cassava responsible for the release of cyanide from the cyanogenic glucoside linamarin

Lulo: A tomato-like fruit

Mafafa: A tropical crop with an edible underground portion, or corm; New World counterpart of taro; also known as yautia

Maize: *Corn* in American English

Makasera: Class of low-cyanide-containing cassava varieties used by Tukanoan Indians in the Amazon

Manioc: *See* cassava

Marantacea: Family of plants with edible roots, one of which is arrowroot, a root with finely textured, highly digestible starch

Marasmus: A severe form of undernutrition in children mainly due to energy deficiency, same as starvation in adults

Masa: Corn meal or dough made from corn used to prepare tortillas, tamales, and *atole*

Mesic: Pertaining to a very dry environment

Metabolism: The sum of all chemical reactions taking place in a living cell. Includes all of the chemical reactions by which the body obtains and uses energy from food

Metate: A flat stone used to grind maize or other grains with a second stone (mano) held in the hands

Micronutrient: Nutrients the body requires in small amounts. Vitamins and minerals are micronutrients.

Milpa: A Spanish term derived from the Nahuatal language meaning field. Used to describe a form of slash and burn agriculture practiced by Mayan farmers in the Yucatan.

Mio-Pliocene: Referring to the late Miocene and first part of the Pliocene between 7 and 4.4 million years ago. During this time period, the earliest hominins are found in the fossil record.

Monoculture: Cultivation of a single crop on a farm or in a region or country.

Natal comuna: Ecuadorian Spanish for "village of birth"

NHANES National Health and Nutrition Examination Survey. Continuous surveys started in the 1960s to assess the nutritional status and health of adults and children in the United States

Night blindness: An early symptom of vitamin A deficiency characterized by the slow recovery of vision after exposure to flashes of bright light at night

Obeseogenic: Related to, or contributing to obesity

Occlusal surface: Refers to the surface of the tooth which comes into contact with the surface of a tooth on the opposite jaw during chewing.

Olmarei: The basic family unit in Maasai social organization. Includes a man, his wives and dependents

Organoleptic: Perceived by a sense organ such as the nose

Orthography: Representation of the sounds of a language by written symbols

Osteomyelitis: Acute or chronic bone infection usually caused by a combination of local trauma to the bone, and bacterial or fungal infection. Characterized by bone lesions upon the skeleton

Oxalate: A salt of oxalic acid that occurs naturally in plants

Palm grubs: The edible larvae of *Rhynchophorus palmarum* sp., invade fallen palms and gorge on the pith and heart of the palm. The Moriche Palm, *Mauritia flexuosa* is a common host, particularly in headwater swamp areas of the Amazon rainforest.

Pangolin: Group of mammals found in Asia and Africa that subsists on ants and termites

Pathogen: Disease-causing agent such as a virus, bacterium, or other microorganism

Peccary: A pig-like mammal found in the New World family Tayassuidae

Pedagogical: Typical of teaching

Pelagic: Used to describe organisms which live in the ocean or open seas as opposed to seashores or inland waters

Pellagra: Disease caused by a deficiency of the B vitamin niacin in the diet and characterized by diarrhea, dementia, and dermatitis (skin disorder) in areas of the body exposed to sunlight

Periosteal: Referring to the periosteum, the layer of dense fibrous connective tissue covering bone and the outer bone

Phenology: The scientific study of the influence of climate on annual phenomena such as bird migration, plant flowering, and so on

Phytates: Compounds commonly found in plant seeds and the husks of grains which bind to minerals and can prevent their absorption

Phytochemical: Naturally occurring chemical compound found in plants

Pica: The craving and consumption of non-food substances such as clay soils, chalkboard chalk, ash, paint chips, paper and soap

Pinnipeds: A group of sea mammals

Plasticity: The ability of an organism to change its biology or behavior in response to environmental changes

Plio-Pleistocene: Referring to the Pliocene and first part of the Pleistocene, between 5 and 1 million years ago. During this time period early hominins from the genera *Australopicthecus, Paranthropus* and *Homo* are represented in the fossil record.

Pluralism: A system which encompasses many different resources

Pollo dorado: Spanish for "fried chicken"

Porotic hyperostosis: A porous, sieve-like appearance of bone, possibly resulting from iron-deficiency anemia

Postprandial: After a meal

Pregravid: Before pregnancy

Proletarianization: Conversion into proletarians (that is, workers, especially in Marxist theory) who do not possess capital or property and must sell their labor in order to survive

Resting Metabolic Rate (RMR): The rate of energy used by the body when a person is awake and at rest. The RMR is slightly higher than BMR

Ruminant: A group of grazing or browsing mammals characterized by a four-compartment stomach and "cud chewing" behavior. Includes cows, sheep, goats, moose, bison, deer and giraffes

Samai: Variety of millet (a grain) traditionally grown and used by farmers in India

Scutellum: A shield-shaped plant part

Seco: Spanish for "dry"; a traditional Ecuadorian dish containing a portion of meat, white rice, potatoes, or other vegetables, and a relish of finely chopped onions and tomatoes

Seco de chivo: A *seco* containing goat meat

Sedge: A perennial grass-like plant of the family *Cyperacea* which typically grow in marsh areas

Simulacrum: A representation or image

Solanine: A toxic alkaloid found in potatoes that have been exposed to light and turned green

Somatization: Transformation of so-called psychological problems into physical symptoms such as aches and pains

Sopa: Spanish for "soup" [or pasta]

Stable isotope: The isotope of an element that does not undergo radioactive decay

Strontium: A chemical element similar to calcium, but not essential to the diet

Supernatant: Something that floats on the surface

Syntagmatic: Refers to elements (usually linguistic) that occur sequentially, as in "the dog" and "is barking"

Tapir: *Tapirus terrestris*. The second largest mammal inhabiting the tropical forests of South America

Terpenes: Naturally occurring chemical compounds of the essential oils which give spices their flavors

Tertiary: Third

Thenai: Variety of millet (a grain) traditionally grown and consumed by farmers in India

Tryptophan: An essential amino acid and the dietary precursor to niacin, a B vitamin

Ungulates: Mammals with hoofs

VO$_2$max: Physiological term: Maximal rate of oxygen uptake

Volatilize: Leave as a vapor

Xerophthalmia: A condition of the eye caused by vitamin A deficiency; characterized by extreme dryness of the cornea. The disease can progress from reversible lesions to irreversible corneal destruction and permanent blindness

Yabbies: Semi-aquatic crayfish found in low-lying swamps, streams and dams throughout Australia

Zingiberaceae: Family of plants with edible underground stems (rhizomes); includes ginger (*Zingiber officinale*) and turmeric (*Curcuma longa)*, the spice that gives curry powder its yellowish color

Z-score: A statistical method which standardizes data into a scale so that many different datasets can be compared

INDEX